COMMUNITY HEALTH NURSING

PROCESS AND PRACTICE FOR PROMOTING HEALTH

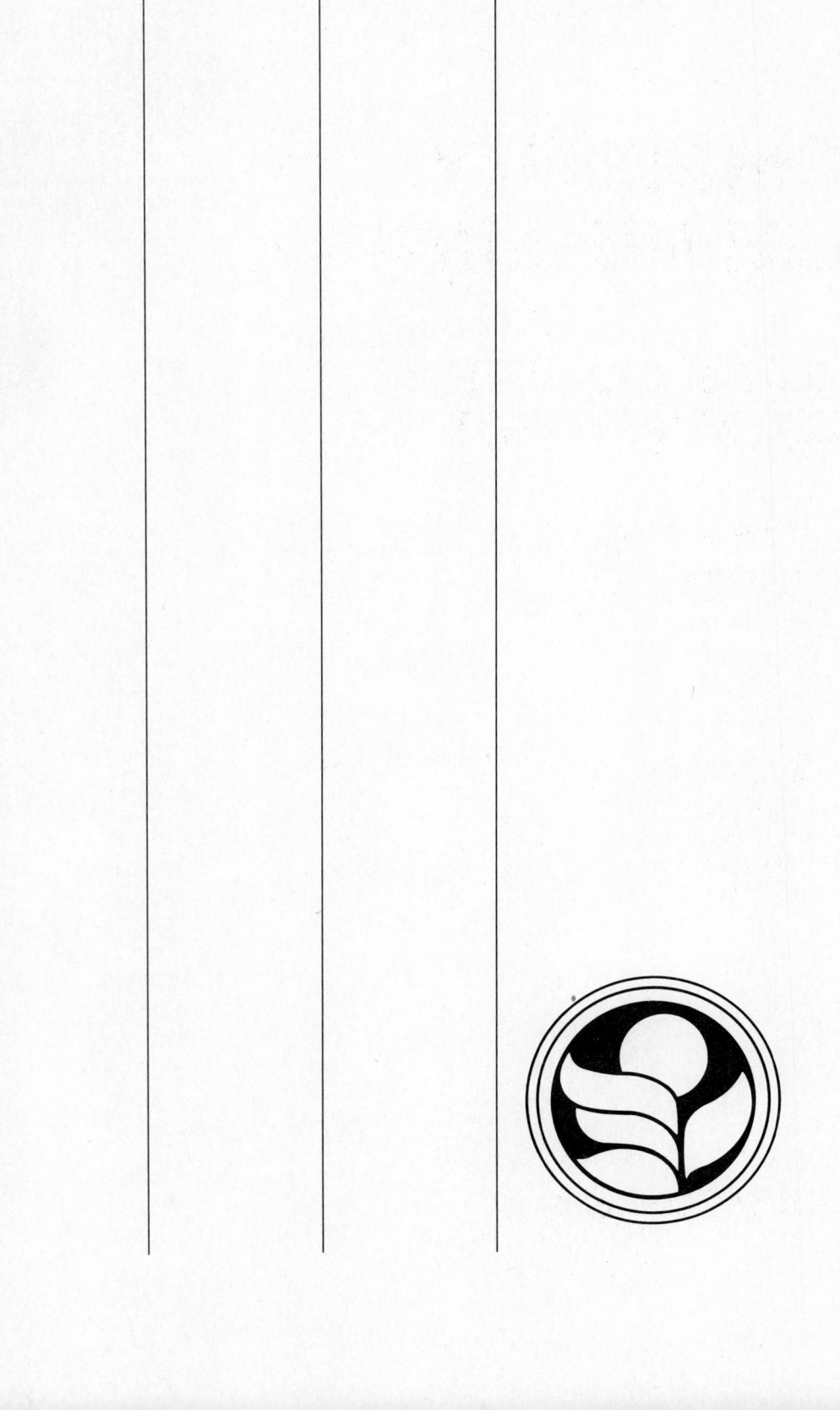

COMMUNITY HEALTH NURSING

PROCESS AND PRACTICE FOR PROMOTING HEALTH

MARCIA STANHOPE, R.N., D.S.N.

Associate Professor and Coordinator,
Family Nurse Practitioner Component,
Graduate Program, College of Nursing,
University of Kentucky,
Lexington, Kentucky

JEANETTE LANCASTER, R.N., M.S.N., Ph.D.

Professor and Chairperson,
Master of Science in Nursing Program,
University of Alabama School of Nursing,
University of Alabama in Birmingham,
Birmingham, Alabama

with 166 illustrations

THE C. V. MOSBY COMPANY

ST. LOUIS   TORONTO   1984

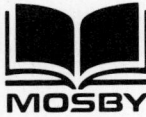

MOSBY

A TRADITION OF PUBLISHING EXCELLENCE

Editor: Alison Miller
Assistant editor: Susan R. Epstein
Manuscript editors: Lois Brunngraber, Selena Bussen
Design: Diane M. Beasley
Production: Carol O'Leary, Barbara Merritt, Jeanne A. Gulledge

Printed in the United States of America

The C.V. Mosby Company
11830 Westline Industrial Drive, St. Louis, Missouri 63146

Library of Congress Cataloging in Publication Data

Stanhope, Marcia.
  Community health nursing.

  Bibliography: p.
  Includes index.
  1. Community health nursing. I. Lancaster,
Jeanette, 1944-   II. Title. [DNLM:
1. Community health nursing—United States. WY
106 C7356]
RT98.S78 1984   362.1′73   83-12161
ISBN 0-8016-4760-6

T/VH/VH 9 8 7 6 5 4 3 2 1   01/D/037

Contributors

Rena Alford, R.N., M.N., P.N.P.

Home Health Service, Pee Dee District I, South Carolina Department of Health and Environmental Control, Florence, South Carolina

Sandra Anderson, R.N., Ph.D.

College of Nursing, University of Arizona, Tucson, Arizona; Community Health Nurse Consultant in International Health

Eleanor Bauwens, R.N., Ph.D., F.A.A.N.

Associate Dean, Baccalaureate Program, School of Nursing, University of Arizona, Tucson, Arizona

Vivienne Brown, R.N., M.S.N.

Hospital Representative, Risk Management Services, St. Paul Fire and Marine Insurance Company, Charlotte, North Carolina

Beverly Flynn, R.N., Ph.D.

Professor and Chairperson, Department of Community Health Nursing, Graduate Program, School of Nursing, Indiana University, Indianapolis, Indiana

Sara Fry, R.N., M.S., M.A.

Assistant Professor, School of Nursing, University of Virginia, Charlottesville, Virginia

Denise Geolot, R.N., M.S.N.

Chief, Nurse Practitioner Programs Sections, Division of Nursing, Health Resources and Services Administration, U.S. Department of Health and Human Services, Washington, D.C.

Jean Goeppinger, R.N., Ph.D.

Associate Professor and Director, Primary Nursing Care in Society, Graduate Program, School of Nursing, University of Virginia, Charlottesville, Virginia

Phyllis Graves, R.N., D.S.N.

Professor, College of Nursing, Northwestern State University of Louisiana, Shreveport, Louisiana

Nancy Dickenson-Hazard, R.N., M.S.N., C.P.N.P.

Executive Director, National Board of Pediatric Nurse Practitioners and Associates, Rockville, Maryland

Cynthia Selleck Henson, R.N., M.S.N., F.N.P.

Assistant Professor, School of Nursing, University of Alabama, Birmingham, Alabama

Rosemary Johnson, R.N., M.P.H.

Professor, Community Health Nursing, Graduate Program, College of Nursing, Arizona State University, Tempe, Arizona

Ellen Kent, R.N., M.S.N., F.N.P.

Instructor, Family Nurse Practitioner Component, Graduate Program, College of Nursing, University of Kentucky, Lexington, Kentucky

David Kerschner, R.N., M.S.N.

Community Health/Family Nurse Clinician, U.S. Public Health Service, Division of Indian Health, Chinle Comprehensive Health Care Facility, Chinle, Arizona

Jeanette Lancaster, R.N., M.S.N., Ph.D.

Professor and Chairperson, Master of Science in Nursing Program, University of Alabama School of Nursing, University of Alabama in Birmingham, Alabama

Wade Lancaster, Ph.D.

Associate Professor, School of Business, University of Alabama, Birmingham, Alabama

Peggye Guess Lassiter, R.N., M.S.N.

Assistant Professor, Primary Nursing Care in Society, Graduate Program, School of Nursing, University of Virginia, Charlottesville, Virginia

Bobbi Lee, R.N., M.P.H.

Assistant Professor, Department of Nursing, Ball State University, Muncie, Indiana

Gwendolen Lee, R.N., Ed.D.

Associate Professor, Graduate Program, College of Nursing, University of Kentucky, Lexington, Kentucky

Margaret Millsap, R.N., Ed.D.

Chairman, Department of Nursing, Birmingham Southern College, Birmingham, Alabama

Cynthia Northrop, R.N., M.S., J.D.

Assistant Professor, Community Health Nursing, School of Nursing, University of Maryland, Baltimore, Maryland; Attorney, Laurel, Maryland

Paula Pointer, M.A., C.A.S.E.

Pointer Associates, Human Resources Development, Birmingham, Alabama

Sharon Sheahan, R.N., M.S.N., F.N.P.

Associate Professor, Family Nurse Practitioner Component, Graduate Program, College of Nursing, University of Kentucky, Lexington, Kentucky

Ann Sirles, R.N., M.S.N., F.N.P.

Assistant Professor, School of Nursing, University of Alabama, Birmingham, Alabama

Delois Skipwith, R.N., D.S.N.

Professor, School of Nursing, University of Alabama, Birmingham, Alabama

Rebecca Sloan, R.N., M.S.N., F.N.P.

Assistant Professor, School of Nursing, University of Alabama, Birmingham, Alabama

Marcia Stanhope, R.N., D.S.N.

Associate Professor and Coordinator, Family Nurse Practitioner Component, Graduate Program, College of Nursing, University of Kentucky, Lexington, Kentucky

Patricia Starck, R.N., D.S.N.

Dean, School of Nursing, Troy State University, Troy, Alabama

Joan Turner, R.N., D.S.N.

Associate Professor, School of Nursing, University of Alabama, Birmingham, Alabama

Barbara Valanis, R.N., Dr.P.H.

Professor of Nursing, Assistant Professor of Epidemiology, University of Cincinnati, Cincinnati, Ohio

Doris Wagner, R.N., M.S.

Chief Nurse, Bureau of Public Health Nursing, Marion County Health Department, Indianapolis, Indiana

Eileen Garvey Wiles, R.N., M.S.N.

Executive Director, Home Health, Inc., Birmingham, Alabama

Carolyn A. Williams, R.N., Ph.D.

Associate Professor, Department of Epidemiology, Research Associate, Health Services Research Center, University of North Carolina, Chapel Hill, North Carolina

Cora Withrow, R.N., D.S.N.

Associate Professor, Parent-Child Health Component, Graduate Program, College of Nursing, University of Kentucky, Lexington, Kentucky

Nannette Worel, R.N., M.S.N.

Director of Hospital Education, St. Vincent's Hospital, Birmingham, Alabama

This book is dedicated to the memory of my parents, Loretta and Clark Stanhope, whose love of family spurred them to struggle for a life quality and quantity that often seemed unattainable. The humility and patience they exhibited in their pursuit to conquer health problems of unquestionable magnitude will serve as a constant reminder of the obstacles confronted and the need for a health care system that is more responsive to client needs and concerns.

Marcia Stanhope

Without the support, encouragement, and loving kindness of five people, my contributions to this book would not have been possible. To my parents, Glada and Howard Miller, thanks for always believing in me and encouraging me to reach for higher levels of accomplishment. Special recognition goes to my husband, Wade, also a source of encouragement but also one who raised issues and questions and urged me to think more critically and carefully about many life pursuits, including writing. To my daughters, Melinda and Jennifer, be aware that I recognize and appreciate your patience as "book work" preempted your time at home. Your help at home and your enthusiasm and interest are special qualities.

Jeanette Lancaster

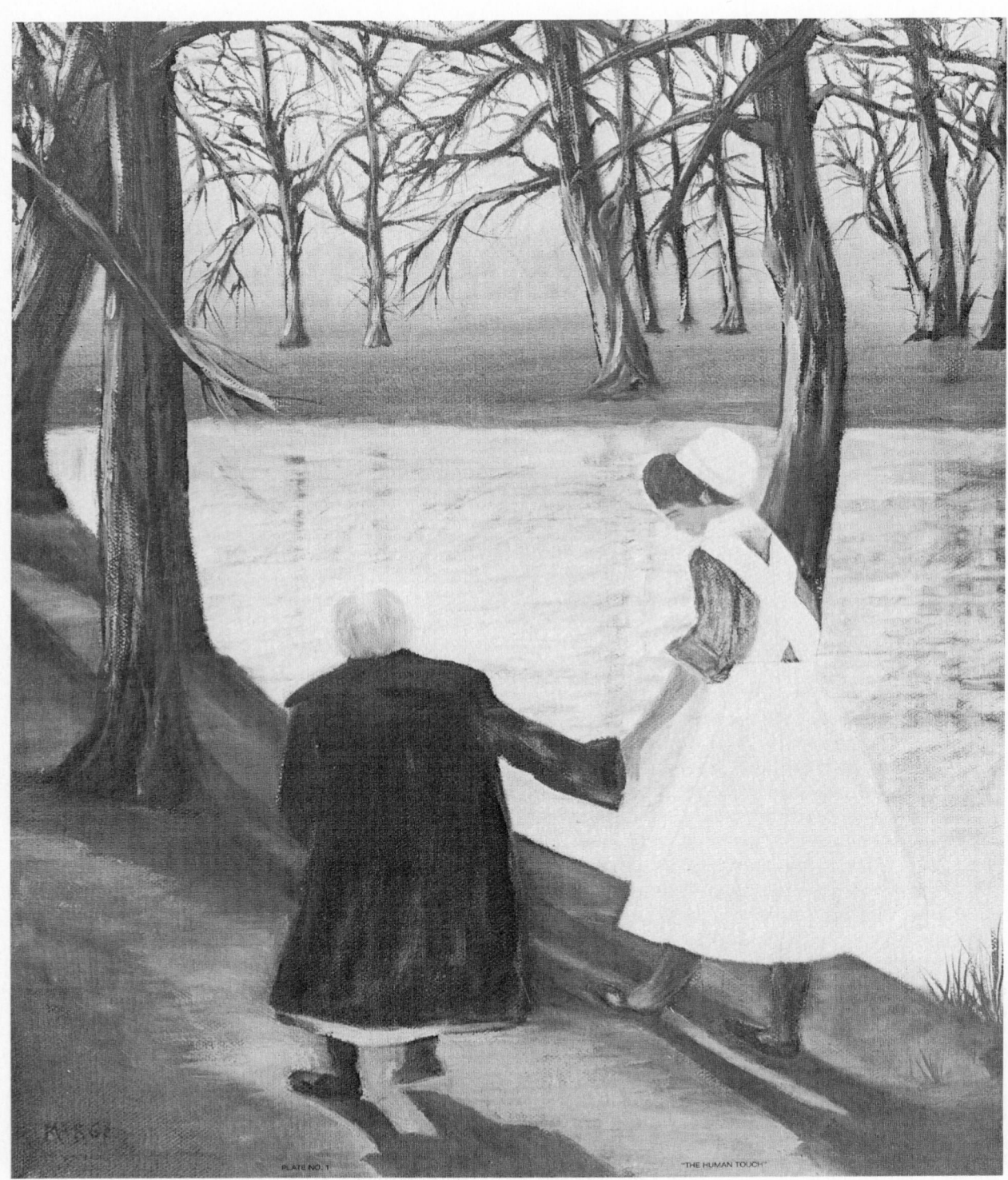

The Human Touch by Marjorie Glaser Binder

Preface

Current health problems increasingly illustrate that human progress has been purchased at a great cost. Indeed, the accounting mechanisms of history may never accurately document the price that has been paid for urbanization, technological advances, and human comforts, since not all societal changes have served to promote health. At present the most well-fed and affluent society in history can document serious signs of health disruption in the form of a severely damaged environment, crumbling and loss of influence of many traditional social institutions, mortality and morbidity statistics that reflect the effects of life-style on health, and an alarming amount of mental illness and crime. People are not effectively responding to the rapidly changing times; the onslaught of societal stimulation and change has affected both physical and emotional coping mechanisms.

Recent estimates indicate that as much as one half of the mortality from the 10 leading causes of death can be attributed to an unhealthy life-style. Also, from 1960 to 1981, total spending on health care in the United States jumped from $27 billion to $287 billion annually, yet the results have not kept pace with the expenditures. Health care monies have largely been allocated to the treatment of disease rather than to prevention. In an era of economic constraints how long will it be feasible to support a "fix-it" orientation to health care?

Seemingly, a refocusing of priorities by emphasizing health promotion is in order. A present-day public health revolution would be timely to recast the nation's health strategy to emphasize disease prevention. The nation's first public health revolution dealt with infectious diseases via major sanitary reforms, the development of effective vaccines, and mass immunization. By the middle of the twentieth century, major health problems were no longer related to the communicable diseases of childhood or those resulting from crowding and poor sanitation, but rather morbidity and mortality resulted from the chronic diseases of the middle and later years.

By and large, medical practices have not markedly influenced the overall decline in mortality in the United States since the early 1900s. In fact, despite the vast amount of money spent on health care, the United States still lags behind several of the industrialized nations, which is readily noted when one compares mortality and morbidity statistics.

Individual health practices such as maintenance of desirable weight, eating and drinking in moderation, engaging in both regular exercise and recreation, and getting adequate rest have been demonstrated to be inversely related to mortality. The solution to life-style–induced health problems involves both individual and social commitment to the facilitation of health promotion choices. People must understand the need for changes in personal health–related practices; society, and especially health care providers, must provide support including education, alterations in health policy priorities, changes in financing, and research to demonstrate the benefits of health promotion.

What does this mean for nurses? Nursing as a caring and helping profession exists because people are not always healthy and self-sufficient. In an era emphasizing health promotion and disease prevention, nursing's challenge is to evolve fully as the central unifying figure in the health care system. Community health nursing is a practice that is continuing and comprehensive, is directed toward all age groups, takes place in a wide variety of settings, and includes health education, maintenance, coordination, and evaluation for individuals, families, groups, and communities.

Society, the health care system, nursing, and health status indicators are all in a state of continuous change. To meet the demands of a constantly changing environment, nursing must become increasingly futuristic in developing roles and practice areas. Such a view encompasses the importance of several key variables including a knowledge of public health tradition and principles, the current and evolving characteristics of the health care system with a keen awareness of the role and responsibilities of nurses, the constraints and facilitators of a health promotion orientation, and the necessity for consumer responsibility for health.

This text was written to provide nursing students and practitioners with a comprehensive source book that provides a foundation for designing community health nursing strategies for individuals, families, and communities. The unifying *theme* for the book is the integration of health promotion concepts into the multifaceted role of the community health nurse. Such a preventive focus emphasizes traditional public health practice with increased attention directed toward the effect of the environment (both internal and external) and life-style–induced health problems.

To achieve this goal, the text is divided into six sections: (1) an introduction to the contemporary health care delivery system, which describes the historical and current status of the health care system including a variety of factors that can promote or constrain the provision of community health nursing services; (2) the conceptual foundations and tools for community health nursing, which describes selected conceptual models for nursing care as well as specific skills inherent in the community health nursing role; (3) the practice of community health nursing, which describes major factors affecting health care, populations needing service, and specific intervention strategies; (4) major community health problems from a developmental approach from birth through senescence; (5) diversity in the role of community health nurses, which describes changing roles, functions, and practice settings; and (6) community health nursing for today and tomorrow, which describes coping strategies for community health nurses as well as future trends toward increased research in the practice role and future practice arenas.

We wish to take this opportunity to express sincere appreciation to our families and friends who supported and encouraged us through this herculean task and to the administration, faculty, and staff of the University of Kentucky College of Nursing and of the University of Alabama School of Nursing in Birmingham who generously contributed their time, effort, and support to this endeavor. The attitudes of cooperation and commitment to quality evidenced by the Mosby staff members who worked with us on this project are greatly appreciated.

Marcia Stanhope
Jeanette Lancaster

Contents

Part Four

**MAJOR COMMUNITY HEALTH PROBLEMS:
A DEVELOPMENTAL APPROACH**

Part Five

DIVERSITY IN THE COMMUNITY HEALTH NURSING ROLE

Part Six

COMMUNITY HEALTH NURSING FOR TODAY AND TOMORROW

Appendixes

Community
HEALTH NURSING

PROCESS AND PRACTICE
FOR PROMOTING HEALTH

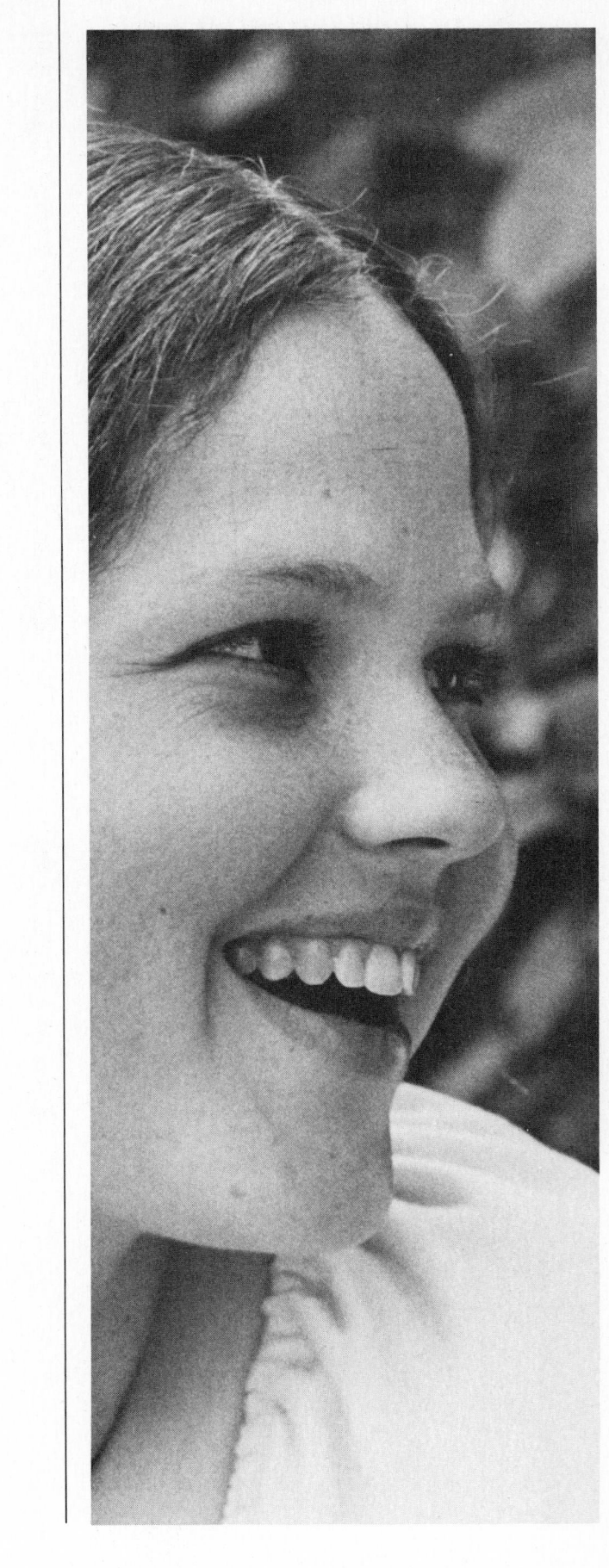

Part One

Contemporary Health Care Delivery System: Effect on Community Health Nursing

Community health nurses have been leaders and innovators in improving the quality of health care for people since the late 1800s. A person would have to look far and wide to find a community health nurse who contributed more creativity, energy, and time to work than Lillian Wald. Over the decades community health nurses have been instrumental forces for change; they have courageously tried many new approaches designed to improve the overall health status of their communities. Early nursing leaders recognized the need for specific preparation for community health nurses and the influence of legal, economic, social, ethical, and political forces on their practice. However, despite many contributions to health care, the system for delivery continues to need major changes to be entirely responsive to the needs of Americans.

Health care providers and consumers have accelerated their demands for a reorientation of the American health care system. In fact, some critics say that there is no system but rather a loosely connected and often fragmented array of providers and facilities that make up a nonsystem. Health care is criticized as being inconsistent in accessibility, affordability, and quality. Simultaneously, the most common causes of death continue to be heart disease, cancer, strokes, and accidents. Each of these killers has been associated with personal behaviors.

Even though the United States spends a larger portion of its gross national

Continued.

Part One

product on health than any other nation, it does not rank in the top 10 countries of the world in terms of overall health status of residents.

If community health nurses are to be effective and be vital forces for promoting the health of Americans, it is necessary to understand the history of community health nursing as well as the current status of the health care system. Too often we fail to learn from our predecessors because we do not appreciate that history often repeats itself. The experiences facing community health nursing in the 1980s may bear some similarity to those facing nurses in earlier times. The approaches that have proved successful in the past often can be modified and implemented to deal with contemporary challenges.

Similarly, effective strategies for community health nurses must be designed so that they are consistent with the total mosaic of health care delivery. The professional must understand the scope and nature of change and the future directions of the health care system to plan effective nursing approaches. The status of the health care system as described in Chapter 2 is determined by a wide range of variables, including the organization for practice, providers, and available resources. Three major influences on the health care system are emphasized in Part One because of their paramount role in influencing the system. Chapters 3, 4, and 5, respectively, described how economics, ethics, and governmental forces influence health care.

Health care has become big business in the United States, and various groups volley for control of the fiscal picture. To date hospitals account for the largest single portion of health care funds. Whether or not this pattern will change as health promotion is increasingly encouraged is a question that is as yet unanswered. The economics of health care are heavily influenced by ethics and governmental regulations. As fiscal resources for health care decrease, more questions are raised about how monies should be spent, and ethical dilemmas continued to cloud the picture of who gets what resources.

Though the government neither owns nor solely finances health care, its influence is felt in all sectors. Currently, governmental funds provide a wide range of direct and indirect health care services. As in all other situations in life, this form of the golden rule applies: "He who has the gold, rules." That is, the government, along with providing funds, has a history of issuing many regulations about the use of the funds. Frequently, only agencies meeting certain standards and following selected guidelines are given governmental funds. Community health nurses must clearly understand the health care system in which they function and recognize the constraints and facilitators of their practice.

Chapter 1

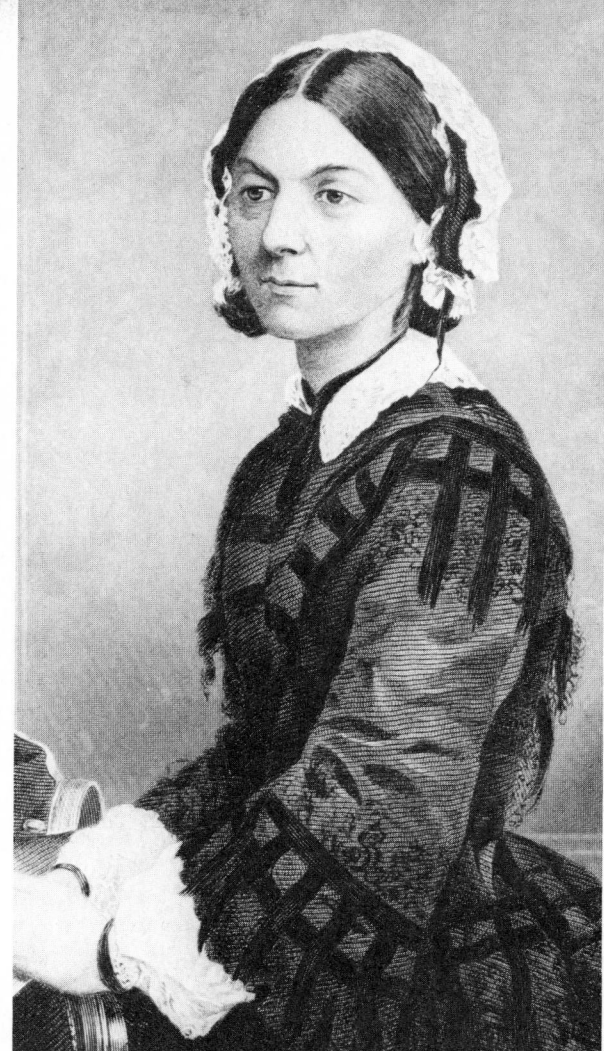

JEANETTE LANCASTER

HISTORY OF COMMUNITY HEALTH AND COMMUNITY HEALTH NURSING

NATURE AND SCOPE
OF COMMUNITY HEALTH

Early definitions of public health* focused on sanitation and community health hazards. Today these problems are under far better control than in previous centuries, freeing public health practitioners to emphasize health promotion for individuals and groups as well as the community. Advances in bacteriology and immunology in the nineteenth and early twentieth centuries led to an appreciation of disease prevention as a major part of public health.

In 1920 Winslow described public health as the

*Historically the term *public health* was used more often than the more recent term *community health*.

science and art of preventing disease, prolonging life, and promoting health through organized community efforts directed toward the following (Winslow, 1920, p. 183):

1. Sanitation of the environment
2. Control of communicable diseases
3. Education regarding personal hygiene
4. Organization of medical and nursing services for early diagnosis and preventive treatment of disease
5. Development of social machinery to insure everyone a standard of living adequate for health maintenance, so organizing these benefits as to enable every citizen to realize his birthright of health and longevity

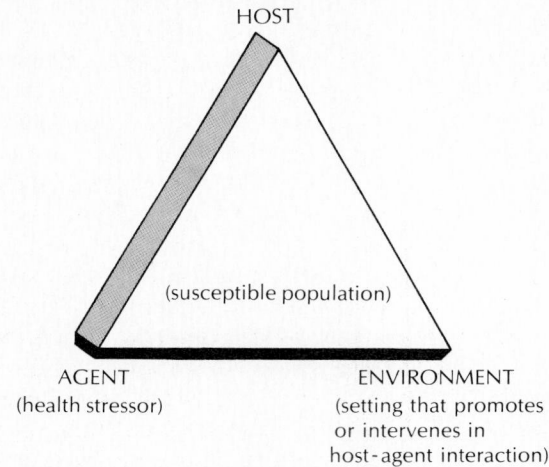

Fig. 1-1. Classic epidemiological triad.

Although the semantics referring to the scope of practice have changed since Winslow defined public health, the focus and scope have remained largely the same. Hanlon and Pickett (1979, p. 4) subsequently defined the relationship of health and public health as follows:

> Health is a state of total effective physiologic and psychologic functioning; it has both a relative and an absolute meaning, varying through time and space, both in the individual and collective, private and public medical, environmental, and social; and it is conditioned by culture, economy, law, and government.

The goal of public or community health is to promote the highest possible level of physical, mental, and social well-being for all people.

The classical epidemiological triad (Fig. 1-1) depicts the role of the environment in health maintenance, thereby emphasizing the holistic or interrelated nature of public health. Although there are many models for viewing person-environment interaction, this model defines the environment as including physical, biological, and sociocultural influences. Adaptation depends on the degree to which hosts can resist disruptive agents. The environment intimately influences host resistance, since the physical and psychosocial setting can either provide strength and support or serve as an additional stressor.

Community health is unique in its use of the word *health*. This term reflects an orientation toward wellness focusing on the maintenance and promotion of the health of the entire population being served. Leavell and Clark (1965, p. 21) have identified three levels of prevention that describe the scope of responsibility of community health. Primary prevention deals with health promotion and specific protection for disease,

and efforts are made to strengthen the organism's coping ability so health is not compromised. Primary preventive activities include health education and counseling, immunizations, family planning services, well-child care, dental prophylaxis, and a variety of classes to prepare people to cope more effectively with various stages of life (parenting, retirement) as well as life crises (divorce, death, and so on.)

The concept of primary prevention was carefully explained by Shamansky and Clausen (1980, p. 106):

> Primary prevention is prevention in the true sense of the word; it precedes disease or dysfunction and is applied to a generally healthy population. The targets are those individuals considered physically or emotionally healthy, exhibiting normal or maximal functioning.

This level of prevention takes place before symptoms appear and is conceived of as promoting optimal health by strengthening existing client resources by "providing the necessary emotional support, information and attitudinal analysis for decision making about a given health condition" (McCance and Reiber, 1982, p. 81).

Secondary prevention begins when a pathological process has been identified and includes early diagnosis and prompt treatment to halt the process. The goal at this stage is to help the person regain normal functioning as soon as possible. For example, early signs of a learning disorder or other developmental delay would receive immediate attention to thwart the process or to intervene with remedial actions.

Tertiary prevention consists of actions to assist in restoring people to their maximal state of functioning once disease and disability occur. At this level the goal is rehabilitation and restoration at the highest level of functioning. These efforts include diet counseling for people with nutritionally related diseases as well as activity restoration in those suffering from conditions such as a stroke.

This section has attempted to briefly outline the scope of public health. Over the years the name has changed from public health to community health more in response to trends in health care delivery than to any conceptual differences. The term *community health* is used throughout the remainder of this text. Often the terms are used synonymously. Regardless of the term used, it reflects a philosophy and set of guiding tenets for practice rather than the setting where care is given, the scope of activity includes an orientation toward the health of the total community.

Because this book is about community health nursing, the last section of this chapter describes the contemporary role of the community health nurse. To do this, it is necessary to trace the historical development of both community health and community health nursing. The historical review demonstrates that nurses have been leaders in the crusade for better health care through an emphasis on the needs of the community as a source of health or illness of residents.

HISTORICAL REVIEW OF THE DEVELOPMENT OF MODERN HEALTH CARE PRACTICES

An understanding of the dominant cultural ideas of each era since early recorded history is useful in understanding the historical antecedents of what is now the system of health care delivery. According to Pellegrino (1963, p. 10), "Medicine and the ideas by which an era lives have an intimate relationship." Hence, the dominant conceptualization of people is determined by the prevailing cultural patterns at a given time. These patterns also influence and in turn are influenced by the prevalent patterns of medical practice. The history of health care is briefly traced from the pre-Christian period to the current era to show the cultural influences and the major developments that have occurred.

Pre-Christian Period

Cause and effect relationships characterized thinking and action during the pre-Christian period. Historical records indicate that people, even in antiquity, were concerned with the events surrounding birth, death, and illness. With few exceptions primitive tribes had a certain amount of both group spirit and a generally accepted sense of hygiene. In their struggles to exist, early people tried to understand disease to devise ways of coping with disease-producing agents. They based health practices on magic and superstition rather than on facts about the cause and effect of certain events and actions on health. Medicine men cared for both health and religious needs and held highly esteemed places in society.

Rudiments of community health can be traced to the earliest recorded civilizations. Over 4000 years ago, a little known civilization north of India apparently planned their cities in rectangular blocks. Excavations have revealed bathrooms, drains, and broad, paved streets equipped with drainage sewers (Rosen, 1958). Additionally, excavations from the Middle Kingdom (2100-1700 BC) reflect community health practices in ancient Egypt. Two thousands years before the Christian era, securing an adequate supply of drinking water was a major consideration. In palaces in Crete magnificient bathing facilities included water-flushing arrangements for the toilets.

Both the Babylonians and Egyptians emphasized *hygiene* and possessed some *medical skills.* The Egyptians

of about 1000 BC, the healthiest of all early civilizations, used principles based on observation and empirical knowledge rather than magic. They also possessed a variety of pharmaceutical preparations and constructed earth closets and public drainage pipes. Their fascination with making elaborate preparations for the next world influenced their ideas about medicine. From their observations in the embalming parlor of putrefaction, or the decay of organic matter, the Egyptians developed complex explanations of the causes of disease. They believed disease resulted from absorption of noxious substances back into the intestine. Based on these beliefs, they developed treatment approaches using cathartics, enemas, purges, bloodletting, and opening of abscesses. Their custom of embalming provided the Egyptians with knowledge about the structure of the human body (Griffin and Griffin, 1973). The Egyptians learned to recognize approximately 250 different diseases and developed a number of drugs and procedures including surgery to treat them.

Unlike the Egyptian cause-and-effect orientation to disease, the Babylonians developed theories of medicine based on religious views. They thought disease was due to spirit intrusion and based their therapies on notions of dream interpretation and astrology.

Greek Era

Philosophy and medicine became intimately related during the Greek era as scientific advances moved medicine beyond the realm of magic. Intrigued with causal relationships, the Greeks greatly advanced the scientific basis of medicine. They viewed people as part of nature and believed health resulted from being in harmony with nature. In contrast, disease resulted from an imbalance of "the good mixture," or according to Hippocrates, health resulted from an equilibrium of the four humors: yellow and black bile, phlegm, and blood. Hippocrates (about 460-370 BC), influential in changing the magic of medicine into the science of medicine, taught physicians to use their eyes and ears and to make judgments based on facts. Likewise, Plato was concerned with medicine as evidenced in his statement that "health is possible only if there is a right order between the different components of the soul itself—its impulses, emotions, and knowledge" (Pellegrino, 1963, p. 13).

Also, the Greeks regarded the delivery of health services as a humanistic responsibility of civilized man, and the medical ethics established in Greece continue to guide medical practice. They also extended concern for hygiene to higher levels than any preceding era, with particular emphasis on personal cleanliness, exercise, diet, and sanitation. In contrast with current community health practices, the weak, sick, or crippled were

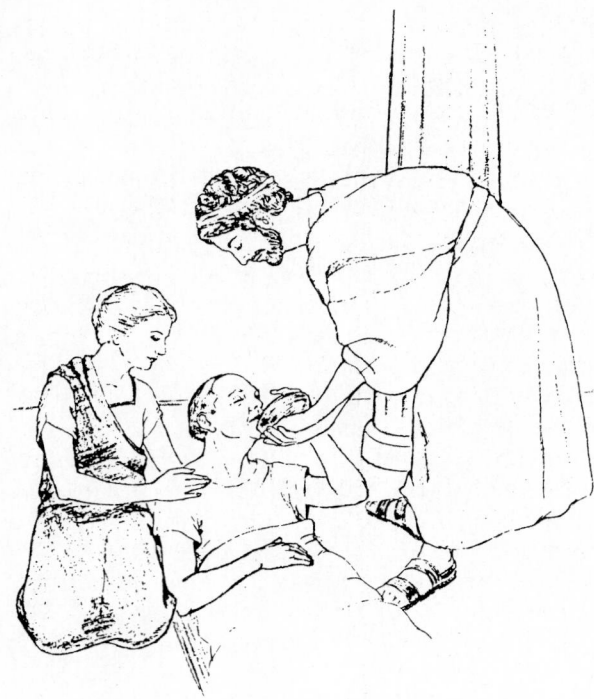

Fig. 1-2. Care of the sick during the early Greek era. (From Griffin, G. J., and Griffin, J. K.: History and trends of professional nursing, St. Louis, 1973, The C.V. Mosby Co.)

either ignored or deliberately destroyed during early Grecian history.

Additionally, the first notation of women being associated with healing is found in connection with the Greek mythological character of Aesculapius who eventually became deified as the god of healing. One of his five children, Hygeia, became the goddess of health and another, Panacea, the restorer of health. In later Greek civilizations, healing largely occurred in shrines where patients congregated and were looked after by attendants called "basket healers" (Deloughery, 1977). See Fig. 1-2.

The first clear-cut evidence of acute communicable disease is recorded in classical Greek literature. There are numerous references to severe sore throats that often ended in death. The Greek word *Kynanche* mentioned acute inflammatory processes of the throat and larynx and probably referred to what is now known as diphtheria. In ancient Greece, medicine was an itinerant vocation with practitioners going from town to town, knocking on doors, and offering their services. Larger cities appointed physicians and paid for their services from funds; these probably were the earliest community physicians in history.

Roman Empire

The Roman view of health shared many concepts with the Greeks yet focused much more on pragmatic application of ideas rather than astute observation and a continual search for new knowledge. The Roman Empire is remembered for its administrative and engineering efforts. According to Pellegrino (1963), Romans viewed medicine from a community health and social medicine perspective. They emphasized regulation of medical practice, punishment for negligence, drainage of swamps, provision of pure water, establishment of sewage systems, and supervision of street cleaning and public food preparation. They also made substantial efforts at census taking. This civilization established laws that provided for the registration of slaves and other citizens as well as the periodic collection of census information.

The Roman censor Appius Claudius Crassus Caecus, who built the first great Roman road, the Appian Way, was responsible for bringing a supply of water to Rome by means of an aqueduct (Rosen, 1958, p. 39). To monitor the purity of water, settling basins were established at points along the aqueduct to allow sediment to deposit. When the water reached Rome, it was received in large reservoirs from which emerged smaller reservoirs so that water could be segregated according to its purpose. The Romans not only valued pure water but also had sewage systems in major cities. The Romans developed community health services with an effective and systematic organization, which continued to function as the Empire disintegrated. Additionally, at the peak of the Roman Empire women visited and cared for the sick. Special hospitals were established when it became impractical to shelter patients in the bishops' houses.

Middle Ages

The decline of the Greco-Roman era led to both a decay of urban culture and a disintegration of community health organization and practice (Rosen, 1958, p. 50). The period between 500 and 1500 AD is referred to as the Middle Ages and represents a heterogeneous phase in history during which superstitions dominated thinking yet advances such as the development of health care facilities originated. As cities grew, they built great walls to protect their inhabitants against invasions by hostile groups. These encircling walls, while necessary for safety and protection, also led to considerable crowding and poor sanitary and hygienic conditions. Clean water supplies and freedom from excessive accumulations of refuse in the streets were difficult to ensure.

With the dawn of the Christian era, a new conceptualization of man influenced health practices. The early

Christian church believed that the Roman and Grecian ways pampered the body at the expense of the soul. Disease was believed to result as a punishment for sin and moral wrongdoing. This philosophy ultimately led to what is known as the Dark Ages. Thinking reverted back to *mysticism and superstition.* Religious persecution of those who tried to introduce new ideas occurred. Progress in medicine as both an art and a science came to a halt. People in this era considered it immoral to even look at their own bodies, hence bathing was an infrequent practice and people often wore dirty garments. They almost totally disregarded sanitation and allowed both refuse and body waste to accumulate near dwellings. Despite this reversal of thinking from earlier eras, the Middle Ages did develop hospitals to care for the poor and neglected. Although the people of this era still believed in magic, the basic tradition of Greek medicine was refurbished and medical education within the university established (Pellegrino, 1963). The onset of plagues forced some changes. Leprosy and bubonic plague were brought into the busy ports and commercial centers. The people practiced what today would seem like a cruel version of quarantine.

Because of the acute and disfiguring nature of leprosy at that time, lepers terrified the people. Laws regulated the activities of lepers, and many were declared legally dead and isolated from others by being forced to wear identifying clothes and to warn of their approach with a bell or horn. These requirements served as effective extinction measures, since lepers often died from hunger, exposure, and lack of treatment (Rosen, 1958). Although inhumane, these efforts virtually eradicated leprosy in Europe and represented the first victory for epidemiology.

No sooner did leprosy wane as a major European epidemic than an even deadlier menace, bubonic plague, spread as a result of trade agreements between Europe, the Near East, and Asia. The first quarantine laws were passed in Marseilles, France, to ban entry of cargo and people from ships suspected of being infected. Although the plague was recognized as a communicable disease, the transmissible agent remained a mystery.

Laymen administered community health, and clerics practiced medicine. However, from the eleventh century on, laymen began to enter medicine, and most were employed by cities. Although during the Middle Ages there were several deficits in implementing a unified public health program, the concept of *social assistance* for illness and other misfortune was well developed. Often hospitals were developed in conjunction with monasteries. From the thirteenth century, hospitals increasingly came under secular jurisdiction. In England between the twelfth and fifteenth centuries more than 750 hospitals were established, and of these, 217 were for lepers (Rosen, 1958, p. 77).

Furthermore, the Middle Ages contributed health education and personal hygiene knowledge, yielding books on healthful living and emphasizing moderation in diet. Three recommended procedures for maintaining health were purging (cleansing the bowels through the use of a purgative medicine), cupping (applying a glass vessel devoid of air to the skin to draw blood to the surface), and bleeding (process used in ancient times for emitting blood to relieve people of disease). Barbers and bath attendants carried out these procedures (Rosen, 1958, p. 79).

The rise of monasteries and convents as places for caring for the sick led to the early existence of nursing activities, since care at that time included meeting both physical and spiritual needs. Between 1091 and 1291, early male and female nurses joined military orders during the Crusades, 200 years of religious wars between the Turks and Christians. As the early Christian church developed, those who had devoted their lives to Christian service cared for the poor, fatherless, and sick. Initially they cared for all three groups under the same roof. However, the knowledge the Crusaders gained from the Arabs led to the establishment of hospitals. Early hospitals were known as a *Hôtel-Dieu* with the best known being in Paris. During this era several orders of nuns provided simple nursing care directed primarily toward meeting the patient's physiological needs (Griffin and Griffin, 1973).

Renaissance

The great epidemics of the Middle Ages led to attitudes of fatalism and a general depressed orientation toward health. However, during the Renaissance people started opening their minds to new ideas, and between 1500 and 1700 medicine began to advance. In general, the Renaissance was characterized by achievements in the arts and scholarly efforts as well as by a rise in commerce and industry. A growing belief in *humanism* developed. Human dignity and worth began to influence health practices. Eventually a group of free thinkers developed in Europe which included Descartes, Voltaire, and Darwin (Rosen, 1958). The combined results of many individuals with enlightened ideas led to a search for scientific truth.

The Renaissance ushered in a new period of history during which community health as currently known was begun (Rosen, 1958). The many technological advances designed to cure the epidemics of the Middle Ages provided the impetus and resources necessary for the changes that took place in the Renaissance. These changes, while not directly influencing community health, supplemented the foundation of modern community health.

There were at least two community health greats during the Renaissance: St. Vincent de Paul and Mademoiselle Le Gras. De Paul is credited as a prominent figure in the history of nursing and social welfare. In 1617 he organized the Sisterhood of the Dames de Charité, which may be the first recorded evidence of home health care. The members visited the sick. As their numbers increased and the demands for their services rose, Mademoiselle Le Gras was appointed as supervisor. This conveyed to community health the belief that home nursing could best be carried out if based on sound principles rather than just kindness and intuition and that nurses needed supervision in their activities. They based their work on a belief in teaching nurses as well as the people they visited how to help themselves (Maynard, 1939).

It was debated whether diseases prominent during the Renaissance including scarlet fever, rickets, scurvy, syphilis, smallpox, and malaria were caused by contagion or constitution. The invention of the microscope by Anton van Leeuwenhoek in the late seventeenth century supported the contagion view by permitting the observation of microorganisms in soil and water.

Although establishment of a systematic national health policy in Europe failed, health problems began to be analyzed and proposals for national action were set forth (Rosen, 1958). William Perry contributed significantly with his belief that communicable disease control would save infant lives and improve the lot of the people. Although this idea made sense, there was no way of enforcing it, since local authorities had no jurisdiction outside their boundaries and ships frequently brought contagious diseases into the ports.

During this time residents supposedly kept the streets clean. They had no system of sewage disposal, and private enterprises supplied water. Towns provided assistance for the sick and lame. Hospitals during this period became places not only to care for the sick but also to study and teach medicine. These advances all were forerunners of later scientific discoveries and gains.

During the Renaissance Leonardo da Vinci produced his anatomical studies and sketches, which are regarded as classics. Andre Vesalius is credited with the scientific development of anatomy, and William Harvey is considered the originator of medical science based on fact rather than on tradition. Further, during this period Harvey established the principle of the physiological experiment and discovered the circulation of blood.

Industrial Revolution

The Industrial Revolution with its emphasis on power and profits reversed many of the gains of the Renaissance. Also, as urban populations grew because of the emphasis on industry and production, the number of people needing health care outpaced the voluntary and often piecemeal efforts to provide services. The 80 years between 1750 and 1830 influenced the future determination of community health because of the upheaval and change as well as the revolution and restoration prevalent at that time.

Population increased dramatically. Major problems included a high infant mortality rate, neglect and often murder of illegitimate infants, poor working conditions, and diseases of certain occupations as well as the growing incidence of mental illness. During the eighteenth century people with mental illness were locked in jails, workhouses, or madhouses. An early defender of the mentally ill, Vincenzo Chiarugi, brought about major reforms at St. Bonifacio in Florence, Italy, where in 1788 he established a system in which properly trained nurses cared for mentally ill people under the direct supervision of a physician. Likewise, the work of William Tuke at York Retreat in England and Philippe Pinel at La Bicetre Hospital in Paris brought about major advances for mentally ill people. Kindness, physical exercise, good food, and fresh air characterized the care at each asylum.

The growth of hospitals paralleled the development of asylums. At the turn of the eighteenth century few hospitals existed in England other than in London. Recognizing the population growth, laymen and physicians worked together to establish many new general hospitals. By 1797, seven general hospitals in London had 1970 beds (Rosen, 1958). Also, by the middle of the century specialty hospitals cared for such groups as seamen and their families; obstetrical patients; children; and patients with special conditions such as eye, chest, and orthopedics disease.

Around the turn of the century urban living conditions improved in England and in 1764 a group of medical police began to create a medical policy regulated by the government. This group advanced the belief that people were responsible for their own health. Health education efforts, largely directed toward the middle and upper classes, grew.

The Industrial Revolution witnessed tremendous advances in transportation, communication, and other forms of technology. Modern public health efforts began in England, the first modern industrial nation. However, to understand how these efforts came into being it is necessary to consider the primary social problem of that era—caring for the poor. The Elizabethan Poor Law of 1601 guaranteed medical and nursing care to the blind, lame, and poor. Table 1-1 chronicles significant community health events beginning with the Elizabethan Poor Law. Each parish cared for its own people, and some parishes established manufacturing centers where the poor could learn to care for themselves. The first project to teach the poor to support themselves began in Bristol in 1696, and the trend led to a steady increase in workhouses until the early nineteenth century. However, the Poor Law Amendment Act of 1834 ushered in a new era of social welfare and community health (Rosen, 1958). This act set up a Commission of Inquiry on the Poor Laws, which was administered by Edwin Chadwick.

Chadwick, educated as a lawyer, devoted his career to helping the poor. In a laissez-faire era characterized by a belief that the state should not interfere with the lives of people, Chadwick attempted to make immediate changes to ensure freedom for all. Two primary points in the Poor Law Amendment Act affected community health. First, the act had established an administrative system based on "unions of parishes run by boards of guardians under a central Poor Law Commission. Each union was to have a medical officer; there would also be medical inspectors" (Swinson, 1965, p. 27). Secondly, this act purported that most pauperism was voluntary. However, Chadwick vigorously campaigned that poverty was a social, not an individual problem and that bad housing, sanitation, and poor water supplies should be corrected to prevent disease. The poor should not be punished for poverty but rather educated to help themselves. He believed that the report of the commission would be enthusiastically received in a Christian country like England. However, the report, which included statements by physicians of the amount of child labor occurring in unhealthy mines, was received as an exaggeration.

Several bills were introduced into Parliament during the first half of the nineteenth century to regulate the working hours of children; however, they were defeated because the millowners exerted more power in Parliament than the proponents of safe working conditions for children. Also, while Chadwick was vigorously campaigning to secure aid to remedy unsanitary conditions, Poor Relief funds were designated to only treat poor people not to remedy social and environmental conditions. Chadwick pointed out that unlimited funds were being spent on treating a filthy, destructive epidemic whereas prevention would be much less costly.

Finally an investigation was approved to study the extent to which typhus was present. It took 2 years to complete the study, which Chadwick detailed in a document entitled "Report on the Sanitary Condition of

Table 1-1. Milestones in the history of community health	
1601	Elizabethan Poor Law written
1765	First American medical school started in Philadelphia
1797	Seven general hospitals in service in London
1789	Marine Service Hospital established
1834	Poor Law Amendment in England sets up a Commission of Inquiry on the Poor Laws administered by Edwin Chadwick
1845	National Institute established
1847	American Medical Association established
1848	Hygiene committee formed by AMA
1850	Shattuck Report prepared on the status of medical education
1855	Quarantine Board established in New Orleans; beginning of tuberculosis campaign in the United States
1864	Factory Act of 1864, which controlled treatment of children in industries, passed; Treaty of Geneva; inauguration of Red Cross
1866	New York Metropolitan Board of Health established
1872	American Public Health Association established
1877	Women's Board of the New York Mission hires Frances Root to visit the sick poor
1878	National Quarantine Act passed by Congress
1879	New York Ethical Society places trained nurses in dispensaries
1880	Division of Child Hygiene established in New York Health Department

the Labouring Population." The commission refused to publish Chadwick's report when they saw how the measures suggested would influence landowners. The report, published under Chadwick's name, became a major social document by emphasizing the destructive effects of filth in the cities, including poor sewage systems and lack of waste disposal facilities. In his report Chadwick established four main conclusions: (1) health depended on sanitation, (2) sanitation was an engineering matter, (3) in each area one authority should administer all sanitary matters, and (4) expert engineering and medical advisers were essential (Swinson, 1965, p. 36). The government reacted to Chadwick's report by establishing a Health of Towns Commission to determine how Chadwick's recommendations could be put into actions.

Not only was sanitation poor but sepsis was the great curse of hospitals. Joseph Lister's contributions to antiseptic surgical techniques made amazing changes in the morbidity and mortality of surgical patients (Swinson, 1965). Despite considerable opposition, Lister introduced a carbolic spray to kill germs in the air, and he also made his students wash and scrub their hands thoroughly. Swinson (1965, p. 57) aptly summarizes the significance of Lister's work when he says "Looking back, it is extraordinary to realize that before Lister introduced his methods, there had been little change in surgical methods in England since the Middle Ages."

The English passed considerable legislation affecting community health. For example, the Factory Act of 1864 controlled the treatment of children in industries. Legislation also was passed dealing with the sale of food to prevent people from consuming polluted foods. Moreover, the Sanitary Act of 1866 gave the Privy Council the power to inspect their districts and suppress nuisances. Duplication of efforts devoted to community health arose, leading to a Local Government Board in 1871 which took up the work of the Privy Council.

As mentioned, during the Renaissance women visited the homes and cared for the sick. Early forerunners of community health nursing are found when one reviews the work of nursing orders in the British Isles. Mary Aikenhead (Sister Mary Augustine) started the Irish Sisters of Charity. In 1812 she and a friend went to the Convent of the Blessed Virgin Mary at York where they observed nuns visiting among the poor. They subsequently began a similar work in Dublin. The Sisters of Mercy were a similar order who founded a home for destitute girls and visited the sick in their homes. These were the first nursing orders in the British Isles.

During the latter part of the Industrial Revolution women performing nursing functions changed from a caring group of women largely supported by a religious order to a group often referred to as the "dregs of the community: dirty, drunken, and dishonest" (Swinson, 1965, p. 22). Charles Dickens (1975) in *Martin Chuzzlewit* provided a lasting impression of nursing in the eighteenth century with his description of Sairy Gamp, a drunk, untrained servant who reportedly provided a semblance of nursing care. However, not all nurses were Sairy Gamps.

About this same time early training schools began to develop in hospitals. The dominant figure in organizing nursing was Florence Nightingale. Her greatest accomplishment, perhaps, was her vigorous crusade for organized training schools for nurses. The legacy of Florence Nightingale is especially significant in light of the social conditions of that period. To fully understand her, it is important to remember that she came from a wealthy, well-educated family. Her parents were opposed to her burning desire to be a nurse because of its poor social image and their desire for better things in life for their daughter. She deferred to her parents' wishes for several years but finally entered nurses' training with Pastor Fliedner at Kaiserwerth in Germany. Books on nursing history chronicle her many accomplishments. However, several of her contributions to nursing need to be summarized to more fully understand the history of community health nursing. Her work during the Crimean War proved that careful, well-planned nursing care could save lives. She demonstrated considerable organizational skill at the hospital at Scutari. When Nightingale arrived, this hospital designed to care for 1700 patients housed 3000 to 4000 men. To run the hospital more effectively, she set up both a central kitchen and a laundry.

She is well remembered for establishing the first modern training school for nurses at St. Thomas Hospital in 1850. This hospital served as an example for Bellevue Hospital, which was established in New York City in 1873. Her insistence on trained nurses is detailed in *Notes on Nursing* (Nightingale, 1946) in which she describes assessment, intervention, and evaluation as nursing activities.

Her interest extended beyond nursing and into many areas. Florence Nightingale was a social worker. She worked to improve the life of soldiers' wives by establishing reading rooms, games, and other entertainment to keep soldiers interested in wholesome activities and away from the "dramshop and loose living" (Griffin and Griffin, 1973, p. 69). She also established a savings bank through which soldiers could forward money to their families in England.

Not only did she provide services for soldiers and their families, but she also worked continuously to reorganize the hospitals at Scutari and in the Crimea and to establish a system for properly training nurses to care for the sick. In 1855 the English established a fund to support nursing education and collected $220,000 in a short time for the Nightingale Fund (Griffin and Griffin, 1973, p. 70).

After the war Nightingale devoted her attention to the slow and exacting process of reforming the army and summarized her work in 1856 as *Notes in Matters Affecting the Health, Efficiency and Hospital Administration of the British Army* (Griffin and Griffin, 1973, p. 71). In the ensuing years people sought her out for advice on hospital administration and construction; she was elected a member of the statistical society for developing a method of uniformly naming and classifying diseases and worked vigorously to reform nursing. See Table 1-2 for additional details about Nightingale.

Nursing During Early American Wars

The need for nurses increases during wartime. Nursing orders came into being with the Crusades. In America the Revolutionary War occurred before Florence Nightingale's many advances were made. However, George Washington asked Congress for a matron and nurses to care for the sick and wounded. During the Revolutionary War (1775 to 1783) hospitals were unsanitary and food, medicine, and trained personnel were sparse. These dismal conditions improved after Nightingale's efforts during the Crimean War (Griffin and Griffin, 1973).

Although the efforts of Florence Nightingale and the work of the Red Cross were known at the time of the Civil War (1861-1865), the system in America for providing nurses for wartime efforts was completely inadequate. Few trained nurses were available, and there were too few well-meaning volunteer women to deal with the onslaught of casualties. "Thus, in the American as in other armies, two types of nursing developed: a regular army nursing service, which was placed under the direction of Dorothea Dix, and an organization sponsored by private citizens, at first tolerated, later supported by the government" (Griffin and Griffin, 1973, p. 85). Although Dix is best known for her work in reform of conditions for the mentally ill, she was highly influential in establishing American wartime nursing efforts.

In 1861 a group of interested women formed the Women's Central Association of Relief out of which grew the Sanitary Commission. This commission brought together the efforts of many scattered organizations and groups to plan health and welfare measures for soldiers. In this same year Dorothea Dix was appointed superintendent of female nurses, whereupon she organized the first army nurse corps. Although her methods were often considered rigid, she recruited approximately 2000 nurses. Despite the recruitment of these nurses, health care during the Civil War was dismal. Equipment and facilities were primitive and overwhelmed by the nearly six million admissions, largely resulting from epidemic or contagious diseases.

At the turn of the century the Spanish-American War seemed inevitable, and Congress authorized the employment of nurses under contract. By this time more than 500 schools of nursing had graduated about 10,000 nurses, and more than 1500 were nurses in the army. The Army Nurse Corps was officially created on February 2, 1901.

Colonial Period

The years of the Colonial period overlap both the span of time from 1750 to 1850 previously referred to as the Industrial Revolution and the period described in the immediately preceding section on nursing during early American wars. While changes described in discussion of the Industrial Revolution were occurring in Europe, other events influential in determining the course of community health were taking place in the Colonies later to become the United States. Epidemics, especially smallpox, characterized the early years of North American settlement. Possibly the Colonists were able to settle in North America because the diseases they brought in were fatal to natives who lacked immunity to them.

Interestingly, the early New England settlers carried on the census-taking activities so highly valued by the Roman Empire. Early Colonial community health efforts included the collection of vital statistics, improved sanitation, and the avoidance of exotic diseases brought in from trade routes. They lacked, however, a continuing and organized mechanism for ensuring that community health efforts would be supported and enforced (Rosen, 1958).

Because of the pressure to establish a federation of states, community health received little attention before the American Revolution. Following the American Revolution, the threat of a variety of diseases, especially yellow fever, led to considerable interest in the establishment of official boards of health. By the end of the eighteenth century New York City, with a population of 75,000, had established a public health committee for monitoring water quality, sewer construction, drainage of marshes, planting of trees and vegetables, construction of a masonry wall along the water front, and interment of the dead (Rosen, 1958).

In July 1798 Congress created a Marine Service Hospital to provide care for sick and disabled seamen. This service was significant for at least three reasons: (1) it served as the stimulus for what later became the United States Public Health Service; (2) it supplied an organized effort to bring about national quarantine efforts and prevent dreaded diseases from entering the United States at its seaports; and (3) it was one of the first recorded examples of prepaid medical insurance, because for twenty cents monthly, merchant seamen were guaranteed medical and hospital care.

Nineteenth Century America

Although the United States grew tremendously between 1800 and 1850, community health efforts by no means kept pace. During this period threats to health escalated as epidemics of smallpox, yellow fever, cholera, typhoid, and typhus entered the country along with the influx of migrants from many parts of the world. By 1850 the living conditions and the average life span in the older American settlements were worse than in

London, which at that time was well known for its deprived living conditions.

The quality of medical care reflected the inadequacies of this period. There had been no medical education until 1765 in Philadelphia when John Morgan patterned the first school after the British model. However, until publication of the Flexner Report in 1910 medical education was taught in a haphazard way with facilities limited both in quality and quantity. Before Abraham Flexner's historical report, many physicians were self-taught with no formal educational or practical experiences. The impact of the movement to reform medical education had far-reaching implications following Flexner's Carnegie Foundation study of medical schools (Schudson, 1974).

In the late eighteenth century medical education followed the pattern originally established by law schools of having lectures and no clinical work in the curriculum. Any applicant who could pay was accepted, and an apprenticeship followed the lecture series. The prestige of medical education reached its lowest ebb; practitioners were disorganized and split by the array of healing philosophies and cults (Schudson, 1974).

At the same time hospitals were generally unsanitary places, staffed by poorly trained workers and with the purpose of providing a place where people, especially the poor, could come to die. Surgery, conducted under highly unsanitary conditions, caused many to develop infections and subsequently die from their treatment.

Just as American cities began establishing community health efforts, an influx of immigrants poured in from the troubled European countries. These immigrants taxed the stability of cities, especially those on the Eastern coast. Housing and sanitation became major problems. As urban communities grew and their sanitary conditions deteriorated, major conflict arose between those wanting health reforms and those wishing to maintain the status quo. A number of voluntary health associations developed to create a base for the mobilization of forces for the community.

From the 1840s on, attention focused on attacking community health problems and improving urban living conditions. The National Institute, a distinguished scientific body, was formed in Washington, D.C., in 1845. Founded in 1847, the American Medical Association (AMA) responded to pressure to form a hygiene committee to carry out sanitary surveys and develop a system for collecting vital statistics. Such a committee established this mechanism in 1848 to secure sanitary surveys for all parts of the country.

Concurrently efforts were being carried out in Massachusetts which produced the famous Shattuck Report. This report, published in 1850 by the Massachusetts Sanitary Commission, reflected massive work by Lemuel Shattuck, a bookseller and publisher. Originally a teacher in Detroit, he became an active member of the school committee in Concord, Massachusetts, and reorganized the public school system of the city. Through an interest in genealogy, Shattuck recognized the need for vital statistics and established statewide registration of vital statistics, which became a model for other states (Rosen, 1957).

Although the Shattuck Report now receives credit as a noteworthy and farsighted document, it fell on virtually deaf ears in its own time. Implementation of the actions recommended by the report came 19 years after its publication. Major recommendations called for the establishment of a state health department and local health boards in every town; sanitary surveys; varying kinds of vital statistics; environmental sanitation, food, drug, and communicable disease control; well-child care including immunizations and health education; and proposals on smoke and alcohol control, town planning, and the teaching of preventive medicine in medical schools. Perhaps his greatest accomplishment was to adapt the ideas and practices of both his predecessors and contemporaries to the needs of America in the 1850s. In the tracing of community health history the themes Shattuck mentioned were also reflected in the sanitary efforts of the Babylonians, the holistic views of the Greeks, the system for health care of the Romans, the social assistance for illness and the development of hospitals in the Middle Ages, the advances in health policy of the Renaissance, and the efforts made to improve sanitary conditions during the Industrial Revolution.

The repeated introduction of yellow fever and other epidemics brought about the inception of a quarantine board in New Orleans in 1855. In determining its range of activities, the New Orleans quarantine board decided to limit its activities to hygiene education efforts, housing, preventable diseases, slaughtering of animals, sale of poisons, and general living conditions of the large population of poor people (Rosen, 1958). This first state board of health also requested information from local boards about their duties and powers as well as about the leading causes of death within their jurisdiction. Interestingly, California, the second state to establish a board of health, was far across the United States from Louisiana. By the end of the nineteenth century, 38 states had health boards.

Between 1857 and 1864 several major cities held National Quarantine and Sanitary Conventions, which prepared the way for the American Public Health Association in 1872. In 1866 the New York Metropolitan Board of Health came into existence. This marked a turning point in community health history in New York as well as in the entire country. The foundation was now established for stable community health advancement.

Era of Bacteriological Investigation and Other Major Advances: 1875 to 1950

Between 1875 and 1950 bacteriology added to the understanding of health and disease. The idea that disease can have a living cause was not totally new but gained considerable attention in the nineteenth century. The work of Jacob Henle in Berlin is viewed as classic in the history of bacteriology and of communicable diseases. Although Henle's book does not contain a single discovery, its relevance is based on the logical consideration of the work of others and a synthesis of ideas to support the notion that living microscopic organisms were the cause of contagious and infectious diseases (Rosen, 1958). Other major contributions included Pasteur's work on fermentation and Koch's work with the anthrax bacilli.

In 1878 Congress passed the National Quarantine Act creating the National Board of Health. This body existed until 1883. The passage of this act reflected national interest in the prevention of epidemic diseases. This law gave authority for investigating the origin and causes of epidemic diseases and for preventing their introduction and spread.

Medical Education

Simultaneous with the advancements in community health, medical education improved in quality and a medical school was established in 1893 at Johns Hopkins University. The Flexner Report provided a boost for medical education when it urged schools to improve the quality of their education through more stringent admission criteria and the closing of financially insolvent schools. Essentially, the Flexner Report is indirectly credited with the elimination of diploma mills and their replacement with approximately 100 medical schools.

These early reforms in medical education of the 1900s also influenced the development of hospitals. Specialization in medical practice existed as early as 485 to 425 BC, as reflected in Herodotus' statement that "every physician is for one disease and not for several, and the whole country is full of physicians; for there are physicians for the eyes, others of the head, others of the teeth, others of the belly, others of the obscure diseases" (Rees, 1968).

By the late 1880s Johns Hopkins University had medical specialties, and the French concept of "interne" was introduced in 1897. By the 1930s it became customary for almost all medical graduates to take a year of internship before beginning a practice. Also, as these new highly educated physicians moved across the

United States, the need for hospitals grew. In 1873 there were only 178 nongovernmental U.S. hospitals compared to 4359 in 1909 (Weinstein, 1968). Poor people who had no other place to go and no one else to care for them typically used the early hospitals. Interestingly, the Phillips House at Massachusetts General Hospital in Boston was that city's first hospital solely designed to care for affluent patients (Freymann, 1977). However, it was not until the 1930s that patients used these hospitals for anything besides surgery.

Immunization

By the end of the nineteenth century people could become resistant to certain diseases by immunization of either live or extracted disease-producing organisms. Because of the German cholera epidemic of 1892, the New York City Health Department created a division of bacteriology and disinfection and made the first application of bacteriology to community health. The 1900s witnessed the disappearance of many infectious diseases. Active immunization of children began in New York City in 1920, and by 1940 an estimated 60% of this age group were protected.

Child Welfare Movement

The child welfare movement, similar in both America and Europe, emphasized the need for clean milk, well-child clinics, and instruction to mothers. The child health movement profited from the establishment of a Division of Child Hygiene in the New York City Health Department in 1880. Led by Dr. Josephine Baker, this division demonstrated that infant deaths could be greatly reduced through prevention. In a congested area of New York's lower East Side community health nurses visited each mother and newborn on the day after birth to teach ways to keep the baby well, as shown in Fig. 1-3 (Rosen, 1958). After 2 months 1200 fewer infant deaths in the district occurred than during the same period a year earlier. Simultaneously with the development of well-baby clinics, clean milk was provided by monitoring sources and by requiring pasteurization.

The New York City activities for improving child health spurred other states and provoked governmental action. In 1912 President Taft signed a bill creating the Children's Bureau to investigate and report "matters pertaining to the welfare of children and child life among all classes of our people" (Rosen, 1958, p. 360). The Children's Bureau was based on the belief that infant health depended on the protection of maternity. The idea for such a bureau came from Florence Kelley and Lillian Wald. Kelley served as the first Chief Inspector of Factories for Illinois and later as General Secretary of the National Consumers League, and Wald

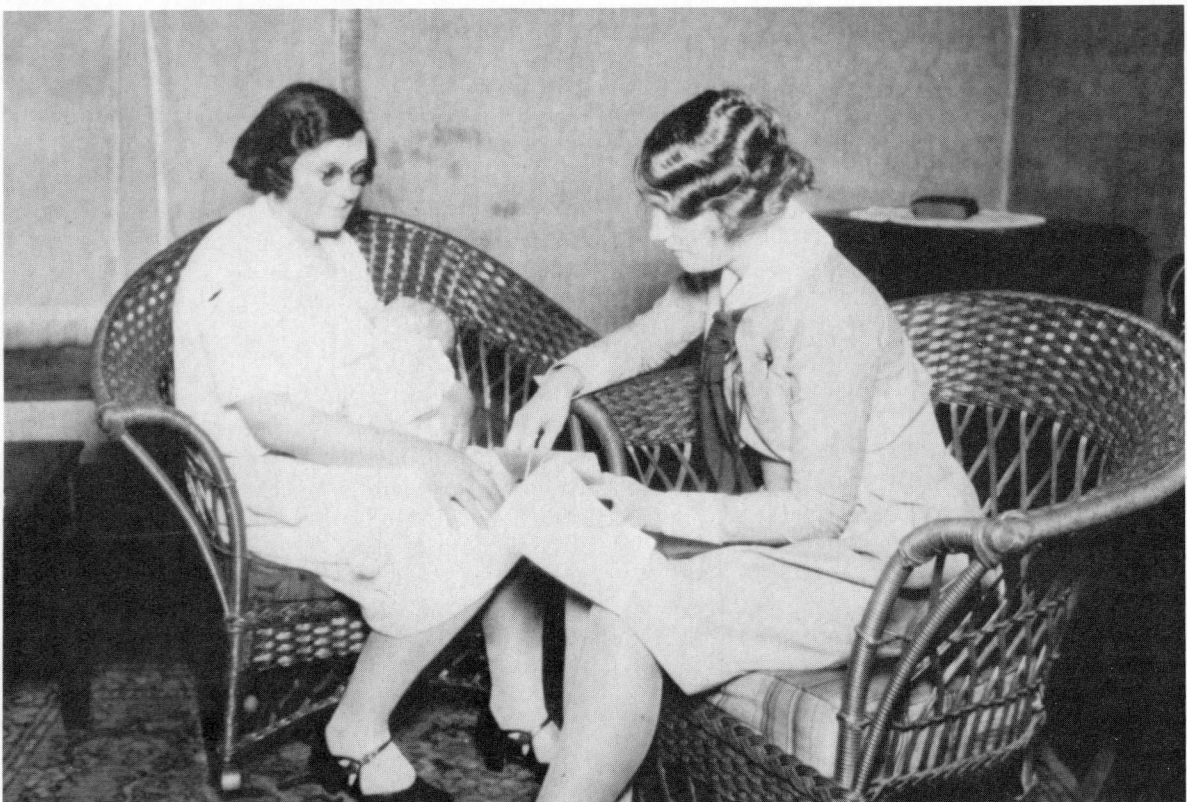

Fig. 1-3. Early public health nurse making home visits to mother and newborn. (Donated by the Jefferson County Department of Health, Birmingham, Ala., Myra Downs, Director, Bureau of Public Health Nursing.)

founded community health nursing in America and established the Henry Street Settlement in New York. Fig. 1-4 is an example of instruction in dietetics in a public school classroom in the early 1900s.

In 1908 the pediatric department of the New York Outdoor Medical Clinic began the first organized prenatal program. Visiting nurse services for pregnant women began in Boston in 1909 and in St. Louis in 1912. The Maternity and Infancy Act (Sheppard-Towner) in 1920 was heralded as landmark legislation and was the first measure to appropriate Federal funds for a health and social welfare program (Rosen, 1958). A successful program ensued for 7 years until funding was discontinued. However, in 1935 Title V of the Social Security Act reenacted the Children's Bureau.

Role of Government

The early twentieth century witnessed multiple improvements that both directly and indirectly affected health status. Organized community health efforts improved simultaneously with changes in medical care and the development of hospitals as treatment facilities

for all people. In 1902 Congress renamed the Marine Hospital Service and gave it an established organizational format under the direction of a surgeon general. The title was again broadened in 1912 to become the United States Public Health Service (USPHS). Table 1-1 lists several events in the history of community health in the United States.

Several significant events influenced the further development of community health efforts, including two major wars followed by an economic depression. In 1917 the National Leprosarium, established at the same time as the USPHS, assumed responsibility for providing health examinations for all immigrants. In 1918 entry into World War I called attention to the need for prevention, detection, and treatment of sexually transmitted diseases, leading to the establishment of the Division of Venereal Diseases within the USPHS. This division cooperated with state health departments to control and prevent these diseases. Subsequently, in 1929 the Narcotics Division, later renamed the Division of Mental Hygiene, became responsible for the confinement and treatment of narcotic addicts.

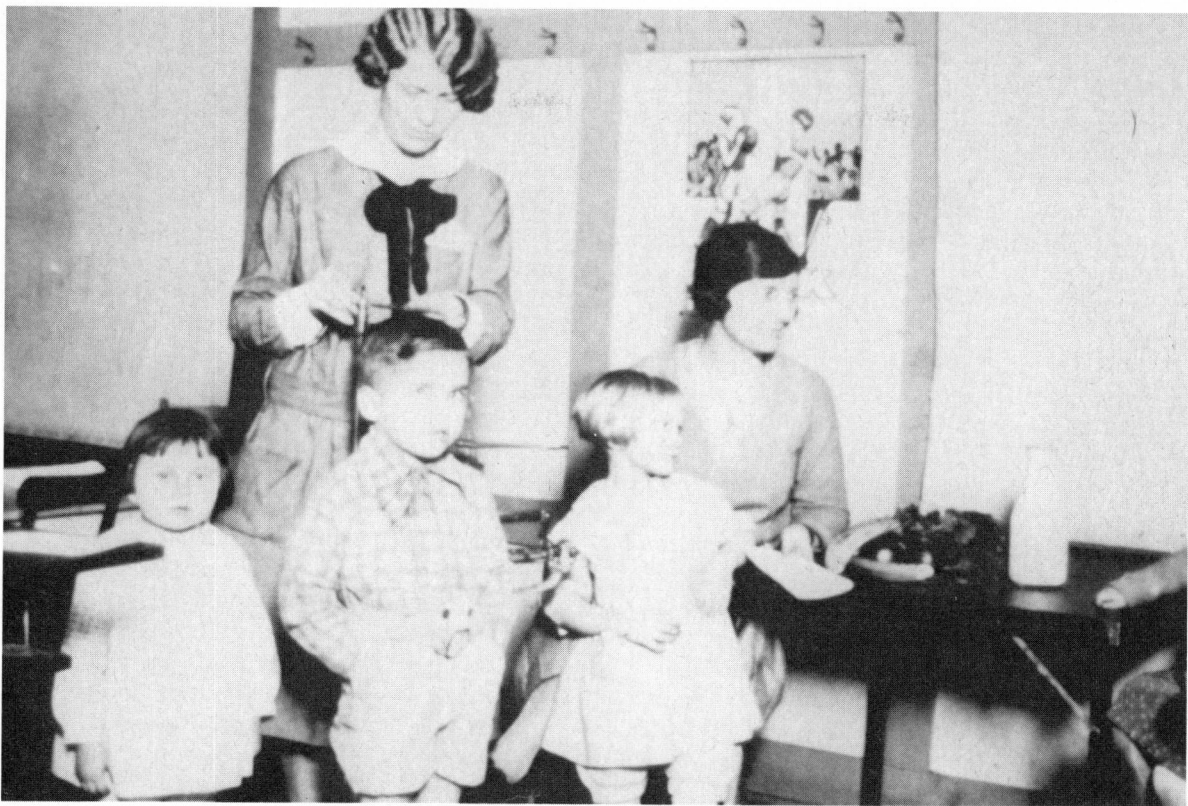

Fig. 1-4. Instruction in dietetics in school in early 1900. (Donated by the Jefferson County Department of Health, Birmingham, Ala., Myra Downs, Director, Bureau of Public Health Nursing.)

During the next several decades substantial changes took place at the Federal level, which affected the structure of community health resources and included the Federal Social Security Act of 1935. Title VI of the act affected the scope of community health through its original mission to assist states and their subdivisions in the establishment and maintenance of adequate community health services including the training of personnel for both state and local health activities. Other influential developments included the passage in 1937 of the National Cancer Institute Act, which provided for research into the cause, diagnosis, and treatment of cancer.

Finally, in 1939 the Public Health Service relocated from the Treasury Department to the newly created Federal Security Agency, which President Roosevelt planned as a major effort to reorganize and consolidate federal services. The Public Health Services had undergone many changes in organization as well as alterations resulting from passage of several health-related acts such as the National Mental Health Act of 1946 and the establishment in 1948 of institutes in the four

areas of heart, microbiology, experimental biology and medicine, and dental research.

In 1949 the Mental Hygiene Division moved from the Bureau of Medical Services to the National Institutes of Health to form the National Institute of Mental Health. Other major institutes formed in the ensuing years included the National Institute of Neurological Diseases and Blindness (1950) and the National Institute of Arthritis and Metabolic Diseases (1959); both the Division of General Medical Sciences and the Institute of Child Health and Human Development were established in 1962, and the Division of Environmental Health Sciences was established within the Public Health Service in 1966. When the Environmental Protection Agency opened in 1970, most of the environmental health activities of the Public Health Service were transferred to it. Additionally, for more effective service to states, the Public Health Service developed 10 regional offices located in Boston, New York, Philadelphia, Atlanta, Chicago, Kansas City, Dallas, Denver, San Francisco, and Seattle.

Both the Hill-Burton Act (1946) and the Children's

Bureau (1912) influenced community health. Each will be discussed in a later section. Other federal agencies whose work influences community health include the Food and Drug Administration, agencies within the Departments of Agriculture and Interior, Office of International Health of the Public Health Service, Agency for International Development of the Department of State, and the Department of Health, Education, and Welfare (which on May 4, 1980, became the Department of Health and Human Services).

Food Control

The first efforts of the federal government to control and supervise the quality of food began in 1879 with a bill introduced into Congress to prohibit the adulteration of food and drink. It took 27 years for this goal to be realized, and ultimately the present Food and Drug Administration grew out of this aim. In 1906 President Roosevelt signed the Pure Food and Drugs Act, and the present Federal Food, Drug, and Cosmetics Act was signed in 1938.

Within the Department of Agriculture several bureaus conduct community health activities. The Bureau of Animal Industry investigates the cause, prevention, and treatment of diseases of domestic animals which have implications for people. The Bureau of Dairy Industry is concerned with the sanitary regulation and handling of milk, and the Bureau of Human Nutrition and Home Economics has made considerable gains in the areas of rural health and nutrition.

DEPARTMENT OF HEALTH AND HUMAN SERVICES (HEALTH, EDUCATION, AND WELFARE)

The Department of Health, Education, and Welfare came into being on April 11, 1953, as part of President Eisenhower's reorganization of the executive branch of the government. The original purpose was to "bring into closer functional relationship and to improve the administration of the important health, education, welfare, and Social Security functions then being carried on by the federal government" (Hanlon and Pickett, 1979, p. 43). These functions have not entirely been attained, since the Department has traditionally been comprised of multiple separate subdepartments with their own goals and objectives. Unity of purpose has yet to be realized. However, on May 4, 1980, the Department of Health, Education, and Welfare was restructured to become the Department of Health and Human Services. A second agency, the Department of Education, was formed to handle selected activities.

VOLUNTARY ACTION FOR HEALTH

Although the government retains a major responsibility for the health and welfare of its citizens, voluntary organizations play key roles in community health. Rapid economic growth in the United States helped to create many of the problems attracting the attention of voluntary health agencies and also provided the resources and leisure time necessary for volunteers to start such organizations. By 1945 there were about 20,000 agencies with 300,000 volunteers in the United States. Currently, there are more than 100,000 voluntary, nongovernmental health and welfare agencies (Wilner et al., 1978). Appendix H describes health organizations used by community health nurses.

Despite the diversity among these agencies they tend to fall into four general categories: (1) those dealing with specific diseases such as tuberculosis, cancer, diabetes, and so on; (2) those concerned with certain organs of the body including heart, lung, eyes, and ears; (3) those involved with the health and welfare of special groups such as the aged or children; and (4) those dealing with health problems that affect the community as a whole, such as accident prevention, mental health, planned parenthood, or human abuse (Rosen, 1958, p. 384). Voluntary agencies obtain financial support primarily from individual contributions and secondarily through business and industry. Some secure funds from payments by clients for services, membership dues, and investment income.

Competition is keen among voluntary agencies to secure donations and service of volunteers. The rapid growth of agencies and the number of individual fundraising efforts led many cities to form community chests or united funds. These agencies carry out a single drive or appeal for funds and then divide the monies received among the participating organizations (Wilner, et al., 1978). The first united fund-raising effort began in 1949 in Detroit as the Torch Drive. Currently most larger cities have a combined fund-raising campaign, which lessens the number of requests made on people.

Although space does not permit a thorough discussion of the history of specific voluntary agencies, the progression of development of two major agencies will be summarized here.

National Tuberculosis Association

The National Tuberculosis Association is the·oldest agency of its type, and its development epitomizes the voluntary health movement. Initially tuberculosis was viewed as hereditary disease, which could only be treated by a change in climate. However, Koch's discovery in 1882 of the tubercle bacillus dramatically changed this view.

The first tuberculosis dispensary was the Victoria Dispensary for Consumption, which was started in 1887 in Edinburgh. The National Association for the Prevention of Consumption and Other Forms of Tuberculosis developed in 1898 to educate people about disease prevention (Rosen, 1958, p. 386). In 1893 the Michigan State Board of Health voted to require the reporting of tuberculosis to local health departments, and similar efforts in Baltimore and Philadelphia followed. The Pennsylvania Society for the Prevention of Tuberculosis, organized by physician Lawrence Fleck, was a pioneer effort in many ways. This marked the first attempt to combine professionals and laymen in combating a specific disease. Secondly, this organization called for coordination among hospitals and boards of health to work toward prevention through community education. The National Association for the Study and Prevention of Tuberculosis was formed in Atlantic City in 1904 (its name was changed in 1918 to the National Tuberculosis Association). Because of financial problems, the Russell Sage Foundation supplemented funding for 10 years.

Red Cross

The Red Cross began accidentally in northern Italy in 1859. At that time, with 300,000 Italian and French soldiers actively fighting, deaths and injuries abounded. Hundreds died from lack of attention. This appalling situation attracted the attention of a Swiss tourist, Jean Henri Dunant, who assembled female volunteers from the town of Solferino, Italy, to care for the wounded. Inspired by Florence Nightingale's work in the Crimea he devoted his life to preventing the horrors he had seen in Solferino. Traveling from country to country he urged the establishment of bands of volunteers to treat wounded men. Finally in 1863 the Society of Public Utility of Geneva, Switzerland, convened with 36 representatives from 14 countries to study Dunant's proposal. This meeting established the basic principles of the Red Cross and developed plans to organize Red Cross societies in selected countries across the world.

Before it could be fully organized, the Red Cross was called into service to care for the wounded of the bloody war between Denmark and newly organized Prussia in 1863 to 1864. The Geneva Convention of 1864 established Dunant's original principles and made the Red Cross an official international group for caring for the wounded. Out of this Convention came the International Red Cross Committee, the coordinating committee of all the Red Cross committees. The international committee aids victims of war and disaster when the magnitude of the problem is greater than the scope of national committees.

During wars the National Red Cross Societies (component parts of the International Red Cross) assist by mobilizing nurses, nurses's aides, and volunteers to establish ambulance services, hospitals, hospital ships, canteens, libraries for soldiers, entertainment, occupational therapy, and so forth. It also aids war refugees and prisoners and may assist citizens in devastated cities. Aid may also extend to families of war victims and to providing housing for disabled men. Nurses have always played a major role in the Red Cross by directly carrying out many of the designated functions (Deloughery, 1977).

American Red Cross

The American Red Cross has its own interesting history. As Red Cross efforts developed in European countries, Clara Barton went abroad to study their functions. She became convinced that such an operation had a definite place in the United States. In 1881 Clara Barton's efforts resulted in the incorporation of an American Association of the Red Cross in the District of Columbia with Clara Barton serving as president. The yellow fever epidemic of 1888 in Florida required that the Red Cross be called into action. Over the years an extensive organization developed with local committees and sections for selecting and training volunteer nurses who could, with little notice, be called into service. In the latter part of the nineteenth century the Red Cross sponsored a nurses' training program lasting two years and 3 months. This was discontinued as nursing education advanced and modern training schools were developed in hospitals.

In 1898 the Red Cross was officially recognized as the American National Red Cross Relief Committee. Lillian Wald recommended that community health nursing be a part of the Red Cross in 1903. Although these efforts originated in New York, they initially served rural areas. By 1913 the towns having populations as large as 25,000 received nursing care through the Red Cross. This activity, called the Town and Country Nursing Service, included "home hygiene and care of the sick, dietetics, public hygiene in rural areas and small towns, disaster nursing and instruction of nurses's aides" (Deloughery, 1977, p. 79) (Fig. 1-4).

Over the years the American Red Cross method of teaching instructors has been adapted to the needs of many countries. Since 1945 the Red Cross home nursing instruction has been part of the curriculum in many secondary schools where it can be taught not only by nurses but also by teachers and volunteers. The blood program began in 1947. Today the Red Cross boasts of nearly 4000 chapters in the United States, each with a voluntary board of directors and voluntary committees to direct its efforts. Chapters plan programs to meet the needs of specific communities, including needs for health education.

Conclusion

Voluntary health agencies accomplish a great deal through their persistent and at times pioneering efforts at research and demonstration projects as well as professional lay education. However, they have been under scrutiny in recent years in connection with the way funds were spent. Critics contend that too little of the dollar contributed goes for research, service, or education. Despite what may seem like shortcomings in their operation, voluntary health agencies remain viable and are a potent force in health care (Wilner, et al., 1978).

INTERNATIONAL HEALTH

The extent and quality of world health problems are influenced by population density, climate, and a variety of biological factors. Most of the preventable diseases to which humans are subject involve other biologic beings, including bacteria, viruses, protozoa, helminths, and insects (Hanlon and Pickett, 1979). Additionally, climatic conditions in warm, moist tropical and subtropical zones of the world provide a rich medium for the transmission of disease. Also, disease is transmitted more readily in densely populated regions than in more sparsely populated areas.

Currently most preventable diseases occur in the warmer regions with malaria still the leading cause of death in the world. Ninety percent of children under 5 years of age in Liberia have positive blood smears for malaria, and 70% of the adults are continuously infected (Hanlon and Pickett, 1979). This disease is rampant in a large part of the lowlands of South and Central America, Africa, and almost all of the south and southeast parts of Asia. Other major world health problems include schistosomiasis, helminth or worm infestation, leprosy, venereal diseases, yaws, tuberculosis, typhoid and paratyphoid fever, diarrheas, and dysenteries. Approximately three fourths of the world's population "drink unsafe water, dispose of human excreta recklessly, prepare milk and food dangerously, are constantly exposed to insect and rodent enemies, and live in a primitive state of insanitation" (Hanlon and Pickett, 1979, p. 62).

One of the most serious aspects of the world's health problems is the shortage of health personnel in most parts of the world. This is especially true in the developing nations, which also have the poorest living conditions and greatest predisposition to disease. The economic and social conditions of a country are directly related to the health of the people, and of course, the levels of health influence social and economic factors. Where living conditions are inadequate, health care primitive or available only at a distant location, food supplies limited, and education minimal, the prospects of rampant disease are great.

Organizations for International Health

Over the years a number of international health programs have been developed to assist less fortunate countries in increasing their standard of living. The first organized effort for international health began in Paris in 1851 with the establishment of the First International Sanitary Conference. Twelve countries participated and each sent a physician and a diplomat to the conference. A series of conferences led to the establishment of a permanent international health agency known as the International Office of Public Health (d'Office International d'Hygiene Publique), which began in Paris in 1909. Referred to as the "Paris Office," the small fulltime staff primarily gathered information, revised international regulations, and arbitrated differences (Wilner, Walkley, and O'Neill, 1978).

The end of World War I witnessed the establishment of the League of Nations. A health section came into being in 1923 and became known as the "Geneva Office." Functioning alongside the Paris Office, both dealt with international efforts to prevent and control disease. In addition, the Geneva office developed an Epidemiological Intelligence Service, conducted studies of rural hygiene, housing, health of school children, health centers, and health insurance (Rosen, 1958). The technical studies of this agency facilitated international consensus on crucial areas such as the serological diagnosis of syphilis and the standardization of biological products employed therapeutically.

The Health Section of the League of Nations created the first mechanism for attacking widespread diseases such as malaria, tuberculosis, syphilis, rabies, leprosy, cancer, and sleeping sickness. Additionally, it provided direct services to individual nations on request. Some of these activities were carried out in conjunction with the Rockefeller Foundation as well as other foundations with health interests. The basic premise of the Rockefeller Foundation through its International Health Division has been the belief that countries need to be aided in helping themselves by supporting research, educating health personnel, and establishing demonstration programs.

World Health Organization

In 1948 the duties and powers of the League of Nations were transferred to a newly created agency, the

World Health Organization (WHO). On June 24, 1948, the first World Health Assembly convened in Geneva, Switzerland, with delegates from 52 member states and observers from 11 nonmember states and 10 international governmental organizations. A nation may be a member of WHO without being a member of the United Nations. The United States has been an active member of WHO since its inception. WHO, founded on the premise that health is a basic right of all people, has become the worldwide coordinating, official agency in international health. Headquarters remain in Geneva with regional offices in four parts of the world including one in Washington, D.C. Its working budget in 1978 of $172 million was financed by contributions from active member nations and from the United Nations Technical Assistance Board.

The functions of WHO can be summarized as follows (Hanlon and Pickett, 1979, p. 69):

1. It is the one directing and coordinating authority on international health work. It is not a supranational ministry of health; rather it is a worldwide cooperative through which the nations help each other to help themselves in raising standards.
2. It provides to member countries various central technical services, that is, epidemiology, statistics, standardization of drugs and procedures, a wide range of technical publications, and so on.
3. Its most important function is to help countries to strengthen and improve their own health service. On request it provides advisory and consulting services through public health experts, demonstration teams for disease control, visiting specialists, and so on.

Priorities are established by the World Health Assembly of WHO; those for the years 1978 to 1983 included the following (Division of Information, 1967):

1. Development of comprehensive health services
2. Disease prevention and control
3. Promotion of environmental health
4. Health manpower development
5. Promotion of biomedical and health services research
6. Program development and support

Pan American Health Organization

The Pan American Health Organization (PAHO) originated in 1902 in Mexico City as the International Sanitary Bureau and was organized by a Pan American Sanitary Conference. This organization has headquarters in Washington, D.C., and is the center of coordination of international public health information and activities in the Western Hemisphere. The Pan American Health Organization became a regional office of WHO in 1949, although it still maintains its own organiza-

tional identity. PAHO holds an annual conference, and since its inception, it has contributed greatly to public health advancement by disseminating information, providing technical assistance, offering financial fellowships, and promoting cooperation in medical research (Hanlon and Pickett, 1979).

United Nations Children's Fund

This agency has worked closely with WHO since its inception at the end of World War II. Its initial purpose was to provide assistance to the war-torn countries. Over the years this agency has spent vast amounts of money on food and supplies to promote maternal and child welfare throughout the world. Often in partnership with WHO, the United Nations Children's Fund (UNICEF) has carried out many programs of BCG vaccination, yaws control, and malaria control demonstrations. In recent years family planning has been emphasized. Also, in the late 1940s this agency established an International Children's Center, which brings together a variety of health disciplines to focus on the physical, mental, and social aspects of child development.

Agency for International Development

The agencies previously discussed have been formed by multination efforts that jointly finance, staff, and operate the agency. Another type of agency is bilateral in nature and exists when two nations agree to work together for improving community health conditions. Prominent among the bilateral agencies is the Agency for International Development (AID), which was organized in 1961 within the U.S. Department of State and which promotes the work of the United States with other nations on a one-to-one basis. The predecessor of AID, the Institute of Inter-American Affairs, was established after World War II to initiate and conduct bilateral technical assistance programs in health, agriculture, education, and other areas. Like its predecessor, AID has made significant contributions in community health training and technical assistance to requesting countries.

DEVELOPMENT OF NURSING IN THE UNITED STATES

During the late nineteenth century women physicians increased in numbers and many aided the advancement of nursing care. In 1867 Dr. Marie Zakrzewska, professor of obstetrics at the New England Female Medical College in Boston, initiated a nursing program at the New England hospital for women and children. Linda Richards, who successfully completed the program is often called America's first trained nurse.

The role of women changed dramatically after the turn of the century. The fight for women's suffrage continued, and many women became involved in the Prohibition movement. Women increasingly sought employment in business and industry and entered college in greater numbers; because of the war effort during Word War I, many secured jobs previously held by men.

Simultaneously with the changes in women's roles, the demand for nurses increased. Hospitals began to be accepted as places for treatment not just as places where people went to die. Hospitals of all sizes developed training schools for nurses with little or no regard for meeting the educational needs of the students. Instead, they viewed pupils as a ready and convenient source of cheap labor. Some of the graduates of these early schools proved to be quite effective, whereas others caused embarrassment because of their inability to provide adequate patient care. In each state, groups of nurses pushed for legislation to control the education and practice of nursing. These efforts led to nursing licensure with the first state licensure law passed in North Carolina in 1903.

Evolution of Nursing Education

The first three training schools for nurses were established in the United States in 1868 at Bellevue Hospital in New York, New Haven Hospital in Connecticut, and Massachusetts General Hospital in Boston. Each of these hospitals used the model developed by Florence Nightingale. However, lack of funds led each to be controlled by the hospital rather than being an autonomous educational unit as Nightingale had advocated. Each school grew and developed in its own individual manner with long classes, no standard curriculum, military-type discipline, and full obedience to physicians.

Although as nursing had developed as an apprentice-style occupation, the field of medicine began to shift from this mode of training to one of autonomy from hospitals and into the academic arena. The first basic nursing program associated with a university began in 1909 at the University of Minnesota. Simultaneously, several hospitals started to affiliate with colleges for the education of nurses. In addition, Teachers College in New York developed college courses for graduate nurses.

Initially community health nursing required special education. Debate ensued as to whether community health nurses needed a basic nursing education or just special training in home care. Nursing leaders decided that all nurses needed some community health content, hence basic undergraduate courses began to include the topic of community health, with Boston leading the

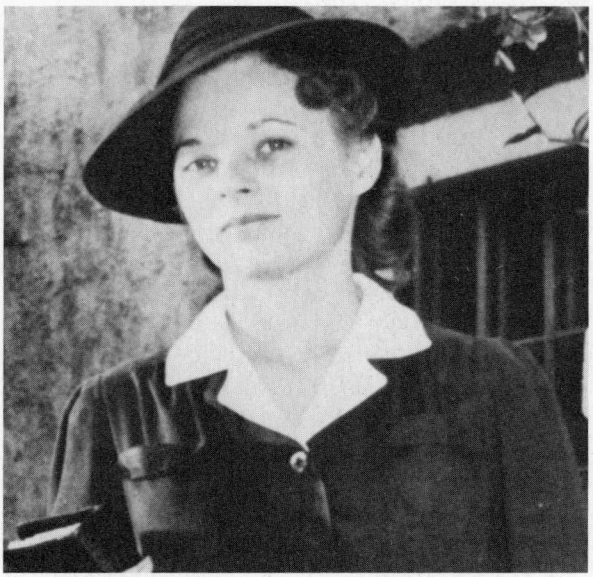

Fig. 1-5. Early public health nurse. (Donated by the Jefferson County Department of Health, Birmingham, Ala., Myra Downs, Director, Bureau of Public Health Nursing.)

way with the first undergraduate community health course.

As community health nursing grew as a specialized and respected area of nursing, it became apparent that the inclusion of this content in basic curricula was insufficient. In 1914 Mary Adelaide Nutting offered the first postgraduate nursing course in community health at Teachers College in affiliation with the Henry Street Settlement (Deloughery, 1977). When this turned out to be successful, Boston began a special training program for community health nurses, which developed into an 8-month course affiliated with Simmons College (Fig. 1-5).

In 1918 during World War I the Vassar Camp School for nurses started as a unique and patriotic aspect of nursing education. The American Red Cross and the Council of National Defense jointly supported this novel program, which proposed that nursing education could be shortened from 3 years to 2 years for college graduates. The Vassar Camp School, modeled after the Plattsburg Military Camp in New York, gave intensive training to college graduates so they could become army reserve officers and meet urgent wartime needs. A total of 435 graduates of this program represented many colleges across the country. The program ended when peace was declared.

Nursing education profited from the landmark study published in 1923 as *The Report of the Committee for Study of Nursing Education.* This study, directed by Josephine Goldmark, led to the Rockefeller Foundation's endowment of the School of Nursing at Yale University. During this same year, the financial support of Frances Payne Bolton, a wealthy Cleveland citizen, established the School of Nursing at Western Reserve University. She had become interested in nursing education on reading the Goldmark report and subsequently contributed significantly to nursing education.

Schools of nursing proliferated during the 1920s amid turmoil and change. In 1925 the three major nursing organizations (National League for Nursing, American Nurses' Association, and National Organization for Public Health Nursing) authorized a program for grading schools, and in 1926 the Committee on the Grading of Nursing Schools began with 21 members. The committee had three major goals: to study the supply and demand for nursing service, to complete a job analysis of nurses, and to grade nursing schools. Grading began in 1929 and was repeated again in 1932, leading to the closing of several hundred weak schools.

About the time of World War II it became evident that graduates of collegiate schools of nursing did not need the same educational preparation in public health nursing as those from diploma programs. Collegiate programs increasingly included content in community health nursing. The first basic program in nursing was accredited in 1944 and included sufficient community health content so that graduates did not need additional training courses in order to practice community health nursing (National Organization for Public Health Nursing, 1944, p. 371).

Over the next 30 years several major changes in nursing education occurred, including the development and rapid expansion of practical nursing programs and the establishment in 1953, with Mildred Montag's doctoral dissertation at Teachers College in New York City, of Associate degree nursing programs. Moreover, starting in 1963 the National League for Nursing required baccalaureate programs to include public health nursing in order to be eligible for accreditation. Additionally, a major conceptual change in nursing resulted from the 1965 American Nurses' Association position paper on nursing practice which proposed that the education of nurses should take place in institutions of higher learning. In recent decades nursing has advanced as a scholarly profession characterized by increased research among practitioners and the development of a conceptual basis for practice.

Organizations for Nursing Education and Practice

By 1893, with 225 schools of nursing in operation, it became necessary to establish some form of standards (Shyrock, 1959). Isabel Hampton Robb assumed the leadership role in establishing the Society of Superintendents of Training Schools of Nurses in the United States and Canada in 1893. This new society sought to establish training standards and promote colleagueship among nurses. This organization later became the National League for Nursing. Two years later the Nurses' Associated Alumnae of the United States and Canada was organized. This group later became the American Nurses' Association with the original purpose of strengthening the union of nursing organizations, elaborating nursing education, and promoting ethical standards (Tinkham and Voorhies, 1977).

Initially the American Society of Superintendents of Training Schools limited its membership to the heads of the larger schools. However, it soon became apparent that it would be beneficial to expand the membership. The first wave of expansion included the superintendents of smaller schools, and later membership became available to all people interested in nursing education.

In 1911 a joint committee was appointed, composed of representatives of the American Nurses' Association and the American Society of Superintendents of Training Schools to standardize nurses' services outside the hospital. Lillian Wald chaired the committee, and Mary Gardner served as secretary. The committee recommended that a new organization be formed to meet the needs of community health nurses. They subsequently invited 800 agencies known to be involved in community health nursing activities to send delegates to an organizational meeting in Chicago in June 1912. A heated debate commenced as to the name and purpose of this organization; however, at noon on June 7, 1912 the delegates unanimously voted the National Organization for Public Health Nursing into existence with Lillian Wald as its first president.

The new organization sought "to standardize public health nursing activities on a high level and coordinate all efforts in the field" (Deloughery, 1977, p. 116). Although primarily a nursing organization, all people interested in community health nursing could be members. Because of its willingness to cooperate with other groups with similar interest, the organization grew rapidly and remained in existence until the American Public Health Association came into being.

Also during 1912 the American Society for Superintendents of Training Schools became the National League for Nursing Education. This new group immediately formed a committee to study the products of nursing education and to identify ways to standardize educational programs. The first major step toward this goal occurred in 1917 with the publication of the Standard Curriculum for Nursing Schools, which established the national League for Nursing Education as the source of information on nursing education.

International Council of Nursing

The first international group of nurses met in London in 1899 as the International Council of Women. Mrs. Bedford Fenwick encouraged nurses to form their own separate group, and 2 years later when the International Council of Nurses met at the World Exposition in Buffalo, New York, she was elected president (Jamieson and Sewall, 1954). In those days matrons of hospitals generally did not know one another. During the World's Fair in Chicago in 1893, Fenwick had met Isabel Hampton Robb, at that time superintendent of the nurse training school at Johns Hopkins Hospital in Baltimore, who invited her to visit the school. This led to a recognition of the need for nurses to meet together on an international level.

Subsequently at the Matrons Council in London in 1899, Fenwick campaigned for an organization to promote the advancement of nursing education. The aim of the International Council of Nursing (ICN) was to "increase the educational level of nurses, to increase professional ethic, to more adequately meet societal needs, and to raise the civic spirit of its members" (Deloughery, 1977, p. 184). As early as 1901 the ICN passed a resolution supporting the nursing role in prevention of illness and restoration of health.

EVOLUTION OF COMMUNITY HEALTH NURSING

Many of the early accomplishments of community health nurses have been interwoven into the preceding sections. However, this section traces the efforts of community health nurses from the first records of visiting nursing sponsored in 1683 by St. Vincent de Paul in Paris and carried out by the Sisterhood of the Dames de Charité. These women, both married and single, visited and provided care to the sick in their homes. During a promised service commitment of usually a year these women associated with a hospital for the supervision of patient care (Bullough and Bullough, 1964). Table 1-2 chronicles the milestones in community health nursing.

Home Health Care

The next significant era for community health nursing is traced to William Rathbone in Liverpool, England. Because of the outstanding care provided to his dying wife, Rathbone in 1859 led in establishing a district nursing service. Based on his experience, Rathbone concluded that many people with long-term illnesses could be better cared for in their own homes than in a hospital. He urged his wife's nurse, Mary Robinson, to begin a program of home nursing care for poor people. Subsequently, at Rathbone's urging the Liverpool Relief Society divided the city into nursing districts, and assigned a committee of "Friendly Visitors" to each district to provide health care to needy people (Kalisch and Kalisch, 1978).

Based on the Liverpool experience, Rathbone wrote a book entitled *Social Organization of Effort in Works of Benevolence and Public Charity by a Man of Business* in which he outlined a philosophy for home health care (Dolan, 1978). England became a forerunner in home health care, and Rathbone's work spurred Florence Nightingale to publish a pamphlet on nursing entitled *Suggestions for Improving Nursing Service,* which recommended steps for nursing care in the home. Rathbone ultimately founded the Metropolitan Nursing Association to provide home health nursing (Bullough and Bullough, 1964). During this time the largest religious organization in London, the Bible and Domestic Mission, sent women into the slums to read the Bible and in 1868 added nursing care to their program (Dolan, 1973).

In Colonial America, the first visiting nurse society began in Philadelphia in 1886 to provide home health care to the sick. Earlier efforts had been noted in New Amsterdam (New York) in the works of the *Krankenbezoekers* (seekers out of sick) and *Ziskentroosters* (ones who gives comfort to the sick). Following the War of 1812, a Ladies Benevolent Society was organized to aid sick and impoverished people. In 1877 the Women's Board of the New York Mission hired Frances Root, a graduate of Bellevue Hospital's first nursing class, to visit the sick poor and provide nursing care and religious instruction (Bullough and Bullough, 1964).

Nurses at the first visiting nursing society in Philadelphia strictly followed physician's orders, gave selected treatments, and kept temperature and pulse records. Since their visits were brief, the nurses soon recognized the need to teach family members basic elements of care. Thus from the very beginning community health nursing included teaching and prevention.

In 1886 two women in Boston approached the Women's Education Association to seek support for district nursing. They used the term *instructive district nursing* to emphasize the relationship to education and to increase their likelihood of receiving support from this group. They then met with representatives of the Boston Dispensary, which was providing free medical care to the poor according to the dispensary district in which they lived. In February 1886 the first district nurse was hired in Boston. As the number of district

Table 1-2. Milestones in the history of community health nursing

1617	Sisterhood of the Dames de Charité organized in France by St. Vincent de Paul; may have been first home health care service
1812	Sisters of Mercy established in Dublin where nuns visited the poor
1813	Ladies' Benevolent Society of Charleston, S.C., founded
1836	Modern Order of Lutheran Deaconesses created by Pastor Fliedner at Kaiserwerth
1851	Florence Nightingale goes to Kaiserwerth
1859	District Nursing established in Liverpool by William Rathbone
1860	Florence Nightingale Training School for Nurses established at St. Thomas Hospital in London
1867	Nursing program started at New England Hospital
1868	Training schools established at Bellevue Hospital, New Haven Hospital, and Massachusetts General Hospital
1872	Training School for Nurses started at New England Hospital for Women and Children
1873	Linda Richards becomes first nurse graduated in United States
1885	District Nursing Association in Buffalo established
1886	First visiting nursing society in Philadelphia provides home health care; instructive district nursing begins in Boston
1889	Chicago Visiting Nursing Association established
1892	School nursing first undertaken in London
1893	Visiting nursing service for the poor in New York organized by Lillian Wald and Mary Brewster; American Society of Superintendents of Training Schools for Nurses organized (became National League for Nursing Education in 1912)
1895	Industrial nursing program initiated at Vermont Marble Works
1897	Nurses' Associated Alumnae of United States and Canada organized (became ANA in 1911)
1898	Public health nurses hired by Los Angeles Health Department; Detroit Visiting Nurse Association formed
1899	International Council of Nurses organized; university education for nurses introduced at Teachers College, New York.
1900	*American Journal of Nursing* begins publication
1901	58 organizations providing public health nursing (about 130 nurses)
1902	School nursing started in New York (Lina Rogers)
1903	First nurse practice acts; tuberculosis nursing in Baltimore
1905	200 organizations providing public health nursing (about 440 nurses)
1906	First post graduate course in district nursing offered by the Instructive District Nursing Association (Boston)
1907	Alabama law permitting employment of public health nurses passed
1908	Detroit Health Department hires public health nurses
1909	The Visiting Nurse Quarterly first published in Cleveland (in 1918 became a monthly, *The Public Health Nurse,* and in 1931 name changed to *Public Health Nursing*); first nursing program affiliated with a university (Minnesota) inaugurated; 566 organizations providing 1413 public health nurses; Metropolitan Life Insurance initiates offer of home nursing to its industrial policy holders
1910	Public health nursing program instituted at Teachers College, New York
1911	First state public health nursing laws passed
1912	National Organization for Public Health Nursing formed with Lillian Wald as first president; Rural Nursing Service of American Red Cross established; National League for Nursing Education started
1913	Division of Public Health Nursing, New York State Department of Public Health, organized
1914	First undergraduate nursing education course in public health offered by Adelaide Nutting at Teachers College
1916	1922 organizations providing 5,152 public health nurses
1917	Publication of the Standard Curriculum for Nursing Schools

Continued.

Table 1-2. Milestones in the history of community health nursing — cont'd

1918	Vassar Camp School for Nurses organized; USPHS establishes division of public health nursing to work in extracantonment zones
1919	*Public Health Nursing* written by Mary S. Gardner
1920	NOPHN approves university programs in public health nursing
1922	4040 public health agencies providing 11,548 nurses
1923	Report issued by Committee for Study of Nursing Education (Goldmark Report)
1924	U.S. Indian Bureau Nursing Service established
1925	Frontier Nursing Service using nurse-midwives organized (Mary Breckenridge); first NOPHN statement of qualifications for public health nurses; John Hancock Mutual Life Insurance Company starts Visiting Nurse Service
1926	Committee on Grading of Nursing Schools begins studies
1931	4,255 public health organizations providing 15,865 nurses
1933	Pearl McIver becomes first nurse employed by USPHS
1934	*Survey of Public Health Nursing* published by NOPHN
1935	*Facts about Nursing* first published by ANA
1942	American Association of Industrial Nurses established
1943	Bolton-Bailey Act for nursing education and Cadet Nurse Program passed; Division of Nursing Education started by USPHS (Lucille Petry appointed)
1944	First basic program in nursing accredited as including sufficient public health content
1946	Nurses classified as professional by U.S. Civil Service Commission
1948	NLN establishes accrediting service
1949	National Federation of Licensed Practical Nurses organized
1950	25,091 nurses employed in public health field
1951	NLN recommends collegiate basic nursing education include content in public health nursing; National Association of Colored Graduate Nurses merges with ANA
1952	Six nursing organizations merge into two: ANA and NLN; associate degree nursing started; Boston University begins program in general nursing approved for preparation of public health nurses
1953	*Nursing Outlook* published
1955	27,112 nurses employed in public health field
1959	NLN votes that no new specialized baccalaureate program be accredited (move toward general education in nursing); after 1963 only baccalaureate programs including public health nursing to be eligible for accreditation
1960	NLN establishes criteria for evaluation of educational programs in nursing that lead to baccalaureate and master's degrees
1964	Nurse Training Act passed
1965	Position paper of ANA proposes that education for nurses take place in institutions of higher learning
1970	National Commission on Nursing and Nursing Education offers Abstract for Action
1971	Nurse Training Act expanded
1974	Nurses Coalition for Action in Politics (N-CAP) formed; first certification exams for excellence in clinical practice offered by ANA
1975	Health Services, Health Revenue Sharing and Nurse Training Acts passed
1978	President Carter vetoes Nurse Training Act

nurses increased, they worked closely with physicians to carry out medical orders. Patients paid no fees, and initially two lay managers of the association supervised the nurses (Tinkham and Voohries, 1977). In 1888 the Instructive District Nursing Association became incorporated as an independent voluntary agency to provide care to the sick poor under the direction of a trained physician and to instruct families to take better care of themselves and their neighbors by living a wholesome life (Brainard, 1922).

Settlement Houses

During this era wealthy people became interested in charitable activities and began to fund settlement houses in the poorer sections of many larger cities. These settlement houses offered a variety of services for members of the community. For example, in 1893 Lillian Wald and her friend Mary Brewster, both trained nurses and wealthy women, organized a visiting nursing service for the poor of New York. In order to be readily accessible to the recipients of their care, these women moved into the neighborhood they served and led in the establishment of the Henry Street Settlement. Although highly diversified, nursing remained at the center of Henry Street activities. Nurses at Henry Street visited patients being cared for by a large number of different physicians and charged for their services according to the patients' ability to pay. From the beginning nurses supervised nurses at Henry Street Settlement.

Lillian Wald was an extremely far-sighted woman, who after graduating from New York Hospital's Training School attended classes at a local medical college while simultaneously conducting classes in personal health care on New York's lower East side (Kalisch and Kalisch, 1978). Because of the inadequate health care and the terrible economic conditions of the area, she campaigned for the establishment of Henry Street Settlement.

According to Christy (1970, p. 50), Wald was the predecessor of the modern public health nurse in the United States. Just as Nightingale chronicled much of her work, Wald wrote *The House on Henry Street*. Not only did she establish the Henry Street Settlement, but she led in the development of payment by insurance companies for nursing services. In 1909, along with Lee Fraskel, Lillian Wald established the first community health nursing program for workers at the Metropolitan Life Insurance Company. Believing that keeping workers healthier meant their productivity would increase, she urged that nurses at agencies such as Henry Street Settlement provide skilled nursing care to ensure healthier workers. Wald convinced the company that it would be more economical to utilize the services of

community health nurses than to employ their own nurses and also that services could be available to anyone desiring them with fees graduated according to the ability to pay. This project existed for 44 years and contributed several significant accomplishments to community health nursing including the following:

1. Providing home nursing care on a fee-for-service basis
2. Establishing an effective cost-accounting system for visiting nurses
3. Using advertisements in both newspapers and the radio to recruit nurses
4. Reducing mortality rates from infectious diseases

Lillian Wald also believed that the nursing efforts at Henry Street Settlement should be aligned with an official health agency, and she arranged for nurses to wear an insignia that signified that they served under the auspices of the board of health. Also, she established rural health nursing services through the Red Cross to provide nursing care to rural people and thereby improve their quality of life. Her other accomplishments included helping to establish the Children's Bureau, fighting in New York City for better tenement living conditions, city recreation centers, parks, pure food laws, graded classes for mentally handicapped children, and assistance to immigrants (Fig. 1-6).

At about this same time a group of women in Los Angeles established the College Settlement. They requested that the City Council give them a monthly allowance so a district nurse could visit the sick poor. In 1898 public funds paid the first nurse to provide nursing care in the home.

Health Departments and Community Health Nursing

Advances in community health nursing paralleled those in both nursing and community health. During the 1920s community health nursing recognized the relationship between health and economic security and began to assume responsibility for community health. By 1920 all states and most large cities had health departments with the majority of the staff being community health nurses. During this period community health nursing assumed a leadership role in establishing standards for nursing practice. As mentioned earlier, community health nurses received advanced preparation and the major community health nursing organization provided for collaboration among citizens, nurses, and other health providers. All who desired community health nursing care received it regardless of their ability to pay. The type of nursing care provided in the community during this era serves as a prototype of contemporary community health nursing. During the early decades of the twentieth century the scope of

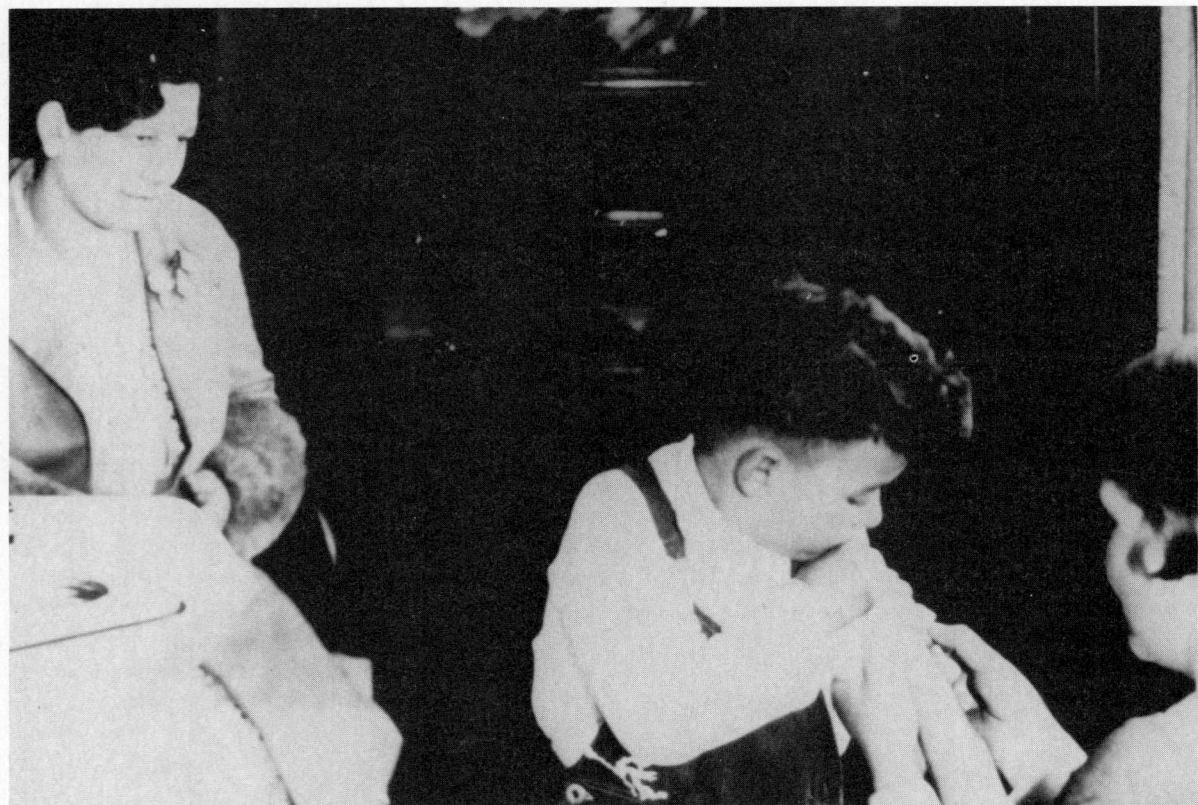

Fig. 1-6. Clinic visit for immunization. (Donated by the Jefferson County Department of Health, Birmingham, Ala., Myra Downs, Director, Bureau of Public Health Nursing.)

community health nursing included disease prevention, health promotion, and family-oriented services.

World War I and Community Health Nursing

As mentioned in the discussion of nursing education, the great demand for nurses created by the onset of World War I in 1915 threatened the role of community health nurses, whose numbers were insufficient to meet the need. However, the American Red Cross helped to sustain community health nursing by establishing a roster of nurses who could be enlisted to supply health care. The Red Cross emphasized educational programs for the community as well as programs directed toward communicable diseases.

During the war the National Organization of Public Health Nurses loaned a nurse to the U.S. Public Health Service to establish a community health nursing program for military outposts, which led to the first community health nursing program sponsored by the federal government (Gardner, 1919, p. 44). After World War I many changes occurred which subsequently affected community health nursing. Despite the economic con-

straints of the depression, this era witnessed many advancements in community health nursing. Because of limited local and national resources many people volunteered to assist others, and these volunteers rapidly learned the value of community health nursing. Also, many federally funded relief projects utilized nurses, which led to the need for governmental consultation to the states. In 1934 Pearl McIver became the first nurse employed by the U.S. Public Health Service to provide consultation services to state health departments. Initially only a few states had budgeted community health nursing positions; by 1936 all states included some type of community health nursing consultation services in their budgets.

Community Health Nursing Between Two World Wars

As the Social Security Act of 1935 attempted to overcome the national setbacks of the depression, it expanded community health nursing. Title VI stimulated protection and health promotion for all people. Two major provisions of Title VI included (1) the appropriation of

$8 million to assist states, counties, and medical districts to establish and maintain adequate health services as well as to train public health workers and (2) the allocation of $2 million for research and the investigation of disease and sanitation. This act also provided funds for the education and employment of public health nurses. Training for Nurses for National Defense, the GI Bill, the Nurse Training Act of 1943, and Public Health and Professional Nurse Traineeships provided additional educational funds (McNeil, 1967). The onset of World War II in 1941 accelerated the need for nurses. The National Nursing Council, comprising six national nursing organizations and assisted by the U.S. Department of Education, received a million dollars to expand facilities for nursing education. The U.S. Public Health Service managed these nursing education funds. During this time community health nursing expanded its scope of practice. Community health nurses moved into rural areas, and many official agencies began to provide bedside nursing care.

The Years Following World War II

During World War II many nurses joined the Army and Navy Nurse Corps. To provide sufficient nurses to meet wartime demands, the Bolton Act of 1943 established the Cadet Nurses Corps and authorized $60 million to recruit and educate 70,000 cadets in 1125 schools between 1944 and 1946. During this time these nurses constituted 90% of the enrollment in basic nursing programs. The chief of this program, Lucille Petry, provided leadership in nursing education during a particularly difficult time.

After the war the need for nurses continued and many utilized the GI Bill to further their education. Before its discontinuation in 1948, the National Nursing Council for War Service, comprising a variety of nursing organizations concerned about the future of nursing, launched what is known as the Brown Report (Brown, 1948). This report recommended that professional nursing education be carried out in institutions of higher learning, that nonprofessional nursing education be the responsibility of public vocational schools, and that inferior diploma schools be closed and good ones strengthened. Subsequently, Mildred Montag's dissertation in 1951 served as a model for the development of nursing education within junior colleges.

The year 1952 witnessed some major changes in professional nursing organizations. The American Nurses' Association (ANA) and the National League for Nursing (NLN) became the two major nursing organizations. The ANA set out to improve professional nursing practice, including economic and general welfare, and limited membership to registered nurses. In contrast, the NLN, open to both nurses and lay people, es-

tablished a goal of providing cooperative relationships between nurses and friends of the profession to work together for quality education and practice. A coordinating council provided collaboration between the two groups. Also, during these years both the ANA and NLN aided in the establishment of the National Student Nurses' Association.

Over the years the NLN has focused on the quality of educational programs and mechanisms for their evaluation. In 1948 the NLN established an accrediting service to evaluate all nursing programs in a systematic fashion. In contrast, the ANA has maintained a major interest in licensure of nursing.

At the end of World War II, President Truman requested that Congress address the following aspects of the health care system (Kalisch and Kalisch, 1977, p. 8):

1. Prepayment of medical costs with compulsory insurance and general revenues
2. Protection from loss of wages as a result of sickness
3. Government aid to medical schools for research
4. Increased construction of hospitals, clinics, and medical institutions

However, only the Hospital Survey and Construction (Hill-Burton) Act of 1946 enacted this last aspect and provided funds to assess the need for hospitals and, if need existed, the planning and construction of hospitals and public health centers. This program, which required state matching funds (two-thirds) and federal funds (one-third), accounted for the widespread development of hospitals in the United States.

Many changes after World War II subsequently affected community health nursing. These included a more prosperous economy, prohibition, and the increasing use of the automobile. Where community health nurses had previously made visits on foot, in horse-drawn buggies, or on bicycles, automobiles made it possible to see far more people.

Additionally, wartime service called national attention to the poor health of young and middle-aged males. Approximately 29% of all men called up for military service were rejected because of poor and often preventable health conditions. This sad state of affairs led to the development of many health programs by both official and nonofficial agencies (Roberts, 1954). Following World War II, community health nurses were accused of being more interested in organizing their practice than in actually providing care to clients. The leadership and maverick spirit of early nursing leaders appeared to wane, and an era began when community health nursing became defensive rather than exhibiting leadership in health care (Tinkham and Voorhies, 1977, p. 88). Some contend that this trend still exists.

In 1946 a committee of representatives from agencies interested in community health met to establish guidelines for this area of nursing (Public Health Nursing, 1946, p. 387). These guidelines became necessary because community health nursing evolved in an unplanned fashion with sponsorship by many voluntary agencies, thereby leading to a great deal of overlap. The guidelines took into account the history of community health nursing and proposed that a population of 50,000 was required to support a community health program and that there should be one nurse for each 2,000 people. Other principles addressed were that (1) the function of community health nursing includes health teaching, disease control, and care of the sick and (2) the community should adopt one of the following three organizational patterns (Public Health Nursing, 1946):

1. All community health nurse services administered by the local health department
2. Preventive health care provided by health departments and home health care by a cooperating voluntary agency
3. A combination service jointly administered and financed by official and voluntary agencies with all services provided by one group of community health nurses

By the early sixties community health nursing began to assume a more active role in society. Practice in community health nursing became a requirement of all baccaleaurate programs in nursing. Also, in 1964 the ANA defined a community health nurse as a graduate from a baccalaureate program in nursing accredited by the National League for Nursing.

In 1966 the American Public Health Association and the NLN jointly developed a program for accrediting community health nursing services. This was the first effort to accredit the delivery of nursing services and continues today as a vital and sought-after program.

Frontier Nursing Service

The Frontier Nursing Service (FNS) was influential in the development of community health programs and characterized by a unique pioneering spirit. Its historical development is detailed here because of its contributions from nurses to improve the health care of a rural and often inaccessible population. The FNS came into being from the commitment of a nurse, Mary Breckenridge, to provide care to isolated and needy people in Appalachian sections of Kentucky. Breckenridge came from a wealthy Southern family and devoted her life to the establishment of the FNS after the death of her first husband, the failure of her second marriage, and the loss of a 4-year-old son and a newborn daughter. The loss of her own children motivated her to devote her life to promoting the health care of disadvantaged women and children (Browne, 1966).

A graduate of St. Luke's Hospital in New York, Mary Breckenridge organized community health nursing activities in France. Working with the American Committee for Devastated France, she saw the tremendous health needs of women and children. Based on her experiences in France, Breckenridge decided that people in rural areas of the United States would benefit from the service of nurses-midwives (Dolan, 1978).

To prepare herself for providing midwifery services in the Kentucky mountains, Breckenridge spent time auditing public health, statistics, and psychology courses at Teachers College in New York. In 1923 she went to England to obtain nurse-midwifery training. The Kentucky committee for Mothers and Babies was organized in 1925, and the name was changed to Frontier Nursing Service when the organization was incorporated in 1928. At the suggestion of a supportive physician, baseline data were obtained as to infant and maternal mortality rates before beginning services.

The reduced mortality rates following the inception of the FNS are especially remarkable considering the environmental conditions in which these rural Kentucky people lived. Many homes had no heat, electricity, or running water; often physicians were over 40 miles from their patients (Tirpak, 1975). During the 1930s nurses lived and saw patients from one of six outposts and often had to make their visits on horseback (Fig. 1-7). However, on completion of the FNS hospital in Hyden, Kentucky, in 1928, physicians began entering service. Payment of fees ranged from labor and supplies to funds raised through annual family dues, philanthropy, and fund-raising efforts of Mary Breckenridge (Holloway, 1975). The inception of Medicaid and Medicare made available a more predictable source of revenue.

In 1939 Mrs. Breckenridge established the FNS School of midwifery. Over the years deliveries increasingly took place in hospitals, thereby reducing the need for midwifery and accelerating the demand for family nursing. By 1975, with only 7% of nursing time devoted to midwifery, the 41 FNS nurses devoted their attention to meeting the primary care needs of the residents of Leslie County, Kentucky (Frontier Nursing Service, 1978). Once admitted to a nurse's district, clients are seen at least once a year until they die or move. This service continues today as a vital and creative mode for delivering public health services to rural families. The role of nurses, similar in many ways to the contemporary nursing role in the FNS, is discussed in detail in Chapter 33.

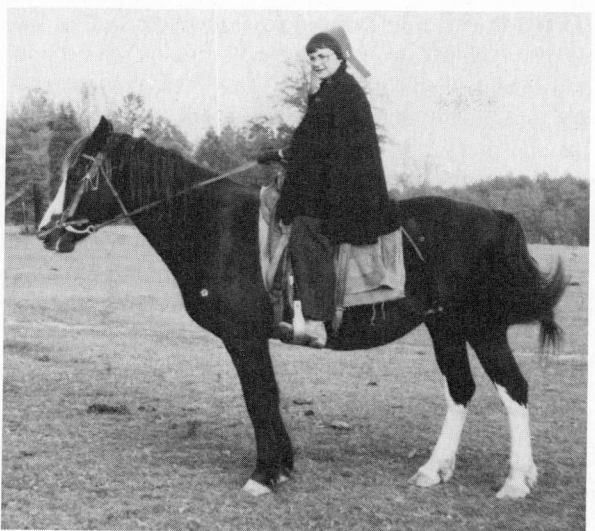

Fig. 1-7. Nurses rode horseback in the Frontier Nursing Service. (Donated by K. Huttlinger, graduate of M.S.N. program at University of Alabama in Birmingham.)

CURRENT STATE OF COMMUNITY HEALTH NURSING

The lack of decisiveness about what constitutes community health nursing is consistent with the controversy and confusion present in the entire profession. Community health nursing has evolved into a focus on care of individuals, families, and communities. While those in other areas of nursing work in the same domain as the public health nurses, the focus and orientation are different. The scope of practice is defined by the nature of community health nursing rather than being dominated solely by the setting. Providing nursing care in the community does not in itself constitute community health nursing. Community health nursing is a specific and specialized orientation to care that embodies principles of public health as guiding precepts. The key difference between community health nursing and the other areas of nursing is the emphasis on the personal and environmental health of the total population not just of selected individuals. Since Chapters 7 and 37 provide more in-depth discussion on community health nursing, this section only highlights the current role to demonstrate how it has evolved from the early days of visiting nursing carried out first by religious orders and then by insightful and energetic leaders like Lillian Wald. Chapter 7 compares the ANA and APHA conceptual frameworks for community health nursing

and supplements this brief review of the current status of community health nursing.

Primary health care is not synonymous with community health nursing. In contrast to community health nursing's focus on the physical, biological, social, psychological, and environmental health of a population group, primary care is a "coordinated system of personal health care, emphasizing first-contact care and continuity" (Ruth and Partridge, 1978, p. 625). Primary care emphasizes ambulatory care that is accessible and coordinated and that addresses total client needs both for curative as well as preventive services. Primary care generally focuses on the individual whereas community health nursing is population based.

Williams (1977, p. 251) has helped to clarify the focus and goals of community health nursing by emphasizing the unit of care as the health of population groups or aggregates of people "who have in common one or more personal or environmental characteristics." Aggregates may be defined at many levels: age, risk for certain health problems, race, and so on. A major factor differentiating community health nursing is the focus on promoting health-related behaviors as well as providing personal health services to members of populations or communities. Rather than serving only the subgroups who need care, community health nurses anticipate, estimate, and design measures to interrupt the onset of personal health problems. Such a focus may sound global or vague; however, it is specific, highly complex, and scientific. It takes considerable skill to estimate the potential onset of a health problem as a result of unsafe living conditions (such as polluted water supplies) and intervene before health problems ensue.

Community health nurses must understand the natural history of disease, recognize potential causative agents and implement intervention as soon as possible. Inherent in a community health philosophy is attention to the influence of environment factors (physical, biological and sociocultural) on the health of populations and priority is given to preventive and health maintenance strategies rather than curative strategies (Williams, 1977).

SUMMARY

As was shown in this chapter, the history of community health nursing can be traced to the earliest recorded history of civilization. Throughout its development there have been numerous progressive campaigns often overshadowed by transient setbacks as health has been alternately given high priority and then ignored. Many of the advances in community health arose out of necessity. Epidemics and other devastating health conditions demanded resolution and could not be postponed until a more propitious time.

Major social, economic, and political developments have influenced community health programs in the United States with many advances made as a result of congressional actions. Citizens have pressed their congressmen to work for better living and health conditions. Community health nursing has been at the forefront in developing and encouraging other groups to institute healthier living conditions and care for all people.

The history of the early Christian church is replete with examples of home health care. Of considerable import was the work of St. Vincent de Paul and Mademoiselle Le Gras who established what was probably the first actual community health nursing program. The life and work of Florence Nightingale influenced all nursing practices including education, hospital development, and the actual delivery of nursing care. Likewise, it is difficult to imagine how one woman, Lillian Wald, could have been so farsighted, energetic, and resourceful in her development of varied and numerous community health nursing efforts. She organized visiting nursing in New York, established the unique program at the Henry Street Settlement, and was responsible for many improvements in living conditions in New York City. She also established the first program of nursing services provided by an insurance company. Had there been more women like Lillian Wald in both the history of nursing and community health nursing, one can imagine the gains that might have been made.

Expansion in nursing education progressed steadily from the first school to train nurses established in Boston at the New England Female Medical College. Only 1 year after this school was established, three additional ones began on the East Coast: Bellevue Hospital in New York City, New Haven Hospital in Connecticut, and Massachusetts General Hospital in Boston. By 1893, just 22 years later, there were 225 schools of nursing in the United States. These early schools were located in hospitals, and it was not until 1909 that the first basic nursing program associated with a university began at the University of Minnesota. The inclusion of community health nursing content was first provided in 1914 under the leadership of Mary Adelaide Nutting at Teachers College in New York. This trend continued and was supported by major nursing organizations. Two landmark studies pertaining to nursing education were completed by Josephine Goldmark and Mildred Montag. In their unique ways each study influenced the future development of nursing education.

Over the years community health nursing has evolved from a home care service characterized as being delivered by caring women who ministered both to the health and spiritual needs of individuals and families to a broadly based, population-focused discipline that considers individuals, families, groups, and communities as the scope of practice.

BIBLIOGRAPHY

Brainard, A.M.: Evolution of public health nursing, Philadelphia, 1922, W. B. Saunders Co.

Breckenridge, M.: Wide neighborhoods, New York, 1952, Harper & Row, Publishers.

Brown, E.L.: Nursing for the future, New York, 1948, Russell Sage Foundation.

Browne, H.: A tribute to Mary Breckenridge, Nurs. Outlook **14**:54-55, May, 1966.

Bullough, V., and Bullough, B.: The emergence of modern nursing, New York, 1964, Macmillan Publishing Co.

Christy, T.: Portrait of a leader: Lillian Wald, Nurs. Outlook **18**:50-54, March 1970.

Deloughery, G.L.: History and trends of professional nursing, ed. 8, St. Louis, 1977, The C.V. Mosby Co.

Desirable organization for public health nursing for family service, Public Health Nurs. **38**:387-389, Aug. 1946.

Dickens, C.: Martin Chuzzlewit, New York, 1975, Penguin Bookstore. (Edited by P.N. Furbank.)

Division of Information: World Health Organization, Geneva, 1967, The World Health Organization.

Dolan, J.: History of nursing, ed. 14, Philadelphia, 1978, W.B. Saunders Co.

Freyman, J.G.: The American health care system: its genesis and trajectory, Huntington, N.Y., 1977, Robert E. Krieger Publishing Co.

Frontier Nursing Service: FNS Q. Bull. **54**(2):3-6, 1878.

Gardner, M.S.: Public health nursing, ed. 3, New York, 1919, Macmillan Publishing Co.

Griffin, G.J., and Griffin, J.K.: History and trends of professional nursing, ed.7, St. Louis, 1973, The C.V. Mosby Co.

Hanlon, J.J., and Pickett, G.E.: Public health: administration and practice, ed. 7, St. Louis, 1979, The C.V. Mosby Co.

Holloway, J.B., Jr.: Frontier Nursing Service—1925-1975, J. Ky. Med. Assoc. **13**:491-492, Sept. 1975.

Jamieson, E.M., and Sewall, M.F.: Trends in nursing history, ed. 4, Philadelphia, 1954, W.B. Saunders Co.

Kalisch, P., and Kalisch, B.J.: Nursing involvement in the health planning process, DHEW Pub. No. HRA 78-25, Hyattsville, Md., 1977, Department of Health, Education, and Welfare.

Kalisch, P., and Kalisch, B.J.: The advancement of American nursing, Boston, 1978, Little, Brown & Co.

Leavell, H.R., and Clark, E.G.: Preventive medicine for the doctor in his community, ed. 3. New York, 1965, McGraw-Hill Book Co.

Maynard, T.: The apostle of charity: the life of St. Vincent de Paul, New York, 1939, Dial Press.

McCance, K.L., and Reiber, G.E.: Prevention: implications for nursing research, Adv. Nurs. Sci. **4**:79-87, Jan. 1982.

McNeil, E.E.: Transition in public health nursing, John Sundwall Lecture, University of Michigan, Feb. 27, 1967.

National Organization for Public Health Nursing: approval of Skidmore College of Nursing as preparing students for public health nursing, Public Health Nurs. **36**:371, July 1944.

Nightingale, F.: Notes on nursing, Philadelphia, 1946, J.B. Lippincott Co. (Originally published in 1859.)

Pellegrino, E.D.: Medicine, history, and the idea of man, Ann. Ame. Acad. Pol. Soc. Sci. **346**:9-20, March 1963.

Rees, W.D.: Personal view: Herodotus, Br. Med. J. **4**:182, Oct. 19, 1968.

Rosen, G.: A history of public health, New York, 1958, M.D. Publications.

Ruth, M.V., and Partridge, K.B.: Differences in perception of education and practice, Nurs. Outlook **26**:622-629, Oct. 1978.

Schudson, M.: The Flexner Report and the Reed Report on the history of professional education in the United States, Soc. Sci. Q. **55**:347-361, Sept. 1974.

Shamansky, S.L., and Clausen, C.L.: Levels of prevention: examination of the concept, Nurs. Outlook **28**:104-108, Feb. 1980.

Shyrock, H.: The history of nursing, Philadelphia, 1959, W.B. Saunders Co.

Swinson, A.: The history of public health, Exeter, England, 1965, A. Wheaton & Co.

Tinkham, C.W., and Voorhies, E.F.: Community health nursing: evolution and process, ed. 2, New York, 1977, Appleton-Century-Crofts.

Tirpak, H.: The Frontier Nursing Service—fifty years in the mountains, Nurs. Outlook **33**:308-310, May 1975.

Weinstein, M.R.: The illness process, psychosocial hazards of disability programs, JAMA **204**:209-213, April 1968.

Williams, C.A.: Community health nursing—what it is: Nurs. Outlook **25**:25-254, April 1977.

Wilner, D.M., Walkley, R.P., and O'Neill, E.J.: Introduction to public health, ed. 7, New York, 1978, Macmillan Publishing Co.

Winslow, C.E.A.: The untitled field of public health, Mod. Med. **2**:183, March 1920.

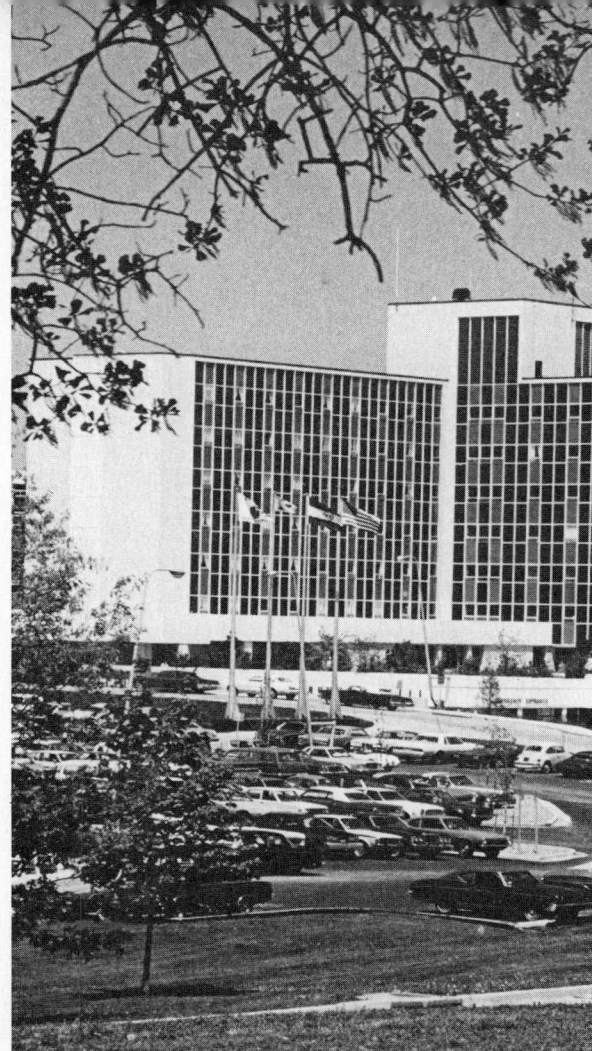

Chapter
2

JEANETTE LANCASTER
WADE LANCASTER

CURRENT STATUS OF THE HEALTH CARE SYSTEM

Health is a topic of concern to all Americans, either directly or indirectly, individually or collectively, consciously or unconsciously. Health, inextricably linked with all aspects of daily living, is a prerequisite for executing the multitude of diverse chores and activities required to maintain a satisfactory level of existence. The concept of health is related to the notion of well-being; health is not an end in itself but represents on-going efforts to enrich one's level of well-being. Health is not just "feeling good," but instead is a broad concept embracing social, emotional, and physical aspects of life. It includes the cognitive, affective, and action domains of human behavior as it refers not only to individuals but also to the capabilities of families, communities, organizations, institutions, societies, and even nations.

Hence, as a concept, health is important, complex, and multidimensional with biological, physical, personal, professional, technical, economic, legal, ethical, political, social, and cultural components. This chapter discusses the current health care system by examining both the concept of health was well as by describing the current structure of the system including consumers, providers, and the current organizational arrangements for delivering services.

WHAT IS HEALTH AND HEALTH CARE?

The term *health* is defined in widely divergent ways. The World Health Organization defines health as "a state of complete physical, mental, and social well-being and not merely the absence of disease or infirmity" (WHO, 1958). In contrast, Brody and Sobel (1981, p. 30), using a systems theory view, define health as "the ability of a system (for example, cell, organism, family, society) to respond adaptively to a wide variety of environmental challenges (for example, physical, chemical, infectious, psychological, social)." From this perspective health is seen as a positive process, not just the absence of symptoms. Additionally, this definition moves beyond the restriction of health as biological or mental well-being and includes a consideration of the surrounding environment.

From a systems view, disease is seen as a "failure to respond adaptively to environmental challenges resulting in a disruption of the overall equilibrium of the system" (Brody and Sobel, 1981, p. 3). Discussing health and creative adaptation, Rene Dubos (1981, p. 6) says that for humans, "health transcends biological fitness. It is primarily a measure of each person's ability to do what he wants to do and become what he wants to become." Thus these views of health and illness imply a necessary awareness of the totality in which people exist and the effect of the environment on total health. This text proposes that a major responsibility of community health is the promotion of health. However, in many ways the current health care system is not oriented in this direction. The health care system typically becomes activated when an illness is detected. To understand the conceptual view of community health as outlined in many of the following chapters, several additional definitions are set forth and the current health care system is described.

The terms health services, health care, health care system, health promotion, and health prevention are defined here to provide an understanding of several contemporary issues surrounding the health care system. *Health services* refers to all "personal and public services performed by individuals or institutions for the purpose of maintaining or restoring health" (Levey and Loomba, 1973, p. 4). Similarly, the *health care system* denotes the "totality of resources a population or society distributes in the organization and delivery of health services" (Levey and Loomba, 1973, p. 4). As such, the health care system is the organized local, state, or national effort designed to deliver services deemed essential to obtain a preestablished set of goals. This chapter discusses the overall structure of the current health care system, examines selected issues, and refers readers to other chapters for details related to topics such as the economics and regulatory mechanisms of the health care system.

Although the terms health care and medical care are often used interchangeably they have distinct differences. *Health care* or the product of health services is delivered through two primary vehicles: personal health services and community health services. Health care encompasses treatment of disease as well as health promotion and disease prevention. *Medical care* is the generic term describing the organization, financing, and delivery of personal or individually oriented health services. It encompasses the services and skills of a variety of providers including physicians, dentists, nurses, and various health therapists as well as the provision of medications, orthopedic appliances, hospital, nursing home, and mental health care and other care and resources from a variety of institutions. A major concern of medical care is the diagnosis and treatment of the disease process, which means that medical care is actually a subset of the broader concept of health care (Levey and Loomba, 1973).

Two additional terms need defining: health promotion and disease prevention; promotion and prevention are often used synonymously, yet there are conceptual differences between them. *Health promotion* refers to "activities directed toward developing the resources of clients that maintain or enhance well-being," whereas *disease prevention* describes "activities that seek to protect clients from potential or actual health threats and their harmful consequences" (Pender, 1982, p. 2). Both health promotion and disease prevention have a different focus from treatment of illness; therefore, they often are not considered a legitimate part of the health care system that focuses on diagnosis and treatment.

As described in Chapter 1 as well as in later chapters, the concepts of health and health care can be divided into three levels. These levels can be described either as models of care or models of prevention. When the terms primary, secondary, and tertiary care are used to describe different levels of care, they refer to efforts provided for people who enter the health care system with an existing or suspected illness. From this perspective *primary care* refers to a person's first contact with the health care system, which results in a decision for a course of action directed toward problem resolution and includes continuity and coordination of care (Institute of Medicine, 1978). In contrast, *secondary care* focuses on cure and restoration, and *tertiary care* is specialized and typically uses sophisticated diagnostic tests and therapy to alleviate health disruption. The terms primary, secondary and tertiary prevention as defined in Chapter 1 are used before health disruption (primary), in efforts to return health status to a stable state if disruption occurred (secondary), and in attempts to reverse, arrest, or delay the progression if disease occurred (tertiary) (Institute of Medicine, 1978).

ISSUES RELATED TO THE HEALTH CARE SYSTEM

Health care issues have attracted a considerable amount of attention in recent years for several reasons. First, because of modern technological and procedural advances, physicians often seem like "miracle workers." Exotic equipment and procedures now keep people alive who in previous decades would have died at a much younger age. Second, spending for health purposes has risen to record levels both in actual dollars spent as well as in the proportion of the gross national product (GNP) devoted to health care. Third, the government's involvement in health care through both regulations and financing has increased. Fourth, the philosophy that "health is a right for all people" has, in recent years, been countered by the belief that individuals are personally responsible for their own health status. Fifth, the health care system's lack of organization seems to lead to duplication, lack of accessibility, and inferior and expensive services. According to Notkin and Meader (1978, p. 19), "to be charitable, the American health care system can be described as chaotic." Notkin and Meader (1978) purport that the chaos pervades the entire system and includes activities directed toward planning, organizational arrangements, personnel, financing, and determinants of quality of care. Several of these components are described later in this chapter in terms of what is currently available and what new directions may be indicated. Before examining these components, it is helpful to examine several characteristics of the health care system which affect its present structure and mode of operation.

Characteristics of the Health Care System

The health care system is composed of consumers, providers, and mechanisms for delivery of health services. Several factors distinguish health services and differentiate the patterns of delivery of health services from those of other services. For example, from birth to death all people are part of the market potential for health care. Thus the number of people needing to enter, and for many to remain in, the system is large. Also, consumers of health care often are unable to determine their need for specific services.

In addition, the consumer of health care services is a client, not a customer. In the purest sense of the word, customers "take title to a good upon purchase, and sellers have no control over the consumption of the product—they can only advise" (Rathmell, 1974, p. 121). In contrast, clients, being in a more dependent position, place themselves in the hands of providers. The client can decide whether to buy the services and treatment offered, but in most instances the provider decides what should be purchased. The provider is a gatekeeper who determines when and how entry into the health care system shall occur. Without a physician, or in some instances a nurse practitioner, clients cannot avail themselves of medications, treatment procedures, nursing care, or hospitalization.

Consumers tend to be less informed about health services than anything else they purchase (see later discussion of consumerism). With most other products and services, people shop around to compare goods and services as to price, availability, and potential usefulness. People who switch physicians more than once are considered neurotics because the expectation is that clients select providers not methods of treatment. In general, health consumers know what product they want—health, but they do not know what treatment will insure this outcome. Most consumers do not know that for many forms of health disruption, certain behaviors such as diet and exercise, are often as useful as expensive medications.

Fuchs (1972) states that the health care sector is not a competitive market. From his perspective, a competitive market consists of (1) well-informed buyers and sellers, no one of whom is powerful enough to influence price, (2) buyers and sellers who act independently, and (3) free entry for other buyers and sellers not currently in the market.

In contrast, the health care system violates the characteristics of a competitive market in a variety of ways. In most small to medium-size towns the market cannot support enough facilities and providers to even be considered a competitive market.

The first ingredient in Fuchs' list—well-informed consumers—merits attention, since it affects the health care system in several ways. In general, the only way people know if they need to see a health care provider is by seeing one. Physicians usually do not advertise and in most states pharmacies continue to do minimal if any advertising on prescription items.

In the health care system sellers have tremendous control over price; because health is such a precious commodity to buyers, most are reluctant to ask health care providers for estimated costs. There are few incentives in the health care system to keep costs at a fixed level. Although insurers often establish price ceilings, physicians then bill clients for the portion of the bill not covered by a third party.

Fuchs (1972) accuses licensure of being a prime form of restricted entry for sellers (a violation of the third element in his list). He advocates voluntary certification rather than compulsory licensure. Providers could be certified at varying levels of expertise and thus increase price flexibility. This idea offers several provocative notions, since certification is currently in evidence and yet entry into the health care system is still predominantly physician controlled. Free entry into the health care system is not available to all people. The poor are typically limited as to which hospitals and providers they can utilize. Hospitals often require proof of third-party payment or personal ability to pay before admitting people. Similarly, most physicians require proof of insurance or payment at the time of treatment.

Fuchs (1972) also holds that providers rarely work in a cooperative spirit to reduce costs and increase client satisfaction, but rather most efforts of a collegial nature lean toward "price fixing" or other ways to maximize profits.

It is often contended that there is no health care system. The health care industry is a "cottage industry" dominated by small, inefficient, and uncoordinated enterprises (physicians, nurses, hospitals, clinics, nursing homes, home health care agencies) that add up to a fragmented and wasteful nonsystem (Ellwood, 1973). According to Ehrenreich and Ehrenreich (1974, p. 36), "proponents of the non-system theory trace the problem to the fact that health care, as a commodity, does not obey the orderly, business laws of economics." For example, with a food commodity like sugar, demand for the product reflects the public's desire to eat sugar as well as the ability and willingness to pay for it. The supply adjusts itself to the demand, and the situation remains reasonably balanced. In contrast, health care is not governed by this type of economic law. For the most part, people buy health care when they have to, not when they want to. Further, once a consumer selects a provider, the range of decisions available for the consumer decreases markedly. The provider decides whether to treat the ailment, not when and where. What this means is that within the medical marketplace, it is the supplier who controls the demand.

ORGANIZATION OF THE HEALTH CARE SYSTEM

Models of Health Care Delivery

The four models presented here depict the organization of the current health care system. Local, state, and national components are only mentioned briefly in this chapter and in much greater depth in Chapter 5.

The most *elementary model* of a health care system is depicted in Fig. 2-1. Two constant and fundamental components of the system are the consumers and the providers. In this simplified model, consumers engage in exchange relationships with providers.

The organization of health care reflects a strange blend of private and public enterprise. The vast majority of providers are in private practice, which means that they can decide where they want to practice, who

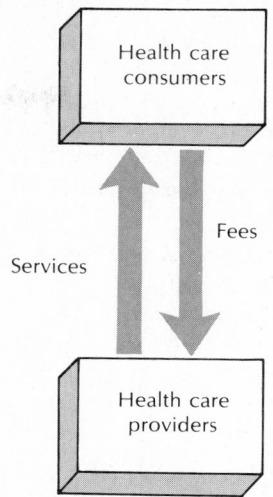

Fig. 2-1. Elementary model of the health care delivery system.

they will accept as patients, and how much they will charge. Also, an increasing number of medical care providers are labeled as specialists, which further complicates the point of entry. If clients do not know what is wrong with them, how can they know which specialist to choose? There is also a great deal of competition among providers. Many physicians are reluctant or refuse to acknowledge the value of other providers such as nurse practitioners.

The health care system is composed of two major groups, clients and providers, and is largely built on a fee-for-service basis. Until recently the prevalent mode of financing health services was personal payment. In recent years third-party payments have increased dramatically and affected the entire system. In Fig. 2-2, the *modified elementary model,* third-party funding agencies are added to the elementary model. The bulk of health care services in the United States are paid for either directly or indirectly by the consumer. Although more Americans are covered by insurance than have been in previous years, approximately one third of all health care costs come directly out of the individual's pocket. As will be discussed in detail in Chapter 3, national health care expenditures have grown monumentally since the 1940s. Much of the increase is caused by inflation, new and expensive technology, larger salaries for health care professionals, increased life span, and regulations (Notkin and Meader, 1978). These factors, especially inflation, technology, and changes in the characteristics of the population, are discussed in Chapter 3. Chapter 5 addresses the organization and financing of the health care system from the viewpoint of regulatory mechanisms.

Fig. 2-3 depicts the *private sector model* and illus-

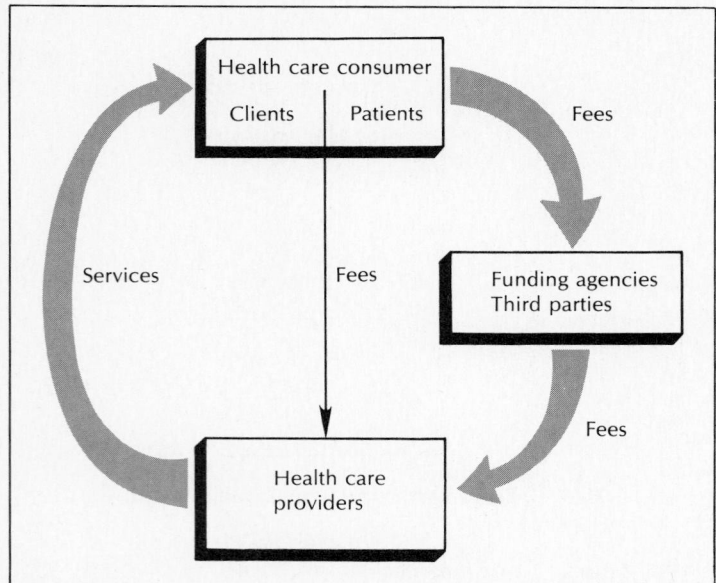

Fig. 2-2. Modified model of the health care delivery system.

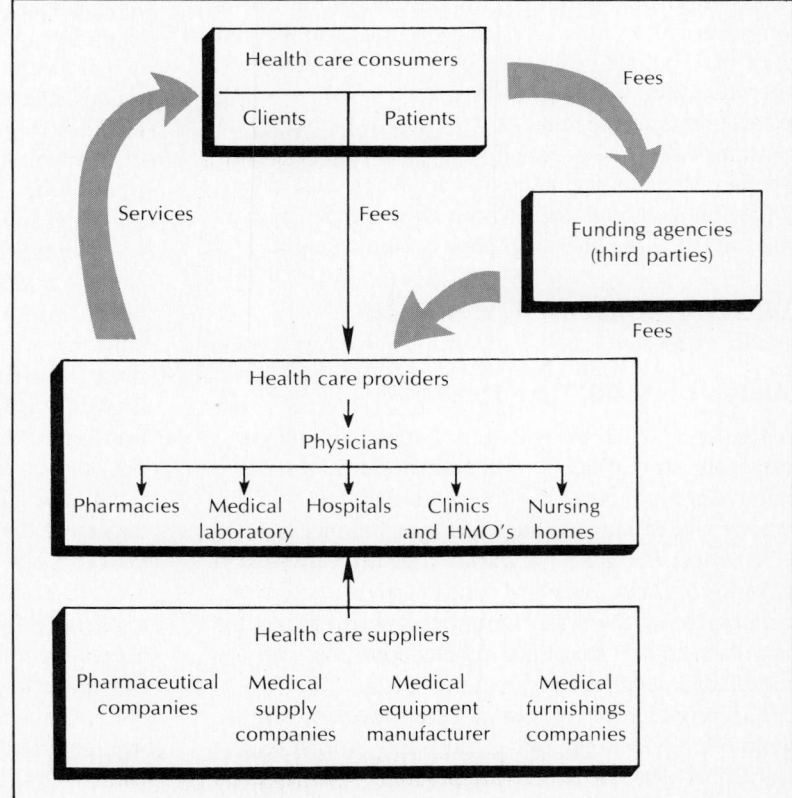

Fig. 2-3. Health care delivery model: private sector.

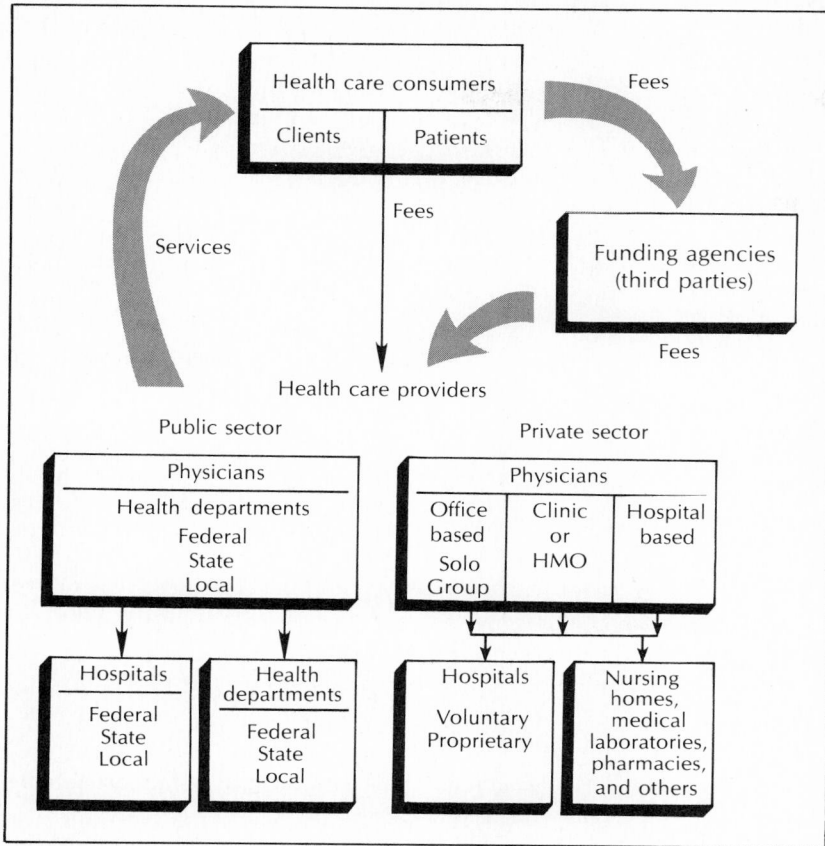

Fig. 2-4. Health care delivery model: public and private sector.

trates an increasing level of complexity by the health care system. The illustration is initially broken down into three components: personnel, facilities, and suppliers. Providers according to this model include both personnel and facilities such as hospitals, clinics, health maintenance organizations, nursing homes, medical laboratories, and pharmacies. The final component is made up of companies that supply health products to providers and consumers such as distributors of pharmaceutical supplies, medical equipment manufacturers, medical furnishing companies, and distributors of general supplies.

The existing health care system as depicted in Fig. 2-3 is called the *professional model* since its most conspicuous ingredient is the physician. In contrast to many other American industries that have changed structurally to keep pace with technological and social advances, the health care industry has largely retained its pre-Industrial Revolution organizational structure. Consequently, as mentioned earlier, it is often referred to as a "cottage industry" relying heavily on small independent firms (Ellwood, 1973).

Fig. 2-3 illustrates the central role of the physician as gatekeeper and, in many instances, navigator of the

health care system. With few exceptions in the private sector, medication, nursing care, laboratory tests, hospitalization, treatments and the use of specialists are determined by the physician.

The *public and private sectors model* is illustrated in Fig. 2-4. Also shown is an alternate conceptual view of the private sector. As seen in the illustration, the public sector is composed of public health agencies, both voluntary and official, which operate at the federal, state, and local level. Voluntary agencies are nonprofit organizations that depend on donations, fees, membership dues, endowments, payments from insurance plans, and contracts. In contrast, official agencies are primarily tax supported. Voluntary agencies were briefly discussed in Chapter 1. Official agencies include the armed forces, Veterans Administration, the United States Public Health Service, and various state and local health departments that provide medical care, preventive services, and environmental control services directly to the public (Reinhart, 1973). Collectively, these agencies carry on a variety of tasks. At the federal level, agencies deal with national and international health as well as the health of specific population groups, such as military personnel, veterans, Indians,

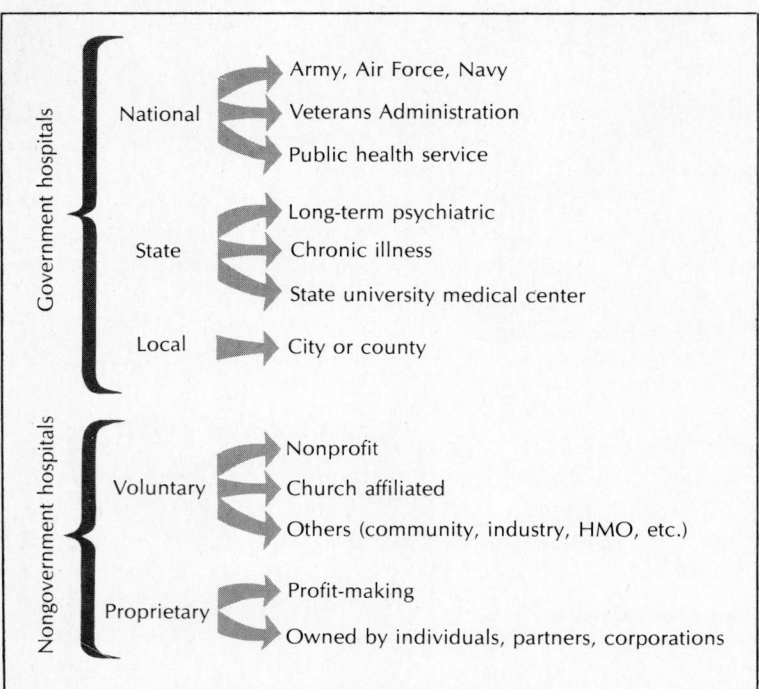

Fig. 2-5. Types of hospitals in the United States.

the aged, the economically deprived as well as people who are physically or mentally handicapped.

At the federal level, the basis of public health lies in the United States Constitution. The authors of the Constitution used broad phrases such as "promote the general welfare" which influence the scope of public health. Additionally, several powers are granted to the federal government which influence health care activities (Wilner, et al., 1978). Further information on the organization of health care from a local, state, and national perspective is found in Chapter 5.

Mechanisms for Health Care Delivery

An enormous number and range of facilities make up the health care delivery system. Facilities include physician's offices, dentists' offices, hospitals, nursing homes and other related inpatient facilities, mental health centers, rehabilitation centers, and local and state as well as federal agencies.

Hospitals

Hospital care constitutes the largest portion of the health care dollar. At present there are more than 7200 hospitals in the United States. They fall into one of two categories: government and nongovernment. Government hospitals are found at all three levels: national, state, and local. Fig. 2-5 illustrates a general categorization of hospital types. A new concept in hospitals is the management contract in which a corporation may op-

erate several hospitals with the goal of increasing both efficiency and revenues.

Historically, hospitals began as institutions to house poor people who were seriously ill and had no family or other resources to care for them. Members of religious groups who saw their work as a form of missionary activity ran many of the early hospitals. The word *hospital* is derived from *hospice*, meaning guest room, and historically referred to a place of refuge for travelers or for the unwanted to go for care. The oldest North American hospital was erected in 1524 in Mexico City as the Hospital of Jesus of Nazareth. The oldest hospital in the United States still operates in New Orleans as the Charity Hospital (Shindell et al., 1976).

Generally, hospitals attempt to carry out no more than four major services: patient care, education, research, and community service. As shown in Fig. 2-5, three predominant forms of ownership of nonfederal, short-term hospitals exist: privately owned, nonprofit; state and county; and proprietary. The majority of hospitals are privately owned, nonprofit institutions and operate under a variety of sectarian and nonsectarian auspices. While the privately owned and proprietary hospitals are increasing in number, state and local government hospitals are decreasing. Traditionally, state and local government hospitals provided care for indigent patients, but Medicare and Medicaid increased the options available for indigent people.

Proprietary hospitals, designed as profit-making ventures, must pay taxes. Because of their profit orientation, proprietary hospitals have been accused of focusing more on making money than on providing quality care. In some instances, charges tend to be higher in proprietary hospitals; however, many are seeking to deliver care in a variety of innovative and possibly cost-effective ways.

Hospitals can also be categorized according to their degree of specialization. In general, two types of specialty hospitals predominate: those treating a specific disease, such as a cancer or diabetes hospital, and those providing care to a special class of individuals, such as children, veterans, or women, with all types of diseases. In general, specialty hospitals are decreasing with the exception of those for a special class of clients such as children's hospitals. In recent years the University Medical Center has become an ever-growing source of care. Teaching hospitals are recognized as the core of the health care system, since they provide education, service, and research to a wide variety of people.

A large proportion of hospitals in the United States are voluntary and run by a board of trustees who are legally responsible for the operation of the hospital and maintenance of acceptable standards (Shindell et al., 1976). The board, primarily composed of businessmen, engineers, attorneys, and physicians, hires an administrator to run the hospital. Although hospital boards are legally responsible for governance, they rely heavily on physicians to govern and monitor their professional care. This expectation is often unrealistic, since the majority of physicians in private practice can devote limited time to this activity.

Most hospitals, functioning as autonomous self-regulating institutions, are subject to a variety of rules and regulations from external sources such as governmental and professional groups. Outside regulation primarily comes from local, state, and federal rules, the American Medical Association, the Joint Commission on Accreditation of Hospitals, and the Medicare and Medicaid programs (Shindell et al., 1976).

Health Maintenance Organizations

A health maintenance organization (HMO) is an "organized system of health care that guarantees to provide high-quality physician services, emergency and preventive treatment and hospital services to individuals who have agreed to obtain their medical care from the HMO for an extended period of time" (Ellwood and Herbert, 1973, p. 100). HMOs are relative newcomers to the health care delivery scene. Much of the credit for this type of delivery system goes to Sidney Garfield who was instrumental in establishing the Kaiser-Permanente system in the 1930s. This program began in southern California in the depression years be-

tween 1933 and 1938 when Garfield tried a prepayment scheme in his own practice in order to make ends meet during such economically barren times (Garfield, 1970). The idea was tried more broadly during the construction of the Grand Coulee Dam between 1938 and 1942 by the Kaiser family. This plan now includes more than 50 clinics, predominantly on the West Coast, and serves as a model or incentive for the development of numerous HMOs. The Health Maintenance Organization Act of 1973 (P.L. 93-222) specified that all companies employing 25 or more people must offer employees the opportunity to have health insurance or membership in an HMO if one is available.

Health maintenance organization legislation attempted to stimulate the establishment of HMOs by providing funds for their development and expansion. The HMO Act of 1973 listed the requirements of a health maintenance organization, defined the basic and supplemental service to be provided to the membership, and determined the basis for fixing the rate of prepayment as well as the organizational structure (National League for Nursing, 1978, p. 2). The legislation was amended in 1976 to require federal qualification and regulation for all HMOs receiving Medicare and Medicaid funds and for consumers to be involved in the policymaking process.

The HMO concept flourished in the last decade because of amendments to the Act of 1973 and subsequent funding allocations. Before 1950, enrollment growth followed a steady pattern with about 26 plans in operation in 1970. However, since 1970 the average rate of growth has been about 22 HMOs per year, as seen in Fig. 2-6. Not only was there a large increase in the number of HMOs, but there was a substantial increase in the number of states having HMOs (*Health: United States,* 1981). Since 1970 enrollment in HMOs has increased from 3.1 million to 9.5 million.

The distinguishing characteristic of HMOs is that all care is provided for a fixed, prenegotiated fee paid periodically and in advance of need. The chief advantage lies in the economic incentive to keep costs under control. Prevention is emphasized to reduce the need for costly services. The greatest potential for savings from HMOs, reduction of the costs of unnecessary hospitalization, also accounts for the greatest fear: that providers will underuse necessary services to save money.

As a part of these services people receive complete and continuous care. Services are provided to all segments of society in exchange for prepayment, and prevention is emphasized. Principles of HMO operation can be divided into the following five primary characteristics (National League for Nursing, 1978):

1. It is an organization that makes a contract with

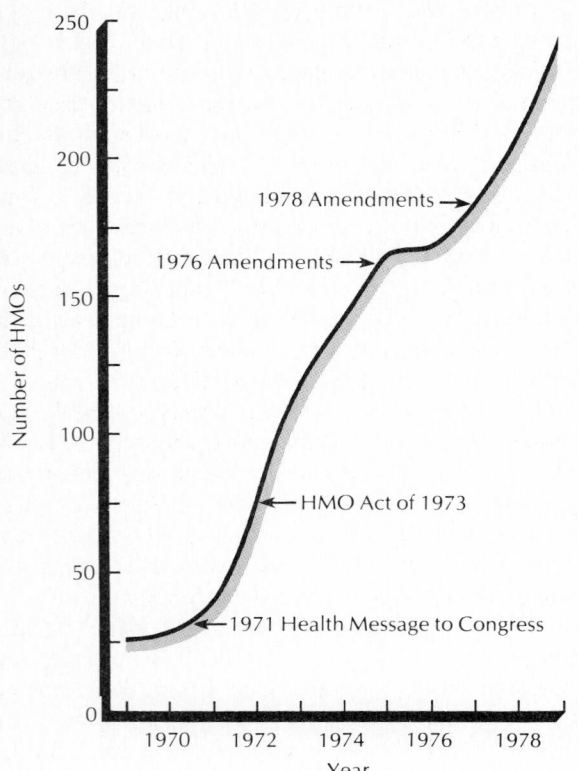

NOTE: California prepaid health plans, which were eliminated by 1977, are excluded.

Fig. 2-6. Number of health maintenance organizations: 1970 to 1980. (From Health: United States, 1981, Pub. No. 82–1232, Hyattsville, Md., 1981, U.S. Department of Health and Human Services, p. 76.)

consumers (or employers on their behalf) to assure the delivery of stated health services.

2. The benefits are comprehensive and include physician's services, hospital care, ambulatory care, and preventive care.
3. There is a voluntarily enrolled population, sometimes referred to as a "defined" population.
4. There is "prepayment," that is, the HMO receives a payment in advance from each enrolled participant.
5. There is an emphasis on preventive medicine, keeping the patient well through primary care services.

Through its own resources or by contracted sources, HMOs should provide comprehensive care including emergency services, hospital care and arrangements for mental health, rehabilitation, and convalescent services. The basic schedule of benefits includes physician services in the office, hospital, and home; hospital care including surgery and obstetrics; and a full range of laboratory services and specialized treatments.

Health maintenance organizations eliminate third-party insurance payments. They emphasize primary care to prevent costly illnesses and hospitalizations. Proponents of the HMO concept believe that traditional medical care practices waste money by overemphasizing hospital care. Health maintenance organizations can reduce the fragmentation and inaccessibility of services by providing the full range needed in one setting or at least in close proximity. Furthermore, they often reduce costs by prevention; the HMOs economic incentive is prevention or at least early detection and treatment. A single hospital day consumes a large portion of a subscriber's fees.

However, faults exist in HMOs. While credited with many benefits, critics contend they undertreat to save money and reduce consumer choice with regard to selection of a physician or a hospital. Some HMOs have been accused of causing clients to wait excessive lengths of time and to provide impersonal care. Several advantages and disadvantages are summarized in the box on the next page.

Community health nurses play a vital role in the success of many HMOs. Nursing care in these organizations emphasizes prevention, and frequently nurse practitioners find them good setting in which to provide primary care from an interdisciplinary team approach. Such settings allow nurses to define health problems, assess client needs, implement, coordinate, evaluate care, & call on the expertise of other providers as needed. In HMOs as in any other collaborative practice, nurses function *with* not *for* physicians. The functions of nurses in HMOs are compatible with those described in Chapter 33 and may include the coordination activities listed in Chapter 32 as well as home health care described in Chapter 34.

The future success of HMOs will depend on their ability to give quality care while maintaining costs; the federal government's attitude and efforts in fostering their growth; their location; marketing successes; and physician willingness to give up the traditional fee-for-service.

Official and Private Agencies

While the topic of visiting nursing or home health care is discussed in Chapter 34, some information is needed here, since these agencies constitute an increasingly important part of the current health care system. At present a wide variety of agencies provide home health care services including official, voluntary, and private (Stewart, 1979).

Official agencies, established by law at either the national, state, or local levels, receive the majority of their funds from the appropriate legislative body and are accountable to the public. The main functions of federal

Advantages and disadvantages of HMOs

Advantages

- Emphasize prevention
- Provide incentives for health maintenance via annual checkups
- Emphasize organizational efficiency — use of nurse practitioners and physicians, shorter hospital stays
- Offer lower costs to consumer than group insurance plan
- Provide higher level of consumer satisfaction
- Reduce fragmentation of care

Disadvantages

- Restrict consumer choice of physician & hospital
- Result in impersonal care
- Omit accident or illness coverage outside service area
- Fail to deliver some services because of cost

and state agencies include "administer and coordinate programs, conduct research, analyze statistics and set standards and qualifications" (Stewart, 1979, p. 25). In contrast, local agencies are charged with carrying out federal and state guidelines as well as providing services that often include health education, health promotion, and direct services to some or all segments of the population of the designated community.

In recent years there has been a phenomenal growth of private home health care agencies that may either be proprietary (profit-making) or be considered private yet nonprofit. More detail on these agencies can be found in Chapter 34. In addition, hospitals have begun to develop home health care agencies to provide continuity of care between the hospital and the patient's home. There are some advantages inherent in these agencies in that they can draw on the services of hospital employees to perform follow-up care.

Voluntary Health Agencies

The voluntary health movement began in Philadelphia in 1892 with the Anti-Tuberculosis Society. Since that time approximately 100,000 voluntary health- or disease-related agencies have been formed and many foster public health goals (Hanlon and Pickett, 1979). Characteristic of voluntary agencies is their structure which is composed of both staff and volunteers. Many utilize volunteers in decision-making, evaluation, fund-raising, and program implementation. Staff members carry out many agency activities, and the entire or-

ganization is responsible to the public for their programs and expenditures.

Voluntary agencies, having no official status or governmental funding, rely on private and community sources of support. The majority of voluntary health agencies have been known as Visiting Nursing Associations, but this is changing. These agencies are autonomous and usually governed by a voluntary board of interested citizens. There is a long history of visiting nursing agencies that have been pioneers in the provision of home health care. In some parts of the United States voluntary and official agencies combined resources to decrease costs and prevent duplication of services.

Operating funds for voluntary agencies come from a variety of sources including contributions, fees for service, membership dues, investment earnings, selling of goods and publications, gifts, grants, contracts for services, and tax funds (Turner, 1977, p. 480). Fund raising is a vital role of voluntary agencies and requires the efforts of many volunteers and staff members.

Voluntary agencies concerned with health fall into four major types. One type relies heavily on citizen contributions and donations. Hanlon and Pickett (1979, p. 49) divide this type of voluntary agency into four subgroups. The first subgroup deals with specific diseases, such as the American Cancer Society or the American Diabetes Association. The second subgroup of health-related agencies, largely dependent on citizen contributions, is concerned with specific organs or bodily structures such as the American Lung Association or the American Heart Association. The third subgroup of agencies deals with the health and welfare of special groups and includes the National Council on Aging. Finally, the fourth subgroup is concerned with particular phases of health and welfare such as the National Safety Council or Planned Parenthood Federation of America.

Private foundations constitute the second large group of voluntary agencies involved in health activities. Supported by philanthropy, these private groups are generally more flexible in their activities than the first group, since they are accountable to a board and not the public. Leading agencies of this type include the Rockefeller Foundation, the W. K. Kellogg Foundation, the Milbank Memorial Fund, and the Carnegie Foundation.

Professional associations such as the American Public Health Association, the American Medical Association, the American Nurses Association, and the National League for Nursing make up the third group of voluntary agencies. Not only do these organizations provide stimulation and enrichment for members, but each has been instrumental in establishing standards for practice and encouraging research; several have funded projects to improve the health of certain segments of their population.

A fourth group includes those agencies that serve as coordination agents, such as the United Fund in major cities. The functions of these agencies are to fund and assist in the local planning of various agencies. In addition to these four groups, some segments of private industry, most notably insurance companies, have been influential in promoting public health efforts in the communities they serve.

Voluntary agencies have served at least seven key functions in the health care area, as follows (Hanlon and Pickett, 1979, pp. 50-51):

1. They have been pioneers in trying out new ideas and methods.
2. They have demonstrated a variety of techniques to improve health.
3. They provide health education functions, including client, public, and medical education.
4. They guard citizens' interests in health by being watchdogs of what is being developed in their area.
5. They promote health legislation.
6. They develop well-balanced community health programs by filling in the gaps left by the service restrictions of other agencies.
7. They provide "seed" money for research.

Areas that need to be addressed by voluntary agencies in the future include examination of the "multiplicity" of agencies available in a community and the need to avoid duplication of services. Cooperative planning with an eye to overall community needs would be one way to coordinate services so that maximal needs are met in the most efficient way possible. Agencies need also to evaluate the success of their programs and to determine if their outcomes were consistent with their stated goals and mission. Voluntary agencies, through effective leadership, can be ever alert to their responsibility to the public they serve and also to their need to include a wide range of volunteers in the implementation of programs and actions.

Nursing Homes

The number of elderly in the United States increased from 9 million in 1940 to 24.7 million in 1979. The greatest rate of increase has been in the group over 85 years of age. This group currently utilizes a disproportionate amount of the health care dollar. In 1978 people over 65 years of age represented 11% of the population and spent 29% of all health care dollars (*Health: United States,* 1981).

In 1977 more than 1.1 million people 65 years of age and older lived in 18,900 nursing homes. These residents accounted for nearly 5% of the population 65 years and older (National Center for Health Statistics, 1979).

Inflation and increased utilization have raised national expenditures for nursing home care more than 100% every 5 years during the last two decades. In 1978 $15.8 billion was spent on nursing home care (*Health: United States,* 1981). Also, a large percentage of the health care costs for this age group is borne by the public through Medicare. In 1978, 46% of the residents in nursing homes were supported by Medicaid.

Because of the high cost of nursing home care, several projects have attempted to demonstrate effective yet less costly ways to care for elderly people who are unable to live independently. One alternative currently being evaluated is to assign elderly people to case managers who can assess their health and social needs and design and implement a plan to meet these needs, which would include various alternatives, one being nursing home care (Federal Register, 1979).

Another group of alternatives includes board and care homes or personal care homes (*Health: United States,* 1980). It is estimated that at present there are over 200,000 state-certified beds in this type of home. Other options for providing long-term care include home health care, chronic disease hospitals, mental institutions, and community-based day care centers (*Health: United States,* 1981).

Hospice Concept

The hospice concept of care, practiced for many years in Europe, has recently become popular in the United States as a "humane alternative in health care delivery for terminally ill patients" (Andreoli, 1982, p. 318). Hospice care is increasingly becoming a component of community health nursing as many agencies develop programs to make the final period before death comfortable, dignified, and productive for patients and their family. The term *hospice* comes from the medieval word for a place of shelter for travelers on difficult journeys. The current use of the term describes programs "designed to control and relieve the emotional and physical suffering of the terminally ill . . ." (Markel and Sinon, 1978, p. 3). These programs are either provided in the home by home care nurses or within a hospital.

Over 200 hospices are developing in the United States, each with unique features (Lack, 1979). Although programs vary considerably, there are several essential characteristics of a hospice. Generally, hospices are autonomous, centrally administered programs with coordinated inpatient and outpatient services; care is planned and directed by an interdisciplinary team and is available around the clock. The client and family are the primary unit of care and psychologi-

Table 2-1. Basic characteristics of hospice programs

1. The hospice program

Autonomous.

Centrally administered.

A program of coordinated outpatient and inpatient services, primarily concerned with home care, with back-up inpatient services when home care is not feasible.

2. Primary unit of care—patient and family

Total patient care includes dealing with family and other significant patient relationships.

3. Symptom control

Physical: pain, nausea, vomiting, and other symptoms are controlled as effectively as medically possible.

Emotional: behavioral sciences are important in helping patient and family cope with emotional distress accompanying impending death.

Spiritual: attention to human spiritual concerns is equally as important as pain care and is integral to a hospice program.

4. Physician-directed interdisciplinary care

All health care is provided under the direction of a qualified physician.

The interdisciplinary areas include: social work, physical, occupational and speech therapy, pastoral care, and a wide variety of consultant services (e.g., psychiatric, radiologic, pediatric, oncologic).

5. Trained volunteers

Volunteers are specially selected and extensively trained; they augment staff services and are not engaged in lieu of staff.

Volunteers provide vital services other than clinical (e.g., transportation, companionship, recreational, and other services).

6. Services available on call

Hospice services are available on a 7-day week, 24-hour basis.

Hospice nursing staff bear primary responsibility and call on other program resources as necessary.

7. Staff support and communications

Opportunities for staff to discuss their concerns — either one-to-one, or in a group, on a structured or unstructured basis — are imperative.

Channels for staff discussion, support, and mutual evaluation are established.

8. Bereavement follow-ups

Hospice services are extended to the family during the period of bereavement. Extent and length of bereavement care are based on factors before and following death of patient.

9. Hospice services based on need

Hospice services are based on need rather than ability to pay.

From Markel, W. M., and Sinon, V. B.: The hospice concept, New York, 1978, American Cancer Society.

cal, sociological, and spiritual services are provided as well as a carefully designed regimen of narcotic and nonnarcotic analgesics to regulate physical symptoms. The home health care nurse is the key to providing services as well as in coordinating the other members of the team. Chapter 34 provides additional information about hospices in relation to home health care.

Hospice care seeks to maintain an individual's quality of life by taking pharmacological, psychological, or spiritual measures to keep terminally ill persons at their optimal level of functioning. The basic characteristics of hospice care as outlined by the American Cancer Society are shown in Table 2-1. Hospice care cannot always be delivered in the home but may require intermittent periods of hospitalization to allow the family to rest from the exhausting task of caring for a loved one around the clock. Also, some hospice programs are provided in an inpatient setting designed solely for that purpose, such as Calvary Hospital in the Bronx, New York; others are provided in the home through a staff who delivers care to the client and family.

Mental Health Services

It is estimated that more than one million people have mental and nervous conditions causing limitation of activity. At present mental health problems constitute the fourth most prevalent cause of disabling chronic conditions, and about one tenth of all health manpower are employed in mental health services. These figures include 23,000 psychiatrists, 16,000 psychologists, and 33,000 psychiatric nurses.

Since the mid-1960s there has been a movement toward community mental health and away from the previous model for delivering mental health services primarily through private office-based practices and hospitalization. Since the original community mental health legislation of 1963, approximately 700 community mental health centers have been established. The major aim of community mental health centers has been to provide a full range of mental health services in the local community while retaining a focus on prevention. Thus at present the major goal of community mental health is to treat patients in their own communities, close to families and other social support systems.

The initial community mental health legislation mandated that the following five essential services be provided: (1) inpatient services; (2) outpatient service; (3) partial hospitalization; (4) emergency care on a 24-hour basis; and (5) consultation and education to community agencies. Five additional services were recommended in order to provide a full range of care: diagnostic, rehabilitation, precare and aftercare, training, and research and development.

Through the years mental health services have been heavily funded by the federal government with matching state and local funds. In 1980 new legislation mandated that in order to receive federal funding, centers must be more flexible in funding, create a more effective partnership with other federal, state, local, and private providers, and serve the priority needs identified in the 1977 President's Commission on Mental Health. These priorities included programs for disturbed children, the elderly, and people with chronic mental illness and a prevention program (President's Commission on Mental Health, 1978). Additional information specific to mental health needs is provided in Chapter 18.

HEALTH WORK FORCE

During the 1960s and 1970s, Congress appropriated considerable sums of money for students in health-related educational programs in order to increase student enrollment. The 1980s brought a new trend when federal policymakers in the Department of Health and Human Services and the Office of Management and Budget became convinced that the demand was limitless and also that a sufficient number of students had already been helped in this way.

The total work force in the health field is approximately 6.7 million. It includes 4.8 million professionals and approximately 1.9 million nonprofessionals, making it one of the nation's largest industries in terms of number of employees (*Health: United States,* 1980). When work force figures are analyzed, there are approximately 17,100 doctors of osteopathy (D.O.) and 432,400 doctors of medicine (M.D.). There are 20.2 professionally active physicians per 10,000 population in the United States (*Health: United States,* 1981). In 1979, of the 389,157 professionally active doctors of medicine, the majority were employed in nonfederal positions (371,788) with 338,328 providing patient care and the remainder engaged in teaching, research, and administration. During this same year 17,369 physicians were federally employed and the majority provided patient care (*Health: United States,* 1981).

Other work force approximations include 140,000 dentists, 120,000 pharmacists, 1,302,000 registered nurses, 213,000 therapists, 59,000 dieticians, 571,000 health technologists and technicians, 1,001,000 nursing aides, and 370,000 practical nurses (*Statistical Abstracts of the United States,* 1981).

The health care industry is labor intensive and for many years has enjoyed an era of expansion and public and private support for education, research, and facilities. As the economic situation in the United States continues to tighten, an increasing amount of attention will be devoted to the work force needs of the health care industry. It is anticipated that funds will be less available to support education of health care providers.

In terms of mechanism of functioning, health care providers can be categorized as independent or dependent practitioners and as supporting staff. Independent practitioners include those authorized by law to provide a designated range of services without supervision or authorization from any other provider. Examples of independent practitioners include physicians, both allopathic (conventional medical practitioners) and osteopathic,.dentists, chiropractors, optometrists, and podiatrists.

Dependent practitioners are allowed by law to deliver a specified range of services that must be performed under the supervision and authorization of independent practitioners. Representatives of the dependent category include nurses, psychologists, social workers, pharmacists, physicians' assistants, dental hygienists, and the various therapists such as occupational, physical, and speech. The line separating dependent and independent practitioners is becoming blurred as many groups, including nurses, strive for more autonomous forms of practice.

Supporting staff members carry out work tasks authorized and often delegated by either independent or dependent practitioners. The work of members of this group is not always regulated by laws directly pertaining to them, in which case they work under the legal sanctions provided by their supervisors. Members of the supporting staff group include research assistants, various types of technicians, and clerical, maintenance, housekeeping, and food processing workers.

Since 1970 the number of active physicians in the United States increased at a rate that outpaced population growth. In fact, Health Resources Administration estimates indicate that there may be a physician surplus by 1990 if current trends continue. Despite this increase, certain segments of the nation, especially rural and urban inner-city areas, still lack adequate primary care. According to a Health Resources Administration report, more than 1000 primary care shortage areas were designated in 1980 (*Health: United States,* 1979,

p. 45). Physicians have in the past been inclined to practice in urban areas, and many seek to remain near their own homes or near the medical center where they trained.

Nurse Practitioners, Physician's Assistants, and Nurse-Midwives

The federal government is actively trying to improve access to health care in physician-shortage areas by supporting the education and employment of health care providers who are not physicians. Two types making major contributions in primary care are nurse practitioners (NPs) and physician assistants (PAs). The primary distinction between these groups is that NPs perform functions previously considered within the domain of physicians as well as their nursing role; in contrast, PAs assist or substitute for the physician in the performance of specific medical tasks. The best utilization of both NPs and PAs is not as a substitute for the physician but rather as members of a collaborative health care team. PAs and NPs perform the following basic functions (*Health: United States,* 1980, p. 83):

1. Take medical histories and do physical examinations to define health and medical problems.
2. Institute therapeutic regimens within established protocols and recognize when to refer the patient to a physician or other health care provider.
3. Provide counseling to individuals, families, and groups in the area of health promotion and maintenance.

The federal government has encouraged the increased preparation of NPs and PAs through substantial financial subsidies since 1969. In 1969 funds for NP and PA training programs was $1 million, whereas 1979 witnessed $21 million in federal funding (Congressional Budget Office, 1979). The first NP program began in 1965 at the University of Colorado to train pediatric nurse practitioners. During the same year, the first PA program was developed at Duke University. Initially both programs were privately funded with the first federal funding going to the MEDEX program at the University of Washington. This program trained PAs to work in under-served rural or urban areas under physician supervision.

In 1971 the President's Annual Message on Health endorsed the use of NPs and PAs to improve access to care and contain costs (*Health: United States,* 1979). The Nurse Training Act (PL 94-63) of 1974 provided funds for increased training of NPs while the Comprehensive Health Manpower Training Act (PL 92-157) provided funds for both NPs and PAs. Further, in 1977 the Health Profession's Educational Assistance Act of 1976 (PL 94-484) was amended by the Health Services Extension Act (PL 95-83) to fund programs to train

NPs who both came from and would agree to practice in health personnel shortage areas. Additional support was given to NPs and PAs when the Rural Health Clinic Services Act of 1977 (PL 95-210) provided for Medicare and Medicaid coverage for medical services furnished by these two groups in certified clinics located in rural physician shortage areas.

Nurse-midwives, like NPs and PAs, emphasize the care of well rather than ill persons. The American College of Nurse Midwives (ACNM) defines nurse-midwifery as "the independent management and care of essentially normal newborns and women antpartally, intrapartally, postpartally, and or gynecologically, occurring within a health care system that provides for medical consultation, collaborative management, or referral . . ." (*Health: United States,* 1979, p. 50). The mother is the primary focus of care for the nurse-midwives with the majority of their time spent on prenatal, labor and delivery, and postpartal care as well as family planning services.

Research findings have indicated that NPs, PAs, and nurse-midwives have a definite place in the health care delivery system. These providers have been judged capable of carrying out a substantial number of tasks previously reserved for physicians without compromising the quality of care. In general, services can be provided at considerable cost savings to consumers while maintaining quality and a high level of consumer acceptance and satisfaction. In recent years, these groups have received considerable pressure to limit their practice so as to avoid infringing on what physicians perceive as their role.

Two factors significantly influence the geographical distribution and utilization of NPs and PAs. The first involves the restrictions placed on their practice by various professional practice acts and rules and regulations in the different states. In many states the acts and rules governing their practice are restrictive because of supervision requirements and the scope of practice permitted. For example, some states require direct (on the premises) supervision by a physician, whereas others allow NPs and PAs to practice in remote sites if on-site physician supervision is regular (weekly or biweekly usually) and telephone supervision is continuously available. In general, supervision requirements for NPs are not as strict as those for PAs. Both groups, however, are prohibited from prescribing drugs in most states.

The second restriction on the practice of PAs and NPs deals with the question of whether reimbursement is made for their services by third-party insurers including Medicare and Medicaid. Traditionally, reimbursement from third-party payers has only been forthcoming when physicians were on-site and services were billed by them. The exception was established in 1977 by Public Law 95-210, which amended Titles XVIII and XIX of the Social Security Act. This legislation provided for Medicare and Medicaid reimbursement for NP or PA services in certified clinics that lacked a full-time physician. An additional threat to the practice of these providers may be the rapidly increasing number of physicians in the United States. Chapter 33 provides detailed information on nurse practitioners.

NONTRADITIONAL HEALTH CARE

Previous sections of this chapter have discussed a variety of traditional health care institutions and providers. At this point the rapidly expanding area of nontraditional health practices and practitioners needs to be addressed, since community health nurses have been part of this movement. Several nontraditional health practices including biofeedback, hypnosis, and progressive relaxation therapy are described in Chapter 38 as ways of relieving stress. These will not be repeated here, but rather additional health alternatives will be addressed including the concept and practice of holistic health, faith healing, chiropractic, acupuncture, and kinesiology.

Many nontraditional health practices arose out of despair with the current health care system. It is well established that modern medicine is limited in what it can do to save lives as well as to enrich the quality of life. Personal health habits, including nutrition, exercise, stress reduction, and cigarette smoking, have been afforded much acclaim as factors influential in the determination of health. Interest has increased dramatically in recent years in the notion that traditional disease-oriented health care is simply insufficient in preventing and controlling the major twentieth century diseases—many of which are life-style induced. Several alternative forms of health care are discussed in the following sections.

Holistic Health Centers

Holistic health centers began in the United States as alternative services in the last two decades. Many of the early centers that developed in the mid to late 1960s focused on the needs of young people. The early workers were activists who resembled earlier settlement house workers in their idealism and humanitarianism. "These activist workers believed that, given time, space, and encouragement, ordinary people could find the strength to help themselves and one another to deal with the vast majority of the problems that confronted them" (Gordon, 1980, p. 468). Starting with a handful of switchboards, free clinics, and houses for runaways, the number has grown to approximately 2,000 hot

lines, 400 free clinics and more than 200 runaway houses.

Although the program offered in holistic health centers varies, there are several commonalities including the following (Gordon, 1980, pp. 470-475):

1. Although implemented in a wide variety of ways, all holistic health centers subscribe to programs that respond to physical, psychological, and spiritual needs.
2. Programs are individually designed for consumers.
3. The philosophy is directed toward personal responsibility for health in contrast to relying on pharmacological and surgical remedies.
4. Centers emphasize education and self-care rather than treatment and dependence.
5. Holistic health centers treat their clients as members of families and of social systems.
6. Holistic health centers view health as a positive state, not merely as being the absence of disease.
7. Diagnostic procedures blend traditional methods with those derived from other healing systems and types of healers.
8. Holistic health centers regard proper diet and exercise as cornerstones of healing.
9. They maximize the therapeutic benefit to be derived from the setting by making facilities as pleasant and inviting as possible for both clients and staff both in physical and interpersonal relations so as to enrich the environmental influence on people.
10. They rely on an active partnership between caregivers and consumers.
11. They include both professional and lay staff.
12. Holistic health centers provide ongoing education and development for members of the community.
13. They view illness as an opportunity for change and growth.

Examples of current centers include the network of Wholistic Health Centers developed in the early 1970s in Springfield, Ohio, by a minister named Granger Westberg. The aim of the first center was to establish a free clinic for low-income people which saved money by operating out of the church. Teams of ministers, nurses, and physicians work together in these centers to develop health programs that include psychological, spiritual, and physical needs. The treatment offered includes traditional medical care, pastoral counseling, biofeedback, education in stress reduction, parent effectiveness training, yoga, meditation, and so on (Gordon, 1980, p. 470).

A similar program is offered at the Pain and Health

Rehabilitation Center on a farm in Wisconsin by neurosurgeon Norman Shealy. Disillusioned with the effects of drugs and surgery, Shealy created a holistic program for sufferers of chronic pain. Beginning with transcutaneous nerve stimulation (TENS), facial rhizotomies, and behavior modification, he has expanded his program to include diet, physical fitness, massage, biofeedback, and biogenics. The latter is a program combining progressive relaxation and other techniques designed to promote peace and relieve pain (Gordon, 1980).

As discussed in Chapter 14, self-care is a topic of interest for many Americans. Self-care activities range from structured individual or group programs to self-treatment manuals. The number and types of groups with a self-care or mutual aid orientation grow annually. Most larger cities have many mutual aid groups such as Alcoholics Anonymous, Synanon, Recovery Inc., Parents Without Partners, and Weight Watchers.

In addition, self-care centers in many cities are identical or similiar to holistic health centers. Self-care centers emphasize consumer-oriented services, diet, exercise, stress management, meditation, and so on. In these centers, the responsibility for obtaining and maintaining a maximal level of health lies with the individual.

Faith Healing

The practice of faith healing has been in effect since the beginning of recorded history. The basis of many religions includes the incorporation of faith healing. For example, members of the Christian Science faith do not believe in using drugs, surgery, or any other form of medical care, including hospitalization, to relieve the suffering of believers. Instead, members of this faith are taught that disease is a state of mind, hence, relief from maladies occurs from altering one's beliefs (Cornacchia and Barrett, 1980).

Faith healing is generally considered to be a belief "that the healer himself has the power to cause cure of or recovery from illness and that God's will gave the healer his power" (Fromer, 1983, p. 111). It has long been recognized that one's state of mind, belief in the care giver, and anticipation of a certain outcome influence responses to care. What differs, however, in faith healing is the belief that another person via one's own faith in God can bring about healing.

Chiropractic

Chiropractic refers to a system of "manipulative treatment which teaches that all diseases are caused by impingement on spinal nerves and can be corrected by spinal adjustments" (Thomas, 1973, p. C-57). Daniel Palmer developed this mode of care and founded a school of chiropractic techniques in 1894 in Davenport, Iowa. Palmer discounted the germ theory and his early followers were generally uniformed regarding realistic ways to treat patients. Chiropractors usually limit their practice to external, physical manipulations of the spine for treating illness.

According to Fromer (1979, p. 106), there are currently two types of chiropractors. The "straights" continue to rely on the correction of subluxated vertebrae to cure disease, whereas the "mixers" combine this technique with procedures that include light, air, water, exercise, diet, and electricity. They are currently licensed to practice in all states except Mississippi and Louisiana following a 4-year apprentice-type training and refer to themselves as "doctor."

While the services of chiropractors in nutritional counseling, physical therapy, psychosomatic counseling, exercise, herbs, and manipulation have value, drawbacks exist. Improper manipulation can dislocate bones and damage blood vessels. Additionally, clients may allow health conditions to go beyond the point of reversibility by delaying the seeking of traditional medical care while seeing a chiropractor. Of course, reputable chiropractors recognize the limits of their skill and refer clients to other health care providers as indicated by the clients' health care needs.

Community health nurses should be informed about the number and availability of chiropractors in the community, since clients may pursue this type of assistance in lieu of more traditional forms of care. Not only do these nontraditional providers have less rigorous educational experiences than do physicians, nurses, and other professionals, but they do not practice in JCAH-accredited hospitals, perform surgery, prescribe medications, or practice obstetrics.

Acupuncture

Acupuncture has some features in common with acupressure. The primary difference is that acupuncture inserts needles into selected parts of the body to control pain, whereas acupressure uses finger pressure on certain parts of the body to control pain. This method of treatment has been used in the Orient for 5,000 years as a form of medical treatment for the entire body. The belief behind acupuncture asserts that pain is relieved when the balance between yin and yang, which flow through the body along 14 meridians, is restored (Fromer, 1979). Acupuncture, performed by people trained in this skill, is effective especially in the relief of pain. Training and skill are required in the placement and twirling of the needles, or otherwise the technique

can cause pneumothorax, hematomas, cardiac ruptur-
ing, infection, and damage to a variety of vital organs
and parts including the spinal cord.

Kinesiology

Kinesiology, or the study of movement, applies principles of anatomy, physiology, and physics to movement (Sutterly, 1979). A variety of specific approaches
make up the overall category of kinesiology including
bioenergetics, polarity therapy, and yoga. Bioenergetics
refers to a "series of exercises designed to bring about
natural healing based upon bringing into harmony the
natural environment and body rhythms" (Sutterly,
1979, p. 11). After muscles are tested and measured, a
variety of techniques and exercises are employed to alter tension and muscular-skeletal postures or align-
ments to bring about the type and amount of harmony
needed to promote healing.

Polarity therapy is based on the presence of polarities
in the human body (Lande, 1976). This therapy calls for
an understanding of the positive and negative energy
patterns in the body, so that massage can be given
which reestablishes bodily harmony.

Yoga blends both kinesiology and meditation and relieves stress for many people.

Other Nontraditional Health Practices

In addition to the nontraditional health practices just
described and those discussed in Chapter 38, several
techniques, while not discussed in detail, are defined
here and references cited for those interested in further
study.

Reflexology is a systematic massage of the soles of
the feet based on principles similar to those relating to
acupressure. Pressure and stimulation to nerve endings
in the soles of the feet relieve pain in other organs of the
body. The major purpose of reflexology is to "relax
nerve tension, increase circulation in the blood and
lymphatic systems, and get the body into top form so
that it will have power to throw off any accumulated
poisons" (Lande, p. 182).

Massage has been used for many years as a treatment, and in the past nurses were quite adept at this
technique. In recent years systematic methods of massage have been employed to relieve tension, enhance
flexibility, and create greater coordination between
mind and body (Lande, 1976, p. 186).

Homeopathy, founded by Samuel Hahnemann, proposes that a variety of herbs, drugs, and chemicals
when used in small quantities can cure or prevent a disease ordinarily caused by a larger dose of the same substance (Cornacchia and Barrett, 1980). The Hahnemann Medical College in Philadelphia still teaches one
course in homeopathy. This technique continues to
form the basis for desensitization to allergies.

Therapeutic touch is a nursing modality pioneered by
Dolores Kreiger (1975) and used by many nurses to aid
healing in their clients. This approach uses "the meditative state to enter the energy field of the client and to
passively visualize or free the flow of energy from practitioner to recipient with the intent to support or promote healing" (Sutterly, 1979, p. 13). Clients are helped
to achieve self-healing by drawing on the energy flow of
the practitioner. Also, practitioners trained in therapeutic touch can assess bodily areas out of harmony in a
client by alterations and sensations in their own energy
flow as they touch the client.

Each of these techniques uses a specific approach to
assist people to cope with pain, stress, disease, and other maladies. When used appropriately and by trained
people, they are often beneficial.

Nurses must be aware of what is available in the
community, the usefulness and credibility of the care
given, and whether the nontraditional care comple-
ments or interferes with the performance of traditional
forms of care.

CONSUMERISM

The consumerism movement is built on the belief
that people have both a right and a responsibility to be
knowledgeable and involved in the choices made about
their health and illness care. This movement presup-
poses that consumers will take time to acquaint themselves with selected health-related information and that
providers will make a concerted effort to disseminate
such information in easily understood forms.

As mentioned in an earlier section of this chapter,
consumers of health care differ from consumers of
many other products and services. Health care consumers typically invest complete, unquestioning trust
in health care providers, especially physicians. Few
consumes devote as much time to researching the relative merits of a proposed medical treatment as they devote to choosing automobiles to buy. Also, health care
consumers are often hesitant to raise questions about
costs or to do any sort of comparative shopping. Several reasons for the lack of informed health care consumers are discussed in this section.

The tendency to passively rely on health care providers to repair one's physical and emotional maladies has
changed considerably in recent years. People increasingly recognize their personal responsibility for health
and realize that many health problems can be avoided
by proper care including preventive maintenance such
as health promotion. Advocates like Bess Myerson and

Ralph Nader continue to diligently inform people of both their rights and responsibilities as consumers. People are encouraged to scrutizine both the products *and* services they purchase by reading about them, asking carefully formulated questions, and thinking critically about what is best for them.

Consumerism, while currently undergoing an impetus in the United States, is not a new concept. Early consumer participation can be traced to medieval times (400-1400 AD) when guilds of workers in Europe joined together to protect their common interests. These guilds developed "sick chests" to provide funds for medical care needed for sickness or disability resulting from accidents. Hence, this early evidence of health insurance was devised by consumers. Likewise, in seventeenth century England, societies such as the Oddfellows or the Ancient Order of Foresters extended the "sick chest" idea to include people outside their guilds. The friendly society concept also developed in the colonies and by 1867 more than 24,000 benevolent societies operated in the United States (Hamilton, 1982). Over the years the consumer movement has taken many forms with the guiding aim being to secure health care that is accessible, effective, and reasonable in cost.

A major hurdle for consumers to overcome is their perceived or actual lack of power. According to Hamilton (1982, p. 14), "Power, or the lack of it, is at the root of all consumer issues." As mentioned earlier in this chapter, the power ratio is unevenly distributed in health care, since physicians largely control entry into the system. Consumerism in health care discounts the basic notions held by economists about the role and influence of consumers. According to classic economic theory, consumers create mandates for producers who then concede to consumer demands. In accordance with this view, in the 1800s W. H. Hutt coined the phrase "consumer sovereign" to describe the power held by consumers in determining the behavior of producers (Hutt, 1936).

For consumer sovereignty to occur the following four conditions must exist (Hamilton, 1982, p. 15):

1. Consumer demand must determine production of goods and provision of services.
2. Consumers must have the information necessary to judge the quality, utility, and safety of products and services.
3. Consumers must choose products and services that give the greatest utility for the lowest prices.
4. Both consumers and providers must have free access to the marketplace.

These conditions do not presently exist in health care. First, demand is not left up to consumers but rather is determined by providers who decide what services and products are needed and in many instances prescribe them by specific company names. One reason providers retain such control is that consumers have not had sufficient information to make informed choices (the second condition for consumer sovereignty). Only recently have unbiased sources of information become available to consumers. In recent years, however, the U.S. Food and Drug Administration (FDA) has taken an active role in informing consumers about the hazards of health care. Consumers now serve on FDA advisory panels and participate in the review of drugs, diagnostic and treatment devices, and radiological equipment (Hamilton, 1982).

In most other consumer-provider interactions advertising plays a much greater role than it does in health care. Advertising, although biased in many instances toward the product being discussed, does inform consumers about the relative merits of products, prices, and locations for purchase. Health care providers look down on advertising as being "below them." While advertising would increase competiveness for products such as eyeglasses and dentures, it probably would not solve the problem of poorly informed consumers. The third condition of consumer sovereignty, which is that consumers spend to get the greatest utility at the lowest price, does not hold true in health care. Because of the fear involved in illness and disability, people do not consistently seek second opinions, negotiate prices, or question the provider's rationale for selecting a proposed treatment. Erroneously, consumers equate quality with high prices. Similarly, because of the fear of a potential malpractice suit, some providers charge far greater fees than others. Consider the dramatically different fee accrued in 1 hour by a neurosugeron compared to that of a psychiatrist. People are more willing to pay very high charges for brain surgery than for the examination of emotional problems. Hence, emotions play a significant role in determining health care costs.

The last condition of consumer sovereignty holds that consumers and providers have equal access to the marketplace. In the present health care system, access is largely influenced by physicians and third-party payers. Physicians prescribe and order services, many of which would be otherwise unavailable. In many instances consumer participation in hospital-sponsored health education provided by nurses must be prescribed by physicians. Further, insurance carriers and Medicare and Medicaid influence what services will be reimbursed and at what rate.

What can and should be done to alter the power ratio in health care? Should consumers become more involved in their care and if so, how do they begin? If one believes in consumer involvement in health, the place to begin is with a recognition of consumer rights. There have been several attempts on the part of providers to draft documents setting forth patient rights. However, consumers *must* assume responsibility for their rights, since they have the most to gain if their rights are acknowledged and respected and the most to lose if their rights are ignored or violated. Consumers are entitled to privacy, confidentiality, and self-determination of care as well as effective and compassionate care. Yet these rights are only realized when providers are sincerely committed to client-centered care.

To become participants in the health care system, consumers must become better informed and also gain more power. Consumers, individually and collectively, need to know what choices are available and what are the potential consequences of selecting one rather than the other. Nurses can play a key role in advancing the cause of consumerism by informing clients of their choices, encouraging them to seek additional information, and motivating them to become involved in consumer issues beyond their personal sphere. Consumers can organize groups to promote health care by approaching and enlisting the support of various power groups in the community.

CRITICISMS OF THE HEALTH CARE SYSTEM

It is often said that no health care system exists in the United States, but instead there is an illness care system in which health is viewed as a renewable resource or a commodity that can be "fixed" if disrepair occurs. Bruhn (1981, p. 29) contends that the "maintenance of health or its enhancement has been largely ignored by health care professionals, claiming that they are too busy taking care of the sick to support greater responsibility on the part of individuals for staying healthy." Major criticisms leveled against the health care industry include skyrocketing costs, fragmentation of services, shortage and maldistribution of providers, lack of quality control efforts, and disparity in availability from one region to another.

Although the United States spends more on health care than any other nation in the world, indexes of health reflect a less than adequate state of health. As can be seen in Table 2-2 several other countries have lower infant mortality rates than the United States. Additionally, the average life expectancy for both males and females in the United States is lower than in many other countries. As seen in Table 2-3 the United States does not rank very high in life expectancy rates when compared to several other countries. It is significant also to note that current projections to the year 2000 anticipate that males will gain only about 2 to 3 years in life expectancy compared to an anticipated gain of 3 to 5 years

for females. The reasons for this gloomy projection in life expectancy gains can be seen when the causes of morbidity and morality are examined. The four most common causes of death continue to be heart disease, cancer, strokes, and accidents. As will be discussed in Chapter 14, the most optimistic view of health relies on preventing illness. As people assume greater responsibility for their health and rely less on the health care system to repair them, major advances can be made. The way people live contributes to several common causes of death, especially the four just listed as major killers.

Despite poor overall ratings in health indexes, significant changes have been made in the United States in heart disease mortality. Between 1950 and 1978 the age-adjusted death rate decreased by about 1% per year. From 1978 to 1980 heart disease mortality rates declined more rapidly in younger age groups and for women. Some possible explanations for the decline in heart disease mortality include decreased smoking, improved management of hypertension, decreased dietary intake of saturated fats, more widespread physical activity, improved medical emergency services, and more widespread use and increased efficacy of coronary care units (*Health: United States*, 1980, p. 25).

Despite large increases in the physician supply as well as that of other providers, access to health care continues to be a matter of national concern. While access in general has improved in recent years, the major problem continues to lie in the differences between rural and urban populations. From 1960 to 1970 the number of physicians practicing in rural counties declined 12.4% while the supply of physicians in urban counties increased 34.8%. However, from 1970 to 1976 the number of physicians in rural counties increased 16.0% and the physician-to-population ratio increased 6.7%. While these increases are noteworthy, they are still less than the urban physician-to-population increases. The number of physicians in urban counties increased during this period 24.8%, and the physicians-to-population ratio increased 18.1% (*Health: United States*, 1980, p. 79). By the end of 1979 there were still 1,710 primary personnel shortage areas representing an underserved population of 22 million people.

In looking back to the 1800s one can see that many of the health problems of the industrial era were really community health issues—waste, unpotable water, poor diet, harsh labor practices, and poor working conditions compounded by crowded and often unsanitary living conditions. These problems have largely been taken care of but new disabling conditions have arisen: stress, air quality, congestion, overindulgence, and lack of personal responsibility for health (Carlson, 1976). Because of noteworthy medical advancements of re-

Table 2-2. Infant mortality rates and perinatal mortality ratios in selected countries in 1973 and 1978

Country	Infant mortality rate (deaths per 1,000 live births)		Average annual change 1973-1978 (%)	Perinatal mortality ratio (deaths per 1,000 live births)		Average annual change 1973-1978 (%)
	1973	1978		1973	1978	
Canada	15.5	12.4	−5.4	17.7	15.1	−5.2
United States	17.7	13.8	−4.9	20.7	15.2	−6.0
Austria	23.8	15.0	−8.8	24.8	15.0	−9.6
Denmark	11.5	8.9	−5.0	14.6	10.7	−7.5
England and Wales	16.9	13.1	−5.0	21.3	17.1	−5.3
France	15.5	10.6	−7.3	18.8	15.8	−3.4
German Democratic Republic	15.6	13.2	−3.3	19.4	15.2	−4.8
German Federal Republic	22.7	14.7	−8.3	23.2	13.8	−9.9
Ireland	18.0	15.6	−3.5	23.1	21.8	−2.9
Italy	25.7	17.7	−8.9	29.6	20.8	−6.8
Netherlands	11.5	9.6	−3.5	16.4	13.0	−5.6
Sweden	9.9	7.8	−4.7	14.2	9.6	−7.3
Switzerland	13.2	8.6	−8.2	15.5	10.7	−7.1
Israel	22.8	17.2	−5.5	21.2	17.4	−3.9
Japan	11.3	8.4	−5.8	18.0	13.0	−6.3
Australia	16.5	12.5	−6.7	22.4	17.8	−5.6
New Zealand	16.2	14.2	−3.2	19.4	14.3	−5.0

From Health: United States, 1981, DHHS Pub. No. (PHS) 82-1232, Hyattsville, Maryland, 1981, U.S. Department of Health and Human Services, p. 115.

Table 2-3. Life expectancy at birth in selected countries in 1973 and 1978

Country	Male life expectancy (years)			Female life expectancy (years)		
	1973	1978	Average annual change	1973	1978	Average annual change
Canada	69.5	70.5	0.3	77.0	78.2	0.3
United States	67.6	69.5	0.4	75.3	77.2	0.4
Austria	67.4	68.4	0.2	74.7	75.7	0.2
Denmark	71.1	71.7	0.1	76.6	77.7	0.2
England and Wales	69.2	70.2	0.3	75.5	76.3	0.2
France	69.5	69.9	0.1	77.3	77.9	0.2
German Democratic Republic	68.9	68.9	−	74.2	74.5	0.1
German Federal Republic	67.8	69.2	0.3	74.4	76.0	0.3
Ireland	68.5	69.0	0.2	73.4	74.3	0.3
Italy	68.9	69.8	0.3	75.2	76.1	0.3
Netherlands	71.2	72.0	0.2	77.2	78.7	0.3
Sweden	72.1	72.5	0.1	77.7	79.0	0.3
Switzerland	71.1	72.0	0.2	77.2	78.9	0.3
Israel	70.2	71.6	0.3	73.2	75.1	0.4
Japan	70.9	73.2	0.5	76.3	78.6	0.5
Australia	68.3	70.0	0.4	75.3	77.0	0.4
New Zealand	69.2	69.4	0.1	74.8	75.6	0.2

From Health: United States, 1981, DHHS Pub. No. (PHS) 82-1232, Hyattsville, Maryland, 1981, U.S. Department of Health and Human Services, p. 116.

cent decades, too many Americans continue to abuse their health, thinking that they can "be fixed" when the need arises.

Rick Carlson, an outspoken critic of the contemporary health care system, asserts that the most significant improvements in health care have come from alterations in the social, economic, and environmental conditions rather than from medical practices. Carlson (1980) advocates a consumer-intensive health care system that places responsibility for personal well-being on the consumer who must maintain good health practices, recognize signs indicating the onset of a crisis, respond immediately to these signs, and be able to establish and maintain a health regimen.

Hence proponents for changing the health care system believe that a major reorientation toward primary care is called for which focuses on prevention and health promotion. Many of the remaining chapters in the book address specific roles which nurses can play in the enactment of an orientation toward health which focuses on promotion of health and the prevention of illness.

SUMMARY

With total health care expenditures exceeding $247.2 billion annually, health care has become one of the largest industries in the United States (*Health: United States,* 1981). Despite vast expenditures, the United States ranks fifth in overall life expectancy and tenth in infant mortality (*Health: United States,* 1981). The health care system continues to be criticized for lack of access of services to all people at an affordable cost. Most writers who address the current dilemmas in the health care system contend that major sources of problems originate with cost, availability, and accessibility of services. In many sections of the country, health personnel and resources are poorly distributed. Some urban areas have an abundance of both providers and facilities, whereas people in many rural areas and some inner cities have virtually no services available within a reasonable commuting distance.

Critics state that major weaknesses in the health care system can only be overcome by a reshaping of national priorities regarding health care. While there is no doubt that the United States possesses some of the finest hospitals, health care providers, and health care facilities in the world, there is no question that additional efforts are essential to reshape the system and move from a focus on restoration of health to one of promoting health. As discussed in Chapter 1, community health providers have consistently advocated that it is less costly to prevent illness than to provide adequate treatment once disruption has occurred. However, the study of the cost of preventive measures has been neglected in the past; therefore, few statistics support the belief in the cost effectiveness of prevention. Nurses who work in preventive care are in a key position to contribute research efforts in this much-needed area.

Additionally, changes in the health care system need to recognize that the community itself is a major determinant of the health of its residents. Clean water, adequate sewage disposal, food, heat, and proper personal health practices are major factors in determining the health of the residents. Nursing has a major role to play in the ultimate restructuring of the health care system by continuing to urge communities and other health care providers to focus on health, personal responsibility for health, and a view that takes into account the needs, sources of support, and resources in a given community.

BIBLIOGRAPHY

Andreoli, K.G.: Future directions: organizational settings for practice. In Lancaster, J., and Lancaster, W.: Concepts for advanced nursing practice: the nurse as a change agent, St. Louis, 1982, The C.V. Mosby Co., pp. 316-333.

Blum, H.L.: Planning for health, New York, 1974, Human Sciences Press.

Brody, H., and Sobel, D.S.: A systems view of health and disease. In Lee, P.R., Brown, N., and Red, I., editors: The nation's health, San Francisco, 1981, Boyd and Fraser Publishing Co., pp. 27-37.

Bruhn, J.: Personal health in a sustainable society, Appalachian Business Rev. **8**(1):29-40, 1981.

Carlson, R.: The end of medicine, Executive **3**:6-9, Fall, 1976.

Carlson, R.J.: The future of health care in the United States. In Hastings, A.C., Fadiman, J., and Gordon, J.S., editors: Health for the whole person, Boulder, Colo., 1980, Westview Press, pp. 483-496.

Congressional Budget Office: Physician extenders, their current and future role in medical care delivery, Congress of the United States, Washington, D.C., April 1979, U.S. Government Printing Office.

Cornacchia, H.J., and Barrett, S.: Consumer health, ed. 2, St. Louis, 1980, The C.V. Mosby Co.

Dubos, R.: Health and creative adaptation. In Lee, P.R., Brown, N., and Red, I., editors: The nation's health, San Francisco, 1981, Boyd and Fraser Publishing Co., p. 6.

Ehrenreich, J., and Ehrenreich, E.B.: The American health empire: the system behind the chaos. In Aaker, D.A., and Day, G.S.: Consumerism: search for the consumer interests, ed. 2, New York, 1974, The Free Press, pp. 36-48.

Ellwood, P.M.: Models for organizing health services and implications for legislative proposals, The Milbank Mem. Fund Q. **51**:76 Spring, 1973.

Ellwood, P.M., and Herbert, M.E.: Health care: should industry buy or sell?, Harvard Business Rev. **51**:99-107, July-Aug. 1973.

Federal Register **44**:75720, Dec. 21, 1979.

Fromer, M.J.: Community health care and the nursing process, St. Louis, 1979, The C.V. Mosby Co.

Fuchs, V.R.: Health care and the United States—economic system: an essay in abnormal physiology, Milbank Mem. Fund Q. **1**:211-237, April 1972.

Garfield, S.R.: The delivery of medical care, Sci. Am. **222**:15-23, April 1970.

Gordon, J.S.: Holistic health centers. In Hastings, A.C., Fadiman J., and Gordon, J.S.: Health for the whole person, Boulder, Colo., 1980, Westview Press, pp. 467-482.

Gunn, S.M., and Platt, P.S.: Voluntary health agencies: an interpretative study, New York, 1945, The Ronald Press Co.

Haag, J.H.: Consumer health: products and services, Philadelphia, 1976, Lea & Febiger.

Hamilton, P.A.: Health care consumerism, St. Louis, 1982, The C.V. Mosby Co.

Hanlon, J.J., and Pickett, G.E.: Public health: administration and practice, St. Louis, 1979, The C.V. Mosby Co.

Health: United States, 1978, DHEW Pub. No. (PHS) 78-1232, Washington, D.C., 1978, Department of Health, Education, and Welfare.

Health: United States, 1979, DHEW Pub. No. (PHS) 80-1232, Washington, D.C., Dec. 1979, Department of Health, Education, and Welfare.

Health: United States, 1980, DHHS Pub. No. (PHS) 81-1232, Washington, D.C., Dec. 1980, Department of Health and Human Services.

Health: United States, 1981, DHHS Pub. No. (PHS) 82-1232, Washington, D.C., Dec. 1981, Department of Health and Human Services.

Healthy people: the Surgeon General's report on health promotion and disease prevention, Pub. No. 79-55071, Washington, D.C., Dec. 1979, Department of Health, Education, and Welfare.

Herzlinger, R.: How can we control health care costs?, Harvard Business Rev. **56:**102-110, March-April 1978.

Hutt, W.H.: Economists and the public, London, 1936, Jonathan Cape Ltd.

Institute of Medicine: A staff paper: perspectives on health promotion in the United States, Jan. 1978, Washington, D.C., National Academy of Sciences.

Kreiger, D.: Therapeutic touch: the imprimatur of nursing, Am. J. Nurs. **75**(5):784-778, May 1975.

Lack, S.A.: Hospice—a concept of care in the final stage of life, Conn. Med. **43**(6):367, 1979.

Lancaster, J.: The nature and scope of community mental health nursing. In Lancaster, J.: Community mental health nursing: an ecological perspective, St. Louis, 1980, The C.V. Mosby Co., pp. 3-8.

Lande, N.: Mindstyles—lifestyles, Los Angeles, 1976, Price/Stern/Sloan Publishers, Inc.

Levey, S., and Loomba, N.P.: Health care administration: a managerial perspective, Philadelphia, 1973, J.B. Lippincott Co.

Markel, W.M., and Sinon, V.B.: The hospice concept, New York, 1979, American Cancer Society.

National Center for Health Statistics: The national nursing home survey, 1977 summary for the United States Vital and Health Statistics, Series 13-No 43, DHEW Pub. No. (PHS) 79-1794, Washington, D.C., 1979, U.S. Government Printing Office.

National League for Nursing: Health maintenance organization, New York, 1978, The League.

Notkin, H., and Meader, L.V.: The American health care system, Personnel Administrator **25:**18-36, May 1978.

Pender, N.J.: Health promotion in nursing practice, Norwalk, Conn., 1982, Appleton-Century-Crofts.

President's Commission on Mental Health: report on the task panel on the nature and scope of the problem, Task Panel Reports, vol. 2, Appendix, Washington, D.C., 1978, U.S. Government Printing Office.

Rathmell, J.M.: Marketing in the health sector, Cambridge, Mass. 1974, Winthrop Publishers, Inc.

Reinhart, U.E.: Proposed changes in the organization of health care delivery: an overview and critique, Milbank Mem. Fund Q. **51:**171, 1973.

Shindell, S., Salloway, J.C., and Obernabt, C.M.: A coursebook in health care delivery, New York, 1976, Appleton-Century-Crofts.

Statistical abstracts of the United States: 1981, ed. 102, 1981, U.S. Department of Commerce, Bureau of the Census.

Stewart, J.: Home health care, St. Louis, 1979, The C.V. Mosby Co.

Sutterly, D.C.: Stress and health: a survey of self-regulation modalities, Top. Clin. Nurs. **1**(1):1-20, April 1979.

Thomas, C.L., editor: Taber's Cyclopedic-Medical Dictionary, ed. 12, Philadelphia, 1973, F.A. Davis Co.

Turner, J.B., editor: Encyclopedia of social work, Washington, D.C., 1977, National Association of Social Workers.

Wilner, D.M., Walkley, R.P., and O'Neill, E.J.: Introduction to public health, ed. 7, New York, 1978, Macmillan Publishing Co.

World Health Organization: The first ten years of the World Health Organization, New York, 1958, WHO.

Chapter 3

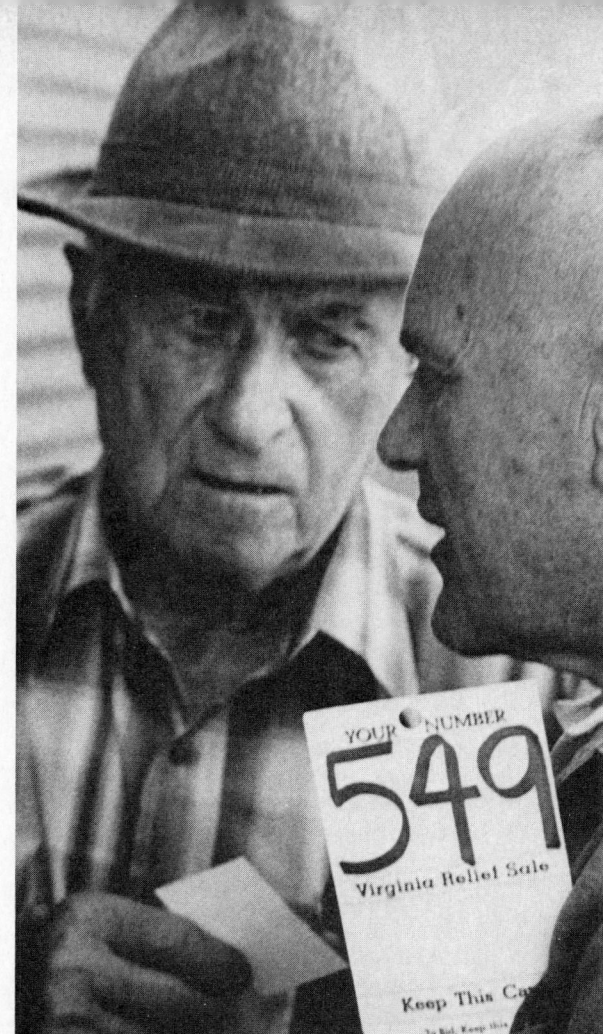

MARCIA STANHOPE

ECONOMICS OF HEALTH CARE DELIVERY

The present health care delivery system, characterized by limited resources, regulatory restrictions, and increased technological advances, is unlike the health care delivery system of the 60s and 70s, which experienced vast expansions, unlimited financial resources, an open job market, and a nursing discipline that was expanding and broadening its responsibilities and influence.

Because of the present system characteristics, the concerns of the 80s, 90s, and twenty-first century will focus on examining the economics of health care delivery, limiting the continuous growth of the largest industry in the United States; and organizing and assigning priorities to the use of available resources at the least cost. Nursing will be concerned with establishing its contribution to the health of the nation and ensuring its economic viability in the market structure in lieu of less costly health care personnel, such as the health care assistant who may be trained by institutions to perform nursing functions.

The purpose of this chapter is to provide an overview of the economic issues of the health care delivery system. Discussion focuses on factors influencing health care, schema for financing health care, economics of primary prevention, methods for evaluating health and nursing costs, and the value of human life in health care spending.

DEFINITIONS

To grasp the importance of the economics of health care and its significance to nursing, a basic understanding of key economic terms is essential.

Economics is the social science concerned with the

problems of using or administering scarce resources in the most efficient way to attain maximum fulfillment of society's unlimited wants (Heider-Dorneich, 1978). *Health economics* is concerned with the problems of producing and distributing the health care resources of the nation in a way that will provide maximum benefit to the most people.

The *goal* of health economics is maximum benefit, or quality care, from the goods that are produced and supplied by health providers and demanded and purchased by the consumer. The availability of health goods (services) requires monies. The spending of monies on health goods limits the benefits derived from other goods available in society, such as food, clothing, shelter, transportation, education, and recreation.

Society must being to make tough decisions about the allocation of monies for available resources. Today the nation allocates approximately one tenth of the gross national product for health goods. This one tenth represented $286 billion spent in 1981 for health care alone. The *gross national product* (GNP) is defined as the total value of all goods and services produced in the economy in one year (*Health: United States,* 1978). The GNP is an important statistical measure because it is the most comprehensive measure of a nation's total output of goods and services; and it is useful for comparing and contrasting expenditures on all of society's benefits, telling us on what we place the most value. The value, or price, of a service is determined by using a U.S. Department of Labor indicator, the consumer price index. The *consumer price index* is a shopping basket approach that compares prices of all consumed goods and services on a monthly or quarterly basis (*Health: United States,* 1978).

HEALTH SERVICES COMPONENTS

From the 1800s to the present, the U.S health care delivery system has experienced three developmental stages. The health services component framework will be used in describing the system's evolution.

Three basic components provide the framework for health services delivery: labor (work force), facilities, and technology. Historically, changes have occurred in the three components as changes have occurred in morbidity, mortality, national health policy and economic and social forces.

The *first developmental stage* of the health care delivery system occurred during the period 1800 to 1900. As mentioned in Chapter 1, the period was characterized by epidemics of infectious diseases, such as plague, cholera, typhoid, smallpox, influenza, malaria, yellow fever, and gastric disorders. The health problems of the

period were related to contaminated food and water supplies, inadequate sewage disposal, and poor housing conditions (Hanlon and Pickett, 1979; Rushmer, 1980; Torrens, 1981; Torrens and Lewis, 1980).

Minimal technology was available to aid in disease control. The doctor's black bag contained the few medicines and tools available for health care in the era, and hospitals were characterized by overcrowding, disease, and lack of cleanliness. Since the sick poor, if cared for in a hospital, usually died because of hospital conditions, most people were cared for at home by family and friends (Lee, 1981; Rushmer, 1980).

During this period the labor force was composed of poorly trained physicians who attained their skills through apprenticeships with practicing physicians. Nurses were typically volunteers recruited from the lower social strata or from religious orders. Their primary focus was to assist the clients with activities of daily living. In 1867 the first nurse training school was established at the New England Hospital for Women and Children to provide formal preparation for nursing in the U.S.; by 1886 organized district nursing (home nursing) had been established (Aiken, 1981; Torrens and Lewis, 1980).

The *second developmental stage* of the health care delivery system dating from 1900 to 1945, was marked by the control of acute infectious diseases. Environmental conditions began to improve, with major advances in water purification, sanitary sewage disposal, milk and water quality, and urban housing quality. The health problems of the era changed from mass epidemics to individual acute infections or traumatic episodes (Hanlon and Pickett, 1979; Rushmer, 1980; Torrens, 1981; Torrens and Lewis, 1980).

The workers of the period were better educated. Physician education evolved from apprenticeships to scientifically based college education; the change occurred after the publication of the Flexner Report of 1910. Clinical medicine was in its "golden age" because of major advances in surgery and childbirth, identification of the cause of pernicious anemia and such technological discoveries as insulin in 1922 for the control of diabetes, sulfa drugs in 1932 for treatment of infectious diseases, and antibiotics such as pencillin in the 1940s (Lee, 1981; Rushmer, 1980; Torrens and Lewis, 1980).

Nurses of the era were primarily trained in hospital schools of nursing. The goal of nurse training was to educate nurses in the dependent function of following physician's orders. Hospitals and health departments were growing in numbers and strength. The public health departments' major emphasis was on quarantine and case finding. These tasks were delegated to the public health nurse. Also, 225 visiting nurse organizations were offering skilled attendance and were focusing on the teaching of cleanliness and the proper care of the sick in the home. Thus health education was identified as a nursing function early in the development of the health care delivery system (Lee, 1981; Rushmer, 1980; Torrens & Lewis, 1980).

The *third developmental stage,* from 1945 to the present, has shown a shift away from acute infectious health problems and a shift toward chronic health problems such as heart disease, cancer, and stroke. Table 3-1 provides a comparison of the leading causes of mortality from 1900 to 1980. With decreasing infant mortality and increasing life expectancy, Table 3-1 indicates that chronic illnesses resulting from environmental and lifestyle influences promise to be the major health threats of the twenty-first century.

Major technological advances of the era have included the development of chemotherapeutic agents, immunological prophylaxis, advances in anesthesia, advances in electrolyte and cardiopulmonary physiology, expansion of diagnostic laboratories and complex equipment, organ and tissue transplants, radiation therapy, specialty units for critical care, coronary care, and intensive care to name a few. The numbers and kinds of health care service facilities have increased and the numbers and kinds of health care providers constitute more than 5% of the total U.S. work force. The health care delivery system has become the largest single employer in the nation, employing 7,186,000 people in 1980. Table 3-2 shows the increase in the number of people employed in the health industry from 1970 through 1980. This table indicates that the three largest employers over the ten-year period have been hospitals, convalescent institutions, and physician's offices, respectively.

Before 1940 there were fewer than 40 titles for health care providers; in 1980 the number of identifiable titles, as reported by the U.S. Department of Labor, had risen to 665. The increase in specialization in the health care system has led to changes in certification, qualifications, education, and standards of care in each professional area. The combination of these factors has contributed to the increased number and kinds of providers to meet the demands of the health care system. As of 1980, there were 449,500 physicians and 1,400,000 nurses providing health care services within a nation boasting a population of 215,723,000. Of the practicing nurses, approximately 6.4% were employed in areas of community health nursing.

Although chronic disease is the health threat of the future, the data presented paint a picture of a system directed toward the care of acute episodic illness. Emphasis in preventive health care is slowly occurring.

FACTORS INFLUENCING THE ECONOMICS OF HEALTH CARE

Three major factors have been instrumental in influencing the growth of the health care delivery system throughout history: inflation, technology, and changes in population demography.

Inflation

Inflation has become the major economic problem of the decade. General inflation has affected the prices of all goods and services in the nation. Fig. 3-1 shows inflation, or cost of all goods and services, outdistancing the real economic growth of the nation from 1960 to 1980 (Fig. 3-1 indicates an increase of 4.9% in inflation and a decrease of 1.2% in real economic growth) while

Table 3-1. Leading causes of death in the United states, 1900 and 1980

Cause	Death rate per 100,000 population
1900	
Influenza and pneumonia	202.2
Tuberculosis	194.4
Diarrhea and enteritis	139.9
Heart disease	137.4
Cerebral hemorrhage	106.9
Nephritis	88.7
Accidents	72.3
Cancer	64.0
Diseases of early infancy	62.6
Diphtheria	40.3
Simple meningitis	33.8
Typhoid and paratyphoid	31.3
All causes	1719.1
1980	
Heart diseases	333.9
Malignant neoplasms	181.6
Cerebrovascular accidents	79.1
Accidents	49.5
Influenza and pneumonia	26.7
Diabetes mellitus	15.0
Cirrhosis of liver	13.7
Arteriosclerosis	13.4
Suicide	12.6
Causes of mortality in early infancy	12.0
Bronchitis, emphysema, asthma	10.1
Homicide	10.0
All causes	882.3

health care costs have grown approximately 12% faster than the consumer price index, resulting in a *900%* increase during this 20-year span (Aiken, 1981).

Table 3-3 depicts the changes in monies spent for health care from 1950 to 1980. Note that Table 3-3 shows a rise in health care expenditures from $12.7 billion in 1950 to $247.2 billion in 1980, while the population has increased from 151.3 million to 216 million. During this 30-year period health services and supplies accounted for 92% to 95% of the total costs while construction costs decreased from 6.7% to 2.5% of the total expenditures; research costs accounted for a mere 0.9%, increasing to 2.2% in 1980.

During these 30 years hospitals and physicians have been the two major recipients of health care expenditures, whereas government-sponsored public health programs have received only 3% of the total health care dollars.

Five major theories have been suggested to explain the rising health care costs (Davis, 1972; Davis, 1973; Davis and Foster, 1972; Feldstein, 1971; McCarthy, 1977):

1. The "demand-pull" theory attributes increasing costs to rising income and the growth of insurance, which have increased purchasing power and demand.
2. The "labor-cost push" theory suggests that expenditures rise in response to increased hospital

Table 3-2. Number of persons, in thousands, employed in the health service industry, according to place of employment, in United States from 1970 to 1980*

Place of employment	1970†	1975	1976	1977	1978	1979	1980
Total	4,246	5,865	6,122	6,328	6,673	6,849	7,186
Offices of physicians	477	607	641	677	753	755	756
Offices of dentists	222	327	325	321	360	385	407
Offices of chiropractors‡	19	30	27	31	33	36	40
Hospitals	2,690	3,394	3,568	3,645	3,781	3,843	3,947
Convalescent institutions	509	884	945	949	1,009	1,035	1,185
Offices of other health practitioners	42	60	68	75	83	84	85
Other health service sites	288	563	548	632	687	747	806

From Gibson, R.M., and Waldo, D.R.: National health expenditures, 1980, Office of Research, Demonstrations, and Statistics. In Health Care Financing Administration: Health care financing review, HCFA Pub. No. 03123, Washington, D.C., Sept. 1981, U.S. Government Printing Office.
*Data based on household interviews of a sample of civilian noninstitutionalized population. Totals exclude persons in health-related occupations who are working in nonhealth industries, as classified by the U.S. Bureau of the Census, such as pharmacists employed in drugstores, school nurses, and nurses working in private households.
†April 1, derived from decennial census; all other data years are July 1 estimates.
‡Data for 1977 to 1980 are from the American Chiropractic Association; data for the preceding years are from the U.S. Bureau of Labor Statistics.

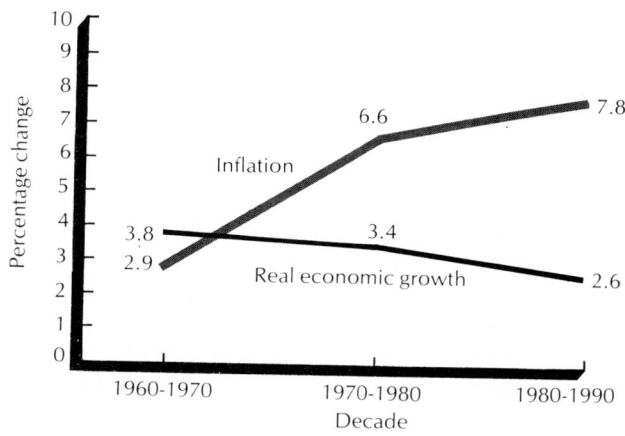

Fig. 3-1. Performance comparison of the U.S. economy over the three decades 1960 to 1990. (From U.S. Department of Commerce: Survey of current business, July 1977, Washington, D.C., July 1978; and Duffy, M.: The future economy and health related issues, Data Resources, Lexington, Mass., July 1979.)

wages and lagging productivity gains in the hospital industry.

3. The "scientific progress" theory indicates that new and costlier methods of care force prices up.
4. The "waste" theory implies that prices rise because of capital investment in costly, expensive-to-maintain facilities that already exist in sufficient supply.
5. The "cost-reimbursement" theory assumes that increases in supply, equipment, and salary expenditures have occurred with the growth and the number of insurance plans reimbursing at cost.

Although all factors mentioned in these five theories have contributed to inflation of health care costs, some have had more effect than others. The availability of insurance to cover health care costs and the development of new and costlier methods of health care technology appear to be the major contributors to increased costs. To the extent that new categories of health care personnel have been introduced into the system, increased wages have contributed to increased costs. In 1960 there were 2.3 employees per client day, whereas in 1980 there were 3.8 employees per client day. The increased numbers of health care facilities and the vast duplication of services offered have contributed to the need for increased numbers of employees and amounts of supplies and equipment and thus to increased costs.

Technology

Medical technology has been defined by the Congressional Office of Technology Assessment as "the set of techniques, drugs, equipment, and procedures used by health care professionals in delivering medical care to individuals and the system within which such care is delivered" (Health: United States, 1978). Included in any discussion of costs of technology is the cost of utilization of technology.

Health care professionals, such as physicians, have become dependent on technologies for diagnosis and treatment and have become the principle purchasing agent of the technologies for the client. The population, with an increasing sophistication about health and health care needs, demands the use of laboratory, radiological, diagnostic, palliative, and therapeutic services for treatment.

One of the most significant examples of a new tech-

Table 3-3. National health expenditures and percent distribution, according to type of expenditure, in United States for selected years from 1950 to 1980*

Type of expenditure	1950	1960	1965	1970	1975	1979	1980
				Amount in billions			
Total	$ 12.7	$ 26.9	$ 41.7	$ 74.7	$132.7	$214.6	$247.2
				Percent distribution			
All expenditures	100.0	100.0	100.0	100.0	100.0	100.0	100.0
Health services and supplies	92.4	93.6	91.6	92.8	93.7	95.2	95.3
Hospital care	30.4	33.8	33.3	37.2	39.3	39.9	40.3
Physician services	21.7	21.1	20.3	19.2	18.8	19.0	18.9
Dentist services	7.6	7.4	6.7	6.4	6.2	6.3	6.4
Nursing home care	1.5	2.0	5.0	6.3	7.6	8.3	8.4
Other professional services	3.1	3.2	2.5	2.1	2.0	2.2	2.2
Drugs and drug sundries	13.6	13.6	12.4	10.7	9.0	8.0	7.8
Eyeglasses and appliances	3.9	2.9	2.8	2.6	2.4	2.2	2.1
Expenses for prepayment	3.6	4.1	3.9	3.6	3.3	4.1	4.2
Government public health activities	2.9	1.5	2.0	1.9	2.4	3.0	3.0
Other health services	4.2	4.1	2.7	2.8	2.8	2.3	2.2
Research and construction	7.6	6.4	8.4	7.2	6.3	4.8	4.7
Research	0.9	2.5	3.6	2.6	2.5	2.2	2.2
Construction	6.7	3.9	4.8	4.6	3.8	2.5	2.5

From Gibson, R.M., and Waldo, D.R.: National health expenditures, 1980, Office of Research, Demonstrations, and Statistics. In Health Care Financing Administration: Health care financing review, HCFA Pub. No. 03123, Washington, D.C., Sept. 1981, U.S. Government Printing Office.
*Data compiled by the Health Care Financing Administration.

nology contributing to increasing cost is renal dialysis. Following the 1972 congressional amendment to the Social Security Act extending Medicare coverage to pay for renal dialysis, approximately 6,000 people received care under this program. By 1976 the program covered 21,500 clients, and by 1981 the clients covered by the program numbered 23,598.

Renal dialysis programs and other new technologies place a demand on institutions for personnel and investments in equipment and facilities, and they add to administrative costs when the federal government is involved in the financing and regulating of the technologies. The boxed material on this page provides a list of a few of the federal regulatory mechanisms that have contributed to the control and cost of technology.

In addition to federal regulations, insurance companies' reimbursement methods for health services are a contributing factor to increased technological costs. Essentially three reimbursement methods are used to pay agencies for health goods and services:

Examples of federal regulatory mechanisms contributing to technology costs

- 1906 Prescription drug regulation passes—Food, Drug, and Cosmetic Act
- 1938 Manufacturers required to prove drug safety—Food, Drug, and Cosmetic Act
- 1952 Hill-Burton Act provides construction monies and requires a specified volume of ''free care'' in exchange
- 1962 Manufacturers required to prove drug efficacy—Food, Drug, and Cosmetic Act
- 1966 Amendments to Social Security Act providing Medicare and Medicaid result in increased use of technologies
- 1972 Social Security Act amendments extending coverage for end-stage renal disease provide payment for use of treatment technologies
- 1972 Social Security Act amendments provide for Professional Standards Review Organizations to review appropriateness of hospital care for Medicare and Medicaid recipients
- 1974 Health Planning and Resources Development Act introduces certificate-of-need authority to limit major capital expenditures at local and state levels
- 1976 Medical Devices Amendments regulates safety and effectiveness of medical equipment, such as pacemakers

---

1. *Cost-plus reimbursement:* an agency is reimbursed for actual costs plus added allowable costs, such as depreciation of facilities and equipment and administrative costs.
2. *Retrospective cost reimbursement:* an agency is reimbursed per unit of service, an agreed-on price usually predetermined by the state insurance departments or departments of health.
3. *Prospective cost reimbursement:* an attempt is made by agencies and insurance companies to predict, using previous experience and current rates, what an agency's cost will be for the coming year. The agency plans an annual budget with projected goals for service units. The insurance company reimburses the agency before provision of service.

Positive and negative incentives are built into the reimbursement system. The cost-plus reimbursement scheme encourages agencies to add depreciation and administrative costs that may inflate actual service costs for the budgetary period. The retrospective cost reimbursement method encourages agencies to pad unit cost prices to cover unexpected cost increases for purchased goods and services during the budgetary period. The prospective cost reimbursement scheme encourages agencies to stay within budget limits and adds an incentive for providing less service units to contain or reduce costs. In 1983 the government has instituted prospective reimbursement for the Medicare program.

Most public agencies operate on an annual budget and plan for costs by estimating salaries, expenses, and costs of inputs for a budgetary period. Public agencies receive primary funding from tax revenues with additional reimbursement for select goods and services through private third party payers. As health care costs increase and as cost reduction becomes the key issue, prospective cost reimbursement and projected annual budgeting for the next fiscal year will likely be the trend of the future for the private sector, as it is now for public agencies.

Along with agency reimbursement, physician reimbursement is a key factor in the use and cost of technologies. The two primary methods for fee-for-service physician reimbursement are:

1. *Benefit schedule:* a list of physician services with monetary or unit values attached by third party payers which specifies the amount third parties must pay for specific services.
2. *Fee screen system:* the usual, customary, and reasonable charge (UCR) that allows physicians to set their own reimbursement levels for units of service. The UCR is based on a regional evaluation of physician charges in all specialities. The

evaluation provides for the establishing of a maximum reimbursement limit on units of service by third parties.

According to Lee (1981), the fee-for-service reimbursement schemes have been shown to be inflationary. The numbers and kinds of services provided a client are physician controlled, and as third party reimbursement increases, physicians' fees increase. The consumer has the burden to cover the costs over and above the third party coverage. Negative experience with fee-for-service physician reimbursement and the inflationary nature of the system may impede progress toward third party reimbursement for other health care providers, such as nurses.

Changes in Population Demography

The third factor viewed as a major contributor to rising health care costs is the changing population demography. Table 3-4 depicts the present distribution of the three factors affecting increased costs of health care delivery from 1965 to 1980. One can see that the level of prices (inflation) has been the major contributor, intensity (technology) has been a secondary contributor, and population has been a significant third contributor. In 1966 prices and intensity had similar effects on health care costs. In 1974 the effects of inflation began to outdistance all other factors influencing health care expenditures, and in 1980 prices contributed 75% to the growth of all health care expenditures.

Between 1970 and 1980 the number of people in the United States aged 17 and under began to decline and the number of people aged 65 and over increased. These data suggest an aging population trend with increased health risks. Projections indicate that the population of the United States will increase to 260 million people by the year 2000 and that death rates will continue to decline. The population had already reached 216 million by 1980, and the crude death rate had declined from 963.8 per 100,000 people in 1950 to 866.2 per 100,000 people in 1980. Projected age-specific population data for the year 2000 suggest there will be 58% more people in the 65-plus age group than in 1970. Table 3-5 gives population data by age group from 1950 to 1980.

Table 3-6 shows changes in per capita expenditures for personal health care by age distribution for the years 1965 to 1978. The data indicate the major increases have been in health care expenditures for the elderly population, whereas the least expenditures have been for people under 19 years of age. Since the Social Security Amendments of 1966, the rate of Medicare expenditures for health care for the elderly has been greater than the rate of increased expenditures for the remainder of the population. Reasons for the increased rate of

Table 3-4. Personal health care expenditures and distribution of factors affecting growth in United States from 1965 to 1980

Year	Personal health care expenditures in billions	Distribution of factors affecting growth (%)		
		Prices	Population	Intensity*
1965-1980	—	58	9	33
1966	$ 39.6	46	11	33
1967	44.4	54	9	43
1968	50.2	43	8	37
1969	56.9	41	8	51
1970	65.1	48	8	44
1971	72.0	58	12	30
1972	80.2	40	10	50
1973	88.7	41	10	49
1974	101.0	66	7	27
1975	116.8	70	7	23
1976	131.8	69	8	23
1977	148.7	64	8	28
1978	166.7	69	9	22
1979	189.1	71	8	21
1980	217.9	75	8	17

*From Health Care Financing Administration: Unpublished data.

Table 3-5. Population data, in millions, for selected age groups from 1950 to 1980

Age (years)	1950	1970	1980
Under 18	47.3	69.7	63.7
18-24	15.1	24.5	30.1
25-44	45.7	48.4	62.9
45-64	30.8	41.9	43.5
65 and over	12.4	20.0	25.5

From U.S. Department of Commerce: Statistical abstract of the United States, 1981, Washington, D.C., 1981, U.S. Government Printing Office.

expenditures are the rapid growth of the numbers of elderly in the United States, the increased number of elderly women who are heavier users of health services than men, the decline in family social support requiring the elderly to seek care and assistance outside the family structure, the increase in surgery rates, the greater use of more complex medical and surgical services, and the increased ability of the elderly to pay for services received.

Table 3-6. Personal health care per capita expenditures, according to age, source of payment, and type of expenditure; in United States for selected years from 1965 to 1978

Year and type of expenditure	All ages			Under 19 years			19-64 years			65 years and over		
	Per capita amount	Source of payment (%)		Per capita amount	Source of payment (%)		Per capita amount	Source of payment (%)		Per capita amount	Source of payment (%)	
		Private	Public		Private	Public		Private	Public		Private	Public
1965												
All expenditures	$188.43	78.9	21.1	$ 83.02	84.5	15.5	$215.58	80.8	19.2	$ 472.31	70.1	29.9
Hospital care	70.46	61.3	38.7	22.51	64.2	35.8	87.24	64.6	35.4	175.52	50.9	49.1
Physician services	42.85	93.1	6.9	22.27	97.7	2.3	49.21	91.6	8.4	92.50	93.1	6.9
Dentist services	14.20	98.3	1.7	10.04	97.5	2.5	17.85	99.0	1.0	11.30	94.4	5.6
Other professional services	5.22	96.4	3.6	1.76	95.5	4.5	6.41	96.4	3.6	12.99	96.7	3.3
Drugs and drug sundries	29.18	96.6	3.4	18.17	98.9	1.1	31.60	98.0	2.0	61.14	89.7	10.3
Eyeglasses and appliances	9.44	98.3	1.6	3.98	98.7	1.3	12.78	98.2	1.8	13.63	99.2	0.8
Nursing home care	10.48	65.6	34.4	—	—	—	2.42	70.0	30.0	97.19	65.0	35.0
Other health services	6.60	32.9	67.1	4.29	12.4	87.6	8.07	45.5	54.5	7.99	8.6	91.4
1970												
All expenditures	315.37	65.9	34.1	137.68	76.1	23.9	337.27	75.4	24.6	853.81	38.8	61.2
Hospital care	133.39	47.6	52.4	45.72	58.2	41.8	153.21	60.2	39.8	348.74	11.4	88.6
Physician services	68.81	78.5	21.5	36.39	89.6	10.4	75.90	89.0	11.0	149.80	38.5	61.5
Dentist services	22.80	95.3	4.7	15.80	93.5	6.5	27.88	96.2	3.8	20.42	93.5	6.5
Other professional services	7.70	86.1	13.9	2.43	78.6	21.4	9.05	92.6	7.4	19.23	73.3	26.7
Drugs and drug sundries	40.34	94.2	5.8	25.03	96.4	3.6	42.42	95.6	4.4	85.63	88.0	12.0
Eyeglasses and appliances	10.07	94.9	5.1	4.11	96.1	3.9	13.16	96.9	3.1	15.03	83.9	16.1
Nursing home care	22.44	51.2	48.8	.81	—	100.0	4.18	29.7	70.3	204.87	54.4	45.6
Other health services	9.90	28.8	71.2	7.39	10.3	89.7	11.48	39.9	60.1	10.09	8.9	91.2
1978												
All expenditures	674.46	61.0	39.0	258.77	71.5	28.5	690.76	71.2	28.8	1,821.14	36.1	63.9
Hospital care	307.13	45.6	54.4	92.84	54.6	45.4	334.95	59.2	40.8	794.72	12.0	88.0
Physician services	141.29	74.1	25.9	67.61	84.4	15.6	148.66	84.5	15.5	320.59	41.8	58.2
Dentist services	52.69	95.7	4.3	35.33	91.4	8.6	62.85	96.9	3.1	49.96	96.1	3.9
Other professional services	16.73	77.3	22.7	4.98	48.9	51.1	18.99	88.5	11.5	39.53	59.0	41.0
Drugs and drug sundries	62.45	91.3	8.7	37.19	94.2	5.8	65.02	93.0	7.0	123.69	84.2	15.8
Eyeglasses and appliances	15.62	91.4	8.6	6.22	95.2	4.8	19.57	95.4	4.6	22.50	69.9	30.1
Nursing home care	60.44	45.5	54.5	.86	3.3	96.7	19.36	20.2	79.8	456.18	51.5	48.5
Other health services	18.11	27.1	72.9	13.72	10.6	89.4	21.36	35.1	64.9	13.96	10.0	90.0

From Fisher, C.R.: Age differences in health care spending, 1978, Office of Research, Demonstrations, and Statistics. In Health Care Financing Administration: Health Care Financing Review, HCFA Pub. No. 03045, Washington, D.C., 1980, U.S. Government Printing Office.

FINANCING OF HEALTH CARE

Health care financing has evolved through the twentieth century from a system primarily financed by the consumer to a system primarily financed by third party payers. Table 3-7 shows changes in the percentage of financing for the consumer, the government, and private third party payers from 1929 to 1980. The data show that from 1950 to 1980 direct consumer payment has decreased by 33%, while third party payments have increased by the same 33%. The total federal and state governments' share of health care payments has increased by 17.2%. The federal government's contributions to health care have actually increased by 18.3% and the state's share has declined by 1.0%. Philanthropic contributions to health care have declined over the 30-year period, and the private health insurance industry has increased its contributions by approximately 17%. Throughout the 30-year period the total governments' contributions have been higher than those of private payers and the federal government's contribution has been similar to the contribution of the private payers. In 1980 third party payers contributed slightly more than twice the amount of the consumer to health care costs.

Government Payments

The federal government became involved in health care financing for population segments early in U.S. history. As mentioned in Chapter 1, in 1798 the federal government created the Marine Hospital Service to provide medical service for sick and disabled sailors and to protect the nation's borders against importation of disease through the seaports. The Marine Hospital Service is deemed the first national health insurance plan in the United States. The original plan cost each sailor 20¢ per month in a payroll deduction for illness care. The average monthly cost for private health insurance today is $50.

Evolving from the first national health insurance plan, the National Health Board was established in 1879. The board was later renamed the United States

Table 3-7. Personal health care expenditures and percent distribution, according to source of payment; in United States, selected years from 1929 to 1980*

Year	All personal health care expenditures in billions†	All sources of payment (%)	Direct payment (%)	Third party payment (%)			Government		
				Total	Private health insurance	Philanthropy and industry	Total	Federal	State and local
1929	$ 3.2	100	‡88.4	11.6	—	2.6	9.0	2.7	6.3
1935	2.7	100	‡82.4	17.6	—	2.8	14.7	3.4	11.3
1940	3.5	100	‡81.3	18.7	—	2.6	16.1	4.1	12.0
1950	10.9	100	65.5	34.5	9.1	2.9	22.4	10.4	12.0
1955	15.7	100	58.1	41.9	16.1	2.8	23.0	10.5	12.5
1960	23.7	100	54.9	45.1	21.1	2.3	21.8	9.3	12.5
1965	35.8	100	51.7	48.3	24.5	2.2	21.6	10.1	11.4
1970	65.1	100	39.9	60.1	24.0	1.6	34.5	22.3	12.2
1971	72.0	100	38.6	61.4	24.1	1.7	35.6	22.3	12.3
1972	80.2	100	38.6	61.4	23.8	1.6	36.0	23.6	12.4
1973	88.7	100	38.6	61.4	23.8	1.5	36.1	23.8	12.4
1974	101.0	100	36.1	63.9	24.2	1.5	38.2	25.5	12.7
1975	116.8	100	33.4	66.6	25.8	1.4	39.5	26.9	12.6
1976	131.8	100	32.6	67.4	26.9	1.4	39.1	27.4	11.7
1977	148.7	100	32.8	67.2	26.9	1.4	38.9	27.6	11.4
1978	166.7	100	32.5	67.5	27.0	1.3	39.1	27.8	11.3
1979	189.1	100	32.8	67.2	26.5	1.3	39.3	28.1	11.3
1980	217.9	100	32.4	67.6	26.6	1.3	39.6	28.7	11.0

From Gibson, R.M., and Waldo, D.R.: National health expenditures, 1980, Office of Research, Demonstrations, and Statistics. In Health Care Financing Administration: Health care financing review, HCFA Pub. No. 03123, Washington, D.C., Sept. 1981, U.S. Government Printing Office.
*Data compiled by the Health Care Financing Administration.
†Includes all expenditures for health services and supplies other than expenses for prepayment and administration, and government public health activities.
‡Includes any insurance benefits and expenses for prepayment (insurance premiums less insurance benefits).

Public Health Service (USPHS). Under the aegis of the USPHS, the federal government developed a public health liaison with state and local health departments for the purpose of controlling communicable diseases and improving sanitation. Additional health programs were also developed to meet obligations to federal beneficiaries, including American Indians (Indian Health Service), the armed forces (Department of Defense), and veterans of wars (Veterans Administration).

Today the federal government is involved in health care research, training, financing, and delivery and provides monies for four aspects of public health: (1) broad national health interests; (2) special groups, such as mothers, infants, and the aged; (3) special problems or programs, such as food and drugs; and (4) international health.

See Appendix H for an overview of the major historical events depicting the federal government's increasing involvement in financing health care delivery.

Third Party Payments

Federal government involvement in health care delivery began in the eighteenth century, and the system of private third party payments started in the nineteenth century. Medical insurance in the private sector was first offered in 1847 by a commercial insurance company. The purpose of the insurance was to provide protection and defray financial losses against disability attributable to accidents. Sickness benefits were later attached to the accident policies as cash payments for income losses caused by specific catastrophic communicable diseases, such as smallpox and scarlet fever.

A comprehensive study in the 1920s by the Committee on the Costs of Medical Care showed that a small portion of the population was paying most of the costs of medical care for the majority of the people. The Depression, rising medical costs, and the need to spread financial risk across communities spurred the development of the third party payment system.

The system began as a major industry in the 1930s with the start of the Blue Cross system. The system initially provided for prepayment for hospital care. The Baylor University prepayment plan to provide teachers with hospital coverage, established in 1929, was the model for the Blue Cross plan (Jonas, 1977; Klarman, 1977; Lee et al., 1981; Richardson, 1980; Williams, 1980).

In 1939 Blue Shield plans to provide physician payment were started. The Blue Cross plans began as tax-free, nonprofit organizations established under special *enabling legislation* in various states. In the 1940s and 1950s major growth in inpatient hospital and medical-surgical coverage occurred. Employee group coverage appeared and profit-making commercial insurance underwriters began offering health insurance packages with competitive premiums.

The commercial insurance companies could offer lower premium rates because of the methods used to set rates. Whereas Blue Cross used a *community rate,* establishing a similar premium rate for all subscribers regardless of illness risk, the commercial companies used an *experience rate* in which the premium paid by a subscriber was based on an estimate of the risk of claims by the subscriber.

The premium competition, the popularity of health insurance packages as a fringe benefit, and the use of health insurance as a negotiable collective bargaining item led to increased numbers of covered benefits, payment of higher portions of inpatient and outpatient expenses, and increased employer-paid premiums. These factors led to higher premium costs, higher health care costs, and plans that could not economically cover high-risk segments of the population such as the aged, poor, and disabled.

Needs of the high-risk population segments led to passage of Medicare and Medicaid legislation to provide these groups with health care coverage. Medicare, Medicaid, and other national health programs were authorized for specific population segments.

Consumer Payments

As previously indicated, direct out-of-pocket payment by the consumer has been declining for the past 30 years. Before 1930 and the beginning of Blue Cross, the consumer had more influence over health care costs because nearly all health bills were paid out-of-pocket.

However, the health care system has always represented a sellers' market. In a sellers' market all goods and services are provided and controlled by the physician once the buyer, the client, makes the decision to enter the health care market. When the health care system was economically controlled by the consumer market, it restricted entrance into the system to those who could afford to pay or to those few who could find care financed by charitable and philanthropic organizations.

After 1930 and through the 1960s, with more third party and government contributions to the health care bill, health care costs increased, quality of care efforts became greater, and consumer demand and availability of services increased. Today the consumer pays directly approximately 40% of all physician fees and 6% of all hospital bills. However, these figures do not reflect the amount of money the consumer pays in taxes to finance government-supported programs like Medicare and Medicaid, the insurance premiums that come from wages thus decreasing the size of paychecks, or the direct insurance premiums paid for supplemental insurance to plug the gaps in the primary health insurance policy.

Consumer demands have increased and strengthened benefits of private health insurance packages, the numbers of government programs available to the aged and poor, and the availability and accessibility of health care services. These consumer demands have contributed to health care inflation and are causing a financial drain on the economic potential of the individual.

NATIONAL HEALTH CARE PLANS

The *Medicare Program,* Title XVIII of the Social Security Act of 1965 provides hospital insurance, Part A, and medical insurance, Part B, to the elderly, to the permanently and totally disabled, and to people with end-stage renal disease (*Health: United States,* 1981).

The hospital insurance package, Part A, is available to the entire elderly population without cost if the individual has paid Social Security taxes. Part A of Medicare provides payment for hospital services, home health services, and extended care facilities. Part A includes an annual deductible that is based on a rate equal to a 1-day stay in the hospital. The deductible has increased over the years as daily hospital costs have increased. Estimates indicate that 98% of the elderly population are covered by Part A.

The medical insurance package, Part B, is available to all people who wish to pay a monthly premium for the coverage. The premium cost was $9.60 per month in 1981. Part B of Medicare provides coverage for other than hospital services, such as physician services, outpatient hospital care, outpatient physical therapy and speech therapy, home health care, laboratory services, ambulance transportation, prostheses, equipment, and some supplies. After a small deductible, up to 80% of reasonable charges are paid for these services. Part B resembles major medical insurance coverage of private insurance carriers. Table 3-8 shows the increasing cost of the Medicare program from 1967 to 1980.

Since the passage of the Medicare amendments to the Social Security Act in 1965, the cost of Medicare has increased dramatically. Hospital care continues to be the major factor contributing to Medicare costs and has prompted many debates about the control of the spiraling costs of the program. Many changes in the Medicare program and the reimbursement methods are being proposed for the 1980s.

The *Medicaid program,* Title XIX of the Social Security Act of 1965, provides financial assistance to states and counties to pay for medical services to the aged poor, the blind, the disabled, and families with dependent children. The Medicaid program is jointly sponsored and financed with matching funds from the federal and state governments.

Full payment for four types of service was provided originally: (1) inpatient and outpatient hospital care; (2) laboratory and radiological services; (3) physician services; and (4) skilled nursing care, at home or in a nursing home, for people over 21. The 1972 Social Security Amendments added family planning to the list of full-pay services. Prescriptions, dental services, eyeglasses, intermediate facilities care, and coverage for the *medically indigent* are allowable program options. By law the medically indigent are required to pay a monthly premium. Any state participating in the Medicaid program is required to provide the five basic services to participants who are below state poverty income levels. The optional programs are provided at the discretion of each state. Federal government takeover and reorganization of the Medicaid program may occur in the 80s. Table 3-9 indicates the increased cost of the Medicaid program from 1967 to 1980 (Health: United States, 1981; Jonas, 1977).

In contrast to Medicare, the major contributor to costs in the Medicaid program has been nursing home care, and with hospital care, it accounts for 78% of all costs to the program.

The *military medical care system* is another federal program providing health care and insurance to a population group—military personnel and their dependents. This program is described as a "well organized system of high-quality health care provided at no direct cost to the recipient" (Torrens, 1981, p. 164).

With Medicare and Medicaid, the federal government purchases goods and services for population segments through existing health care systems. With the military medical care system, the government is in the health care business providing military personnel with health care wherever they are located. This health care system has several important characteristics: (1) the system is all-inclusive and ever-present; (2) coverage is effective at all times; (3) prevention, early case finding, and health promotion are emphasized; and (4) dependents and families are served by a subsystem that combines military and civilian health services (Torrens, 1981).

The Civilian Health and Medical Program of the Uniformed Services (CHAMPUS) allows families and dependents to purchase private sector care if service is unavailable in the military system. The program is provided, financed, and supervised by the military system. In 1981 the CHAMPUS Program began direct, independent reimbursement of nurse practitioners and physician assistants for services to military dependents.

The *Veterans Administration health care system,* linked to the military health care system, is operated

Table 3-8. Medicare expenditures and percent distribution, according to type of service, in United States for selected years from 1967 to 1980*

Type of service	1967	1970	1975	1978	1979	1980†
			Amount in billions			
Total	$ 4.5	$ 7.1	$ 15.6	$ 24.9	$ 29.3	$ 35.6
			Percent distribution			
All services	100.0	100.0	100.0	100.0	100.0	100.0
Hospital care	69.0	71.8	74.8	73.9	73.1	73.9
Physician services	24.7	22.5	21.3	21.7	22.1	21.6
Nursing home care	4.6	4.2	1.9	1.2	1.4	1.1
Other services‡	1.7	1.4	1.9	3.2	3.4	3.4

From Gibson, R.M., and Waldo, D.R.: National health expenditures, 1980, Office of Research, Demonstrations, and Statistics. In Health Care Financing Administration: Health care financing review, HCFA Pub. No. 03123, Washington, D.C., Sept. 1981, U.S. Government Printing Office.
*Data compiled by the Health Care Financing Administration.
†Preliminary estimates.
‡Other services include home health agencies, home health services, eyeglasses and appliances, and other professional services.

Table 3-9. Medicaid expenditures and percent distribution, according to type of service, in United States for selected years from 1967 to 1980*

Type of service	1967	1970	1975	1978	1979	1980†
			Amount in billions			
Total	$ 2.9	$ 5.2	$ 13.5	$ 18.8	$ 21.7	$ 25.3
			Percent distribution			
All services	100.0	100.0	100.0	100.0	100.0	100.0
Hospital care	42.3	42.9	34.6	37.2	37.2	37.7
Physician services	10.9	13.3	14.0	10.6	9.8	9.1
Dentist services	4.4	3.2	2.9	2.1	1.9	2.0
Other professional services	0.9	1.4	1.5	2.1	1.9	2.0
Drugs and drug sundries	7.2	7.9	6.6	5.9	5.6	5.2
Nursing home care	31.7	27.2	36.0	38.8	40.5	40.9
Other health services‡	2.6	4.1	4.4	3.2	3.3	3.2

From Gibson, R.M., and Waldo, D.R.: National health expenditures, 1980, Office of Research, Demonstrations, and Statistics. In Health Care Financing Administration: Health care financing review, HCFA Pub. No. 03123, Washington, D.C., Sept. 1981, U.S. Government Printing Office, unpublished data.
*Data compiled from state and federal government sources. Medicaid expenditures from federal, state, and local funds under Medicaid. Includes per capita payments for Part B of Medicare and excludes administrative costs.
†Preliminary estimates.
‡Other services include laboratory and radiological services, home health, and family planning services.

within the United States for retired, disabled, and other specified categories of military service veterans. The system has a hospital orientation. The system, comprising 171 hospitals and 200 outpatient departments, is one part of a benefit package received by veterans. Eligibility for health care is often tied to other financial benefits within the system structure.

A discussion of national health care programs should include a look at the federal government's interest in providing an integrated comprehensive system for the total U.S. population. To spur the development of a comprehensive system, the *Health Maintenance Organization Act* became law in 1972. As discussed in Chapter 2, health maintenance organizations (HMOs) are prepaid systems providing comprehensive health care services to participants for a basic monthly premium. Prepaid group practice plans existing in the United States since the 1940s served as models for the HMO Act.

HMO plans usually provide more coverage to an enrollee without copayment or deductible than is typical of other health insurance schemes. Federal and state governments continue to encourage the development of HMOs by providing grants and loans for planning and operation, and some states are encouraging employers to offer HMOs as health insurance options in benefit packages. There are more than 200 HMOs existing in the United States, thereby offering a competitive system to other health insurance schemes.

• • •

Since 1847 health care coverage by governmental and private third party payers has greatly increased. At the beginning of the 80s estimates indicated that 90% of the U.S. population were covered by a health insurance plan. Approximately 98% of the elderly had Medicare hospital insurance coverage and 97% had Medicare medical insurance. Over 21 million American poor were covered by Medicaid; over 1 million veterans obtained health care through the Veterans Administration system, 10 million military personnel had access to care through the military system; and 9.5 million people were enrolled in HMOs. The population groups finding health care inaccessible were the working poor, low-income childless couples, low-income families with an unemployed father present, the medically indigent (persons who have monies to buy the necessities of life, but who cannot afford an acute illness crisis or catastrophic illness). These groups constituted 10% of the total population.

The third party pay system is often blamed for rising health care costs. To summarize, many reasons are cited for the relationship between the third party payer system and increasing costs (Lee et al., 1981).

1. The cost-plus reimbursement scheme used to pay hospital care for Medicare-Medicaid patients asks few questions about the "plus."
2. Payment for laboratory and other tests is limited to in-hospital "sick" patient charges.
3. Lack of incentive exists to hold down or reduce costs, since government or private insurers pay most medical bills.
4. The usual, customary, and reasonable charge pay system provides physicians with incentive to charge all clients maximum fees so they can boost the U.C.R. charge schedule.
5. The number of unnecessary surgeries and other tests performed increases because third parties will pay.

Health care costs have been rising faster than the costs of goods and services generally, but there is no definitive answer to the questions of cost containment or cost reduction. A number of plans for future payment of health care have been introduced.

FUTURE HEALTH CARE FINANCING PLANS

To solve the problems of rising health care costs, several suggestions have been proposed: (1) the present system should continue but call for voluntary cost containment by providers and organizations; (2) the present system should be replaced by a totally competitive market with provider and agency regulation reduced, thereby allowing providers and agencies to advertise package deals for health care and permitting the marketing of services; (3) the federal government should provide a national health care plan.

Problems are apparent in these three proposals for reducing health care costs. First, voluntary cost containment has been in effect since 1978, and health care costs continue to rise. Second, a totally competitive market may reduce health care costs, but it may also lead to poor quality of health care because health professionals and health care institutions may be deregulated; if deregulation occurs, there would not be any control over the health care provider, the quality of health provider education, or the kinds of services institutions may offer. Third, if the federal government offers a fully paid national health care plan, health care costs will probably increase because of a greater demand for service by the consumer. Cases of fraud and abuse and the economic problems in the Social Security system, including Medicare, are prime examples of what may happen with a national health care plan.

Since the suggestions for solving rising health care costs are problematical, four approaches to future financing of health care delivery have been suggested (Enthoven, 1981; Jonas, 1977; Klarman, 1977; Richardson, 1980):

1. One approach to future financing of health care is greater reliance on copayment or cost sharing with a large deductible for consumers. This approach would require the consumer to pay a larger share of the total health care bill at the time of illness. The consumer will be led to make more decisions on what and how many services to buy at what cost. Consumers presumably would shop around for the lowest price. The major problem with the approach is the consumer's ability to judge quality of service and the consumer's implicit need to rely on the provider to act in the best interests of the patient.
2. The approach advocated by the American Medical Association (AMA) and Health Insurance As-

sociation of America (HIAA) would provide a broadened benefit package financed through Social Security taxes for the elderly, employer-employee financing for employees and families, and general taxation for all other people.

3. The American Hospital Association (AHA) proposes abolishing Medicare and providing financing for employed workers and families through employee-employer contributions and providing for all others through general taxation.

4. The Committee for National Health Insurance proposes one plan to cover all persons to be financed through a combination of general taxation and employee and employer Social Security contributions.

The advocates of copayment plans argue that the full coverage plan of financing will result in overutilization and increasing costs of health care delivery. The multiple plans recommended by the AHA, AMA, and HIAA are viewed as requiring increasing tax subsidies because the aged and poor, covered by tax subsidies, tend to be sicker than employed workers. All arguments suggest that copayment plans will reduce service demand and thus health care costs.

Four major cost study methods are used to determine efficacy of the health care delivery system today and will be discussed next.

COST STUDIES APPLIED TO HEALTH CARE DELIVERY

Excessive and inefficient use of goods and services in health care delivery is viewed by many as the major cause of rising costs in health care delivery. For this reason Congress established in 1978 the Center for National Health Care Technology and mandated the center to define the safety, efficacy, efficiency, and cost effectiveness of medical procedures. A recent study released by the center presents a strong argument for the cost effectiveness of nurse practitioners (LeRoy and Solkowitz, 1981).

Many studies appear in the literature about the cost effectiveness of nurse practitioners and cost benefit, efficiency, efficacy, and effectiveness of medical procedures and programs; however, minimal data are available about the cost benefit, efficiency, and effectiveness of nurses generally.

A recent statement issued by the American Nurses' Association indicates that nurses should receive third party reimbursement and that nursing care should become a separate budget item in all organizations so that cost studies can show the efficiency and effectiveness of the nursing profession. Presently hospitals include nursing care costs in daily patient hotel costs (room charges), whereas other agencies, such as home health care agencies, include administrative costs, supplies, and equipment costs with nursing care costs. Little effort is made to show actual costs of nursing care in most places where nurses are employed.

At present a movement exists in the United States to provide third party reimbursement for nurses. Medicare and Medicaid provide *indirect nurse reimbursement* to agencies offering home health care services. The Rural Health Clinic Services Act of 1977 provides for indirect reimbursement for the services of nurse practitioners in rural health clinics; and a 1980 Medicaid amendment to the Social Security Act provides for direct reimbursement of nurse-midwives. In 1978 Maryland was the first state to provide *direct reimbursement* for nurse practitioners and nurse-midwives; Maryland extended the legislation in 1979 to provide direct reimbursement for "any duly licensed health care providers" for services within their lawful scope of practice. Presently there are six states providing direct reimbursement for nurse practitioner or nurse-midwifery services and many others are pursuing reimbursement legislation. Such a trend will provide impetus for separating general nursing care costs from other program costs. Such a trend will give an adequate environment for performing cost studies in nursing.

The four major types of cost studies primarily applied in the health care industry are cost accounting, cost benefit, cost efficiency and cost effectiveness.

Cost Accounting

Cost accounting studies are performed to find the actual budgetary cost of a program, procedure or technique. A question answered by this method could be, What is the cost of providing a family planning program in Anytown, U.S.A.? To answer the question, the total costs of equipment, facilities (rental), personnel (salaries and benefits), and supplies are figured. The total program costs are divided by the number of clients participating in the clinic for a set time period; the total program cost per client is the end product. Thus a cost accounting study can provide data about total program costs and about total cost per client.

Cost Benefit

Cost benefit studies are a way of assessing the desirability of a program, procedure, or technique by placing a specific quantifiable value, a dollar amount, on all costs and all benefits of the variable to be evaluated. If benefits outweigh the costs, then the program is said to have a net positive impact. The major problem with cost benefit analysis is placing a quantifiable value on all benefits of a program. The question is, Can a dollar value be placed on human life, on safety, on the relief of pain and suffering, or on prevention of illness? If an attempt is made to perform cost benefit analysis of a hospice program, can a quantifiable value by placed on the family and client support and comfort provided or on the relief of pain of the terminally ill? Can such benefits be weighted against costs to justify program existence (LoGerfo and Brook, 1980; Prest and Turvey, 1965; Schwartz and Joskow, 1978)?

Theoretically, it is recognized that public health programs have net positive impacts, or high cost benefit ratios, because in preventing future causes of morbidity with illness prevention programs, such as hypertensive screening, the future cost of chronic long-term illness from stroke or cardiovascular disease is averted or reduced. Yet the cost benefit of investments in such programs can only be shown with multiple longitudinal studies and time. To initiate a cost benefit study for a program, it must be decided which costs and which benefits are to be included, how the costs and benefits are to be valued, and what constraints are to be considered—legal, ethical, social, and economic. For instance, if the length of a client's life or the disease incidence after program participation are considered benefits, will client morbidity or mortality during or after the program be considered negative impacts on the program and will placing values on these benefits favor higher socioeconomic groups over lower ones, men over women, those of working age over those younger and older (Lo Gerfo and Brook, 1980)?

Cost Efficiency

Cost efficiency analysis for purposes of this discussion is the analysis of actual costs to perform a number of services at different volumes if the same standards are applied. Volume implies numbers of clients. To determine cost efficiency of a program or procedure, productivity must be analyzed. Productivity is the relationship between the output and the input of a process. The concept of nurse productivity encompasses the effectiveness, the quality, and the efficiency of nursing care (nursing output with minimal resource waste, for example the number of clients served at the least cost).

To determine the nursing inputs for a given output (clients served) in a cost efficiency analysis, one is primarily concerned with a nurse's workload, including direct client care, administrative functions, coordinating functions, and educational activities. The functions are then related to the client load, client need, nursing organizational structure, and staff mix.

Fig. 3-2 shows an example of the cost efficiency of a home health agency. The graph indicates that as the number of client visits per year increases, the cost per client visit decreases. The graph assumes that there are the same number of nurses from the beginning to the

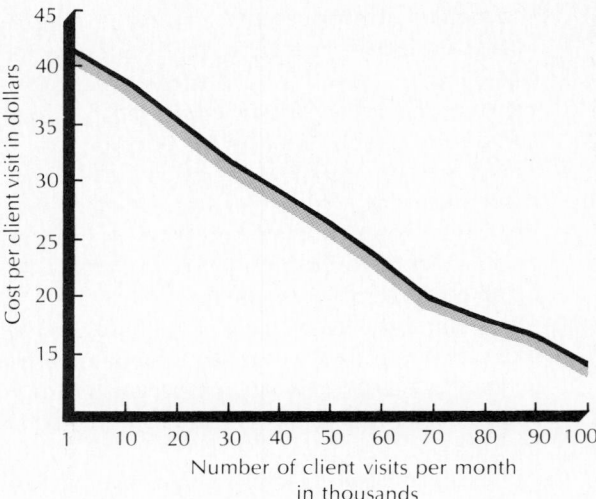

Fig. 3-2. Average cost per client visit at home health agency.

end of the time period, that the nurses' workloads were essential to provide home health services, that caseloads were predicated on staff mix and client need, and that organizational structure was conducive to maximize nursing input to produce identified output.

Cost Effectiveness

Cost effectiveness analysis, a measure of the quality of a program procedure or technique as it relates to cost, is the most frequently used analysis in nursing. Cost effectiveness is a subset of cost benefit analysis and is designed to provide an estimate of costs incurred in achieving a given outcome. A cost effectiveness study can answer two questions: what are the outcomes of a single program relative to its costs, and what are the costs and effectiveness of two programs directed toward the same outcome (Enthoven, 1981; LoGerfo and Brook, 1980; Prescott, 1979)? In cost benefit analysis both costs and outcomes are quantitative, whereas in cost effectiveness analysis the outcomes are qualitative. Outcome measures addressed by cost effectiveness studies might be increased client knowledge after health teaching; changes in client's condition after treatment; differences in graduates of two programs with similar goals, and the ability of two hearing screening programs to detect hearing loss.

The boxed material on the next page shows the procedure for completing a cost effectiveness study. A cost effectiveness study requires collection of baseline data on clients before implementing the study and the testing or evaluation at a predetermined time after the study is completed.

There are several potential outcomes of a cost effectiveness study. For example, a community health nurse

---

Steps in cost effectiveness analysis

Step I	Identify the treatment goals or client outcome to be achieved.
Step II	Identify at least two alternative means of achieving the desired outcomes.
Step III	Determine client's pretreatment level on desired outcomes.
Step IV	Determine the costs associated with each treatment.
Step V	Determine amount of treatment given to each group of clients.
Step VI	Determine the posttreatment level on desired outcome variables.
Step VII	Combine the costs (Step IV), amount of treatment (Step V), and outcome information (Step VI) to express costs relative to outcomes of treatment.
Step VIII	Compare cost outcome information for each treatment type to present cost effectiveness analysis.

From Prescott, P.: Nurs. Outlook. **29**(11):722-728, Nov. 1979. Copyright, American Journal of Nursing Co.

---

is interested in comparing two methods for teaching diabetic clients self-care techniques. The nurse chooses self-teaching modules and a group formal instruction program for comparison. There are nine potential outcomes the nurse may find in comparing the two teaching methods. One teaching method may be: (1) less costly and less effective than the other; (2) less costly and equally as effective; (3) less costly and more effective; (4) equal in cost but less effective; (5) equal in cost and equally effective; (6) equal in cost and more effective; (7) more costly and less effective; (8) more costly and equally effective; and (9) more costly and more effective than the other. Of the nine potential outcomes in a cost effectiveness study, the program of choice would be the most effective teaching method for the least cost (outcome three), unless the most costly program demonstrates superior effectiveness (outcome nine) or the least costly program demonstrates less quality (outcome one).

All of the cost studies have three major tasks: financial, research, and statistical. The financial tasks involve identifying total program costs and breaking them down into smaller parts. To identify the costs of a nurse's participation in a teaching program, the costs for facilities, equipment, supplies, and salaries would have to be examined. All costs associated with the teaching program, such as nurse's time and use of facilities, equipment, and supplies, should be compared to the total program costs. The statistical tasks involve the identification of appropriate quantifiable measures for analyzing data, and the research tasks involve setting up an appropriate study design to answer the questions of benefit, efficiency, or effectiveness.

Nurses of all educational preparation may be involved in cost studies with the assistance of people knowledgeable in research statistics and accounting techniques. Nurses with undergraduate preparation may be involved in the actual implementation of a cost study, whereas nurses with graduate preparation may be involved in planning, designing, implementing, analyzing, and evaluating study results.

Although cost studies are essential to show the worth of nursing in the marketplace of the future, nurses must be ready to provide input so that sound decisions may be made from the study results. Nurses must be ready to identify appropriate program outcomes, client outcomes, total dimensions of roles of graduates, and total dimensions of nursing procedures so that appropriate decisions about nursing services delivery will be made using adequate information.

PREVENTION

An area in the health care delivery system that needs to show cost effectiveness is the area of primary prevention. *Primary prevention,* distinguished from secondary and tertiary prevention, consists of activities that prevent a disease from occurring. Primary prevention has three major aspects: personal health services, such as immunization against infectious diseases; environmental services, such as adequate water and sewage treatment to prevent parasitic diseases or water fluoridation to prevent dental caries; and health behavior practices, such as nonsmoking programs to prevent lung cancer, use of seat belts to prevent accident fatalities, and good nutrition to prevent obesity and ensuing complications. *Secondary prevention* consists of activities designed to detect disease before need for treatment (early casefinding). Secondary prevention consists primarily of screening for disease before complaint of symptoms, such as hypertensive screening, hearing and vision testing, glaucoma screening, and Pap tests and breast examinations for cancer. *Tertiary prevention* is the activity engaged in by most health providers, that is, the treatment, care, and rehabilitation of people with acute and chronic illnesses (*Health: United States,* 1978; Kristein et al., 1978).

Although estimates indicate that 98% of the health care dollars are spent on secondary and tertiary prevention, the major causes of morbidity and mortality in our adult population have shown little net decline. Several assumptions can be made about the causes of the slight decline in morbidity and mortality in the past decade: The slight decline in heart disease mortality rates, about 2% per year, may be caused by changes in smoking habits, diet, and increased awareness of health risks. Slight declines in stomach cancer may be related to nutritional factors. Injuries from auto accidents, reduced by 20% since 1973, may be due to seat belts, lower speed limits, and higher gasoline prices. Decreases in infant and maternal mortality rates may result from declining birth weights, prenatal care, and family planning. All of the reasons cited for declining problems are primary preventive measures.

Given that primary preventive measures could reduce the risk of early death, disease, disability, and discomfort from disease, why then do the federal and private third party payers not provide coverage for such measures? The answer is in the following discussion. In addition to the benefit of improved health status of the population, a focus on prevention could mean a reduction in the need for and use of medical, dental, hospital, and health provider services. This would mean for the largest industry in the United States that the market would be reduced in size and become more controlled by the consumer of goods and services than by the seller of these services. Medicare, Medicaid, and private insurance carriers encourage a sickness-oriented system. Although there are existing data to indicate that primary preventive care is cost effective, most of our dollars continue to be spent for secondary and tertiary prevention (Breslow, 1978; Kristein, 1977; Kristein et al., 1978; Mortimer, 1978; Rabkin and Struening, 1978).

Hanlon and Pickett (1979) have postulated that a potential savings of lives and money could be made by using all existing knowledge pertaining to the causes of death. Table 3-10 shows the projected percentage of reduction in death rates for major causes and the suggested actions to reduce mortality.

In 1979 the Surgeon General of the United States published a report entitled *Healthy People.* The report called for a renewed preventive health care commitment through the identification of priorities and specific goals. The central theme of the report was that the health of the nation could be significantly improved through actions taken by individuals and by policy makers to promote a safer, healthier environment for all at home, at work, and at play.

The report suggested that most people could improve their personal health by observing the following practices:

- Elimination of cigarette smoking
- Reduction of alcohol abuse
- Moderate dietary changes to reduce intake of excess calories, fat, salt, and sugar

- Moderate exercise
- Periodic screening for major causes of morbidity and mortality, such as blood pressure and cancer
- Adherence to speed laws and use of seat belts

The report also emphasized the link between physical and mental health and the need to maintain strong family ties, assistance of supportive friends, and use of community support systems.

For the policy makers, the report suggested a need to recognize the relationship between health and the physical environment which could lead to the reduction of morbidity and mortality caused by air, water, and food contamination, accidents, radiation exposure, excessive noise, occupational hazard, dangerous consumer products, and unsafe highway design.

Subsequently the Secretary of DHHS in 1980 presented a report, *Promoting Health/Preventing Disease—Objectives for the Nation,* outlining the national health status and objectives to be attained by the health care system by 1990. The following target areas were identified in the report: control of high blood pressure; pregnancy and infant health; immunization; sexually transmitted diseases; toxic agents; occupational health; flouridation and dental health; surveillance of infectious disease; smoking; misuse of alcohol and drugs; nutrition; physical fitness and exercise; and stress. The objectives of the report are aimed at reducing death rates and related measures of poor health, reducing measurable risks, increasing public and professional awareness of risk and reduction possibilities, and improving services (*Health: United States,* 1980).

Reducing the burden of avoidable illness and disability will reduce the human and economic costs imposed on the U.S. population. To accomplish the goals of prevention, changes will have to occur in environmental protection, life-styles, and orientation of health providers and institutions toward health promotion. Support will have to be gained from employers, schools, product designers and manufacturers, food distributors, and the insurance industry for preventing injury and promoting healthier life-styles.

THE VALUE OF HUMAN LIFE

The concept of human capital has evolved in economics as a way of measuring the value society places on the worth of the individual. The value is quantified and expressed in dollar amounts, and it constitutes a real limit on how much money either people or society will pay for personal health care (Spratt, 1975).

The human body has often been compared to a machine, with proper functioning dependent on its various physical and biochemical components. To maintain proper functioning and productivity, the machine must be nurtured, protected, housed, educated, and

Table 3-10. Postulated percentage reductions in deaths, by cause, if all available knowledge were used*

Cause of death	Reduction (%)	Suggested action
Typhoid and paratyphoid	100	Environmental measures Immunization Epidemiologic control
Meningococcal infections	100	Control of epidemics Adequate and early chemotherapy Antibiotics
Streptococcal infections	100	Chemotherapy Antibiotics Antitoxin
Pertussis	100	Early and thorough immunization Hyperimmune serum, chemotherapy, and antibiotics for secondary infections
Diphtheria	100	Early immunization and adequate antitoxin
Tuberculosis — all forms	100	Intensive early case finding Hospitalization and treatment Adequate diet and housing
Dysenteries	100	Environmental control Chemotherapy
Malaria	100	Environmental control Chemotherpy
Syphilis	100	Intensive early case finding Treatment Epidemiologic control
Measles	100	Imunization Chemotherapy Antibiotics
Poliomyelitis	100	Immunization
Neoplasms	50	Early cancer detection and treatment centers Best possible physician and surgeon Chemotherapy Radiation therapy Surgery Circumcision Elimination of smoking
Rheumatic fever	95	Best possible physician Prophylactic antibiotics
Diabetes mellitus	60	Best possible physician Intensive early case finding Diet Insulin Applied genetics
Diseases of thyroid gland	100	Best possible physician Newer drugs Surgery Iodization of all salt
Nutritional diseases	100	Adequate diet Diagnosis and treatment

From Hanlon, J.J., and Pickett, G.E.: *Public health: administration and practice*, ed. 8, St. Louis, 1983, The C.V. Mosby Co.
* Where chemotherapy and/or antibiotics have been listed as the explanations for the reductions in deaths, objection on the basis of the development of drug-resistant organisms will no doubt be raised. Gains possible today might be much less in a few years. It is believed that research will be able to remain one or two drugs, at least, ahead of the organisms.

With the one exception (all other causes), no variation of effectiveness of therapy and other control measures with age of the individual has been postulated. Since any scheme of correction would probably have been as liable to criticism as no correction, the latter course was followed.

Continued.

Table 3-10. Postulated percentage reductions in deaths, by cause, if all available knowledge were used — cont'd

Cause of death	Reduction (%)	Suggested action
Alcoholism and addictions	25	Psychiatry Nutritional therapy Sociology Education
Intracranial vascular lesions	10	Best possible physician Antihypertensive drugs and diet Anticoagulants Avoidance of infections Antibiotics
Diseases of the heart	10	Best possible physician Surgery
Pneumonia, broncho-	75	Chemotherapy Antibiotics
Pneumonia, lobar	90	Chemotherapy Antibiotics
Pneumonia, unspecified	75	Chemotherapy Antibiotics
Influenza	85	Immunization Chemotherapy and antibiotics for complications
Peptic ulcer — stomach and duodenum	50	Psychiatry Best possible physician
Diarrhea, enteritis, etc.	95	Environmental controls Chemotherapy Antibiotics
Appendicitis	100	Surgery Chemotherapy Antibiotics
Hernia, intenstinal obstruction	95	Best possible physician and surgeon
Cirrhosis of the liver	25	Newer nutritional knowledge
Biliary calculi	25	Best possible physician and surgeon
Nephritis and nephrosis	25	Chemotherapy Antibiotics Best possible physician
Diseases of the prostate	50	Best possible physician and surgeon
Complications of pregnancy	87	Complete elimination of deaths from toxemia and sepsis, and reduction of deaths from hemorrhage by 50%
Congenital malformations	10	Diet during pregnancy Avoidance of viral infections during pregnancy Surgery
Premature births	70	Adequate prenatal care and diet
Suicide	50	Psychiatry Sociology
Homicide	50	Psychiatry Sociology, including gun control
Accidents — motor vehicle	50	Education Psychiatry Engineering Traffic planning and control Safety measures
Accidents — other	50	Education Psychiatry Safety measures Engineering
All other causes	50	Better medical care (except for under 1 year, where deaths from congenital debility, birth injury, and others peculiar to the first year of life could be reduced by 75%), genetic counseling, family planning, adequate prenatal care and diet, and adequate care during first year of life

Table 3-11. Estimated costs of illness, according to type of cost and major disease category, in United States, 1975*

Disease category	All costs		Direct costs	Indirect costs		
	Amount in billions	Percent distribution		Total	Morbidity	Mortality
				Amount in billions		
Total	$238.9	—	$118.5	$120.4	$57.8	$62.5
				Percent distribution		
All diseases	—	100.0	100.0	100.0	100.0	100.0
Diseases of the circulatory system	45.7	19.1	13.5	24.7	15.1	33.5
Stroke	6.1	2.5	2.2	2.9	0.6	5.0
Heart and other	39.6	16.6	11.3	21.8	14.5	28.5
All neoplasms	18.9	7.9	4.4	11.3	1.9	20.1
Accidents, poisonings, and violence	27.5	11.5	5.8	17.1	9.8	23.9
Diseases of the respiratory system	18.7	7.8	6.4	9.2	14.8	4.2
All other	128.1	53.6	69.9	37.7	43.3	18.3

From Paringer, L., Berk, A., and Mushkin, S.: Economics of cost and illness, fiscal year 1975, Report BIA, Georgetown University, Washington, D.C., 1977, Public Services Laboratory.
*Discounted at 10 percent. All costs in 1975 dollars.

trained. These goals can only be accomplished by investing time and money in the potential capital (Hanlon and Pickett, 1979; Spratt, 1975).

Since the dollar value of individual productivity is also a function of time, the potential capital worth of an individual is a function of longevity and functional capacity during a lifetime. The values the market places on different levels and types of education and work capability are basic determinants of the capital value of a human being. It has been shown that an individual's current market value increases to age 25 and steadily declines thereafter and that the value of the male in society is greater than the value of the female (Cooper and Broady, 1975).

A major goal of the health care delivery system today is to preserve and maximize human capital by offering health-preserving and social practices that result in avoidance of disease, that is, primary prevention, and by offering diagnosis, treatment, and rehabilitative services for existing diseases, that is, secondary and tertiary prevention. The past goal of the health care delivery system has been to emphasize the "sickness system." DHHS health goals suggest a higher value should be placed on primary prevention. Table 3-11 shows the direct dollar costs and the indirect human capital costs in 1975 from diseases which might have been preventable.

The outcome of health care goals should be the provision of a quality of life which will promote happiness, productivity, efficiency, and the capacity to engage in and enjoy life activities. Quantifying life is meaningless to the person unless the quality of life can be maximized and unless functional days become more valuable than dollars spent. An emphasis on primary prevention may hold the key to reducing dollars spent while increasing the quality of life.

FACTORS AFFECTING HEALTH LEVELS

The goal of health economics is quality care leading to health and wellness of the population. Four major factors are known to affect health levels: personal behavior, environmental factors, human biology, and the health care system.

Society's investment in the *health care system* has been based on this premise: more health services equal better health. The increasing investment society has made in health care delivery is shown in Table 3-12. Although the investment has been a major one, medical services are said to have the least effect on health (McKeown, 1981; McKinlay and McKinlay, 1977).

As first documented in England and Wales in the nineteenth century, health has improved throughout history resulting in an increased life expectancy for infants and children. The reductions in deaths from the early nineteenth century causes of death—infectious diseases—were attributed to improved nutrition from increased food supplies. Major advances in hygiene and safe food and water contributed to continuing declining death rates after the 1850s. The World Health

Table 3-12. Gross national product and national health expenditures in United States for selected years from 1929 to 1980*

Year	Gross national product in billions	National health expenditures		
		Amount in billions	Percent of gross national product	Amount per capita
1929	$ 103.4	$ 3.6	3.5	$ 29.49
1935	72.2	2.9	4.0	22.65
1940	100.0	4.0	4.0	29.62
1950	286.5	12.7	4.4	81.86
1955	400.0	17.7	4.4	105.38
1960	506.5	26.9	5.3	146.30
1965	691.0	41.7	6.0	210.89
1970	992.7	74.7	7.5	357.90
1971	1,077.6	83.3	7.7	394.23
1972	1,185.9	93.5	7.9	437.77
1973	1,326.4	103.2	7.8	478.34
1974	1,434.2	116.4	8.1	534.63
1975	1,549.2	132.7	8.6	603.57
1976	1,718.0	149.7	8.7	674.14
1977	1,918.0	169.2	8.8	754.81
1978	2,156.1	189.3	8.8	835.57
1979	2,413.9	214.6	8.9	936.92
1980	2,628.8	247.2	9.4	1,067.06

From Gibson, R.M., and Waldo, D.R.: National health expenditures, 1980, Office of Research, Demonstrations, and Statistics. In Health Care Financing Administration: Health care financing review, HCFA Pub. No. 03123, Washington, D.C., Sept. 1981, U.S. Government Printing Office.
*Data compiled by the Health Care Financing Administration.

Organization contends that experience in Third World countries today supports the premise that adequate diet reduces risk of infection, thereby leading to decreased morbidity.

Health problems of the twentieth century are being attributed primarily to *personal behavior* and *environmental* factors. These problems may be preventable by controlling personal behavior and environmental factors. Although these two factors are coming to the forefront as major influences on health, answers to the question of genetic, or human biological, influence on health are still being explored. For instance, risk factors for heart disease and stroke are being related to life-style influences such as smoking, diet, and exercise and to genetic influences such as family history of heart disease, stroke, and hypertension. The federal health goals of the 1980s focus on control of *behavioral influences* thought to be the major determinants of health, such as alcohol and drug abuse, smoking, nutrition, exercise, and stress, and *environmental influences* thought to be the major determinants of illness, such as pollution of air, water, noise, and foods. The goals also address control of and risk reduction from human *biological influences* and the improvement of *health care services.* Parts Three and Four of the text will focus on the personal, environmental, and biological influences affecting the nation's health.

SUMMARY

Economics is concerned with the most efficient use of resources to fulfill society's unlimited wants. Economics operates under the law of supply and demand; since our society is primarily composed of competitive organizations, when demand goes up, supply goes down and cost goes up, or vice versa.

Health economics is concerned with the distribution of health care resources to provide maximum benefit to the most people. Since the health care delivery system is largely monopolistic, the laws of supply and demand do not hold true. As demand goes up for health care services, the supply of services also increases and costs go up. As long as the health care system remains in the control of the health provider, the usual economic principles will not hold true.

As the cost of health care services increases, the consumer has less money to spend for other needs and wants. Economic indicators show that the health care costs continue to increase per year and have risen to a cost of $286 billion, or over $1000 per person per year.

The major factors influencing the costs of health care delivery are inflation, technology, and population changes. The availability of insurance and government monies to cover health care costs, the method of reimbursement, and the development of new and costlier methods of health care technology appear to be the major contributors to rising health care costs. The rising numbers of elderly in the population, the increasing proportion of women, and the decline in family support systems are viewed as the major population changes contributing to increased demand for services and increased costs of services.

Several health care financing schemes have been suggested for the future: greater reliance on copayment with a large deductible for consumers; a broadened benefit package financed through Social Security taxes for the elderly, employer-employee financing for employed families, and general taxation for all others; and a package financed only through employer-employee contributions and general taxations.

One of the major problems in health care delivery is determining the efficacy of health care services and health care providers. To say whether health care costs are unreasonable, one must be able to compare the costs of those services to client benefit and to the efficiency and effectiveness of services delivered. Four methods are employed for performing cost studies in the health care system: cost accounting, cost benefit, cost efficiency, and cost effectiveness. Nursing has given minimal time to demonstrating its worth in health care delivery. Since nursing has not shown its contribution to the client in health care, the discipline has had difficulty proving that nursing services should be reimbursable and autonomous, whereas other disciplines, such as physical therapists, occupational therapists, and psychiatric social workers, have moved ahead in establishing themselves in both areas.

Another identifiable problem in health care delivery is establishing the value of primary preventive care. Today 98% of health care dollars are spent on illness care. Although history and recent studies indicate that changes in nutrition, the environment, and life-styles would provide a healthier future society, the cost studies are not readily available to show the savings society could have with a preventive emphasis in its health care delivery system. The large amount of dollars society annually spends on health care indicates that society values human life. However, the focus of this society's future investment should be to provide more than longevity. The goal of health economics should be to provide a quality of life that offers happiness, productivity, and the capacity to engage in life activities, through the provision of reasonably priced quality services focused on illness prevention and health promotion.

BIBLIOGRAPHY

Aiken, L.H.: The practice setting: an overview of health policy issues. In Aiken, L.H., editor: Health policy and nursing practice, New York, 1981, McGraw-Hill Book Co.

Breslow, L.: Abelson, editor: Health care:regulation, economics, ethics and practice. Washington, D.C., 1978, American Association for the Advancement of Science.

Cooper, B., and Broady, W.: Lifetime earnings by age, sex, and educational level,(Social Security Administration, Research and Statistics note, Sept. 30, 1975, Washington, D.C., 1975, U.S. Government Printing Office.

Davis, K.: Community hospital expenses and revenues:pre-medicare inflation, Social Security Bull. 35(10):3-19, Washington, D.C., Oct. 1972., U.S. Government Printing Office.

Davis, K.: Hospital costs and the medicare program, Social Security Bull. 36(7):18-36, Washington, D.C., Aug. 1973, U.S. Government Printing Office.

Davis, K., and Foster, R.: Community hospitals:inflation in the pre-medicare period, Social Security Administration Research Report No. 41, Washington, D.C., 1972, U.S. Government Printing Office.

Enthoven, A.: Health plan:the only practical solution to the soaring cost of medical care, Reading, Mass., 1981, Addison-Wesley Publishing Co. Inc.

Feldstein, M.S.: The rising costs of hospital care, Washington, D.C., 1971, Information Resources Press.

Hanlon J., and Pickett, G.: Public health administration and practice, St. Louis, 1979, The C.V. Mosby Co.

Health: United States, 1978, DHEW Pub. No. (PHS) 78-1232, Washington, D.C., Dec. 1979, Department of Health, Education, and Welfare.

Health: United States, 1980, DHHS Pub. No. (PHS) 81-1232, Washington, D.C., Dec. 1980, Department of Health and Human Services.

Health: United States, 1981, DHHS Pub. No. (PHS) 82-1232, Washington, D.C., Dec. 1981, Department of Health and Human Services.

Healthy People: the Surgeon General's report on health promotion and disease prevention, DHEW Pub. No. (PHS) 79-55071, Washington, D.C., 1979, Department of Health, Education, and Welfare.

Heider-Dorneich, P.: Social control in health economics, Rev. Soc. Economy. 36(1):1-18, April 1978.

Hill, D.: Economic constraints in the health care delivery system. In Lancaster, J., and Lancaster, W., editors: Concepts for advanced nursing practice: the nurse as change agent, St. Louis, 1982, The C.V. Mosby, Co.

Jonas, S.: Health care delivery in the United States, New York, 1977, Springer Publishing Co. Inc.

Klarman, H.E.: The financing of health care. In Knowles, J., editor: Doing better and feeling worse:health in the United States. New York, 1977, W.W. Norton & Co. Inc.

Kristein, M.M.: Economic issues in prevention, Prev. Med. 6(2):252-H264, June 1977.

Kristein, M., Arnold C.B., and Wynder, E.L.: Health economics and preventive care. In Abelson, P., editor: Health care:regulation, economics, ethics, and practice. Washington, D.C., 1978, American Association for the Advancement of Science.

Lee, P.R.: Technology and the cost of medical care. In Lee, P., Brown, N., and I., Red, editors: The nation's health, San Francisco, 1981, Boyd & Fraser Publishing Co.

Lee, P., Brown, N., and Red, I.: Health costs:what limit? The nation's health, San Francisco, 1981, Boyd & Fraser Publishing Co.

LeRoy, L., and Solkowitz, S.: The implications of cost-effectiveness analysis of medical technology, Congress of the U.S., Office of Technology Assessment, case study no. 16, Washington, D.C., 1981, U.S. Government Printing Office.

LoGerfo, J., and Brook, R.: Evaluation of health services and quality of care. In Williams, S., and P., Torrens, editors: Introduction to health services, New York, 1980, John Wiley & Sons Inc.

McCarthy, C.: Financing for health care. In Jonas, S., editor: Health care delivery in the United States, New York, 1977, Springer Publishing Co. Inc.

McKeown, T.: Determinants of health. In Lee, P., Brown, N., and I., Red, editors: The nation's health, San Francisco, 1981, Boyd & Fraser Publishing Co.

McKinlay, J.B., and McKinlay S.M.: The questionable contribution of medical measures to the decline of mortality in the United States in the twentieth century, Milbank Mem. Fund Q. **55**(3):405–H428, 1977.

Mortimer, E.A., Jr.: Immunization against infectious disease. In Abelson, P., editor: Health care:regulation, economics, ethics, and practice, Washington, D.C., 1978, American Association for the Advancement of Science.

Prescott, P.A.: Cost-effectiveness:tool or trap? Nurs. Outlook, **27**(11):722–H728, Nov. 1979.

Prest, A., and Turvey, R.: Cost-benefit analysis:a survey, The Economic J. **75**(300):683-735, Dec. 1965.

Rabkin, J., and Struening, E.: Life events, stress, and illness. In P., Abelson, editor: Health care:regulation, economics, ethics, and practice, Washington, D.C., 1978, American Association for the Advancement of Science.

Richardson, W.: Financing health services. In Williams, S., and Torrens, P., editors: Introduction to health services, New York, 1980, John Wiley & Sons Inc.

Rushmer, R.: Technological resources for health. In Williams, S., and Torrens, P., editors: Introduction to health services, New York, 1980, John Wiley & Sons Inc.

Schwartz, W.B., and Joskow, P.L.: Sounding Board—Medical efficacy versus economic efficacy:a conflict of values, N. Eng. J. Med. **299**(26):1462–1464, Dec. 1978.

Spratt, J.J.: The relation of human capital preservation to health costs, Am. J. Economics Sociol. **34**(3):295-307, July 1975.

Torrens, P.: Overview of health services in the United States. In Lee, P., Brown, N., and Red, I., editors: The nation's health, San Francisco, 1981, Boyd & Fraser Publishing Co Inc.

Torrens, P., and Lewis, C.: Health care personnel. In Williams, S., and Torrens, P. editors: Introduction to health services, 1980, New York, John Wiley & Sons.

Williams, S.: Ambulatory and community health services. In Williams, S., and Torrens, P., editors: Introduction to health services, 1980, New York, John Wiley & Sons Inc.

Your Medicare handbook: Social Security Administration Pub. No. 05-10050, Washington, D.C., July 1980, Department of Health and Human Services.

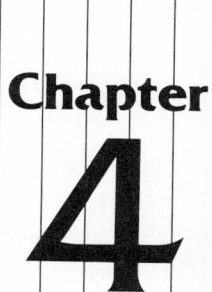

Chapter 4

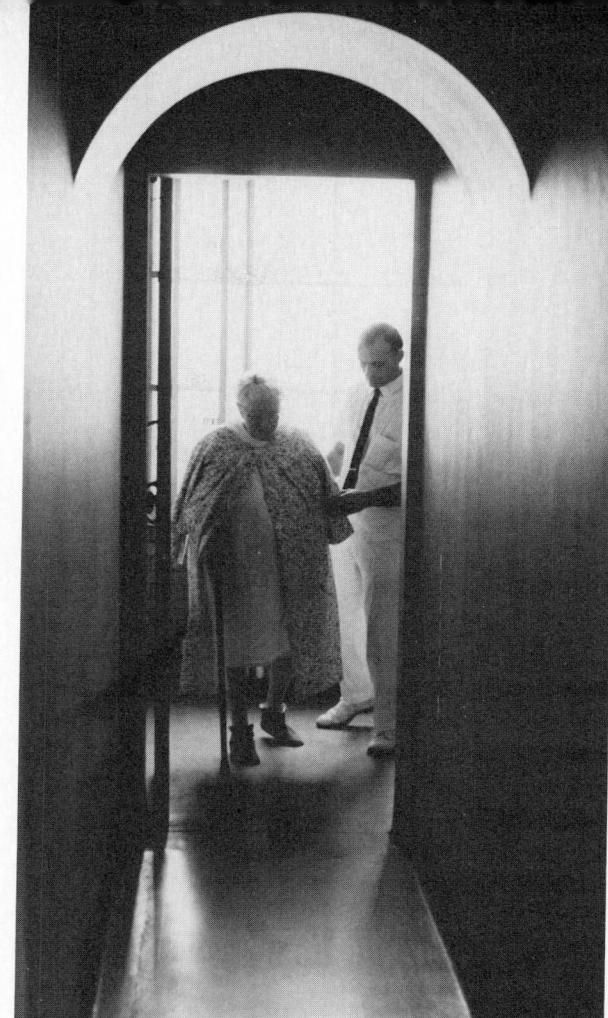

SARA T. FRY

ETHICS IN COMMUNITY HEALTH NURSING PRACTICE

Community health nurses experience many ethical conflicts in today's health care delivery system. The nursing profession has traditionally upheld the rights and human needs of the individual client. Yet in today's community health care system, this traditional focus is difficult to maintain when nursing services have the additional goal of maximizing the health of aggregate populations at risk. The traditional focus is also difficult to maintain in systems where nursing resources are influenced by legislation and funding for specific population groups. One result of this latter difficulty is that other populations identified as being at risk are not adequately served by community health nursing efforts because of the lack of funds to meet their needs. Nurses who experience this conflict between the individualistic focus of the professional ethic and the aggregate focus of community health recognize the dilemma of professional nursing in community health settings.

The purpose of this chapter is to analyze traditional ethics of professional nursing and apply these principles to the practice of community health nursing. Since the client is the focus and end of all nursing actions, a discussion of clients' rights will be the first task. Clients' rights to health and health care and other rights are examined from the viewpoint of traditional ethics and the expression of individual client needs, interests, and rights in community health situations.

Since clients have rights that are recognized by professional statements of ethics as well as by public documents, professionals have responsibilities or duties. These duties—telling the truth, respecting confidentiality, client advocacy, and accountability—are discussed in depth. The conflicts between these professional duties are also explored and possible solutions are suggested.

Not all nursing actions, however, are simply correlative to clients' rights. There is a relationship between general ethical principles and moral rules and the various theories of social justice which influence health care delivery and nursing services. These principles, their definitions, and applications in community health nursing are presented in terms of the moral requirements of the principles and their potential conflicts in the planning, implementation, and evaluation of nursing services.

Finally, the priority of the ethical principles in community health nursing, including the meaning of accountability, is discussed. Accountability—being answerable to someone for what has been done in the nursing role—is a strong, prescriptive value in nursing, directing the nurse to practice professional skills and expertise in a certain way. Thus the development of methods to measure accountability is a high priority in community health nursing. It is a priority in that community health nursing must not only demonstrate the cost-effectiveness of its services in promoting health and preventing illness but also show how it meets moral requirements for professional practice. If community health nursing can, indeed, demonstrate its ability to increase the community's health while meeting requirements for accountability to clients, then great gains will be made in the name of community health nursing services.

CLIENTS' RIGHTS AND PROFESSIONAL RESPONSIBILITIES IN COMMUNITY HEALTH CARE

Clients' Rights

There is historical background for the assertion and recognition of clients' rights in today's health care delivery system. One of the earliest recognitions of clients' rights concerning health was made by the National Convention of the French Revolution in 1793. Underscoring the theme of basic human rights, the leaders of the revolution declared that there should only be one patient to a bed in hospitals (the usual practice at that time was to assign two to eight patients per bed), and hospital beds were to be placed at least 3 feet apart (Annas, 1978). This kind of direction by a government or legislating body in the recognition and assertion of clients' rights has continued to be prominent in considerations of the right to health and the right to health care as extensions of basic human rights. However, the rec-

ognition of other clients' rights—such as rights to informed consent, to refuse treatment, or to privacy—have apparently been aided by consumer groups and health care providers such as the American Hospital Association (Annas, 1978).

Right to Health

A right to health has been historically recognized as one of the basic human rights of all persons. When introducing the Public Health Act of 1875 to the British Parliament, Prime Minister Disraeli noted that "the health of the people is really the foundation upon which all their happiness and all their powers of state depend" (Brockington, 1956, p. 47). In modern times, the right to health has been considered comparable to the rights to life and to liberty, which obligates "the State to prevent individuals from depriving each other of their health" (Szasz, 1976, p. 478). As a natural human good, health is a fundamental right and the state is obligated to protect it, although it is the responsibility of all persons to monitor their own health state.

In the United States recognition of a right to health is indicated in eighteenth century quarantine laws and early nineteenth century laws granting citizens the right to obtain, free of charge, effective cowpox vaccine (Beauchamp and Faden, 1979). These laws and early nineteenth century public health measures such as sanitation and water supply regulations to control the spread of disease demonstrate early protective laws in matters of human health and hygiene. However, most of these measures protected a negative right to health—the right to not have one's health endangered by the actions of others. The state or government recognized its obligation to enact those measures that prevent the actions of others from adversely affecting the health of an individual.

It is important to note that positive obligations to provide services may seemingly "flow from negative rights" (Beauchamp and Faden, 1979, p. 124). In other words, the negative right to be free to enjoy good health may lead to the positive right to obtain certain services or community health safeguards. For example, the negative right to not have one's health endangered by others led to the provision of public health measures concerning sewage disposal, water supplies, and the regulation of prostitution in the past (Brockington, 1956).

The negative right to not have one's health affected by social conditions has even led to regulations concerning housing and measures to protect the health of children. In modern times, this latter view of the negative right to health has encouraged some community health advocates to propose broad, federally supported programs and services to protect citizens against preventable diseases and disability (in particular, alcoholism and smoking-related illnesses) caused, in part, by social conditions (Beauchamp, D.E., 1976, 1980).

Thus advocacy—in the guise of protecting a negative right to health—has helped open the door to consideration of the right to health as a positive right: a rights claim against the state and its agencies to provide actions in the form of services and programs to improve health. It has been aided by documents such as the Universal Declaration of Human Rights of the United Nations Assembly. Noting the right of all persons to a standard of living adequate to provide for health and well-being and the right "to food, clothing, housing, and medical care" (UNESCO, 1949), this document suggests that persons not only have a strong negative right to health but a strong positive right to health (or medical) care as well. It suggests that persons are entitled to certain services, programs, and goods in order to maintain or achieve health as a basic human right.

Right to Health Care

Even though it is sometimes claimed that the "right to health" is an elliptical term for the expression "the right to health care" (Daniels, 1979), the two terms denote different kinds of rights and should be kept separate. The right to health is a negative right to a natural human good which can be of various degrees. It is a right to not have one's health interfered with by others. However, the right to health care is a positive right to goods and services in order to maintain and improve whatever state of health exists. It is a rights claim against the state or its agencies to provide specific health care services that one requests or is entitled to receive. For example, immunizations, kidney dialysis services, home health services for Medicare and Medicaid recipients, and federally funded prenatal and family planning services all recognize the positive right to specific health care services.

The distinction between the two terms is often blurred for two reasons. First, the World Health Organization defines *health* as "a state of complete physical, mental, and social well-being and not merely the absence of disease or infirmity" (World Health Organization, 1958). The emphasis on complete physical, mental, and social well-being in this definition tends to suggest that one is unhealthy without complete well-being. Since persons experience, as a result of the natural lottery, various degrees of health (but are not necessarily "unhealthy"), this would mean that services must be provided to bring about physical, mental, and social well-being for one to possess complete health. Thus, in recognizing a right to health, the right to health care ser-

vices to achieve complete health would also have to be recognized.

This is obviously a mistake. The World Health Organization's definition of health should merely be considered as an ideal state of health—one which very few persons actually possess or maintain over a long period of time. As a definition of an ideal state of health, it has no bearing on the provision of health care services as a right of all persons and should not be construed as a state that must, in fact, exist.

A second reason why the distinction between the two terms has become blurred stems from the recent advancements of modern medicine and the willingness of government to subsidize medical treatment for specific disorders such as renal disease (Public Law 92-603, 1972) and some genetic disorders (Public Law 92-278, 1976). This tendency has created a rising escalation of expectations in terms of services to achieve optimal health. It seems as if government, in recognizing a right of citizens to be as healthy as possible, must necessarily recognize a right of citizens to those services to achieve optimal health. Therefore, by subsidizing treatment of some diseases and genetic disorders, government has created the idea that the right to health means a right to good health, a state that can only be achieved through the provision of specific health care services.

Yet this is clearly wrong. In an analysis of Szasz's position (1976), Bell points out that "the right to health does not entail a right to health care because it does not entail a right to good health (only a right to good health if I already have it)" (1979, p. 162). Recognition of the right to health simply does not mean that the state is obligated to initiate health services to maintain health or improve it. Although there may be other reasons why the difference between the right to health and the right to health care are not very clear, these two reasons are certainly pertinent.

Other Rights

The right to health and the right to health care are not the only rights of clients recognized by the health care delivery system. Other basic human rights are recognized as well.

In the United States the general issue of client rights in health care did not receive widespread recognition until the early 1970s. At that time, a commission of the Department of Health, Education, and Welfare was studying medical malpractice. In its final report the commission recommended that "hospitals and other health care facilities adopt and distribute statements of patient's rights in a manner which most effectively communicates these rights to all incoming patients" (DHEW, 1973, p. 71). It is important to realize that this recommendation was intended for community health agencies as well as for acute care centers.

During the same period of time the American Hospital Association was also studying the issue of patients' rights. In 1972 this organization issued the results of its study, entitled "The Patient's Bill of Rights." The use of this document in health care facilities soon became the means by which many health care providers communicated rights to their clients. Recognizing that "the traditional physician-patient relationship takes on a new dimension when care is rendered within an organizational structure," this document affirmed the basic human rights of all clients who seek health care services (American Hospital Association, 1973). It included the rights to (1) considerate and respectful care, (2) obtain complete medical information, (3) receive information necessary for giving informed consent, (4) refuse treatment, (5) considerations of privacy, (6) confidential treatment of personal information and medical records, (7) request services, (8) information on other institutions and individuals related to care and treatment, (9) refuse participation in research projects, (10) expect reasonable continuity of care, (11) examination and explanation of financial charges, and (12) know institutional regulations.

The Patient's Bill of Rights has been criticized for several reasons. First, it seemingly grants rights to clients that have always belonged to clients (Gaylin, 1973). Second, the bill asserts a number of rights that clients have legal claims against whether or not an institution supports the document. Third, the statement "takes the circuitous route of speaking to the patient of his rights, rather than to the hospital of its duties . . ." (Gaylin, 1973, p. 142). These criticisms indicate that the problem of client rights in health care is not actually with the client. As Gaylin points out, health clients do not need to be reminded of their basic rights. Instead, health care providers ought to consider what their responsibilities are to the client. The issue of client rights has been problematical in health care delivery because health care providers fail to recognize and protect basic rights of clients. If this is the case, what kind of responsibilities do health care providers have in response to client rights?

Professional Responsibilities

In response to clients' rights, health care professionals incur particular duties or responsibilities as illustrated in Fig. 4-1. Some of these duties are supported by professional codes of ethics and are correlative to basic liberty rights of the client.

Codes of Ethics

Professional codes of ethics are statements encompassing rules that apply to persons in professional roles. Two questions generally arise concerning the importance of these codes in health care delivery: (1) what is their relation to universal moral principles? and (2) what is their relation to legal requirements for professional practice? (Beauchamp and Walters, 1978).

In answering the first question, we should consider the rules contained in professional codes of ethics for nurses to be specific applications of more universal moral principles. While some professional codes of ethics are merely statements about professional etiquette or conduct between professional groups and have no relation to external ethical principles, this is not the case in nursing. The professional code of ethics for nurses prescribes moral behavior and actions based on moral principles (Fry, 1982). Thus the professional nurse has a moral obligation to follow the rules in a code of ethics such as the *Code for Nurses with Interpretive Statements* of the American Nurses' Association (1976).*

In answering the second question, we should consider many of the rules in the *Code for Nurses* to be morally obligatory and legally required. Some of the rules may even have legal ties to licensure requirements concerning professional acts. For example, the rules of respecting client confidentiality and accountability are mentioned as both morally obligatory and legally required by the *Code for Nurses*.

Codes of ethics also prescribe duties that are required of the professional in response to rights of the client.

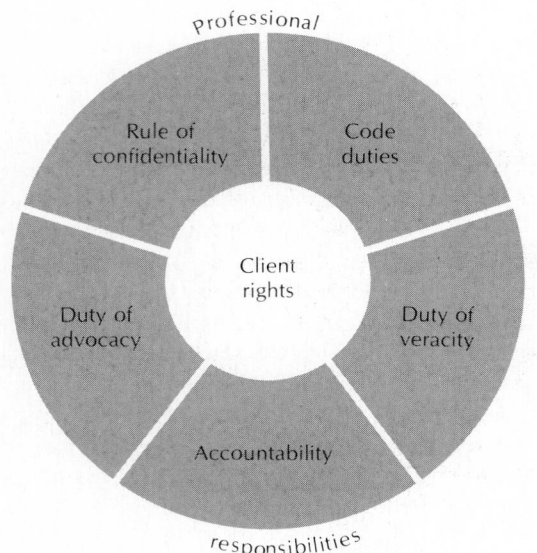

Fig. 4-1. Client rights and professional responsibilities.

*Hereafter referred to as *Code for Nurses.*

The duties of veracity and advocacy are specifically mentioned in the *Code for Nurses* as being correlative to clients' rights.

Duty of Veracity

Truthfulness has long been regarded as fundamental to the existence of trust among human beings. Persons have a duty of veracity—a duty to tell the truth and not lie or deceive people. In health care relationships several arguments are usually given for a duty to tell the truth (Beauchamp and Childress, 1979).

One argument claims that we tell the truth and forbear from lying or deceiving because this is part of the respect we owe persons. We respect persons because they are self-determining, or autonomous, individuals with all the rights and privileges of autonomous persons including the right to be told the truth and not be lied to or deceived. Because we respect persons and their autonomy, we have a duty of veracity. For example, in community health nursing we respect persons and uphold a duty of veracity by not deceiving clients as to the nature of the care they are receiving.

A second argument claims that the duty of veracity is derived from or is a way of expressing the duty of promise-keeping (Ross, 1930). Health care professionals have a duty of veracity because in communicating with the client, an implicit contract is created that engenders a duty to tell the truth and not lie or deceive. The contract between client and community health nurse creates the expectation that nurses will, in interacting with the client, speak truthfully.

A third argument claims that relationships of trust or the dependence on truthful interactions in relationships are necessary for cooperation between clients and health care professionals. After all, to not tell the truth or to deceive clients will, in the long run, undermine relationships and bring about undesirable consequences for future relationships with clients. Thus the community health nurse has a responsibility to maintain truthful relationships with clients in order to protect and to strengthen other health care relationships in general.

Yet community health nurses often have difficulty heeding or observing a duty of veracity. Information is sometimes withheld from the client or he is deceived because the nurse may think certain information will cause the client anxiety. This tendency is illustrated by responses to a 1975 survey in which over 15,000 nurses responded to questions relating to how knowledge of the client's condition should be handled by the nurse. In response to the question, "When a patient who has a terminal illness bluntly asks you if he is dying and his physician does not want him to know, what do you usually do?"; 1% would tell him; 1% would avoid the question or try to distract him; 1% would reassure him that he is not dying, just ill; 2% would lie, saying they did not know; 14% would tell him that only the physician can answer the question; and the majority (81%) would ask why he brought up the question or try to get him to talk about his feelings (Popoff, 1975, p. 24).

Nurses also withhold information because they think that clients, particularly if very sick or dying, do not really want to know the truth about their condition. But this belief is not substantiated by surveys of the sick and dying. In a survey of 100 cancer patients, 89% preferred knowing their condition; in a survey of 100 non-cancer patients, 82% said they preferred knowing; in a survey of 740 patients being diagnosed in a cancer detection center, 98.5% said they wanted to know their condition (Veatch, 1978).

Regardless of the various reasons for not telling the truth to clients or withholding information, it is clear that community health professionals have a duty of veracity. As the *Code for Nurses** notes, "Each client has the moral right to . . . be given information necessary for making informed judgments; to be told the possible effects of care . . ."(American Nurses' Association, 1976, p. 4). In fact, the duty to not lie or deceive is a stronger moral duty than the duty to disclose information.† The duty of veracity is a duty correlative to the patient's right to know and includes a strong moral obligation not to lie or deceive.

Rule of Confidentiality

In general social interaction certain information is regarded as confidential. Regarding information as confidential enables us to control the disclosure of personal information and to limit the access of others to sensitive information.

In community health care relationships, confidentiality of information is maintained for several reasons. First, if health care professionals did not follow a rule of confidentiality, clients might not seek help when they needed it. They would not reveal necessary information relating to their illnesses which would facilitate treatment for illnesses or disease processes. For example, if community health nurses could not be trusted to hold personal information in confidence, family planning clients might not reveal information relating to their reproductive history that would facilitate ap-

---

*Quotations from *Code for Nurses* reprinted with permission of ANA.
†The duty to disclose information evolves from special relationships between agents. In such relationships, one agent can claim a right to information that the other agent would not be obligated to provide to a stranger. The duty to not lie, however, does not depend on special relationships. Lying threatens any relationship because, as Beauchamp and Childress point out, ". . . lying means that an agent asserts what he believes to be false in order to deceive another" (1979, p. 205).

propriate and safe nursing care and follow-up treatment. In short, maintaining confidentiality helps protect the functioning of professional and client relationships.

A second reason for maintaining confidentiality is derived from the sphere of privacy we recognize as a basic human right of all persons. Because persons are self-determining moral agents, they have a right to determine how personal information, especially health information, is communicated. As the *Code for Nurses* points out, "The nurse safeguards the client's right to privacy by judiciously protecting information of a confidential nature" (American Nurses' Association, 1976, p. 6). Because of respect for persons, nurses respect clients' rights to privacy by maintaining the moral rule of confidentiality.

In health care relationships, however, the duty to observe the rule of confidentiality is not always an absolute duty; it is merely a *prima facie* duty, meaning that it may be overridden when in conflict with other duties that are morally stronger. The duty to observe confidentiality may be overridden for several reasons:

1. When in conflict with other duties toward the client. For example, the duty to preserve life may outweigh the duty to respect confidential information concerning self-destructive wishes of the client.

2. When in conflict with duties toward identified others. For example, if a mental health client tells the nurse of intent to harm or even kill another member of the community, regardless of the confidential nature of the mental health nurse/client relationship, the nurse's duty to protect others from harm by warning the intended victim of the client will override the duty to keep confidentiality. This action may even be required by law (Tarasoff, 1976).

3. When in conflict with duties toward nonidentified others or the rights and interests of society in general. For example, communicable diseases such as tuberculosis or venereal disease are required to be reported by law regardless of the confidential nature of that information; this is done to protect the health of others. Another example concerns the right to keep information in one's health record private which may be overridden by duties to others in society. This occurs when health records are used for epidemiological research without the client's knowledge. There are, of course, stringent constraints placed on the use of this information by epidemiologists in health research (Gordis and Gold, 1980; Kelsey, 1981). But in general, the duty to increase or protect the health of the community through research outweighs the duty to respect the confidentiality of health records.

Duty of Advocacy

The nursing profession recognizes a strong duty of advocacy where the care or safety of clients is concerned. As the *Code for Nurses* states, "... the nurse must be alert to and take appropriate action regarding any instances of incompetent, unethical, or illegal practices by any member of the health care team or the health care system itself" (American Nurses' Association, 1976, p. 8). In the role of advocate, the nurse speaks for or in support of the best interests of the individual client or vulnerable client populations.

This is a strong protect-the-client-from-harm duty which is derived from a general ethical principle of beneficence or the "duty to help others further their important ... interests" (Beauchamp and Childress, 1979, p. 136). Yet the role of advocate can be difficult for the community health nurse. First, it must be recognized that clients should always determine what is in their best interests. Acting on the basis of what the nurse thinks is in the best interests of clients can lead to paternalism when the wishes of clients are never ascertained.

Second, the duty of advocacy extends to populations at risk, which may bring the community health nurse into conflict with health policy or established professional practices within a community or institution. Nurse advocates who have experienced this kind of conflict have sometimes found their jobs and other professional relationships in jeopardy (Smith, 1980). Needless to say, positions of advocacy can be difficult to maintain when they conflict with accepted professional practices.

Third, it has been questioned whether the duty of advocacy requires the community health nurse to put one's own job, health, or professional standing at risk on behalf of advocacy for the client. According to Beauchamp and Childress, this is not a moral requirement of the principle of beneficence (1979). What is required is that the nurse fulfill the primary commitment to client care and safety by protecting the client from harm. While the implicit contract of the nurse/client relationship does, in general, require positive acts of benefiting in terms of care rendered, this does not extend to the role of advocate. Thus the community health nurse is only required, in the role of advocate, to protect, speak for, and support the interests of the client to *not* be harmed in the provision of health care services.

Accountability: Moral Obligation or Moral Virtue?

The need for moral accountability within nursing practice in response to basic human rights has long been recognized. Even Florence Nightingale reputedly made strong objections to the overriding of a person's will for the benefit of others in the performance of nursing care (Palmer, 1977). Believing in the creativity and self-determining rights of man, Nightingale apparently included humanistic orientations in her early training programs for nurses. These orientations became the foundations on which accountability requirements in nursing were eventually constructed.

Modern leaders in nursing have also noted that means must be sought to promote progress in health care delivery while simultaneously protecting the rights of the individual (Berthold, 1969). Noting the need for scientific accountability within the performance of nursing functions, Gortner called for a standard of accountability in nursing as the means by which the quality of nursing services will be provided (1974).

Yet it is uncertain what is meant by a "standard of accountability" in nursing. Furthermore, what does the standard of accountability require of the nurse? In the *Code for Nurses,* accountability is defined as "being answerable to someone for something one has done" (American Nurses' Association, 1976, p. 10). It includes providing an explanation to one's self, to the client, to the employing agency, and to the nursing profession for what one has done in the role of nurse. It is an obligation that has both moral and legal components and implies a contractual agreement between two parties. This means that when a community health nurse enters into a contractual agreement to perform a service for a client, the nurse will be held answerable for performing this service according to agreed terms, within an established time period and with stipulated use of resources and performance standards. The nurse as contractor is responsible for the quality of the services rendered and is accountable to the individual client, the health service agency, the nursing profession, and even one's own conscience for what has been done.

Referring to accountability in nursing as a moral obligation means that being answerable for what one has done is correlative to clients' rights to a certain level of competent nursing care and their rights to self-determination in health care. As a moral obligation, accountability directs the professional to act in a particular way according to moral norms (Fry, 1981). But is accountability merely a moral obligation? Because of the central role of accountability in nursing care and its grounding in the trust relationship shared by client and nurse, accountability may also be a moral virtue, one that is peculiar to the practice of nursing.

Moral virtue may be characterized in different ways. According to Carney, moral virtue is "an ideal of human personhood at which to aim" (1978, p. 435). This statement indicates that moral virtue is apparently an

ideal standard of human behavior and may help one to discern the morality of human acts.

It is generally believed that people develop virtues that support the types of moral obligations already acknowledged in daily actions. These virtues then enable people to carefully perform their duties, thus increasing the probability that performance in practice settings will closely approximate professional standards (Carney, 1978). According to this view, there is a close relationship between moral obligations already operating in a practice and moral virtues. Hence, it might be quite natural to view accountability as moral virtue.

MacIntyre has called virtue an "acquired human quality the possession and exercise of which tends to enable us to achieve those goods which are internal to practices" (1981, p. 178). MacIntyre further points out that since every practice requires a certain kind of relationship between those who participate in it, virtues are how we define our relationships to those with whom we share practices. Thus he concludes that virtues (such as justice, courage, and honesty) are essential to practices like medicine and nursing. They help define the kind of relationships we have with persons in practices and sustain the traditions that provide historical context to both practices and individual lives (MacIntyre, 1981).

In nursing, and especially in community health nursing, accountability appears to be the quality that defines the kind of relationships between client, nurse, other professionals, and the public at large which form the moral foundations of the professional ethic in nursing. Furthermore, since accountability is correlative to clients' rights to competent levels of nursing care, it is responsive to the humanistic traditions that permeate nursing's history. Viewed in this manner, accountability, as a moral virtue (being derived from moral obligation), enables the nurse to achieve what is internal to the practice of community health nursing: the protection of the client's human dignity and right to self-determination in matters of health.

ETHICAL PRINCIPLES IN COMMUNITY HEALTH

Relationship of ethical rules, principles, and theories

In making moral decisions we usually appeal to various rules, principles, or theories (see Fig. 4-2). *Rules* state that certain actions should (or should not) be performed because they are right (or wrong). An example would be that "nurses ought to always tell the truth to clients." *Principles* are more abstract than rules and serve as the foundation of rules. For example, the ethical principle of autonomy is the foundation for such

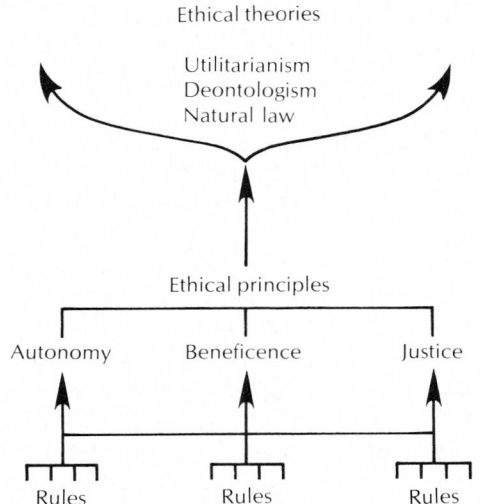

Fig. 4-2. The relationship of ethical theories, principles, and rules.

rules as "always get informed consent," "tell the truth," and "protect the privacy of the client." Likewise, the principle of justice serves as the foundation of rules such as "treat equals equally" and "divide your time on the basis of needs." *Theories,* however, are collections of principles and rules. They provide theoretical foundations for deciding what to do when principles or rules conflict. Examples of a few major theories are *utilitarianism, deontologism,* and *natural law* (see Glossary for exact definitions).

Within theories, the various moral rules and principles are arranged according to their importance or justifiability. For example, in utilitarianism, the principle of beneficence often carries more weight than the ethical principles of autonomy or justice. But this does not mean that beneficence cannot be overriden by either the principle of autonomy or the principle of justice in many circumstances.

In deontologism the ethical principle of autonomy generally carries more weight but still can be overridden by the principles of beneficence or justice.

In natural law theory, that principle which most conforms to the view of human nature adopted in the theory will carry more weight than the other principles. But again, other ethical principles can override the predominate principle in many circumstances.

Ethical principles are thus *prima facie* principles and not absolute. Each ethical principle is always morally significant but may not always prevail when in conflict with other principles. Ethical theories simply suggest which ethical principles will more likely prevail when moral decisions have to be made.

But what makes some judgments moral while others are considered nonmoral? Moral judgments are evaluations of what is good or bad, right or wrong, having certain characteristics that separate them from other evaluations such as personal preferences, beliefs, or matters of taste. The difference between the evaluations lies in the reasons for or the grounds on which the judgments are being made and according to the characteristics of the judgments themselves (Frankena, 1973).

Moral judgments are generally made of human actions, institutions, or character traits. What makes them moral (instead of nonmoral) is that they have the characteristics of (1) being ultimate or preemptive, meaning that other values or human ends cannot, as a rule, override them (Fried, 1978); (2) having universality, meaning that they apply to everyone under relevantly similar circumstances (Baier, 1958); and (3) having an other-regarding focus, meaning that they treat the good of everyone alike and do not give a special place to one's own welfare (Beauchamp and Childress, 1979). Judgments that have these characteristics are moral judgments.

It is obvious that community health nurses frequently make moral judgments. When the nurse decides to arrange a home visiting schedule on the basis of need or seriousness of illness, a moral judgment is made. When the nurse decides to refer a client to a physician for further evaluation based on the expressed wishes of the client and his condition, a moral judgment is made. When a nurse decides, regardless of personal beliefs about abortion, to inform a client of all the options available concerning a request for abortion, a moral judgment is made. When a nurse decides not to participate in political activities urged by others that might lessen health care coverage for vulnerable populations, a moral judgment is made. What makes these decisions moral rather than nonmoral are the reasons for which the judgments were made and their stated characteristics.

Principle of Beneficence
Definition

The principle of beneficence states that "we ought to do good and prevent or avoid doing harm" (Frankena, 1973, p. 45). It includes the idea that beneficence is a duty to help others gain what is of benefit to them but does not carry the obligation to risk one's own welfare or interests in helping others. In fact, some theorists maintain that beneficence does not morally require us to always benefit others even when we can do so. Rather we are only morally required to prevent harm to people. This may be true in general social interactions among persons. But in special relationships, the implicit contract underlying the nature of the relationship seems to indicate that positive benefiting or acts of beneficence should take place. This seems to be the case in nursing.

The need for health care forms the basis of the relationship between community health nurse and client and imposes a moral duty on the nurse to benefit the client through nursing actions. However, there may be limits on the amount of beneficial nursing care a client should expect. Certainly no nurse should be expected to provide nursing care to individual clients or client populations at physical risk to oneself or when clients' needs infringe on one's personal life or responsibilities to other clients, to oneself, or to one's own family. While the duty to prevent harm occurring to clients is a stringent one in nursing, the claim to positive benefiting is limited.

Applications in Community Health

In community health nursing, the principle of beneficence can be applied in (1) balancing harms and benefits to client populations and (2) in the use of cost benefit analyses in decisions affecting client populations.

Balancing Harms and Benefits. Acting so as to bring about the greatest balance of good over evil, or value (benefit) over disvalue (harms), is acting in accordance with a *rule of utility*. This rule is derived from the principle of beneficence and includes the moral duty to weigh and balance benefits against harms in order to increase benefits and reduce the occurrence of harms (Beauchamp and Childress, 1979).

In community health a rule of utility may be appealed to in deciding whether to fund certain health programs more than others, whether to conduct screening programs for communicable disease after several cases have been found in vulnerable populations, and whether to conduct research projects where individual rights to privacy may be concerned. In each example, the decision is made by balancing the possible harms and benefits of several alternative courses of action. The community health nurse facilitates this process by accurately assessing the known benefits and harms to clients from a nursing care point of view and presenting them along with other relevant facts that might enter into the decision-making process.

Cost Benefit Analysis. Cost benefit analysis is a specific application of the principle of beneficence. It is a device for measuring the harms and benefits of providing various methods of care or health programs while also figuring the cost of the relative trade-offs that might have to be made in selecting certain courses of actions. All of the units taken into consideration, such as lives saved, costs averted, taxes saved, and illness prevented, are eventually converted into one common

unit—usually money—to measure the benefits and costs of alternative approaches to a problem or to decide how to distribute health program monies.

Problems and Conflicts

Decision making in community health settings on the basis of a principle of beneficence and the weighing of harms and benefits raises moral questions concerning (1) paternalism in health care decisions and (2) the extent of the rule of utility in decision making.

Paternalism. Paternalism is a liberty-limiting principle that is frequently invoked to override people's actions or expressed wishes for their own good or best interests. Parents may override a child's desire to play with the interesting knobs on a stove because they do not want the child to get burned. Community health nurses may override clients' expressed wishes "not to hear any bad news" by telling them the results of laboratory testing so that their health states can be treated and improved. Nurses do this because they feel it is in clients' best interests in the long run to know the state of their health.

In general, it is morally justified to restrict a person's liberty when the harm to be caused is a physical harm, possibly life-threatening, and is caused by those whose liberty is restricted. However, it is more difficult to justify paternalistic actions for perceived psychological harms. For example, it might seem morally justified to override a teenager's desire to participate in a potentially risky (to health) research project but not seem morally justified to withhold information of a defective fetus from a woman who is 6 months pregnant because it might cause her psychological harm and grief during the remaining months of pregnancy.

It is also difficult to justify paternalistic actions for the purpose of benefiting the person whose liberty is restricted. For example, it is hard to morally justify restraining and forcibly giving medication to a mental health client who has refused chemotherapy because the medication will benefit him by reducing his paranoia or irrational fears. Yet we recognize that health care practitioners often carry out paternalistic actions. If this is the case, are there some acts of paternalism which are morally justified and if so, what are the criteria for justified paternalism in community health decisions?

Since paternalism always violates the moral principle of autonomy and the moral rule to treat persons as self-determining moral agents, justified paternalism is a very limited area. According to Gert and Culver (1979), paternalism is justified only if (1) the evils that would be prevented are much greater than the evils, if any, that would be caused by the violation of the moral rule and (2) we would be willing to universally allow the violation of the moral rule in these same circumstances and be able to publicly advocate this kind of violation. Thus acts involving justified paternalism seem to be limited to those acts that prevent a person from committing some grave bodily harm to himself—self-mutilating or self-destructing behaviors and acts committed out of ignorance such as the ingestion of harmful substances unknowingly. Beyond these and similar acts, it is hard to justify paternalism in community health. Few situations meet the previously stated criteria for justified paternalism.

Extent of the Rule of Utility. Attempting to bring about the greatest possible balance of benefit over harm in community health may lead to two problems. The first is the potential overriding of individual liberties and values for the common good. For example, in calculating the benefits of a health policy to citizens in terms of tax savings and other economic benefits, the health needs of individual citizens may be overlooked or simply not deemed as important when entered into the calculations for aggregate utility. Human needs and wants that cannot be easily or accurately converted into monetary units may simply be left out in deciding for the greatest amount of overall benefit. As pointed out by MacIntyre, the methodology of cost benefit analysis in particular cannot truly represent the value choices of individuals (1979). Incommensurable value choices pertaining to health and life are distorted or ignored in figuring perceived harms and benefits into the calculations of the analysis. Thus policy decisions on the basis of the rule of utility as expressed in cost benefit analysis may be inaccurate as well as irrelevant to the health needs of individuals.

A second problem arises when the rule of utility is applied in health policy decisions having long-term effects. For example, it is often unclear how short-term harms and benefits ought to be weighted against long-term consequences in cost benefit analysis. If the benefits and harms to individual health or economic savings in the future are judged more important than present savings or health conditions, then individual and collective interests in health may be sacrificed for future benefits.

Principle of Autonomy
Definition

Autonomy refers to freedom of action as chosen by an individual. Persons who are autonomous are capable of choosing and acting on plans they themselves have decided on.

To respect persons as autonomous individuals is to acknowledge their personal rights to make choices and act according to individual determinations; they are respected as self-determining moral agents or persons.

Thus when nurses respect persons as moral agents, they are acting in accordance with the requirements of the moral principle of autonomy.

Applications in Community Health

The principle of autonomy is applied in community health through considerations of (1) respect for persons, (2) the protection of privacy, (3) the provision of informed consent, (4) freedom of choice including treatment refusal, and (5) the protection of diminished autonomy.

Respect for Persons. In community health, clients are respected for no other reason than because they are persons and have the right to determine their own plan of life. Community health nurses acknowledge respect by seriously considering the opinions and choices of clients while not, at the same time, obstructing their actions unless they are harmful to themselves or others. Denying clients freedom to act on their own judgments or withholding information necessary to make judgments demonstrates a lack of respect for clients.

For example, consider the elderly client who may not be treated with the respect accorded younger clients. Community health nurses often find it easier and quicker to communicate with family members or simply "tell" the client what treatment has to be performed. The elderly client may not be given a choice or even considered in the treatment plan. Age, however, does not render a client less worthy of our respect (Fig. 4-3). The elderly have the right to determine their life and health plans insofar as they have the capacity to do so. To deny them the opportunity to choose according to their capacities demonstrates a lack of respect for persons and is an infringement of the principle of autonomy.

Protection of Privacy. The nature of community health nursing care involves close observation of clients, physical touching, and access to personal health and economic information about clients and their families. All of these aspects of nursing care may invade the privacy of clients or threaten their right to control personal information.

Since the relationship between nurse and client is built on trust, the nurse has a responsibility to protect the privacy of clients and their families insofar as clients' health is concerned. This means that personal information gathered in the initial home assessment of clients must be recorded in a manner that acknowledges respect for clients' privacy and is communicated only to those directly concerned with client care.

When personal economic information must be shared with third parties for payment of nursing care, clients have the right to authorize or withhold disclosure of information. Even though the information may

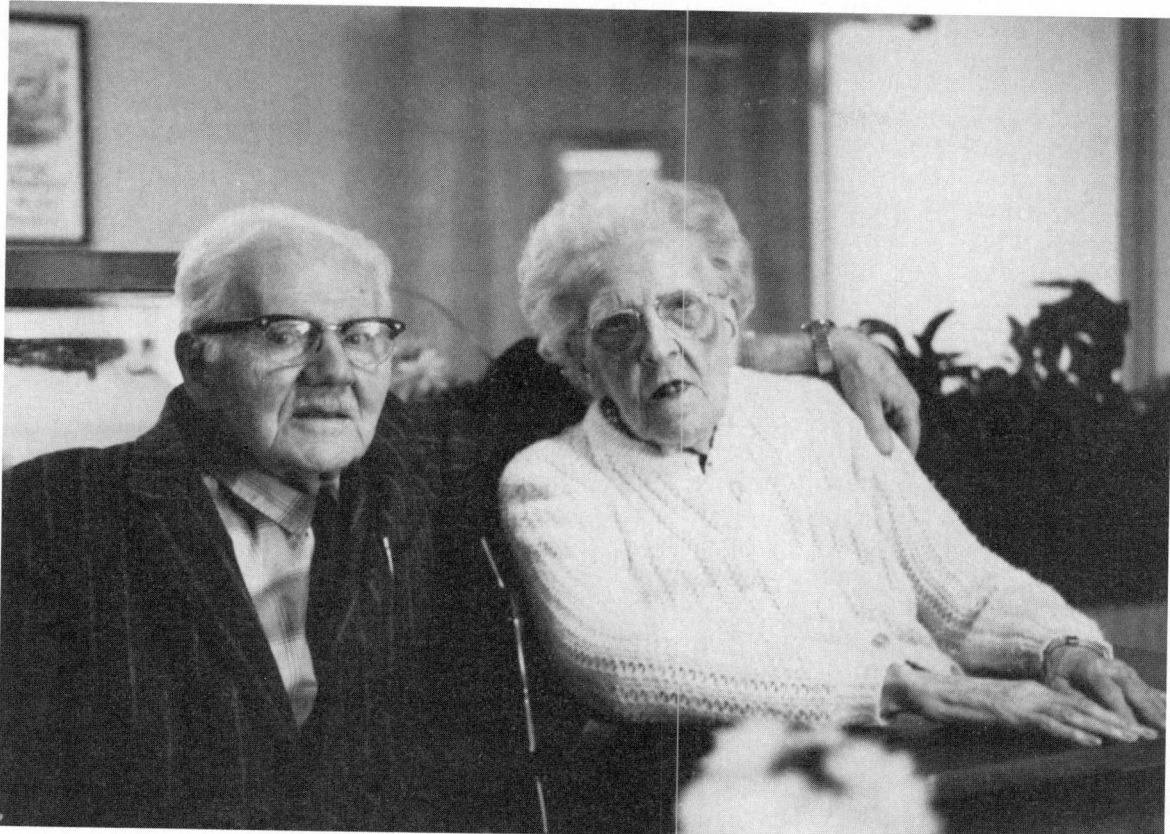

Fig. 4-3. Age does not render clients less worthy of our respect.

be essential for continuity of nursing care services, the client retains control of all information generated by the nurse/client relationship.

When clients' records are examined for quality assurance purposes or notes about home or clinic visits are included in research studies to assess the effectiveness of community health nursing services, the protection of privacy may be a genuine problem. Utilization of health records in determining funding levels for community health nursing services does not justify the use of nurse-generated information about the client without the client's knowledge and permission. Health record information can only be used for quality assurance purposes or research studies and shared with others under clearly defined policies and written guidelines that protect client privacy. In addition, community health nursing services are responsible for making sure that policies and guidelines appropriately protect client privacy and that clients are informed of this protection *before* information about them is released to any source. Only when measures to protect the privacy of clients are fully carried out can it be said that community health nursing meets the requirements of the ethical principle of autonomy.

Provision of Informed Consent. The principle of autonomy requires that clients be given "the opportunity to choose what shall or shall not happen to them" (National Commission, 1978, p. 10). Clients are provided this opportunity when consent is voluntarily made and when adequate disclosure standards for informed consent are included in the contract for community health nursing services. Three elements are essential for adequate informed consent: information, comprehension, and voluntariness.

1. *Information.* For clients to have adequate information, the nurse must disclose information pertaining to treatment procedures, their purposes, any discomforts and anticipated benefits, alternative procedures for therapy, and the opportunity to question procedures or end the contract at any time. Clients should also be adequately informed as to how confidentiality of their health records will be maintained.

2. *Comprehension.* The manner and context in which information is conveyed to clients is also important for informed consent requirements. Clients must be allowed time to consider information provided by the community health nurse as well as time to ask questions. If the client is unable to comprehend because of a

language barrier, such as between an English-speaking nurse and Spanish-speaking client, the nurse must provide an interpreter to remove such barriers. This, of course, implies that the client is competent to understand and can make decisions based on rational reasons. Competent clients are those able to understand a treatment procedure or proposed care plan, weigh its discomforts and benefits, and then make decisions about undertaking the procedure or plan.

3. *Voluntariness.* This element of informed consent is so important that any contract or agreement with the client constitutes valid consent only if voluntarily given, free of coercion and undue influences by other persons or the health agency. The notion of voluntariness includes the ability to choose one's own health goals and the ability to choose among several goals when offered a choice of options (Beauchamp and Childress, 1979). Again, the principle of autonomy is the main ethical principle guiding this provision.

These three elements—information, comprehension, and voluntariness—constitute informed consent in community health nursing practice. Informed consent is not valid without all elements and no contract between client and nurse is ethically acceptable without valid, informed consent.

Individual Freedom of Choice. Respecting the client's right to self-determination includes respecting potential treatment refusal. The client's interest in personal freedom to follow one's own will, the potential harm to the client or other citizens, the cost of treatment refusal, and the values of society are all factors that usually enter into the nurse's acknowledgement or acceptance of treatment refusal (Capron, 1978). However, as long as a client is judged competent to make this kind of decision, it is difficult to infringe on autonomy by not allowing treatment refusal.

Some of the most interesting and difficult legal cases involving treatment refusal have involved the exercise of religious beliefs (*In re estate of Brooks,* 1965). Others have involved the autonomy of the teenage minor to refuse lifesaving treatment such as kidney dialysis (Veatch, 1976). More recent cases affecting the values of entire communities have involved the right of parents to refuse lifesaving treatment for their defective newborns, (Will, 1982).

In community health nursing, respect for the client's or guardian's right to refuse treatment may hinge on nurse judgment of the competency of the client to make such choices. The physical competency of the elderly or severely ill client, the psychological competency of former mental patients as well as the maturity or legal competency of minors may, in part, rely on the assessment of client abilities as made in the home environment by the community health curse.

In situations of questionable competency, decisions have generally opted for the preservation of life (Beauchamp and Childress, 1979). In situations where competency to make decisions has been established, other factors such as obligations to others (such as dependent children) may determine whether or not autonomy of choice will be respected. No hard and fast rule on treatment refusal can be made. Yet community health nurses should recognize that respect for persons may involve allowing clients and their legal guardians to make decisions concerning their life and health which may be very difficult for the nurse to accept.

Protecting Diminished Autonomy. The principle of autonomy is generally applied only to persons capable of autonomous choice. Persons who have diminished autonomy, whether from physical or psychological incapacities or immaturity, are not considered fully autonomous persons. Thus it is thought justifiable to interfere with the actions of those not fully autonomous to protect them from harmful results of their choices and actions without infringing on the principle of autonomy. This interference, however, requires appeals to other principles, such as beneficence, as the source of special duties toward those not fully autonomous.

The community health nurse may have difficulty recognizing when clients are not capable of self-determination because of diminished capacities. The capacity for self-determination is relative to maturity, chronological age, the presence or absence of illness, mental disability, or other social situations that restrict a person's liberty to be self-determining. Yet respect for the principle of autonomy requires that practitioners recognize when persons lack the capacity to act autonomously and therefore are entitled to protection in health care delivery (Fig. 4-4).

Problems and Conflicts

Respecting the ethical principle of autonomy can be difficult in community health nursing practice. Those areas creating the most conflict for nurses have included (1) the carrying out of coercive health measures and (2) invasions of privacy for health reasons.

Coercive Health Measures. Clients consulting a community health agency for nursing services may have a communicable disease that is not only harmful to themselves if untreated but may affect the health of family members, neighbors, or coworkers. The client may not want to receive treatment and may even refuse to take medications or attend follow-up care recommended for the illness. For example, many areas of the United States still require clients diagnosed with active tuberculosis to be confined to a state institution until their disease process is no longer considered active or communicable to others. When diagnosed, clients must

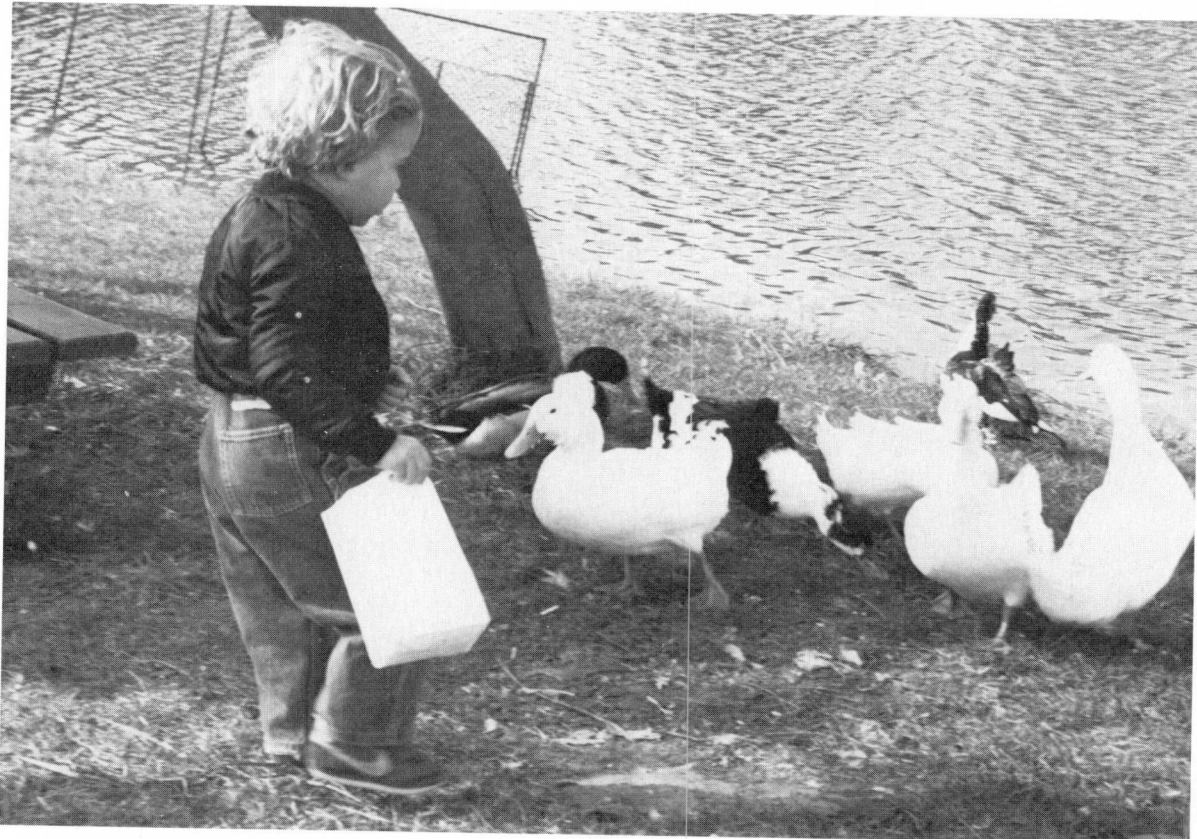

Fig. 4-4. Children have diminished autonomy and are entitled to protection in health care delivery.

leave their jobs and families and incur the results of social stigmatization that still accompanies the diagnosis of tuberculosis. Clients have no choice in the matter. They must be admitted to the state institution and must take treatment, regardless of their own wishes, choices, or life plans.

The community health nurse may be the one to enforce these regulations or be the agent to override a client's expressed wishes in this matter. Thus nurses may find the conflict between individual rights to self-determinations in health matters and the protection of the community's health to be especially difficult when they are the agents carrying out this kind of coercive health measure.

Invasions of Privacy. In protecting the health of vulnerable populations, the community health nurse may infringe on rights to privacy by actively gathering information of a private nature from those unwilling to give this information. For example, a sharp rise in the incidence of venereal disease among a high school population may require interviewing of teenagers diagnosed with disease and the accurate follow-up of all named contacts. This action may lead to invasions of individual privacy through discussion of sexual habits and preferences and potential disclosures to adults, including parents.

All of these actions are infringements of self-determining behavior but are considered justifiable on the basis of potential harms to others. Regardless, it is incumbent on the nurse to inform those whose privacy is invaded that information will be recorded and communicated in a way that does not infringe on the future privacy of the individual.

Privacy may also be invaded by the assessment and recording of personal client information. For example, the community health nurse may record information about the social habits and life-styles of pregnant women, which may subsequently be used in retrospective research studies correlating neonatal mortality and morbidity with social habits (particularly drug and alcohol use during pregnancy). This type of personal information is often freely communicated on the basis of the trust relationship between nurse and client. It may also be recorded in the client's record without full understanding of the potential impact of this information if, in fact, a child is born with anomalies related to social habits or life-styles during pregnancy. The presence of this information in prenatal records may mean that it might eventually be shared with other health professionals and members of the client's family constituting further invasions of the client's right to privacy of personal information.

In community health these invasions may be justified on the basis of preventing harm to innocent third parties (the defective child), but the actual communication of this information in a way sensitive to the client's right to privacy may create many conflicts of interest for the nurse.

Principle of Justice
Definition

The formal principle of justice claims that equals should be treated equally and that those who are unequal should be treated differently according to their differences (Beauchamp and Childress, 1979). In considerations of community health we appeal to a principle of justice in determining the manner in which social burdens and benefits, including health goods, ought to be distributed among all individuals in the community.

Applications in Community Health

Different theories of justice may be appealed to in deciding how to distribute health care resources. These theories include: (1) the entitlement theory, (2) the utilitarian theory, (3) the maximin theory, and (4) the egalitarian theory. Each theory has its advantages and disadvantages in terms of the distribution of health goods in the community.

Entitlement Theory. The entitlement theory claims that everyone is entitled to whatever they get in the natural lottery at birth and there is no responsibility for government or its agencies to improve the lot of those less fortunate than others. If people have good health, are rich, and have been able to acquire possessions by purchase, gift, or legitimate exchange, they are entitled to what they have. They may also increase their possessions in any way possible as long as they do not cheat others or acquire possessions unjustly (Nozick, 1974).

It is, of course, considered unfortunate that some people are mentally or physically handicapped in society, yet others have no obligation to give some of their monies to the handicapped to make their lives more comfortable. Aiding the unfortunate is simply an act of charity on the part of members in the community.

In this theory, inequalities between individuals in matters of health, position, and wealth are tolerated. Only aggressions or harms against others and the unjust acquisitions of goods are prohibited. Thus the actual distribution of goods seems more in line with a princi-

ple of autonomy or the exercise of the right to liberty than a principle of justice (Veatch, 1981).

Utilitarian Theory. This theory of justice claims that the best way to distribute resources among the citizenry is to decide how expenditures or the use of resources will achieve the greatest net total of good and serve the largest number of people (Mill, 1957). In times of limited resources, when all that is needed or wanted cannot be provided in the community, this method of distribution is appealing. While it does tend to overlook the needs and wants of individuals, it manages to maximize net benefits over costs and serves the greatest number of people.

In this theory the needs and wants of some individuals will not be satisfied, and they may, indeed, be harmed in the process. This would be considered unfortunate, but in distributing limited resources so that "the greatest good for the greatest number" is achieved, government and its agencies would have fulfilled their obligations to citizenry. It is easy to see that the principle of beneficence dominates other considerations in utilitarianism. Justice is served by benefiting the greatest number at the least cost.

Maximin Theory. The maximin* theory of justice first identifies the least advantaged members of the community (for example, the economically poor, the elderly, the mentally retarded, and children below one year of age) and decides how they might be benefited rather than deciding on greatest net aggregate benefit. It then permits free exercise of liberty on the part of all citizens and allows social and economic inequalities to evolve in such a manner that these inequalities are of benefit to the least advantaged or least well-off members in society (Rawls, 1971). Many kinds of inequalities in terms of health, health care resources, and possession of economic benefits will be tolerated and considered just as long as the position of the least advantaged is improved or benefited. For example, health professionals can charge high fees or receive substantial salaries just as long as they also serve the interests of the disadvantaged. In a similar manner costly health care resources, such as kidney dialysis, CAT scans, and artificial hearts, can be developed and purchased by those who can afford them as long as the lot of the least advantaged is also improved in the process.

Obviously, distributing health goods according to this theory will create problems in times of limited resources or monies. Even though the maximin theory advocates distribution in accordance with a principle of justice, providing benefit to the least advantaged first is

---

Maximin is a short term for maximizing the minimum position in society.

a constraint on the expansion of health care resources and technological advancement unless some way can be figured out to benefit the least advantaged in the process. Thus it is possible that technological advancement and the development of more sophisticated health care goods cannot be made widely available to the public in times of limited economic resources. The result is that interests and needs in matters of health may not be satisfied within this system of justice.

Egalitarian Theory. The egalitarian model of justice claims that justice requires the "equality of net welfare for individuals" (Veatch, 1981, p. 265). In this theory the distribution of good in the community takes the needs of all citizens into account equally. Thus everyone would have a claim to an equal amount of all goods and resources, including health care.

Clearly, this is a goal which cannot be achieved. It would be virtually impossible for any system of justice to guarantee equality of goods and resources for everyone, let alone equal health care. The egalitarian theory must necessarily be emended. Instead of health care being a good that everyone should have an equal amount of, basic health care should be viewed as a good that all should have equal access to. In short, everyone should have equal access to those basic health goods and resources to improve their health according to need (Green, 1976; Veatch, 1981).

This is a system that respects the autonomy of individuals to seek those health services they need or want and gives equal consideration to the positive benefiting of individuals in terms of improved health. Most important, it is just in that it follows the dictates of a principle of justice while not, at the same time, limiting the liberty of anyone in terms of basic health needs. It treats equals equally and unequals unequally and provides a just manner for the distribution of health resources in the community.

Problems and Conflicts

The application of a principle of justice in community health nursing creates conflicts in two areas: (1) establishing priorities for the distribution of basic goods and health services in the community and (2) determining which populations or individuals shall obtain available health goods and nursing services.

Distributing Basic Goods and Services. In deciding how to distribute basic health care assets or resources within a community, the first decision is to set the priorities for distribution. Should the protection and promotion of health be the main consideration? Or should a major portion of resources be set aside for other social goods, such as housing or education? If community leaders agree that everyone has a right to equal access to basic health care according to need and this right must be satisfied for justice to be served, then enough community assets and financial resources will be allotted to meet the requirements of this basic right (Milio, 1975).

A second decision concerns the most effective and efficient methods of meeting this basic right while preventing death and disability among citizenry. Should the emphasis be placed on direct health care services (such as clinics and programs) or should indirect services (such as health education and transportation services) receive equal emphasis?

Third, decisions will have to be made for the appropriate relationship between rescue services and preventive services (Beauchamp and Childress, 1979). In other words, is it more effective to concentrate on kidney dialysis and terminal cancer services or should concentrated effort and economic resources be devoted to prevention of disease and disability through, for example, hypertension and diabetic screening?

Fourth, decisions will need to be made as to whether certain diseases or categories of illness receive more emphasis than others. For example, should the prevention and treatment of coronary heart disease take precedence over the prevention and treatment of venereal disease? Decisions in this area may well allocate monies and services to certain socioeconomic groups or racial groups and will have to be given careful consideration to avoid conflicts of interest in matters of health.

Fifth, in establishing certain priorities, it is necessary to ascertain whether these priorities will compromise important values or principles. For example, preventive strategies aimed at discouraging alcohol consumption or smoking may well involve emphasis on behavioral change or the altering of life-styles by members of the community. The nurse might question whether priority setting in terms of these preventive strategies would have a substantial impact on the autonomy of community members, particularly their choice to engage in health risky behaviors.

Clearly, the prioritizing of health interests and the various ways to carry out these priorities may create conflicts of interests among health care providers with subsequent influence on the actual delivery of needed nursing care. These conflicts of interests continue in the next area of decision making.

Distributing Nursing Resources. Once the priorities for health within a community are designated along with the multiple ways these priorities will be carried out, community health nursing services need to decide who will receive services and what criteria can be used to distribute services equally in accordance with client needs.

One strategy may be to focus services on those who

have the most reasonable chance of benefiting from services; for example, children and childbearing families (Beauchamp and Childress, 1979). Clearly, this is a utilitarian approach to distributing services aimed at providing the greatest net benefit overall. Even though it is also an approach that accommodates an interest in disease prevention, we might question whether this strategy meets the moral requirements of a principle of justice which holds that everyone has a claim of equal access to basic health care services according to health care need. Certainly a strategy that focuses on one age group in the community will overlook many individual wants and needs in terms of health care services and cannot be considered just.

A second strategy is to provide basic services in all categories in limited amounts and accommodate requests for nursing care services on a first come, first served basis. This approach may certainly cost more in terms of services provided and may even overlap with similar services provided in the community through health maintenance organizations or group practices of private family physicians. It does meet the basic requirement of providing the opportunity for everyone to have equal access to services even though they may have to wait a long time to be served. Yet it may not be the most efficient means of disbursing nursing resources according to the needs of clients.

A third strategy is to focus nursing services on those who are most able to pay for services, an approach that is all too frequently used in today's health care delivery system. This approach has been fostered by legislation and funding by government and its agencies. Unfortunately, this approach may have limited relevance to the needs of a particular community. For example, focusing the majority of nursing resources in a home health care program because of Medicare reimbursements in a community that has a small elderly population seems unjust when considering the health needs of other populations.

A fourth approach is to categorize those in the community according to health needs and decide who should receive first priority. Those who cannot survive without nursing resources (those receiving kidney dialysis or respiratory therapy at home) would have first priority. Those who can be assisted so as to prevent long-term disability (populations at high risk; the preeclamptic client; children with minor cardiac anomalies; close contacts of tuberculosis clients, and so on) would come next. Those who do not have an acute disabling illness or are not at risk of long-term disability (school-aged children, the elderly, and some persons with chronic diseases) would come last. Other groups whose health needs can be easily met and who can ben-

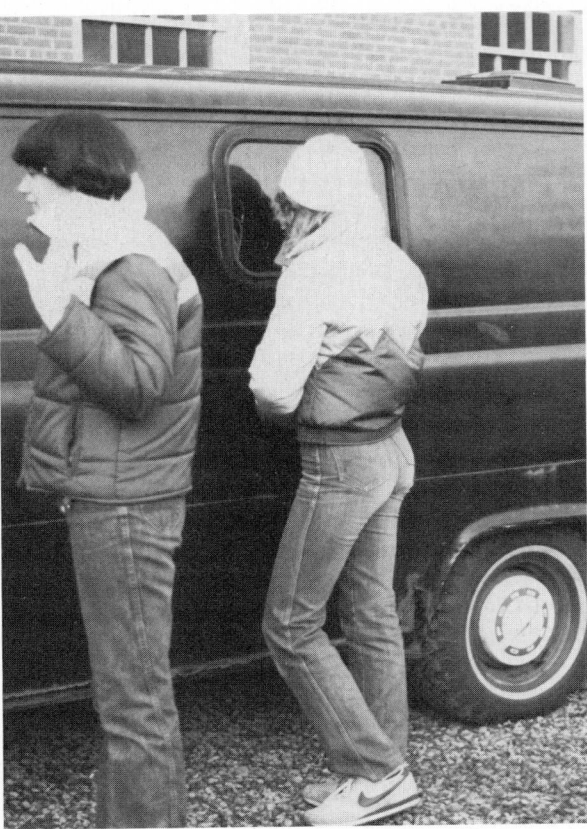

Fig. 4-5. Teenage populations have a low priority in the allocation of health and nursing resources.

efit the health of others (women with uncomplicated pregnancy, mothers with children under 2 years of age) may also be accorded a high priority in this system.

This approach has a decided utilitarian twist to it and limits the access of some groups to nursing services according to their priority in the schema (Fig. 4-5). While it does distribute nursing resources according to who can benefit the most, some clients (such as dying cancer clients) wind up with no access to the system at all. This can hardly be considered just if we adopt the principle of justice (rather than a utilitarian principle of beneficence) as the guiding principle for distributing health goods.

As can be demonstrated by all of these various approaches to distributing nursing care resources, the moral requirements of justice create numerous conflicts of interest for health practitioners when it comes to specific choices.

APPLICATION OF ETHICS TO COMMUNITY HEALTH NURSING PRACTICE

The Priority of Ethical Principles

In community health nursing, ethical principles direct and guide nursing actions with individuals and aggregate groups. The professional ethic, in general, places a greater emphasis on the observance of the principles of autonomy and beneficence than the principle of justice in most nursing actions (Fry, 1982). For example, in the *Code for Nurses,* respect for the principle of autonomy is emphasized by such statements as "the nurse provides services with respect for human dignity and the uniqueness of the client," that "each client has the moral right to determine what will be done with his/her person," and that "the nurse's respect for the worth and dignity of the individual human being applies irrespective of the nature of the health problem" (American Nurses' Association, 1976, pp. 4,5). All of these statements indicate a high respect for client autonomy or claim that the nurse has a strong, primary duty to respect the client's right to self-determination.

The ethical principle of beneficence is given slightly less emphasis in the *Code for Nurses.* For example, the code claims that "the nurse's primary commitment is to the client's care and safety"; also "The nurse safeguards the client's right to privacy by judiciously protecting information of a confidential nature," and "It is the responsibility of the nurse to advise clients against the use of dangerous products. This is seen as discharge of nursing functions when undertaken in the best interest of the client" (American Nurses' Association, 1976, pp. 8, 6, 18). Acts of beneficence may even include overriding the autonomy of individuals in the interests of other clients. The *Code for Nurses* describes the occurrence of this nursing action when "The nurse must also recognize those situations in which individual rights to self-determination in health care may temporarily be altered for the common good" (American Nurses' Association, 1976, p. 4).

However, the principle of justice is not strongly emphasized in the professional code of ethics. It is noted in passing that nursing practice is not influenced by age, sex, race, color, personality, or other personal attributes or individual differences in customs, beliefs, or attitudes. The code also states that "The nurse adheres to the principle of nondiscriminatory, nonprejudicial care in every employment setting or situation and endeavors to promote its acceptance by others," and ". . . the nurse's readiness to . . . render or obtain needed services should not be limited by the setting, whether nursing care is given in an acute care hospital, nursing home, drug or alcoholic treatment center, prison, pa-

tient's home, or other setting" (American Nurses' Association, 1976, p. 5). It is clear that these statements related to the moral requirements of the principle of justice are not as strong as those related to the moral requirements of the principles of autonomy and beneficence.

In community health nursing, nursing actions are guided not only by the professional ethic and its priority of ethical principles; the *public health ethic,* which has a different priority of principles, exerts considerable influence as well. This ethic is strongly modeled on the priority of the principle of beneficence and follows the rule of utility in disease detection and prevention and in health maintenance (Beauchamp, D. E., 1976; Shindell, 1980). This emphasis certainly influences the practice of community health nursing as is evidenced by the recent statement of the definition and role of public health nursing from the Public Health Nursing Section, American Public Health Association (1980). In this statement public health nursing accomplishes its goal of improving the health of the community by identifying aggregates and by moving "away from solely meeting the needs of consumers as individually presented and toward practicing public health nursing for the 'sum' of individuals or families within the program" (American Public Health Association, 1980, p. 9).

This statement indicates an orientation in community health nursing toward following a rule of utility in matters of health pertaining to clients. The needs of aggregates as groups of individuals is determined for the purpose of providing net benefit to population groups over possible health harms. This emphasis on the moral requirements of the principle of beneficence does not align with the highly individualistic respect-for-client-autonomy emphasis of the *Code for Nurses.*

Accountability in Community Health Nursing

Moral accountability in nursing practice means that nurses are answerable for how they promote, protect, and meet the health needs of clients while respecting individual rights to self-determination in health care. In community health nursing, where the greater emphasis is on aggregates rather than individual clients, moral accountability means being answerable for how the health of aggregate groups has been promoted, protected, and met (Fig. 4-6). Thus meeting accountability requirements in community health nursing will be different than meeting accountability requirements in other spheres of nursing practice.

For example, whereas the professional ethic clearly indicates that nurses are morally accountable for how they respect the client's right to self-determination and provide health services with respect for "the unique-

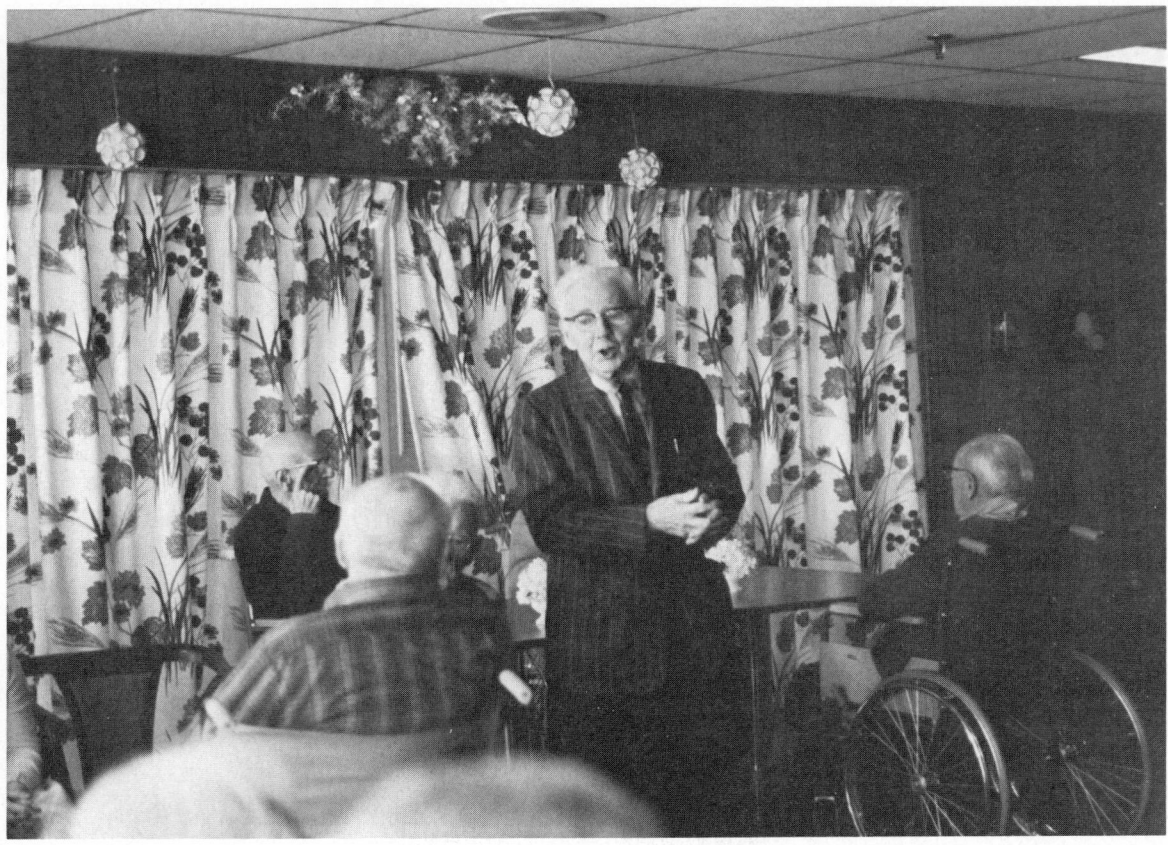

Fig. 4-6. Community health nurses are accountable for the health of aggregate groups such as the elderly in a nursing home.

ness of the client," the application of this ethic in community health nursing indicates that community nurses are morally accountable for how they provide health services so as to maximize total net health in population groups. It further indicates that they are accountable for demonstrating the increased health of aggregate groups through various research methods and studies while containing costs (Schlotfeldt, 1976). This is the meaning of accountability in community health nursing. Rather than being primarily accountable for how the moral requirements of the principle of autonomy are met, the community health nurse is primarily accountable for how the moral requirements of the principle of beneficence are met by nursing services.

The moral requirements of the principles of autonomy and justice are still important in community health nursing. Yet they are less important than the requirements of the principle of beneficence. In community health nursing, the emphasis of the professional ethic is slanted toward benefit to aggregates, which implies following a rule of utility in planning, implementing, and evaluating community health nursing services.

Future Directions

The emphasis on the moral requirements of a principle of beneficence in community health nursing has two implications. The first implication is heralded by the position paper, *The Definition and Role of Public Health Nursing in the Delivery of Health Care,* which defines public health nursing as deriving its theoretical direction from both the public health sciences and professional nursing theories and has as its goal "improving the health of the entire community" (American Public Health Association, 1980, p. 4). If this is how community health nursing is to be defined, then it is important that the planning, implementation, and evaluation of nursing services in the community be clearly differentiated from the provision of nursing services in other spheres of health care delivery. While community health nursing is a synthesis of both the sciences of public health and nursing (Archer, 1982), there needs to be a clear understanding of how the ethical components of professional practice, including the observance of clients' rights and professional responsibilities, are considered in the provision of nursing services. There is also a need for clarity and agreement on the priority of ethical principles in community health nursing. The goal of improving the health of the entire community by identifying aggregates and directing resources to them indicates an orientation toward meeting health needs according to the rule of utility. Is the ethical principle of beneficence the principle that should primarily guide community health nursing practice? Clearly, the moral underpinnings of community health nursing need to be given careful consideration in any statement defining the role of the discipline.

The second implication concerns the evaluation of accountability in community health nursing practice. Just as community health nursing has been affected by changes in both the health care delivery system and nursing practice in recent years, accountability requirements have likewise been affected by changes in public and professional expectations and the scope of nursing practice. For example, the expanded role of the nurse has increased the legal accountability of the nurse practitioner who is certified to function as an independent care giver. Thus there is a current and future need for periodic assessment of the moral and legal requirements of accountability in community nursing services.

There is also the need to determine how accountability will be measured in community health nursing and how existing programs and services will be evaluated to determine the effectiveness of various nursing services in meeting accountability requirements. This is a task that has yet to be accomplished by today's community health nursing leaders.

SUMMARY

The practice of community health nursing is influenced by both traditional ethics of professional nursing and the aggregate focus of community health. In providing nursing care services to individuals as well as aggregate groups within the community, the nurse must necessarily balance both of these influences. Clients' rights to equal access to health care services as well as aggregate groups' needs and interests in matters of health will often compete for the attention and services of the practicing community health nurse. Thus the nurse must become familiar with the moral requirements of the practice of nursing in general and the practice of community health nursing in particular.

Community health nursing practice, as a synthesis of both public health science and nursing science, is theoretically responsive to our prevailing ideas of social justice and the methods of distributing health care resources as chosen by the community. Yet community

health nursing practice, as a composite of the individualistic ethic of nursing and the aggregate ethic of public health, is also responsive to the moral requirements of ethical principles as prioritized within these ethics. How the individual community health nurse and community health nursing services view these moral requirements may well determine the future direction and influence of the discipline in meeting the health needs of communities.

BIBLIOGRAPHY

American Hospital Association: Statement on a patient's bill of rights, Hospitals **47:**41, Feb. 16, 1973.

American Nurses' Association: Code for nurses with interpretive statements, Kansas City, Mo., 1976, The Association.

American Public Health Association, Public Health Nursing Section: The definition and role of public health nursing practice in the delivery of health care: a statement of the public health nursing section, Washington, D.C., Nov. 1980, The Association.

Annas, G.J.: Patients' rights movement. In Reich, W.T., editor: Encyclopedia of bioethics, vol. 3, New York, 1978, The Free Press, pp. 1201-1205.

Archer, S.E.: Synthesis of public health science and nursing science, Nurs. Outlook **30:**442-46, Sept.-Oct. 1982.

Baier, K.: The moral point of view, Ithaca, N.Y., 1958, Cornell University Press.

Beauchamp, D.E.: Public health and social justice, Inquiry **13:**3-14, March 1976.

Beauchamp, D.E.: Public health and individual liberty, Ann. Rev. Pub. Health **1:**121-36, 1980.

Beauchamp, T.L., and Childress, J.F.: Principles of biomedical ethics, New York, 1979, Oxford Press.

Beauchamp, T.L., and Faden, R.R.: The right to health and the right to health care, J. Med. Philos. **4:**118-31, June 1979.

Beauchamp, T.L., and Walters, L.: Patients' rights and professional responsibilities. In Beauchamp, T.L., and Walters, L., editors: Contemporary issues in bioethics, Belmont, Calif., 1978, Wadsworth Publishing Co.

Bell, N.K.: The scarcity of medical resources: are there rights to health care? J. Med. Philos. **4:**158–69, June 1979.

Berthold, J.S.: Advancement of science and technology while maintaining human rights and values, Nurs. Res. **18:**514-22, Nov.-Dec. 1969.

Brockington, C.: A short history of public health, London, 1956, Churchill.

Capron, A.M.: Right to refuse medical treatment. In Reich, W.T., editor: Encyclopedia of bioethics, vol. 4, New York, 1978, The Free Press, pp. 1498-1507.

Carney, R.S.: Theological ethics. In Reich, W.T., editor: Encyclopedia of bioethics, vol. 1, New York, 1978, The Free Press, pp. 429-437.

Daniels, N.: Rights to health care and distributive justice: programmatic worries, J. Med. Philos. **4:**174-91, June 1979.

Department of Health, Education, and Welfare, Commission on Medical Malpractice: Report of the secretary's commission on medical malpractice, vols. 2, DHEW Pub. Nos. (OS) 73-88, (OS) 73-89, Washington, D.C., 1973, U.S. Government Printing Office.

Feinberg, J.: Social philosophy, Englewood Cliffs, N.J., 1973, Prentice-Hall Inc.

Frankena, W.K.: Ethics, Englewood Cliffs, N.J., 1973, Prentice-Hall Inc.

Fried, C.: Right and wrong, Cambridge, Ma., 1978, Harvard University Press.

Fry, S.T.: Accountability in research: the relationship of scientific and humanistic values, Adv. Nurs. Sci. **4:**1-13, 1981.

Fry, S.T.: Ethical principles in nursing education and practice: a missing link in the unification issue, Nurs. Health Care **3:**363-68, Sept. 1982.

Gaylin, W.: The patient's bill of rights, Sat. Rev. Sci. **1:**22, Feb. 24, 1973.

Gert, B., and Culver, C.M.: The justification of paternalism. In Robison, W.L., and Pritchard, M.S., editors: Medical responsibility: paternalism, informed consent, and euthanasia, Clifton, N.J., 1979, Humana Press, pp. 1-14.

Gordis, L., and Gold, E.: Privacy, confidentiality, and the use of medical records in research, Science, **207:**153-56, Jan. 11, 1980.

Gortner, S.R.: Scientific accountability in nursing, Nurs. Outlook **22:**764-68, Nov. 1974.

Green, R.: Health care and justice in contract theory perspective. In Veatch, R.M., and Branson, R., editors: Ethics and health policy, Cambridge, Ma., 1976, Ballinger Publishing Co.

In re estate of Brooks, 32 I11. 2d 361, 205 N.E. 2d 435, 1965.

Kant, I.: Groundwork of the metaphysic of morals, New York, 1964, Harper & Row Publishers Inc. (Translated by H.J. Paton; originally published in 1785.)

Kelsey, J.L.: Privacy and confidentiality in epidemiological research involving patients, IRB **3:**1-4, Feb. 1981.

MacIntyre, A.: Utilitarianism and cost-benefit analysis. In Beauchamp, T.L., and Bowie, N.E., editors: Ethical theory and business, Englewood Cliffs, N.J., 1979, Prentice-Hall Inc.

MacIntyre, A.: After virtue, Notre Dame, Ind., 1981, University of Notre Dame Press.

Milio, N.: The care of health in communities: access for outcasts, New York, 1975, Macmillan Publishing Co. Inc.

Mill, J.S.: Utilitarianism, New York, 1957, The Bobbs-Merrill Co. Inc. (Edited by O. Priest; originally published in 1863.)

National Commission for the Protection of Human Subjects of Biomedical and Behavioral Research: The Belmont report: ethical principles and guidelines for the protection of human subjects of research, DHEW Pub. No. (OS) 78-0012, Washington, D.C., 1978.

Nozick, R.: Anarchy, state, and utopia, New York, 1974, Basic Books Inc. Publishers.

Palmer, I.S.: Florence Nightingale: reformer, reactionary, researcher, Nurs. Res. **26:**84-89, March-April 1977.

Popoff, D.: What are your feelings about death and dying? Part 1, Nursing **5:**15-24, 1975.

Public Law 92-603, Social Security amendments of 1972, 92nd Congress, Oct. 30, 1972.

Public Law 92-278, The national sickle cell anemia, Cooley's anemia, Tay-Sachs and genetic disease act, Title IV, 90 stat., Section 410, 1976.

Rawls, J.: A theory of justice, Cambridge, Mass., 1971, Harvard University Press.

Rosen, G.: Preventive medicine in the United States: 1900-1975, New York, 1975, Science History Publishers.

Ross, W.D.: The right and the good, Oxford, 1930, Oxford University Press.

Schlotfeldt, R.M.: Accountability: a critical dimension in health care, Health Care Dimen. **3:**137-48, 1976.

Shindell, S.: Legal and ethical aspects of public health. In Last, J.M., editor: Maxcy-Rosenau public health and preventive medicine, ed. 11, New York, 1980, Appleton-Century-Crofts, pp. 1834-1845.

Smith, C.S.: Outrageous or outraged: a nurse advocate story, Nurs. Outlook **28:**624-25, Oct. 1980.

Szasz, T.: The right to health. In Gorovitz, S., et al., editors: Moral problems in medicine, Englewood Cliffs, N.J., 1976, Prentice-Hall Inc.

Tarasoff, V.: *Regents of The University of California,* 131 Cal. Rptr. 14, 551 P.2d 334, 1976.

UNESCO: Human rights, a symposium, New York, 1949, Allan Wingate.

Veatch, R.M.: Death, dying, and the biological revolution, New Haven, Conn., 1976, Yale University Press.

Veatch, R.M.: Truth-telling: attitudes. In Reich, W. T., editor: Encyclopedia of bioethics, vol. 4, New York, 1978, The Free Press, pp. 1677-1682.

Veatch, R.M.: A theory of medical ethics, New York, 1981, Basic Books Inc. Publishers.

Will, G.F.: The killing will not stop, The Washington Post, April 22, 1982, p. A-29.

Williams, C: Community health nursing: what is it? Nurs. Outlook **25:**250-52, 1977.

World Health Organization: The first ten years of the World Health Organization, New York, 1958, WHO.

Chapter
5

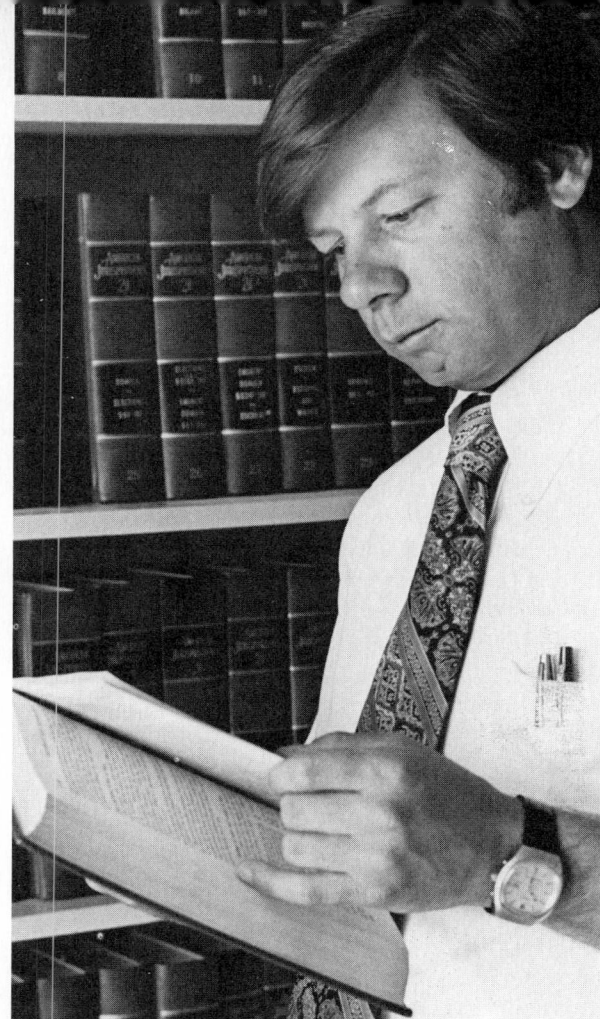

CYNTHIA NORTHROP

GOVERNMENT AND LEGAL INFLUENCES ON THE PRACTICE OF COMMUNITY HEALTH NURSING

Community health nurses are an integral part of the health care system and are significantly affected by the government and the legal system. This chapter will provide descriptions of these institutions, including organization and primary functions of governments, governmental regulation, and professional self-regulation. The chapter concludes with an overview of laws affecting community health nursing practice.

GOVERNMENT ROLE IN HEALTH CARE

Many nurses who select community health nursing as an area of practice are intrigued by the interdependence of law, health, nursing practice, and government.

They often seek additional coursework beyond their initial degree and unique work experiences to further their understanding of how law and government relate to health care.

An understanding can be gained from one major body of literature, that of political science. Within this field one can gain insight into how government, law, philosophy and political viewpoints have emerged as important factors in our health care system and how they have greatly shaped the care that is delivered. For example, when the U.S. Constitution was created, the writers shaped and envisioned a system of government that would support and promote the general welfare of its citizens.

The Constitution, a primary source of law, defines the powers and abilities not only of the branches of government (legislative, judicial, and executive) but also of the different levels of government (federal, state, and local). All community health nurses should read the Constitution in order to understand their role better.

Government as Democracy

The essence of our American government is linked to two key concepts: equality and consent of the people. Dahl (1972), a leading writer on democracy in the United States, describes these concepts in great detail. Government activities in the health care arena can only be carried out if those actions reflect these concepts. As will be highlighted later, Congress has enacted laws, for example, which involve the issue of equal access for Americans to health care services. It is a constitutional grant of power which enabled Congress to enact such a law. Such must be the case with each federal law; it must be grounded in a power found in the U.S. Constitution.

Democracy functions as a delicate balance between levels and branches of government and between governments and individuals. Individuals have certain rights and governments have certain powers; the governments themselves are set up as a system of checks and balances. Possessing rights and powers carries responsibilities as well. Individuals may participate in democracy in many ways, including voting, lobbying, leading, and representing. Change within a democratic system is inevitable as individuals and human needs change and vary.

Fig. 5-1 shows the key components of the U.S. government. A very complex system, the federal government includes a legislative, executive, and judicial branch. As created by the U.S. Constitution, this governmental structure of three branches consists of multiple subcomponents. The executive branch alone has 13 cabinet departments and over 70 independent agencies.

Table 5-1 is a summary of the functions and powers of the three branches of the U.S. government. The federal government is granted specific powers in the Constitution and all other powers are left to the states. The Tenth Amendment to the U.S. Constitution says that the federal governmental powers are limited and explicit powers. Any action taken by the federal government must be justified within the U.S. Constitution. Selected powers of each branch of the federal government are listed in Table 5-1. These powers generally include making laws and regulations, setting policy, interpreting and enforcing laws, and coordinating the efforts of federal activities including preparation of a budget.

State and local governments are also organized into three branches: legislative, judicial, and executive. Each state has its own constitution that provides the framework of powers and privileges within that jurisdiction. Because federal powers are explicit, state powers are much broader in nature. The system of government was designed so that states were given all other powers not explicitly mentioned as federal powers. Therefore, a limitation on the federal government is state power. Another limitation would be the statements in the Bill of Rights reaffirming to individuals certain guarantees. These rights limit the power of state, local, and federal governments. For example, the Fourth Amendment limits governmental action by granting the right against unreasonable searches and seizures. Notice that the individual right does not prohibit government action entirely but requires governments to act with reason. Hence, the individual right is not absolute but does place a limitation and restraint on governmental activities. Also notice that although the Bill of Rights is attached to the federal constitution, the Fourteenth Amendment says that these rights are limitations on state governments as well. No state shall make or enforce any law that shall abridge the privileges or immunities of citizens.

The Constitution, governments, and individuals are the primary factors in the democratic system in the United States. Including the impact of political parties which will be discussed later, all such factors form a pluralistic approach to the governmental role in health care and other parts of our society. Each factor expresses an opinion as to what the role should be. Each contributes to the shape of that role.

Legal Basis for Governmental Role in Health Care

One of the first constitutional challenges to congressional legislation in the area of health and welfare came in 1937. Although Congress had created other health programs, the challenge to its legal basis for doing so did not arise until it established unemployment compensation and old-age benefits. The Supreme Court decided that such federal government action was within congressional powers to promote the general welfare found in Article I, Section 8, of the U.S. Constitution. Most legal bases for congressional action in health care are found in Section 8. They include the following:

1. Provide for the general welfare
2. Regulate commerce among the several states
3. Raise funds to support the military
4. Provide spending power

These statements within Section 8 of Article I have been interpreted by the Courts to include a wide variety of federal powers and activities.

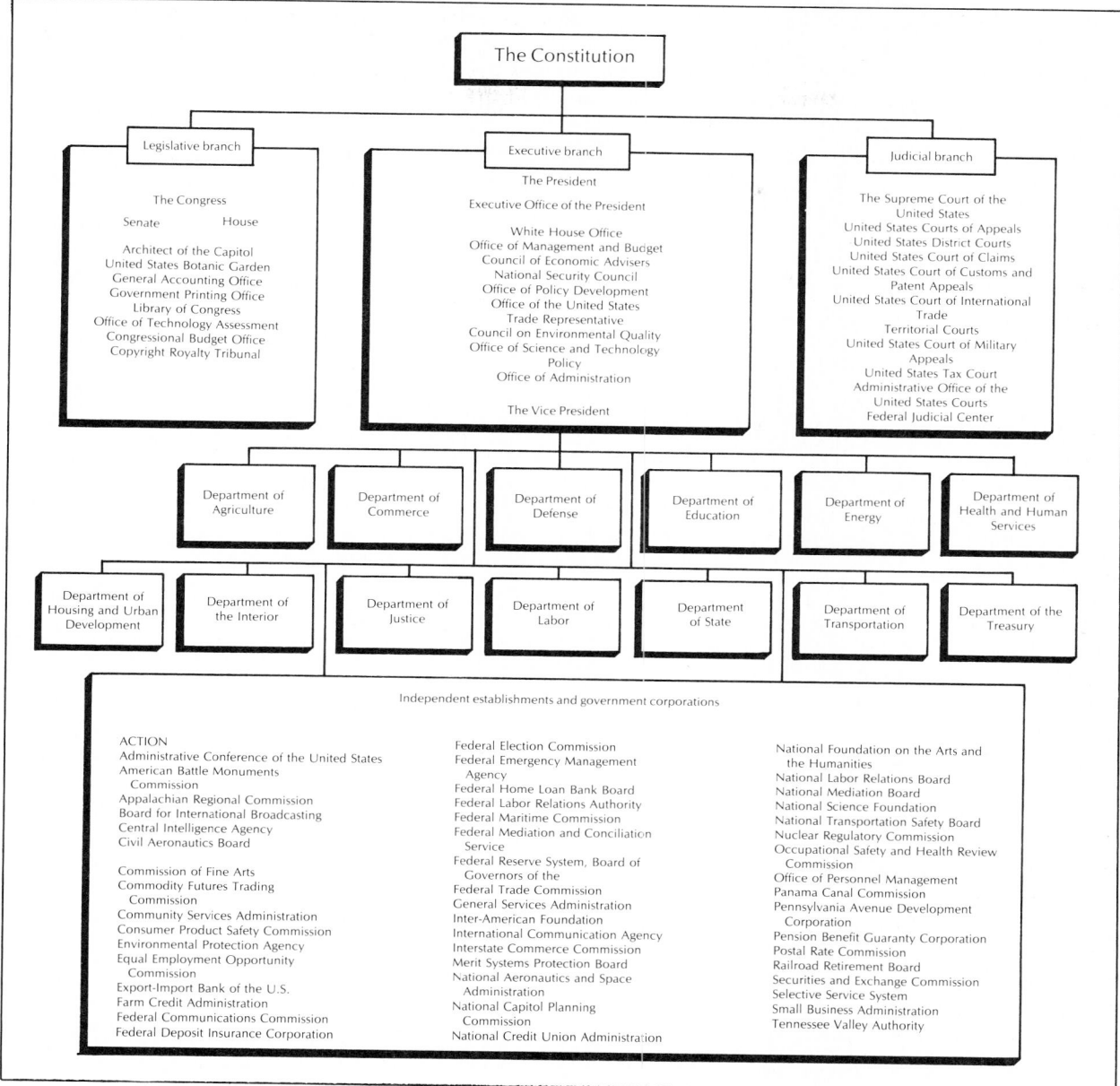

Fig. 5-1. Key components of the government of the United States. (From Office of Federal
Register: United States Government Manual, Washington, D.C., 1981, U.S. Government Printing
Office, p. 813.)

The legal basis for state and local activities in the
area of health does not require the identification of an
explicit power within a state constitution. Most state
power than has to do with health care is referred to as
the state's police power. This broad power means that
states may act to protect the health, safety, and welfare
of their citizens. Such police power must be reasonably
exercised, and the state must demonstrate that it has a
compelling interest in taking actions, especially those
actions that might infringe on individual rights.

An example of a state exercising its police powers is
that of a state legislature requiring immunization of
children before school admission. The state's reasonable actions must be to protect the health, safety, and
welfare of its citizens. In the immunization of preschool
children the state government is attempting to elimi-

Table 5-1. Summary of functions and powers of the three branches of U.S. government

Legislative branch	Judicial branch	Executive branch
All legislative (law-making) powers granted in the U.S. Constitution are vested in the Congress which consists of two bodies	The judicial (law-interpreting) power is vested in the Supreme Court and in Inferior Courts established by Congress	The executive (law-enforcing) power is vested in a president.
Senate	**Supreme Court**	**The President**
100 members (two from each state) 6-year terms (one third elected every 2 years)	Chief justice and 8 associate justices (9 members) Term each year is usually October to June	Head of the branch that includes the vice president and three executive departments; advised by the Cabinet, which consists of the heads of 13 departments
House of Representatives	**Inferior Courts** (Lower Courts)	**The Cabinet**
435 members (determined by population) 2-year terms	U.S. Courts of Appeals (all states and territories are assigned to one) U.S. District Courts (determined by population) Territorial Courts Special Courts (i.e., Claims, Tax, Customs, and Patents)	Agriculture Commerce Defense Education Energy Health and Human Services Housing and Urban Development Interior Justice, Attorney General Labor State Transportation Treasury
Selected powers of Congress Assess and collect taxes Regulate commerce Coin money Establish post offices and post roads Establish courts inferior to Supreme Court Declare war Raise and maintain an army and navy Make laws necessary and proper for carrying out above powers Make amendments	*Selected powers of these courts* Hear and decide cases within their jurisdiction (delineated in the Constitution) Make rules of procedure	*Selected powers of the President* Those granted by Congress Management of structure and budget of the executive branch Issuing of executive orders, plans, and initiatives

nate communicable diseases and to prevent death and disability. These goals involve activities that protect the health, safety, and welfare of state citizens.

Trends and Shifts in Government Roles

Governmental involvement in health care at both the state and federal level began gradually. Many historical events align closely with the role that has developed. Wars, economic instability, depression, plurality of viewpoints, and political parties all have shaped the governmental role. Postdepression plans to revive the country, Roosevelt's New Deal, established major precedents for government spending on health care for Americans. In 1930 federal laws were passed to promote the public health of merchant seamen and American Indians. The Social Security Act of 1935 was a substantial piece of legislation, which has grown since that time to include not only the aged and unemployed but survivors' insurance for widows and children, child welfare, health department grants, and maternal and child health projects. In 1934 Senator Wagner of New York initiated the first national health insurance bill. Today debate still continues on the extent of governmental responsibilities in health care.

Before the 1930s the only major governmental action relating to health was the creation of the Public Health Service in 1798. The Department of Health and Human Services (DHHS), known until 1979 as the Department of Health, Education, and Welfare (DHEW), was not created until 1953. It had a small predecessor that was established in 1941, the Office of Defense, Health, and Welfare Services. In 1946 Congress enacted a mental health bill and the Hospital Survey and Construction Act and created the National Institutes of Health. These legislative acts created entities that became part of the executive branch, now within the DHHS.

In a democracy, what governments should and can do for the citizens in the area of health care depends on the beliefs of those citizens. Strong beliefs of self-determination and self-sufficiency mixed with beliefs about social responsibilities are hallmarks of a pluralistic approach to solving societal problems. Political party platforms provide the best example for demonstrating how different beliefs yield different approaches to problems. Appendix H contains the 1980 national political party platforms on health. These statements from Democrats and Republicans give their views of what governments should be doing in health. Goldsmith (1973) studied 12 health platforms written by these two parties between 1948 and 1968 and found them to be predictable of future governmental direction in health care. In particular, Goldsmith stated that the platform pointed to areas of future health legislation. He recommended that influential health policy leaders in each party be identified and that health care providers and others examine the party platforms.

The two statements on health in Appendix H reflect differences in beliefs about governmental involvement. For example, the Democrats strongly support a national health insurance program and have identified its major characteristics. The Republicans reject all proposals for compulsory national health insurance. On the other hand, both parties support alternatives to institutional care. The 1980 elections brought into office a Republican president and a majority of Republican senators. This represented a shift not only in party control but in viewpoint. Changes in viewpoint of those making, enforcing, and interpreting law directly relate to the priorities and actions taken by government.

A major thrust of the 1980 Republican administration was to shift federal government activities to the states. Therefore, many of the federal functions are being given to states. Control and regulation of programs in some instances are being shifted to the state and local governments without federal money to support them. States are dealing with the role changes in their own individual ways.

This shift of responsibilities from one level of government to another is no guarantee that, depending on future platforms and elections, other kinds of shifts will not occur. One example of a health program shifting

between states and federal government is Medicaid. The financial responsibility for Medicaid, one of the social and health care programs, is shifting. In past years Medicaid was financed equally by state and federal funds; changes in funding have increased the state's contribution greatly.

This discussion has focused primarily on trends and shifts among and within government levels. An additional aspect of governmental responsibilities is the relationship between government and individuals. Freedom of individuals must be balanced with government powers. Citizens also express their views of what amount of governmental interference will be tolerated. For example, the issue of sex education in public schools delineates at least two viewpoints on the governmental and individual relationship:

1. Since the government through the legislative branch established a system of education, some citizens believe that education should include content on sex
2. Some citizens believe sex education belongs in the family and should not be interfered with by a governmental body (public schools)

These are only two of the views expressed in the public literature. To summarize, is sex education an appropriate governmental power or should a parent be able to decide voluntarily when to teach his or her child about sex? Although many have strong feelings about this issue, the purpose of the example is to stress how responsibilities of governments and individuals can shift back and forth between them as well as between levels of government.

Major Governmental Health Care Functions

Although the amount and degree of health care functions that governments carry out may shift and vary, there are four general categories of functions:

1. Direct services
2. Financing
3. Information
4. Policy setting

These four functions are found at all levels of government—federal, state, and local.

Direct Services

Federal, state and local governments provide direct health services to individuals and groups based on certain criteria, although provision of direct services is not the major function of government in health care. Examples of this governmental function are provision of health care for American Indians, members and dependents of the military, veterans, and federal prisoners. State and local governments employ community health nurses to deliver services to individuals and families, usually based on financial need. However, state and local governments also may provide direct services to all individuals for particular purposes, such as hypertension screening, tuberculosis screening, and well-child immunizations. Health services are also provided for prisoners in local jails or state prisons by state and local governments.

Financing

Governments pay for health care services, training of personnel, and research. Financial support in all three areas has made a significant contribution and major impact on consumers and health care providers. State and federal governments finance the direct care of clients through Medicare, Medicaid and Social Security programs. Many nurses have been educated with government funds; schools of nursing have been built and equipped through federal capitation funds. Other health care providers have also been supported financially by governments. Finally, monies in the form of grants have been given by governments for specific research and demonstration projects. Probably one of the best known centers of medical research is the federally funded National Institutes of Health.

Information

All branches and levels of government at one time or the other have collected, analyzed, and made available data about health care and health status in this country. An example is the annual report, *Health: United States*, compiled by the DHHS (1981). Collection of vital statistics, including mortality and morbidity data, gathering of census data, and health care status surveys are all governmental activities. Table 5-2 lists available international and federal government data sources on the health status of the total U.S. population. These sources are available in government documents section in most large libraries.

Policy Setting

Policy setting, the last major category of government functions to be discussed, relates to all of the functions. Decisions about health care are made by the government at all levels and within all branches of government. Decisions that shape health care are policy-making and policy-setting activities. As mentioned earlier, governments often give financial support to one group of individuals rather than to another group. Such a decision influences health care resources for both groups and is a policy setting function of government as well. Health policy decisions usually have broad implications for economic growth, resource allocation, and development in the health care field. Examples of policy

Table 5-2. International and national sources of data on the health status of the U.S. population

Organization	Data source
International	
United Nations	Demographic Yearbook
World Health Organization	World Health Statistics Annual
Federal	
Public Health Service	National Vital Registration System
	National Survey of Family Growth
	National Health Interview Survey
	National Health Examination Survey
	National Health and Nutrition Examination Survey
	National Master Facility Inventory
	National Hospital Discharge Survey
	National Nursing Home Survey
	National Ambulatory Medical Care Survey
	Medical Specialist Supply Projections
	National Morbidity Reporting System
	U.S. Immunization Survey
	Surveys of Mental Health Facilities
	Estimates of National Health Expenditures
Department of Commerce	U.S. Census of Population
	Current Population Survey
	Population Estimates and Projections
Department of Labor	Consumer Price Index
	Employment and Earnings

setting include the Health Planning, Resources and Development Act and the Professional Standards Review Organization.

ORGANIZATION OF GOVERNMENTAL AGENCIES

Community health nurses are actively involved with many parts of the government. The structure in which governments function will be discussed in this part of the chapter. In addition, information about international organizations and their activities in the health care field will be included. Roles of community health nurses in different governmental agencies will be discussed.

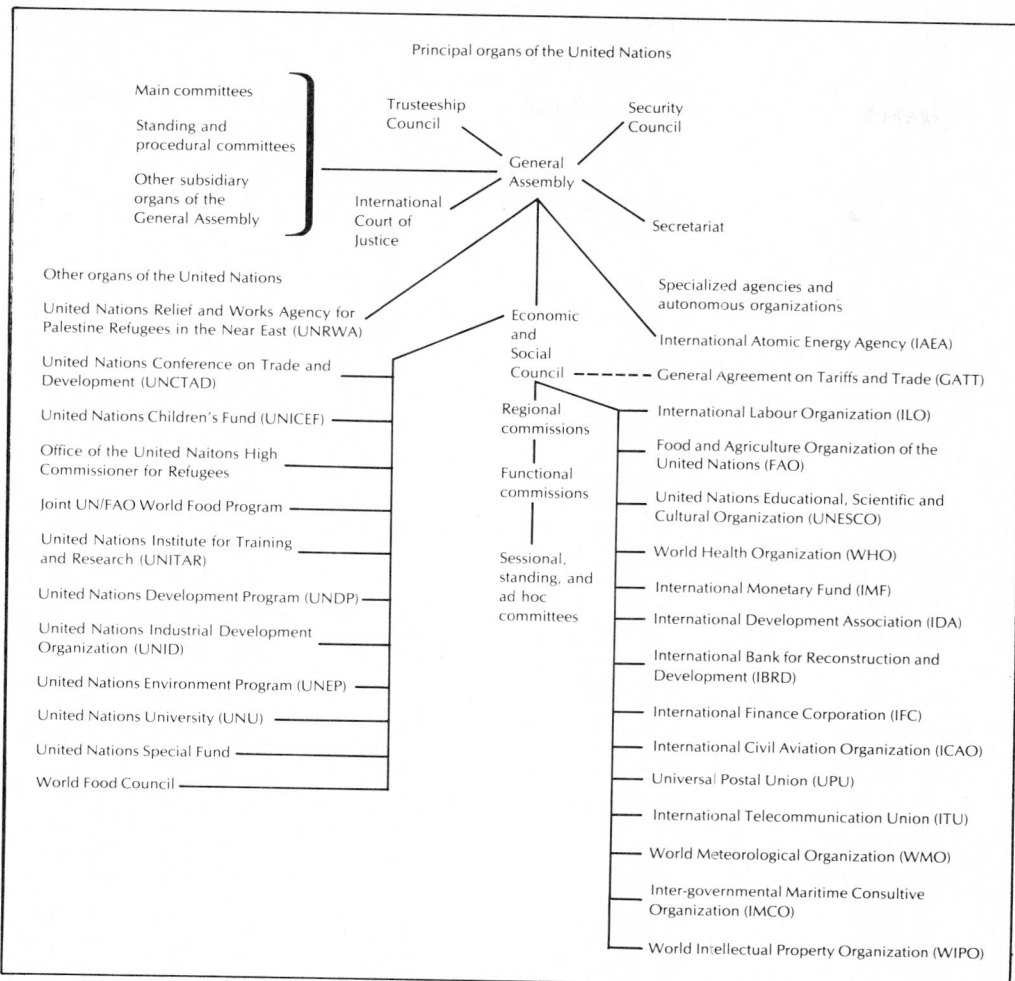

Principal organs of the United Nations

Fig. 5-2. The United Nations system (From United Nations: Basic facts about the U.N., New
York, 1977, UN.)

International Organizations

In June of 1945 many national governments joined
together to create an international organization, the
United Nations. Its charter describes its aims and goals.
Several goals deal with human rights, world peace, and
security, and promotion of economic and social advancement of all people. The United Nations (Fig. 5-2)
is headquartered in New York City and made up of six
principal organs. Several other organs and many specialized agencies and autonomous organizations are
also within the system. One of these special, autonomous organizations is the World Health Organization
(WHO).

Established in 1948, WHO relates to the United Nations through the Economic and Social Council. Its goal
is the attainment by all people of the highest possible
level of health. Headquartered at 20 Avenue Appia,
1211 Geneva, Switzerland, WHO is composed of three
main organs: the Assembly, Executive Board, and Secretariat. The Secretariat is described in detail in Fig. 5-
3. The organization has six regional offices. The office
for the Americas is located in Washington, D.C. It is
known as the Pan American Health Organization, or
PAHO. Glancing over Fig. 5-3 one can get an idea of
the variety of activities of this organization.

The World Health Assembly, to which all United
Nation members belong, meets annually. It is the
policy-making body of WHO. Consisting of 30 members elected by the assembly, the executive board meets
at least twice a year. WHO provides worldwide services
to promote health, cooperates with member countries
in their health efforts, and coordinates biomedical re-

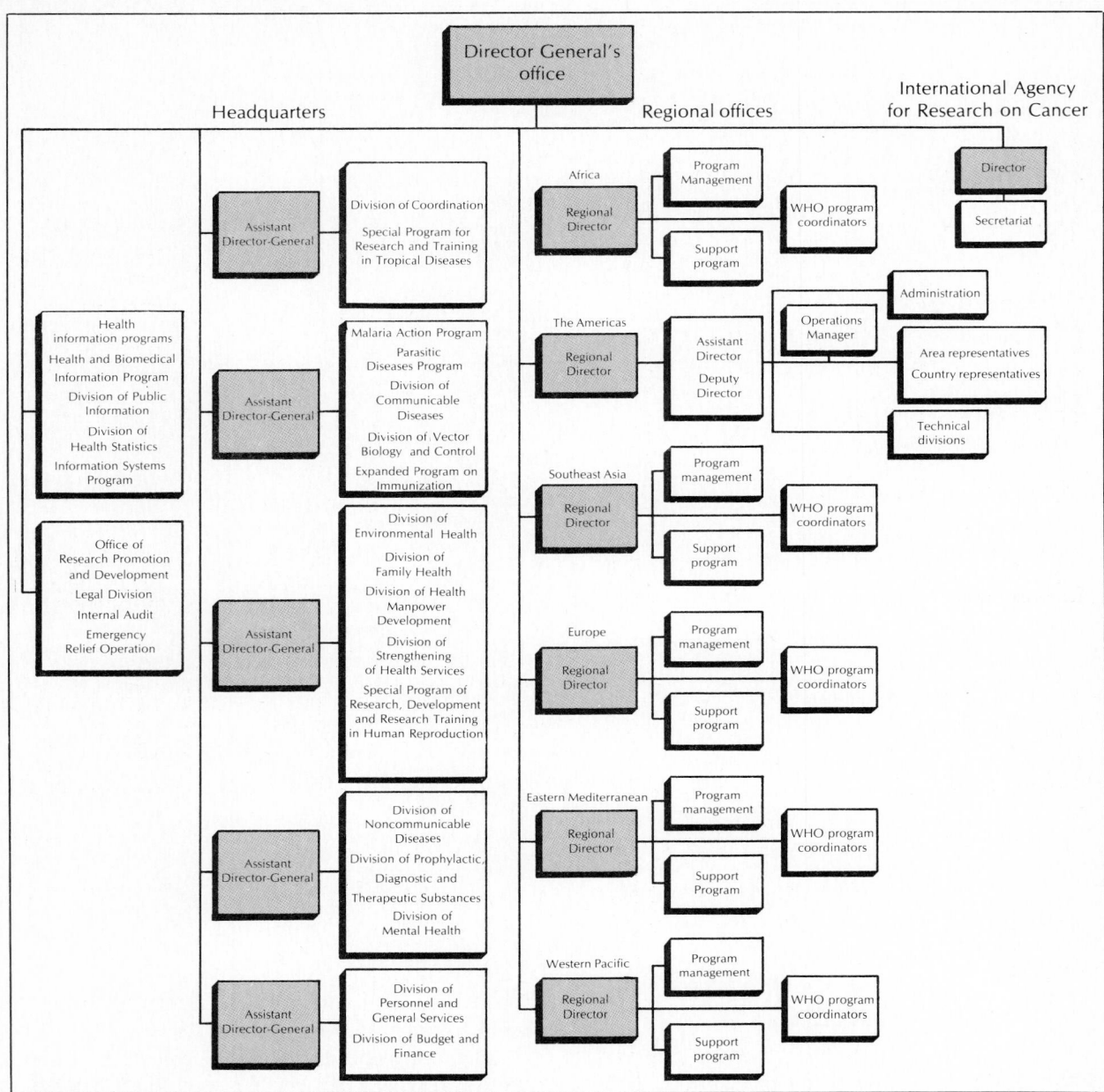

Fig. 5-3. Structure of the World Health Organization. (Used with permission of the Office of Publication, WHO, Geneva, 1982.)

search. Its services, which benefit all countries, include a day-to-day information service on the occurrence of internationally important diseases; publication of the international list of causes of disease, injury, and death; monitoring of adverse reactions to drugs; and establishment of world standards for antibiotics and vaccines. Assistance rendered to individual countries at their request includes support to national programs to fight disease, train health workers, and strengthen health services. An example of biomedical research collaboration is a special program for research in six widespread tropical diseases—malaria, leprosy, "snail-fever," filariasis, leishmaniasis and "sleeping sickness."

The number of community health nursing roles in international health are varied and growing. Besides offering direct health services, nurses serve as consul-

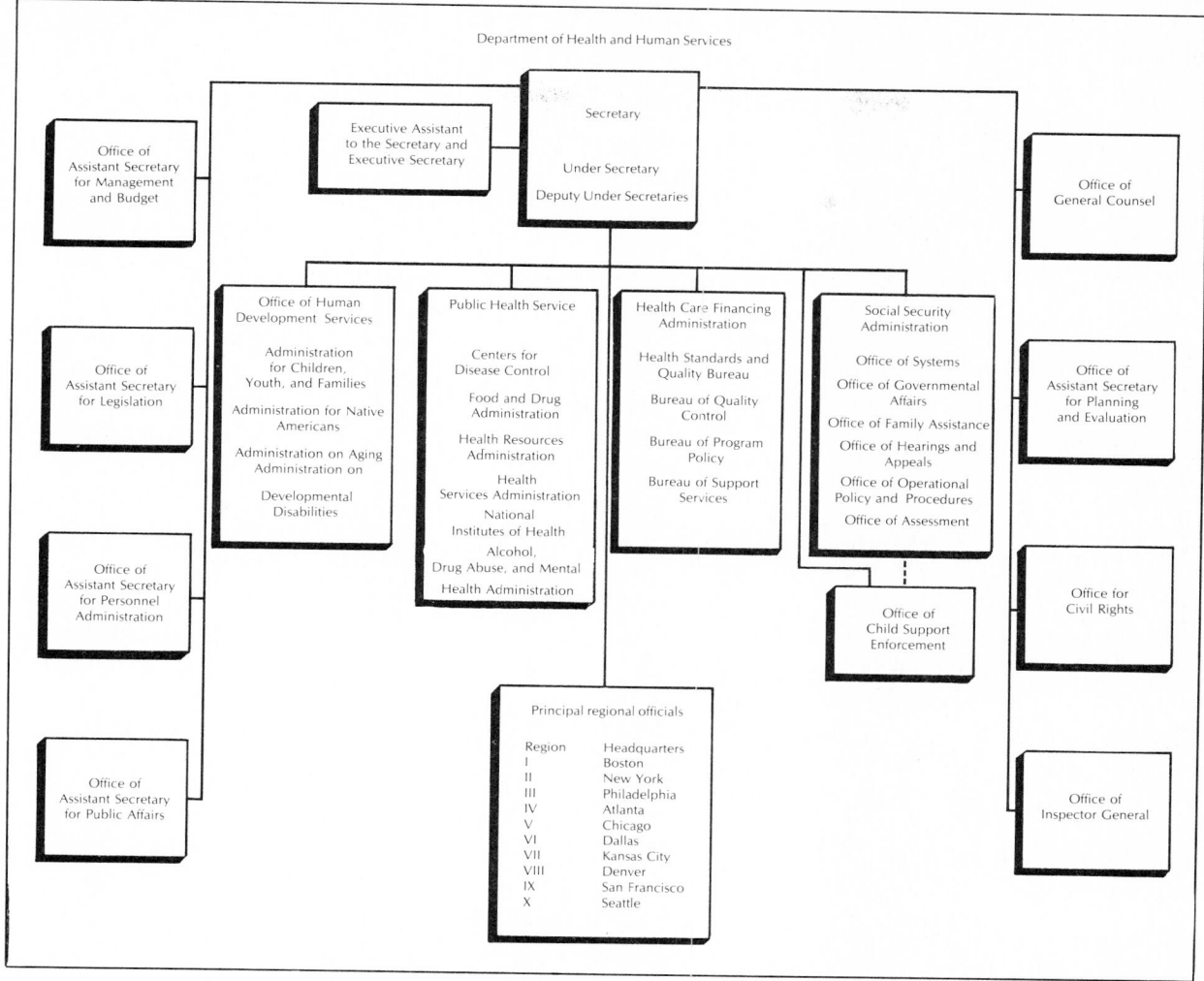

Department of Health and Human Services

Secretary
Under Secretary
Deputy Under Secretaries

Executive Assistant
to the Secretary and
Executive Secretary

Office of
Assistant Secretary
for Management
and Budget

Office of
General Counsel

Office of Human
Development Services

Administration
for Children,
Youth, and Families

Administration for Native
Americans

Administration on Aging
Administration on

Developmental
Disabilities

Public Health Service

Centers for
Disease Control

Food and Drug
Administration

Health Resources
Administration

Health
Services Administration
National
Institutes of Health
Alcohol,
Drug Abuse, and Mental
Health Administration

Health Care Financing
Administration

Health Standards and
Quality Bureau

Bureau of Quality
Control

Bureau of Program
Policy

Bureau of Support
Services

Social Security
Administration

Office of Systems
Office of Governmental
Affairs
Office of Family Assistance
Office of Hearings and
Appeals
Office of Operational
Policy and Procedures
Office of Assessment

Office of
Assistant Secretary
for Planning
and Evaluation

Office of
Assistant Secretary
for Legislation

Office of
Assistant Secretary
for Personnel
Administration

Office of
Child Support
Enforcement

Office for
Civil Rights

Office of
Assistant Secretary
for Public Affairs

Principal regional officials

Region	Headquarters
I	Boston
II	New York
III	Philadelphia
IV	Atlanta
V	Chicago
VI	Dallas
VII	Kansas City
VIII	Denver
IX	San Francisco
X	Seattle

Office of
Inspector General

Fig. 5-4. Organizational chart of the Department of Health and Human Services. (From Office of
Federal Register: *United States Government Manual*, Washington, D.C., 1981, U.S. Government
Printing Office, p. 830.)

tants, educators, and program planners and evaluators.
They focus their work on a variety of community
health concepts, including environment, sanitation,
communicable disease, wellness, and primary care.

Federal Agencies

Many federal agencies are involved in governmental
health care functions. Legislation passed by Congress
may be delegated to any agency within the executive
branch for implementation, surveillance, regulation,
and enforcement. Congress decides which agency will
monitor specific laws. For example, most health care
legislation is delegated to the DHHS. However, legislation on the environment or on occupational health
may be within another agency's realm, for example, the

Environmental Protection Agency or Labor Department. Examples of those most involved with health
care will be included in the following discussion.

Department of Health and Human Services

DHHS is the agency most concerned with people
and most involved with the human concerns of Americans. It touches more American lives than any other
federal agency. As mentioned earlier, it was created in
1953 as the Department of Health, Education, and
Welfare and renamed DHHS in 1979 when a separate
cabinet department, the Department of Education, was
established. The organizational chart of DHHS (Fig.
5-4) depicts an office of the Secretary and four principal
operating components: Social Security Administration,

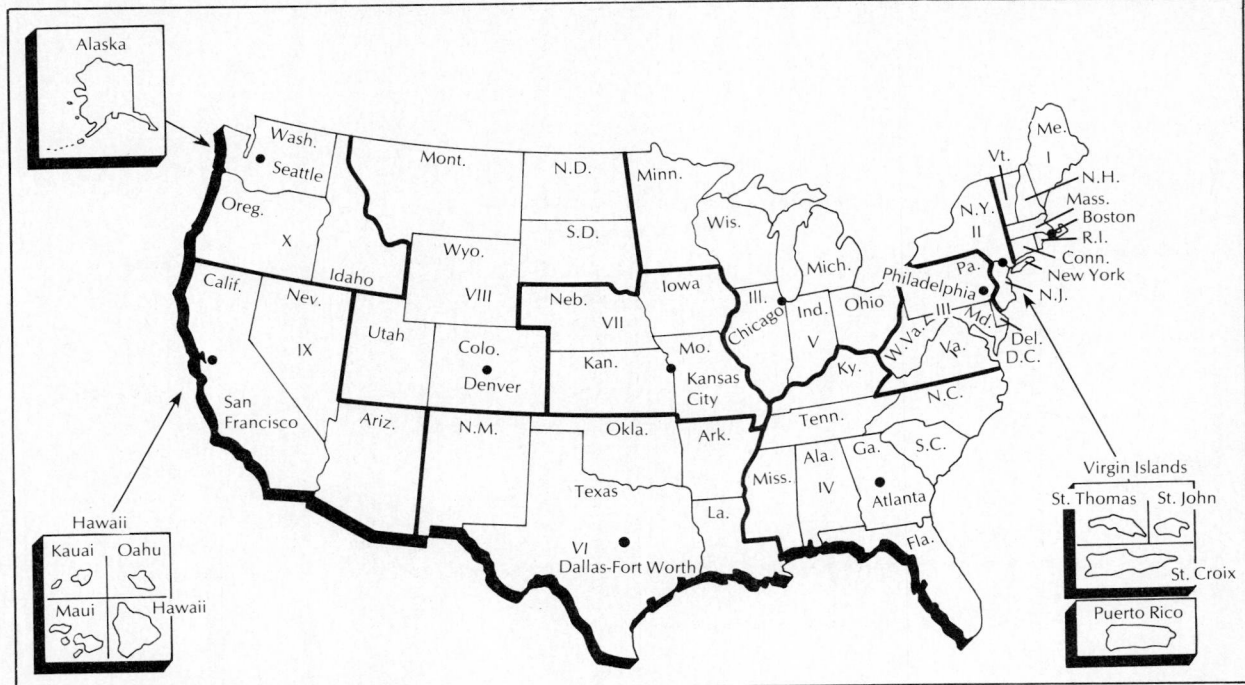

Fig. 5-5. Standard federal regions. (From Office of Federal Register: United States Government Manual, Washington, D.C., 1981, U.S. Government Printing Office, p. 867.)

Health Care Financing Administration, Office of Human Development Services, and the Public Health Service. The last component is highly involved with health care and health status of Americans. The 10 regional offices of DHHS are identified in Table 6 and further delineated in Fig. 5-5.

Public Health Service

The major components of the Public Health Service (PHS) include the following (Office of Federal Register, 1982):

1. Office of the Assistant Secretary for Health and Surgeon General
   a. National Center for Health Statistics
   b. National Center for Health Services Research
   c. National Center for Health Care Technology
2. Alcohol, Drug Abuse and Mental Health Administration
   a. National Institute on Alcohol Abuse and Alcoholism
   b. National Institute on Drug Abuse
   c. National Institute of Mental Health
3. Centers for Disease Control
   a. Epidemiology Program
   b. International Health Program
   c. Laboratory Improvement Program
   d. Center for Prevention Services
   e. Center for Environmental Health
   f. National Institute for Occupational Safety and Health
   g. Center for Health Promotion and Education

   h. Center for Professional Development and Training
   i. Center for Infectious Diseases
4. Food and Drug Administration
   a. Biologics
   b. Drugs
   c. Foods
   d. Radiological Health
   e. Veterinary Medicine
   f. Medical Devices
   g. Toxicological Research
   h. Regional Operations
5. Health Resources Administration
   a. Bureau of Health Professions
   b. Bureau of Health Facilities
   c. Bureau of Health Planning
6. Health Services Administration
   a. Bureau of Community Health Services
   b. Indian Health Services
   c. Bureau of Medical Services
   d. Bureau of Health Personnel Development and Service
7. National Institutes of Health
   a. National Cancer Institute
   b. National Heart, Lung, and Blood Institute
   c. National Library of Medicine
   d. National Institute of Arthritis, Metabolism, and Digestive Diseases
   e. National Institute of Allergy and Infectious Diseases
   f. National Institute of Child Health and Human Development

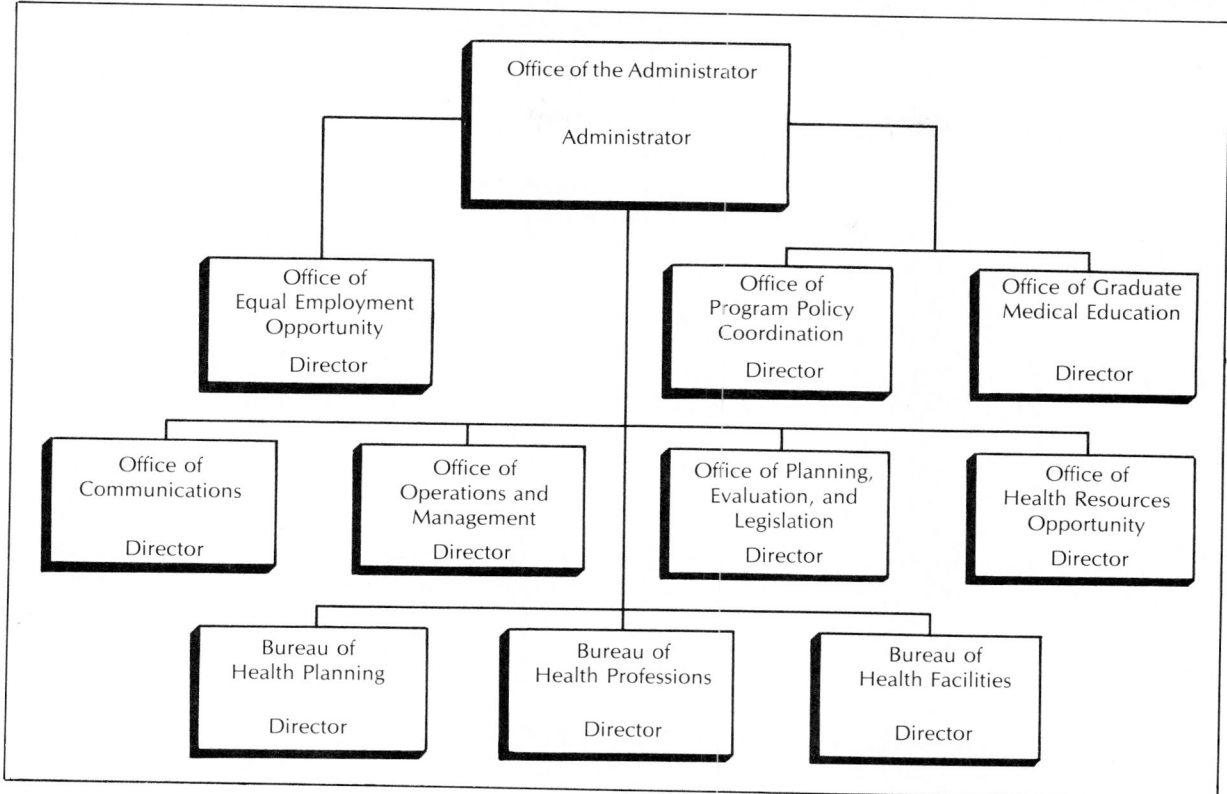

Fig. 5-6. Organizational chart of the Bureau of Health Resources Administration, Public Health
Service, Department of Health and Human Services (1982).

g. National Institute of Dental Research
h. National Institute of Environmental Health Sciences
i. National Institute of General Medical Sciences
j. National Institute of Neurological and Communicative Disorders and Stroke
k. National Eye Institute
l. National Institute on Aging
m. Clinical Center
n. Fogarty International Center
o. Division of Computer Research and Technology
p. Division of Research Resources
q. Division of Research Services
r. Division of Research Grants

The PHS has been a long-standing, significant contributor to the improved health status of Americans. The fifth component listed in the preceding list is the Health Resources Administration. Its components, including several offices and bureaus, are identified in Fig. 5-6. One of these bureaus particularly important to nursing is the Bureau of Health Professions, which is outlined in Fig. 5-7. Nursing and other health disciplines are part of this bureau. Medicine, dentistry, and nursing have divisions of their own. In addition, a divi-

sion exists for associated health professions. Fig. 5-8 is the organizational chart of the Division of Nursing. Jo Eleanor Elliott is the director of the division and holds the highest nursing position in the federal government.

The Division of Nursing has the following specific goals: (1) provides the professional nursing expertise and leadership required by the Bureau of Health Professions in planning, coordinating, evaluating, and supporting development and utilization of the nation's health work force resources; (2) supports and conducts programs on the development, use, quality, and awarding of credentials of nursing personnel, including registered nurses, practical or vocational nurses, and nursing aides; (3) in cooperation with others, assists state and local areas in planning, developing, and improving nursing services and educational programs; (4) conducts and supports programs related to the provision of nursing care to advance the health status of individuals, families, and communities; (5) engages with other bureau programs in cooperative efforts of research, development, and demonstration on the interrelationships between individual members of the health care team, their tasks, education requirements, and related train-

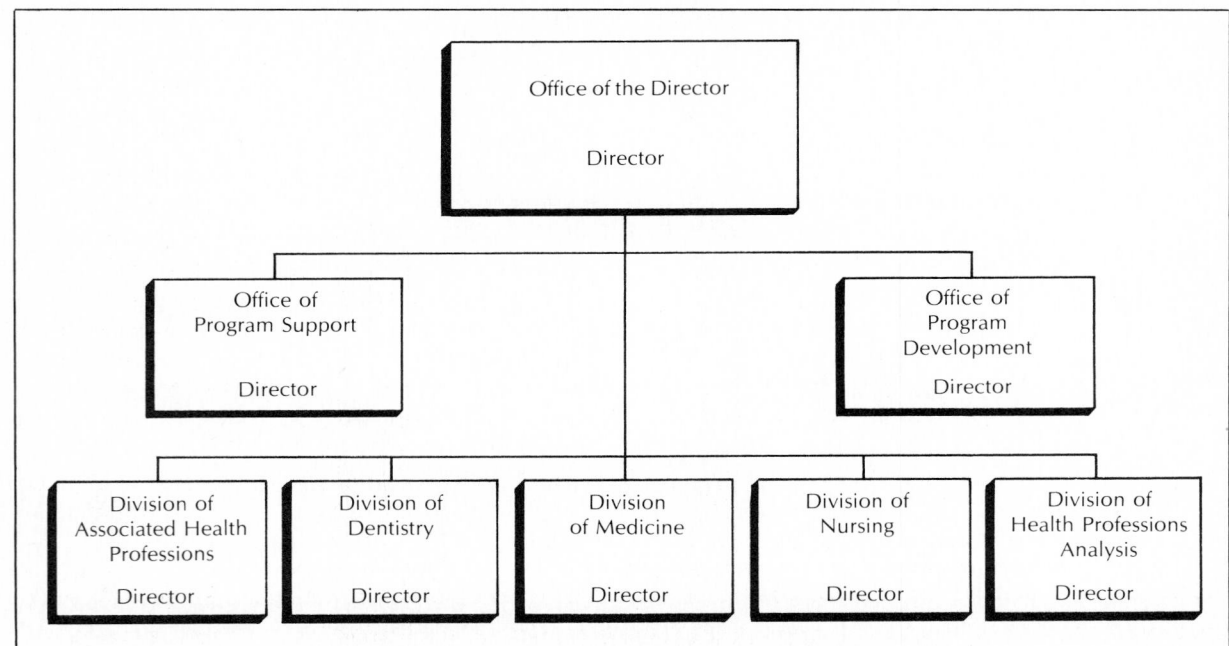

Fig. 5-7. Organizational chart of the Bureau of Health Professions, Public Health Service, Health Resources Administration, Department of Health and Human Services (1982).

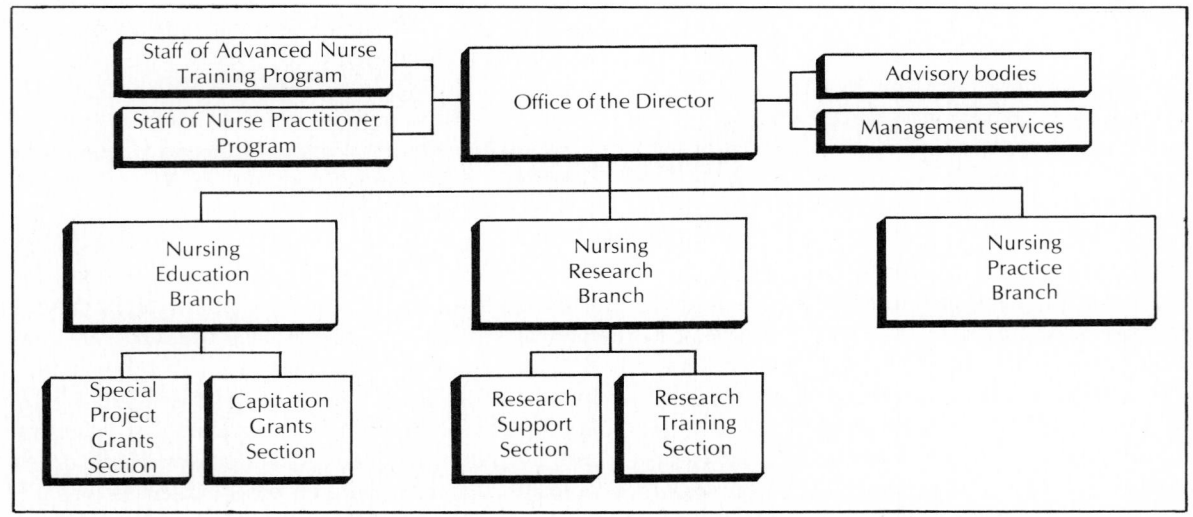

Fig. 5-8. Organizational chart of Division of Nursing (1982). Current director is Jo Eleanor Elliott.

ing modalities; (6) maintains liaison with health professional groups and others, including consumers, having common interest in the nation's capacity to deliver nursing services; (7) fosters, supports, and conducts projects to expand the scientific base of nursing practice and role reformulation and to develop and incorporate new knowledge into practice and education; and (8) provides consultation and technical assistance to public and private organizations, agencies, and institutions, including the PHS regional offices and other agencies of the federal government, on all aspects of nursing relevant to the division's functions (Division of Nursing, 1982).

Other Federal Government Agencies

DHHS has primary responsibility for federal health functions. However, the cabinet departments of the federal government have been delegated by Congress to carry out certain other health functions. Those departments that will be described in this chapter are Commerce, Defense, Labor, Agriculture, and Justice.

Department of Commerce. Within the Department of Commerce (DOC) is the Bureau of the Census, which carries out an information function in health care. Established in 1902, this bureau is responsible for taking a census of the population every 10 years. Information collected from individual persons and households is confidential and used only for statistical purposes. Also a part of the DOC is the National Oceanic and Atmospheric Administration, which provides special services in support of urban air quality control.

Department of Defense. The Department of Defense (DOD) delivers health care to members of the military and their dependents. The Assistant Secretary of Defense for Health Affairs administers the Civilian Health and Medical Program of the Uniformed Services (CHAMPUS). Established in 1974, CHAMPUS has the mission of delivering civilian health care services primarily for spouses and dependents of active, retired, or deceased service members. The departments within Defense (Army, Navy, Air Force & Marines) each have a surgeon general. Health services, including community health services for members of the military, are delivered by a Health Services Command in each department. In each command nurses of high military rank, including brigadier general, are part of the administration of health services.

Department of Labor. The Department of Labor has two administrations with health functions: Occupational Safety and Health Administration and the Mine Safety and Health Administration. Both are charged with writing safety and health standards and ensuring compliance in the work place, including inspections, investigation of complaints, and citations if necessary.

Each coordinates its activities with state departments of labor and of health.

Department of Agriculture. The Department of Agriculture is involved in health care primarily through administering the Food and Nutrition Service. Although plant, product, and animal inspection by the Department of Agriculture is also related to the health of Americans, the Food and Nutrition Service established in 1969, oversees a variety of food assistance activities. In collaboration with state and local government welfare agencies, food stamps are provided to needy persons to increase their food purchasing power. Other programs include school lunch and breakfast programs; Supplemental Food Program for Women, Infants, and Children (WIC); and grants to states for nutrition education and training.

Department of Justice. Health services to federal prisoners are administered within the Department of Justice. The Bureau of Prisons, Medical and Services Division includes medical, psychiatric, dental, and health support services along with environmental health and safety, farm operations, food service, commissary, laundry, and other personal services for inmates.

The fact that many federal executive branch agencies are involved in direct service, funding, collecting and disseminating information, and setting policy reinforces the pluralistic approach of American government to health care.

State and Local Government Departments

Most state and local (county and city) jurisdictions have governmental activities that affect the health care field. At the state level three executive branch departments will be described: health, education, and corrections. The organization of a local health department will also be described and community health roles will be included.

State Health Departments

Selected programs within a typical state health department are as follows:

Legal services
Services to the chronically ill and aging
Juvenile services
Medical assistance: policy, compliance, operations
Mental health and addictions
Mental retardation and developmental disabilities
Environmental programs
Departmental licensing boards
Division of vital records
Health services cost review
Health planning and development
Preventive medicine and medical affairs

Community health nurses serve in many capacities throughout most state health departments. These capacities are similar to those in international and federal agencies: consultation, direct services, research, teaching, supervision, planning, and evaluation of health programs. Most health departments have a division or department of community health nursing. Most also have a board of examiners of nurses which usually is found in the department of licensing boards. Created by state legislation known as a state nurse practice act, the examiner's board is made up of nurses and consumers. A few states have other providers or administrators as members. The functions of this board are described in the practice act of each state and generally include licensing and examination of RNs and LPNs; approval of schools of nursing in the state; revocation, suspension, or denial of licenses; and promulgation of regulations about nursing practice and education. Nurse practice acts will be discussed later under a section on scope of nursing practice.

State Education Departments

Some state departments of education coordinate health curricula and services provided within local school systems. Other state legislatures mandate coordination of services solely within the health department or jointly between health and education departments. Often liaison groups or councils are formed to facilitate joint coordination. Consisting of members from state health departments and state departments of education, these councils develop policy and guidelines for school health services and health education. Community health nurses often represent health and education departments at these councils and help shape health policy. Community health nurses also serve in departments of education in similar capacities as in health departments.

State Departments of Corrections

Community health nurses also work in state departments of corrections as planners, implementors, coordinators, and in some cases, supervisors of health and nursing services for inmates in state prisons. Community health nurses in such state positions may also coordinate the health service efforts of local jails. Some local jails hire a nurse directly whereas others use the services of community health nurses in local health departments.

Local Health Departments

Depending on funding and other resources, programs offered by local health departments along with state departments vary greatly. A fairly comprehensive list of such programs, taken from an urban-suburban county health department in a mid-Atlantic state, includes the following:

Addictions and alcoholism clinics
Adult health
Birth and death records
Child day care and development
Child health clinics
Crippled children's services
Dental health clinic
Environmental health
Epidemiology and disease control
Family planning
Geriatric evaluation
Health education
Home health agency
Hospital discharge planning
Hypertension clinics
Immunization clinics
Information services
Maternal health
Medical social work
Mental health
Mental retardation and developmental disabilities
Nursing
Nursing home licensure
Nutrition division
Occupational therapy
Physical therapy
School health
Speech and audiology
Vision and hearing screening

At the local level, as at the state level, coordination of health efforts is essential between health departments and other county or city departments. For example, local boards of education and departments of social services are an integral part of activities of local governments. More often than at the other levels of government, community health nurses at the local level provide direct services. Some community health nurses deliver special or selected services, such as tuberculosis or venereal disease contact studies or child immunization clinics. Other community health nurses have a more generalized practice, delivering services to families in certain geographic areas called census tracts; this method of delivery of community health nursing services involves broader needs and a wider variety of nursing interventions.

Impact of Governmental Health Functions and Structures on Community Health Nursing

Thus far one of the main themes of the chapter has been the variety of structures in which the major governmental functions are carried out. This variety and range of functions has had a major impact on community health nursing. Funding, in particular, has shaped

Government and Legal Influences on the Practice of
Community Health Nursing   **111**

roles and tasks of community health nurses. The categorization of money by governments to special needs has led to special, more narrowly focused community health nursing roles. Generalized community health nursing practice usually declines with more specifically identified funding. For example, funds earmarked for communicable disease programs usually will not pay for and support home care services.

Many community health nursing roles have been influenced by federal, state, or local government. Training grants for nurse practitioners in primary care have provided incentives to individual nurses to attend programs and develop new community health nursing roles within the health care system. Family, school, adult, or pediatric nurse practitioners emerged primarily because of the funding provided by governmental agencies. Education in public health has also been changed by governmental policies and funding.

Other health policy information, funding, and direct service functions of government have influenced community health nursing. Health care to special populations such as migrant workers, pregnant women, or at-risk children has taken the form of law. Legislatures have identified special needs and programs to meet those needs. Often community health nurses are called on to implement these programs. Vital statistics and other epidemiological data collected by governmental agencies have influenced the location, work force, planning, and evaluation of community health nursing services.

According to the policies evolving from Reaganomics, whatever federal money is given to the states will be in the form of block grants. A sum of money with no specific program tags, the block grant may have a great impact on community health nursing. Having less money in special programs will mean a shift of community health nursing roles toward more generalized practice. Whether community health nursing should be a specialty or a generalized practice is an age-old debate. The purpose of mentioning the debate here is to show how government funding has clearly shaped the functions of community health nurses within all levels of government.

PRIVATE SECTOR INFLUENCE ON REGULATION

Most of the roles of government in health care previously discussed were related to legislation passed by the legislative branch and administration of the laws by the executive branch. One power that the legislature grants to the executive branch agencies when it passes a law and delegates the law's administration to an agency is the power to make regulations. Laws precede and dic-

tate who writes what kind of regulation. Because regulations flow from legislation, they have the force of law.

The private sector, which includes anyone who is not part of the government or public sector, can influence and shape legislation through many means. These same means can be used by the private sector to influence the writing of regulations. This part of the chapter will describe the process of regulation writing and ways to influence it. This section concludes with a discussion of self-regulation activities in the private sector.

Process of Regulation

In each level of government the executive branch can and in most cases must prepare regulations. These rules are more detailed than the law they are based on and relate to the subject of the executive department. These rules establish, fix, and control standards and criteria for carrying out a certain law. Fig. 5-9 gives the steps in the usual regulation-writing process.

After receiving a legislative directive, the department in the executive branch begins the process of regulation by studying the topic or issue. Advisory groups or special task forces including nondepartment members sometimes are formed to provide early input on the content of the regulations. As the work of the groups or individual department members progresses, initial drafts of the proposed regulations are written.

After refinement, the proposed regulations are placed in final draft form and published in the legally required document. At the federal level that document is called the *Federal Register*. Similar state registers exist in most states where regulations from state departments are published. The publication of proposed regulations includes notice about a time period within which public comment will be accepted. Public comment in this situation usually is written. The notice may also give a date, time, and place for a hearing that is open to the public. Anyone may attend; if one wishes to speak at the hearing, published rules for that procedure must be followed. Usually, speaking involves some type of notification and the limiting of testimony to a certain amount of time of which the speaker is informed ahead of time.

Revisions to the proposed regulations are made based on public comment and public hearing. Depending on the amount and content of the public reaction, final regulations are prepared or more study is done of the area and issues involved. Final published regulations carry the force of law. The date of when regulations become effective is also published.

Surveillance, or close monitoring, and participation of the private sector in regulation writing can begin as soon as a law is passed and delegated to an executive branch agency. Government manuals, updated at least

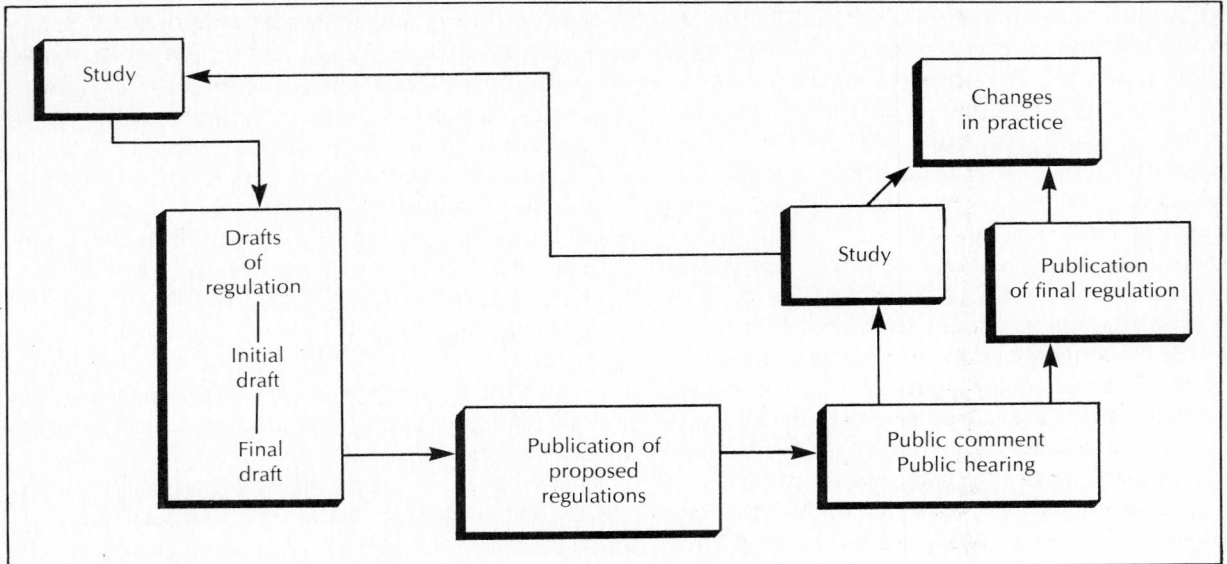

Fig. 5-9. Process of regulation writing.

yearly, list names and phone numbers of individuals within the executive branch. Early contact and expression of interest on how a particular law gets administered may result in membership on a task force or advisory board. If not, the membership of such groups is public information, and one could contact these members to determine their thoughts on what shape the regulations will take.

Surveillance of the *Federal Register* or state registers on a regular basis is essential. Once proposed regulations are published, members of the private sector may influence regulations by attending the hearings, providing comments, testifying, and engaging in lobbying aimed at individuals involved in the writing. Concrete, written suggestions for revision submitted to these individuals is usually a persuasive manner in which to proceed.

Final regulations, published in a *Code of Regulations* (both federal and state), usually mean changes in practice. Regulations need to be disseminated to all individuals whose practice is affected by them. This dissemination can be effectively helped along with private sector involvement. Regulations need to become part of policy and procedure manuals of agencies affected by them.

Self-Regulatory Activities

Self-regulation is an essential characteristic of a profession (American Nurses Association, 1976). It can involve many activities that have as their goals overseeing the rights, obligations, responsibilities, and relationships of a nurse to society, to nursing as a profession, and to clients. On entering the profession of nursing, an individual assumes a position of responsibility and trust. That position involves accountability for all outcomes of nursing practice. The importance of professional responsibility cannot be underrated. It has been said that as a last resort a profession should regulate itself before others (the government, for example) impose regulation. It is with this idea that suggested self-regulatory activities are made in this chapter.

Not only should community health nurses devote energies to monitoring and participating in regulation writing and other political processes (lobbying, voting, working for candidates, running for offices), but they should develop and participate in self-regulatory activities. These activities emanate from the private sector (nongovernmental groups and individuals) and, as mentioned above, are devoted to governing one's own actions. However, self-regulation is never the only activity that governs one's own actions. Other activities discussed in this chapter, law and government, are also governing or controlling practices of the professions.

Examples of self-regulation are listed in the box on p. 113. Belonging to an organization is not enough; contributing to the policy statements, attending meetings, and so on give essential support to organizations providing self-regulation. Activities listed in the box are divided into those that individual nurses are accomplishing and those that, with support of individuals, organizations are accomplishing. This is a selected list, and additional areas of self-regulation can be identified.

Selected Self-Regulatory Activities

Individual nurses

Being knowledgeable about the Nurse Practice Act

Initiating reports of nursing misconduct according to the Nurse Practice Act to state boards

Being knowledgeable about the *Code for Nurses*

Initiating reports of nursing misconduct according to the *Code for Nurses* to state nursing associations

Supporting organizational activities of self-regulation

Encouraging consumers to register legitimate complaints

Private nursing organizations

Accreditation of nursing education

Certification of excellence in nursing

Ethics committees

Continued development of ethical guidelines

Research committees on human rights

Peer review systems, audits, and quality assurance activities

---

LAWS AFFECTING COMMUNITY HEALTH NURSING PRACTICE

The practice of community health nursing is the synthesis of nursing practice and public health practice applied to promoting and preserving the health of populations (American Nurses' Association, 1973). This abbreviated definition recognizes the diversity of community health nursing and the inherent relationship of law to that practice. Not only are there legal aspects that relate to nursing practice, but nurses are also subject to legal aspects of public health practice.

This part of the chapter examines selected legal aspects of community health nursing, including those aspects that are unique to the practice. How laws and regulation have shaped community health nursing will be addressed, including examples of different kinds of laws. These examples are organized according to those that relate to general community health nursing practice and to those that relate to special areas of community health nursing practice. It is difficult to provide a complete "cookbook" on laws having an impact on community health nursing practice because of the breadth and variety of these roles. However, the chapter concludes with a section on legal research, which provides information on sources for keeping informed and for getting legal advice for questions and areas not addressed. The importance of these sources cannot be overemphasized. Getting advice and review by legal counsel of the community health agencies where nurses are employed should be an integral part of the decision-making process. If a nurse is in private practice or self-employed, a lawyer in the community should be sought for assistance.

Types of Laws

Several definitions of law are available. Many of these tend to describe what law is *not* rather than what it is. However, as a beginning point and as background, definitions of law include the following:

1. A rule established by authority, society, or custom
2. The body of rules governing the affairs of people within a community or among states; social order; the common law
3. A set of rules or customs governing a discrete field or activity, for example, criminal law, law of contracts
4. The system of courts, judicial process, and legal officers giving effect to the laws of a society; profession of a lawyer

These definitions reflect the close relationship of law to community and to society's customs and beliefs. Since community health nursing practice in the community reflects society's beliefs and customs, law has had a major impact on it. While, historically, community health nursing practice emerged out of individual voluntary activities, soon society recognized the need for it and, through legal mandates, created positions and functions for nurses in community settings. These functions in many instances carry with them the "force of law." For example, if the community health nurse discovers a person with smallpox, the law directs that the nurse, along with others legally designated in the community, take specific direct action. The law provides mechanisms whereby if the person with smallpox does not comply, other, more invasive interventions can be carried out. This is just one example of how the law has shaped community health nursing practice. Although this example probably involves a nurse employed in an official community health agency, there are other employment situations that also point to how laws have shaped practice. After giving an overview of differing types of laws, examples of laws having an impact on both general and special areas of community health nursing practice will be presented.

There are five types of laws that are part of our society, but for discussion purposes they have been placed into three groupings. Each type has a different source or legal base that will be described in the following discussion:

1. Constitutional law
2. Legislation and regulation
3. Judicial and common law

Constitutional Law

Constitutional law emanates from federal and state constitutions. As discussed earlier in this chapter, both documents describe, among other things, the powers and duties of officials; the responsibilities and division of government into three branches (executive, legislative, and judicial), and the rights of individuals. From this type of law community health nurses can get answers to questions in selected practice situations. For example, on what basis can the state require quarantine or isolation of individuals with tuberculosis? The answer to this question can be found in constitutional law.

The U.S. Constitution contains explicit and limited functions of the federal government. All other powers and functions are those that the individual states hold. The major power of the states which relates to community health nursing practice is that a state may intervene in a reasonable manner to protect the health, safety, and welfare of the citizenry. As described earlier in this chapter, the state's "police power" is not without limitation. First, it must be a "reasonable" exercise of power. Second, if the power interferes or infringes on individual rights, the state must demonstrate that there is a "compelling state interest" in exercising its power. Hence, isolating an individual or separating one from a community because they have a communicable disease has been deemed an appropriate exercise of state powers. The state can isolate even though it is an infringement on individual rights (freedom, autonomy) under the following conditions:

1. If the isolation is done in a reasonable manner
2. If a compelling state interest exists in the prevention of an epidemic
3. If the isolation is necessary to protect the health, safety, and welfare of individuals in the community or the public as a whole

Legislation and Regulation

Legislation is the type of law that comes from the legislative branches of government at different levels; state, local, or federal. Much legislation has an impact on community health nursing. In the previous situation dealing with the person with a communicable disease, the state exercised its power through legislation. As mentioned above, regulations are very specific statements of law that relate to individual pieces of legislation.

Community health nurses are often employed within the executive branch. The state or local health department is part of this branch. Hence, nurses become an instrument of the state's police power, in that nursing interventions often are done to implement legislation and regulations. Nurses employed in other community settings, those with no governmental responsibilities or legal mandates, are still often subject to legislation and regulations. For example, community health nurses rendering home health care in a private agency must deliver care according to Medicare (federal law) legislation and regulations or Medicaid (state law) legislation and regulations in order for the agency to be reimbursed for those services. Private and public health care services rendered by community health nurses are subject to many government regulations.

Judicial and Common Law

Judicial and common law is the last group of laws having an impact on community health nursing. Judicial law is that law based on court or jury decisions. Federal or state legal procedure, depending on the jurisdiction, outlines the details of how disputes are to be settled. Representatives from both sides of an issue present evidence, written or oral, before a court and/or jury who decide the outcome. Either party may have a basis on which to appeal the first decision; a higher court reviews that decision and renders a second one. Other appeal routes may be sought, depending on the outcome and issue. Special legislatively designed processes of settling claims may exist, depending on the jurisdiction. For example, medical malpractice panels exist in many states and may be the body that reviews a claim first.

The opinions of the courts are judicial opinion and also referred to as "case law." The court uses other types of laws to make its decision, including previous court decisions or cases. Precedent is one principle of common law. Judges are bound by previous decisions unless they are convinced that the "old law" is no longer relevant or valid. This process is called "distinguishing" and usually involves a demonstration of how the currently disputed situation differs from the previously decided situation. Other principles of common law are part of a court's rationale and the basis of making a particular decision. Such principles include justice, fairness, respect for individuals, autonomy, and self-determination. These common law principles are part of our traditions and heritage as a society and play an important role in decisions made by courts.

Judicial opinions and common law exist for a wide variety of types of legal disputes. Disputes and their opinions usually involve several categories of law. Categories of law most relevant to community health nursing are tort, contract, and criminal law. While there are other categories of law, most cases involving all of nursing practice include several torts, contract disputes, and criminal acts.

Categories of Law

Torts are civil wrongs between private individuals. Criminal wrongs are behaviors that the state, through the legislature, deems to be of such a degree and nature as to carry charges and penalties. *Torts* are either intended or unintended actions, such as negligence, false imprisonment, or invasion of privacy. *Criminal actions,* on the other hand, are wrongs that usually involve malicious intent to do harm to another's person or property. Selected criminal wrongs are homicide, manslaughter, burglary, and theft.

Contracts are mutual agreements between two or more individuals, referred to as parties. Elements of a contract are the offer, acceptance of that offer, and consideration. One of the best examples of nursing disputes based on contracts is found in the employment area. For example, a community health nurse agrees to work in a particular agency. An offer of employment is made and the nurse accepts the offer. The consideration is that the agency gains a nurse and the nurse receives compensation. Money is exchanged for nursing services as consideration for the contract. Should a dispute arise over the job between the nurse and the employer, the key to solving it lies with the contract. What was the mutual understanding of the nurse and the agency? Often contracts are written, but contracts can be made without writing them. A written contract is advisable if an agreement is complex or if it will make the parties' agreement easier to prove. Verbal agreements are valid agreements if the elements of a contract are present.

Contracts are created in other areas than employment situations. In community health nursing, agreements are made with clients almost everyday. For example, the nurse contracts a client to arrange a home visit. Discussion ensues and both agree on a mutual time, place, and purpose for the visit. The nurse offers a visit and the client accepts that offer; the consideration is that the nurse gains access to the client in order to plan better care or intervention and the client schedules the visit in lieu of other opportunities or uses of that time.

General information and background has been presented on the types of laws affecting community health practice. Discussion, including examples, of laws having an impact on general and special areas of community health nursing practice, follows this section.

General Community Health Nursing Practice and the Law

Despite the broad nature and the varied roles of community health nursing practice, there are two legal aspects that apply to most of these practice situations. The first aspect is the tort of professional negligence or malpractice; the second is the scope of practice defined by custom and state practice acts. Each of these aspects will be discussed in some detail.

Professional Negligence

Negligence was mentioned earlier as one of several torts that can be involved in all of nursing practice. Professional negligence or malpractice is defined as an act or failure to act when a duty is owed to another which was not reasonable and which leads to injuries compensable by law. For a client to succeed in persuading the judge or jury that a nurse was negligent, one has to prove *all* of the following:

1. The nurse owed a duty to the client
2. The duty to act as a reasonable, prudent nurse under the circumstances was breached or not fulfilled
3. The failure to be reasonable under the circumstances lead to or was the proximate cause of the alleged injuries
4. The injuries claimed are compensable through usual legal remedies

Reported cases, those cases appealed to higher courts, involving negligence and community health nurses are almost nonexistent. As one example, a case involving an occupational health nurse will be discussed.

The California case of *Cooper vs National Motor Bearing Co.* 288P 2d 581, 1955, involved an occupational health nurse who negligently implemented standing orders on an injury involving a puncture wound. The nurse, by her own testimony, admitted that she did not examine or probe the wound or refer the injured worker to the physician but just swabbed and bandaged it. Only after a 10-month period, documented by many visits to the dispensary and the worker's complaints of the wound not healing, did the nurse refer the worker to the company doctor. On referral basal cell carcinoma was found and surgery followed.

The fact that the nurse was employed by the industry to render first aid established the first element of negligence: a duty was owed the worker. By her own testimony the nurse stated that it was her duty to refer any condition or injury she was not familiar with, or not sure about, to the doctor for diagnosis. The standard of good nursing care in the community was to examine the wound for foreign bodies. The nurse knew the normal healing time was 1 to 2 weeks. If a wound persisted and did not heal, proper nursing care would indicate referral to a physician. Testimony was given that the practice of an occupational health nurse in this particular type of industry is to probe wounds for foreign bodies. According to the nurse's education and experience, she should have been aware of the possibility of foreign objects in such a wound.

In this case the nurse's failure to detect the foreign body was the proximate cause of the basal cell carcinoma. The injuries were compensable through existing legal remedies. The pain, suffering, loss of wages or time from work, and bodily disfigurement were all injuries that could be calculated and totaled as a monetary amount. The nurse and the company were found negligent by the California Court.

An integral part of negligence suits is the question of who should be sued. Obviously, those who made the mistakes should be sued, but part of the consideration of who to sue relates to who can best compensate for the injuries. When a nurse is employed and functioning within the scope of that employment, the employer is responsible for the nurse's negligent actions. This is referred to as the doctrine of *respondeat superior*. By directing a nurse to carry out a particular function, the employer becomes responsible along with the individual nurse for the negligence. The scope of employment is usually more inclusive than a job description and does not include criminal activities. Because employers are usually better able to compensate for the injuries suffered, they are most often sued and not nurses.

Community health nurses employed by governmental agencies need to ascertain whether that agency has sovereign immunity. Under this doctrine, the agency may be exempt from suit for particular kinds of actions, such as negligence. However, sovereign immunity will not shield from suit certain individuals within an agency, including nurses, who are acting under the auspices of the government when the negligence occurs.

Scope of Practice

The scope of practice issue involves differentiating between the practices of physicians, nurses, and other health care providers. Scope of practice is assessed (1) by examining the usual and customary practice of a profession and (2) by taking into account how the legislation defines the practice of a particular profession in a jurisdiction. The issue is particularly important to community health nurses who have traditionally practiced in a wide scope.

The usual and customary practice of community health nursing can be determined through a variety of sources, including the following:

1. Content of community health nursing educational programs, general and special
2. Experience of other practicing nurses (peers)
3. Activities and statements, including standards, of community health nursing professional organizations

4. Policies and procedures of agencies employing nurses
5. Needs and interests of the community
6. Literature, including books, texts and journals

All of these sources can describe the usual practice of a community health nurse and the scope of that practice.

Every community health nurse should know and follow closely the proposed changes in nursing, medicine, and other related practice acts. As mentioned earlier, these pieces of state legislation define a scope of practice for these professionals. The nurse should always examine *all* related definitions to nursing practice. For example, the definitions of practice of registered nursing, medicine, and pharmacy in Maryland are given in the box on the next page.

These three definitions along with customary practice are pertinent, for example, to the question of whether a community health nurse is "dispensing" medications in a methadone clinic in a local health department when following physician prescription and preparing several identical doses for the client to take between clinic visits. The question of scope forces one to clarify both independent and dependent community health nursing functions. The failure to know one's limitations may lead to charges of practicing another profession without a license, fines, and possible suspension or revocation of the license. Because practice acts vary, so does the scope of practice issue. It is best to refer directly to practice acts for a particular state code.

This section has examined two legal aspects that generally have an impact on community health nursing practice. Because of the variety of work experiences of community health nurses and hence the variety of legal aspects, the following section will deal with areas of practice with a special focus.

Special Community Health Nursing Practice and the Law

The field of community health nursing includes nurses prepared as generalists who practice in community health settings and nurses prepared as community health nursing specialists. An essential component of community health nursing practice is knowledge of community resources and other health professionals. The community health nurse typically delivers care to clients or groups where they live, work, play, or go to school. In addition, the nurse encompasses further specialization in clinical areas such as family health, school and college health, occupational health, and community mental health and fulfills functional roles in administration, education, research, and consultation (American Nurses Association, 1980). Legal aspects of community health nursing vary, depending on (1) the set-

---

Practice of Registered Nursing, Medicine, and Pharmacy in Maryland, 1982

Registered Nursing—Health Occupations 7-101 (f)

Practice registered nursing means the performance of acts requiring substantial specialized knowledge, judgment and skill based on the biological, physiological, behavioral or sociological sciences as the basis for assessment, nursing diagnosis, planning, implementation and evaluation of the practice of nursing in order to: maintain health; prevent illness; or care for or rehabilitate the ill, injured or infirm.

For these purposes, practice registered nursing includes: administration; teaching; counseling; supervision, delegation and evaluation of nursing practice; execution of therapeutic regimen, including the administration of medication and treatment; independent nursing functions and delegated medical functions; and performance of additional acts authorized by the Board under section 7-205.

Medicine—Health Occupations 14-101 (i)

Practice medicine means to engage, with or without compensation, in medical: diagnosis; healing; treatment; or surgery. Practice medicine includes doing, undertaking, professing to do and attempting any of the following: diagnosing, healing, treating, preventing, prescribing for, or removing any physical, mental, or emotional ailment or supposed ailment of an individual: by physical, mental, emotional, or other process that is exercised or invoked by the practitioner, the patient, or both; or by appliance, test, drug, operation, or treatment; ending of a human pregnancy; and performing acupuncture.

Practice medicine does not include: selling any nonprescription drug or medicine; practicing as an optician; or performing a massage or other manipulation by hand, but by no other means.

Pharmacy—Health Occupations 12-101 (j)

Practice pharmacy means to engage in any of the following activities: selecting, preparing, and dispensing drugs, medicines, or devices; providing information and explanation to patients and health care practitioners about the safe and effective use of drugs, medicines, or devices; or identifying and appraising problems concerning the use or monitoring of drug therapy.

In general, this title does not limit the right of an individual to practice a health occupation that the individual is authorized to practice under this article. Preparing of prescriptions by authorized prescriber. This title does not prohibit an authorized prescriber from personally preparing and dispensing the authorized prescriber's prescriptions.

Nonprescription sales by general merchants. This title does not limit the right of the general merchant to sell: any nonprescription drug, medicine, or device; any commonly used household or domestic remedy; or any farm remedy or ingredient for a spraying solution, in bulk or otherwise.

---

ting where care is delivered, (2) the clinical specialty, and (3) the functional role.

For the purposes of this chapter, four special areas of community health nursing practice and their respective legal aspects will be highlighted. Those four areas are school and family health, occupational health, home care and hospice services, and correctional health. Examples of legislation and judicial opinions affecting community health nurses within these selected areas will be included.

School and family health nursing may be delivered by community health nurses employed by health departments or boards of education. School health legislation provides a framework for nursing functions. The legislation establishes a minimum of services that must be provided to children in school systems including public and private schools. For example, most states require that children be immunized against certain communicable diseases before entering school. Children must have had a physical examination at that time, and

most states require at least one physical at a later time in the course of their schooling. Legislation also specifies when and what type of health screening will be conducted in schools, such as vision and hearing testing. Many jurisdictions carry out these activities specified by the legislature plus many other activities. In financially "good times" there is usually an increase in the services community health nurses render in school and family health nursing. When the economic situation deteriorates, usually the services delivered are only those specified by the legislature.

A major area of legislation impacting community health nursing practice with schools and families is child abuse and neglect. Most states require nurses to report to police or a social service agency any situation in which they suspect a child is being abused or neglected. This is one instance in which society has said a professional may breach confidentiality in order to protect someone who may be in a helpless and harmful position. There is civil immunity for such reports and nurses may be called as witnesses should a hearing follow the investigation made by a social service agency.

Much federal legislation affects community health nursing practice with schools and families; Head Start, early diagnostic screening programs, nutrition programs, services for the handicapped, and special education are just a few examples. Most of this legislation, although written by Congress, requires cooperative federal and state funding, planning, and implementation. Each nurse working within a service based on legislation should be oriented to the legislation. It is advisable that the legislation and its regulations become part of the agency's nursing policies and procedures so that the nurse may refer to it.

Occupational health is another special area of practice which is greatly affected by state and federal laws. The Occupational Safety and Health Act (OSHA) places many requirements on industries. These requirements shape the types of services given to workers and functions of community health nurses. OSHA also established a reporting system for workers exposed to toxic agents in the work place. A record-keeping system required by OSHA greatly affects health records in the work place. Each state has an agency similar to the federal agency which also monitors and inspects industries, including the health services rendered by nurses. Access to records, confidentiality, and the use of standing orders are legal issues of great significance to nurses employed in industries.

Home care and hospice services rendered by community health nurses is greatly affected by state laws that require licensing and certification. Compliance with these laws is integrally linked to the method of payment for the services. For example, a service must be licensed and certified in order to obtain payment for services through Medicare, which is federal law. Federal regulations implementing Medicare have had an impact on much of community health nursing practice including how nurses record the details of their visits.

Many states have passed laws requiring nurses to report elder abuse to proper authorities. In some states there is an impact on home care and hospice services through legislation related to rights to death with dignity, rights of residents of long-term care facilities, definitions of death, and use of living wills. The legal and ethical dimensions on community health nursing practice are particularly important in this area of practice. Individual rights, such as the right to refuse treatment, and nursing responsibilities, such as the legal duty to render reasonable and prudent care, may often be in conflict in delivering home and hospice services. Much case discussion, sometimes including outside consultation, is required when rights and responsibilities are in conflict and a decision must be made to resolve that conflict.

Nursing practice in correctional heath systems is controlled by state and federal law and regulation as well as by recent Supreme Court decisions. The laws and decisions relate to the type and amount of services that must be given or made available to incarcerated individuals. For example, physical examinations of each prisoner after they are sentenced are required. Prisoners must be provided minimal care, especially care when they are sick. Court decisions requiring that health services be adequate are based on constitutional law. If minimal services are not provided, it is a violation of a prisoner's right to be free of cruel and unusual punishment. Such decisions provide a framework that strongly influences the setting of nursing priorities. For example, providing sick calls would be a first priority rather than nutrition classes.

Each area of special community health nursing practice mentioned in this chapter and other areas are significantly shaped by legislation and judicial opinion. Those nurses responsible for setting and implementing program priorities need to identify and monitor laws related to each special area of practice. Suggested legal resources that might be used to stay current with laws will be described in the following section.

Legal Resources

In addition to seeking legal counsel, one can find many resources in public libraries as well as law libraries which can help community health nurses find laws pertinent to their practice. Possible legal resources include the following:

State bar associations
State code
State annotated code
Indexes to codes
Supplements to codes and indexes
Federal Register and state registers
Codes of regulations (federal and state)
Administrative agency rules and decisions
Case law
Opinions of attorney generals
Legal dictionaries
Legislative histories
Legal periodicals

In using these legal resources, begin by reviewing the topical index to each source. As the headings are reviewed, several can be identified as having something to do with the content areas of practice (such as immunizations or family planning) and the types of clients (for example, minors, adolescents, and children) served by the community health nurse. Computer search tools are often available to one looking for laws and regulations relevant to one's practice. One legal computerized search is called Lexis. The Library of Congress has a

service called Scorpio. Both services will not only
search books and journals but recent case law, bills,
amendments, and legislation. One of the best ways to
stay informed is to monitor and read the area newspaper.

SUMMARY

This chapter has presented information about the
governmental and legal influences on the practice of
community health nursing. The influence of government
and law on community health nursing is significant. However, community health nurses can be part of
the influence on government through regulation writing and lobbying. Organization, functions, and structures of government and the process of regulation writing are all important areas for community health nurses
to know. Legal aspects of the roles and functions of general and specific areas of community health nursing, especially scope of practice and negligence will prove to
be useful information for nurses in community health.

BIBLIOGRAPHY

Altman, S., and Sapolsky, H.: Federal health programs, Lexington, Mass., 1981, D.C. Heath & Co.

American Nurses' Association: Standards of community health nursing practice, Kansas City, Mo., 1973, The Association.

American Nurses' Association: Code for Nurses, Kansas City, Mo., 1976, The Association.

American Nurses' Association: A conceptual model of community health nursing, Kansas City, Mo., 1982, The Association.

American Public Health Association: The definition and role of public health nursing in the delivery of health care, Washington, D.C., 1981, The Association.

Aroskar, M.A.: Ethical issues in community health nursing, Nurs. Clin. North Am. **14**(1):35-44, March 1979.

Beauchamp, T., and Childress, J.: Principles of biomedical ethics, ed. 2, New York, 1983, Oxford University Press.

Blum, H.: Planning for health, New York, 1981, Health Sciences Press.

Bullough, B.: The law and the expanding nursing role, ed. 2, New York, 1980, Appleton-Century-Crofts.

Campazzi, B.: Nurses, nursing and malpractice litigation, Nurs. Adm. Q. **5**(1):1-18, 1981.

Curtin, L., and Flaherty, M.: Nursing ethics theories and pragmatics, Bowie, Md., 1982, Robert J. Brady Co.

Dahl, R.: Democracy in the United States: promise and performance, ed. 2, Chicago, 1972, Rand McNally & Co.

Davis, A., and Aroskar, M.: Ethical dilemmas and nursing practice, ed. 2, New York, 1983, Appleton-Century-Crofts.

Division of Nursing, Bureau of Health Professionals, Health Resources Administration, Public Health Service: The Division of Nursing, Hyattsville, Md., 1982, The Division.

Fox, J.: Controversial and legal issues, Family Comm. Health **2**(3):62-68, Nov. 1979.

Fromer, M.: Ethical issues in health care, St. Louis, 1981, The C.V. Mosby Co.

Goldsmith, S.: Political party platform health planks: a mechanism for participation and prediction? Am. J. Public Health **63**(7):594-601, 1973.

Health: United States, 1981, DHHS Pub. No. (PHS) 81-1232, Washington, D.C., Dec. 1981, Department of Health and Human Services.

Healthy People: the Surgeon General's report on health promotion and disease prevention, DHEW Pub. No. (PHS) 79-55071, Washington, D.C., 1979, Department of Health, Education, and Welfare.

Hemelt, M., and Mackert, M.: Dynamics of law in nursing and health care, ed. 2, Reston, Va., 1982, Reston Publishing Co., Inc.

Miles, R.: The Department of Health, Education, and Welfare, New York, 1974, Praeger Publishers Inc.

Murchison, I., Nichols, T., and Hanson, R.: Legal accountability in the nursing process, ed. 2, St. Louis, 1982, The C.V. Mosby Co.

Northrop, C.: Promotion of ethical conduct in nursing research through legislation and self-regulation, Proceedings of the First Annual Scholarly Nursing Leadership Conference: Ethical dimensions of nursing research, Baltimore, 1980, University of Maryland.

Northrop, C., and Mech, A.: The nurse as expert witness, Nurs. Law Ethics **2**(2):1,2,6,8, March-April 1981.

Office of Federal Register: United States government manual, 1981-1982, Washington, D.C., 1982, U.S. Government Printing Office.

United Nations: Basic facts about the UN, New York, 1978, UN.

Weaver, J.: National health policy and the underserved, St. Louis, 1976, The C.V. Mosby Co.

Wiley, L.: Liability for death: nine nurse's legal ordeals, Nursing '81. **2**(9):34-43, 1981.

Wing, K.: The law and the public's health, St. Louis, 1976, The C.V. Mosby Co.

World Health Organization: The work of WHO, 1978-79: biennial report of the Director-General, Geneva, 1980, WHO.

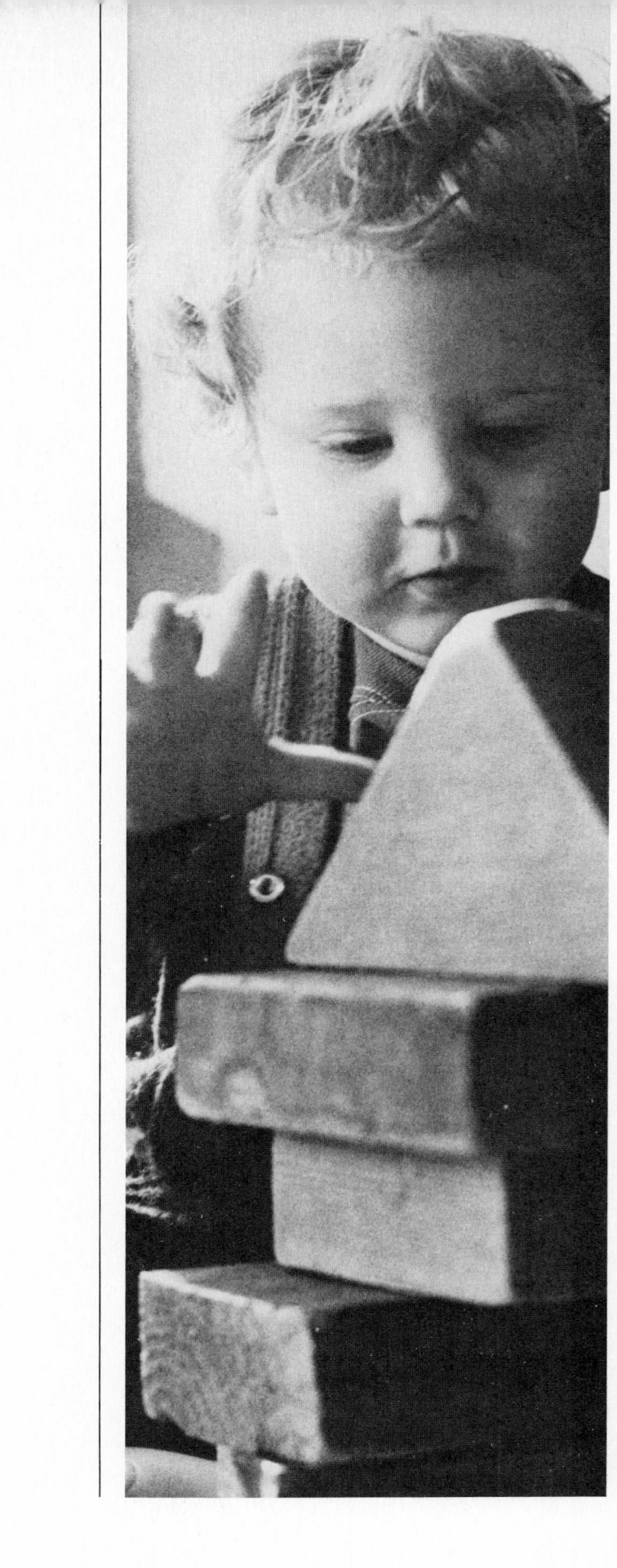

Part Two

Conceptual Foundations and Tools for Community Health Nursing Practice

There is no question that nursing is struggling in its quest for a scientific base for practice. Community health nursing must make clear its body of knowledge lest overriding economic and political forces determine the scope of practice. Community health nurses must continue to develop and evaluate conceptual models and move forward in theory development. No one conceptual model fits all needs and demands in community health nursing practice. Chapter 6 provides an overview of a wide variety of conceptual models from nursing and the social sciences, which offer promise of usefulness for practice. In addition, because of its integral role in community health nursing, the epidemiological model for practice is detailed in Chapter 7.

Chapters 8, 9, and 10 describe three key tools community health nurses use in implementing their role. To effectively provide health promotion, community health nursing largely relies on educational strategies. Clients, whether individuals, families, or groups within the community, benefit from the educational aspect of community health nursing. Education for health promotion is based on a careful assessment of client needs. Similarly, as pointed out in Chapters 8 and 9, programs must be based on consumer perception of needs and be consistent with the consumer's goals and preferences for action.

Likewise, as programs are developed in all aspects of community health nursing, effective methods of evaluation are essential. As funds decrease in the health sector, the need for programs to be cost effective will increase. Planning, evaluation, record keeping, and quality assurance are integral tools for effective community health nursing practice.

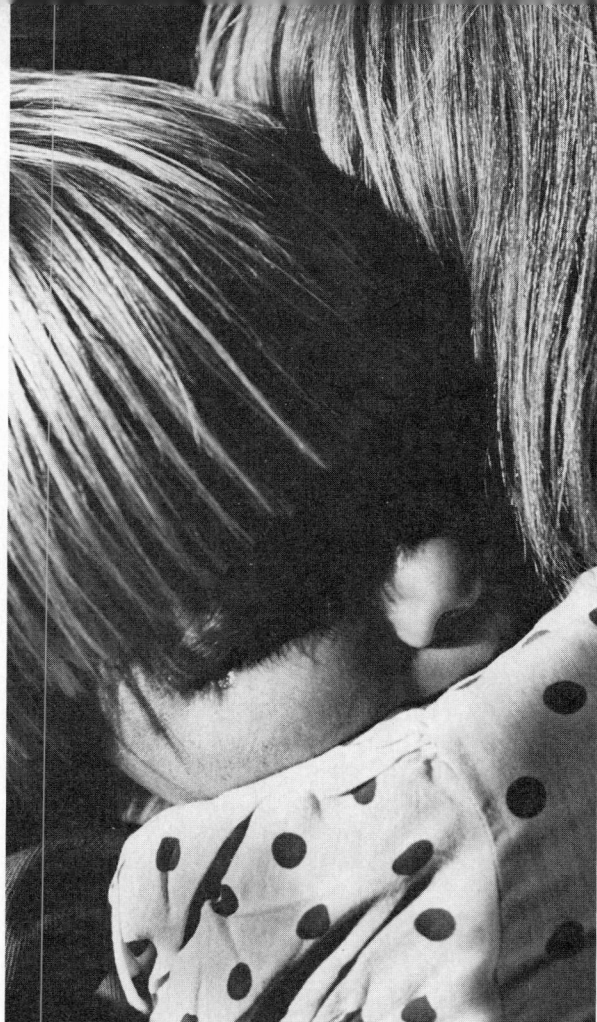

Chapter 6

GWENDOLEN LEE
JEANETTE LANCASTER

CONCEPTUAL MODELS FOR COMMUNITY HEALTH NURSING

Nursing has been described as both an art and a science. In recent years there has been considerable argument as to the extent of a scientific basis for nursing. As described in Chapter 1, community health nursing has historically reflected the qualities of both art and science in the early accounts of home visiting, health teaching, and drawing on epidemiological concepts to determine the focus of actions. Since the development, refinement, and ultimate autonomy of a profession rests on the uniqueness of the knowledge gathered by scientific inquiry, these activities are being emphasized in nursing (Fuller, 1978).

"For the first hundred years of its existence, nursing established itself as an indispensable helping profession with little emphasis on substantiating its scientific foundation" (Andreoli and Thompson, 1977, p. 32).

However, since the 1950s the concept of nursing as a science or as a profession with a scientific base has received increasing attention. There has been an urgency for nurses to systematically test, organize, and expand the body of knowledge on which practice is derived.

As nursing has progressed toward the goal of establishing itself as a scientific discipline, there has been a burgeoning interest in both research and theory development. These two goals are interrelated, since many advances in theory development are based on findings derived from careful and systematically completed research. The purpose of research is that of delineating and advancing the theoretical base of nursing.

Donaldson and Crowley (1978, p. 113) caution that not all inquiry undertaken by nurses is research contributing to the discipline of nursing; "to be nursing research, studies must be undertaken from a nursing perspective." They stated that since the days of Florence Nightingale there have been three general themes of inquiry in nursing:

1. Concern with principles and laws that govern the life processes, well-being, and optimum functioning of human beings—sick or well. (This trend can be seen in Nightingale's work as summarized in Chapter 1.)
2. Concern with the patterning of human behavior in interaction with the environment in critical life situations. (The writing of Dorothy Johnson in the 1960s focused on systems of behavior as have the more recent works of Martha Rogers with the emphasis on life rhythms.)
3. Concern with the processes by which positive changes in health status are affected. (Peplau described nursing as an interpersonal process.)

To develop and refine these concerns, nursing must advance as a theory-based profession. A study of theory calls attention to relationships and interactions which influence the practice of nursing. The development of conceptual models has provided impetus to the refinement of theory and the process of research. Throughout this chapter some theories will be discussed that are based on classic writings, these theories are presented to reflect current thinking in theory development in nursing.

This chapter discusses selected conceptual models that can be used to guide community health nursing practice. Interdisciplinary, nursing, and selected psychosocial models will be described with application of their potential usefulness to community health nursing. In order to describe these models, it is first necessary to construct the essential background information useful in understanding the use of models in research, practice, and education. To do this, several terms need to be defined and the usefulness of conceptual models for guiding practice requires explanation. Additionally, the Division of Community Health Nursing of the American Nurses' Association has developed a "Conceptual Model of Community Health Nursing," and the American Public Health Association has written a position paper entitled "The Role and Definition of Public Health Nursing in the Delivery of Health Care." Each of these models will be summarized, and they will be compared as to major themes and inherent differences. The second half of the chapter will look at selected interdisciplinary and psychosocial theories applicable to community health nursing, such as systems, developmental, interactional, motivation, change, communication, and leadership theory. Also to be discussed are nursing models applicable to community health nursing including the Roy Adaptation Model of Nursing, Rogers' Science of Unitary Man, Johnson's Behavioral Systems Model, Orem's Self-care Nursing Model, Neu-

man's Health-Care Systems model, and King's systems, concepts, and process model.

USEFULNESS OF CONCEPTUAL MODELS FOR GUIDING COMMUNITY HEALTH NURSING PRACTICE

In order both to advance the scientific basis of community health nursing practice and to gain recognition within the health care system, nurses must develop theoretical bases for their practice. Chinn and Jacobs (1978) have described a four-stage set of operations for moving toward a theoretical basis of practice, which includes (1) concept examination and analysis, (2) formulation and validation of relational statements, (3) theory construction, and (4) the practical application of theory. Although each of these stages certainly needs attention, the most critical at the present is the first stage, since it establishes the basis for the remaining three stages. A model is a tool useful in examining and analyzing concepts. The function of a model is to define or describe something, assist with analysis of systems, specify relationships and processes, and represent situations in symbolic terms that may be manipulated to derive predictions.

In recent years the use of conceptual models has been adapted as a "system for observing, ordering, clarifying, and analyzing events" (Bush, 1979, p. 13). As such, models provide a useful way of communicating what a person has in mind when speaking of an abstract entity, structure, or process that cannot be directly observed. Models are used to solve both simple and complex problems by concentrating on one or more segments instead of the entirety. This approximation or abstraction of reality that is constructed on paper, in one's mind, or as a representative structure depicts the designer's idea of a model. As Hazzard (1971) pointed out, no one segment of the human universe is so simple and easy to understand that it can be grasped and controlled without the use of abstraction. Because of the complexity usually involved, models do not represent every aspect of reality, but instead they focus on those details perceived as having the greatest relevance to the situation (Lancaster and Lancaster, 1981). A model is useful because of its ability to order, clarify, and systematize selected aspects of the phenomena it attempts to replicate.

DEFINITION OF KEY TERMS

To fully appreciate the usefulness of models, it is necessary to sort through the semantic jungle surrounding this topic. Frequently the terms *model* and *theory* are used interchangeably. All theories are models, but the converse is not true; all models are not theories, since not all models have the requisites of theoretical construction. A model expresses structure, whereas a theory adds substance to that structure. According to Kerlinger (1973, p. 9), "A theory is a set of interrelated construct (concept) definitions and propositions that present a systematic view of phenomena by specifying relations among variables, with the purpose of explaining and predicting the phenomena."

Several additional terms need to be defined to fully understand the use of conceptual models and their relationships to theory. Basic to the preceding definition is the term *concept,* which refers to a category or class of objects or phenomena that represent either an abstract version of the real world (such as an idea) or a concrete idea such as a chair or bench (Fawcett, 1980; Williams, 1979). Concepts that refer to phenomena not directly observable are usually considered *constructs.* In contrast, *hypothesis* or *proposition* specify the relationship between two or more concepts (Williams, 1979). Examples of concepts include nurse, chair, and house, whereas less observable constructs might be society, intelligence, and age. A hypothesis might be "the more information hypertensive clients have about their disease, the more they will adhere to the therapeutic regimen." The last term to be defined to describe theory is *variable,* which is a concept that takes on more than one value. A theory then has certain attributes: clearly defined concepts and hypotheses tying the concepts together which are interrelated and also testable.

An additional term that needs to be defined is *conceptual framework,* or "a group of concepts plus a set of propositions which spell out the relationships between those concepts . . ." (Williams, 1979, p. 93). By this description all theories are conceptual frameworks. As can be seen, the terms *conceptual model* and *conceptual framework* are essentially the same. For the purposes of this discussion conceptual model will be the term of choice.

A *conceptual model* can be defined as "a set of concepts and those assumptions that integrate them into a meaningful configuration" (Fawcett, 1980, p. 10). A model might call attention to the environmental forces or stressors acting on a person to motivate adaptive change as well as the resources available for the maintenance of equilibrium while coping with stressors. As will be seen in the nursing models reviewed in a later section, the concepts to date are highly abstract and many are not directly observable in the real world. Likewise, the hypotheses linking the concepts tend to be abstract generalizations not always immediately testable. These models do provide a way of looking at concepts and of describing the phenomena and their interrelationships.

At the present time most of what are referred to in nursing as theories actually fall within the realm of conceptual models or sets of concepts and a group of statements that explain how these concepts are interrelated. The aim of nursing research is to clarify, test, and refine the current models so that they reach the specificity of theory. Conceptual models, then, constitute a key stage in theory development by providing focus, ruling some variables in as relevant and others out as unrelated.

Contemporary conceptual models of nursing specify varying relationships and interactions among four essential components: person, environment, health, and nursing. Each of the nursing models discussed in this chapter has a unique view of the four primary concepts and each conceives of the interactional pattern in a different fashion; however, several commonalities do exist. Most nursing models view people as holistic beings who have biopsychosocial qualities. People are viewed also as being interactive and part of a family, community, and society. Each model views health and nursing in a different way and delineates the nursing process in accordance with its unique tenets. Conceptual models having the greatest application to community health nursing view people as being in continuous interaction with their environment. The environment affects its inhabitants and vice versa. Additionally, environment refers to that which is internal as well as the more easily observable external environment. The environment in community health is dynamic and ever-changing and can be either a positive or negative force in health.

In community health nursing, the major focus of attention is on health. The unique feature of this area of nursing is its emphasis on assisting individuals, families, groups, and communities to maintain health. To do this, the community is viewed from a holistic perspective as a motivator or disruptor of health care. The nursing goal is to assess, plan, implement, and evaluate ways to make the designated community a healthy place to live. The aim of community health nursing is also directed toward assisting recipients of care assume personal responsibility for their health; teaching, counseling, and advocacy are essential features of the nursing role.

USING CONCEPTUAL MODELS

To some extent everyone has a conceptual model since all people have assumptions and beliefs about how the world operates. Everyone has a unique set of concepts guiding the categorization of ideas and information within their belief system. In nursing practice, people view situations differently and have personalized ways of responding to others. Whether implicit or explicit, people's conceptual models play a major role in determining behavior. For example, two psychiatrists, one coming from a psychoanalytical framework and the other from an interpersonal view, would perceive the treatment goals differently if each were seeing the same 29-year-old woman who became mute upon moving from her parents' home to her own apartment. The psychoanalytical therapist may attach the muteness to unresolved dependency on the parents and recommend that she go into analysis to uncover any deep-seated problems. In contrast, the interactionally oriented therapist would be more likely to encourage her to talk about the here-and-now and explore what she fears about the new living situation. Conceptual models guide actions and are either consciously or unconsciously recognized. As will be seen in the latter part of this chapter, a variety of conceptual models have potential usefulness in community health nursing, and many nurses already practice in accordance with a model such as systems theory or a developmental framework.

Conceptual Models in Nursing Education

Since conceptual models serve to provide focus, they have for several years been used to guide curriculum design in nursing programs. The usefulness of conceptual models in curriculum development is embodied in the *Criteria for the Appraisal of Baccalaureate and Higher Degree Programs,* which holds that programs leading to both the first (baccalaureate) and second (master's) professional degree should evidence that "the curriculum implements the philosophy, purpose, and objectives of the program and is developed within a conceptual framework" (National League for Nursing, 1977, p. 13). According to this document, a conceptual framework is "a distinct, systematic organization of concepts which stems from the philosophy and purposes of the program and gives direction to the curriculum" (p. 17).

For many years educational programs have employed a wide range of conceptual models to organize content. Originally, curriculum models were either eclectic (synthesizing many theories into a unique one) or drew on psychosocial or physiological theories (motivation, human interaction, and so on) to guide curricular design. In recent years as nursing models have been increasingly tested in research and practice, they have provided additional sources for guiding curriculum choices. Bush (1979) noted that educational models serve three primary purposes: they guide student-teacher interaction, aid in planning the curriculum, and assist in selecting instructional materials. Readers will later have the opportunity to evaluate the merits and potential of several conceptual models.

Conceptual Models in Research

Nursing research has received a major impetus to include a conceptual basis for study. Just as in education, conceptual models focus the study design and also guide in the delineation of variables to be included and those which can logically be omitted. However, there are some differences in the ways conceptual models are used in research and in curriculum design. In research the use of models must be more explicit and precise, whereas in curriculum design it can be broader to allow flexibility and creativity in the delineation of content. To verify the effectiveness of the research process, concepts must be clearly defined and carefully developed to allow for accurate measurement.

Conceptual models help to define and guide research questions and tasks and also provide for focusing on the overriding goals or anticipated outcomes of the research (Bush, 1979). The researcher may elect to use an existing model or develop one specifically for the study. It must be cautioned that a conceptual model may serve as a "blender" and keep some sparks of creativity from emerging, since the purpose of the model is to order, clarify, and analyze selected concepts. Additional research usually selects one aspect of a conceptual model to test. If one were to attempt to evaluate the entire scope of the Roy Adaptation Model of Nursing or Orem's Self-Care Nursing Model, the task would be unending. Instead, one aspect or tenet is subjected to investigation. As research accumulates, the body of knowledge about nursing models will inevitably lead to their refinement and ultimate usefulness. Currently, many models convey more of a philosophy of care than a model of care, since the relational statements have not clearly been delineated. Most models do have carefully articulated concepts, and once they have been tested and relationships documented, the models will offer greater usefulness for education, research, and practice.

Conceptual Models in Nursing Practice

In practice just as in education and research, conceptual models give direction, simplify, and help to organize information. Models assist nursing practitioners to think about clinical situations by utilizing concepts to sort out events. If models are to be used in nursing practice, consideration must be given to values, beliefs, assumptions, goals of nursing action, and the recipient of nursing care.

Nurses have historically used models in their actions. Look back to the work of Florence Nightingale and Lillian Wald for clear evidence of an epidemiological model for practice. Nightingale in her early work in the Crimean War recognized both the role of the environment on health and the destructiveness of disease patterns. Similarly, Wald devoted much of her life to campaigning for better living conditions in New York City so that disease would not run rampant among the people she served.

Historically, community health nurses have relied heavily on an epidemiological model to guide practice. Because of its key role in community health, the epidemiological model is discussed in depth in Chapter 8. The next two sections focus on two recently developed and in many ways similar models for practice: that of the ANAs Division on Community Health Nursing Practice and that of the APHAs Public Health Nursing Section. In using models for practice be aware that some are not carefully developed and can confuse rather than guide practice.

THE ANA CONCEPTUAL MODEL OF COMMUNITY HEALTH NURSING PRACTICE

In the fall of 1978 the executive committee of the ANA Division on Community Health Nursing Practice appointed a task force and charged this group "to define the scope of community health nursing practice; to delineate the specialty areas; to identify the levels of practice; and to recommend the educational levels and areas" (American Nurses' Association, 1980, p. 1). This model was developed and presented to ANA members at the 1979 convention in Houston, Texas.

This document is divided into five sections: definitions, assumptions and beliefs, nurses in community health nursing, scope of practice, and implications. Because of their importance to an understanding of this model, the definitions are reviewed here in depth and the assumptions and beliefs are listed below. The scope of practice is also described here in some detail because it essentially constitutes the conceptual framework.

The definition of community health nursing set forth in the ANA *Conceptual Model of Community Health Nursing* is futuristic in focus with its emphasis on health promotion and consumer involvement and its consideration of health as being influenced by multiple factors within people as well as by the environments in which they seek to live. The definition reads as follows (American Nurses' Association, 1980, p. 2):

Community health nursing is a synthesis of nursing and public health practice applied to promoting and preserving the health of populations. The practice is general and comprehensive. It is not limited to a particular age group or diagnosis, and is continuing, not episodic. The dominant responsibility is to the population as a whole; nursing directed to individuals, families, or groups contributes to the health of the total population. Health promotion, health maintenance, health education, and management, coordi-

nation, and continuity of care are utilized in a holistic approach to the management of the health care of individuals, families and groups in a community.

This definition encompasses both direct and indirect services to individuals, families, groups, and communities. Its scope is concerned with both wellness and illness in providing as well as facilitating the delivery of services. A set of assumptions and beliefs further elaborate on the goal of community health nursing and describe the scope of practice.

Assumptions and Beliefs

The following assumptions and beliefs about community health nursing are set forth* (American Nurses' Association, 1980):

Assumption 1: The health care system is complex.
Assumption 2: Primary, secondary, and tertiary health care are components of the health care system.
Assumption 3: Nursing, as a subsystem of the health care system, is the product of education and practice based upon research.
Assumption 4: The provision of primary care predominates in community health nursing practice, with lesser involvement in secondary and tertiary health care.
Assumption 5: Community health nursing occurs principally in primary health care settings.
Belief 1: Health care should be available, accessible, and acceptable to all persons.
Belief 2: The making of health policy should include participation by recipients of health care services.
Belief 3: The nurse as a provider and the client as a consumer of health care services can form a conjoint relationship to advocate and effect change in health policies and services.
Belief 4: The environment affects the health of populations, groups, families, and individuals.
Belief 5: Prevention of illness is essential to promote health.
Belief 6: A health axis intersects with the life span axis.
Belief 7: The client is the only constant member of the health care team.
Belief 8: Individuals within a community are ultimately responsible for their own health and must be encouraged and taught to be active participants in their own health care.

Scope of Practice

According to the ANA conceptual model, the focus of community health nursing is on the prevention of illness and promotion and maintenance of health. Nursing activities to achieve these goals include client

*Reprinted with the permission of ANA.

education, counseling, advocacy, and management of care. The major emphasis in community health nursing is on primary care, which begins when clients enter the health care system and continues throughout the duration of the client's care. Secondary and tertiary care are afforded less emphasis than is primary care. Clients are considered to be active members of the health care team, and the goal of care is to assist clients assume self-responsibility for health care.

The specific functions viewed as priorities in the role of the community health nurse are seen in the eight standards identified by the Division on Community Health Nursing Practice and given in Appendix G (American Nurses' Association, 1980).

The major goal of the community health nurse, as pointed out in Chapter 1, is the preservation and improvement of the health of the community. This overall objective is accomplished through two major modes or routes. The first community health nursing mode is direct care to individuals, families, and groups within a designated community. The second mode directs attention to the health of the total population and considers how community health problems and issues affect individuals, families, and groups. For example, the problem of improper waste disposal or stagnant water near a residential area would be considered a community health nursing problem in terms of how the residents of that area were affected.

Practicing in the first mode, community health nurses work directly with clients to promote optimal health, and where health has been disrupted, to assist in restoration and stabilization of chronic conditions. The pattern of practice takes place through clinics, home health care, and group work with clients having common health needs. Practice is collaborative with other members of the health care team, is holistic in orientation, and emphasizes the evaluation of nursing care to individuals, families, and the community.

In the second mode the focus is on the community as client, and the aim is to assist communities to identify health needs, establish priorities, plan and implement actions, and identify and intervene in factors affecting the health of the community. This mode emphasizes the ongoing interaction between people and their environment in which each is affected by the other. The role of the community health nurse embraces all three levels of prevention: primary, secondary, and tertiary with emphasis on primary. As will be noted in the following discussion, many similarities exist between the ANA *Conceptual Model of Community Health Nursing* and the definition and role delineation established by the APHA Public Health Nursing Section.

THE APHA DEFINITION OF PUBLIC HEALTH NURSING AND ITS ROLE IN THE DELIVERY OF HEALTH CARE

Like the ANA, a work group of the APHA Public Health Nursing Section was established as an ad hoc committee to define public health nursing* and delineate its scope of practice. Specifically, this ad hoc committee was charged by the membership of the Public Health Nursing Section with the following:

1. Exploration of the current dimensions of public health nursing practice and their theoretical frameworks
2. Development of a position paper that clarifies the definition and role of public health nursing in the delivery of health care

The work of the ad hoc committee was accepted by the membership of the Public Health Nursing Section in October 1980 and subsequently published as *The Definition and Role of Public Health Nursing in the Delivery of Health Care* (American Public Health Association, 1981). This position paper acknowledges the complex and rapidly changing nature of the health care system including such factors acutely affecting public health nursing practice as early patient discharges from the hospital to the home, the movement toward health promotion, the plethora of federally mandated services bombarding public health agencies in order to qualify for funds, the increasingly political nature of health care, and the changes in nursing education and practice which have evolved in response to changes in the health care system.

The overall purpose of the position paper was to clarify the "role of public health nursing in the delivery of health care" (American Public Health Association, 1981) in regard to expected client outcomes, prevention of illness, health promotion and maintenance, determination of public health nursing priorities and appropriate utilization of skills, and clarification of the ways in which public health nursing practice interrelates with other components on the health care system. In order to state a clear and concise position, the following definition of public health nursing was recommended (American Public Health Association, 1981, p. 4):

> Public health nursing synthesizes the body of knowledge from the public health sciences and professional nursing theories for the purpose of improving the health of the entire community. This goal lies at the heart of primary prevention and health promotion and is the foundation for public health nursing practice. To accomplish this goal, public health nurses work with groups, families, and indi-

*The term *public health nursing* will be used in this section of the discussion instead of *community health nursing* because this is the term used by the APHA to refer to their nursing clinical section.

viduals as well as in multidisciplinary teams and programs. Identifying the subgroups (aggregates) within the population which are at high risk of illness, disability, or premature death and directing resources toward these groups is the most effective approach for accomplishing the goal of public health nursing. Success in reducing the risks and in improving the health of the community depends on the involvement of consumers, especially groups experiencing health risks, and others in the community, in health planning, and in self-help activities.

The position paper further noted that public health nursing practice is a systematic process in which the following occur (American Public Health Association, 1980, pp. 4-5):

1. The health and health care needs of a population are assessed by nurses or in collaboration with other disciplines in order to identify subpopulations (aggregates), families, and individuals at increased risk of illness, disability, or premature death.
2. A plan for intervention is developed to meet these needs that includes available resources and those activities that contribute to health and its recovery and to the prevention of illness, disability, and premature death.
3. A health care plan is implemented effectively, efficiently, and equitably.
4. An evaluation is made to determine the extent to which these activities have an impact on the health status of the population.

As can be seen, there are many similarities in the definition of community health nursing offered by the ANA and that of public health nursing offered by the APHA. Specifically, both emphasize the blending of nursing and public health knowledge as a foundation for determining the scope of practice. They both acknowledge that community health nursing efforts are directed toward all people whether they are cared for as individuals, as part of a family, in a community, or as a community at large. Each definition emphasizes a multidisciplinary role for the successful implementation of public health practice and they both focus on the increasing priority of health promotion. The APHA definition does emphasize primary care more than does the ANA definition, and it also clearly points out the need to determine within a community those groups at greatest risk for health disruption so that nursing interventions can be targeted toward them to prevent the onset of disease.

A knowledge of the definition of community health nursing offered by ANA and that of public health nursing offered by APHA is essential for the community health nurse. These models were developed for use by community health nurses, and they are specific in their direction and emphasis for community health nurses.

The next section introduces conceptual models that are interdisciplinary and consequently very broad. They can be useful for application across disciplines including nursing and to community health nursing in particular. This will be followed by a section on nursing models and then a section on models derived primarily from the psychosocial sciences.

INTERDISCIPLINARY MODELS APPLICABLE TO COMMUNITY HEALTH NURSING

Several models exhibit and retain their basic structure and order even though they cross interdisciplinary lines, that is, they can be used or adapted appropriately by more than one of the physical, biological, and social sciences as well as by the professions. These are generally referred to as "types" or "categories" of models. Those interdisciplinary models to be considered here are the systems, developmental, and interaction models.

Systems Theory

Systems theory, also referred to as General Systems Theory (GST) was described as a conceptual model to illustrate the unity in the sciences. Advocating an organismic (as opposed to a mechanistic) view, Bertalanffy (1952, p. 11) wrote that "every organism represents a *system*, by which term we mean a complex of elements in mutual interaction"; the elements in interaction to which he referred were wholeness, organization, openness, and feedback (pp. 9-13), and he delineates how these concepts are important phenomena in the realms of physics, biology, psychology, and philosophy (pp. 176-204). The rationale for such a model was that it allowed for the transfer of laws from one realm (or science) to another. Just as Bertalanffy had thought, the model has proved useful, since it almost universally permeates the literature of many disciplines and many professions.

Characteristics

Wholeness refers to that property of a system in which an aggregate of units responds as an integrated single unit, or a collection of parts responds as an integrated single part. A given element will not show the same properties in isolation that it will show when it is part of a larger whole: for example, the response of a single nerve can be different depending on whether it is isolated or a part of an intact nervous system.

Organization implies that the elements or parts in the system are arranged in a specific way that accommodates or facilitates their relationship to each other. Whether one is speaking of a biological system or a communication system, stimuli or messages, which-ever the case may be, move in a specific direction through the parts. The arrangement of the elements and the order of their relationship to each other refers to their *organization*. It is the organization that permits the whole to show properties that are nonexistent in the isolated parts. Gestalt psychologists referred to this as a property that could not be obtained by adding up all the components and adopted the universal phrase that "the whole is greater than the sum of its parts."

Openness of a system refers to the extent to which it exchanges energy in any form with the environment. An open system is affected by the environment (receives input) and in turn affects the environment by its output. In a closed system there is no exchange of energies. The early writers on systems theory, for example, Bertalanffy, emphasized that living systems are open systems that are in constant and dynamic interchange with the environment.

Several concepts, generally discussed in relation to general systems theory, are intricately related to the openness of a system, and it is appropriate to define them under the characteristic of openness. These concepts are boundary, entropy, negentropy, and equifinality.

Boundary refers to a line or border that shows what elements constitute the system; that is, what elements are inside the system. In biological phenomena the cell membrane is a boundary regulating what goes in and comes out of the cell. In social systems the boundary is more like an imaginary line used in referring to given individuals as a group. *Entropy* is a concept based on a major implication of the second law of thermodynamics which states that elements in a closed environment will proceed toward greater randomness or less order. Entropy is also described as disordered energy, or energy that is bound and cannot be converted to work. *Negentropy* is the energy that is "free," can be used for work, and tends toward order. Since living systems are open systems, they do not adhere to the implications of the second law of thermodynamics. The final term is *equifinality*, which means that the end state of the open system is independent of the beginning state or starting point.

Feedback is the process whereby the output of the system is redirected as part of the input of the same system. The regulation of the body as a physiological system utilizes feedback to regulate temperature, heart rate, and respiration, to mention only a few. However, the discussion of input, throughput, output, and feedback characterizes all explanations of systems.

Advantages and Disadvantages

There are several advantages to systems theory. It can be applied (1) across disciplines so that universal laws are identified and useful, and (2) to individuals, groups, and communities. Furthermore it emphasizes how each isolated variable affects the whole and how the whole affects each part. A disadvantage is that it does not explicitly emphasize growth and change toward a higher level of organization.

Application to Community Health Nursing

Wholeness. The community as a whole is a social system made up of interrelated and interdependent subsystems. The subsystems include the economic, educational, religious, health care, political, welfare, law enforcement, energy (heat, light, and water), and recreational systems. When any one of the subsystems are affected, it affects the community as a whole.

A subsystem whose changes are seen immediately and obviously in the whole community is the economic system. For example, in the early months of 1980 the United States was involved in an economic recession. As the recession grew, people began to cut back on unnecessary health care like routine trips to the doctor. Welfare recipients found it more difficult to qualify for food stamps, the crime rate increased, and law enforcement had to increase its surveillance of crimes against individuals, such as home burglaries, car theft, and purse snatchings. With less money available for educational support, some community colleges cut recreational programs to concentrate funds on academic pursuits. The political subsystem was faced with the problem of keeping the community functional by spending monies on primary services like community fire safety, while cutting programs like rape crisis centers, and still keeping the voters happy. In this economic crisis the religious subsystem worked to increase the morale of the community and meet the needs of the unemployed, the homeless, and the hungry.

Organization. All of the subsystems of the larger social system, the community, are organized and related to each other in a specific way. There are specific communication channels for the organizations to relate to each other and to the whole.

Openness. The community is an open system that exchanges materials, such as energy and goods, but also services, values, and ideals with the environment outside the community. The community as a system has boundaries, the most obvious being geographical lines. The imaginary line–type boundary is one that encompasses all the subsystems in the community and identifies what is inside and outside the community. Entropy can be compared to the landfill garbage dumps (waste) or the problems such as crime, violence, and poor health in the community, whereas negentropy can be compared to the resources, health, wealth, and altruistic values of the people. Equifinality indicates that wherever the community begins, for example, with the poor and unattractive, given the necessary resources and energy, it may attain economic balance and beauty.

Feedback. An excellent example of feedback in the community is in the economic system. If the output is good, it provides good input and further contributes to the growth of the economy in the community.

Developmental Theory

Developmental theory as a way of thinking about how changes occur is based on theories of development of the human organism. Lewis (1982, p. 10) classifies theories of child development as reactive and structural. Reactive theories emphasize the influence of the environment on the development of the child. These include stimulus-response theory, learning theories, classical conditioning, and operant conditioning. Structural theories emphasize the genetically determined program for development and are usually described in stages. Examples of structural theories given by Lewis (1982, pp. 12-13) include Freud's psychosexual stages (oral, anal, phallic, latency, and genital), Erikson's psychosocial phases (trust vs. mistrust, autonomy vs. shame and doubt, initiative vs. guilt, industry vs. inferiority, identity vs. role confusion, intimacy vs. isolation, generativity vs. self-absorption, and integrity vs. despair), and Piaget's stages of cognitive development (sensorimotor, period of preoperational thought, stage of concrete operations, and formal operations). Although Lewis refers to these as structural theories, they are generally referred to as developmental theories.

Characteristics

Chin (1980, pp. 30-31) describes the major characteristics of developmental models as direction, stages or phases, progression, potentiality, and forces. These characteristics refer to the process of growth or change.

Direction refers to the fact that growth proceeds in a specific direction toward an end state or goal. In development of the individual a direction of physical growth is toward being taller and a direction of mental growth is toward complexity in thought and language.

Stages or phases and levels are terms used to describe periods when the individual or group is concentrating on a particular task or developmental milestone. Each stage has facets of growth or behavior that are unique to it. For example, the development of motor capabilities at different ages proceeds sequentially, such as when an infant crawls, pulls to a standing position, and then walks over a period of months.

Progression suggests that the way in which changes occur over time has a characteristic form. Chin (1980, p. 31) describes four forms of progression: linear, spiral, oscillation, and differentiation. Linear refers to changes such as aging, which proceeds in a unidirectional manner. Spiral refers to the fact that some behaviors when performed again are similar but are at a more complex level, for example, thinking and problem solving are behaviors that are repeated but performed at higher levels. Oscillation refers to the fact that individuals may go back and forth for a period of time between behaviors of a stage they are growing out of and behaviors of a more complex stage they are growing toward. Differentiation refers to changes in which the functions of the individual becomes more specialized.

Potentiality refers to the capabilities offered by the genetic endowment of the individual when given a supporting and nurturing environment.

Forces include genetic and environmental factors. Individuals are genetically programmed for growth and development. The environmental forces can enhance or deter the development.

Although it is easier to understand these characteristics in the development of the individual organism, one should remember that the developmental model is also applied to change in groups or social organizations such as health care delivery systems.

Advantages and Disadvantage

Advantages of developmental models are (1) characteristics are easy to understand and when considered in relation to the human organism, it is possible to observe the developmental changes, and (2) there is emphasis on growth, which is viewed as a positive event and which may be experienced psychologically even when physical growth has ceased. A disadvantage of developmental models is that environmental or circumstantial factors may be minimized.

Application to Community Health Nursing

The usefulness of developmental theory in working with infants and children is evidenced by the fact that growth and development is an inherent part of every nursing curricula. A major part of the nurse's role in working with infants and children is that of assessing their developmental progress and of helping parents to promote that progress by a stimulating environment. One of the most widely used screening tools that assess child development is the Denver Developmental Screening Test (DDST). The DDST was developed and tested to yield a developmental profile in the areas of gross motor, language, fine motor-adaptive, and personal-social skills (Further details of the DDST can be found in Chapter 30 and Appendix K). The developmental approach has also been widely discussed and written about as a way of working with families. Duvall (1977, p. 144) described the family life cycle in eight stages: beginning, early childbearing, preschool, school, teenagers, launching center, middle years, and retirement. The nurse can use each of these stages of development and their respective tasks for each stage in the assessment and in the promotion of family development. The application of developmental models can probably be best illustrated by pointing out the widespread use of Peplau's development model (Blake, 1980), Maslow's hierarchy of needs, and crisis intervention (Thibodeau, 1983).

Interaction Theory

Interaction models are based on theories that stem from philosophical writings early in this century, such as those of Cooley (1909) and Mead (1934). Mead, influential in the developmental of social psychology, viewed man as a reflection of human society, that is primarily a social and cultural being. Furthermore, he contended that a newborn develops a self as a consequence of relationships with others and the environment (Butts and Cremin, 1953). Contemporary social psychologists such as Rose (1962) use the term symbolic interactionism, and Burr et al. (1979) use the framework of interactionism to encompass role theory and self-theory.

Characteristics

Communication in simple terms is the act of giving and receiving information. Communication between humans consists of both verbal and nonverbal language but also uses symbols. Interaction theory emphasizes that symbols, whose meanings and values are important in communication, are learned through the process of socialization, and they influence the development of personality (Rose, 1962).

Role refers to the performance or enactment of behaviors that are set or defined by the person's position or status (Burr et al., 1979). A given individual may have the role of parent, spouse, nurse, friend, and sibling all within a few hours of time; this is referred to as multiple roles. Each role brings expectations, and sometimes role strain occurs as a result of role conflict.

Self-concept refers to the way in which persons visualize and think about themselves. Some writers such as Fitts (1965) subdivide the concept of self into such categories as physical self, social self, family self, moral-ethical self, and personal self. The picture that we have of ourselves influences the way we interact with others.

Perception is the way a person perceives a situation or an event. It is influenced by antecedent, cognitive, and emotional factors already present in the person's background.

Advantages and Disadvantage

Interaction theory calls attention to how elements affect each other and especially the individuality of human beings. However, one can focus on the interaction to the exclusion of other variables.

Application to Community Health Nursing

Nursing literature frequently addresses the phenomena of family dynamics. The interaction model can be useful in analyzing family dynamics.

Communication. Community health nursing presents many occasions when, in order to be more helpful to a family, assessment of the communication patterns is indicated. The reason for the contact with the nurse may be health related, but the manner in which the family is coping with the health problems may be intricately related to the communication patterns. That is, who talks to whom about what and in what way? Furthermore, it is important to know who listens, what is heard by the person listening, if the message sent is the message received, and finally what kind of feedback the members of the family give to each other.

Role. Assessment of the role structure is also important in working with families. As previously described, role refers to a set of expected behaviors by virtue of occupying or holding a given position, and every person assumes multiple roles. The person who enters the health care system inevitably has multiple roles: problems or illnesses that generally bring the person to the health care system will affect the person's ability to function in many of the roles. The person may worry about the inability to function in all the roles. An obvious example is the mother who worries that illness such as a heart defect will interfere with her childbearing role in the family. In the health maintenance function of the nurse, one uses knowledge about roles to identify such things as role conflict, a situation in which a person is confronted with incompatible expectations, or role strain, anxiety, work and stress associated with the role. The nurse will also have contact with first-time parents who are undergoing the role transition from couple to parents and adding the roles of mother and father to that of husband and wife.

Self-Concept. Self-concept, or the way one sees oneself, is an important aspect of health and well-being. It influences health-seeking behaviors and how one adapts to problems of a health/illness nature. The change from being a well person to someone who is not in total control of one's life and especially one's health may result in a lower self-concept. Thus, it is important that the nurse listen for cues and help the person use the self-concept positively.

Perception. Just as perception of isolated events and situations such as auto accidents differs from one person to another, persons' perceptions of events and situations happening to them are affected by previous experiences, as well as attitudes, beliefs, and socialization into a particular culture. It is useful to the nurse to recognize the differences in perception. The perception of the client of their situation may not be the same as that of the nurse.

NURSING MODELS APPLICABLE TO COMMUNITY HEALTH NURSING

A number of conceptual models have been developed and described by nurses for use in nursing. Authors who are prominent in the literature include Roy, Rogers, Johnson, Orem, Neuman, and King; all of their models will be described briefly.

One way to examine the similarities and differences in nursing models is to consider how each define the terms *person, environment, health,* and *nursing* (Table 6-1). These four concepts were described by Fawcett (1978) as essential units based on a review of conceptual frameworks in baccalaureate programs by Yura and Torres (1975). Some of the authors have not defined all these terms even though they use them in their models.

Roy

The Roy Adaptation Model of Nursing was first presented in the periodical literature in 1970 (Roy, 1970) and has since been used as a conceptual framework for nursing curricula, nursing practice, and nursing research. This model has some of the characteristics of a systems theory and some of the characteristics of interaction theory, and Roy (Riehl and Roy, 1980, p. 179) describes it as a "systems theory though it also contains interactionist levels of analysis."

Characteristics and Key Assumptions

Man is viewed as an adaptative system. Changes occur in the system in response to stimuli (input). If the changes promote integrity of the individual such as growth or self-mastery, it is an adaptive response. Otherwise it is considered a maladaptive response. The system has two major mechanisms for adapting or coping: the regulator and the cognator. The regulator mechanism is concerned with the neural, endocrine, and perception-psychomotor processes, and the cognator mechanism is concerned with the processes of perception, learning, judgment, and emotion (Roy and Rob-

erts, 1981, pp. 60-63). Additionally, four modes for effecting adaptation of the system include physiological needs, self-concept, role function, and interdependence.

Application to Practice

Goal. The goal of the nurse is to "promote man's adaptation in situations of health and illness" (Roy, 1976, p. 23). The nurse achieves the goal by manipulating or changing the stimuli causing the stress to help the person cope more effectively. When people encounter more than the usual amount of stress, such as that caused by illness, their established coping mechanisms may be ineffective. Thus a nursing intervention is required.

Nursing Process. The nursing process according to Roy consists of first- and second-level assessment, problem identification, nursing diagnosis, setting of priorities, goal setting, intervention, and evaluation (Roy, 1976, p. 22). In the first-level assessment, client behaviors in each of the adaptive modes (physiological, self-concept, role function, and interdependence) are observed and described. In the second-level assessment, the nurse identifies the focal, contextual, and residual stimuli influencing client behavior. The focal stimulus is the situation such as stress, injury, or illness immediately confronting the individual. The contextual stimuli are the other factors present such as family milieu or environment. The residual stimuli are influencing factors from the client's previous background: beliefs, attitudes, experience, and traits. Following the second-level assessment, problems are identified, nursing diagnoses are made, priorities are set, and then goals are formulated. The next step, intervention, manipulates the stimuli to promote adaptation, and the evaluation is used to judge the effectiveness of the nursing approach.

Strengths and Limitations

Strengths of the model include the following: (1) most of the terminology is familiar or is clearly described; (2) the nursing process is similar to the standard process of assess, plan, implement, and evaluate; (3) the focus is on behaviors, thereby offering greater individuality to the client assessment; and (4) assessment of psychosocial needs is emphasized.

Limitations of the model are that (1) there is overlap of the adaptive modes, especially in the modes of self-concept, role function, and interdependence; (2) the judgment of behavior as adaptive or maladaptive will be influenced by the value system of the nurse assessing the client; and (3) the term *adaptation* generally does not convey a meaning of growth as intended in the model.

Rogers

Rogers' Science of Unitary Man first appeared in the literature in 1970. It has been used as the conceptual base for the curriculum at New York University, for several research projects, and to a lesser extent in nursing practice.

The Rogers model (1970, pp. 49-77) has strong ties to general systems theory, which are reflected in her basic assumptions, and there are elements of the developmental model inherent in her models.

Characteristics and Key Assumptions

Energy fields, universe of open systems, pattern and organization, and four dimensionality are described by Rogers as the four building blocks for her conceptual system (Rogers, 1980, p. 330). *Energy fields* refers to the conceptualization of humans and their environment as matter or energy evidenced by wave patterns. She emphasizes the energy field as part of a person's wholeness: "the human field is more than and different from the sum of its parts" (Rogers, 1980, p. 330). *Openness* refers to the view of persons as open systems who interact continuously with the environment. The term *pattern and organization* refers to the way the energy fields emerge, characterized by wave pattern and organization. *Four dimensionality* is another characteristic of energy fields, which is described by Johnson and Fitzpatrick as "transcendence of the time-space interaction" (Johnson and Fitzpatrick, 1982, p. 10). Four dimensionality is easier to understand by thinking of the phenomena of clairvoyance, because a person who sees the future transcends time for an instant.

Rogers postulates the development of unitary persons by use of three principles of homeodynamics. *Helicy* refers to life as proceeding in one direction and rhythmically along a spiral. *Resonancy* refers to the wave pattern and organization of the energy fields. *Complementarity* refers to the simultaneous mutual interaction of the human and environmental fields.

Application to Practice

Goal. Rogers' background in community health (M.A. at Columbia University and M.P.H. at Johns Hopkins University in public health) obviously influenced her statement of nursing's goal: "Maintenance and promotion of health, prevention of disease, nursing diagnosis, intervention, and rehabilitation encompass the scope of nursing's goals" (Rogers, 1970, p. 86). She also emphasizes that nursing is for the well and the sick, rich and poor, in all settings: home, school, work, and play.

Nursing Process. Rogers (1970, p. 86) made the goal of nursing clear: that individuals achieve their maximum health potential. However, it was others who turned her model into an operational framework for the nursing process. Whelton (1979, pp. 10-14) illustrates areas of assessment and nursing process in the areas of wholeness, openness, pattern and organization, unidirectionality, and sentience and thought.

Falco and Lobo (1980) illustrated the process of assessment using the principles of homeodynamics: complementarity, resonance, helicy. Whall (1981, pp. 33-34) made Rogers' theory operational by illustrating the assessment of families under the categories of (1) individual subsystem (developmental biological, psychological, or social), (2) interactional patterns, (3) unique characteristics of the whole, and (4) environmental interface synchrony.

Strengths and Limitations

Strengths of this model are (1) emphasis on the total context of the universe, (2) the goal of maximum health potential, and (3) emphasis on the effect of environment (not only such factors as air pollution but also lifestyle) on a person's health. Limitations of the model are (1) terminology is not easily understood and (2) it has not been made operational for practice.

Johnson

Dorothy Johnson's Behavioral Systems Model was first presented as an unpublished paper at Vanderbilt University in 1968. It was subsequently used in the graduate program at the University of California at Los Angeles. It has also been tested to some extent by research studies (Holaday, 1974) and has been applied in practice (Grubbs, 1980). It is clearly a systems model with the behavioral system having subsystems that are both linked to each other and open.

Characteristics and Key Assumptions

Johnson assumed that the person can be viewed as a behavioral system in the same way that physicians view man as a biological system. The behavioral system consists of seven subsystems: achievement, affiliative, aggressive, dependency, eliminative, ingestive, and sexual. Each subsystem has four structural elements: drive or goal, set or predisposition to act, choices of action alternatives from which he can choose, and the person's action or behavior. The behavioral system as a whole and each of the subsystems has functional requirements: protection, nurturance, and stimulation. The outcome of the behavioral system is the patterned, repetitive, and purposeful ways of behaving, which if efficient and effective are orderly, purposeful, and predictable.

Application to Practice

Goal. "The goal of nursing action in each case is to restore, maintain, or attain behavioral system balance and stability at the highest possible level for the individual" (Johnson, 1980, p. 214). The nurse must be concerned with promoting efficient and effective behavior related to health.

Nursing Process. Assessment to begin the nursing process consists of listing all significant behaviors in each of the seven subsystems. The behaviors are identified as being functional or dysfunctional. The variables influencing or causing the behaviors are also identified. The nursing problem (diagnosis) is made and is placed in one of four diagnostic classifications: (1) insufficiency, which indicates the subsystem is not functioning because of inadequacy of functional requirements; (2) discrepancy, which indicates the behavior is not meeting the intended goal; (3) incompatibility, which indicates that goals or behaviors of two subsystems are in conflict; and (4) dominance, which indicates that the behavior in one subsystem is used more than any other.

Before the implementation, long- and short-term goals are set. There are four intervention modes used in nursing implementation: (1) restrict or place limits on behavior, (2) defend or protect from negative stressors, (3) inhibit or suppress ineffective responses, and (4) facilitate or give nurturance and stimulation. Following implementation, evaluation is made in terms of long- and short-term goals.

Strengths and Limitations

The conceptualization of man as a behavioral system gives an alternative to the medical model as a way of viewing man. In this way the nursing role can be differentiated from medicine's role. Johnson has demonstrated how the model can be used as a system for nursing care. However, some of the terminology is unfamiliar to nurses and the nursing literature, and one has to become oriented to a new terminology.

Orem

Orem's Self-Care Nursing Model began in 1959 when Orem (1980, p. 5) described the nurse's role as giving assistance to the person experiencing inabilities in self-care. It was further developed in 1965 by the nursing-model committee of the School of Nursing Faculty of the Catholic University of America (Nursing Development Conference Group, 1973). The first full description, *Nursing: Concepts of Practice,* was published in 1971. The model is also described in later works (Nursing Development Conference Group, 1973; and Orem, 1980). Orem's model was categorized by Riehl and Roy (1980) as a systems model; however,

Bush (1979) characterizes it as an interaction model. Orem uses the concept of nursing systems (Orem, 1980, p. 92) and discusses role (Orem, 1980, pp. 8-16) and self-concept (Orem, 1980, p. 88), but the analogy between the model and systems theory or the model and interaction theory is somewhat tangential.

Characteristics and Key Assumptions

Orem's model evolves from the way she conceptualizes nursing and especially from her belief that nursing is concerned with self-care. Important terms in the model are self-care, self-care agency, therapeutic self-care demand, and self-care deficit.

Self-care consists of those activities that an individual does for himself to maintain life, health, and well-being. *Self-care agency* refers to the person who provides the self-care. Every individual has need of a composite of self-care actions called *therapeutic self-care demand.* If the therapeutic self-care demand is greater than the self-care agency, there exists a *self-care deficit.* When this occurs, there is a need for nursing intervention.

Application to Practice

Goal. The goal of nursing is to meet client's self-care demands until the family is capable of providing it.

Nursing Process. Orem categorizes self-care into three types: (1) universal, which consists of self-care to meet physiological and psychosocial needs, (2) developmental, the self-care required when one goes through developmental stages, and (3) health deviation, the self-care required when an individual has a deviation from health. Using the Orem model, assessment is made of the therapeutic self-care demand, the self-care agency, and the self-care deficits in the areas of knowledge, skills, motivation, and orientation.

Following the nursing assessment, a plan is formulated for the nursing system, which is the approach the nurse uses to meet the client's self-care deficit. These plans are categorized into three systems: (1) wholly compensatory, in which the client has no active role; (2) partly compensatory, in which the client and the nurse have an actual role; and (3) educative development, in which clients can meet their need for self-care with some assistance from the nurse.

To implement the nursing system, the nurse uses one of the following actions: (1) acting for or doing for, (2) guidance, (3) supporting, (4) providing, and (5) teaching.

Evaluation is not presented as a step in the nursing process (Orem, 1980, p. 202). However, in a later discussion of nursing actions, Orem (1980, p. 216) describes monitoring patients to determine the effects of self-care and making judgments about the sufficiency and efficiency of nursing action. Therefore, she does advocate evaluation.

Strengths and Limitations

Orem's model builds onto self-care a function that nurses have assumed responsibility for historically, especially since Henderson (Harmer and Henderson, 1955, p. 4). Orem emphasized the client's role in planning and implementing care according to their capability. There is structure in the model to focus on the client as a learner and the nurse as a teacher. A limitation in using the model is that the terminology can be confusing.

Neuman

Neuman's Health-Care Systems Model was first introduced as a total-person approach to viewing client problems (1972). She refers to her conceptual framework as an "open systems model of two components—stress and reaction to it" (Neuman, 1980, p. 122). Her model also draws from the Gestalt and field theories in psychology (Fagan and Shepherd, 1970).

Characteristics and Key Assumptions

Neuman's model was designed to bring together simultaneously the behavioral, biological, developmental, and interacting components of the person. Man is depicted graphically as a series of concentric circles that have stressors impinging on them. The basic structure (factor common to all organisms) is viewed as the center of the concentric circle. Surrounding the basic structure are (1) flexible lines of resistance, or the organism's internal mechanisms for defense against stress, (2) normal line of defense, or what the individual has become over time, (3) flexible line of defense, which is a protective buffer around the normal line of defense.

Stressors and reaction to stress can be viewed as intrapersonal, interpersonal, or extrapersonal. Intrapersonal refers to those factors within the individual, interpersonal refers to factors between individuals, and extrapersonal refers to factors outside the individual.

Application to Nursing Practice

Goal. The goal of nursing is to assess all the variables (physiological, psychological, sociocultural, and developmental) which affect the individual's response to stress and to intervene appropriately.

Nursing Process. Implementation of nursing intervention is carried out through primary prevention such as reducing stress, secondary prevention such as early case finding, and tertiary prevention such as reeducation.

Strengths and Limitations

The model builds on the function of primary, secondary, and tertiary prevention, which is supported by the discipline of community health and has been a major contribution of the nursing profession. Furthermore, it emphasizes the total person as opposed to viewing man in one dimension. However, it fails to delineate a distinct role or function of nursing that other health professionals do not also encompass in their work. Nursing should provide some service that is unique to nursing.

King

King's theory (1968) for nursing was first introduced as a "conceptual frame of reference." The framework was used in the curriculum at Ohio State University when King was director of the School of Nursing, and King has reported its use in her own research (1978). King refers to her work as a systems theory, and it does reflects some properties of the system model. It also reflect properties of an interaction model and is sometimes described as an interaction model (Bush, 1979).

Characteristics and Key Assumptions

Man/person. Man is a social, sentient, rational, reacting, perceiving, controlling, purposeful, action-oriented, and time-oriented being (King, 1981, p. 143). King describes her conceptual framework as a general systems theory with three subsystems: personal system, interpersonal system, and social system. The *personal* system is made up of the concepts of perception, self, growth and development, body image, space, and time. The *interpersonal* system is made up of the concepts of human interactions, communication, transactions, role, and stress. The *social system* is made up of the concepts of organization, authority, power, status, and decision making. The three systems—personal, interpersonal, and social—are dynamic and interacting (King, 1981).

Application to Nursing Practice

Goal. The goal of nursing is health.

Nursing Process. Implementation of nursing interventions is carried out through the process of action, reaction, interaction, and transaction between the client and the nurse. King also described a theory of goal attainment which is implemented through a goal-oriented nursing record. This consists of five major elements: a data base, a problem list, a goal list, a plan, and progress notes (King 1981, p. 165).

Strength and Limitation

The model emphasizes the participation of clients in planning their own care by King's emphasis on the

Table 6-1. Definitions of person, environment, health, and nursing

Nurse-author	Person (Client)	Environment	Health	Nursing
Roy	"An adaptive system with cognator and regulator acting to maintain adaptation in regard to the four adaptive modes" (Roy and Roberts, 1981, p. 44)	Conditions, circumstances, and influences surrounding, and affecting the development of an organism or group of organisms (Roy and Roberts, 1981, p. 43)	The implied definition is that health exists if that person has adaptive responses that "promote the integrity of the person in terms of the goals of survival, growth, reproduction, and self-mastery" (Roy and Roberts, 1981, p. 43)	Manipulating stimuli so that a person's coping mechanism can bring about adaptation (Roy and Roberts, 1981, p. 46)
Rogers	"Unitary man—a four-dimensional, negentropic energy field identified by pattern and organization and manifesting characteristics and behaviors that are different from those of the parts and which cannot be predicted from knowledge of the parts" (Rogers, 1980, p. 332)	"A four-dimensional, negentropic energy field identified by pattern and organization and encompassing all that outside any given human field" (Rogers, 1980, p. 332)	Health not specifically defined; however, she does state that disease and pathology are value terms (Rogers, 1980, p. 336) and since values change, phenomena perceived as disease such as hyperactivity may change over time and not be perceived as disease	Goal of nursing is that individuals achieve their maximum health potential through maintenance and promotion of health, prevention of disease, nursing diagnosis, intervention, and rehabilitation (Rogers, 1970, p. 86)
Johnson	Behavioral system composed of patterned, repetitive, and purposeful ways of behaving (Johnson, 1980, pp. 208, 209)	Malfunctions in the behavioral systems are frequently due to "sudden internal or external environmental change" (Johnson, 1980, p. 212)	It seems reasonable to assume that health would be considered behavior that is orderly, purposeful, predictable, and functionally efficient and effective (Johnson, p. 209)	"External regulatory force which acts to preserve the organization and integration of the patient's behavior at an optimal level under those conditions in which the behavior constitutes a threat to physical or social health, or in which illness is found" (Johnson, 1980, p. 214)
Orem	"A unity that can be viewed as functioning biologically, symbolically, and socially" (Orem, 1980, p. 120)	Although not explicitly defined, the role of the nurse in providing a developmental environment is discussed (Orem, 1980, p. 66)	"A term that has considerable general utility in describing the state of wholeness or integrity of human beings" (Orem, 1980, p. 118)	"A service, a mode of helping human beings" (Orem, 1980, p. 5); "nursing is contributed effort toward designing, providing, and managing systems of therapeutic self-care for individuals or multiperson units within their daily living environments" (Orem, 1980, p. 117)

Continued.

Table 6-1. Definitions of person, environment, health, and nursing — cont'd

Nurse-author	Person (Client)	Environment	Health	Nursing
Neuman	"Man is a system capable of intake of extrapersonal and interpersonal factors from the external environment. He interacts with this environment by adjusting it to himself" (Neuman, 1982, p. 14)	"Environment consists of the internal and external forces surrounding man at a point in time" (Neuman, 1982, p. 9)	"Health or wellness is the condition in which all parts and subparts (variables) are in harmony with the whole man" (Neuman, 1982, p. 9)	"Nursing can . . . assist individuals, families, groups to attain and maintain a maximum level of total wellness by purposeful interventions . . . aimed at reduction of stress factors and adverse conditions which affect optimal functioning" (Neuman, 1982, p. 11)
King	A social, sentient, rational, reacting, perceiving, controlling, purposeful, action-oriented, and time-oriented being (King, 1981, p. 143)	Refers to human being interacting with the environment (King, 1981, p. 66) but does not define it	Dynamic life experiences of a human being, which implies continuous adjustment to stressors in the internal and external environment through optimum use of one's resources to achieve maximum potential for daily living (King, 1981, p. 5)	"Nursing is perceiving, thinking, relating, judging, and acting vis-a-vis the behavior of individuals who come to a nursing situation" (King, 1981, p. 2)

transaction but fails to explain how the intervention is carried out following the transaction.

Similarities and Differences of Models

Similarities in the models in Table 6-1 include their consideration of the impact of environment on man and man's interaction with the environment. Behavioral patterning, holistic man, and maximum functioning of the organism are common themes. The differences are more in their emphasis for the most part, although there are some unique views, for example, Rogers' emphasis on energy fields and Johnson's conceptualization of man as a behavioral system. In other models there is particular attention to themes previously introduced in nursing. Neuman's emphasizes primary, secondary, and tertiary prevention, but that content is recognized as essential for any nursing student. Orem's model is organized around self-care, but that is also content recognized as essential in nursing programs. Roy's recognizes man as a psychosocial human being. King's emphasis on transaction fits with more recent literature on contracting.

PSYCHOSOCIAL THEORIES APPLICABLE TO COMMUNITY HEALTH NURSING

Motivation

The influence of motives on behavior and the influence of motivation on achievement or work productivity has long been recognized (Hersey and Blanchard, 1977, p. 5). Between 1900 and 1930 classical theory, also referred to as "scientific management," postulated that the basic motive of man was economic gain: the emphasis in organizations was on tasks. However, following the studies at the Hawthorne Plant of the Western Electric Company, the classical theory was abandoned for the human relations theory. The human relations theory advocated the importance of job satisfaction and the feeling of belonging to a group (interpersonal relations); thus in the work settings the emphasis in organizations should be on relationships (Hersey and Blanchard, 1977, p. 91).

An early advocate of the human relations movement was Elton Mayo who noted that the assumptions of many managers about workers was that workers wanted to make as much money as possible for as little work as possible (Hersey and Blanchard, 1977, p. 54). Douglas McGregor developed this thesis further and is now widely known for his list of assumptions about human nature and human motivation, called Theory X and Theory Y. McGregor (1960) drew heavily from the work of Maslow on motivation. Although there are other motivation theories, including that of Herzberg (1976), Maslow's will be described, since his writings have been most widely used in nursing.

Chief Characteristics

Maslow's theory (1970) postulates that the basic driving force or basic motive of people arises from a hierarchy of needs. When needs of the lower hierarchy are met, the need at the next higher level becomes the basic motivating need. The hierarchy of human needs progresses from lower to higher needs as follows: physiological requirements → safety and security → social affiliation (love and belonging) → esteem → self-actualization.

Advantages and Disadvantages

Maslow's writings, perhaps more than any other single work, have given nursing the impetus to view clients as human beings with needs beyond those that are physiological. His writings promoted a movement to look beyond the pathophysiology of disease to the psychosocial needs of clients. However, the broad categories may obscure individuality of clients and their unique reaction to illness.

Application to Community Health Nursing

Many nursing programs have used Maslow's hierarchy of needs as a model for curriculum. An example of how it generally is applied to nursing care planning is as follows: (1) problem: failure to thrive; (2) interference with basic human need: social affiliation or love and belonging; (3) nursing plan and implementation: set goals for mother or mother surrogate to meet need of social affiliation; and (4) evaluation: assess alleviation of problem.

As mentioned above, the categories of needs are broad, and often one has to further delineate how the need is being interfered with before action can be taken.

Change

Change is constant and inevitable; some changes are planned, others are unplanned. Since it is an objective of most baccalaureate programs that their graduates be change agents, it is planned change that is of concern here. "Planned change is a conscious, deliberate, and collaborative effort to improve operations of human systems . . . through the utilization of valid knowledge" (Bennis et al., 1976, p. 4). Lewin (1951), the noted psychologist, applied concepts from field theory to the process of change.

Chief Characteristics

According to field theory, change occurs in a three-step process: unfreezing, moving, and refreezing. Unfreezing begins with dissatisfaction with the present system or a feeling that there is a need for things to be different. The dissatisfaction may first occur among or within the group members. The leader must promote the unfreezing process or the willingness of the group members to give up their old or familiar ways of doing things and to be willing to consider alternatives to the present situation. A major part of unfreezing is called force field analysis, or identifying those forces in support of the change (driving forces) and those forces that fail to support or are against the change (restraining forces) (Bernhard and Walsh, 1981, p. 143).

The second step in the change process, moving, involves implementing the change. Three change strategies are empirical-rational, normative-reeducative, and power-coercion (Chin and Benne, 1976, p. 23). The empirical-rational strategy provides people with knowledge that the change will make things better, for example, chlorine added to the water supply makes it safe for drinking. The normative-reeducative strategy goes beyond an increase in knowledge to include change in values and attitudes. For example, a change in format of a nursing procedure or a nursing process would require a change in the nurse's value and attitude that the change was for the better. The power-coercive strategy implements change by the use of power. An administrator may make a change without any input from the staff members, that is, the individual uses the power base for the change.

The final stage in the change process is called refreezing. In refreezing, the newly acquired behavior has been practiced and is stable.

Advantages and Disadvantages

An advantage of this model for change based on field theory is that it delineates a systematic process for identifying elements in a situation which should be assessed and known before proceeding with the change process. It also describes how to stabilize the change. A disadvantage is that it does not address how the change agent can deal effectively with individual differences of people in the group involved. For example, offering a variety of incentives for change may meet an individual's needs, thereby motivating the person to support the change.

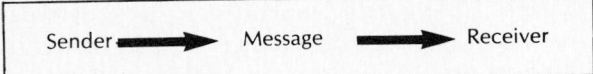

Fig. 6-1. Linear model of communication.

Application to Community Health Nursing

Suppose a community health nurse in a middle management position has just attended a conference on problem-oriented records and thinks that system would be an improvement over the system currently being used. According to the first stage in change theory, unfreezing, the manager would need to determine if any of the staff were dissatisfied with their own method. If dissatisfactions about the existing method exist, the unfreezing process has begun. The nurse then needs to ask the staff members to discuss their views on the process currently used. In this way the nurse can identify the driving and restraining forces in the staff and move toward presenting the proposed change to the administration to see whether it supports the change. If there is enough support for the next stage, then it is time for the moving stage. This stage may mean sending others to a conference on problem-oriented medical records or inviting someone to come in and present a conference. This would be the normative-reeducative strategy. Then the change would be implemented, and the refreezing phase would begin.

Communication

Communication or the act of transmitting, giving, or exchanging information can be described by the use of two simple models. The first model (Fig. 6-1) is linear and consists of a sender, a message, and a receiver. The second model (Fig. 6-2) is circular and includes a sender, message, receiver, and feedback.

More elaborate models exist in the literature, and Lancaster (1982, pp. 111-112) has described four models of communication theory: (1) The systems approach, which consists of input, processing, output, and feedback. (2) The questioning approach, which consists of asking the questions Who? What? How? To whom? and To what effect? (feedback). (3) A human relations model, described as generation of idea, encoding, transmission, receipt of message, decoding, and action. (4) A composite model, which consists of generation of idea, encoding, transmission, receipt of message, decoding, action, and feedback to encoding. The model described here (Fig. 6-2) is simplistic but contains the most essential elements and fits better with the basic description of communication, which follows.

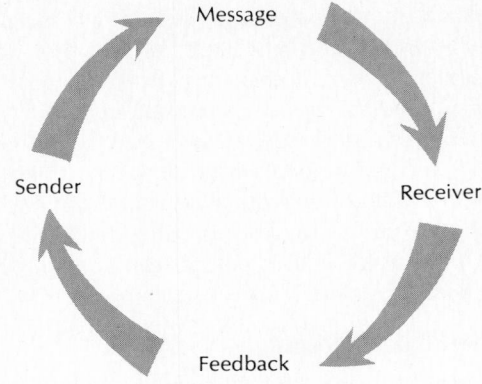

Fig. 6-2. Circular model of communication.

Chief Characteristics

Form. Communication is the expression of a message in any one of four forms: art, writing, verbal, and nonverbal. Music, art, poetry, and literature are all ways of expression and communication. Written words in the form of books, articles, and letters are another way of communicating. Verbal communication is through language or symbols, and the most obvious example is television. The nonverbal form of communication includes body movements and facial expression, voice tone and quality, allocation of personal space, touch, and personal expression through things such as style of dress.

Purpose. Human communication is generally carried out for the following purposes: (1) to give information, (2) to obtain information, (3) to release tension, and, (4) to solve problems.

Situational Variables. Variables that affect communication and have a part in whether it is successful or unsuccessful include (1) relationship between those communicating, (2) communication of a persons' perception of the topic, and (3) beliefs, values, and attitudes of those involved in the communication.

Advantage and Disadvantage

An advantage of the communication model in Fig. 6-2 is that, although simple, it illustrates that communication is a circular process, an exchange, that requires processing and interpretation. An obvious disadvantage is that, because of its simplicity, it does not explain in detail factors that influence communication.

Application to Community Health Nursing

The community health nurse is most often a person who elicits information from a client and consequently is the receiver of information. Some general guidelines or techniques for more effective communication are as follows:

1. Attend and receive the message as an active listener.
2. Clarify the message by asking for an illustration.
3. Reflect and paraphrase to check accuracy of message received.
4. Validate and summarize at the close of the session.

Leadership

Leadership refers to the "process of influencing the activities of an individual or a group in efforts toward goal achievement" (Hersey and Blanchard, p. 85). Two ways of describing leadership are generally used. One way is to describe styles of leadership. Style refers to the way in which a person practices leadership, or the way of acting. Although there are others, the three most recognized styles of leadership are autocratic, democratic, and laissez-faire. The second way of describing leadership is by theories of leadership. As defined previously, the purpose of a theory is to describe, predict, and explain. Thus theories on leadership attempt to describe the concepts in leadership and the relationship between them. In other words, they try to answer the question of what elements constitute leadership, or in some cases, what elements constitute a leader.

Chief Characteristics

Styles. Style refers to the amount of control the leader exerts over subordinates versus the amount of freedom allowed to them. The autocratic leader uses maximum control, makes decisions, and tells the subordinates what to do, when to do it, how to do it, and then how well they did it in either the form of praise or criticism. The democratic leader invites input from the group in decision making and allows some flexibility in how and when to implement the decision. The group receives feedback from the leader in a more factual way rather than in a judgmental way. The democratic group also receives feedback from each other. The laissez-faire leader gives the group total freedom and is sometimes seen as a person who abdicates leadership responsibility. Stogdill (1974, p. 365-370) reported that autocratic and democratic groups show about the same productivity, whereas the laissez-faire group showed less productivity, less satisfaction, and less cohesiveness. The democratic group showed more group cohesiveness, and the autocratic group demanded more attention from the leader.

Theories. Earlier theories of leadership can be considered descriptive in that they describe a single factor as the key to effective leadership. The first of these was the *great man theory,* which postulated that some are "born leaders." This was consistent with the practice of passing the leadership role from the king who was father and leader to his son.

A second descriptive theory of leadership is *trait theory.* This theory aimed at putting together all the traits that make a good leader. These traits included physical stature, intelligence, education, personality, charisma, and socioeconomic status.

A third theory of leadership, called *situation theory,* used the idea of the right man being in the right place at the right time. The question often asked of some leaders is one such as this: Did Napoleon make history or did history make Napoleon? If one subscribed to situation theory, it could be said that history made Napoleon.

A fourth theory, called *interaction theory,* postulated that it was neither the person's personality nor the situation, but a combination of the two. Thus anyone could become a leader in the right situation (Bernhard and Walsh, 1981).

More recently, especially since the early 60s, theories of leadership have evolved which emphasize that multiple factors must be considered in determining effective leadership. These theories reflect influence from motivation theories but have also considered the styles of leadership, the followers themselves, and the situation. Studies at the University of Michigan identified two important aspects of leadership, which they called employee orientation and production orientation. The employee-oriented leader is a leader who is concerned with relationships among the workers whereas the production-oriented leader is one who is concerned with task-oriented behaviors of workers which result in increased production of the product or service.

Leadership studies at Ohio State University identified the two dimensions of leadership as initiating structure and consideration. *Structure* was concerned with task behavior and *consideration* was concerned with relationship behavior. During the Ohio State studies, these dimensions were plotted on vertical and horizontal axes to form four quadrants. Blake and Mouton (1964) also used this way of showing leadership dimensions, referred to it as a managerial grid, and used the terms *concern for people* and *concern for production.*

The outcome of these and other studies led Hersey and Blanchard (1977, p. 100) to conclude that it was unrealistic to think of a single ideal type of leadership behavior. They used the two axes to plot leadership, using task behavior on the horizontal axis and relationship behavior on the vertical axis. They added maturity of followers on the horizontal axis and projected effectiveness on the vertical axis, calling it the Tri-Dimensional Leader Effectiveness Model (Hersey and Blanchard, 1977, p. 105).

The effectiveness of the leadership behavior demands that the leader use the appropriate style of leadership for the appropriate situation. This meant that the leader's style varied from one situation to another. This has led to the general acceptance that effectiveness of leadership depends on the leader's ability to behave according to the situation and the followers.

Advantages and Disadvantages

The Tri-Dimensional Leader Effectiveness Model by Hersey and Blanchard supports the position that leadership skills can be taught and learned. It does not give credence to the idea that leadership is a bit of magic and that only certain individuals are born with the necessary characteristics. Every nurse is a leader in some arena and will be a more effective leader by taking into consideration all the variables that influence leadership effectiveness. A disadvantage of the model is that it does not address the role of authority and power in the effectiveness of leadership.

Application to Community Health Nursing

There are a large number of health professionals involved in the delivery of health care, and the nurse is often expected to offer the needed leadership. The leader has to take into consideration the task or goal to be accomplished, group needs including their relationship needs, and the situation.

The nurse brings to the situation personal knowledge about change theory, motivation theory, group process skills, and interactional skills. All of these are needed for effective leadership.

SUMMARY

This chapter has presented selected conceptual models and indicated their usefulness in guiding the practice of community health nurses. The importance of theory development and scientific inquiry to nursing was reviewed, key terms were defined, and the usefulness of conceptual models to nursing education, nursing research, and nursing practice was described. The ANA and APHA conceptual models specific to community health nursing were included as well as interdisciplinary, nursing, and psychosocial models.

Interdisciplinary models applicable to community health nursing presented included systems, developmental, and interaction. For each model an evaluation was made as to its main characteristics, general advantages and disadvantages, and its application to community health nursing. Only through clear understanding of such models, including their good and bad points,

can they ultimately become useful in practice, education, and research.

In addition, the psychosocial theories of motivation, leadership, communication, and change were explored. As in the discussion of both nursing and interdisciplinary models, the reader's attention was directed toward a general overview, chief characteristics, advantages and disadvantages, and application to community health nursing.

BIBLIOGRAPHY

American Nurses' Association: Standards: community health nursing practice, Kansas City, Mo., 1973, The Association.

American Nurses' Association: A conceptual model of community health nursing, Kansas City, Mo., 1980, The Association.

American Public Health Association: The definition and role of public health nursing in the delivery of health care, Washington, D.C., 1981, The Association.

Andreoli, K., and Thompson, C.: The nature of science in nursing, Image 9:32-37, June 1977.

Bennis, W.G., et al., editors: The planning of change, New York, 1976, Holt, Rinehart & Winston.

Bernhard, L.A., and Walsh, M.: Leadership—the key to the professionalization of nursing, New York, 1981, McGraw-Hill Book Co.

Bertalanffy, L.V.: Problems of life, New York, 1952, Harper & Brothers.

Blake, M.: The Peplau developmental model for nursing practice. In Riehl, J.P., and Roy, S.C., editors: Conceptual models for nursing practice, ed. 2, New York, 1980, Appleton-Century-Crofts, pp. 53-73.

Blake, R.R., and Mouton, J.S.: The managerial grid, Houston, 1964, Gulf Publishing Co.

Burr, W.R., et al., editors: Contemporary theories about the family, New York, 1979, Free Press.

Bush, H.A.: Models for nursing, Adv. Nurs. Sci. 1:13-21, Jan. 1979.

Butts, R.F., and Cremin, L.A.: A history of education in American culture, New York, 1953, Holt, Rinehart & Winston, Inc.

Chin, R., and Benne, K.D.: General strategies for effecting changes in human systems. In Bennis, W.G., et al., editors: The planning of change. New York, 1976, Holt, Rinehart & Winston.

Chin, R.: The utility of system models and developmental models for practitioners. In Riehl, J.P., and Roy, S.C., editors: Conceptual models for nursing practice ed. 2, New York, 1980, Appleton-Century-Crofts, pp. 21-37.

Chinn, P.L., and Jacobs, M.K.: A model for theory development in nursing, Adv. Nurs. Sci. 1:1-11, Oct. 1978.

Cooley, C.H.: Social organization, New York, 1909, Scribner's.

Donaldson, S.K., and Crowley, D.M.: The discipline of nursing, Nurs. Outlook 26:700-704, 1978.

Duvall, E.M.: Marriage and family development. ed. 5, Philadelphia, 1977, J.B. Lippincott Co.

Fagan, J., and Shepherd, I.L.: Gestalt therapy now, Palo Alto, Calif., 1970, Science & Behavior Books.

Falco, S.M., and Lobo, M.L.: Martha E. Rogers. In George J., editor: Nursing theories: the base for professional nursing practice, Englewood Cliffs, N.J. 1980, Prentice-Hall, Inc.

Fawcett, J.: The "what of theory development." In National League for Nursing: Theory development: what, why, how?, New York, 1978, The League.

Fawcett, J.: A framework for analysis and evaluation of conceptual models of nursing, Nurse Educator, pp. 10-14, Nov.-Dec. 1980.

Fitts, W.H.: Tennessee self-concept scale manual, Nashville, Tenn., 1965, Counselor Recording and Tests.

Friedman, M.M.: Family nursing: theory and assessment, New York, 1981, Appleton-Century-Crofts.

Fuller, S.S.: Holistic man and the science and practice of nusing, Nurs. Outlook **26**: 700-704, 1978.

Grubbs, J.: An interpretation of the Johnson Behavioral System model for nursing pratice. In Riehl, J.P., and Roy, S.C., editors: Conceptual models for nursing practice, ed. 2, New York, 1980, Appleton-Century-Crofts, pp. 217-249.

Harmer, B., and Henderson, V.A.: Textbook of the principles and practice of nursing, ed. 5, New York, 1955, Macmillan Publishing Co.

Hazzard, M.E.: An overview of systems theory, Nurs. Clin. North Am. **6**:385-393, Sept. 1971.

Hersey, P., and Blanchard, K.H.: Management of organizational behavior: utilizing human resources, ed. 3, Englewood Cliffs, N.J., 1977, Prentice-Hall Inc.

Herzberg, F.: The managerial choice: to be efficient and to be human, Homewood, Ill., 1976, Dow Jones-Irwin, Inc.

Holaday, B.J.: Achievement behavior in chronically ill children, Nurs. Res. **23**(1):25-30, Jan.-Feb. 1974.

Johnson, D.E.: The behavioral system model for nursing. In Riehl, J.P., and Roy, S.C., editors: Conceptual models for nursing practice, ed. 2, New York, 1980, Appleton-Century-Crofts, pp. 207-216.

Johnston, R.L., and Fitzpatrick, J.J.: Relevance of psychiatric mental health nursing theories to nursing models. In Fitzpatrick, J.J., et al. editors: Nursing models and their psychiatric mental health applications, Bowie, Md.,1982, Robert J. Brady Co.

Kerlinger, N.: Foundations of behavioral research, New York, 1973, Holt, Rinehart & Winston.

King, I.: A conceptual frame of reference for nursing, Nurs. Res. **17**(1): 27, Jan.-Feb. 1968.

King, I.: The "why" of theory development. In National League for Nursing: Theory development: what, why, how? New York, 1978, The League.

King, I.: A theory for nursing: systems, concepts, process. New York, 1981, John Wiley & Sons, Inc.

Lancaster, J., and Lancaster, W.: Models and model building in nursing, Adv. Nurs. Sci. **3**:31-42, April 1981.

Lancaster, J., and Lancaster, W.: Concepts for advanced nursing practice, St. Louis, 1982, The C.V. Mosby Co.

Lewin, K.: Field theory in social science, New York, 1951, Harper Brothers.

Lewis, M.: Clincal aspects of child development, ed. 2, Philadelphia, 1982, Lea & Febiger.

Maslow, A.H.: Motivation and personality, ed. 2, New York, 1970, Harper & Row Publishers, Inc.

McGregor, D.: The human side of enterprise, New York, 1960, McGraw-Hill Book Co.

Mead, G.H.: Mind, self and society, Chicago, 1934, University of Chicago Press.

National League for Nursing: Criteria for the appraisal of baccalaureate and higher degree programs in nursing, ed. 4, New York, 1977, The League.

Neuman, B.: The Betty Neuman health care systems model: a total person approach to patient problems. In Riehl, J.P., and Roy, S.C., editors: Conceptual models for nursing practice, ed. 2, New York, 1980, Appleton-Century-Crofts, pp. 119-134.

Neuman, B.: The Neuman systems model: application to nursing education and practice, Norwalk, Conn., 1982, Appleton-Century-Crofts.

Neuman, B.M., and Young, R.J.: A model for teaching total person approach to patient problems, Nurs. Res. **21**:264, May-June 1972.

Nursing Development Conference Group: Concept formalization in nursing:process and product, Boston, 1973, Little, Brown & Company.

Orem, D.: Nursing: concepts of practice, ed. 2, New York, 1980, McGraw-Hill Book Co.

Owens, R.G.: Organizational behavior in education, ed. 2, Englewood Cliffs, N.J., 1981, Prentice-Hall, Inc.

Riehl, J.P., and Roy, C.: Conceptual models for nursing practice, ed. 2, New York, 1980, Appleton-Century-Crofts.

Rogers, M.E.: An introduction to the theoretical basis of nursing, Philadelphia, 1970, F.A. Davis Co.

Rogers, M.E.: Nursing: a science of unitary man. In Riehl, J.P., and Roy, C.S., editors: Conceptual models for nursing practice, New York, 1980, Appleton-Century-Crofts, pp. 329-337.

Rose, A., editor: Human behavior and social processes: an interactionist approach, Boston, 1962, Houghton Mifflin Co.

Roy, C.: Adaptation: a conceptual framework for nursing, Nurs. Outlook **18**:42-45, March 1970.

Roy, C., editor: Introduction to nursing: an adaptation model, Englewood Cliffs, N.J., 1976, Prentice-Hall, Inc.

Roy, S.C., and Roberts, S.L.: Theory construction in nursing: an adaptation model, Englewood Cliffs, N.J., 1981, Prentice-Hall, Inc.

Stogdill, R.N.: Handbook of leadership: a survey of theory and research, New York, 1974, Free Press.

Thibodeau, J.A.: Nursing models: analysis and evaluation, Monterey, Calif., 1983, Health Sciences Division, Wadsworth Publishing Co.

Whall, A.L.: Nursing theory and the assessment of families, Psychiatr. Nurs. **19**(1):30-36, Jan. 1981.

Whelton, B.J.: An operalization of Martha Rogers' theory throughout the nursing process, Int. J. Nurs. Stud. **16**:16-20, 1979.

Williams, C.A.: The nature and development of conceptual frameworks. In Downs, F.S., and Fleming, J.W., editors: Issues in nursing research, New York, 1979, Appleton-Century-Crofts, pp. 89-106.

Wilson, H.S., and Kneisl, C.R.: Psychiatric nursing, Menlo Park, Calif., 1979, Addison-Wesley Publishing Co., Inc.

Yura, H., and Torres, G.: Today's conceptual framework within baccalaureate nursing programs. In National League for Nursing: faculty-curriculum developmental. III. Conceptual framework—its meaning and function, New York, 1975, The League.

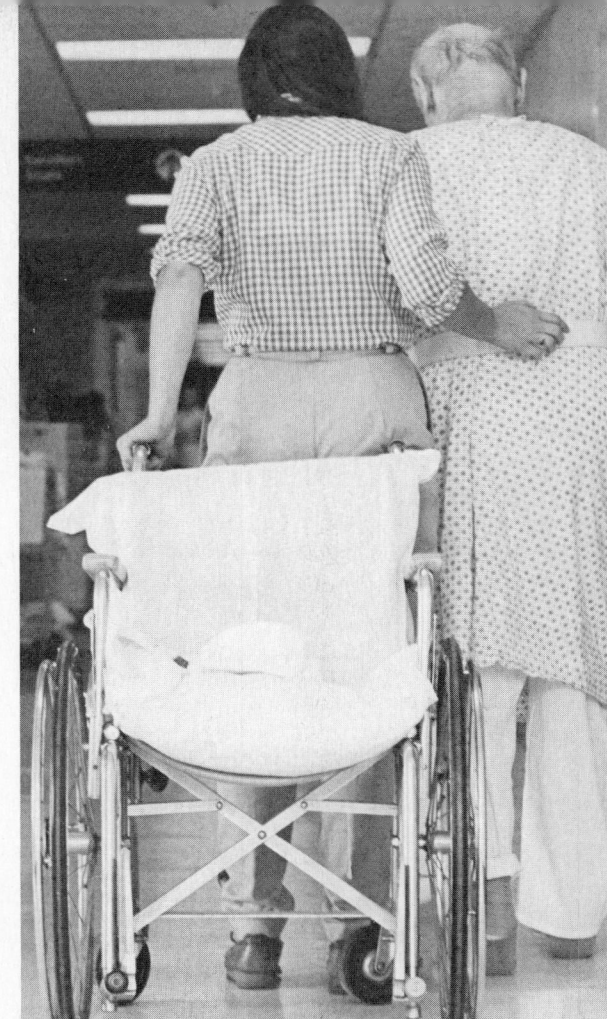

Chapter 7

BARBARA VALANIS

THE EPIDEMIOLOGICAL MODEL AND COMMUNITY HEALTH NURSING

Epidemiology is a community health science and is essential to nursing practice. This chapter describes the science of epidemiology, its concepts, principles, and methods. The emphasis is not on how to do epidemiological research but on understanding the conceptual framework of epidemiology for approaching community health problems. First epidemiology is defined and its uses are discussed. Subsequently basic concepts are developed, followed by a brief presentation of methods which focus on identifying measures of health and delineating characteristics of the three basic approaches to epidemiological research. Finally, the role of epidemiology in community health nursing practice is illustrated through application of an epidemiological model to a specific community health nursing problem.

HISTORY AND DEFINITION

The term *epidemiology* is derived from three Greek words: (1) *epi,* upon; (2) *demos,* the people; and (3) *logos,* science. Thus it is the science of events that occur (come upon) in a community (the people). Health-related events are the focus of epidemiology. Epidemiologists study a variety of factors related to the environment and the people in that environment in an attempt to identify the determinants of observed patterns of health. Epidemiologists function as detectives concerned with the entire spectrum of health status from health to serious illness. They seek to identify the who, what, where, when, and how of disease causation. By comparing the characteristics of persons, places, and

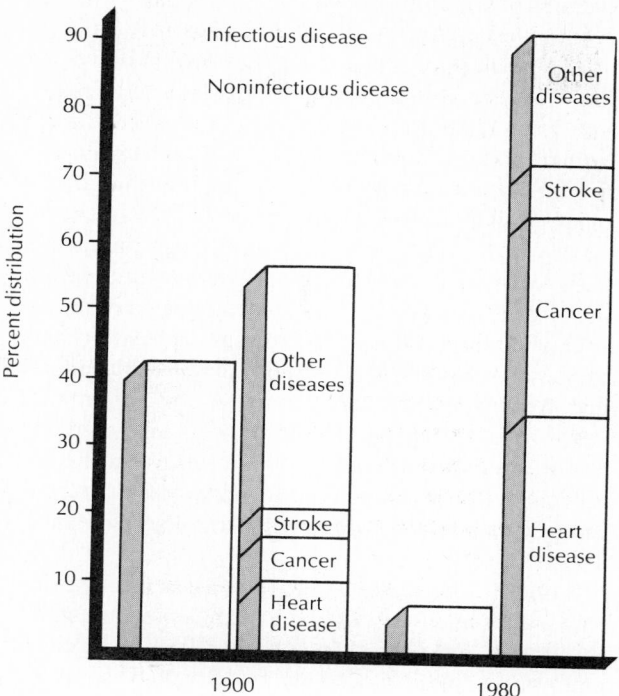

Fig. 7-1. Proportional distribution of deaths from
infectious and major noninfectious diseases in the United
States in 1900 and 1982.

time associated with a particular illness with these same characteristics for those who do not have the illness, epidemiologists narrow down the suspected causal agents of that illness. Once an agent is identified and the susceptible population recognized, epidemiologists attempt to identify the means by which the agent is transmitted to the susceptible human population. This information provides a basis for intervention by community health officials who can act to prevent or control occurrence of the disease by removing the agent, by reducing the susceptibility of the population, or by interfering with the transmission of the agent to the human population.

Epidemiology is an ancient science and, for the most part, observational in nature. People have been trying for thousands of years to determine what causes disease. Supernatural events were one of the first factors used as an explanation of the occurrence of illness. As long ago as 460-377 BC, Hippocrates, considered by some to be the first epidemiologist, tried to explain disease occurrence on a rational rather than a supernatural basis, pointing out that environment and life-style are related to the occurrence of disease.

During Biblical times, public health measures were instituted on the basis of observations about occurrence of disease, even when the actual disease agent was unknown. The ancient practice of isolating lepers, for example, arose from the observation that the disease

often developed in those persons who came in close physical contact with a leper.

In more recent years the investigative observations of John Snow in England resulted in the initiation of intervention measures to prevent the use of certain water supplies. His work in the 1850s led him to suspect contaminated water as the source of cholera outbreaks. By measuring the frequency of cholera deaths in relation to the number of people living in a geographical area (mortality), he determined that rates of cholera were much higher among certain parts of the city with a common water supply than among other sections with a different water supply. Thus measures could be taken by public health officials to limit the occurrence of cholera by control of contaminated water even though the actual agent, the cholera vibrio, was as yet unknown (Snow, 1936). Koch finally isolated the cholera vibrio in 1883.

Most early epidemiological observations and investigations were related to occurrences of infectious disease and lacked a systematic approach to investigation. The development of rates such as Snow's mortality observations provided a scientific basis for the growth of systematic epidemiological methods in the study of health and illness distributions. As data on infectious diseases accumulated and led to public health intervention, infectious diseases were largely controlled. Subsequently, disease of a chronic nature with noninfectious origins became more common, taking over as major causes of morbidity and mortality, particularly in industrialized nations (Fig. 7-1).

As a result, epidemiological investigations today include infectious disease; noninfectious, chronic conditions such as heart disease, cancer, and stroke; acute events such as spontaneous abortion or accidents; and a wide spectrum of emotional and mental health conditions such as depression or alcoholism. In addition, epidemiology is no longer limited to the study of diseases or patterns of ill health; it also focuses on description of normal characteristics of populations. Instances of such focus include studies of body weight in relation to height and of blood group subtypes in different population groups. By extending its scope to include mental and social conditions in addition to disease, epidemiology has helped behavioral scientists, social workers, community health planners, and all those concerned with the health and well-being of human populations. It is truly multidisciplinary, both providing information to the medical, social, and behavioral sciences and drawing on these sciences in its research.

There has been considerable discussion among epidemiologists in recent years attempting to formulate a single best definition of the science as it is practiced today (Abramson, 1979; Evans, 1979; Frerichs, 1978; Lillienfeld, 1978; Rich, 1979). The following definition reflects the major components of the modern discipline: *Epidemiology is the study of the distribution of states of health and of the determinants of deviations from health in populations.* The purpose of epidemiology is to identify the etiology of deviations from health and to provide the data necessary to prevent and control disease through community health intervention.

COMPONENTS OF EPIDEMIOLOGY

The term *epidemiology* has come to refer both to the particular methods applied in studies of disease causation and to the body of knowledge that arises from such investigations. The collection of epidemiological knowledge is usually termed substantive epidemiology, although some authors may refer to it as descriptive epidemiology. For purposes of this chapter, the term *descriptive epidemiology* refers to the first phase of epidemiological research, which includes observations and recordings of the existing patterns of a disease occurrence. The term *substantive epidemiology* refers to the body of knowledge, the known epidemiological characteristics of a particular disease or illness. This epidemiological description of a particular disease, which constitutes the substantive epidemiology for that condition, includes the natural history of the disease,

patterns of occurrence, and factors associated with high risk for developing the disease (risk factors).

The methods of epidemiology are used to derive the knowledge base of the discipline, just as a physiologist uses methodological tools to study the physiology of the human body and produce a knowledge base in that field. In the same way that knowledge of human physiology provides a basis for diagnostic and treatment decisions in medical practice, epidemiology provides a basis for diagnosis and treatment in community health practice. That is why we call epidemiology a basic science of community health. Whereas a physician uses the basic medical science of physiology in diagnosing and treating an individual patient, the community health practitioner uses epidemiology in diagnosing and treating a community. The unit of application is different for the two sciences: the individual is the focus in medicine and the group in epidemiology (see Table 7-1).

Similarly, there are two levels for describing a disease—the clinical description and the epidemiological description. The clinical description relates to the onset and progression of symptoms in individuals similarly affected. The epidemiologist has to single out in terms of probabilities, averages, and means those demographic and physiological characteristics that are most common in the diseased population. Hence statistics are a crucial tool for the epidemiologist.

An episode of food poisoning illustrates the distinction between a clinical and epidemiological approach to illness. Clinicians (nurse practitioners, physicians) record the signs and symptoms such as elevated temperature, presence of nausea and vomiting, or diarrhea which are experienced by the patient. After taking a careful history and performing a thorough physical examination, supplemented if necessary by laboratory tests, clinicians consider the differential diagnoses and come to the conclusion that the most likely diagnosis is gastroenteritis attributable to food poisoning. They then institute treatment and record the patient's progress in terms of when symptoms were relieved.

Epidemiologists, by contrast, describe this event in terms of how it affects the group. They note the time and place of onset of symptoms in all the sick individuals who can be identified, preferably including those with symptoms too mild to require medical treatment. They also assemble data on the circumstances related to the illness for all individuals in the group to determine if they share a common circumstance. This may lead to a suspected common source of infection, such as food at a church supper. To identify the likely food item responsible for the poisoning, precise information is gathered on all the various foods eaten by those present

Table 7-1. Comparison of epidemiology and physiology

	Epidemiology	Physiology
	Scientific method	
Tools	Epidemiological methodology	Physiological methodology
Knowledge	Trends in disease occurrence	Physiology of human body
Outcome	Distribution of populations at high risk of disease	
	Social, economic, biological, and genetic determinants of disease	
	Natural history of disease	
Purpose	Diagnosis and treatment in community health practice	Diagnosis and treatment decisions in medical practice
Focus	Group	Individual

and a comparison is made of illness rates among all those present at the supper who ate each food and those who did not. Once the contaminated food is identified, attempts can be made to determine the source of the contamination. Often the source is someone involved in the food preparation. Once the source is identified, community health measures such as treatment of the person carrying the organism and instruction in hygienic food practices must be instituted to assure that the event does not recur.

BASIC EPIDEMIOLOGICAL CONCEPTS

Causality

In common usage the term *cause* is generally understood to mean a stimulus that produces an effect or outcome. Cause in epidemiology also deals with something that produces an effect or outcome. However, since an epidemiologist must investigate causal relationships between a stimulus and an outcome by use of statistical measures of association, it is important to understand ways in which events or circumstances may be related in statistical terms. The first level of relationship to be ascertained is that of statistical association or independency. In statistical terms, two events are said to be independent if the probability that the two events occur together is equal to the probability that one occurs times the probability that the other occurs. For example, in Table 7-2 under Independent Factors, we find that in a given community 20% of the adult population is overweight and 10% of this population has high blood pressure. If the proportion of individuals exhibiting both characteristics (overweight and high blood pressure) is exactly 2% (the product of 20% $\times$

10% = 2%), these two events are considered statistically independent of each other. The cell for high blood pressure and overweight does, in fact, contain 2% of the population. By contrast, in Table 7-2 under Nonindependent Factors, although the percent who are overweight remains at 20% and the percent who have high blood pressure remains at 10% of the population, the proportion of individuals who are overweight and also have high blood pressure is 7%. This is more than three times the 2% that we calculated would be expected by chance alone. In this case these two factors are not independent. A variety of statistical tests for independence of factors is used in analysis of epidemiological data. The type of test is dependent on the structure of the data. Thus in statistical terms, before a relationship between two factors is considered for further investigation of causality, the distribution of the two factors must be one that cannot be accounted for by chance alone, that is, they have a statistically significant association.

It is important to stress that statistical associations are determined for *categories or groups* and not for individual instances. In the example given in Table 7-2, under Independent Factors it is not possible to say that high blood pressure and overweight caused any individual to have heart disease. However, the information under Nonindependent Factors may suggest the likelihood of causal association in an individual instance. This is particularly true if the association between two categories of events is strong.

Once it has been determined that two factors are not independent but that they have a significant association, the next step is to determine whether the relationship is causal. As illustrated in Fig. 7-2, nonindependent associations may be causally or noncausally relat-

Table 7-2. Distribution of blood pressure and weight as independent and nonindependent factors

Weight	Independent factors			Nonindependent factors		
	High blood pressure (%)	Low blood pressure (%)	Total (%)	High blood pressure (%)	Low blood pressure (%)	Total (%)
Overweight	2	18	20	7	13	20
Not overweight	8	72	80	3	77	80
TOTAL	10	90	100	10	90	100

ed. *Direct causal associations* are those in which a factor causes a disease with no other variables intervening.

$$A \longrightarrow B$$

Apparent directness depends on the limitations of current knowledge, and what is considered a direct association may become indirect, since further studies of causal mechanisms may reveal a new, more direct cause for the association. For example, the early studies of toxic shock syndrome implicated tampons as the probable cause. More recent research has indicated that the presence of staphylococcal organisms in the vagina is the actual direct cause. The tampons are a contributing cause in that they create an ideal environment for proliferation of the organism (Centers for Disease Control, 1980).

In *indirect causal associations* a third variable called *intervening variable* occupies an intermediate stage between the cause and effect. If A in the model below is causally related to D (A is the cause and D the effect) but only through the interposition of one or several linked factors such as B and C, the association between A and D is one of an indirect causal relationship.

$$A \longrightarrow B \longrightarrow C \longrightarrow D$$

For example, breathing air polluted by cigarette or other smoke (A) causes damage to the respiratory epithelium (intervening variable B); this damage increases the susceptibility of the epithelium of infection (intervening variable C); this results in chronic bronchitis (D).

Finally, as illustrated in Fig. 7-2, although an association may be nonindependent, it may also be *noncausally associated*. This type of variable rides with the causal variable and varies systematically with it. It is called a *confounding variable*. When uncontrolled, its effect cannot be distinguished from the effects of a hypothetical causal variable under study with which it is highly correlated. As mentioned later, age, if uncontrolled, is a confounding variable for an association between parity and spontaneous abortion.

The ultimate determination of whether an association is causal is through an epidemiological experiment. Thus for practical purposes a factor is considered causal if reducing the amount or frequency of occurrence of the suspected cause reduces the frequency of the effect, in this case the frequency of the illness of interest. For example, if treating hypertensive individuals to keep their blood pressure low reduces the frequency of stroke compared to the frequency of stroke in an equivalent, untreated group of hypertensive individuals, hypertension would be considered a cause of stroke.

There are instances when an epidemiological experiment is not feasible or desirable. In these instances, criteria are needed for making decisions regarding intervention based on available epidemiological data. The five criteria generally used for assessing causality in such instances were presented in the 1964 Surgeon General's report, in which they were used for assessing the causal relationship between smoking and a variety of health outcomes. They are (1) correctness of temporality, (2) strength of the association, (3) specificity of the association, (4) consistency of the association, and (5) biological plausibility.

Correctness of temporality refers to the evidence that exposure to the causal factor did, in fact, occur before the initiation of the disease process. In diseases such as cancer it may be difficult to prove definitively that the exposure occurred before the first cell transformations, since there is a long period of latency during which cell replication and growing continue. It may be 20 to 40 years before the tumor is diagnosed. This makes it difficult to assess the temporal relationship. Clearly, however, if exposure did not occur before onset of the disease, the relationship cannot be causal.

Strength of the association is usually measured by the relative risk ratio. In general, the larger the ratio, the stronger the association and the greater the likelihood that the association is causal. In some studies that do not report risk ratios, significance levels of the statisti-

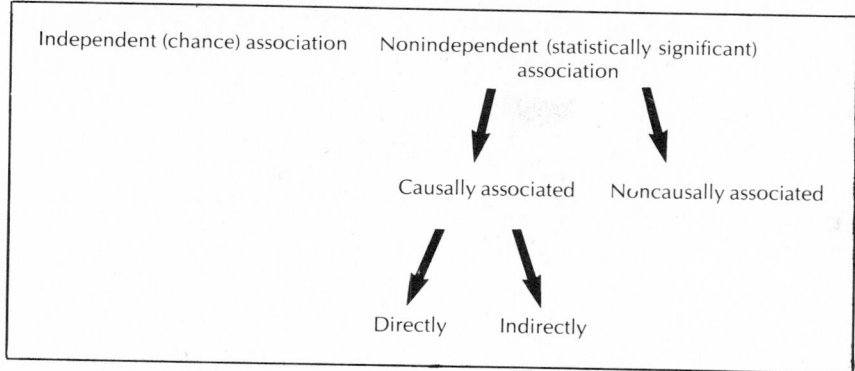

Fig. 7-2. Types of statistical associations.

cal test must be used to assess the strength of the association.

Specificity of the association refers to the uniqueness of the relationship. The terms *necessary* and *sufficient* can be used to clarify this concept. If the disease can occur without the presence of a particular agent, the agent is not necessary. Cardiovascular disease can occur in nonsmokers; tuberculosis, however, cannot occur without exposure to the tubercle bacillus. Sufficient refers to whether the agent is always able to produce the outcome. Although asbestos fibers are necessary to produce asbestosis, the fibers may not be sufficient; it is possible to be exposed to asbestos and not develop asbestosis. Fire exposure is always sufficient to produce a burn, although severity may vary. However, fire is not necessary to produce a burn as burns may result from chemical exposures as well. A highly specific and therefore unique association exists when an agent is both necessary for disease occurrence and sufficient by itself to produce the disease. This association would be causal. The closer an agent comes to meeting these criteria, the greater the likelihood of causality. As discussed in a later section about the web of causation, however, meeting both the necessary and sufficient criteria simultaneously is incompatible with the concept of multiple causes.

Consistency of the association refers to the findings of various epidemiological studies. Because of a variety of design factors, there may be conflicting results among reported studies on the association of a specific agent with a specific disease. Some studies may find no association. Others may find a positive association. The strength of association may vary widely in the positive studies. Barring major flaws in study designs, consistent positive findings would be expected for a causal association.

Biological plausibility implies that a reasonable biological mechanism exists which can explain how an agent could produce the specific disease of interest.

Documentation of biological plausibility is dependent on a variety of other scientific disciplines such as physiology, microbiology, toxicology, and pharmacology. Causality demands a reasonable biological mechanism to explain the association.

A cause can be any of a large number of characteristics relating to time, place, person, or events. Modern epidemiology has moved ahead from the "single-cause idea" and recognizes the presence of multiple causes in any biological phenomenon. However, the single-cause model of the past has its usefulness, particularly in the control of infectious diseases in which the identification of the source of infection leads the way to the isolation of the putative organism and provides a means for eliminating or controlling the frequency of disease occurrence by restricting exposure of noninfected, susceptible individuals to the bacillus. The tubercle bacillus, for instance, was identified as *the* cause of tuberculosis because this organism must be present for tuberculosis to occur. This does not necessarily mean that it will always cause clinically recognizable disease. There are circumstances when the bacillus is present and no disease occurs. The host has to be susceptible to the organism; susceptibility reflects previous exposure to the organism, immune response, and so on. If the host is not susceptible, no disease occurs. The environment is also important, since the likelihood of exposure to the organism may vary greatly in different geographical areas.

In the case of noninfectious disease agents, the single-cause model is of somewhat limited usefulness, since there is no single factor or agent that must be present to cause the disease. For example, even though smoking is recognized as a major cause of lung cancer, nonsmokers and individuals who have never been exposed to the cigarette smoke of others do get lung cancer. Clearly, there must be other substances that cause the disease. Nonsmokers exposed to asbestos may develop lung cancer. Also, smokers who are exposed to other substances, such as asbestos, are much more likely to de-

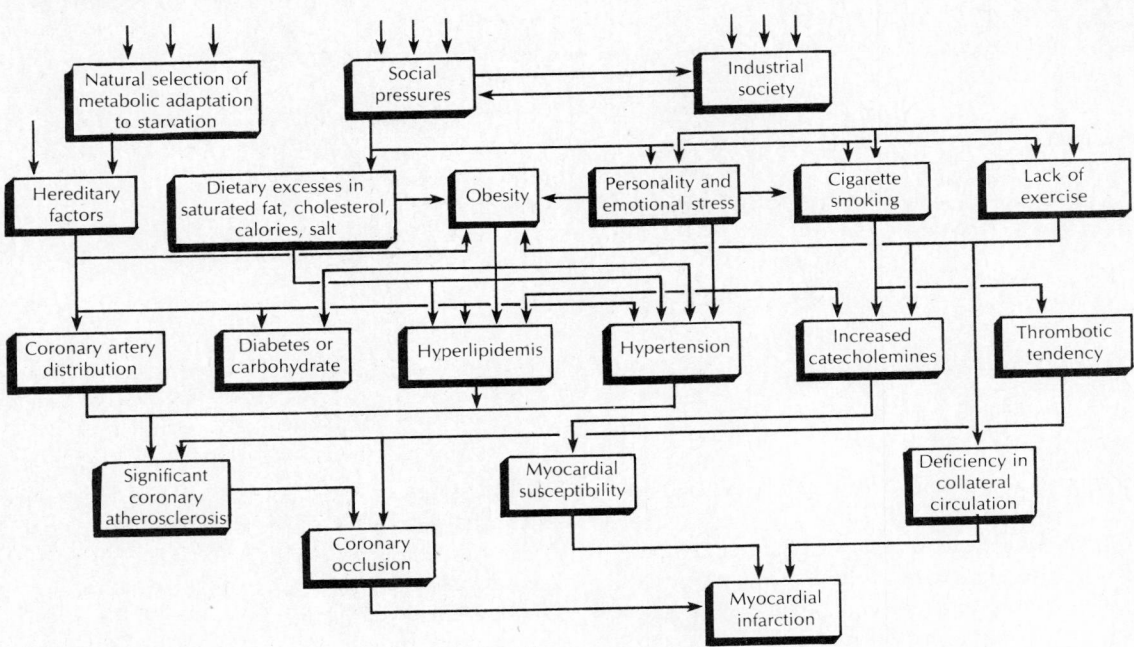

Fig. 7-3. Web of causation for myocardial infarction: a current view. From Friedman, G. O.: *Primer of epidemiology*, ed. 2, New York, 1980, McGraw-Hill Book Co.

velop lung cancer than are those smokers not exposed to these substances. Exposure to multiple causal factors may have an additional or multiplicative effect.

In a different example automobile accidents may result from numerous factors such as speeding, faulty equipment, heavy traffic, poor visibility, driver inexperience, or drinking and driving. Any of these factors could cause an accident. All are amenable to intervention through public education, better engineering design, better vehicle maintenance, and so on. Several of these together increase the risk of an accident. Such interrelationships between a multitude of factors, some known and some unknown but all bearing ultimately on the cause of the disease, constitute the *web of causation*. Fig. 7-3 illustrates the web of causation for myocardial infarction, based on our current understanding of interrelationships among factors. It is, fortunately, not necessary to understand completely the intricacy of relationships between factors to institute adequate preventive measures.

As seen in Fig. 7-3, numerous factors such as smoking, obesity, blood cholesterol level, and stress are causes of heart attack by our earlier definition. The more of these factors present in an individual, the greater the risk of heart attack. Since presence of these factors increase the risk for contracting a disease, we call them *risk factors*. While we do not understand how these factors work or how they interact with each other, we can

intervene and reduce the risk of heart attack by persuading individuals to give up smoking, to lose weight, or to change their diet to reduce cholesterol. Planning of such interventions is based on understanding the natural history of disease.

Natural History

Natural history of the disease, the process by which diseases occur and progress in humans, involves the interaction of three different kinds of factors: the causative agent(s), a susceptible host (man), and the envi-ronment. The web of causation is one model of the interrelationship among these factors. Another model illustrating the relationship among these factors, the ecological model, is shown in Fig. 7-4. Man is seen as surrounded by his social, biological, and physical environments. Change in any of these environments may initiate change in the others, affecting the relationship between man and agents in these environments. As long as a state of equilibrium exists between host, agent, and environment, a state of health is maintained. For example, an increase in the amount of the agent resulting from a change in environmental conditions increases the likelihood that a susceptible host will be exposed. An increase in host susceptibility resulting from lack of sleep, malnutrition, excessive stress, aging, or a variety of other factors also increases the risk of disease. Changes in the environment contribute to changes in

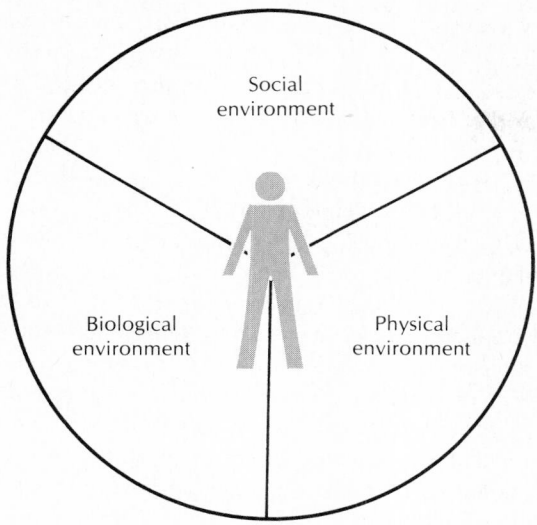

Fig. 7-4. Ecological model of host, agent, and environment relationships.

host susceptibility as well as to the conditions for viability of the agent.

The Agent

An *agent* can be either a factor whose presence causes a disease or one whose absence causes disease. An example of the former is the tubercle bacillus, which causes tuberculosis; an example of the latter is insufficient intake of vitamin C, which may lead to scurvy. Categories of causative agents include physical, chemical, nutrient, biological, genetic, and psychological agents. Physical agents include various mechanical forces or frictions that may produce injury as well as atmospheric abnormalities such as extremes of temperature or excessive radiation. Chemical agents include substances that may occur as dusts, gases, vapors, fumes, or liquids. Nutrient agents are chemical in nature, but the term refers specifically to basic dietary components. All living organisms including insects, worms, protozoa, fungi, bacteria, rickettsia, and viruses are biological agents; it is the last class of agents which is infectious in nature. Genetic agents are agents transmitted from parent to child through the genes. Psychological agents are stressful circumstances in the environment.

Certain characteristics of agents affect their ability to produce disease in the host. For infectious agents these characteristics are infectivity, pathogenicity, and virulence. Measures of these characteristics (i.e., the infection rate, pathogenicity rate, and case fatality) provide a means of population surveillance, allowing public health officials to assess the nature of the problem they are dealing with in order to plan for intervention. These characteristics are discussed further in Chapter 12. The important characteristics of the noninfectious agents include toxicity for chemical agents, size and shape of physical agents, chronicity or suddenness of psychological agents, and homozygocity or heterozygocity of genetic material.

The Environment

Environment refers to all external conditions and influences affecting the life of living things. Physical, socioeconomic, and biological environments provide reservoirs and modes of transmission for agents. The physical environment includes the geological structure of an area and the availability of resources such as water and flora which influence the number and variety of animal reservoirs and arthropod (i.e., insects) vectors. Weather, climate, and season are important influences on these factors.

The socioeconomic environment contributes to the types of infectious agents in a location, since social and economic conditions relate to the extent of environmental sanitation, pasteurization of milk, disposal of garbage and excreta, and the availability of medical facilities for immunization and medical care. The socioeconomic environment may also influence the noninfectious agents; that is, more psychological stressors may be found in poorer socioeconomic environments than in better ones. Poor socioeconomic neighborhoods are more likely to be located near industrial plants, which may produce dangerous chemicals or emit physical particles of agents such as asbestos or coal tar.

Finally, there is the biological environment, including other living plants and animals, which may serve as either the reservoir or as the vector for transmission of an infectious agent. Since these agents are living organisms, they require a place to live and multiply. The habitat of these agents are called reservoirs and may be any human, animal, arthropod, plant, soil, or inanimate matter that provides an environment for survival or reproduction. The reservoir is thus intimately related to the transmission cycle of the agent in nature. The *transmission cycle*, or life cycle, refers to where the agent resides and to how it is transported from here to a susceptible host.

The Host

Disease can only occur in a susceptible human host. Basic to the understanding of host resistance to disease caused by infectious agents is the concept of immunity. *Immunity* refers to the increased resistance on the part of a host to a specific infectious agent. Immunity can be humoral (antibodies in the blood) or cellular (specific to each type of cell). The role of each of these varies with the infectious agent and with the immune response of the host. Immunity can be passive or active. Passive immunity is attained either naturally (maternal transfer of antibodies to the fetus) or artificially (inoculation of specific protective antibodies, e.g., immune serum globulin for infectious hepatitis or diptheria antitoxin for diptheria prevention). Passive immunity is temporary; in the newborn it usually last 6 months during which time the infant is only protected against infection experienced by the mother and for which she has made antibodies. By contrast, active immunity is long lasting and may protect an individual for life. It is attained naturally by infection, with or without clinical manifestations, or artificially by the inoculation of vaccine obtained from fractions of products of the infectious agent or of the agent itself in killed, modified, or variant form. The principle of active immunity is used in many of the major vaccination programs such as for diphtheria and polio. It was also the basis for the successful program to eradicate smallpox from the world through an international vaccination and surveillance program.

In contrast to immunity, the term *inherent resistance* refers to the ability to resist disease independently of antibodies or of specifically developed tissue response. It commonly rests in anatomical or physiological characteristics of the host; it may be genetic or acquired, permanent or temporary. The concept of inherent resistance is useful in understanding host resistance both to infectious agents as well as to other types of agents. For example, factors such as general health status or nutrition may affect resistance to disease. Someone in good health who maintains good nutrition and a regular schedule of rest and exercise may be exposed to the tubercle bacillus and resist infection even though he is not immune to the organism. Similarly, this individual, if exposed to psychological stress, may resist ulcers better than someone in poorer general health.

The Disease Process

Table 7-3 gives the stages of the natural history of any disease and lists points of intervention for each stage. Basically, there are three stages in the natural history (Leavell and Clark, 1958). The first of these is the stage of *prepathogenesis,* or *susceptibility.* In this stage, disease has not developed, although the groundwork has been laid through the presence of factors that favor its occurrence. For example, the poor eating habits and fatigue resulting from lack of sleep which are often present among college students during exam week represent risk factors that favor the occurrence of the common cold.

The second stage in the natural history is the stage of *pathogenesis.* Within this stage there are two substages:

the first substage is *presymptomatic disease,* sometimes called *early pathogenesis.* At this substage, the individual has no symptoms indicating the presence of illness. However, pathogenic changes have begun. In the second substage, *discernible early lesions,* there are changes that may be detectable through sophisticated laboratory tests. These changes are called *subclinical* because they are below the level of the *clinical horizon,* which is an imaginary line dividing the point where there are detectable signs and symptoms from that where there are not. In this substage the client may develop early signs and symptoms. For example, premalignant changes or early malignant tissue changes in the cervix may be detected by a Pap smear long before a woman would experience symptoms and before signs would be visible to an obstetrician on visual examination.

Stage three in the natural history is the stage of *advanced disease.* By this stage, sufficient anatomical or functional changes have occurred to produce recognizable signs and symptoms. This stage includes disease so advanced that death is inevitable. Once a client has entered this stage, possible outcomes may be complete recovery, residual defect that produces some degree of disability, or death. In an attempt to further understand this stage, clinicians and researchers have developed classification schemes for varying degrees of disease severity, including the staging systems used for malignancies, and the functional and therapeutic classifications used for cardiac disease.

Exposure of the host to an agent occurs during the stage of prepathogenesis. In the case of infectious agents, exposure is followed by an *incubation period,* a time when the organism multiplies to sufficient numbers to produce a host reaction and clinical symptoms. This time period is relatively short, usually hours to months. For diseases caused by noninfectious agents, however, this time period from exposure to onset of symptoms, called the induction period or latency period, may be from years to decades. Accidents resulting from a severe psychological stressor may happen shortly after initial exposure to the stressor. By contrast, ulcers as a consequence of psychological stress may require years of exposure.

One of the shorter known latency periods for cancer is the 5-year latency period of leukemia in children resulting from radiation exposure. On the other hand, lung cancer resulting from asbestos exposures may have a latency period of 40 years between exposure and detection of the disease. Exceptions to the general rules governing latency periods as just described, do occur— for example, some chemical agents cause almost instantaneous, acute episodes of poisoning.

In contrast to diseases caused by infectious agents,

Table 7-3. Natural history of disease and application of preventive measures

Stage	Events	Level of application of preventive measures	Specific interventions
Prepathogenesis	1. Interrelations of various host, agent, and environmental factors bring host and agent(s) together 2. Disease-provoking stimulus is produced in the known host	Primary prevention	Health promotion (health education, nutrition counseling, adequate housing, personal hygiene, etc.) Specific protection (immunizations, sanitation, removing occupational and environmental hazards, use of specific nutrients, etc.)
Pathogenesis Early pathogenesis	1. Interaction of host and stimulus 2. Stimulus or agent becomes established (if infectious agent, increases by multiplication) 3. Beginning tissues and physiological changes	Secondary prevention	Early diagnosis and prompt treatment (screening, case-finding, selective examination)
Discernible early lesions	1. Clinical recognition of disease is possible through laboratory or other tests that detect early physiological changes 2. Patient develops early symptoms	Tertiary prevention	
Advanced disease	1. Acute illness 2. Disability 3. Defect 4. Chronic state 5. Death		Disability limitation (treatment to arrest disease process) Rehabilitation (retraining for maximum use of remaining capacities, facilitating reentry to the family unit and to the workplace)

Adapted from Leavell, H.R., and Clark, E.G.: Preventive medicine for the doctor in his community, New York, 1958, McGraw-Hill Book Co.

those diseases caused by noninfectious agents or by still unidentified agents are more likely to be conditions of a chronic nature. Most, but not all, diseases with infectious causes are of relatively short duration. The patient is usually ill for a period ranging from a few days to several months and generally recovers without any residual disability or, if the illness was severe, may die from the illness. The patient who has recovered rarely requires long-term follow-up, although there are exceptions. Tuberculosis and rheumatic heart disease, which result from a staphylococcal infection, are examples of diseases caused by infectious agents that are chronic in nature. In the case of noninfectious agents, there is often residual disability requiring ongoing medical treatment and rehabilitation programs. For example, patients with cardiovascular disease are likely to require ongoing supervision of prescribed medications such as

digitalis, control of diet, and modification of life-style indefinitely.

Levels of Prevention

The natural history of a disease provides the basis for community health intervention. Since a disease evolves over time and pathological change becomes less reversible as the disease process continues, the ultimate aim of intervention programs is to halt or reverse the process of pathological change as early as possible, thereby preventing further damage. A three-level model for intervention, based on the stages of disease natural history, has been developed (see Table 7-3). The goal of intervention at each of the three levels is to prevent the pathogenic process from evolving further. The three levels of prevention are called primary, secondary, and tertiary prevention.

Primary prevention is aimed at intervention before pathological changes have begun and during the natural history stage of susceptibility. Primary prevention seeks to keep the agent away from contact with the host or to eliminate host susceptibility. Primary preventive efforts are of two types, general health promotion and specific protection.

General health promotion includes all activities that optimize the environment and favor healthy living. Thus efforts to improve the physical environment, whether that of the outdoors, the home, school, or work, would be included. Health education aimed at educating the population about good nutrition, the need for rest and recreation, preparation for retirement, hygiene, or the harmful effects of smoking or drug use is a form of general health promotion.

Specific protection refers to measures aimed at protecting individuals against specific agents such as immunization against polio or to attempts to remove agents from the environment such as sewage treatment, pasteurization of milk, or chlorination of water.

Since 1900 effects of primary prevention can be seen in the dramatic reduction in mortality from infectious disease resulting largely from environmental manipulation and immunization programs (Fig. 7-1). This reduction in infectious disease mortality, particularly among infants, young children, young women, and the elderly, has led to an increased size of the total population as well as to the advent of chronic disease as a major community health concern. Although fewer people die of infectious disease, more live to older ages at which chronic diseases are common. Also, industrialization and changes in life-style have increased exposure to potential causal agents for noninfectious disease.

Secondary prevention efforts seek to detect disease early and treat promptly to cure disease at its earliest stage or to slow its progression, prevent complications, and limit disability when cure is not possible. Thus secondary prevention is focused primarily on the stage of presymptomatic disease or very early in the stage of clinical disease. Screening is the most common form of secondary prevention. Many screening tests can detect early physiological indicators of disease before the people have any indication that they are ill. Examples include cervical cancer tests, hearing tests for deafness, the tuberculin test for tuberculosis, and the phenylalanine test for PKU in infants. Such screening programs have become popular in recent years as improved technology has led to a proliferation of available test procedures.

Detection and treatment of conditions at the stage allowed by screening tests provide benefits ranging from prevention of mental retardation in children with PKU by use of a special diet maintained until adulthood to preservation of life for cancer patients whose disease is detected while in the early stage where it is curable. In the case of communicable diseases, not only do early detection and treatment benefit those who are affected through secondary prevention, but the screening program provides primary prevention for those in proximity to affected individuals who will no longer be exposing these others to the infectious agent. For example, the VDRL as a screen for sexually transmitted diseases identifies clients who are then referred for further diagnostic follow-up and for treatment. Once treated, they cannot transmit the disease to others.

A word of caution must be given. Screening tests are given to individuals who presume themselves to be well. Since they are not diagnostic tests, they merely separate persons who are more likely to have the disease from persons who probably do not. Individuals screened as positive require a diagnostic follow-up to determine if they actually have the disease. For example, in a routine physical examination a complete blood count may be performed to screen the person for potential health problems such as the presence of infection or anemia. A low hemoglobin count may require further diagnostic follow-up to ascertain the kind of cause of anemia. A high white blood count may require further diagnostic follow-up to determine the location of the infection. Thus, from an ethical point of view, certain criteria should be met before a screening test is indiscriminately administered:

1. An effective treatment that will change the course of the disease must be available.
2. There must be evidence that the test does, in fact, detect the disease at an earlier stage in the natural history than when symptoms are present.
3. The test must have the ability to screen as positive those individuals with the disease *(sensitivity)* and the ability to screen as negative those persons without the disease *(specificity)*.
4. Follow-up services must be available and accompanied by an adequate notification and referral service for those positive on the screening.

These criteria are necessary because the sensitivity of screening tests is always less than 100%. Conversely, individuals without the disease are not necessarily screened as negative because the specificity of a screening test is never 100%. It is therefore useful to teach clients about early symptoms as a part of the screening program so they will be alerted to the significance of symptoms that might appear several months later.

Tertiary prevention includes limitation of disability for persons in the earlier stages of illness and rehabilitation in those persons for whom residual damage already exists. Tertiary prevention activities are focused on the middle to later phases of the stage of clinical disease when irreversible pathological damage produces disability. For a client recovering from a stroke, exercise therapy to preserve muscle tone, restore motion, and prevent contractures is a form of tertiary prevention, since it both limits disability and begins the process of rehabilitation by maximizing the individual's residual capacities. Psychosocial and vocational services are usually part of a rehabilitation program as well.

Measures for the control of communicable disease are aimed at preventing the spread of the infectious agent from those environments harboring it to individuals who are susceptible and who may be exposed. This can be achieved by modifying or eliminating the environment in which the infectious agent lives, by interfering with the means of transmission to the human host, or by increasing host immunity—all measures aimed at primary prevention. Control is facilitated by maintaining surveillance programs that quickly identify new cases for follow-up with isolation methods to prevent exposure of those susceptible or by instituting specific treatments to limit the period of communicability and progression of pathological conditions (secondary prevention). Tertiary prevention plays a smaller role in infectious disease programs than in noninfectious programs, since infectious disease less often results in permanent disability.

In infectious diseases, illness can be prevented if the agent is destroyed or otherwise removed from the environment or if specific protection is instituted through vaccination programs. This works because the infectious agent is necessary to produce the disease. As previously noted, for chronic conditions caused by noninfectious agents there is no single necessary agent. Chronic obstructive pulmonary disease, for example, may result from smoking, from asbestos exposure, from air pollution, or from a variety of other agents. Each agent must be eliminated to assure control of disease incidence. Measures aimed at specific protections, such as removal of hazardous substances from the workplace, will reduce occurrence of the disease but will not eliminate it.

Synergistic effects or the combined effects of two or more agents are frequently seen in instances of causation by noninfectious agents. For example, nonsmoking workers exposed to asbestos do not have a statistically significant increase in the risk of dying from lung cancer when compared to nonsmoking, nonexposed individuals. However, workers who smoke and are exposed to asbestos are estimated to have 92 times the risk of the nonsmoking, nonexposed individuals (Kleinfeld et al. 1967). This is of concern because control efforts often must settle for minimizing rather than eliminating workplace exposures. The synergistic effect of other exposures could mean that substantial risk remains even with low-level exposures. It was hoped that if exposures to harmful environmental agents were kept low, the latency period before onset of symptoms would be so long that the average individual would not develop problems until old age. Since synergism may shorten latency periods and produce illness in the prime of life at low exposure levels, reducing behavioral risks like smoking is crucial.

Efforts aimed at primary prevention of chronic, noninfectious diseases such as heart disease must focus on such things as maternal diet during pregnancy, the diet of the child during early life, regular exercise, and education programs regarding the hazards of smoking. Although success cannot be guaranteed, prospects for success are greatest if intervention occurs early in life, before physiological risk factors such as obesity and elevated cholesterol levels are permitted to develop. These physiological states involve cellular changes that are steps in the development of disease, and therefore reduction of these risk factors is already secondary prevention.

EPIDEMIOLOGICAL METHODS: SOURCES OF DATA

Epidemiological investigations use data from a variety of existing sources, such as census data collected by the government or records maintained by hospitals. In other instances the data may be generated for a specific study through surveys that include interviews, physical exams, and so on. Basically, there are three types of data required: population statistics, mortality data, and morbidity data.

Data from a population census, carried out every 10 years in many countries, is the main source of population statistics. Census data include information about the geographical and economic characteristics of the population and the personal and demographic characteristics of individuals and households. Certain of these data provide the denominator for routine health statistics.

Mortality statistics are generally based on the numbers and causes of death listed on death certificates, since in most of the world registration of deaths is required by law. As a result, this provides a fairly complete record of the number of deaths. Accuracy of the reported cause of death varies from place to place, but the reported data are probably adequate indicators of the mortality count for major causes of death.

Morbidity data as a rule are not routinely recorded and therefore are less accurate than are mortality statistics. Probably the two major sources of morbidity data

Table 7-4. Rates most frequently used as indexes of community health

Mortality and morbidity	Usual population factor
General mortality	
Crude rate = $\dfrac{\text{No. of deaths during a year}}{\text{Average (midyear) population}}$	Per 100,000 population
Cause-specific rate = $\dfrac{\text{No. of deaths from a stated cause in a year}}{\text{Average (midyear) population}}$	Per 100,000 population
Age-specific rate = $\dfrac{\text{No. of deaths among persons in given age group in a year}}{\text{Average (midyear) population in same age group}}$	Per 100,000 population
Proportional rate = $\dfrac{\text{No. of deaths from a specific cause in given time period}}{\text{Total deaths in same time period}}$	Per 100 population
Morbidity	
Incidence = $\dfrac{\text{No. of new cases of disease in a place from time}_1 \text{ to time}_2}{\text{No. of persons in a place at midpoint of time period}}$	Per 100,000 population
Prevalence = $\dfrac{\text{No. of existing cases in a place at given time}}{\text{No. of persons in a place at same time}}$	Per 100,000 population
Maternal and infant mortality	
Maternal (puerperal) rate = $\dfrac{\text{No. of deaths from puerperal causes in a year}}{\text{No. of live births in same year}}$	Per 100,000 live births
Infant rate = $\dfrac{\text{No. deaths of children less than 1 year of age during a year}}{\text{No. of live births in same year}}$	Per 1,000 live births
Neonatal rate = $\dfrac{\text{No. of deaths of children in a year}}{\text{No. of live births in same year}}$	Per 1,000 live births
Fetal rate = $\dfrac{\text{No. of fetal deaths during year}}{\text{No. of live births and fetal deaths in same year}}$	Per 1,000 live births and fetal deaths
Perinatal rate = $\dfrac{\text{No. of fetal deaths at 28 weeks or more and infant deaths under 7 days of age during a year}}{\text{No. of live births and fetal deaths at 28 weeks or more in same year}}$	Per 1,000 live births and fetal deaths

are hospital records and notification systems, such as the reporting of some 37 infectious diseases decreed as reportable in most states in the United States (see Appendix H) or reporting required by disease registries such as cancer registries or birth defects registries. Surveys are often conducted when data are not otherwise available. Birth certificates provide information for the numerator and for the denominator of various rates measuring health aspects of childbirth and infancy.

Summary statistics for a community are frequently available from organizations that routinely use them for health planning purposes. These organizations include the health department, regional planning agencies, hospitals, and a variety of government agencies.

The rates most frequently used as indexes of community health are listed in Table 7-4.

Concepts of Rates

In epidemiology a count or frequency of events is of limited interest by itself. However, when frequency is used as the numerator of a fraction that expresses a proportion, it is of great value and is called a rate. The reporting, for example, of three cases of infectious hepatitis without indicating if they occurred among 1000 students in a school ($3 \div 1000 = 0.3\%$) or among 20 in a dormitory ($3 \div 20 = 15\%$) is of little practical value to the epidemiologist or to community health practitioners except for the fact that the number of cases of this

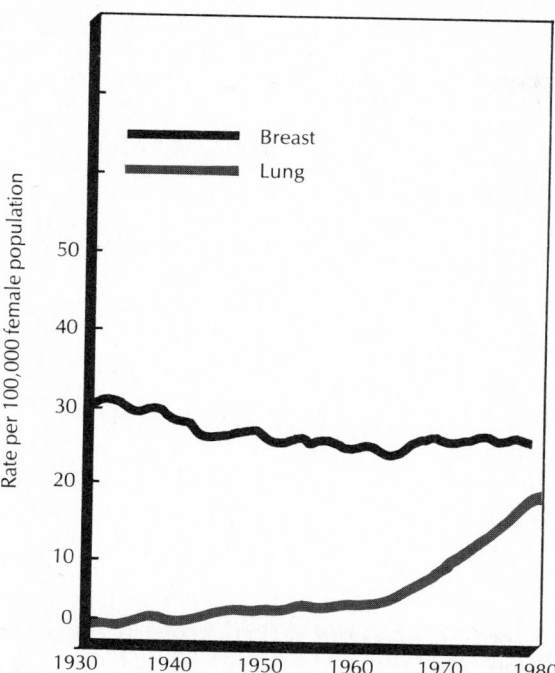

Fig. 7-5. Age-adjusted death rates for women with breast and lung cancer in the United States from 1930 to 1980.

disease may be useful to estimate the need for additional medical services. The rates, however, can be compared to rates for other times or places to assess trends and identify excesses of disease occurrence or to evaluate progress in control efforts. For example, public health officials have recently observed that the rates of lung cancer deaths among females have been increasing rapidly since 1965 (see Fig. 7-5). It has been estimated that if these rates continue to rise at the present rate, lung cancer will overtake breast cancer as the leading cause of cancer mortality for women by 1985. Another example is that smoking concurrent with use of oral contraceptives leads to higher rates of death resulting from heart disease. In an attempt to reduce these preventable deaths, public health officials have instituted antismoking campaigns aimed heavily at young women of reproductive age.

In Cook County, Illinois, in 1976 high rates of measles were observed among high school students by school nurses. Measles are unusual among this age group and highest rates usually occur among primary school children. When these cases were reported to the county health department, an investigation was begun. As a result of an investigation of the exposure and immunization histories of these cases, it was learned that these cases were among the earliest

groups vaccinated after the measles vaccine first became available. They had been vaccinated before 6 months of age. Since there was residual maternal antibody still present in their blood, the vaccination did not stimulate active antibody production as intended. Thus when maternal immunity waned, these persons were susceptible to the disease. As a result, such susceptible individuals were actively sought by county officials so they could be revaccinated before a new epidemic occurred.

Both the increase in female lung cancer mortality and the increase in measles rates among the students in Cook County represent epidemics. *Epidemics* are defined as rates of disease significantly higher than the usual frequency. The usual frequency represents the *endemic* level. A third term, *pandemic*, is used to describe epidemics that include large areas of the world—a worldwide epidemic. Fig. 7-6 illustrates the endemic fluctuation of rates. The peak in 1976 represents an epidemic as it is clearly in excess of normal rates.

Rates are expressed by a *numerator*, a *denominator*, and specification of *place* and *time*. Both the numerator and denominator have to be similarly restricted by population characteristics (age, sex, race) and by time. When the denominator refers to a population that includes the numerator, the relative frequency is expressed as a *rate*, as in the following example:

$$\frac{\text{No. of new cases of cervical cancer in Cincinnati in 1983}}{\text{No. of women in Cincinnati in 1983}} \times 100,000$$

Since cervical cancer can only occur among women, only women are included in the denominator. The women in both the numerator and denominator are those living in Cincinnati in 1983. The resulting rate is generally multiplied times some constant value, usually 100,000, so that rates for different-sized populations can be compared.

By contrast, if the numerator is not included in the denominator, a *ratio* is obtained. The annual fetal death rate is the number of fetal deaths in a year related to the total number of annual births plus fetal deaths. The annual fetal death *ratio* is the number of fetal deaths in relation to only the total number of live births. Here the denominator does not include both the total population of affected and unaffected persons (live births and fetal deaths) but only the unaffected.

The numerator and denominator of rates may be *general* or *specific*. General rates refer to rates that include the total population whereas specific rates apply only to the population subgroup specified, for example, women, children under 17 years of age, or black males.

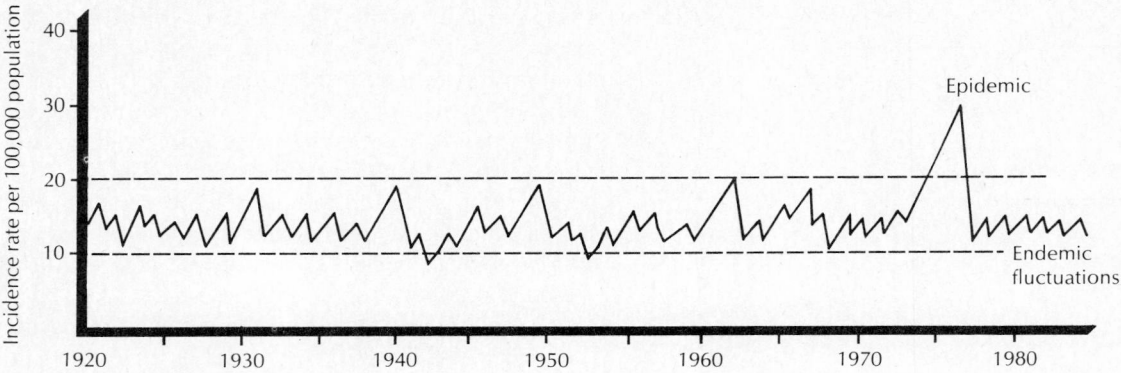

Fig. 7-6. Schematic representation of endemic and epidemic rates.

Death Rates (Mortality)

The numerator of death includes all deaths that occurred in the population during a defined period of time, usually one year. Rates in which the denominator is the entire population from which cases in the numerator are obtained are general rates, often termed *crude rates*, for example, crude rate for deaths in Ohio in 1983. The numerator may be specific for a disease or condition, for example, the crude death rate for coronary heart disease (CHD) includes only deaths from CHD rather than from all causes, whereas the denominator remains general (the entire population). In this example the rate is calculated as follows:

$$\frac{\text{No. of deaths from CHD in Ohio in 1983}}{\text{No. of persons in population of Ohio in 1983}} \times 100,000$$

These crude rates provide one measure for the experience of the entire population. A crude rate of death from CHD, for example, includes deaths among males and females and among young and old. *Specific rates*, on the other hand, allow us to assess the experience of subgroups of a population. Sex-specific rates give us one rate for males, calculated as follows:

$$\frac{\begin{array}{c}\text{No. of males who died from}\\\text{CHD in Cincinnati in 1983}\end{array}}{\text{No. of males in population of Cincinnati in 1983}} \times 100,000$$

If a similar rate is calculated for females, we can compare the rate for males with that for females. A similar procedure for specific age groups would allow us to compare the experience of younger persons with that of older persons. In this example, were we to look at actual age-specific rates, we would see that CHD mortality increases with age.

Crude rates, which provide one rate for the experience of a total population, can present a problem if we wish to compare the population experience of one location with that of another, because the distribution of characteristics within the population may vary. For example, suppose we wanted to compare population A and population B. As seen in Table 7-5, the age-specific death rates are the same in the two populations. However, the crude rates would lead us to believe that the experience of these populations is quite different. This occurs because population B has a large percentage of its members in the older age groups in which heart disease mortality is high, whereas population A has a heavier concentration of members in the younger age groups in which heart disease mortality is low. We might observe such a situation in comparing a state with a young population such as Alaska with a state with a substantial elderly population such as Florida.

A *standardized*, or adjusted, rate can be calculated, which adjusts for the difference in age distributions of populations. Essentially, age-adjusted rates allow one to answer the question, "If these populations had the same age distribution, how would their overall experience with this disease compare?" Calculation of these rates uses two pieces of basic information: (1) the actual specific rates for each population being compared and (2) a population distribution to which the specific rates are applied. The resulting absolute number obtained will differ, depending on the population distribution used. However, the resulting number, although "fictitious" because of the way it is calculated, nonetheless represents a valid way to compare the experience of these two populations, since it is not the absolute level but the relative position that is important. Therefore, it does not matter what population is chosen as the standard. For example, in Table 7-5 if we use the population distribution of population A in calculating the standardized rate for B, we obtain a rate of 22 for population B. Because the age-specific rates for the two populations are the same, this adjusted rate is the same as the crude rate for population A. If the distribution of

Table 7-5. Comparison of death rates in two populations by age-specific rates, crude rates, and adjusted rates

Age (years)	Population No.	%	Annual age-specific death rate per 1,000	Annual no. of deaths	Crude death rate per 1,000	Calculation of adjusted rate for B*	Adjusted rate for B	Calculation of adjusted rate for A†	Adjusted rate for A
Population A									
< 25	4,000	.40	2.0	8				2.0×1,500 = 3	
24-44	3,000	.30	4.0	12				4.0×3,500 = 14	
45-64	2,000	.20	50.0	100				50.0×4,000 = 200	
65+	1,000	.10	100.0	100				100.0×1,000 = 100	
All ages	10,000	1.00		220	$\frac{220}{10,000} = 22.0$			$\overline{317}$	$\frac{317}{10,000} = 31.7$
Population B									
< 25	1,500	.15	2.0	3		2.0×4,000 = 8			
25-44	3,500	.35	4.0	14		4.0×3,000 = 12			
45-64	4,000	.40	50.0	200		50.0×2,000 = 100			
65+	1,000	.10	100.0	100		100.0×1,000 = 100			
All ages	10,000	1.00		317	$\frac{317}{10,000} = 31.7$	$\overline{220}$	$\frac{220}{10,000} = 22.0$		

* A as standard population, using age-specific rates:

$\frac{\text{Population B}}{1,000} \times \text{Population A} = $ Expected no. of deaths

† B as standard population, using age specific rates:

$\frac{\text{Population A}}{1,000} \times \text{Population B} = $ Expected no. of deaths population B is used for the calculation, we obtain a standardized rate of 31.7 for population A, the same as the crude rate for B. In both cases, we find that population A and population B have the same rate of heart disease. It should be remembered that these numbers are meaningful only as comparison and mean nothing alone.

This leads us to the same conclusion we would have drawn by examining the age-specific rates: these two populations have the same experience for heart disease mortality. You may ask—why not just compare the age-specific rates rather than going to so much trouble? This is a reasonable approach if you are trying to compare only two or three populations. However, if your aim is to compare rates for the 50 states or for 20 neighborhoods in a city, you might find the task of making sense of so many rates overwhelming. Use of a single standardized rate to represent the experience of each state makes the task manageable. In addition to standardization for age, rates can be standardized for differences in racial and sex distribution and for other factors distributed differently in the populations being compared.

Another kind of mortality is the comparison of the number of deaths from a particular illness, such as cancer, to all other deaths. Such a rate, called a *proportional mortality,* is calculated as follows:

$$\frac{\text{No. of cancer deaths in a place in year}}{\text{No. of total deaths from all causes in a place in year}}$$

The denominator could also be the total number of deaths from cancer if one were interested in what percent of all cancer deaths are caused by breast cancer, in which case the numerator would be the number of breast cancer deaths. In either instance, if the numerator is specific for certain age, sex, or race groups, the denominator has to be likewise restricted to these same groups. For instance, for the proportional mortality from CHD in white males over 50 years of age in relation to all CHD deaths, the numerator includes all deaths in this restricted group of the general population and the denominator includes all CHD deaths.

Morbidity

The two most commonly used morbidities are incidence and prevalence. *Incidence* is a measure of all new cases arising during a defined period of time, usually 1 year in a population at risk, and is calculated as follows:

$$\text{Incidence} = \frac{\begin{array}{c}\text{No. of new cases of disease in a}\\ \text{place from time}_1 \text{ to time}_2\end{array}}{\begin{array}{c}\text{No. of persons in a place at}\\ \text{midpoint of time period}\end{array}}$$

For this rate the denominator uses the population size at the midpoint of the time period. This rate, called a *cumulative incidence,* is the one commonly used for large general population estimates. Other measures of incidence such as incidence density are modifications of this rate, used in cohort studies where a defined group of persons is followed over time. To account for persons who die, who are lost to follow-up, or who have contracted the disease and are therefore not at risk, a measure called person-years is used as the denominator of these incidence rates. A *person-year* is one person at risk for 1 year. The numerator is the total number of cases accumulated over the study period. The rate yielded by dividing the numerator by the denominator is subsequently divided by the number of follow-up years to yield an average incidence.

Incidence represents the risk of developing a particular disease. Thus these rates are useful in studies of disease etiology where incidence for groups exposed to a putative etiological agent is compared with incidence for groups not exposed. This measure comparing the risk for two groups is the relative risk ratio discussed earlier.

Incidence is useful for monitoring occurrence of a disease in defined populations over time. Incidence is preferable to mortality for this purpose, since incidence reflects only diagnosed occurrence of the disease and unlike mortality, no additional factors such as improvements in treatment leading to improved survival. Such monitoring of disease can alert community health personnel to the presence of new hazards in the environment. A sudden increased in a particular congenital malformation, for example, could indicate an environmental hazard recently introduced to that geographical area.

Special rates expressing incidence, called *attack rates,* are frequently used in surveillance and control of infectious diseases. Attack rates are calculated when a clearly defined population has been exposed to an infectious agent; the rate represents the incidence of illness among that exposed population. An example is the incidence of hepatitis B among a classroom of children at a day-care center exposed to a contagious classmate. Changes in attack rates may indicate a change in the immune status of a population, as in the Cook County measles epidemic discussed earlier, or may be an indication of a more virile strain of an organism. These rates are discussed further in Chapter 12.

Prevalence is a measure of the existing number of cases present in a population at a given time:

$$\text{Prevalence} = \frac{\text{No. of existing cases in a place at given time}}{\text{No. of persons in a place at midpoint of year}}$$

This rate is a function of incidence and duration of the disease. The number of cases of disease that is chronic in nature and that has low mortality will tend to accumulate and will result in an increasing prevalence. Death and recovery are the two most common factors that remove cases from the case load requiring care. A less common factor is substantial out-migration from the community. To evaluate adequacy of existing services and to plan for future needs, public health officials require a measure of the case load requiring care. Prevalence is the measure generally used. Not only does prevalence provide a measure of current case load but future prevalence can be projected by using incidence, recovery, and mortality to estimate changes in prevalence over time.

THE SEQUENCE OF EPIDEMIOLOGICAL INVESTIGATION

Epidemiological investigations generally proceed in an orderly fashion, beginning with observing and recording the existing patterns of occurrence for the condition under study. These observations are recorded in terms of person, place, and time characteristics. From these recorded observations, a description of which specific characteristics are associated with high versus low frequency of disease occurrence is generated. This first phase of investigation, called *descriptive epidemiology,* suggests hypotheses concerning etiology.

Consider the approach of investigators interested in trying to learn what causes breast cancer. The first step is to obtain the rates of breast cancer for groups of people with different characteristics, rates in different geographical locations, and rates at various points in time. Although epidemiologists would prefer to have the rates of newly occurring cases, *incidence,* these are not generally available without a special survey or a disease registry, so the rates of death from the disease, mortality, are generally used in early stages of the investigation.

In examining these rates, it is observed that breast cancer is rare among males compared with females and more frequent among whites than nonwhites, among single women than married women, and among those in higher socioeconomic groups than those in lower socioeconomic groups. Breast cancer occurs with increasing frequency in successively older age groups and shows a decreasing frequency as number of liveborn children increases and age at first full-term pregnancy decreases. By geographical area, rates of breast cancer are higher in the developed, Western countries than in less developed countries. Rates are lowest in Asian countries such as Japan. In the early 1900s breast can-

cer mortality was increasing steadily, but these rates have leveled off during the past 50 years or so, reflecting improvements in early detection and treatment. Incidence now shows little change for whites but continues to rise for nonwhites.

Hypotheses suggested by the descriptive epidemiology of a condition are tested in the second investigative phase, called *analytic epidemiology.* Since these analytic studies are based on observational data, the suspicion exists that the observed association of a suspected causal factor with occurrence of a particular disease may be caused by other factors, such as genetic self-selection of individuals for use of harmful substances or the presence of other factors, called *confounding variables,* which interact in some unknown way with the factor under study to cause the disease. Genetic self-selection in this discussion refers to hereditary chemical imbalances that are thought to predispose an individual to craving for substances like alcohol and cigarettes. Confounding variables may be identified at a later stage of investigation. Suppose that a researcher noted that rates of spontaneous abortion increased with the number of pregnancies. Having babies might not be a causative factor; the number of pregnancies may be related to age of the mother. If physiological aging leads to a decreased capacity for carrying a pregnancy to term, then age would be confounding the original association between parity and spontaneous abortion rates. Because of this problem, multiple analytic studies on the same hypotheses are usually required.

Analytic studies may be done on either an ecological level or a relational level. *Ecological studies* compare large aggregates of people, usually of a defined geographic area, with another such large population. For example, cancer rates may be compared for the population of a town with polluted drinking water and that of a town with pure drinking water to assess whether water pollution is associated with elevated rates of cancer. Or, per capita data on fat consumption may be compared for countries with high and low rates of colon cancer to investigate a hypothesized causal role for fat consumption in development of colon cancer. Such studies, while a useful first step in the analytic phase of investigation, are subject to the *ecological fallacy.* There is a fallacy in assuming that relationships observed among groups can be assumed for individuals. Although there may be a striking relationship between high cancer rates and polluted drinking water in the populations studied, there is not necessarily the same relationship observed on individual levels. Imagine for example, that the majority of residents of the town with polluted water who developed cancer were men who worked in another town where they were exposed to

Table 7-6. A comparison of ecological and relational studies

Level of studies	Types of studies	Other common terms for study design	Basic design
Ecological	Cross-sectional	Correlational Ecological correlational	Rates of disease frequency are correlated with frequency of factor at various points in time
	Case-control	Retrospective	Places with high rates of a disease are compared with places with low rates for levels of factors thought to be related to causing that disease
	Cohort	Prospective Longitudinal	Rates of disease occurrence are compared into the future for places with current environmental exposures and places known not to have such exposures
	Historical cohort	Retrospective-prospective Nonconcurrent cohort	Rates of disease occurrence are compared for places with known past exposure to an environmental factor and places known not to have such exposures; tracking of rates begins in the past at the time of exposure and continues to the present
Relational	Cross-sectional	Correlational	Current rates of exposure among individuals are correlated with current rates of disease frequency among these same individuals
	Case-control	Retrospective Case comparison	Individuals with the study disease are compared with a group of individuals without the disease, who are similar in regard to other characteristics, for frequency of prior exposure to the study factor
	Cohort	Prospective Longitudinal Prospective population	A group of individuals known to be exposed to a factor and a group of similar individuals not exposed are followed into the future for occurrence of the study disease and comparison of its incidence
	Historical cohort	Retrospective-prospective Nonconcurrent cohort Retrospective cohort Retrospective mortality Retrospective incidence	A group of individuals known to have been exposed to a factor at a time in the past is compared with a group of individuals not exposed and their disease incidence or mortality is compared from the time of exposure to the present

carcinogens in the workplace. They actually drank less of the polluted water than did the individuals remaining in the town.

Relational studies, on the other hand, do relate exposure and disease in the same individuals. The presence or absence of exposure and disease is determined for each individual. Then the frequency of joint presence of disease and exposure are assessed.

Four basic types of studies are commonly used: (1) cross-sectional studies; (2) case-control studies; (3) cohort studies; and (4) historical cohort studies. Other names used synonomously with these terms are listed in Table 7-6 along with the design of each.

Cross-sectional and case-control studies are generally used as first steps in the analytic phase of investigation as they can be done quickly, require small samples, and are relatively inexpensive. Cohort and historical cohort studies generally require large samples, take longer to complete, and are expensive. On the other hand, they do yield measures of incidence or risk; no incidence can be derived from the cross-sectional or case-control studies, and any risk measures must be obtained by an indirect means.

When sufficient evidence from analytic studies has accumulated in support of a specific factor being causally related to the occurrence of a particular disease, the experimental phase of epidemiological investigation is begun. This is the third phase of the investigation, which uses an experimental design to confirm the causal nature of relationships identified through observational studies.

Since it would be unethical to expose human subjects to an agent thought to be harmful, in most epidemiological experiments the study sample is chosen from individuals already exposed to the causal agent under study. The suspected causal factor is then taken away from one study group and their disease experience is compared with that of the group who remains exposed to the suspected factor. For example, if hypertension is thought to be a causal agent for stroke, patients with hypertension may be randomly assigned to a treatment group that is given medication to reduce blood pressure, while the remaining subjects receive either no treatment, or diet treatment only. The two groups are then compared for the incidence of stroke. Since in the experimental phase the investigator has control over who is or is not exposed as well as over the experimental conditions, the problems of the analytic studies are not generally present. As a result, data from experimental studies are typically used to prove causal relationships.

USES OF EPIDEMIOLOGY

Investigation of Disease Etiology and Determination of the Natural History of Disease

Since the purpose of epidemiological investigation is to delineate the etiology of disease, thus providing the data needed for control or eradication, etiological studies represent a major use of epidemiological methods. *Natural history* refers to the processes normally leading to disease occurrence before any intervention and to the course and outcome of the disease process. It includes description of the disease process beginning with the first forces creating the disease stimulus in the environment or elsewhere, through the time of host-agent interaction, to the resulting response of man, including illness, recovery, permanent disability, or death. To prevent disease, one must identify the cause(s) of the disease and understand the means by which causal agents are transmitted to the human host. In contrast to epidemiological studies, which emphasize the prepathogenic or early pathogenesis of disease, research carried on by clinicians, whether by physicians, nurses, or other groups, is largely concerned with patient responses to treatment (physiological and psychological) during the later stages in the natural history, since the patients usually studied have sought treatment for symptoms of illness.

Although there are numerous epidemiological studies based solely on hospitalized cases, the body of knowledge that evolves from the compilation of epidemiological studies is necessarily concerned with the spectrum of ascertainable cases in a population. Without this spectrum of disease severity, it is impossible to understand the natural history. Thus epidemiological research often produces a different picture of the disease than do studies derived only from hospital data. As an example, recent data show that half or more of the deaths of middle-aged men from CHD occur in the initial days of the first clinical attack of coronary thrombosis. A substantial portion of these deaths occur in the first hours before the patient reaches the hospital, so these cases are never part of clinical research. In addition, there are many cases of silent myocardial infarction (MI) that are generally unknown to the clinician. However, these data provide important information that can be used for planning early intervention directed toward identification and treatment of the silent MI group. In addition, the data on the high early mortality of clinical attacks suggest the need for lifesaving squads trained in cardiopulmonary resuscitation with readily available equipment.

Identification of Risks

Risk refers to the probability of an unfavorable event. In epidemiology, the term generally refers to the likelihood that people who are without a disease but who come in contact with certain factors thought to increase disease risk will acquire the disease. Those factors associated with an increased risk of acquiring disease are called *risk factors*. These factors may be part of the physical environment, such as toxins, infectious organisms, and radiation, or part of the social environment, for example, stressful life events such as divorce or death of a spouse. They may also be behavioral, such as smoking and lack of exercise, or inherited, like hemoglobin S, which increases risk for infection.

In general, the risk to an individual of developing a particular disease can be estimated only on the basis of the experience of whole populations of individuals. Once this experience is known, the relevant risks can be calculated for persons who are similar to those in that population. Further, population data on disease occurrence can provide data for estimating the effect on disease rates of a community intervention. Epidemiological methods are used to collect the appropriate data and to estimate these risks.

Risk to an individual of developing a disease caused by a particular exposure is derived by comparing the occurrence of disease in a population exposed to the causal agent to the occurrence of disease in a nonexposed population. This measure, called a *relative risk ratio,* estimates how much the risk of acquiring a disease increases with exposure to a particular causal agent or known risk factor. Thus, a relative risk ratio of 5:1 implies that the risk of acquiring that disease is five times greater for someone exposed to an etiological agent than for someone not exposed.

Relative risk ratios are a useful tool for identifying factors that represent increased risk for development of a disease. Diabetes, obesity, hypertension, and smoking are considered risk factors for cardiovascular disease because populations with these characteristics show a rate of that disease several times greater than that of populations without those conditions or behaviors. Once these risk factors are identified, community health programs can be instituted to change high-risk behaviors such as smoking and to identify high-risk individuals through comprehensive screening programs that ensure medical treatment to reduce risk. In addition, nurses and other clinicians can counsel high-risk individuals regarding methods to reduce their risk by adopting healthier life-styles.

An estimate of the effect on disease occurrence of community intervention to eliminate exposure to a causal agent is provided by a measure called *attributable risk.* This measure subtracts the rate of disease occurrence (incidence) in the nonexposed population from the rate of disease occurrence (incidence) in the exposed population. If a nonsmoking population develops cardiovascular disease at a rate of 350 cases per 100,000 population and a smoking population develops cardiovascular disease at a rate of 685 cases per 100,000, then 335 cases per 100,000 population are attributable to cigarette smoking and should be preventable if cigarettes were banned.

Identification of Syndromes and Classification of Disease

Identification of syndromes and disease classification relate directly to clinical medicine. Broad descriptive clinical and pathological categories often include very different elements. Their different statistical distribution and the different ways in which the disease progresses or behaves in a population may make it possible to distinguish one element from another and thus to identify characteristic syndromes. Previously all vascular diseases were classified together. As epidemiological data accumulated, it became clear that cerebrovascular disease and cardiovascular disease were distance conditions, although both shared the characteristic narrowing or occlusion of a blood vessel as a preceding mechanism. However, populations with high rates of cerebrovascular disease, such as the Japanese, had low rates of cardiovascular disease and the converse was true (Morris, 1975). The rubella syndrome was identified as a collection of malformations and functional problems common to offspring of mothers infected with rubella during pregnancy, particularly during the first trimester (Gregg, 1941). A more recent example is the identification of toxic shock syndrome as a definable group of symptoms characterized by fever of greater than 39°C, rash, desquamation of skin, particularly on the extremities, hypotension, and involvement of three or more of the following organ systems: gastrointestinal, muscular, mucous membrane, renal, hepatic, hematological, and central nervous (Centers for Disease Control, 1980).

Differential Diagnoses and Planning Clinical Treatment

Descriptive data on, for example, the age and sex incidence of disease, aid the clinician in understanding the condition and in sorting through multiple possible diagnoses with the same or similar symptoms. Recognizing the association of age with prognosis for long-term survival in breast cancer will probably influence treatment and may influence control programs. Breast cancers diagnosed premenopausally tend to be more lethal than postmenopausal breast cancer, thus requiring more aggressive treatment and closer follow-up. Mumps may be a mild, self-limiting disease in childhood, but in adult men it can lead to infertility. Thus community health intervention to reduce susceptibility or to prevent exposure of males who did not acquire infection during childhood is important.

Surveillance of the Health Status of Populations

Surveillance means keeping watch over. Epidemiological descriptions of diseases provide data regarding who is at high risk of contracting a disease, in which geographical locations it is more likely to occur, and when in time it was most frequently observed. This information alerts health workers to situations that should be monitored for early indication of a disease outbreak so that early detection programs may be set up and intervention promptly instituted. As an example, influenza rates tend to increase during late fall and early winter. Specific types of influenza are likely to recur in 2- to 3-year or 4- to 6-year cycles (Benenson, 1975). Groups at high risk of becoming seriously ill and dying of influenza are infants, young children, and the elderly. By monitoring the population for early cases of influenza through reports of deaths from influenza, of increases in cases seen at emergency rooms, or of increased rates of absence from schools or work because of respiratory illness, public health officials can identify the signs of an outbreak early and can take steps to immunize susceptible, high-risk populations to prevent occurrence of the illness.

In an additional example, the descriptive epidemiology of measles indicates that it occurs most frequently among school-age children, that rates vary by season with highest rates in the fall, and that there are long-term cycles with increased rates every other year in large communities and at less frequent intervals in smaller communities, where outbreaks tend to be more severe. Measles is transmitted from person to person by close contact; it therefore tends to occur in locations where children congregate (Benenson, 1975). Armed with this information, the school nurse can be alert to signs and symptoms of measles during the fall and can follow up on absences to determine if measles caused the absence. Numerous such absences may indicate a need to review the immunization status of the school population. Although most schools, in theory, require up-to-date immunizations for a child to enter, all too often monitoring does not occur and follow-up programs must be instituted to obtain immunizations for the susceptible children.

Monitoring of newly diagnosed cancer cases or of birth defects can alert officials to clusters of cases that may suggest clues as to their causes. The occurrence of several cases of adenocarcinoma of the vagina of young girls was noted by physicians in Boston. They realized that the occurrence of several cases in a short period of time in this age group was a highly unusually event. Their follow-up investigation led to identification of diethylstilbesterol, a drug given to the mothers of the girls during their pregnancies, as the probable causal agent (Herbst and Scully, 1972).

Community Diagnosis and Planning of Health Services

Epidemiology provides the facts about community health. It describes the nature and relative size of the health problems to be dealt with, as well as how they are distributed in terms of geographical location, age group, socioeconomic group, and so on. This kind of information forms the basis for planning the number and types of services required to meet the needs of a particular community. A neighborhood with a high proportion of elderly individuals is likely to have high rates of cardiovascular disease, cancer, and other chronic, debilitating diseases. Particularly if it is a low-income neighborhood, elderly residents may lack the financial resources to travel to a distant source of medical care. Thus health planners need to consider setting up a satellite clinic the the neighborhood or providing transportation or home services. Maternity and child health services can be planned to meet the needs of a community with a young population with a high birth rate. Family planning facilities, well-child centers that include immunization services, and health education programs aimed at prevention of disease through promotion of good health habits may be appropriate.

Evaluation of Health Services

Since many health services are initiated as an effort to treat a community problem identified by epidemiological data, these same data, used as a monitoring device, are useful in the evaluation of these services. For example, one means of evaluating the effectiveness of a maternity and child health center established to reduce the rates of morbidity and mortality among mothers and children is to follow closely the morbidity or mortality to see whether they drop and remain low after the health center is in operation.

APPLICATIONS OF EPIDEMIOLOGY IN COMMUNITY HEALTH NURSING

Most nurses working in community health are employed by agencies that interact directly with individual clients and families, such as visiting nurse associations, community-based maternity and child health or mental health centers, alcohol and drug intervention programs, health maintenance organizations, or nursing centers. Nursing in occupational health settings, although usually limited to contact with the individual client, requires consideration of the family resources and needs in planning care. Some nurses will be employed as health planners or administrators involved in planning and evaluating services of their agency, for example, the director of a visiting nurse association. Nursing administrators in a health department, in contrast, may be involved both in planning services of that agency and in coordinating the services of a variety of community agencies. Similarly, nurses serving on community boards need to be concerned with coordination of existing services and planning to meet currently unmet needs. Regardless of the agency or the nurses position, they will be involved in some phase with the epidemiological process.

Care of patients and families is based on the following steps of the nursing process: (1) assessment, (2) planning, (3) implementation, and (4) evaluation. The same process is used in providing care for communities. In both instances, epidemiology provides the baseline information for assessment of needs, for setting priorities in developing a plan of care, and for evaluating the effectiveness of care.

Agencies providing care to communities through surveillance of health indicators for planning, provision, and evaluation of services interrelate through referrals, required reporting, and feedback mechanisms with agencies such as visiting nurse services whose primary purpose is provision of direct services to clients.

Because of the interrelationships between the various levels of health agencies, observations of need based on a common baseline of information are necessary if nurses at various levels and in various settings are to provide appropriate care. If such a baseline of information is not shared, each nurse would collect only the data considered important; interpretations of the data would vary from nurse to nurse. Epidemiological concepts, such as natural history of disease and primary, secondary, and tertiary prevention, provide a unifying approach for defining which data should be collected and how they should be interpreted.

If such common information is available at all levels and common interpretation is likely, then the referral and reporting system within a community is facilitated and effective response of the system to a need should result. To assess needs, the nurse providing direct care requires data on the presence or absence of risk characteristics, including family composition and relationships, socioeconomic and cultural factors, environmental factors, and medical and health history (incidence, prevalence, and mortality, both current and over a period of time). The nurse involved in planning services for the community requires parallel data for the community: presence and distribution of risk characteristics for the community, including composition by age, race, socioeconomic and cultural factors, environmental factors, and rates measuring the medical and health history.

The following situation illustrates the use of epidemiological data by nurses providing direct services and by those involved in planning at the community level:

A nurse at the Visiting Nurse Service receives a referral for a home visit to a 15-year-old mother whose premature infant has just been discharged from the hospital. The mother of the infant lives with her 40-year-old mother, a heavy smoker who is 50 pounds overweight, and her 45-year-old father, who has high blood pressure and is employed by a company that manufactures pesticides. On her way from the bus stop to the house, the nurse passes overturned trash cans with garbage strewn in the street and numerous teenagers lounging on the doorstep of a neighboring house. When she arrives, she finds that the baby has a temperature of 39°C and diarrhea but no signs of an upper respiratory infection. The grandmother reports that the temperature was normal late yesterday when the infant was discharged from the hospital. The baby's mother has returned to school and the grandmother is caring for the baby. She states that she quit a part-time job so she could do this and that they can just scrape by on her husband's salary of $12,000 a year.

The apartment is hazy with cigarette smoke but appears clean and tidy. Grandmother has a hacking cough and appears slightly short of breath. Her pulse is 96. She had been preparing a dinner of baked ham, canned green beans, and boxed macaroni and cheese when the nurse arrived. An inter-

view with the grandmother reveals a family history of CHD on both sides of the family. The nurse also learns that the baby's mother is continuing to see the baby's father and that she is irritable and impatient when the baby cries. About this time the grandfather arrives home from work, tired and hungry. His clothing and hair are sprinkled with a light but visible dusting of powder. After being introduced, he has a beer, then excuses himself to shower and change.

Table 7-7 lists the observations of the nurse, the pertinent epidemiological facts that facilitate interpretation of the observation, the implications for nursing care, and the possible courses of action based on her assessment. For example, the nurse has observed an elevated temperature in the infant accompanied by diarrhea. The infant was fed once during the night and once in the morning with bottles of milk sent home from the hospital. Only the afternoon feeding was from formula mixed in the home. The nurse's knowledge of the natural history of infectious diseases reveals these important facts: (1) an elevated temperature and diarrhea in the absence of respiratory symptoms suggest a milk-bone infection or some other infection transmitted by oral entry, and since the temperature is elevated, the symptoms are probably caused by an infection rather than by a toxin; (2) most infections have incubation periods longer than 24 hours and most feedings were from hospital-supplied formula. The nurse concludes that the infection may have originated in the hospital and initiates appropriate action, both to secure treatment for the infant and to notify appropriate persons who can evaluate and control any infection problem at the hospital.

Similar assessment processes are illustrated in Table 7-7 for the other observations of the nurse. In each instance the nurse can evaluate her care by referring back to the epidemiological risk factors that suggested the approach to care and can assess whether her actions have been effective by determining whether the risks have been eliminated.

Her interventions with this family will bring her into contact with nurses in other community agencies—the health department nurse, the school nurse, and the occupational health nurse at the grandfather's workplace. Knowledge of the epidemiological risk factors and assessment data by nurses in each of these settings facilitates communication of the needs identified for intervention. Facilities such as the family planning center and an adolescent mothers group are available for referrals because nurses and other professionals engaged in health planning monitored births in the community. Because they observed that the rate of illegitimate births was increasing, particularly among adolescents, they established family planning centers in high-risk neighborhoods. Also, because they were aware of the

Table 7-7. Example of use of epidemiological data

Observation(s)	Relevant epide-miological data	Assessment of implications	Intervention(s)
Baby			
Elevated temperature accompanied by gastrointestinal symptoms less than 24 hours after hospital discharge	Elevated temperature indicates infection, not toxin as source of gastrointestinal symptoms, since most infectious agents have incubation periods longer than 24 hours	Infection could have originated in hospital	Refer to pediatrian for culture and treatment; report possible hospital-related infection in premature nursery to health department nurses who may need to follow up on other recent discharges and to work with hospital epidemiologist to identify source of infection
Mother			
Still dating father of baby; not using birth control	Teenage pregnancies are at high risk for low birth weight and perinatal and infant mortality; close spacing of pregnancies increases risks to physical health of both mother and fetus	Teenage mother remains at high risk of becoming pregnant; such a pregnancy would be at high risk of complications; additional infant would increase pressures on mother and her parents and disrupt family interactions, creating a high-risk environment for child abuse	Counsel mother regarding birth control options and referral to family planning center
No short-term or long-term goals	Low socioeconomic status and multiple pressures are risk factors for child abuse		Assess plans for future; counsel grandparents regarding helping role; refer for family counseling if indicated; contact school nurse for counseling with mother and referral to community adolescent mothers group
Grandmother			
Heavy smoker; obese with shortness of breath; family history of coronary heart disease	Smoking and obesity are risk factors for coronary heart disease (CHD); sidestream smoke can increase risk of other family members for CHD and of premature infant for infection; family history is also associated with elevated risk for CHD	Grandmother is at high risk for developing CHD and/or emphysema; she is experiencing additional stress because of demands for infant care; stress also is a risk factor for CHD	Check blood pressure; refer to physician for physical examination; counsel regarding risk factors for CHD and measures for personal and family risk reduction and techniques of stress reduction; reduce infant exposure to cigarette smoke by smoking only outside infant's room
Cooking meal high in sodium	High sodium diet is risk factor for elevated blood pressure		Counsel regarding nutrition 1. Calorie and sodium reduction 2. Nutritional needs of adolescents 3. Nutrition and child development
Grandfather			
High blood pressure; stress related to current financial responsibilities and demands of job	High blood pressure and stress are risk factors	Grandfather has elevated risk for stroke because of high blood pressure and stress	Counsel regarding stress reduction and low sodium diet to reduce risk of stroke
Pesticide exposure at work — dust on clothing exposes family	Pesticides are associated with increased risk of cancer; infants may be more susceptible than adults; both dermal and respiratory absorption are routes of exposure	Pesticides are introduced into home on clothes; remainder of family is thus exposed; infant may already have had in utero exposure	Counsel grandfather regarding hazards of pesticides, advantages of changing clothes at work; contact occupational health nurse at company regarding possibility of reducing workplace exposures to pesticides and instituting a policy of changing out of dusty clothing at work and having company assume responsibility for cleaning work clothes

increased risk among adolescent mothers for child abuse and for continuation of a cycle of poverty, counseling groups for adolescent mothers were organized. Because the health planners were monitoring appropriate epidemiological indicators, the services needed for appropriate intervention with this young mother were available & the nurse providing direct services could make appropriate referrals.

SUMMARY

Epidemiology, the study of the distribution of states of health and of the determinants of deviations from health in populations, is a community health science essential to nursing practice. Epidemiology refers to both the methods used in the study of disease causation and to the body of knowledge that arises from such investigations. Knowledge of the methods of epidemiology is useful to the community health nurse, both as a tool in conducting the investigation to evaluate and to explain phenomena observed in the course of work and as a basis for interpreting and evaluating the epidemiological research literature. Epidemiological methods, such as measures of health, serve on a community level as tools for assessing community needs, monitoring changes in health status of the community, and evaluating the impact of community programs of disease prevention and health promotion.

The body of knowledge derived from epidemiological studies, including the natural history of diseases, patterns of disease occurrence, and factors associated with high risk for developing disease, serves as an information base for community health nursing practice. This knowledge provides a framework for planning and evaluating community intervention programs aimed at primary, secondary, and tertiary prevention, which respectively consist of prevention of illness, early detection and treatment of disease, and minimization of disability. Programs of primary prevention try to keep disease agents away from susceptible hosts, decrease agent viability, increase host resistance, or alter in other ways the established host-agent-environment relationships. Screening and risk factor reduction programs are exam-

ples of secondary prevention. Vocational retraining and rehabilitative exercises for the disabled are tertiary prevention.

For the individual nurse, the body of knowledge derived from epidemiological research serves as a basis for assessing individual and family health needs and for planning nursing interventions. It also provides tools for evaluating the success of the interventions.

BIBLIOGRAPHY

Abramson, J.H.: Re: definitions of epidemiology (letter), Am. J . Epidemiol. **109:**99-102, 1979.

Benenson, A., editor: Control of communicable diseases in man, 1975, Washington, D.C., American Public Health Association.

Centers for Disease Control, Follow-up on toxic shock syndrome, Morbidity and Mortality Weekly Reports. **29:**441-444, 1980.

Evans, A.S.: definitions of epidemiology (letter), Am. J. Epidemiol. **109:**379-382, 1979.

Frerichs, R.R., and Neutra, R.: Definitions of epidemiology (letter), Am. J. Epidemiol. **108:**74-75, 1978.

Gregg, N.M.: Congenital cataract following german measles in the Mother, Trans. Ophthalmol. Soc. Australia. **3:**35-46, 1941.

Herbst, A.L., and Scully, R.E.: Adenocarcinoma of the vagina in adolescence: report of 7 cases including 6 clear-cell carcinomas (socalled mesonephromas), Cancer **25:**745-757, 1970.

Herbst, A.L., Ulfelder, H., and Poskanzer, D.C.: Association of maternal stilbestrol therapy with tumor appearance in young women, N.Engl. J. Med. **284:**878-881, 1971.

Kleinfeld, M., Messite, J., and Kooyman, O.: Mortality experience in a group of asbestos workers, Arch. Environ. Health **15:**177-180, 1967.

Kuter, B.: The epidemiology of a measles epidemic: suburban Cook County, Ill., 1976-1977, unpublished master's thesis, New York, 1977, Columbia University.

Leavell, H.R., and Clark, E.G.: Preventive medicine for the doctor in his community, New York, 1958, McGraw-Hill Book Co.

Lilienfeld, A., and Lilienfeld, D.: Foundations of epidemiology, New York, 1980, Oxford University Press, p.37.

Lilienfeld, D.: Definitions of epidemiology, Am. J. Epidemiol. **107:**87-90, 1978.

Morris, J.N.: Uses of epidemiology, ed. 3, London, 1975, E & S Livingstone, Ltd.

Rich, H.: More on definitions of epidemiology (letter), Am. J. Epidemiol. **109:**99-102, 1979.

Smoking and Health: Report of the advisory committee to the Surgeon General of the public health service, USDHEW, Pub. No. (PHS) 1103, Washington, D.C., 1964, U.S. Government Printing Office.

Snow, J.: On the mode of communication of cholera, New York, 1936, The Commonwealth Fund, pp.1-175.

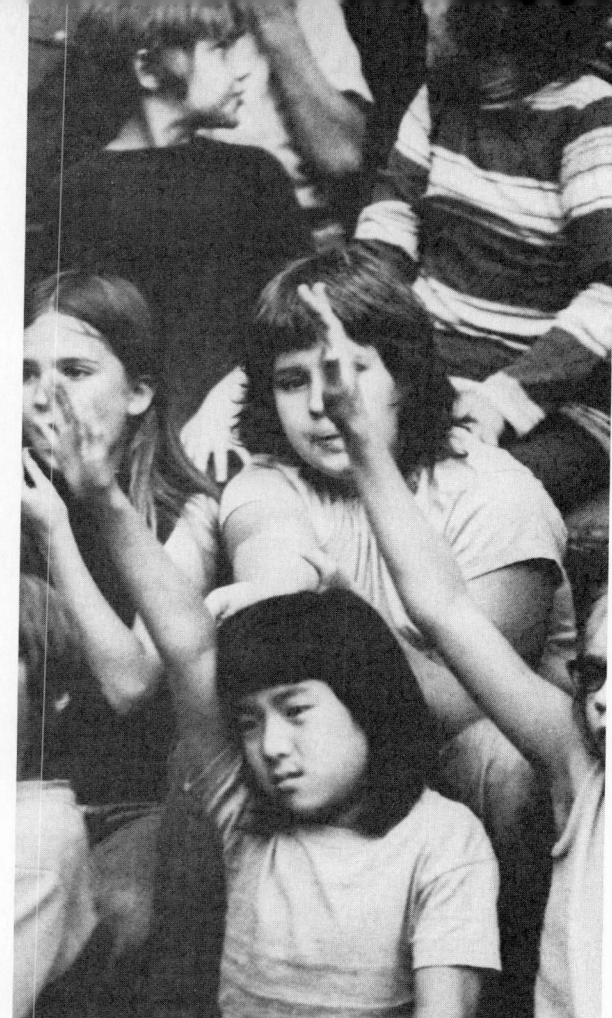

NANNETTE WOREL
JEANETTE LANCASTER

EDUCATIONAL ASPECTS OF COMMUNITY HEALTH NURSING

Health education is a vital part of community health nursing, since the promotion, maintenance, and restoration of health rely on the client understanding health care requirements. Early nursing leaders, such as Florence Nightingale and Lillian Wald, demonstrated creativity, initiative and understanding of the educational needs of their clients. Today health education is equally vital, and community health nurses are in key positions to enact such a role, since they see clients in multiple settings and with varying needs and abilities.

To effectively teach people to care for themselves, nurses must be familiar with key theories of learning, how learning takes place, and principles and concepts of teaching and learning. This chapter focuses on the nursing role in client education and is primarily directed toward adult learners. However, many of the

theories and principles presented are also applicable to students and children. The first section of this chapter discusses selected theories of learning with particular application to community health nursing. Succeeding sections present the nature of learning, principles of teaching learning, assessment of learner needs and interests, definition of learning purposes and objectives, and strategies for effective health education, including sources for, barriers to, and evaluation of learning.

THEORIES OF LEARNING

The study of learning is a critical area of investigation for community health nurses. To promote the health of individuals, families, and communities it is necessary to teach the requisite self-care and health-promotion skills. Generally one person cannot promote the health of another. People are responsible for working toward higher levels of health status through their behavior as individuals as well as in groups. To understand the skills needed to teach concepts of health promotion, it is first necessary to briefly summarize selected learning theories.

Learning is defined in a variety of ways; most definitions include a change in behavior that persists over time, is practiced, and is repeatedly reinforced. Though there are innumerable theories of learning potentially applicable to community health nurses, only a sample of the most prominent ones is included. To enrich understanding and promote clarity, the selected theories are grouped into three general categories: stimulus-response (SR), cognitive-discovery, and humanistic.

SR Theories

SR theorists believe that students should learn in a structured, systematic manner with stimulus situations planned to arouse specific types of responses. This theory builds on the *tabula rosa* (blank slate) view of the mind proposed by John Locke in 1690 (Biehler, 1978). According to Locke, the mind comprises ideas that come from experience. Infants are born with a blank tablet for a mind, on which experiences leave their imprints.

Ivan Pavlov

One of the early SR theorists, Ivan Petrovich Pavlov, left an indelible mark on learning theories primarily by demonstrating SR effects with involuntary reflex actions. His work served as a precursor for later SR theories, although it was not directly applicable to adult learning. His original experiments dealt with digestion; he performed surgery on dogs so that gastric juices were allowed to flow through a fistula to the outside of their bodies where the juices were collected. While carrying out this procedure, he noted that the sight of food caused the dogs to salivate as did the sound of the experimenter's footsteps (Hergenhohn, 1982). Based on what he originally considered a "psychic" reflex, Pavlov demonstrated that dogs can be taught to behave in certain ways when they associate a response with a specific stimulus.

In his most famous experiment, Pavlov taught a dog to salivate when a bell was rung by correlating the ringing of the bell with food. By presenting food immediately after the bell was rung, the response was reinforced. He further determined that if food was not consistently supplied the response was extinguished. In addition, he demonstrated that generalization from one stimulus to another could occur. For example, if a dog that was conditioned to salivate at the sound of a bell heard a whistle, it experienced what Pavlov labeled *stimulus generalization*. However, such generalized responses could be overcome by supplying reinforcement after the bell was rung but never after a whistle was sounded. When this occurred, he said that discrimination had taken place (Biehler, 1978). Over the years it has been recognized that Pavlovian conditioning is successful only for involuntary reflex actions, such as salivating or responding with fear, and requires periodic reinforcement.

John Watson

Another early SR theorist, John B. Watson, was a behaviorist who believed that psychologists should base their conclusions on their observations of overt behavior. In a classic experiment Watson showed how human behavior could be conditioned. To do this he had an 11-month-old boy play with a white rat. When the child began to enjoy this activity, Watson hit a steel bar with a hammer so that the sudden noise would frighten the boy. The child soon began to associate not only his previously enjoyable rat but everything white and fuzzy with the frightening sensation (Watson and Rayner, and 1920).

Edward Thorndike

Some authors consider Edward L. Thorndike to be the "greatest learning theorist of all time" (Hergenhohn, 1982). Thorndike's contributions covered a wide span of interest ranging form comparative psychology, intelligence testing, transfer of learning, educational practices, and application of quantitative measures to sociopsychological phenomena. His research began with the study of mental telepathy in young children. Since the scope of Thorndike's research is vast, only selected concepts are summarized. However, he is especially well-known for his theories of connectionism, the law of exercise, and the law of effect.

Thorndike called the association between a sense impression and the impulse to respond a connection. Earlier theories of association linked ideas to actions, whereas Thorndike made a radical departure by linking sensory impulses to actions. *Connectionism* means that the connection is the neural joining between stimulus and responses. He believed trial and error was the most basic form of learning. In one of his classic experiments, Thorndike put an animal in an apparatus that was set up so that certain responses allowed the animal to escape. Based on this work, he concluded that learning occurs in small, step-by-step gains rather than in large jumps.

The law of exercise states that connections between a stimulus and a response are strengthened as they are used. Strengthening means that there is an increased probability that a response will be made when the stimulus recurs. If a bond between a stimulus and a response is strengthened, there is greater likelihood that the response will take place when the stimulus occurs again. Further, connections between situations and responses are weakened when practice is discontinued.

The law of effect originally was conceived as the strengthening or weakening of a connection between a stimulus and a response as a result of the consequences of the response. However, this law was attacked as being circular in logic. Thus after 1930 Thorndike described the law of effect as stating that "reward increases the strength of a connection, whereas punishment does nothing to the strength of the connection" (Hergenhohn, 1982, p. 74). This law has numerous implications for the way in which the behavior of people, especially children, is shaped.

B.F. Skinner

Burrhus Frederic Skinner began his career as a writer, but when this proved unsuccessful, he pursued the study of psychology at Harvard University. His work is similar to Thorndike's since both emphasize the effect of a stimulus on a response. Skinner, like Thorndike, believed that rewards influence the probability of a response recurring, whereas punishment does not. He was prolific in his writings and theoretical propositions.

The underlying philosophy of the Skinner view is that "scientists have been most successful when they have traced the causes of events and found ways to alter behavior in predictable ways" (Biehler, 1978, p. 229). Skinner differentiates between respondent behavior (elicited by a known stimulus) and operant behavior (not elicited by a known stimulus but simply emitted by the organism). Examples of respondent behavior include jerking the hand when jabbed with a pin, raising the knee when the reflex is tapped, and constriction of the eye in response to a bright light. Operant conditioning is not associated with known stimuli and appears to occur spontaneously. Examples of operant conditioning include beginning to whistle, discarding one book and picking up another, and starting to tap fingers on a desk or table.

According to Skinner, reinforcement is the key to controlling behavior. To test this view Skinner worked with rats and pigeons to demonstrate that actions followed by a reward are likely to be repeated, whereas those that go unrewarded are not likely to recur. The apparatus for conducting these experiments became known as the *Skinner box*. The original box was a small enclosure containing only a bar and a small tray. There is a hopper outside the box that contains a supply of food pellets that are dropped onto the tray when the bar is pressed under specific conditions, such as a tone be-

ing sounded. A hungry rat can be placed in the box, and while exploring its new environment, it bumps into the bar and is rewarded with food. From this experiment Skinner coined the term *operant conditioning* to describe the way the rat operates on the environment. This type of learning also includes instrumental conditioning, since what the animal does is instrumental in securing reinforcement. Skinner believes that children initiate behavior on their own, but the tendency to repeat certain actions depends on whether their behavior has been rewarded.

Summary of SR Theories

Critics contend that SR approaches give instructors excessive power and control and that such an approach requires the instructor to determine what is right and reward that behavior. Further operant conditioning or behavior modification can be used to guide learner behavior not only to increase learning but also to make the instructor's job easier. Programmed learning and computer-assisted instruction have applied SR concepts to aid adult learners by giving them immediate feedback on their learning needs.

Cognitive-Discovery View of Learning

In the early to middle 1900s a substantial number of American psychologists, dissatisfied with the pragmatic views of SR explanations of behavior, turned to European theorists for guidance in their thinking. Historically, European scholars have been more inclined to ponder nonobservable and nonmeasurable forms of behavior rather than to observe overt behavior and attempt to change it without grasping the thoughts and feelings motivating the behavior. Sigmund Freud proposed that people are influenced by behavior that is not only nonobservable but is also unconscious. Similarly Jean Piaget devoted his entire career to investigating children's thinking.

Jean Piaget

Many of the assumptions of the cognitive-discovery view are illustrated by the principles derived by Piaget in his theory of cognitive development. After devoting over 50 years to the study of children's minds, Piaget concluded that people have an innate tendency (equilibration) to bring stability and coherence to their perception of the world. Piaget contended that "children develop coherent and stable conceptions as they incorporate (assimilate) experiences" (Biehler, 1978, p. 289). Because every child has unique life experiences, each one conceives the world in a highly personalized way.

In his early career Piaget determined that the thought processes of younger children are basically different from those of older children and adults. In evaluating

Table 8-1. Piaget's stages of cognitive development

Age	Name	Major tasks or abilities
Birth to 2 years	Sensorimotor	Deals directly with environment by using innate reflexes
2 to 7 years	Preoperational	Begins elementary concept formation
7 to 11 years	Concrete operational	Uses interiorized actions or thoughts to solve problems in immediate life experiences
11 to 14 years	Formal operational	Can ponder hypothetical situations and consider possibilities and alternatives

Summarized from Biehler, R.F.: Psychology applied to teaching, ed 3, Boston, 1978, Houghton Mifflin Co., pp. 115-119.

thought processes, Piaget found that children of the same age tended to make the same mistakes, whereas the errors of children of other ages were qualitatively different. Based on these observations, Piaget opposed the definition of intelligence as the number of correct answers on a test. Instead he proposed that an "intelligent act is one that allows the organism to respond effectively to the environment." He believed that organisms are born with two basic processes: organization or the tendency to systematize and combine processes into coherent systems (Biehler, 1978) and adaptation or the tendency to adjust to the environment.

Piaget believed that people are born with a general potential to perform certain behaviors, such as sucking, looking, and grasping (Hergenhohn, 1976). The schemas available to people determine how they respond to their environment.

Concepts that assist in explaining how people respond to their environment are assimilation, accommodation, equilibration, and interiorization. *Assimilation* is the process of responding to surroundings in accordance with a person's cognitive structures so that elements in the environment are incorporated into the child's cognitive structure. In contrast, *accommodation* refers to the ways children modify their conception of the world as they have new experiences that influence their response. Further, Piaget believed that intellectual processes seek a balance through *equilibration*. Young children respond in a reflex fashion to the environment. As they have more experiences, they become capable of thinking and thereby are able to respond to more complex situations. This merging of reflex and cognitive processes as a response to the environment is known as *interiorization*. As this process develops, the child's adaptive reactions become more covert and include internal and external actions. Piaget called these internal covert actions *operations* and basically equated them with thinking (Piaget, 1952).

Although Piaget thought that intellectual development was continuous throughout childhood, he established four stages as seen in Table 8-1. Piaget's work significantly influenced the education of children, especially his conclusion that children should be allowed to organize and adapt information in their own ways.

Gestalt Theory

According to Piaget, children are innately motivated to learn by built-in desires to make sense of what they see and experience. His work explains much about the cognitive aspect of learning, which is discussed in the next section, whereas Gestalt theory helps to explain discovery in learning and in many ways can be likened to affective learning. *Gestalt* is the German word for configuration or organization. Gestaltists believed that people experience the world in meaningful wholes; they do not see isolated stimuli but rather stimuli gathered together into meaningful configurations or Gestalten (plural of Gestalt). We see people, animals, and furniture rather than lines and patches of color. The key principle of Gestaltists became "the whole is more than the sum of the parts" or "to dissect is to distort" (Biehler, 1978). As is noted, Gestalt psychology is an attempt to apply field theory from physics to answering psychological questions.

Max Wethmeimer is considered the founder of Gestalt psychology. From its inception he worked closely with two colleagues, Wolfgang Kohler and Kurt Koffka. The entire Gestalt movement was conceived as Wethmeimer observed two blinking lights while riding a train. He realized that if two lights blink on and off at a certain rate, they give the observer the impression that one light was moving back and forth (Hergenhohn, 1976). He purchased a toy stroboscope and conducted numerous experiments to determine whether or not there would be an illusion of motion if the eye sees stimuli in a certain way. He called this apparent motion the *phi phenomenon*.

Gestalt theorists were interested in the way in which people interpreted what they sensed and observed.

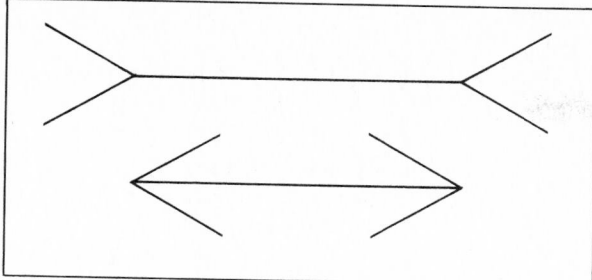

Fig. 8-1. Different arrangements of lines of identical length alter perception. (From Biehler, R.F.: Psychology applied to teaching, ed. 3, Boston, 1978, Houghton Mifflin Co. p. 290. By permission.)

> ### Selected Principles of Perception
>
> - Principle of continuity: Elements that seem to flow in the same direction or follow the same pattern stand out from the background as a figure.
> - Principle of proximity: When stimuli are close together, they tend to be grouped in our perceptual field.
> - Principle of inclusiveness: The figure most likely seen is the one that includes the greatest number of stimuli.
> - Principle of similarity: Similar objects tend to be grouped together in our perceptual field.
> - Principle of common fate: Elements grouped together if they move simultaneously or in a similar manner.
> - Principle of closure: We have a tendency to complete incomplete experiences.
> - Principle of perceptual constancy: An object is seen in the same way under varying circumstances.

From Hergenhahn, B.R.: An introduction to theories of learning, ed. 2., Englewood Cliffs, N.J., 1982, Prentice-Hall Inc., pp. 250 and 252.

When individuals were asked to look at illusions of various kinds, they interpreted what they saw in terms of the arrangement of stimuli. For example, Fig. 8-1 depicts two different arrangements of lines the same length; however, the line on the left appears longer than the one on the right because of the converging lines at the ends of the first line.

Additionally, Gestaltists decided that perceptions are influenced by both past experiences and current interests. For example, people generally conjure up different interpretations of the word joint, depending on their background and experiences. For some this word means a place; others think of a body part, and still others think of a joint as something to smoke.

To explain how various kinds of physical forces operate, physicists developed the concept of a field of forces that can be illustrated by placing iron fillings and magnets on a table and then tapping the table. The fillings are attracted to the magnets in differentiated and symmetrical ways. Early German psychologists, including the Gestaltists, believed that this same basic idea, termed *field theory,* explained behavior.

Kurt Lewin. Kurt Lewin was one of the foremost developers of field theory. He developed a system for diagramming how behavior is influenced by positive and negative valences (forces) and by the direction of these forces (vectors). He also developed the life-space concept, which means that the life space of a person consists of all that is needed to be known about a person to understand his behavior (Biehler, 1978). Essentially the life-space concept says that it is not always possible to draw accurate conclusions about a person's behavior by simply observing overt actions. Lewin demonstrated this concept by placing a group of children in a room with several old, well-used toys. The children selected toys and played peacefully. After a few minutes a partition was removed, and the children found themselves in a room with new and shiny toys. They ecstatically

delved into these new toys and played happily until they were led back to the old toys. On their return to the old toys, the children were not content with them as they had been previously, and their behavior regressed to a less constructive fashion. An observer at this point, not realizing the sequence of events, might consider these children as immature. Hence behavior is not always what it appears on the surface. Health educators must search for underlying feelings, values, beliefs, and past experiences, all of which influence and guide behavior.

Gestalt principles of perception. Although Gestalt psychologists have identified over 100 principles of perception, only a few of the more vital ones to learning theory are summarized in the following box. In addition, they devised the notion of *perceptual constancy,* which means that an object is seen in the same way under varying circumstances. A door is seen as a door when it is open and when it is closed.

Gestalt principles of learning. Because of the Gestalt emphasis on perception, it is not surprising that learning was viewed as a special problem in perception. "They assumed that when an organism is confronted with a problem, a state of cognitive disequilibrium is set up and continues until the problem is solved" (Hergenhahn, 1982, p. 248). A major motivational emphasis came from cognitive disequilibrium. Thus learning is a cognitive phenomenon whereby the individual "comes to see" the solution after pondering the problem. The ingredients are assembled in a variety of ways until the problem is solved. The problem can exist only as solved or unsolved with no in-between state possible. A person or an animal mentally runs through a variety of ways to solve a problem until coming up with one that can be tried, and it works.

Summary of Gestalt Theory. Gestalt theory is useful in community health nursing because of its emphasis on perception and individual differences and needs. From this perspective, learning needs are uniquely assessed for each learner who occupies a specific life space and sees the world from a personal view. In the next section humanistic learning concepts are summarized, and it is seen that the humanistic view is not totally in opposition to Gestalt thinking.

Humanistic View of Learning

There is more diversity within the humanistic view of learning than either the SR or cognitive-discovery view. Humanistic theorists come from varying backgrounds, and their concepts are not based on experimental data as are theorists, such as Skinner, but instead are based on observations, impressions, and speculations. In many respects humanistic views resemble those of the cognitive-discovery view. Humanists agree with cognitive-discovery theorists that observing behavior is not sufficient to explain and predict responses; however, they place greater emphasis on the importance of feelings, emotions, and personal relationships in determining behavior.

Humanistic thinkers contend that it is a mistake to separate actual classroom behavior into categories such as cognitive, psychomotor, and affective. They agree that such categorizations are useful when discussing complex topics but should be avoided in dealing with actual behavior. They also believe that learners should be encouraged to explore their feelings and engage in varying forms of self-expression. Additionally, humanists support the belief that people need to become aware of and able to clarify their values. Notable among humanistic thinkers who have influenced educational processes are Maslow, Rogers, and Combs.

Abraham Maslow

Abraham Maslow concluded from studying and working with animals and people that healthy children seek fulfilling experiences. The first two major forces in psychology were SR and psychoanalysis. Maslow (1968) devised what is known as *third force psychology,* which purports that if people are given free choice, they will do what is best for themselves. Thus educators are urged not to be overly controlling and restrictive with learners but rather to help them grow and develop according to their natural inclinations.

In his book *Toward a Psychology of Being* (1968) Maslow described 43 basic propositions that summarized his views. Some of his key assumptions were that all people are born with an essential inner nature. This inner nature is shaped by experiences and unconscious thoughts and feelings but is not dominated by such forces. Maslow believed that people have the ability to control their own behavior; thus educators should assist learners in satisfying their needs for physiological resources, safety, love, belonging, and self-esteem. Specifically Maslow described a hierarchy of human needs starting with physiological requirements that have the highest strength and must be satisfied before people can look at ways for meeting their other needs. The hierarchy does not necessarily follow the pattern just described, but Maslow believed that this was a typical pattern that operated most of the time.

Carl Rogers

Like Maslow, Rogers is a psychotherapist who previously used psychoanalytic techniques but later enthusiastically embraced and contributed to the development of humanistic thinking. He decided that psychoanalysis encouraged dependency, and over a period of years Rogers developed a new, nondirective mode of therapy that he called *client-centered.* In this mode the client is the central figure rather than the therapist. What Rogers finds most successful on the part of the therapist is to be warm, positive, accepting, and able to empathize with clients' feelings and thoughts. He believes that when clients are so treated, they become more accepting of themselves.

Rogers (1969) transfers his beliefs about therapy to the learning situation and proposes that learning be learner-centered. The outcome of learner-centered education is that students become more self-directed and capable of guiding their own education.

Arthur Combs

Arthur Combs arrived at some of the same conclusions about human behavior as Maslow and Rogers. However, rather than beginning with motivation (Maslow) or psychotherapy (Rogers), Combs began with the cognitive view of behavior. He assumed that "all behavior of a person is the direct result of his field of perceptions at the moment of his behaving" (Combs, 1965, p. 12). Combs advocated that educators should try to understand learning situations by seeing them from the learner's point of view. To help students learn it is necessary to assist them to modify their beliefs and perceptions so that they see things differently and thus behave differently.

He also purported that a person's self-concept is critical to learning. A basic purpose of teaching is to aid learners develop a positive self-concept. Combs proposed that all human behavior is the result of the need for adequacy. The role of the teacher is to provide a learning situation in which students can be encouraged and aided to develop a feeling of competence or adequacy. He identified six characteristics of good teachers that have relevance for community health nursing educators (1) They are well-informed about their subject (2) They are sensitive to the feelings of students and colleagues (3) They believe that students can learn (4) They have a positive self-concept (5) They believe in helping all students to do their best (6) They use many different methods of instruction (Combs, 1965, pp. 20-23).

Summary of Humanistic View

Humanistic psychologists and educators propose that learners should not only acquire knowledge and psychomotor skills (discussed in the next major sections of the chapter) but should also "examine their emotions, explore their feelings, learn how to communicate with others, engage in many forms of self-expression, and clarify their attitudes and values" (Biehler, 1978, p. 339). As is seen in the following sections, humanistic beliefs are consistent with Bloom's taxonomy of learning needs.

Humanistic beliefs are not universally applauded. Some contend that they convey a "holier-than-thou attitude." Others say that they make too much use of games and also at times lapse into providing therapy and not learning. However, despite these criticisms, humanistic concepts of teaching and learning play key roles in nursing. As a profession, nursing is humanistic in orientation and focuses on the needs of individual learners. Although we may not subscribe to the entire humanistic view and all the methods of implementation, the notions should not be discounted without review.

NATURE OF LEARNING

The goal of all teaching is learning. It is discouraging to labor over the preparation of an educational unit and at the conclusion have a participant say, "I'm sorry, but I did not understand much of what you said; could you repeat your key points?" Giving information does not guarantee that learning takes place. To understand the nature of learning it is helpful to discuss three domains of learning: cognitive, affective, and psychomotor (Bloom, 1969). Each domain has specific behavioral components that are arranged in hierarchical levels with each level building on the one before and requiring greater cognitive, affective, and psychomotor abilities.

Cognitive Domain

The cognitive domain deals with the "recall or recognition of knowledge and the development of intellectual abilities and skills" (Bloom, 1969, p. 7). It is divided

---

Verb List for Writing Objectives in the Cognitive Domain

Knowledge

cite	name
define	record
identify	state
list	write

Comprehension

classify	distinguish
compare	explain
contrast	interpret
describe	predict
differentiate	report
discuss	restate

Application

apply	predict
calculate	relate
complete	report
demonstrate	restate
examine	review
interpret	solve
practice	utilize

Analysis

analyze	differentiate
contract	distinguish
criticize	question
debate	summarize

Synthesis

assemble	integrate
compose	organize
construct	plan
design	prepare
formulate	prescribe
generalize	specify

Evaluation

assess	measure
choose	rank
critique	recommend
determine	revise
evaluate	test

into a hierarchical classification of behaviors that Bloom refers to as a taxonomy. Learners master the first and each succeeding behavior in the following order of difficulty: knowledge, comprehension, application, analysis, synthesis, and evaluation. These levels or classes of learning behavior are discussed according to their position in the hierarchy. The following box presents a verb list for use in writing educational objectives for each level of cognitive learning.

Knowledge

Knowledge, the lowest level of cognitive learning, primarily requires recall or bringing to mind the appropriate material. Nurses often impart knowledge in health education efforts. For example, an education goal of community health nurses might be to teach diabetic clients to recognize the signs and symptoms of hypoglycemia. The task is to ensure that clients can accurately recognize symptoms. Other behavioral tasks consistent with knowing are defining, recalling, and listing. Knowledge precedes comprehension.

Comprehension

Comprehension, the second level of cognitive learning, combines recall and understanding. To comprehend is to grasp the meaning of the information provided. The goal of teaching clients is to provide sufficient information and understanding so that they can appreciate the significance of health education. At the knowledge level of cognitive learning, a diabetic client is expected to recognize the symptoms of hypoglycemia. However, at the comprehension level the client is expected to describe the relation between hypoglycemia, diet, and insulin. The behavioral tasks required to assess comprehension include asking learners to (1) state the information taught to them in their own words (2) give examples to demonstrate a grasp of information and (3) be able to describe or summarize what has been learned.

Application

Application is the third level of cognitive learning. Mastery occurs when the learner takes the information provided and uses it in new, particular, and concrete situations. Application is a desirable level of learning in health promotion and self-care activities for it allows clients to apply information to their unique situation. Several behavioral tasks consistent with application include choosing appropriate procedures, applying the principles learned to the person's unique situation, and discussing a specific approach to be used based on the general information presented in a learning experience.

For example, a diabetic client might be asked to review the standard American Diabetic Association's 1200-calorie diet and choose specific foods to be included based on personal preferences and cooking habits. In this situation the client would apply general information to specific personal needs. This level of learning goes beyond asking a client to recite the amount and type of food cited on the standard diet. The next step is to apply this information in such a way that compliance with the dietary regimen is likely to occur.

Analysis

The fourth level of cognitive learning, analysis, requires the learner to break down communication into constituent elements to distinguish between the parts as well as understand the relationship among them (Bloom, 1969). The behavioral tasks consistent with analysis include identifying, discriminating, discovering, detecting, and analyzing. This stage requires mastery of knowledge, comprehension, and application. For example, if a diabetic client experiences a hypoglycemic reaction when the blood glucose level falls below 60 mg per 100 ml of blood, the analysis task is to determine the precipitating factors of the reaction. The nurse might ask the person to look back over the past day or two and determine if any meals were missed or if the client vomited or was involved in considerable exercise and exertion. The goal is to assist in analyzing behavior and events to correlate them with the symptoms of hypoglycemia.

Synthesis

In the fifth level, synthesis, learners are required to build the previous four levels by putting the parts or elements together in a unified whole. They go beyond analyzing to create something new (Spradley, 1981). Not only do clients at this level analyze situations but they find solutions for them. The behavioral tasks at this stage include creating, developing, writing, and designing. In the example of the diabetic client who experienced a hypoglycemic reaction, the nurse might ask the person to describe the symptoms (comprehend), relate them to previous behaviors (analyze), and design a new way to deal with this situation should it recur. Thus if the client undertakes a strenuous activity only to finish and begin experiencing general muscular weakness, restlessness, sweating, trembling, and hunger pains, the synthesis level of learning would indicate the action to be taken; eat a piece of candy or drink some juice immediately. At this level the person knows not only what caused the problem but also what to do about it to seek immediate relief. Thus questions to be asked when a problem arises include "What do you think led to this event?" and "What can you do to treat this occurrence?"

Evaluation

Evaluation, the final level of cognitive learning, occurs when learners judge the value of ideas, procedures, and methods using appropriate criteria. During this stage the learner questions whether or not the intervention strategy worked and its effectiveness. Behavioral tasks for this level include comparing one situation or procedure to another; judging the choice made and suggesting that the event be repeated or altered in future occurrences; and applying selected criteria to determine the result and to plan for a maximally effective outcome for the next time. The diabetic client would judge how effectively and quickly the 4 ounces of orange juice relieved the symptoms of hypoglycemia.

It is not difficult to measure the levels of learning in the cognitive domain because behavior generally changes in the direction of the particular level. Clients evidence information taught when they can do a repeat demonstration of the learning, adapt it to their own situation, and explain the information or skill to someone else. For health education to be effective it is important to assess the cognitive abilities of the client so that the nurse's expectations and plans are directed toward that level. Teaching above or below the client's level of understanding may lead to frustration and discouragement if the client perceives that his needs are not clearly understood.

Affective Domain

The affective domain describes "changes in interest, attitudes, values, and the development of appreciations and adequate adjustment" (Bloom, 1969, p. 7). This domain is particularly called for in the cognitive-discovery view of learning, the Gestalt theory, and the humanistic view.

Learning in the affective domain is more difficult to assess, since affective behavior is often internalized and hence not readily measurable. In this type of learning nurses influence what clients, families, and students think, value, and feel. The values and attitudes of nurses may run counter to those of clients, thus careful, astute listening and willingness to teach what clients are willing and ready to learn is essential. For example, food preferences differ from one culture to another. Counseling about a diabetic diet would be unique for clients who have different cultural backgrounds, such as Mexican, Italian, American Indian, and black and should take into account cultural diet preferences.

Just as with cognitive learning, a series of steps is involved in the affective domain. First, it is important to realize that affective learning occurs on varied levels as learners respond with varying degrees of involvement and commitment (Spradley, 1981). At the first level the learner must simply be willing to *receive* the information. This level coincides with knowledge in the cognitive domain and includes willingness to listen, pay attention, and show awareness of what is being discussed (Krathwohl et al., 1971).

At the second level of affective learning the participant *responds* (or comprehends as in the cognitive domain) to what is being taught by reacting first with compliance and later more willingly and with greater satisfaction. The behavioral tasks expected during this stage include obeying, complying with, enjoying, willingly doing what is required, and accepting responsibility. During this level the diabetic might agree to read educational materials on diets, keep a diet record, and voluntarily seek further assistance and/or information.

During the third level the person begins to *value* the information being taught by accepting the worth of what is being presented, responding to the information, and developing a commitment to change behavior. This level corresponds to application in the cognitive domain. The behavioral tasks expected at this level include choosing from alternatives, stating or demonstrating a preference, desiring to behave in a specific way, and conveying a new level of commitment to what is being espoused. The diabetic black woman might listen to the information about dietary control of her disease, evaluate her diet habits, and select several alternatives to make her diet conform more closely to the recommended standards. She might agree to try cooking her greens in chicken bouillon, broiling rather than frying meats, and limiting her sweets to fruit, sponge cake, or pound cake.

The fourth level, *conceptualization*, corresponds to analysis and synthesis in the cognitive domain (Krathwohl et al., 1971). At this point learners make sense of the values encountered and try to find out more about them.

The fifth level of affective learning occurs when learners *organize* the information by adopting behavior to fit their modified value system. Corresponding to the evaluation level, practice at this stage is crucial to reinforce the modified value system.

Because of the elusive nature and difficulty in modifying such deep-seated qualities as values, attitudes, beliefs, and interests, affective learning is difficult to measure and concretize. Without support, encouragement, and feedback clients can easily step back into old ways of doing things. Praise is useful, since people are often asked to give up cherished habits. Group support can be important because the physical evidence of attitude and behavior change is often only slowly noticed. For example, the visible outcome of conscientious adherence to a diet and exercise regimen may take weeks; thus reinforcement of compliance and devotion to the goal is extremely important.

Psychomotor Domain

The psychomotor domain includes observable performance of skills that require some degree of neuromuscular coordination. Community health nursing clients are taught a variety of psychomotor skills, including injecting oneself, determining blood pressure, bathing infants, changing dressings, and walking on crutches. The psychomotor domain can be found in other areas of learning, which have been previously discussed, depending on the task to be learned.

Three conditions must be met before psychomotor learning can take place: (1) the learner must have the necessary ability, (2) he must have a sensory image of how to carry out the skill, and (3) there must be opportunities for practice (Spradley, 1981). Further there are three prerequisites for skill learning. First, the learner needs to see the process either in person, with video resources, or through clear, pictorial illustrations. Second, there must be a desire, willingness, and need to report the process, and third, there must be an evaluator who will correct any deficits in the return demonstration of the process (Stevens, 1976).

In assessing a client's capability to learn the skill, physical, intellectual, and emotional ability must be evaluated. An elderly, tremulous person may not be capable of seeing well enough or of being sufficiently steady to accurately learn insulin self-injection. To teach a procedure requiring considerable precision to such a client could disrupt health. Similarly some clients do not have the intellectual capability to grasp all the details of a complex procedure. The steps in teaching the skill should be presented in a manner consistent with the client's intellectual capability. It is not desirable to teach above the level of the client's comprehension or to demean the person's ability by oversimplifying the explanation.

There are instances in which clients are perceived to be both intellectually and physically capable of learning a skill, but their emotional status causes questions to be raised about the wisdom of such teaching. Some people are highly anxious and frightened about self-injections. They may know the process but fear fainting if they see a drop of blood. In such a situation an attempt is made to slowly help the person overcome these fears, but in the meantime a family member might need to be taught the procedure. The behavioral tasks to be used in assessing readiness or ability to learn a skill include determining whether or not clients are able and ready to perform the skill and are aware of the steps required for mastery.

The second condition prerequisite to psychomotor learning is the person's ability to visually construct an image of the procedure. Once clients have observed the process, paying careful attention to the steps or techniques, can they visualize themselves actually doing the same thing? To help people acquire this ability, the steps should be explained and demonstrated slowly, one point at a time, and repeated (or the entire process repeated) until they can picture the sequence in logical progression.

Clients must practice new skills with supervision until they have mastered the steps and have become comfortable with and confident of their ability. They observe, imitate, and practice what has been demonstrated. During practice sessions the teacher should provide feedback immediately as to the accuracy of the skill. Any errors should be corrected promptly so that only correct behaviors are reinforce. When teaching skills in the psychomotor domain, the nurse must be alert to capability and readiness to learn, and the teaching should match this assessment.

Summary of Nature of Learning

Each of the three learning domains must be taken into account in effective health education. Teaching strategies must be based on an assessment of learner needs, abilities, beliefs, values, and readiness to learn.

PRINCIPLES OF TEACHING AND LEARNING

Clients in community health nursing vary in age, background, learning needs, and ability to learn. Not only are clients considered to be learners but students are also learners in community health nursing. The varying needs, goals, and abilities of potential learners necessitate that nurses in educator roles have broad knowledge bases from which to select instructional content and teaching strategies. Since a considerable amount of the teaching done by community health nurses is directed toward adult learners, emphasis is placed on the unique characteristics and needs of this group.

Characteristics of Adult Learners

Knowles (1980) sets the stage for a discussion of the unique characteristics of adult learners by differentiating between pedagogy and andragogy. He contends that most of what is known about learning has been derived from the study of animals and children. Further, much of this information has been generated by experiences with children whose attendance at the learning event was compulsory. He perceives that the technology of pedagogy has been derived from the teaching of children. Since the Greek stem *paid* means child and *agogos* means leading, the literal definition of *pedagogy* has been the art and science of leading children. Over time the referent to children has been dropped. Knowles (1980) attributes the current problems with adult education as having derived from this early view of education as an activity for children.

A further problem with pedagogy is that it is based on a belief that the purpose of education is the transmittal of knowledge. In past generations this premise held true, but with the current rapid advances in knowledge and technology information becomes obsolete in a relatively short time. Hence education cannot be defined as the process of transmitting what is known but rather as a lifelong process of discovering what is not known. A new technology for the education of adults has been developed called andragogy, based on the Greek word *aner* meaning man. Broadly translated *andragogy* means helping people learn. According to Knowles, andragogy is based on four assumptions that differentiate it from techniques directed specifically toward children. These assumptions are that as people grow older their concept of self shifts from one of dependency to one of self-direction; they accumulate an enlarging supply of experiences that serve as resources for their own learning; their readiness to learn increasingly becomes consistent with their developmental milestones; and their orientation of learning shifts from future to present and from subject to problem. Adult learners tend to have a greater investment and interest in what they are learning; they see immediate relevance in the information. Hence they want to learn it now in the most painless way possible. Nurses attending continuing education programs exhibit this tendency toward eagerness to have information presented *now*.

Self-Concept

As mentioned, children are initially highly dependent creatures. Their feelings of self-esteem are derived from satisfaction and security in having their needs met. Society defines the normal role of the child as being that of a learner. As children mature, their self-concepts move from the dependency of childhood to the self-direction of adolescence. Adults, in contrast to children, view themselves as doers rather than passive receivers of information. The adult role is one of productivity, self-sufficiency, and independent decision making. The adult self-concept is enriched when the person is treated with respect, allowed to make his own decisions, and seen as a unique person. Adults tend to resist situations in which they perceive that they are being treated like children, and are being told what to do.

Consistent with Knowles' beliefs about adult learners, Knox (1977) postulates that adults are more interested in changing their performance level than in learning information. Most adults come to the educational situation with some expectations in mind. As is discussed more fully later, effective learning approaches begin with an assessment of learner needs, drives, resources, and abilities.

Experience

The vast amount of experience and knowledge of adults affects their learning needs. The concept of experience is different for children versus adults. For children an experience is something that happens to them, whereas to an adult, "his experience is him" (Knowles, 1980). Experience defines who adults are, establishes their unique identity, and represents a vast investment of the person. Adults are more likely than children to contribute to their own learning because of their rich reservoir of personally acquired information. However, because of their experiences, adults are often less open-minded than children. They have felt inconvenience and discomfort from some of their experiences, which may have dulled their desire to try new things.

Because adults are rich resources for learning, greater emphasis can be placed on approaches that draw on their unique experiences, such as group discussions, case presentations, projects, and seminars. Knox recommends three approaches for assisting adults to acquire a more positive attitude toward education. These approaches include encouraging learners to participate in the establishment of their own learning objectives and specific activities for obtaining them; assisting adults in identifying people who have met similar goals and using these people as role models; and providing educational settings that are flexible and encourage the exploration of a variety of educational goals and objectives. The experiences of adults may also require the use of "unfreezing" techniques in which activities are directed toward helping adults look at themselves more objectively and free their minds from misconceptions derived from previous experiences.

Readiness to Learn

It is well accepted that children learn best in accordance with their developmental tasks. That is, there are specific times and stages when learning is easier for people because of their developmental readiness. Like children, adults have "their phases of growth and resulting developmental tasks, readiness to learn, and teachable moments" (Knowles, 1980). In contrast to children whose developmental readiness largely depends on physiological and psychological maturation, adult readiness relates to the evolution of social roles. These social roles or developmental tasks are discussed in detail in Chapter 25. However, Havighurst (1961) identified specific adult milestones. A person in early adulthood is much more interested in learning what is essential to a specific job rather than learning the skills of supervision. Adults also need to learn ways to cope with job demands while they are simultaneously learning how to perform expected job functions.

Hence the timing of learning is as important for adults as it is for children. The teachable moment for adults is when the content and skills to be taught are consistent with the developmental tasks. An example would be a community health nurse's decision on when to commence a weight reduction class devoted to instruction in exercise and nutrition. Immediately before Christmas might be a good time in terms of people needing to carefully monitor their weight. However, many potential members would most likely prefer to focus their attention on which pastry to bake, what new candy recipe to try, and how many casseroles are needed for the holiday meals, rather than to concentrate on a new diet. Similarly many may believe that they get sufficient exercise shopping for holiday gifts, cleaning the house, and getting ready for guests. A health promotion program might be much more successful immediately after the first of the year. Also, as described in Chapters 25 through 27, the teaching of health promotion activities should be related to the learner's developmental stage. For adults exercise can be taught as a leisure-time activity.

Assumptions about Learning and Teaching

Knowles (1980) believes there are three additional assumptions about learning and teaching that form the basis for an andragogical approach. First, he emphasizes the fact that adults can learn; he refutes the myth "you can't teach an old dog new tricks" by countering that the unimpaired basic ability to learn remains throughout life. If people do not perform well in learning situations, it is not that they are unable to learn but rather that learning conditions are not consistent with their needs, motivation, or style of learning.

For example, because of inexperience with the learning process, adults may doubt their ability to learn. They may avoid attending classes or group sessions devoted to education for fear of embarrassing themselves. Likewise, methods of teaching may have changed since adults were in a learner's role, and they must adjust to the new situation. Adults do experience some physiological changes that influence the learning process. For example, visual acuity may decline, necessitating larger visual aids. Adults also tend to have a reduced speed of reaction so that health educators need to pause and provide learners with an opportunity to assimilate information or redirect their attention to a new activity.

Second, Knowles contends that learning is an internal process. Contrary to popular opinion, the most useful type of learning is not the "sponge approach" when learners sit quietly with fixed smiles on their faces while educators pour out the facts for the learners to soak up.

In contrast to this view, learning involves the total person, including intellectual, emotional, and physiological functions. Adults are motivated to devote their energies to those things perceived as priority learning needs. The most critical part of adult learning is the interaction between the person and the environment. The critical function of the teacher is to create a rich environment in which students are motivated to learn. Because of the internal nature of learning, most adults do best in self-paced situations where they have the freedom to choose the type of method best suited to their needs (Roberts, 1981).

The third assumption of andragogical learning is that there are superior conditions of learning and principles of teaching. In accordance with a belief in adult stages of development, certain conditions are more supportive to learning than others. These conditions as described by Knowles are summarized in the following box.

The general purpose of andragogy is to help people realize their full potential. To do this adult learners should be involved in assessing their own needs, formulating their learning goals and objectives, participating in the learning activity, and evaluating their progress toward goal attainment followed by ongoing reevaluation of learning needs. Adults learn better in situations in which they are treated with respect and their experience in life is viewed as a rich resource. Moreover, learning experiences that build and make use of previous learning are the most meaningful (Rosendahl, 1974). However, learning is affected by degree of illness and fear of possible illness. Sensitivity to a client's ability to incorporate new information is essential. If a person is in acute pain, there will be little interest in learning about exercise as a health promotion activity.

Motivation

Adults come to new learning situations with many experiences that influence their motivation to seek additional learning. If past experiences were rewarding and if the learning event made them feel better about themselves, they will bring a far more positive attitude than if they were previously bored, angered, or embarrassed. For example, if a young woman previously attended a preparation for childbirth class in which she felt as though the leader thought she was dumb and clumsy, she is not likely to be highly motivated to attend parenting classes provided by the same agency.

What can be done if it is perceived that some of the learners have had poor experiences in the past? Initially an attitude of warmth and acceptance helps learners feel that their presence is valued, and their needs are important to the leader. Also, begin the first session by asking participants what they hope to obtain from the

There Are Superior Conditions of Learning and Principles of Teaching

It is becoming increasingly clear from the growing body of knowledge about the processes of adult learning that there are certain conditions of learning that are more conducive to growth and development than others. These superior conditions seem to be produced by practices in the learning-teaching transaction that adhere to certain superior principles of teaching as identified below:

Conditions of learning	Principles of teaching
The learners feel a need to learn.	1. The teacher exposes students to new possibilities for self-fulfillment. 2. The teacher helps each student clarify his own aspirations for improved behavior. 3. The teacher helps each student diagnose the gap between his aspiration and his present level of performance. 4. The teacher helps the students identify the life problems they experience because of the gaps in their personal equipment.
The learning environment is characterized by physical comfort, mutual trust and respect, mutual helpfulness, freedom of expression, and acceptance of differences.	5. The teacher provides physical conditions that are comfortable (as to seating, smoking, temperature, ventilation, lighting, decoration) and conducive to interaction (preferably, no person sitting behind another person). 6. The teacher accepts each student as a person of worth and respects his feelings and ideas. 7. The teacher seeks to build relationships of mutual trust and helpfulness among the students by encouraging cooperative activities and refraining from inducing competitiveness and judgmentalness. 8. The teacher exposes his own feelings and contributes his resources as a colearner in the spirit of mutual inquiry.
The learners perceive the goals of a learning experience to be their goals.	9. The teacher involves the students in a mutual process of formulating learning objectives in which the needs of the students, of the institution, of the teacher, of the subject matter, and of the society are taken into account.
The learners accept a share of the responsibility for planning and operating a learning experience, and therefore have a feeling of commitment toward it.	10. The teacher shares his thinking about options available in the designing of learning experiences and the selection of materials and methods and involves the students in deciding among these options jointly.
The learners participate actively in the learning process.	11. The teacher helps the students to organize themselves (project groups, learning-teaching teams, independent study, etc.) to share responsibility in the process of mutual inquiry.
The learning process is related to and makes use of the experience of the learners.	12. The teacher helps the students exploit their own experiences as resources for learning through the use of such techniques as discussion, role playing, case method, etc. 13. The teacher gears the presentation of his own resources to the levels of experience of his particular students. 14. The teacher helps the students to apply new learnings to their experience, and thus to make the learnings more meaningful and integrated.
The learners have a sense of progress toward their goals.	15. The teacher involves the students in developing mutually acceptable criteria and methods for measuring progress toward the learning objectives. 16. The teacher helps the students develop and apply procedures for self-evaluation according to these criteria.

From Knowles, M.S.: The modern practice of adult education: andragogy versus pedagogy, ed. 2, Chicago, 1980, Follett Publishing Co., pp. 57-58.

class(es), what format they prefer (if the leader is willing and able to be flexible) and also what kind of educational programs they have participated in previously. An attitude of acceptance and interest in meeting learner needs can be built by responding honestly to their questions even when the answer is "I don't know, but I'll check for you."

Setting attainable goals and objectives assists people to feel confident and successful in their accomplishments. It may also be important to pace the educational program to the group's ability to move. Each group of learners has a cumulative personality and an ability to grasp information. It should be determined if the learners need detailed, slow, repetitive instruction consistently or only on some topics or whether they are continually one step ahead of you so that the teaching can be paced to their tempo if possible.

Adults have a different time perspective for learning than children. For children the application of what they learn seems distant, whereas adults can generally perceive an immediate application. Though children enter the learning situation with a subject-centered orientation, adults tend to be problem centered. Adults engage in learning largely in response to stimuli or pressures they feel at the moment. The goal of adult educators is to help them learn what is most relevant at the time. Adults, because of their problem-centered orientation, are motivated by immediate application of the learning. Immediate application provides direct feedback and reinforcement of learning. Errors are corrected as soon as possible, and accurate information or skills are provided (Tarnow, 1979).

Individual Differences

People not only vary in their experience, motivation, and level of readiness but perceptions, culture, and language also influence learning deficits: how people view the opportunities available to them affects their learning. Many times potential learners simply are unaware of needs or refuse to learn information or skills that would assist them in promoting or at least maintaining health. It is not rare for diabetics to refuse to learn to inject insulin themselves. It is as if they were saying "If I don't take insulin, I must not have diabetes." Denial often interferes with accurate perception.

Many factors affect perception, including values, culture, age, past experiences, education, emotional status, religion, and socioeconomic level. Rarely do two people perceive a situation exactly the same way. For example, if while walking down a busy city street on a cold day, a man suddenly fell against the building and slumped to the ground, what would seem to be the problem? Would the conclusion be that he had been drinking and was a degenerate, or would his heart be checked to see if it was beating and whether or not cardiopulmonary resuscitation was indicated?

Clients often use what Sullivan (1953) referred to as selective inattention. They simply screen out the part of the message they do not want to hear. This may not be a conscious process, but rather the person may block out a feared or painful message. For example, after suffering a massive heart attack, a 40-year-old man was told to watch his diet, exercise regularly and moderately, and avoid alcohol and cigarettes. Because he had been a heavy smoker and drinker, liked fried foods, and detested exercise, the message he heard was to drink and smoke moderately, avoid exercise, and not eat cheese. The message was misperceived to meet what he viewed as his ability to cope at that time. Such potential for misinterpretation accompanies any health education and increases the need for home health care where information provided in the hospital can be monitored and corrected if misperception does occur.

Culture also affects learning. Each cultural group has unique values, beliefs, and perceptions that must be taken into account when planning health educational offerings. In particular, diets and health attitudes vary considerably. The specific foods recommended on a 1200-calorie diet would be different for middle-aged women who were black, Mexican, American Indian, or Italian; their preferences would differ as would cooking style. Similarly, cultural groups have specific views about health practices, including the role of endogenous practitioners. For many cultures medicine men still provide health care and should not be disparaged but rather collaborated with to ensure consistent and acceptable health advice and care.

Likewise language varies among clients. Many do not understand medical jargon yet are embarrassed to ask for clarification. Thus it is important to observe signs of recognition such as nods, appropriate questions, and directly asking clients to repeat the meaning in their own words. Simply asking "did you understand" may be insufficient because of a hesitancy to reveal what they may view as deficiencies on their part.

DETERMINING LEARNER NEEDS AND INTERESTS

The first and often overlooked step in health education program planning is the determination of learner needs. Often health educators enthusiastically conceive an idea for an exciting program and develop it only to have it poorly received by potential learners. This may be the result of many factors, but often such failures occur when the needs-assessment step is short-circuited. Frequently educators fall into the trap of providing what they think learners ought to know rather than what they want to know. This does not negate the reality in the health care sector that there is some crucial information that clients must know to ensure their survival. For example, diabetics must know how to regulate their diet to control their disease and many must know how to inject insulin themselves because of a lack of family.

Nature of Needs

The process of needs assessment is discussed in Chapter 9 in relation to program planning and evaluation. Thus this section addresses needs assessment specific to health education. In general, adult learners have two types of needs: (1) basic or organismic needs and (2) educational needs. Although different theorists conceive of organismic needs in slightly variant ways, the common themes include physical safety, security, love and affection, self-esteem, and recognition. People need to be physically safe by having proper nutrition, warmth, water, and safety. In addition, to develop fully people need to feel secure in their environment and to perceive that they are accepted by others as individuals of worth. Every person needs stimulation and opportunities to succeed and be recognized as a capable, contributing member of society and of his social group.

In contrast, an educational need is "something a person ought to learn for his own good, for the good of an organization, or for the good of society" (Knowles, 1980, p. 88). An educational need represents a gap between what a person knows and what knowledge is needed to perform effectively according to personal, organizational, or social expectations. The goal of health educators is to help people assess their key educational needs and determine ways to secure the needed information.

Nature of Interests

Interests are related to needs in that they reflect personal preferences for learning activities. People may have multiple educational needs, yet only one or two of these are of keen interest. A student may have three papers due at the end of the term. Thus an educational need would be to go to the library and thoroughly research each of the three topics. However, the student is keenly interested in one topic, moderately interested in the second one, and actually finds the third topic boring. How does the student proceed? He would probably go to the library and begin with the interesting topic and save the worst (or most difficult) for last.

As expected, interests are highly personal and vary considerably from one person to another and within a person from time to time. Interests, like needs, change as people move through the life cycle. Eighteen-year-olds are not generally interested in the same areas as are 50-year-olds.

Assessing Needs and Interests

Three sources of needs and interests need to be considered in planning adult education programs: those of the people to be served, those of the sponsoring agency, and those of the community or society (Knowles, 1980). According to Roberts (1981), assessment of needs can be done either intuitively or systematically through a conscious evaluation process or a combination of the two. Most people rely on intuition to guide many of their actions; however, health educators must be skilled in the systematic process of needs assessment. Since community and agency assessment is covered in Chapter 17, this discussion is limited to individual needs assessment.

The importance of needs assessment cannot be overemphasized, for with it lies the answer to the first question in health education, "What should be offered?" There are many ways of gaining information from individuals about their perceived educational needs, including surveys, questionnaires, interviews, task forces, and professional literature and the media.

To elaborate on questionnaire usage, Knowles (1980) describes two variations of the projective questionnaire, which were developed by graduate nursing students. One of these, the card sort, uses situations typed on 3- by 5-inch cards to elicit responses. For example, a graduate student developed cards for 52 typical problem situations often encountered by nurses. Respondents were asked to sort the cards into three stacks: those in which perfect confidence and security could be anticipated, those with potentially great insecurity, and an in-between category. By tabulating the results of these cards, it was possible to identify several educational needs of the respondents. Another student devised a picture sort, based on the same procedure as the card sort.

Needs assessment also includes an exploration of participants' backgrounds, including their ability, skill, and experience. Nothing is worse than to develop a program that is more complex and sophisticated than the learners' capabilities. Likewise if a program is too simplistic, learners generally get restless and bored. Hence as in the nursing process, the first step is assessment on which the program plan, implementation, and evaluation are built. Principles of needs assessment apply to developing teaching programs for individuals and for groups. In the following section objectives for educational programs are discussed. Although the discussion uses group examples, objectives also must be established for teaching individuals.

DEFINING OBJECTIVES

The formulation of program objectives is described in detail in Chapter 9. However, the purpose here is to briefly discuss health education objectives, followed by a more detailed elaboration of ways to translate learning needs into objectives and principles for writing learning objectives. Program objectives provide guidance and direction in specifically defining the goals to be established. These objectives help determine what learning activities are indicated for a particular group of learners and what content is presented in each learning activity.

Transformation of Needs into Program Objectives

As expected, the starting point for determining program objectives is to identify the needs that have evolved. Knowles (1980) arranges this process in a series of three steps: (1) organizing needs according to priority, (2) screening the needs through designated filters, and (3) translating the remaining needs into program objectives.

Organizing Needs According to Priority

Once learning needs are identified, they can be arranged according to their perceived importance. In planning group educational programs for an agency, a strong advisory committee can help in defining priorities. For example, if a staff group wants to plan three different programs yet has the resources to only plan one at a time, the advisory committee can assist in identifying priorities based on its personal knowledge of the needs of the population served by the staff. The staff may want to teach nutrition, well-child care, and exercise. However, if the population is primarily an aging one, the advisory committee might encourage them to focus on either nutrition or exercise, depending on the unique characteristics of the aging persons served by the agency.

Also, the frequency with which certain programs are mentioned in an assessment of learning needs indicates the need felt for content to be provided in this area. Another factor affecting setting priorities involves the resources available; the facilities, personnel, supplies, and expertise required to meet certain needs may determine the feasibility at a given time. A specific program may be highly desired in a community, yet no agency has personnel with the needed expertise.

Screening the Needs through Designated Filters

Needs can also be screened to determine whether or not they fit provider goals and purposes. Most health education programs attempt to avoid duplication of other programs in the community; thus identified needs may be referred to the provider who sees that need as a program purpose. For example, most cities have residents who want to participate in smoking cessation clinics. However, if the local chapters of the American Cancer Society and the American Lung Association have frequently scheduled classes, there is probably no need for the health department to become involved.

Other programs are screened out because of a lack of resources or a lack of interest in moving in a certain direction. No health educator or agency can be all things to all people. Thus priorities must be established as to program direction. The staff must be knowledgeable about appropriate referral sources. Nothing is more discouraging to a potential learner than to be told "we don't do that, and we don't know who does."

Translating the Remaining Needs into Program Objectives

The next step is to translate the learning needs into objectives that are stated clearly and specifically and define the expected outcomes in measurable terms. Since learning is described as a change in behavior that can include shifts in performance, knowledge, and/or attitudes, objectives are written statements of the intended outcome or change in behavior. Four parts to an objective are addressed in the following questions:

1. Who is to exhibit the behavior?
2. What behavior is expected?
3. What are the conditions?
4. What are the minimally accepted performance standards (criteria)?

The first component, who, refers to the person or group expected to perform the desired behavior. In community health education, clients, family members, or students are generally the learners. Thus a statement, such as "the client demonstrates correct insulin injection," describes a learner activity.

The expected behavior is a task statement of what the learner can be expected to do following the educational experience. The task statement usually has two components: the actual behavior to be performed in demonstrating mastery of the objective and the result of that behavior. For example, the statement "the client appreciates the need for aseptic technique" is a vague objective and does not contain an observable behavior that can be measured. In contrast, verbs such as define, describe, outline, or demonstrate identify a specific action to be taken by the learner. A better objective would be "the client demonstrates aseptic insulin injection technique."

The third component refers to the conditions under which the learner is expected to demonstrate mastery of the task. Examples of conditions include the experiences the client is expected to have had before performing the task. For example, "after reading the booklet on insulin injections, the client is able to use aseptic technique in administering the medication." Not all objectives require that conditions be stated, but when they clarify what is expected, they should be included.

The last part includes the criteria or standards for minimal acceptance that the objective has been achieved. Criteria are standards to evaluate whether or not the behavior demonstrated by the learner shows that he learned what was taught. Criteria may be stated in a variety of ways including the time limit in which the person must accomplish the task to be considered successful ("client learns insulin injection technique in 2 weeks"); the amount of information the client is expected to retain ("client lists four principles of insulin injection technique"); the accuracy of performance ("client injects insulin without contaminating surface"); and the degree of consistency with the method taught ("client injects insulin using aseptic technique as taught in class"). Regardless of how they are stated, criteria should explain how well the learner is expected to perform the task.

Principles for Writing Learning Objectives

A learning objective is a description of an intended outcome rather than a summary of content (Mager, 1975). Objectives must be stated in measurable, behavioral terms. The verbs listed in the following box help to differentiate between words open to few versus many interpretations. In general, it is advisable to use the former, since their attainment can be more precisely determined than those open to many interpretations.

STRATEGIES FOR EFFECTIVE HEALTH EDUCATION

Group Versus Individual Education

Although the first portion of this chapter focuses on principles of teaching and learning that can be applied to both individuals and groups, it should be noted that groups do have unique characteristics that must be taken into consideration when planning educational activities. Information on working with groups in the community is given in Chapter 16.

Groups may arise spontaneously and require the assistance of the community health nurse in meeting their common educational needs. For example, adolescent mothers may seek one another in the waiting area of an outpatient clinic. The adolescents may share common concerns regarding parenting, returning to school, and resuming social activities. The social support derived from the group by individual members may facilitate the dissemination of information by the nurse. More commonly, however, individuals are channeled into groups according to disease states, such as hypertension, diabetes, or cancer. As is discussed in Chapter 16, membership in a certain group may also arise from certain characteristics of the individual, such as obesity, age, or use of alcohol or tobacco. Regardless of the input the community health nurse has in the composition of the group of learners, it is helpful to bear in mind the positive aspects of group education for the client and nurse alike.

Planning educational activities for groups of learners offers several advantages to the nurse. First, it may be an economical way to present the same material to more than one individual. By using the same teaching plan for more than one client, resources in terms of time and money are preserved. In addition, by reducing the number of identical individual teaching plans produced, the nurse can greatly increase efficiency in patient teaching. No longer must the nurse "reinvent the wheel" each time client teaching is attempted, but rather groups of learners can be reached with one teaching plan.

Next, group teaching provides the nurse with a mechanism for ensuring that education is incorporated into and implemented through the nursing care plan. Group instruction assists in eliminating the all-too-common practice of providing educational activities only as time allows, thus resulting in "happenstance" teaching. Group activities offer the nurse and client a

---

Differentiation Between Verbs with Few Versus Many Interpretations

Verbs open to few interpretations

write	define
recite	outline
identify	demonstrate
differentiate	plan
solve	recall
construct	state
list	classify
compare	
contrast	

Verbs open to many interpretations

know (recall, relate, understand, identify)
understand (realize, know)
appreciate
believe (have faith in)
value
feel

structured time for the teaching aspect of the nursing role (Evans, 1980).

Finally, group teaching can increase the relevance of educational programs. Because group instruction often allows the nurse to plan the content well in advance, programs are frequently based on identified rather than presumed learning needs. As mentioned previously, programs based on the identified needs of a population group are most likely to be well received by the target group.

Group teaching offers many positive features to members. It can meet a person's need for security in a learning situation, or it may provide a means through which feelings can be explored and needs met (Murray and Zentner, 1975). The small-group approach (usually fewer than 15 members) to client learning provides each individual with an opportunity to contribute and share resources, such as life experiences and knowledge, with other members of the group. By encouraging group members to learn from one another, each individual is recognized as having something unique and valuable to contribute to the knowledge base of the other group members. In addition, group teaching provides social support to individuals. Learners discover through group interaction that others are struggling with problems similar to their own, such as losing weight or coping with a dying relative. A knowledge of group dynamics as is presented in Chapter 16 is helpful to the nurse in group teaching.

In working with any group, it is the responsibility of the nurse-leader to set the climate for the educational experience. For example, if a lecture format is to be used with the group, the seating arrangement may be quite different from one used for a group discussion. As with individual teaching, the objectives of the teaching program greatly influence the strategy used.

Teaching Effectiveness

The key to effective teaching lies in planning the approach for the specific situation. Though no "hard and fast" rules exist for effective teaching, the following suggestions provide a guide for implementing the educational aspect of community health nursing (Murray and Zentner, 1975):

1. Providing consistency and trustworthiness to the learners.
2. Being enthusiastic and letting the learner know there is something of value being offered.
3. Being careful not to discuss one's personal life with the learner.
4. Paying attention to the image presented and the messages given with the posture, clothes, gestures, hair, and tone of voice of the nurse.
5. Being organized, which helps to convey a sense of competence to the learner.
6. Evaluating the effectiveness of teaching methods routinely.
7. Varying teaching strategies and resources as appropriate.
8. Recording teaching experiences, successes and failures may be helpful to others in similar situations.
9. Expecting good and bad days in teaching and learning; not all educational endeavors have the expected results, so realism is essential.
10. Remembering that the learner is an individual worthy of respect and not a disease process or procedure.
11. Explaining the reason when asking the learner to do something.
12. Never equating intelligence level with educational level. Cultural, religious, and ethnic variables, as well as lack of intelligence may contribute to misunderstandings.
13. Attempting to motivate the learner through recognition of need not outward pressure.
14. Learning to sense the appropriate moment for learning and acting on it.
15. Writing instructions legibly.
16. Allowing time for interruptions.
17. Being careful not to overwhelm the learner with technical terms.
18. Providing feedback about learner progress.
19. Correcting errors with information, not judgments.
20. Being careful not to allow racial bias to interfere with the learning process.
21. Not reinforcing destructive thinking but focusing on constructive thoughts.

In addition, effective teaching depends on a variety of factors, including creativity, communication, the learning format, and the learning climate.

Creativity

Nurses are constantly encouraged to be creative when teaching, but what exactly does that mean? Creativity includes the ability to find gaps in available information and locate ideas and facts to fill them. It also includes organizing and modifying ideas into a new and unique format that is relevant to the needs of the learners. A variety of attributes enable nurses to be imaginative, innovative, and inventive.

Murray and Zentner (1975) offer several suggestions to enhance creative learning:

1. The learner should be allowed an opportunity for creative behavior. Independent learning through

audiovisual materials or questions helps to promote creativity.

2. The nurse should develop skills in creative learning through participation in such activities as role playing, experimentation, and problem-solving discussions.

3. The learner should be rewarded by carefully considering unique ideas. An idea should not be evaluated until it has been thoroughly tested.

4. The nurse needs to maintain a constructive attitude toward new information and to avoid being critical of unique ideas.

5. Creative relations with others, particularly children, should be formed. Such an approach allows the nurse to embark on the unknown yet maintain the position of a resource or an organizer.

6. Provisions need to be made in the teaching plan for continuity in the creative development of solutions.

By developing a creative attitude toward teaching, the nurse is able to approach the learner with effective and unique ways of meeting needs rather than rigid boundaries. Creativity offers a spark to teaching effectiveness and is best implemented through clear communication. In many ways creativity is similar to receptivity and willingness to listen to new ideas and try new approaches. The creative instructor is constantly seeking new learning techniques to interest the recipients in the process of learning. New ideas, strategies, and approaches are tried and revised or discarded, based on suggestions from the learners about the effectiveness of the new materials and techniques.

Sending Clear Messages

Often messages nurses hope to deliver to clients never reach the intended learner because of the use of jargon, cultural influences, or perhaps the present situation of the learner. In presenting educational programs, it is essential that the nurse not only assess learner readiness (as discussed earlier in this chapter) but also be aware of possible barriers to effective communication. Emotional stress and physical illness are only two factors that may limit the amount of information a learner is able to absorb. The nurse must be aware of limitations affecting the learner and plan educational activities accordingly.

In addition to ensuring that the material presented is useful to the client, the community health nurse must assume the responsibility for offering information that is understandable. Though medical jargon and technical terms are comfortable for the nurse to use, they may interfere with the clarify of the intended message. For example, in helping clients understand the need for diet

---

Do's and don'ts for effective communication in teaching

Do

- Watch for learner clues indicating the message is unclear.
- Rephrase the message, repeat the content, and ask for feedback until you are certain the learner has received the intended message.
- Be familiar and comfortable with the content before attempting to teach it.
- Use terms with which you and the client are comfortable.
- Be careful in teasing and joking with clients.

Don't

- Be afraid to ask clients to teach you the terms with which they are comfortable.
- Be condescending. Clients quickly pick up such an attitude and resent it.
- Allow language to alienate you form the learner.

Adapted from Archer and Fleshman (1979); Narrow, B.W.: Patient teaching in nursing practice, New York, 1979, John Wiley & Sons, Inc.

---

control in hypertension, the nurse might use the term *high blood pressure* rather than hypertension to increase clarity for the learner. Thus skill must be developed in fitting the message to the learner. The box above offers do's and don'ts that may be helpful to the nurse in developing communication skills (Archer and Fleshman, 1979; Narrow, 1979).

Selecting the Learning Format

Simply stated, the learning format describes the way participants are organized for an educational activity. The variety of formats (or methods) available to the nurse is vast, and selection of the most effective method is at times difficult. To choose the best format the objectives of the teaching program should be kept firmly in mind, and the advantages and limitations of each method must be carefully weighed. Thoughtful consideration of available methods facilitates meeting program objectives, heightens learner interest, and encourages active participation.

Although formats or methods of learning can be divided into individual and group methods, the nurse practicing in the community is most often required to select learning formats appropriate for use with groups. Table 8-2 describes the most commonly used group formats and lists the potential advantages and disadvantages of each.

Table 8-2. Common formats used with groups

Format	Brief description	Materials required	Advantages	Limitations
Open forum	Public meeting in which participants are provided with opportunity to air their views; generally opens with introduction of subject by speaker, panel, or film, a moderator keeps discussion moving	Microphones	1. Allows audience participation 2. Stimulates thought 3. Raises questions 4. Identifies concerns	1. May delay reaching consensus by group 2. Success often rests on ability of moderator
Role playing	Acting out of situations to gain insight by placing oneself in another's position; usually done in front of group with time allotted at conclusion for discussion	None	1. Provides concreteness to learning situation 2. Encourages use of problem-solving skills 3. Requires learner participation	1. Group members may be too shy to participate 2. Intended content (or points) may or may not surface
Skits	Brief, rehearsed, dramatic presentation; usually requires script and more than one actor	Props according to script	1. May evoke emotional involvement 2. Stimulates discussion	1. May distract from intended message 2. Time is required for obtaining necessary props 3. Requires rehearsal time
Field trip or tour	Visit by group to object or place for first-hand observation and study	1. Adequate transportation 2. Advance arrangements	1. Entertains learner 2. Enables learner to view object or place in context of larger community 3. May motivate learners to seek additional learning experiences 4. Sharpens observational skills 5. Traveling time facilitates participant interaction	1. Time is required to make advance arrangements 2. Potential cost may inhibit participation 3. Amount of time required to make trip may not be feasible 4. Finding appropriate agency may be difficult 5. Schedules are difficult to maintain 6. Possibility of injury to participants is ever present
Interview	Presentation in which one or more individuals answer questions posed by one or more interviewers	1. Microphones 2. Seating arrangements so all learners can see and hear individual(s) being interviewed 3. Tape recorder if transcript is desired later	1. Provides common learning experience for all participants 2. Allows audience to hear differing points of view 3. May be used in eliciting audience involvement 4. Requires less preparation time than formal presentation	1. Requires skill on part of interviewer 2. Interviewer must possess knowledge of subject at hand
Lecture	Formal, oral presentation of subject	1. Seating arrangements so all learners can see and hear speaker 2. Podium and any audiovisual materials desired by speaker	1. May be organized easily 2. May be used with groups of any size	1. Requires speaking ability and expertise on subject 2. Audience is passive 3. Feedback is limited

Table 8-2. Common formats used with groups—cont'd

Format	Brief description	Materials required	Advantages	Limitations
Committee or task force	Small group organized to achieve goal that cannot be efficiently reached by larger group or individual	1. Chalkboard is often helpful for recording ideas or decisions 2. Seating arrangement that facilitates group interaction	1. Relieves members of larger group of tasks at hand 2. Permits variety of interests to be represented 3. Facilitates communication and decision making 4. Provides opportunity for leadership to group members	1. Members of committee may be unable to effectively work together 2. Committee members may not have necessary time to devote to group 3. Larger group may not support actions of committee
Discussion group	Group that meets to discuss predetermined topic; generally governs itself, and may meet as long and as often as is desired by members	Seating arrangement that permits face-to-face interaction of all participants	1. Permits participation of all members 2. Pools abilities and expertise toward reaching common goal	1. Time consuming 2. One member may dominate group 3. Extraneous discussions may divert group's efforts from task at hand
Demonstration	Presentation that shows in detail how to perform certain act or procedure	1. Materials necessary for demonstration 2. Area visible to all group members	1. Learners may be more likely to believe what they see as opposed to what is read or heard 2. Pace is flexible and permits instructor to repeat if necessary	1. Materials needed for demonstration may be expensive, limited, or difficult to transport 2. Number of participants is limited by space and materials available
Brainstorming	Participants "throw out" as many ideas as possible on given subject; ideas are recorded as they are given and are discussed later; all ideas are encouraged without giving thought to practicality of suggestion; requires a moderator	1. Seating arrangement to facilitate group process 2. Blackboard or newsprint on which ideas can be recorded in plain view of entire group	1. Allows participation by all members 2. Allows freedom of expression 3. Encourages creativity 4. May present solutions to previously unsolved problems	1. Suggested ideas may be impractical for implementation 2. Ideas may be criticized during following discussion period 3. Participants may be unable to develop novel approaches to identified problem
Buzz sessions	Large group is divided into several small groups to simultaneously meet for limited time and discuss assigned topic; each group should be small enough to facilitate discussion and may report back to large group at end of session	1. Movable chairs to facilitate formation of small groups 2. Pencils and paper in case notes are desired	1. Allows participation of each member 2. Encourages thought about assigned topic 3. Provides mechanism for generation of "fresh ideas"	1. Reports of small groups may be tedious or contradictory 2. Time may limit contributions each individual may make 3. May be time consuming to organize small groups 4. Small groups may not discuss assigned topic
Case study	Detailed account of one or more events that is presented to group of learners orally or in written form; discussion or written activity usually follows presentation of case study	1. Depends on whether case study is to be presented in written or oral form	1. Assists in developing problem-solving skills 2. Enables learner to consider alternative solutions 3. Presents many concepts on several levels in interesting fashion	1. Learner may not find case study relevant 2. Requires considerable time to prepare 3. Does not require all learners to participate in discussion 4. Requires skill in preparation

Setting the Learning Climate

Carefully planned programs quickly lose their effectiveness if the environment is not conducive to learning. The nurse may not have direct control over certain aspects of the learning environment, such as the condition and location of the building or the reputation of the agency. Fortunately, however, the nurse can take simple measures to manipulate the learning climate of the program.

The nurse can first start to set the learning climate for an educational endeavor when the announcement of the program is made. The tone and appearance of the letters, fliers, and media messages that announce the program draw a mental picture for participants of what the activity is apt to be like. By carefully considering the program objectives and information gained in the assessment phase about the culture, beliefs, and educational level of the learners, the nurse can develop preparatory materials appealing to the target population. When advance registration is required, the program announcement may include an activity to encourage participants to think about the subject matter before the program (Knowles, 1980). For example, a request could be made that participants in a stress management workshop complete a physical activity analysis before arrival. The tool could then be discussed in the workshop to provide continuity and feedback.

Creativity can improve the physical setting. For example, chairs can be moved from traditional rows into circles or semicircles to facilitate interaction, or they may be discarded and pillows, mattresses, or sofas used as substitutes. It helps to arrive early to arrange the seating, adjust the temperature, and organize audiovisual materials. Ashtrays, a coffeepot, and soft music often convey to learners that their comfort is important (Knowles, 1980).

The opening session of any educational activity affects the learning climate. Each participant should be greeted cordially and oriented to the objectives. Attention needs to be paid to unique learner characteristics. The degree of formality and privacy created in the learning environment should reflect the information gathered in the needs assessment.

Organizing Learning Experiences

Planning a teaching program requires that the nurse make decisions about the sequence of the learning activities, beginning with consideration of the traits of the learner rather than the nurse's interpretation of a logical organization of the material to be presented. Several principles for organizing learning experiences aid nurses in educational program planning.

First, *continuity* must be incorporated into the teaching plan. The concept of continuity involves placing repeated emphasis on particular components of the educational experience. For example, a community health nurse working with a group of obese people may wish to emphasize the concept of individual responsibility in weight control. Learning activities would then be planned to ensure that the concept was repeated or reinforced as the group progressed.

Second, *sequence* means that each learning experience builds on the previous one and requires a higher level of functioning. This principle is consistent with Bloom's taxonomy of learning domains. For example, when teaching exercises to a weight control group, the learning activities should be sequenced so that participants touch their toes after they touch their knees.

Finally, the concept of *integration* is helpful in organizing learning experiences. Integration of the various components of the teaching plan enables learners to discover how each aspect fits into the "big picture." Participants in a weight control class may find it helpful to understand how proper diet and exercise are related in controlling weight. Thus, basic principles of organization allow individualization of the "learning design model" (or plan for accomplishing the program objectives) to the learning situation (Knowles, 1980).

Participative Learning

Learning in either the psychomotor domain or at the application level demands that the instructor use action or participative learning as a teaching strategy. In participative learning, learners are responsible for acquiring and actualizing affective, cognitive, and behavioral changes that learning entails whereas the instructor provides the means for this process to take place (Tarnow, 1979). Thus when the objectives of a teaching program require that the learner be actively involved in the learning process, it is the leader's responsibility to structure the learning activities and teaching strategies accordingly. For example, learning the proper technique for injecting insulin requires that the learner have an opportunity to observe a demonstration, practice the procedure, and finally perform a return demonstration for the nurse. The learner's responsibilities can involve observing the demonstration (cognitive domain), practicing the skill (psychomotor domain), and returning the demonstration (psychomotor domain).

The nurse, on the other hand, is responsible for ensuring that proper teaching materials are available (such as alcohol, cotton, insulin, and syringes) and that the learner is provided with adequate information in the demonstration to repeat the procedure. By structuring the learning environment, the nurse is able to allow

Table 8-3. Suggested guidelines for selection of audiovisual materials for use with handicapped clients

Deficit	Suggested guidelines
Auditory	Use of visual and tactile techniques in teaching; films, demonstrations, printed materials, and slides enable learner to rely on senses other than hearing to receive messages
Visual	Use of auditory and tactile techniques in teaching; audiotapes, demonstrations with verbal explanations, and specially prepared printed materials, such as large type, boldface lettering, and generous spacing, assist in allowing client to learn in spite of physical handicap

learner participation, thereby making the learning "more real" than lectures, films, or reading materials (Tarnow, 1979).

Audiovisual Materials

The term *audiovisual materials* is defined in varying ways. Specifically the term is most often used to designate teaching materials, such as printed material, films, videotapes, television, radio, records, and audiotapes.

Advantages

Audiovisual materials allow educators to transcend barriers to learning, such as accessibility, limitations of the human body, and limitations of space and time. Such aids can transport the learner to places previously inaccessible, such as an operating room, research laboratory, or foreign city. Additionally, sights not visible to the naked eye or sounds inaudible to an unaided ear, such as the fertilization of an ovum or fetal heart tones, are available to learners through audiovisual technology. Special events and speakers can be brought to the learner through audiovisual means, thus transcending time and space boundaries. Instructional materials also provide the learner with the opportunity to slow down, move ahead, repeat, or even stop and examine a specific event or procedure to clearly understand the material.

Selection

When used properly, audiovisual materials can enhance and facilitate learning by creating interest, by motivating and stimulating learning and by using otherwise nonproductive time, such as in the waiting area of an outpatient clinic. Used inappropriately, however, they are expensive and may inhibit or interfere with learning by overloading the learner with stimuli, for example. Proper selection of audiovisual materials requires consideration of the characteristics of the learner, objectives to be achieved, and characteristics of the audiovisual materials.

Characteristics of the Learner. The audience must be considered when selecting educational media by determining possible physical handicaps, age, educational level, knowledge of the subject, and size of the group. An understanding of the role that vision, hearing, and to a lesser extent touch, taste, and smell play in the learner's ability to comprehend messages from the media enables appropriate selection of materials to enhance rather than inhibit learning. Any sensory deficit must be carefully considered when selecting educational media. For example, learners with poor vision require different audiovisual aids than those with hearing deficits.

In view of the increasing number of people over 65 years old, cognizance of sensory changes that occur with the aging process is necessary. An awareness of these changes enables nurses to adapt teaching strategies and media presentations to the target population. Table 8-3 demonstrates ways in which the community health nurse can select media appropriate to clients with physical handicaps.

An often overlooked aspect of any teaching endeavor is the amount of reading the learner is asked to do. Films, slides, pamphlets, videotapes, and filmstrips often require learners to read to obtain the full impact of the message. Unfortunately, many clients with whom community health nurses come into contact are unable to read the messages contained in the educational media. Although an individual's level of completed formal education is one guide to the level of reading comprehension, such an indicator may be misleading. For example, in a 1969 study conducted by Wingert et al. in the pediatric emergency room of the Los Angeles County Southern California Medical Center, it was shown that of 255 randomly selected mothers, 45% were unable to read beyond the sixth grade level. Of that 45%, 37% were high school graduates, and 27% had some college. In misjudging the reading ability of the learner, the nurse risks not only embarrassing the client but may also close the door to any future teaching. Thus the community health nurse must be constantly alert for client feedback, indicating an inability to comprehend the material presented.

When selecting educational media requiring reading for a group, the task becomes more complex. The educational level and the occupations of group members provide some estimations of the reading level the presentation should contain. If unfamiliar with group members, another excellent estimation of their reading level is the local newspaper. Learning at what reading level the local newspaper is written and which portion of the community subscribes to the paper, enables educators to determine with some degree of accuracy the level on which the program should proceed.

Several readability formulas are available for determining the difficulty of reading materials. Readability formulas are mechanical procedures, which through the use of vocabulary lists, count syllable length or average sentence length and provide an estimate of reading difficulty level.

Two well-known readability formulas are the Spache Readability formula and the Dale-Chall formula. Both of these formulas use lists of common words against which 100-word samples from the text are compared.

Each word in the sample is compared to the list to determine which of the sample words are on the list. Any word not found on the list is termed *unfamiliar*, and the percentage of those words is found and entered into a mathematical formula along with the average sentence length to calculate the grade level of the printed material. The Spache formula covers reading levels appropriate for grades 1 to 4, whereas the Dale-Chall formula deals with grades 4 through 16.

Another popular formula for determining the reading level of educational materials is that presented by Fry. This formula covers reading levels from grade 1 through college, and as Fig. 8-2 demonstrates, it involves plotting points on a graph. The Fry formula is simple to use and allows the nurse to select three 100-word passages from a teaching aid, such as a pamphlet, a film, or a slide presentation, and then taking the average sentence length and number of syllables per 100 words. These variables are then plotted on a graph to determine readability.

The readability of educational materials can be affected by the legibility of the printed words as well as by illustrations. The size of the type used, the shape of the letters, the amount of space between letters, and supple-

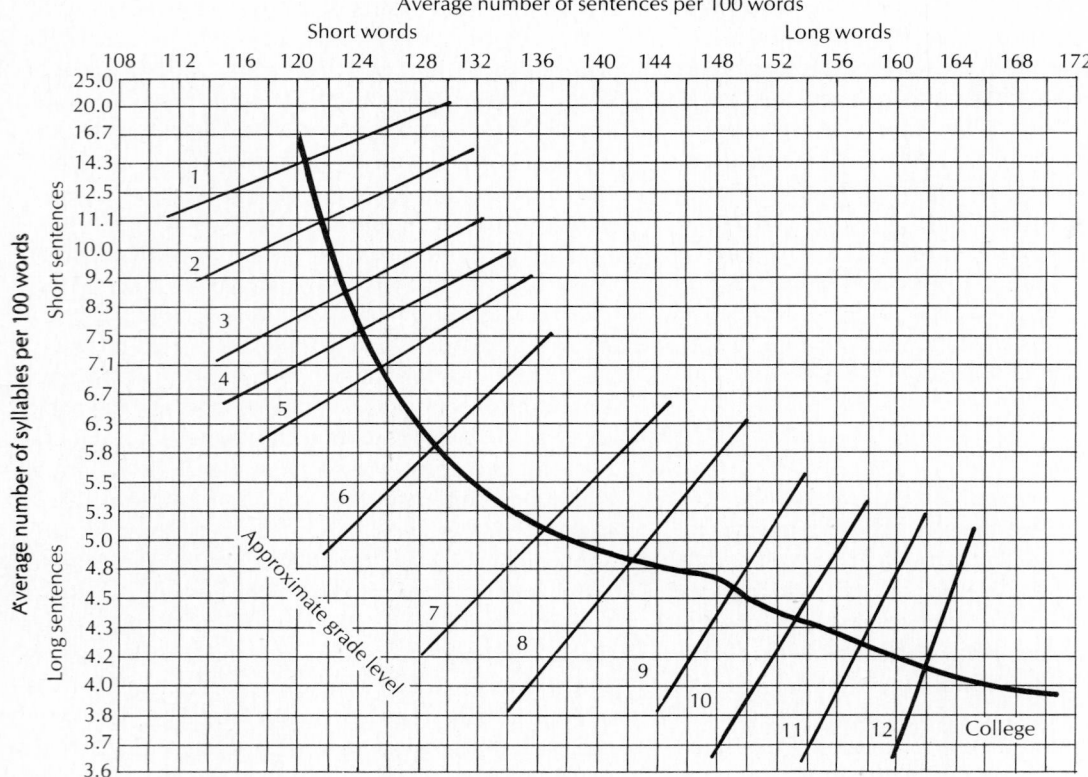

Fig. 8-2. Fry readability formula. (From Fry, E.: Elementary reading instruction. Copyright 1977. Used with the permission of McGraw-Hill Book Co., New York.)

mental illustrations can enhance the readability of printed materials.

Objectives to be Achieved. Earlier in this chapter, writing behavioral objectives is discussed. Well-written objectives are invaluable to the nurse when selecting audiovisual materials. Behavioral objectives specify the learning domain and relative complexity of behavior and therefore are an effective tool in selecting educational media.

Characteristics of Audiovisual Materials. Audiovisual materials are often selected on the basis of what the instructor is comfortable using or what is currently available rather than by considering the specific advantages and disadvantages of each material. Table 8-4 outlines the various audiovisual materials available and compares the advantages and limitations of each type.

Table 8-4. Advantages and limitations of selected audiovisual materials

Audiovisual material	Advantages	Limitations
Books and other printed material	1. May be used for individual instruction 2. Allow learner to proceed at individual pace 3. Require no special equipment or setting for use 4. May be used to supplement other media	1. Useful only with literate learners 2. Reading level of printed material must match that of learner 3. Not suitable for use with groups 4. Useful only when in language of learner
Chalkboard	1. May be used for audiences of up to 100 members 2. Requires no advance preparation 3. Enhances verbal communication 4. Is inexpensive 5. Is reusable	1. Learner cannot control pace of presentation 2. No way of preserving images
Photographic print series	1. Is inexpensive 2. Is widely available 3. Is easily manipulated 4. Permits close-up study 5. Allows learner to progress at individual pace 6. Requires no equipment for use 7. May be used for self-study	1. Black and white pictures may limit proper interpretation 2. Sizes and distances may be distorted 3. Difficult to use with large groups 4. Photographic skill and equipment required for preparation
Slide series	1. May alter sequence to meet specific needs 2. Can be easily revised 3. Is convenient to handle, store, and use 4. Is appropriate for individual or group instruction 5. Is easily prepared with 35 mm camera 6. May upgrade presentation over period of time by gradually replacing single slides 7. Provides sharp image to learner	1. Special equipment is required for preparation and projection 2. Slides may get out of sequence and be inappropriately projected
Filmstrips	1. Are in same sequence 2. Can be held on screen as long as desired 3. Handle easily; compact 4. May be used for individual or group instruction 5. Projected with simple equipment 6. Learner controls projection rate	1. Fixed sequence limits revision 2. Difficult to produce
Audiotapes	1. Can be used in individual or group instruction 2. Prepared and played back easily with simple, inexpensive equipment 3. Economical to duplicate 4. Can be used alone or in conjunction with video materials 5. Stored easily 6. Selected easily (reel-to-reel tapes)	1. Fixed rate for information giving 2. Possible to erase recording if tape is mishandled 3. May be difficult to locate specific portions of tape for playback purposes

Continued.

Table 8-4. Advantages and limitations of selected audiovisual materials — cont'd

Audiovisual material	Advantages	Limitations
Overhead transparencies	1. May be used in front of room, thus permitting eye contact between instructor and learner 2. Prepared easily and inexpensively 3. Operated and maintained easily 4. Are especially effective with large groups 5. Require limited planning; can be written on during presentation 6. May highlight, reinforce, or supplement verbal presentation 7. May be used in lighted or semidarkened room 8. Can be produced for minimal cost 9. Can be used repeatedly 10. Instructor can control speed of presentation 11. May be easily filed for future reference	1. Storage of equipment may be problematic 2. Equipment may block learner's view 3. Ordinary typewriters may produce images too small to be seen
Films or videotapes	1. May be used with individuals or groups 2. May be used in demonstrating motion or relationships 3. Ensure consistency of presentation 4. Enable learner to transcend limitations of time, space, and human body 5. Provide realism in terms of shapes and structures	1. Expensive to prepare, maintain, and purchase 2. Difficult to revise 3. Expense may limit accessibility and cause material to be dated 4. Subject to damage with each use 5. Projection equipment may be cumbersome or difficult to operate 6. Different sizes of reels require special projectors (i.e., 8 mm, 16 mm, etc.) 7. Difficult to keep updated

It is beyond the scope of this text to discuss methods of preparation of audiovisual materials. However, the nurse should be aware of the resources available in the agency and the community for production and loan of audiovisual materials. Whether the nurse develops, borrows, or purchases audiovisual aids, no presentation should begin until the material has been previewed, the equipment has been checked to ensure that it is in working order, and the nurse is familiar and comfortable with the use of the instructional medium.

In selecting audiovisual aids for a specific presentation, the following questions should be asked:
1. Is audio and/or visual necessary? If so, why?
2. Is color or motion necessary? How will it help the presentation?

Because of the cost and time involved, audiovisual materials should be used only when they are essential to convey a message.

Mass media (radio, television, and newspapers) is especially effective in community health. The same process is used in preparing information for dissemination through the mass media as for selecting media for individual presentations. Characteristics of the intended audience must be assessed, objectives written, and a vehicle for the message selected before teaching begins. The nurse must recognize that, "while the use of the media in community settings is no panacea . . . it can be effective in delivering new information, in setting agendas, and in producing simple behavior changes" (McAlister and Berger, 1979). Improper use of mass media, as with any audiovisual aid, may not only fail to communicate to the target audience the intended message, but may also deter any future participation in desired health-related activities.

RESOURCES FOR COMMUNITY HEALTH NURSING

Resources for planning and implementing educational programs include libraries, health departments, and chapters of national organizations (i. e., the Ameri-

```
┌─────────────────────────────────────┐
│ ▌▌▌▌  Community Resource Card        │
│                                      │
│     Date:                            │
│                                      │
│     Agency name:                     │
│     Address:                         │
│     Telephone:          Hours:       │
│     Contact person(s):               │
│     Materials available:             │
│                                      │
│                                      │
│                                      │
│     Cost:                            │
│     Comments:                        │
│                                      │
│                                      │
└─────────────────────────────────────┘
```

can Cancer Society and the American Heart Association). Such agencies have books and printed materials as well as films, filmstrips, and slide presentations that can be borrowed. It is essential that the community health nurse keep abreast of the audiovisual materials available for use and the means for obtaining them. This can be done by maintaining a file of index cards on which various community resources are indicated. On each card the name, address, and telephone number of a potential resource is recorded along with specific information regarding the types of materials available, potential costs, and persons to contact for the materials. At the top of this column is an example of such a resource card.

Keeping the file of community resources up dated saves many hours of searching for just the right resource. Each card enables the community health nurse to know at a glance if a particular agency has the desired materials at a cost that is within budgetary limitations. Many agencies maintain a mutual agreement that says essentially, "our materials are yours as long as we may have access to your selection of resources."

Some communities publish a community resource directory that would supplement the previously suggested card file. Such directories often provide information as to the purpose of an agency, the services offered, eligibility requirements, and referral procedures. Tools such as a resource card file and community resource directory provide nurses with handy overviews of resources that are available for assistance in planning educational programs.

BARRIERS TO IMPLEMENTING THE EDUCATIONAL ASPECT OF COMMUNITY HEALTH NURSING

Historically nurses in the community have played a large role in client education. Individual teaching was done by visiting nurses, and preventive measures were taught by nurses in a variety of settings. The educational aspect of nursing's role in the community has become widely accepted and is now an expected component of the nursing care plan.

Successful implementation of the educational aspect of community health nursing requires that the nurse be aware of and plan for potential barriers. Such barriers include lack of time, money, space, energy, confidence, organizational support, and equipment.

In planning a teaching program there is rarely enough time to adequately plan and implement the activities. The nurse must establish a schedule that allows flexibility yet ensures that deadlines are met. A good rule is to allow an extra 2 weeks in any schedule to accommodate unforeseen delays. Time management is essential to successful program planning.

Lack of money to implement a desired program is an obstacle that is constantly faced. Organizations, businesses, and industries in the community may grant funds for educational projects if benefits to them in terms of employee health can be demonstrated. The assessment phase of the educational process provides nurses with valuable information regarding individual learners' willingness and ability to pay for educational activities.

The amount and type of space available for teaching projects present another barrier to the nurse. Consideration must be given to the size of the group, or if individual instruction is to take place, the need for privacy should be taken into account. Problems with space limitations can be resolved through several means. Teaching strategies that consider the lack of space can be used. Room size may necessitate that programs are repeated to accommodate all interested learners. Nurses must become increasingly assertive in negotiating for space. The educational aspect of nursing's role is so inherent in the nursing process that to eliminate it because of space limitations is to shortchange the nursing profession and clients. Finally, nurses must become involved when possible in the planning of new facilities to meet the educational needs of the community.

Team management is essential to successful program planning. Likewise, most programs require considerable energy and the nurse must have sufficient personal energy to devote to the task without feeling overwhelmed by the magnitude of the program. Self-confidence is also required for a successful program. Community health nurses must believe they have a message to convey and the ability to provide information in a useful, interesting manner.

With the present push for cost-effectiveness, the nurse may encounter a lack of organizational support in implementing teaching projects. Many agencies are forced because of economic pressures to encourage staff members to see as many clients as possible within a fixed period of time. The educational component of care is often viewed as a nice extra that is to be included only if time permits. The nurse must devote careful attention in the assessment phase to demonstrating the need for educational endeavors. For example, if an industry were reluctant to grant employees time from work to participate in preventive or health-promotion activities, the nurse could gather information to demonstrate to management that such activities would be not only beneficial to the individual employees but would be cost-effective in terms of fewer days lost as a result of illness. The nurse could involve key people from each agency in the planning process. Such participation often helps to soften negative attitudes and promotes support of educational endeavors.

A final barrier nurses frequently encounter is the lack of necessary equipment for implementing programs. The nurse should be aware of organizations in the community willing to loan or donate the needed equipment. Grants are often available for the purchase or development of audiovisual materials, and the nurse should be familiar with application procedures. In any event, the planning phase of the teaching project must include taking into account the equipment available and developing teaching strategies accordingly.

Teaching and program effectiveness must be evaluated if an educational program is to succeed.

EVALUATION OF TEACHING EFFECTIVENESS

Never take for granted that because an individual has attended an educational program, learning has taken place! All too often nurses and other health professionals assume that because the information has been transmitted to the learner, all program objectives have been met. Unfortunately, this is not generally the case. Evaluative and feedback mechanisms are necessary throughout the teaching-learning process to ensure final attainment of the program objectives.

Ongoing feedback and evaluation are valuable to the learner and teacher alike. For the learner feedback reinforces desired behaviors and allows for the correction of misinformation. Feedback to the instructor allows for modifications in the teaching process so that the learner can be assisted in meeting the program objectives. Because feedback is most effective when it is immediate, it can be considered a learning tool for both the instructor and the learner (Tarnow, 1979).

Evaluation of the teaching process occurs continuously to assist in redirecting teacher and learner activities. The instructor may receive feedback from the learner (as to teaching effectiveness) in written form, such as a test or evaluation sheet; verbally in the form of questions asked or responded to; or nonverbally as in return demonstrations and expressions on the faces of the learners. If evaluation is done as teaching is in progress, the nurse will be able to predict with a large degree of accuracy the extent to which the program objectives will be met and the time required for their attainment. By waiting until the end of the teaching session to obtain feedback, the nurse may miss opportunities to correct misinformation, dispel confusion, or alter the instructor to enhance learning. Redman (1980) suggests that it is unwise to teach for a long period of time without requiring learners to respond so errors can be corrected.

If for some reason evaluation reveals that the desired learning objectives have not been met, the nurse must consider several questions to try to determine the basis for the ineffectiveness of the teaching. How familiar and comfortable was the instructor with the subject matter? Often the learner may perceive the instructor as not understanding the subject, which in turn may leave the learner hopelessly confused. The client may think that the nurse could not understand this, how could he?

The nurse must next ask "how motivated was the learner?" Factors that influence learner readiness and motivation have already been discussed in this chapter and must be reassessed if teaching seems to be ineffective. Finally the nurse must ask if the desired behavior change is really necessary. Such a question inevitably leads back to the original learning objectives and encourages the nurse to rethink the practicality and merit of each of the unattained objectives (Redman, 1980).

EVALUATION OF PROGRAM EFFECTIVENESS

Before a nurse or other educator can determine the extent to which teaching programs are evaluated, the individual must determine the view of the educational process. For example, if making changes in a human being is viewed as the major responsibility, the evaluation would be concerned with the measurement of behavioral changes within a specified time frame. On the other hand, if the facilitating of self-development of the learner is viewed as the major responsibility, the focus of the evaluation would be on the involvement of the learner.

It is helpful for the nurse to become familiar with the purpose of program evaluation before attempting to judge the effectiveness of a teaching endeavor. Knowles (1980) identifies two main purposes of program evaluation: (1) to improve the organization of the operation, which includes such aspects as the physical facility, personnel, planning process, and decision-making process, and (2) to improve the actual program, which involves the objectives, teaching strategies, and materials. Both purposes serve to stimulate the learner and promote growth and improvement.

Once the purpose and focus of the program evaluation are determined, the evaluation process follows in a series of several simple steps. First, the questions to be answered must be developed and if possible pretested. Then data must be collected to answer the questions, and third, the data must be analyzed. Finally, the teaching program must be modified as a result of the findings of the evaluation. The preceding steps require that decisions are made repeatedly in regard to when the evaluation should take place and who should participate in the process.

The importance of ongoing evaluation to the learner and the nurse is discussed previously in this chapter. The nonverbal cues and unsolicited complaints or compliments often result in spontaneous changes or improvements in the teaching program. Though such informal evaluation is important, it does not take the place of systematic, preplanned evaluations. By building in an evaluation mechanism at the end of predesignated program units, the nurse is able to determine the overall morale and satisfaction of the learners as well as suggestions for improvements in the program. In addition, a continuous evaluation process aids in detecting trouble spots before a crisis occurs (Knowles, 1980).

The frequency of evaluation depends on the subject matter, the amount of time available, the amount of material to be presented, and the nature of the learners. For example, a nurse wishing to assess the effectiveness of teaching insulin injection skills may include different evaluative "check points" in the teaching plan than would a nurse attempting to teach the physiology of human reproduction. Whatever form of evaluation is used, the nurse is responsible for communicating to the learner in advance how and when evaluation is to take place (Narrow, 1979). Many times the nurse chooses not to use the word *evaluation* when talking to clients but instead may say something like, "I'll demonstrate a breathing exercise, and then you can show me how to do it."

Who Should Do the Evaluation?

Every person in a position to make a judgment regarding a program should be included in the evaluation process. The learners and instructors; the program director and management personnel, outside experts, and

Table 8-5. Advantages and disadvantages of common data collection methods

Method	Advantages	Disadvantages
Direct observation of behavior	1. Product and process of learned behavior can be observed	1. Time consuming 2. Does not evaluate cognitive skills underlying psychomotor acts
Interview	1. May be formal or informal, structured or unstructured 2. Data obtained from structured interview may be uniform and easy to analyze 3. Allows for full range of views	1. Time consuming 2. Unstructured may be difficult to analyze 3. May have interviewer bias in results
Questionnaires	1. Obtain reliable information from specific questions 2. Avoid interviewer bias	1. May be misinterpreted by respondent 2. May interfere with activity 3. Time consuming 4. Answers may be misinterpreted by evaluator
Standardized tests	1. Provide an opportunity to compare data from one group with national norms	1. May remind adult learner of childhood schooling 2. Group may not be representative of national norm
Tailor-made tests	1. Produce data about changes for which tests were designed 2. May demonstrate student progress	1. May lack validity and reliability

community representatives provide unique observations, perceptions, and suggestions about the program. The nurse seeking to determine the adequacy of a program for a given community would do well to collect data from as many sources as possible and to include the evaluators in the process of analyzing the data and modifying the program accordingly.

Evaluative Questions

As has already been pointed out, the first step in the evaluation process is to develop questions. The nurse can develop questions to be answered in the evaluation process from the program objectives. For example, an objective of a teaching program may be to provide a physical environment conducive to adult learning. Such an objective lends itself to the formation of such questions as the following: Is the room large enough for the group? Does the room have adequate ventilation and lighting? Can the chairs be rearranged to facilitate group process? These and similar questions provide the nurse with a starting point from which to determine how well program objectives are attained.

Methods of Data Collection

There are a variety of data collection methods available to the nurse, and the specific method used is determined by the objectives of the program being evaluated, the variables to be measured, and the time and cost involved (Shortell and Richardson, 1978). The most common methods of data collection have been summarized in Table 8-5 along with some identified advantages and disadvantages of each. Because each method is subject to error and bias, an ongoing evaluation program requires a combination of methods.

Whichever method of evaluation the nurse chooses to use to determine teaching and program effectiveness, a helpful concept to keep in mind is that of the curve of normal distribution (Fig. 8-3). In any group of learners about 2% will be extremely negative, and 2% will be extremely positive in their evaluation of the program. Another 14% will be fairly negative with 14% quite enthusiastic. The majority of participants (68%) will be somewhat neutral in their responses (Knowles, 1980).

Therefore even though the nurse should consider the extremely negative responses, alarm or discouragement should not appear until the proportion of extremely negative criticism goes above 16%.

SUMMARY

This chapter has described several components of the educational aspects of the community health nursing role. Since the major aim of community health nursing is directed toward health promotion and disease prevention, the value of educational strategies is inherent. To provide effective educational offerings to students, clients, and colleagues, it is imperative for community health nurses to understand the nature of learning. Not all learning experiences require that participants be able to synthesize the information provided. In a number of instances it is appropriate for learners to comprehend or apply information without being accountable for higher levels of cognition. Learning also has cognitive, affective, and psychomotor components. It is insufficient to simply give clinic clients a sheet of diet instructions without paying some attention to their ability to cognitively understand the material and affectively accept the implications of the instructions.

Planning effective health education programs necessitates drawing on theories of learning. People learn in different ways, and there are varying beliefs about how learning occurs. In some situations the most effective mode for health education follows SR tenets. Other learners and educators are more comfortable with cognitive-discovery, Gestalt, or humanistic views of learning, or some combination thereof.

Effective health education programming takes into account a variety of principles of teaching and learning. The majority of clients seen by community health nurses are adults; hence special characteristics of adult learners have been noted as have other learner qualities such as self-concept, experience, readiness to learn, assumptions about learning and teaching, motivation, and individual differences.

Assessment of learner needs and interests followed

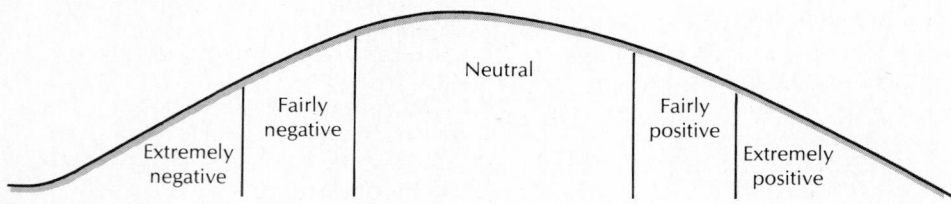

Fig. 8-3. Curve of normal distribution.

the section on principles of teaching and learning. Without a careful assessment, how can educators plan? Historically educators have often tended to develop splendid programs albeit of no interest to learners. Whose time is wasted? To develop educational programs suited to learner needs and wants, a thorough assessment is required. What do learners want or need? How can these needs and desires be most efficiently and effectively met? Who, when, where, and how can an effective program be developed? These questions are answered through careful assessment, planning (including development of purposes and objectives), implementation, and evaluation.

A primary tool of health education is effective teaching. This ability is not inborn. Some people do seem to have a flair for holding the attention of audiences; all people can learn the skills of effective teaching. Many strategies are available to arouse the interest of participants; the careful program planner matches the teaching method to the resources available, the information being presented, and the needs and abilities of the learners. Creativity is an ingredient of health education, which sparks the attention of participants and livens the format of most programs.

In planning health education programs it is necessary to determine whether individual or group strategies will be used. As budgets are cut, emphasis on education often drops noticeably. Thus group approaches are emphasized, since they tend to be less expensive than individual counseling. The value of group education need not be discounted just because it is less costly than other methods.

Any health education offering should ensure clear communication so that learners accurately grasp the message being conveyed. A variety of do's and don'ts for communication were given. For example, educators should know their material before they attempt to teach it. The learning format should be appropriately selected to meet the needs of participants and to be consistent with educator preferences and resources available. The learning climate is also an important consideration. People learn more effectively when their attention is not diverted by being cold, cramped, and unable to hear or see the speaker. Attention to small comfort details yields big dividends in learner satisfaction with programs.

Additionally, learning experiences cannot be simply "thrown together" to be maximally effective. Audiovisual aids must add to and not detract from the learning experience which can be enhanced by appropriate films, videotapes, or other materials, but each must be selected with the program objectives in mind.

Finally evaluation methods must be incorporated into the learning process. Without evaluation the nurse has no means by which to judge the effectiveness of the teaching. In addition, evaluation assists the learner in determining the extend to which program objectives have been met by the teacher and the learner. In short, the educational aspect of the community health nursing role has several components. Each is a vital part in ensuring that every educational endeavor produces maximal learning.

BIBLIOGRAPHY

Adcock, M., et al.: Community health education: the development of effective program strategies. In Lazes, P., editor: The handbook of health education, Germantown, Md., 1979, Aspen Systems Corp., pp. 17-35.

Archer, S., and Fleshman, R.: Community health nursing: patterns and practice, ed. 2, North Scituate, Mass., 1979, Duxbury Press.

Barrett, N., and Schwartz, M.D.: What patients really want to know, Am. J. of Nurs. **81**:1642, 1981.

Bavaro, J.A.: Questioning: the key to learning, Superv. Nurse **11**(6):26-28, 1980.

Biehler, R.F.: Psychology applied to teaching, ed. 3, Boston, 1978, Houghton Mifflin Co.

Bloom, B.: Taxonomy of educational objectives: handbook 1: cognition domain, New York, 1969, David McKay Co., Inc.

Carpenter, W.L.: Twenty-four group methods and techniques in adult education, Unpublished, Florida State University, Tallahassee, 1967.

Cassidy, S.: The ins and outs of presenting a program, Superv. Nurse **11**(4):66-67, 1980.

Combs, A.: The professional education of teachers, Boston, 1965, Allyn Bacon Inc.

Cooper, S.S.: Methods of teaching—revisited. Field trips and study tours. Part II, J. Contin. Educ. Nurs. **11**(3-4):50, 1980.

Cooper, S.S.: Methods of teaching—revisited. The incident process. J. Contin. Educ. Nurs. **11**(3):56, 1980.

Cooper, S.S.: Methods of teaching—revisited. Role playing. Part 10, J. Contin. Educ. Nurs. **11**(1):36, 1980.

Cooper, S.S.: Methods of teaching-revisited. Films and videotapes, J. Contin. Educ. Nurs. **12**(1):34-37, 1981.

Cooper, S.S.: Methods of teaching—revisited. The incident process, J. Contin. Educ. Nurs. **12**(6):22-24, 1981.

Cooper, S.S.: Methods of teaching—revisited. The interview. J. Contin. Educ. Nurs. **12**(4):34-36, 1981.

Cooper, S.S.: Methods of teaching—revisited. Open forum: buzz session, J. Contin. Educ. Nurs. **13**(1):38-40, 1982.

Evans, L.K.: Health education from a group perspective, Top. Clin. Nurs. **2**(2):45-55, 1980.

Frantz, R.A.: Selecting media for patient education, Top. Clin. Nurs. **2**(2):77-83, 1980.

Fry, E.: Elementary reading instruction, New York, 1977, McGraw-Hill Book Co.

Gerlach, V.S., and Ely, D.P.: Teaching and media: a systematic approach, ed. 2, Englewood Cliffs, N.J., 1980, Prentice-Hall, Inc.

Havighurst, R.J.: Developmental tasks and education, New York, 1961, David McKay Co., Inc.

Hergenhahn, B.R.: An introduction to theories of learning, ed. 2, Englewood Cliffs, N.J., 1982, Prentice-Hall Inc.

Hochbaum, G.M.: Patient counseling vs. patient teaching, Top. Clin. Nurs. **2**(2):1-7, 1980.

Kemp, J.E.: Planning and producing audiovisual materials, ed. 3, New York, 1975, Thomas and Crowell Co., Inc.

Knowles, M.S.: The modern practice of adult education: andragogy versus pedagogy, ed. 2, Chicago, 1980, Follett Publishing Co.

Knox, A.B.: Adult development and learning: a handbook on individual growth and competence in the adult years for education and the helping profession, San Francisco, 1977, Jossey-Bass Inc., Publishers.

Krathwohl, D.R., Bloom, B.A., and Masia, B.B.: Taxonomy of educational objectives: handbook 2: affective domain, New York, 1971, David McKay Co., Inc.

Krawczyk, R.M.: Well persons: their importance to nursing education and practice, Nurs. Forum **18**(3):220-230, 1979.

Lewin, K.: Field theory in social science, New York, 1951, Harper & Row Publishers.

Mager, R.F.: Preparing instructional objectives, ed. 2, Belmont, Calif., 1975, Pitman Learning Inc.

Maslow, A.: Toward a psychology of being, ed. 2, New York, 1968, Van Nostrand Reinhold Co., Inc.

McAlister, A., and Berger, E.: Media for community health promotion. In Lazes, P., editor: The handbook of health education, Germantown, Md., 1979, Aspen Systems Corp., pp. 163-173.

Murray, R., and Zentner, J.: Nursing concepts for health promotion, Englewood Cliffs, N.J., 1975, Prentice-Hall, Inc.

Narrow, B.W.: Patient teaching in nursing practice, New York, 1979, John Wiley & Sons, Inc.

Piaget, J.: the language and thought of the child, London, 1952, Routledge & Kegan Paul of America Ltd.

Piaget, J.: Psychology of intelligence, Totowa, N.J., 1966, Littlefield, Adams & Co.

Pohl, M.: The teaching function of the nurse practitioner, Dubuque, Iowa, 1973, Wm. C. Brown Group.

Redman, B.K.: The process of patient teaching in nusring, St. Louis, 1980, The C.V. Mosby Co.

Roberts, F.B.: A model for parent education, Images **13**:86-89, Oct. 1981.

Rogers, C.: Freedom to learn, Columbus, Ohio, 1969, Charles E. Merrill Publishing Co.

Rosendahl, P.: Self-direction for learners, Nurs. Forum. **13**(2):136-146, 1974.

Schultheis, J.G., and de Wolfe, Z.: From academia to practice—realities of delivering nursing education in a medical center, J. Contin. Educ. Nurs. **13**(1):21-23, 1983.

Shortell, S., and Richardson, W.: Health program evaluation, St. Louis, 1978, The C.V. Mosby Co.

Shropshire, C.O.: Group experiential learning in adult education, J. Contin. Educ. Nurs. **12**(6):5-9, 1981.

Spradley, B.W.: Community health nursing: concepts and practices, Boston, 1981, Little, Brown & Co.

Starpoli, C. and Waltz, C.: Developing and evaluating educational programs for health care providers, Philadelphia, 1978, F.A. Davis Co.

Stevens, B.J.: The teaching-learning process, Nurse Educ. **1**:9-20, May-June, 1976.

Sullivan, H.S.: The interpersonal theory of psychiatry, New York, 1953, W. W. Norton and Co., Inc.

Tarnow, K.G.: Working with adult learners, Nurse Educ. **4**:34-40, Sept.-Oct., 1979.

Watson, J.B., and Rayner, R.: Conditioned emotional reactions, J. Exp. Psychol. **3**:1-14, 1920.

Wingert, W.A., and Grubbs, J.P., and Friedman, D.B.: Why Johnny's parents don't read, Clin. Pediatr. **8**(11):655-660, 1969.

Wise, P.: Adult teaching strategies, J. Contin. Educ. Nurs. **11**(6):15-17, 1980.

Wise, P.: Methods of teaching—revisited. Character play and role play, J. Contin. Educ. Nurs. **11**(1):37-38, 1980.

Chapter 9

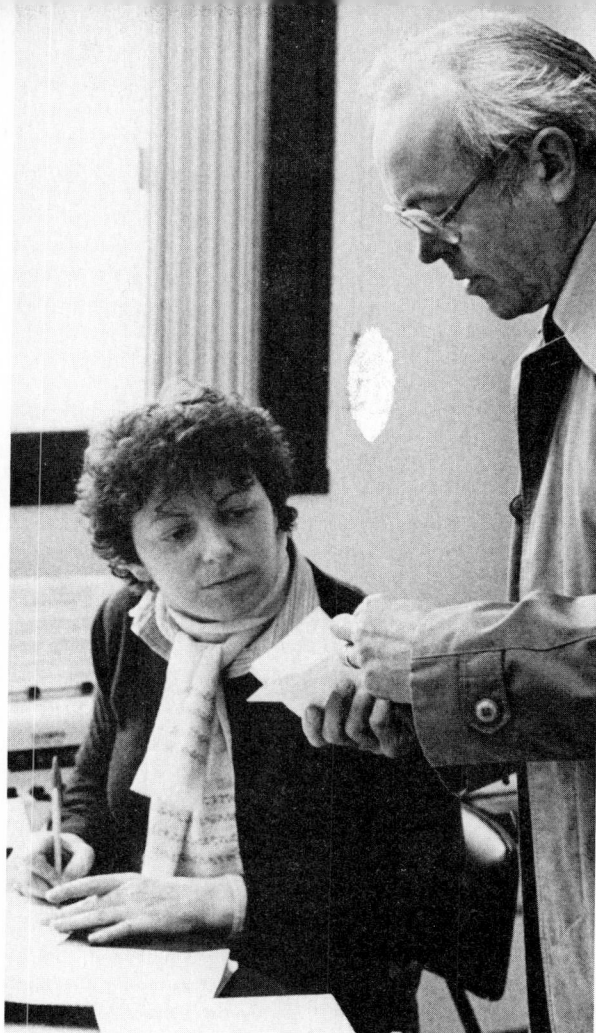

MARCIA STANHOPE
GWENDOLEN LEE

PROGRAM PLANNING AND EVALUATION IN COMMUNITY HEALTH

Many of the authors of chapters in this text have referred to the importance of *planning* before *implementing* nursing activities for clients in homes, clinics, groups, and communities. These same authors have talked about the need for the nurse to *evaluate* activities engaged in on behalf of clients. To do this, say the authors, one must have measurable objectives that evolve from the *assessment* of the needs of the client population. In other words, all community health nurses should be applying the total nursing process to all activities in which community health clients participate.

One may ask, Why is there so much emphasis on planning and evaluation in nursing today? Do nurses constantly need to be reminded that these activities are essential to the delivery of nursing care? Do not all nurses engage in these activities as an integral part of their day-to-day practice?

Planning and evaluation are essential elements of a quality assurance program for the health care system and the nursing subsystem. As economic resources become scarce, nursing and the health care system must be able to justify their purposes for existence, show the responsiveness of their services to consumer needs, and show their concern for professional accountability.

Previous history indicates that with seemingly unlimited resources, health care services and nursing services developed in a primarily unplanned manner in reaction to perceived crises or needs. Nurses continue to be told that they "react instead of act," implying that perceived crises or needs continue to be the basis for nursing care delivery instead of "planning to act" based on assessed needs for nursing care delivery.

This chapter will focus attention on how nurses can "act" instead of "react" by planning programs that can be evaluated for their effectiveness and efficacy in meeting their social purpose. This discussion will focus on the historical development of health planning and evaluation, program planning and evaluation models, the benefits of planning and evaluation, and the elements of planning and evaluation.

PROGRAM PLANNING

Definitions and Goals

A *program* is defined as a set of activities occurring within the health care system, which have specific inputs, with organization and processes for establishing relationships among the inputs and output that can be evaluated against standards (Schulbert and Baker, 1979). Programs are designed to meet the assessed needs of individuals, families, groups, or communities. Examples of specific programs in community health nursing are home health programs for individuals and families in the home setting, immunization programs for children in the school, health risk screening programs for workers in industry and family planning clinic programs. These specific programs are usually conducted under the aegis of the total program plan of the local health department. Broader-based group and community programs are the community school health program, the occupational health and safety program, the environmental health program, and community programs directed at specific illness entities and special interest groups such as the American Heart Association programs, the American Cancer Society programs, and the March of Dimes.

Planning is defined by Rakich et al. (1977, p. 92) as "anticipating and making decisions about the future." Bice (1980, p. 326) calls *planning* "a symbolic process" leading to alternative means and ends, and the choices among them. The Institute for Health Planning (1981, p. 2) defines *planning* as "a conscious design of a desired future state . . . " which includes a description of selection of alternative means to achieve and the activities necessary to attain the future state. The *goal* of health planning is rational, effective, and efficient functioning of health care organizations (Rakich, 1977).

Evaluation is defined as the process of determining the value or amount of success in achieving predetermined (planned) objectives (American Public Health Association, 1960); as applied research whose major objective is determining the effectiveness of the application of knowledge (Hyman, 1962); and as the "followup" of results of the effectiveness of a program. *Program evaluation* is defined as "a collection of methods, skills and sensitivities necessary to determine whether a human service is needed and likely to be used, whether it is conducted as planned and whether the human service actually does help people" (Posavac and Carey, 1980, p. 6). Determination of *effectiveness* lies in the fulfillment of program objectives. The major *goal* of program evaluation is to provide support for the legitimacy and effectiveness of the program to justify society's continued support (Suchman, 1967).

Historical Overview of Health Care Planning and Evaluation

Historically society, primarily through government, has financed health program planning and evaluation. As the health care delivery system has grown in the past 60 years, emphasis in health planning and exploration has increased. Factors that have fostered increased interest in planning and evaluation are advances in health care technology, consumer education and increased health care expectations, third-party payers, unionization of health care workers, urbanization, increased health risks, manpower shortages, and increasing health care costs (McCarthy, 1977; McCarthy and Jonas, 1981).

In the 1920s the American Public Health Association's Committees on Administrative Practice and Evaluation emphasized the need for public health officers to engage in better program planning to change the "topsy-turvy" method by which public health programs were begun (Hanlon and Pickert, 1979). During this same period the Committee on the Costs of Medical Care was established to study the economic and social aspects of health services. The committee recognized the need for comprehensive health care planning, citing the rising costs and the inequitable distribution of health services across the nation (Anderson, 1966; Committee on Costs of Medical Care, 1970).

As a result of the committee report, a few states began to attempt to coordinate medical services for area residents. However, regionalized planning for health services nationwide was not attempted until the American Hospital Association established its Committee on Postwar Planning in 1944. From this committee's efforts came the establishment of a commission on hospital care charged to work closely with each state's designated official health planning agency to coordinate the regionalization of hospital services, equipment, and personnel (Commission on Hospital Care, 1947).

The post–World War II era also brought an interest in evaluating program effectiveness. As government and third party payers began to finance health care services and money became more plentiful, public demand for health services grew. As demand grew, numbers and kinds of health agencies increased, legislation was passed to increase the scope and control over health care, and the health care delivery system was beginning to be held accountable for its actions (Hanlon and Pickett, 1979).

The federal government's first attempt to legislate health planning was the passage of the Hospital Survey and Construction Act in 1946 (Hill-Burton Act). This act was passed to improve the hospital bed-to-population ratio in rural areas and to upgrade facilities and hospital standards. States were authorized to survey their needs and develop state plans for hospital facilities and to adopt minimum standards to be met in hospitals for state licensure. The federal government would then provide matching funds to construct and equip public and voluntary nonprofit hospitals (Public Law 79-725, 1946). Amendments to the Hill-Burton Act in 1956 appropriated additional monies to the Public Health Service for research and demonstration projects for the development, utilization, and coordination of hospital services, facilities, and resources.

From 1949 through the 1970s the Hill-Burton Act was continually amended to expand the scope of the legislation to include grants and loans to improve geographic bed distribution; to construct, modernize, and replace health care facilities; and to develop comprehensive plans for health and facilities regionally and locally.

The 1960s were marked by the Great Society programs of President Johnson. The social, economic, and health programs that grew out of the Great Society concept were designed primarily to meet the needs of the U.S. population and to show that the federal government could be efficient in delivering services to the population at large. During this time the Office of Health Planning was established in DHEW, and research abounded in the areas of cost benefit, program planning, and evaluation. Because the scope and functioning of the Office of Health Planning was limited and had no direct line authority for national health planning, the 89th Congress, in an attempt to develop a national health planning system, passed the Comprehensive Health Planning (CHP) and Public Health Services Amendments in 1966 (Public Law 89-749). Approval for project monies from the Hill-Burton program were tied into this first major U.S. health planning legislation (McCarthy, 1977; McCarthy and Jonas, 1981).

The CHP legislation was intended to establish comprehensive planning for each state and for designated regions within the state. The law provided formula grants to a single official state agency for state health planning; project grants to develop comprehensive health plans for coordinating facilities, manpower and services at the regional level; project grants to train health planners and to develop health services; and formula grants to provide public health services. The law provided for the establishing of two types of agencies within each state. The "A" agencies were the state level health planning agencies charged with the responsibility of developing a statewide plan from the needs data provided by the "B" agencies, which were the local or regional agencies.

Although all of the United States and its territories eventually developed A and B agencies, there were many problems with the CHP amendments of 1966. The legislation did not provide monies to support the administrative functioning of the agencies, and the agencies had to get budgetary monies from local support. The agencies were not given legal power to enforce their decisions about the health needs within the states, and hospitals and other health care facilities were free to build new facilities or expand services without the approval of the health planning agencies. Although the law required 51% consumer membership on the CHP boards, poor training of staff, volunteers, and the consumers led to less than adequate input from these persons into the planning process. Poor orientation of board members resulted in continued provider control over the health plans.

Many other problems existed with this first piece of comprehensive health legislation. The law exempted "private professional practice of medicine, dentistry and related healing arts" as well as the principal of the federal government, such as veterans' hospitals, from the health planning system. The actual responsibilities of the CHP agencies related to Hill-Burton programs and to the regional medical programs (see Chapter 3) were unclear, and although the agencies were asked to "review and comment" on projects submitted for funding under 13 different federal programs, their authority to reject a project was nonexistent. In other words, the Comprehensive Health Planning Amendments of 1966 were less than comprehensive.

The CHP amendments did, however, provide a basis for the development of future planning legislation. From the CHP experience the states and federal government developed a functional method for organizing planning agencies. Data on existing needs and resources were collected, procedures for reviewing facilities and program changes were established, and methods for interorganizational cooperation were developed.

Before the passage of PL 89-749 (1966) several states were working on the development of a new concept called *certificate-of-need*. This concept was to be utilized as a tool for approving new facilities and programs under PL 89-749 and under future health planning legislation. The certificate-of-need program began in New York in 1964 as a regulatory mechanism that set forth criteria outlining public need for health care facilities and programs. Under the certificate-of-need concept, facilities and programs were reviewed, approved, or disapproved and for many years state licensure of new and existing agencies was predicated on the state certificate-of-need review (Curren, 1974; Dorsey, 1973; Havighurst, 1974).

Although PL 89-749 proved to be an inadequate law for comprehensive health planning, the strengths of the planning legislation led Congress to pass a new law in 1974, the National Health Planning and Resources Development Act (PL 93-641). The new law will be cited historically for the specificity of the legislation relative to the structure, process, and functions of a national health planning system. Usually Congress writes legislation that is broad in scope, leaving the writing of specific regulations to the regulatory agencies such as DHHS. Perhaps because of the problems with past health planning legislation, Congress saw a need to provide some regulations within the body of this new legislation.

PL 93-641 established a national health planning structure that required state governors to designate health services areas to be approved by the secretary of DHHS to include a population of 250,000 to 3,000,000. The health services areas were to be the major planning bodies of the national system, and each area was to have a Health Systems Agency (HSA) accountable to the secretary for establishing a local health plan and for adhering to the national health priorities and standards.

Throughout the United States there were to be 200 HSAs. A state health planning and development agency and a state health coordinating council were to be established in each state, and there was to be a National Council on Health Planning and Development to advise the secretary of DHHS and to adopt national standards for health services. By 1978, all agencies of the national system had been established and were functional except for the statewide health coordinating councils.

PL 93-641 stipulated that each HSA was to develop a health systems plan for its health services area and an annual implementation plan. The plans were to be submitted to the Statewide Health Coordinating Council (SHCC), composed of representatives from each HSA, who would review (and coordinate) all of the states' HSA plans to reflect one state health plan. The councils also had the responsibility of reviewing and commenting on HSA budgets and state applications for federal health funds.

The governors, with the approval of the secretary of health, were to designate a State Health Planning and Development Agency (SHPDA) to be aided by the SHCC in developing the state health plan, to plan the state government's role in the health plan, to review institutional services in the state, and to operate the certificate-of-need program. The 1978 Health Planning Amendments called for the approval of the state health plan by the governor before the plan was submitted to the secretary of health for approval. Fig. 9-1 shows the organizational structure for PL 93-641.

The new health planning legislation provided a federal funding mechanism for establishing the system structure using a per capita and matching fund formula; abolished the Hill-Burton program and the regional medical programs, described in Chapter 3, incorporating some of their goals into the new structure; and provided the states with approval authority over project applications for federal funds except for federal monies used to pay for direct medical services received and supported by Medicare and Medicaid.

Although Pl 93-641 provided a more comprehensive structure and more power over federal program funds than the Partnership for Health Program of 1966 (CHP), the HSAs had limited authority to carry out some of the more critical tasks of improving the health of residents, increasing accessibility and quality of services, restraining costs, and preventing unnecessary duplication of services. Power over the private health care sector continued to be limited.

As "New Federalism" became the catch phrase of the 80s and emphasis was placed on cost shifting, cost reduction, and more competition in the health care system, President Reagan proposed the abolition of the federal government's role in health planning. In 1981, with cutbacks in federal funding, states were beginning to plan for the takeover of the HSAs and were establishing their own health systems or they were dismantling their health systems as established under PL 93-641 (Institute for Health Planning, 1981). The future of a continuing macrolevel federal and state cooperative partnership for health planning became questionable in the early 80s.

From the beginning of the federal government's involvement in national health planning, the structure emphasized external planning and evaluation. Confusion about the authority for internal agency program planning and evaluation was paramount. However, Hanlon and Pickett (1979) emphasize the responsibility of community health personnel to participate in internal planning and evaluation once they are given the charge to resolve the problems of a client population. This chapter will focus on methods that the community

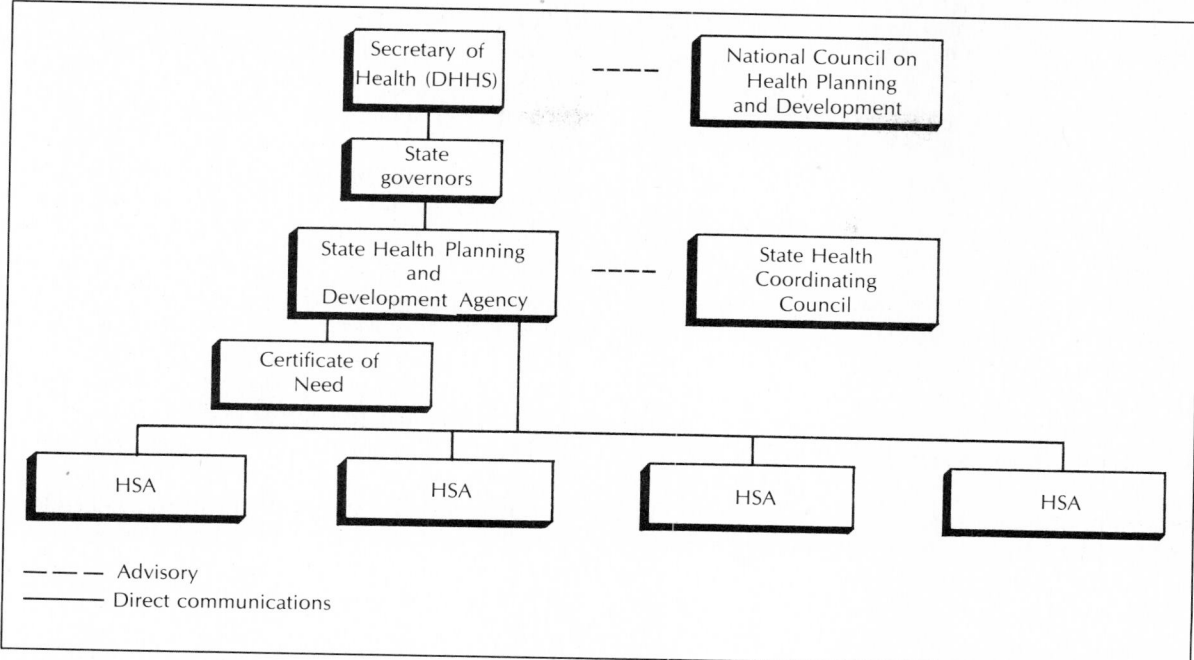

Fig. 9-1. Organizational structure for health planning in the United States, 1974-1982..

health nurse may use to initiate or to participate in internal microlevel program planning and evaluation.

Elements of Planning

Health planning is described as a continuous social process by which data about a client(s) are collected and evaluated for the purpose of creating "a plan." Such planning serves the purposes of generating new ideas, meeting identified client needs, solving health problems, and guiding change in health care delivery (Ruybal, 1978).

Health program planning is affected by governmental control over licensure and funding, by the social structure, and by the cultural and belief system in which the program must function. Program planning is essential to meet federal, state, and local government planning mandates for funding, philanthropic organizations' funding guidelines, and internal organizational planning requirements. Program planning is equally essential for the health care organizations' rational, effective, and efficient functioning.

There are times when programs are developed and implemented because of an interest of a health provider, because federal or philanthropic funds are made available to establish specific programs, or because health providers have identified a program need for a client group without the clients' awareness of the exist-

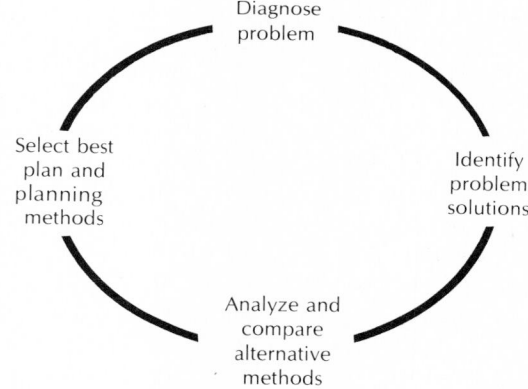

Fig. 9-2. Essential elements of program planning.

ing need. To avoid the development of such programs, planning should include four essential elements (Fig. 9-2): (1) problem diagnosis—assessment of need, (2) identification of problem solutions, (3) analysis and comparison of alternative methods, and (4) selection of the best plan and planning methods.

Assessment of Need

The initial and most critical step in planning for a health program is the assessment of client need. Pro-

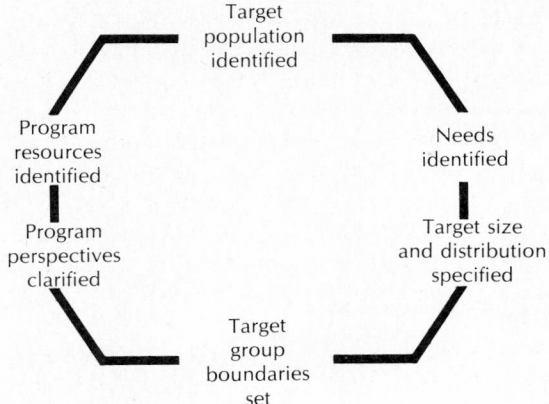

Fig. 9-3. Steps in needs assessment process.

gram planners must verify the existence of a current health problem that is being ignored or being unsuccessfully treated in a client group. These data will provide the rationale to establish a new program or revise existing programs to meet the needs of the client group. The *assessment of need,* defined as "verifying and mapping out the extent and location of a problem and its attendant target population" (Rossi and Freeman, 1982, p. 93), provides data to determine place, person, and time requirements of a health program.

Six basic steps exist in the needs assessment process (Fig. 9-3): (1) identify the target population, (2) identify the needs to be met, (3) specify the size and distribution of the target, (4) set boundaries for the target group, (5) clarify the perspectives on the program target, and (6) identify the program resources (Posavac and Carey, 1980; Rossi and Freeman 1982).

The *target population* may be identified as a community or group, as families or individuals. The target population should be defined specifically by its biological and psychosocial characteristics, by geographical location, and by the problems to be addressed. For example, if the target population is a community with a large number of preschool children who require immunizations to enter school, the target population may be described as all children between the ages of 4 and 6 who reside in central county who have not had up-to-date immunizations by the start of the school year.

The *needs to be met* for the target population must be identified by the target as well as by the health provider. *If the target population does not recognize the need, the program will usually fail regardless of the amount of assessing and planning before program implementation.* To assist the population toward awareness of the existing need, a health education program may be necessary before a program is implemented. In the example of the

need for immunization of preschool children, public service media may be used to alert parents to laws requiring immunizations, to the continued existence of communicable diseases, and to the communicable diseases successfully eradicated by immunization programs, such as smallpox.

Specifying the size and distribution of a target population for a program involves not only the counting of the number of persons in the community who may be eligible for the program but also finding out the number of persons with the problem who are unserved by existing programs and the numbers of eligible persons who have and have not availed themselves of existing services. In planning the preschool immunization program, the estimates of numbers of preschool children in the county may be obtained from census data. One must then decide if the program will serve all children in the county, children of one school district, or only children who do not attend existing health facilities. The decision will be based on the program's overall goal.

Boundaries for the target population are primarily established by defining the size and distribution of the target population. The boundaries will stipulate who is included and who is excluded in the health program. If the immunization program was designed to serve only preschool children of low-income families, all other preschool children would be excluded. If the program was designed to serve all children without immunization, children partially immunized may be referred to the health care facility that initiated the child's immunization program. If the community is composed largely of middle class families, limiting the program to low-income children may make the population size so small that the program would not be cost efficient.

Perspectives on the program target may be found to differ between health providers, organizational administrators, policymakers, and potential clients. Collecting data on the opinions and attitudes of all persons directly or indirectly involved with the program's success is essential to deciding on the program's feasibility, the need to redefine the problems, or the decision to abandon a new program or expand an existing program. For example, in 1982 in one state, all funding for prenatal programs was cut from state, district, and local health budgets. The policymakers had determined that prenatal care was no longer a health priority in spite of existing research that correlates prenatal care with reduction in maternal and infant health problems. A program planner working on expansion of prenatal programs found all work had become meaningless when budgetary requests for program funding were refused. Similarly, policymakers in the 70s, who determined that neighborhood health clinics were the answer to service accessibility for low-income residents, found that their perspectives did not correspond to the perspectives of most health providers or clients. The neighborhood health clinic concept failed as a viable program.

Before implementing a health program, one must also *assess available resources.* Program resources include manpower, facilities, equipment, and financing. The numbers and kinds of personnel available to implement a program must be determined. The availability of supplies and up-to-date equipment is as essential a resource for implementing a program as are the source and amount of funds to implement the program. If one of the essential resources is unavailable to the program, it will be deemed grossly inadequate to meet the needs of the target population.

Needs Assessment Tools

A number of tools exist to assist the program planner in the needs assessment process. The major tools utilized for needs assessment are census data, key informants, community forums, surveys of existing community agencies with similar programs, surveys of residents of the community to be served (target population), and statistical indicators (Posavac and Carey, 1980; Rossi and Freeman, 1982).

Census data are considered valid, reliable, and inexpensive data which are available to the public in several forms. The U.S. census data, updated every 10 years, provide excellent composite data on the population of states, local and political jurisdictions, and census tracts in urbanized areas. The census data may be used to locate target populations by age, sex, race, socioeconomic status, and housing conditions. Census data may be used to compare trends in states and the nation or between states and localities. A word of caution is necessary about the use of census data for program planning. If programs are being planned for rapidly expanding localities, census data may be outdated before they are published. Census data may also be incomplete or otherwise incorrect for such population groups as rural, underserved communities or unincorporated communities.

The *key informants approach* to needs assessment is described as a "simple and inexpensive survey technique that involves identifying, selecting, and questioning knowledgable leaders and experts . . . " in the community about target populations (Rossi and Freeman, 1982).

The use of key informants affords the program planner the opportunity to obtain the perspectives of professional experts, such as nurses, educators, physicians, and social workers, and the community leaders, the politicians and entrepreneurs who are in touch with the needs of the community and who are in a position to support new community programs. The major problem with the key informant approach is that the planner may obtain biased data from the informants because of bias these persons have about the community problems or because of the informants' interests in directing projects to certain ends. A program planner may avoid some bias by using a structured interview guide when communicating with key informants. The structured interview guide also provides an easy mechanism for collating and summarizing the data gathered from the key informant.

The *community forum* is another economical approach to gathering data about needs, size, and characteristics of a target group. The community forum is an open meeting for members of a particular community or group. For example, if the community health nurse is interested in assessing the health needs at Apple School, the administration, teachers, parents, and children could be invited to an open forum to provide input about the health needs of the school children. Of course, the specificity of the topic at a forum meeting will make the difference in the usefulness of the data. If the program planner wishes to assess the need to provide an eye screening program in the school, the participants would direct their input to eye problems and eye screening only. The discussion could be focused on the size, extent of need, and characteristics of the population in need of an eye care program. A discussion of health needs would provide valuable information about general health needs but may not be as helpful for program planning as a more specific topic.

The disadvantages to the forum are (1) that a population cross-section may not attend the meeting, thereby biasing the data with the interests of the population segment in attendance, (2) that the forum may become a political arena for a few and may limit the kinds of information offered by others who do not feel free to speak out. The forum is valuable in obtaining the perceptions of the participants and the target population about specific problems and about methods of health services delivery.

Surveys of existing community agencies providing similar services are essential to the development of a new or expanding an existing program. If the community health nurse has identified a need for a home health care program for the elderly population of the community, the nurse should initially conduct an inventory of the number of facilities within the community providing home health services. Once the numbers of agencies providing services have been identified, the numbers of personnel employed by the agencies and the numbers of persons served by the agencies should be determined. These data can usually be obtained through direct requests of the provider agencies.

The program planner may be interested in determining the kinds of persons served by the existing agencies by disease category, age, socioeconomic level, payment mechanism and so on; the ratio of persons served to the estimated numbers that could be served by the agencies; and the number of persons referred to other agencies for service. This information will provide the planner with data to compare to the population identified in need of home health care. The data may suggest that the target population could potentially be served by all existing agencies, that existing agencies are not employing enough personnel to serve the population and thus a new program may be warranted, that existing agencies are not providing services to certain segments of the target population, and that a new program directed toward the identified population segment would have more potential for success.

The community resident survey serves the purposes of assessing the need of a community for a service, the acceptability of the service to the community, and the willingness of the people to use and pay for a program or service. The community resident survey may be conducted by surveying the total population of a target community or by surveying a sample of the target community. The community health nurse may want to elicit the assistance of a statistician to choose the appropriate sample and size for the resident survey.

The community resident survey should be directed to the specific population the program intends to serve. If the program planned is home health care for the elderly, the survey should be directed to the elderly, to the physicians who will refer to the agencies, and to the social and health provider institutions who will refer to the agencies. If the program is a parenting program, the survey should be directed to pregnant families or families with new babies. In this instance, a survey of the elderly population would skew the data and bias the survey results.

Statistical indicators of disease incidence, prevalence, and mortality, and other rates such case-specific, age-specific, and adjusted rates are useful in estimating the nature of the problem, size of the problem, and need for a program within a target population. *Estimation of risk* is also useful in determining the preventive program needs for specific population (see Chapter 7 for additional information about statistical indicators). Statistical data about a community are readily available through local and state health departments and from the Health Statistics of the United States.

As the community health nurse begins to assess the program needs of the target population, the nurse should consider that a program based on need does not guarantee program success. The demands of the target population for the planned program must be considered. Thus the use of several of the tools just discussed is essential to (1) estimate the need and (2) to assess the demand within the target population to validate that the need is real and a program is desired.

PLANNING METHODS

The need and demand for a program have been determined through the needs assessment process. The next step in the development of the program is to choose a procedural method that will assist the community health nurse in planning the program to be offered. Four planning methods will be discussed in this section: (1) the Planning, Programming, and Budgeting System; (2) Program Evaluation Review Techniques; (3) the Critical Path Method; and (4) the Multi-Attribute Utility Method.

Planning, Programming, and Budgeting System

The Planning, Programming, and Budgeting System (PPBS) is a procedural tool initially developed for use by the Department of Defense and other governmental agencies. PPBS is an outcome-oriented accounting system, the extent of which is to determine the most efficient method of resource allocation to attain measurable objectives (LaPatra, 1975; Rakich et al., 1977).

The steps involved in PPBS are (1) setting program goals, (2) defining measurable program objectives, (3) identifying and evaluating alternatives to accomplish program objectives, (4) choosing the method for accomplishing the objectives, and (5) developing a program budget with justification for minimizing costs while maximizing program benefits (Fig. 9-4).

PPBS is an economic method of expressing a program plan. In PPBS, *planning* represents formulation of objectives and identification of alternatives and methods for accomplishing objectives, *programming* represents delineation of resources (manpower, facilities, equipment, and financing) for each identified alternative, and *budgeting* represents the assignment of dollar values to resources required for the program implementation.

PPBS is widely used at the macro level for planning broad-scale programs of government. It is a system that can also be used at the micro level to plan programs for an agency or for client groups. PPBS in the use of objectives that are operationally defined by standards or performance criteria is a system that lends itself to effective program evaluation. For example, PPBS could be used to develop the annual program plan for the local health department or a prenatal program for the local

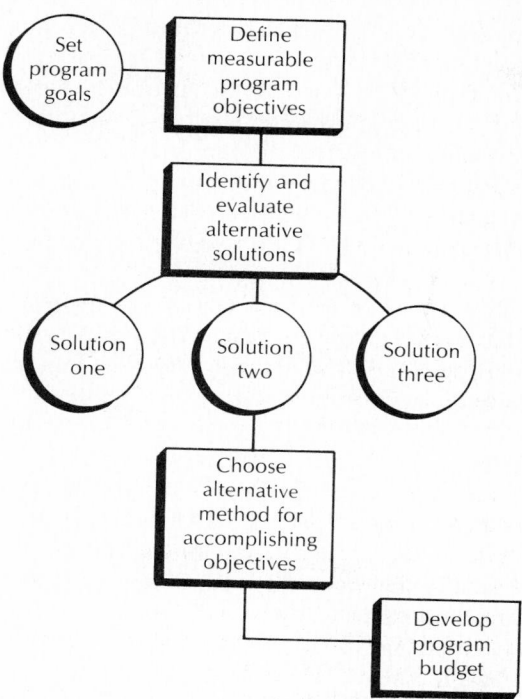

Fig. 9-4. Planning, programming, and budgeting system.

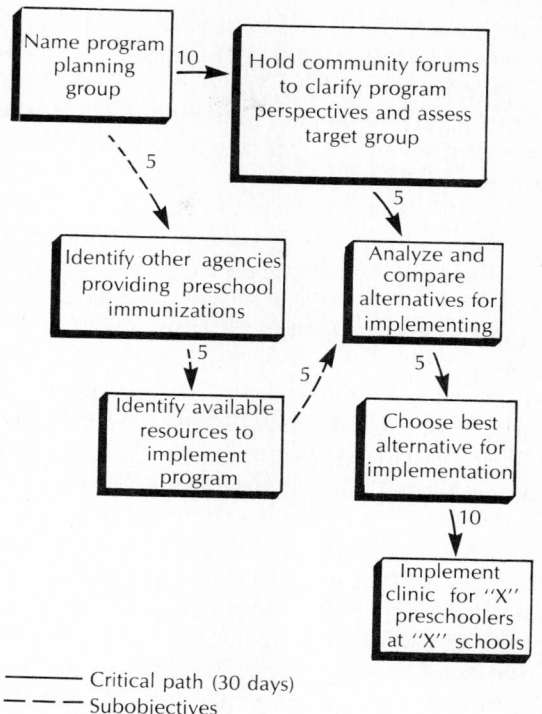

——— Critical path (30 days)
- - - - Subobjectives

Fig. 9-5. Simplified PERT network for planning a preschool immunization program. Numbers represent days required for completion of activities.

community. A community health nurse could also use this method for developing a health education program for the school population on sexually transmitted diseases.

Program Evaluation Review Techniques

The Program Evaluation Review Techniques (PERT) is a network programming method developed in the 1950s through a joint effort of the United States Navy, Lockheed Aircraft Corporation, and Booz-Allen and Hamilton, Inc. The method was developed for the purpose of planning and controlling the program activities involved in developing the Polaris missile.

The PERT procedural planning method is primarily useful for large-scale projects that require the planning, scheduling, and controlling of a large number of activities. PERT is mentioned here to introduce the reader to the concept of network programming.

The major objectives of PERT are to: (1) focus attention on the key developmental parts of a program; (2) identify potential program problems that could interfere with movement toward program goals; (3) evaluate program progress toward goal attainment; (4) provide a prompt reporting method; and (5) facilitate decision making (Roman, 1969).

The PERT technique involves the concept of *time* and *events.* The basic tool used in the technique is the network or flow plan. The flow plan is a series of circles, ovals, or squares representing the program events, or goals, and their interrelationships with the activities of the program. The program activities are the time-consuming elements of the program and are represented by arrows that connect the program accomplishments or goals (Fig. 9-5). The events in the flow plan represent the program goals. Note in the flow plan that it may take several activities to attain a program event (goal) and that some events (goals) must be accomplished before other events may be attained. The interrelationship of several program events (subgoals) may be essential to attain the ultimate program event (goal).

Another element in the PERT technique is the estimation of the time it will take to implement activities leading to program goals. In the PERT system three estimates of activity time are given: the optimistic time it will take to complete activities, given minimal difficulties; the most likely time it will take to complete activities, given past experiences with normal development of said activities; and the pessimistic time it will take to complete activities, given maximum difficulties. From the time estimates a simple formula can be applied to indicate the probability of completing a project in a given time period (Barentson, 1970; Griffith, 1972; Roman, 1969; Wiest and Levy, 1969). The numbers appearing along the arrows in Fig. 9-5 are the estimated number of days required for completion of activities leading to a particular event.

The PERT method embodies three major steps: (1) identification of specific program activities; (2) identification of resources to accomplish the activities; and (3) determination of sequencing activities for the accomplishment of program events.

Critical Path Method

The Critical Path Method (CPM) is a network programming planning method that is described by some authors as a procedural technique entity (Rakich et al., 1977; Wiest and Levy, 1969) and is described by others (Roman, 1969) as an element of the PERT technique.

The CPM is a technique that focuses the program planners attention on the program activities, the sequencing of activities for the best use of time and resources, and the estimated time it will take to complete the project from beginning to end. Using this method the planner can determine the amount of time it will take to accomplish each activity and can identify those activities that may take longer. The planner can then determine the amounts of resources needed (manpower, money, facilities, and supplies) to accomplish tasks at given points in time along the program's "critical path."

The CPM allows for frequent review of progress by program planners. Problems can be identified early in program implementation, and corrective action taken or alternative activities substituted for activities that are not meeting program requirements. The amount of time and the resources being used during program implementation can be assessed, and time and resources can be increased or decreased as necessary and can be compared to initial estimates of program need.

The Multi-Attribute Utility Method

The Multi-Attribute Utility Method (MAUT) is a planning technique based on decision theory (Edwards, Guttentag, and Snapper, 1975). This method can be adapted for making decisions about the care of one client or for making decisions about the national health care programs. The purpose of MAUT is to separate all elements of a decision and to evaluate each element separately for its impact on the overall decision.

Ten basic steps to the MAUT method are described by Edwards, Guttentag, and Snapper (1975):

1. *Identify the person or aggregate whose utilities are to be maximized.* In other words, who is the client for whom the program is being planned?

2. *Identify the issue(s) or decisions to which the utilities are relevant.* This step involves the identification of the program objectives.

3. *Identify the entities to be evaluated.* The program planner identifies the available options or action alternatives to accomplish the program goals.

4. *Identify the relevant dimensions of value.* The program planner places a value on or identifies criteria to be considered to make a choice between competing options or alternatives.

5. *Rank the value dimensions in order of importance.* The program planner will decide which of the criteria are most important and which are the least important for meeting the program goals.

6. *Rate dimensions in importance.* In this step the program planner assigns an arbitrary rating of 10 to the least important value dimension. In considering the "next least important" dimension, the planner decides how many times more important it is than the "least important" dimension. If it is considered twice as important, the dimension will be assigned a 20. If it is only considered half again as important, it will be assigned a 15. If it is considered four times as important, it will be assigned a 40. The process is continued until all dimensions have been rated.

7. *Add the importance weights, divide each by the sum, and multiply by 100.* Edwards refers to this process as "normalizing" the weights. This step is considered to be a purely mechanical step that provides a clearer picture of the relative values of the dimensions by the program planner. A note of caution. If too many dimensions are identified in Step 4, the computational process underestimates the value of some actions while overestimating the value of others. Six to fifteen dimensions are recommended to avoid this problem. Therefore, in this initial process the planner can only be concerned with general criteria for choosing action alternatives.

8. *Measure the location of the entity being evaluated on each dimension.* The planner may ask a colleague or expert to estimate the probability on a scale of 0 to 100 that a given option from Step 3 will maximize the value dimensions (criteria) from Step 4. An option thought to have a low probability of meeting the criteria may be assigned a value of 20 whereas an option thought to have a high probability of meeting the criteria may be assigned a value of 80.

9. *Calculate utilities for entities.* The program planner will obtain the utility of each action alternative identified by multiplying the weight for each dimension (Step 7) by the rating of an option for each dimension (Step 8) and summing the products. The sum of the products for each action is termed the *aggregate utility.*

10. *Decide on best alternative to meet program objectives.* The action alternative with the highest aggregate

utility is considered the best decision for meeting the program objectives. If cost was not considered as one of the criteria on which to evaluate the action alternatives, then the utility of each option may need to be considered in relation to cost.

If money is no object, then the option with the highest utility is the best decision. However, if the highest utility option exceeds the budget, then the next highest utility option may be the alternative to choose. Appendix I presents an example of the application of MAUT to a program decision in community health nursing.

BENEFITS OF PROGRAM PLANNING

Program planning involves two essential steps: (1) a needs assessment that assists the planner in diagnosis of client problems and (2) choice of an organized planning method that assists the planner in identifying problem solutions (program goals), in analyzing and comparing alternative actions for resolving problems, and in selecting the best alternative to attain problem resolution.

Systematic planning for meeting client needs benefits clients, nurses, and the employing agencies. The act of planning focuses attention on what the organization and the health provider is attempting to do for clients. Planning assists in identifying the resources and activities that are essential in meeting the objectives of client services and directs the attention of the organizations and providers toward making sound decisions to attain common objectives. Planning reduces role ambiguity by allowing for assignment of responsibility for the planned activities required to meet program objectives.

Planning also reduces uncertainty in the internal program environment and enhances the abilities of the provider and the agency to cope with the external environment. All persons involved with the program can anticipate what will occur during program implementation and what will be needed to implement the program and can project the program outcomes. Planning assists the provider and the agency to *act* on rather than react to events. Finally, planning allows for quality decision making and better control over the actual program results.

The planning process includes the identification of program goals, the interventions, the resources required, and a schedule of activities for program implementation. Planning is usually reflective of a desire on the part of the planners to reduce the gap between the program goals and the realities of program implementation and to diminish the unanticipated occurrences that may result during program implementation. Inherent in the planning process is the desire to implement a reality-based program that can be readily evaluated.

PROGRAM EVALUATION

Definitions

A program may be defined as "an organized response to reduce or eliminate one or more problems" (Deniston, Rosenstock, and Getting, 1969, p. 222) or "a standing arrangement that provides for a social service" (Cronbach, 1980, p. 14). Programs are established to fulfill a need or eliminate or reduce some recognized problem.

Evaluation may be defined as "a collection of methods, skills, and sensitivities necessary to determine whether a human service is needed and likely to be used, whether it is conducted as planned, and whether the human service actually does help people in need" (Posavac and Carey, 1980, p. 6) or "the provision of information through formal means, such as criteria, measurement, and statistics, to provide rational bases for making judgments that are inherent in decision situations" (Beatty, 1969, p. 53). Evaluation precedes and provides data for decision making about a program.

Suchman (1967, p. 32) defines evaluation as "the determination (whether based on opinions, records, subjective or objective data) of the results (whether desirable or undesirable; transient or permanent; immediate or delayed) attained by some activity (whether a program, or part of a program, a drug or a therapy, an ongoing or one-shop approach) designed to accomplish some value goal or objective (whether ultimate, intermediate, or immediate, effort or performance, long or short range)."

In summary then, the term *program* refers to what exists to serve a purpose and *evaluation* refers to a process to determine whether the program is achieving its purpose.

Planning and the Evaluative Process

Planning for the evaluative process is an integral part of program planning and should *not* be considered something begun after the program has been in operation for several months. As a part of the planning process, Posevac and Carey (1980) describe six steps to use in planning for program evaluation (Fig. 9-6):

The *first step* is to identify the relevant people for evaluation. Program personnel, program sponsors, and the recipients of the program should be included in planning for the evaluation.

The *second step* is to arrange preliminary meetings to discuss the questions of whether the group wants an evaluation, and if so, why, what kind, and when. If the program planners and others agree on an evaluation, the resources for conducting the program evaluation must be identified.

The *third step* is to make a decision about whether

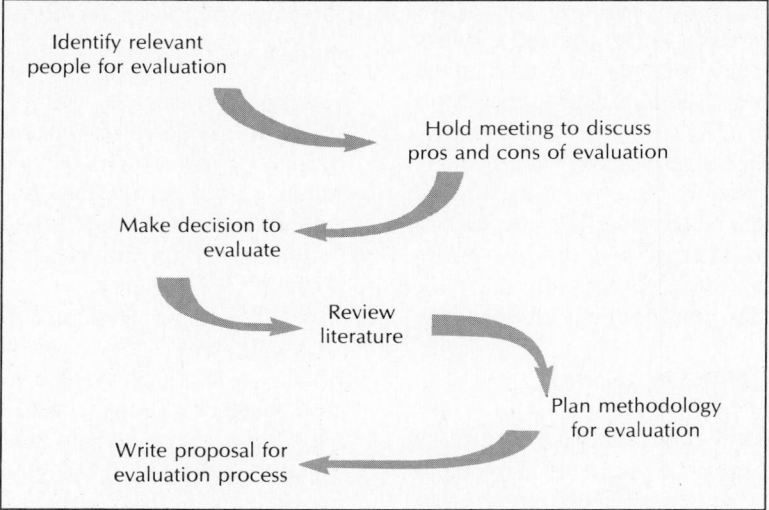

Fig. 9-6. Six steps in planning for program evaluation.

the evaluation should be carried out. After the relevant people have met and considered the questions in the previous steps, they are ready to decide whether the evaluation should be carried out. The decision to conduct the evaluation may be an administrative one, may be based on availability of resources, or may be determined by the existing circumstances. For example, if a program evaluation were attempted in a situation where program personnel or clients chose to be uncooperative, evaluation efforts would fail.

The *fourth step* is to examine the literature. This step is particularly helpful if the organization has chosen an evaluator who is external to the program. If the evaluation is internal, the evaluators may already know the literature.

The *fifth step* is to plan the methodology, which includes decisions about what parameters will be measured, how they will be measured, and on what population the measures will be obtained.

The *sixth* and final step is to write a proposal for the evaluation that outlines the purpose and goals of the overall program, the type of evaluation to be done, the operational measure to be used to evaluate the program goals, the choice of internal or external evaluators, the available resources for conducting the evaluation, and the readiness of the organization, personnel, and clients for program evaluation.

As previously stated, the evaluative process should be operational at the onset of the program. The evaluative process as described by Suchman (1967) is modified and explained here, but the reader will find it to be very similar to steps in the planning process.

The first step in the evaluative process is *goal setting,* which is preceded or concurrent with the value clarification. The statement that children should not be exposed to the illness and suffering of early childhood diseases and polio because they can be prevented is a value statement. It would be followed by a program goal such as a decrease in the incidence of early childhood diseases and polio in the county where the program is planned.

The second step is *determining goal measurement.* In the case of the previous goal, the recording of disease incidence would be an appropriate goal measurement. The third step is *identifying goal attaining activities,* and again in the same case would include such things as media presentation to encourage parents to have their children immunized. The fourth step is *making the activities operational,* actually administering the immunizations, and the fifth is *measuring the goal effect,* reviewing the records and summarizing the incidence of early childhood disease and polio before and after the program. The final step is *evaluation of the program,* or a judgment about whether the program goal was achieved. Keep in mind that only one program goal was used in the example, and the program undoubtedly has more than one goal (Fig. 9-7).

Formulation of Objectives for Evaluation

Specification of Objectives (Goals). According to Mager (1962), objectives should include the specific behavior, the conditions under which the behavior is shown, and the minimum standard of performance. According to Deniston et al. (1969), an objective should specify the following: the *what* or condition to be achieved, the extent or *how much, to whom* or what

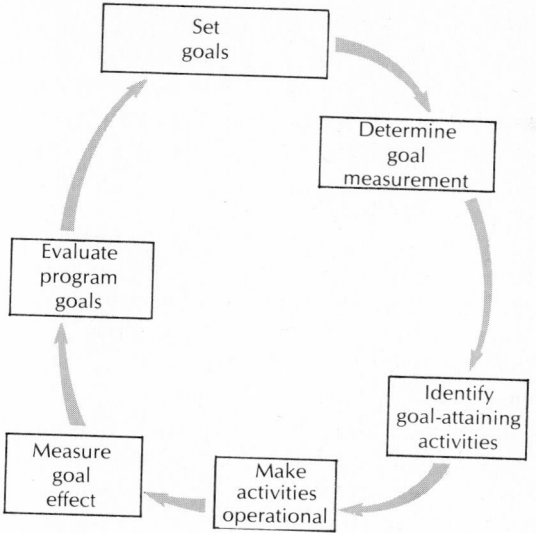

Fig. 9-7. The evaluative process.

group, *where,* and *when.* The population and geographical area may be included in the general description of the program, but the *when* can be an important part of the program objective.

Levels of Program Objectives. It is customary for objectives to be stated in levels. The first level at which the objective is stated is general and broad. Some refer to these as goals. The purpose of the goal or general objective is to focus on the major thrust of the program. The subobjectives or subgoals are more specific; that is, they describe a measurable behavior, the circumstances under which the behavior is observed, and the minimal acceptable standard for the execution of the behavior.

Some general guidelines for writing objectives are that (1) they should describe program recipients behavior, (2) they should be stated as a product or outcome, and (3) they should state only one outcome per objective (Gronlund, 1970).

Program activities are planned to insure attainment of each subobjective or each subgoal; resources are planned for each of the activities. Program assumptions are that attainment of the subobjectives are in sequence and will result in attainment of the general objective, that the planned activity will facilitate or assure the attainment of the objective, and that the resource will be provided for the planned activity.

Benefits of Program Evaluation

The major benefit of program evaluation is that it determines whether the program is fulfilling its purpose. It should answer the question of whether the needs for which the program was designed are being met or whether the problems that it was designed to solve are being solved. Evaluation is a way of demonstrating that the program is fulfilling its purpose. This is critical information for funding agencies, top-level decision makers, accreditation reviews, or the community at large. Evaluation data may be used to justify expanding the program or they may be used to justify reducing the program or even closing it (Knutson, 1969; Soumelis, 1977).

Program Evaluation Versus Evaluative Research

Program evaluation collects information in a systematic way to assess the effectiveness and efficiency of a program under consideration. The purposes of program evaluation are to provide information to assist in decisions about initiating, continuing, expanding, modifying, terminating, or certifying a program. It also provides evidence to oppose or support a program. The evaluation is directed to particular individuals or agencies related in some way to the particular program. Its uses are for problem solving or practical purposes.

Evaluation research collects information according to the rigors of systematic inquiry. All the steps must be precise and explicit enough to allow replication, the variables must be recognized or controlled, and the findings must be analyzed through appropriate statistical techniques. These steps are aimed at obtaining findings that are generalizable beyond the population under study, and optimally the report is available in the literature to other researchers, the profession, and the public at large (Bloch, 1980; Hegyvary, 1980; Krueger, 1980; Phaneuf, 1980).

EVALUATION MODELS AND TECHNIQUES

Evaluation of Program Effectiveness

According to the plan for program evaluation formulated by Deniston et al. (1969), programs consist of objectives (including subobjectives), activities, and resources. Assumptions are made that program objectives are met through planned activities (specific for those objectives) and with planned resources (specific for those activities). This plan addresses the question of whether the program is effective. It does not specifically address whether the program is adequate, appropriate, or efficient. The question of effectiveness asks to what extent are the preestablished objectives attained as a result of the planned activity. Evaluation of program effectiveness consists of three steps: (1) describing the program, (2) measuring the objectives, and (3) determining effectiveness.

Describing the program consists of naming the program and stating the program objective(s), subobjectives, activities, and resources. First, program objectives are specified, including measurement of the condition of the objectives and measurement of as many subobjectives as possible under the time constraints. Measurement of too many subobjectives is too time consuming and costly, and measurement of too few will result in failure to collect enough data to support any statements about whether the objectives are being met.

Second, program activities are specified and linked to the objective or subobjective for which the activity was designed. This permits the evaluator to determine the extent to which activities were performed as planned. Third, resources are specified in order to determine the extent to which resources were used as planned for the activities.

After the program has been described, the next stop is to *measure* whether the objective(s) and subobjectives of the program have been attained. Valid and reliable measuring instruments are essential. The measures must be made at the time specified in the objective(s) and subobjectives. Care must be taken to avoid bias and to use proper sampling techniques.

Effectiveness refers to what extent achievement of the objective(s) can be attributed to the activities of the program. This is accomplished by comparing the program variables of resources, activities, and objectives by using a set of ratios. The first ratio is actual use of resources to planned use of resources, the second ratio is actual program activities to planned program activities, and the third ratio is attainment of the objective attributable to program activity to attainment desired less the attainment that existed in absence of the program. These ratios answer the question of whether the program was conducted according to the plan and whether the achievement of the objectives was the result of the program or the result of chance.

Structure-Process-Outcome Evaluation

The method for evaluation of programs by Donabedian (1966) was initially directed primarily toward medical care but is applicable to the broader area of health care. He described three approaches to assessment of health care: structure, process, and outcome (see Chapter 10).

Structure refers to settings in which care occurs and includes materials, equipment, qualification of the staff, and organizational structure (Donabedian, 1978). This approach to evaluation is based on the assumption that given a proper setting with good equipment, good care will follow, but this assumption is not strongly supported.

Process refers to whether the care that was given was "good" (Donabedian, 1966), competent, or preferable practice, given a particular patient or client. Use of process in program evaluation may consist of observation

of practice but more likely consists of review of medical records. The review may focus on pathology reports to ascertain whether the percentage of surgeries were strongly indicated or questionable. The review could focus on whether documentation of preventive teaching was on the clinical record. Audits using specific criteria are examples of the use of process.

Outcome refers to client recovery and restoration of function and of survival (Donabedian, 1966) but is also used in the sense of changes in health status or changes in health-related knowledge, attitude, and client behavior (Donabedian, 1978). Thus program outcomes may be expressed in terms of mortality, morbidity, and disability for given populations such as infants, but could be expressed in a broader sense through health promotion behaviors such as weight control, exercise, and abstinence from tobacco and alcohol.

Donabedian supports the use of the process approach when possible, followed by outcome, and finally by structure. There is more use of process and outcome than of structure in evaluation of care. Donabedian's model of evaluating program quality is a popular model, which is widely used for evaluation in the health care field.

Tracer Method

The Board on Medicine of the National Academy of Sciences developed a program to evaluate health service delivery called the tracer method (Kessner and Kalk, 1973). The tracer method for evaluation of programs is based on the premise that health status and care can be evaluated by viewing specific health problems called "tracers." Just as radioactive tracers such as iodide are used to study the thyroid gland, specific health problems are selected for use to evaluate the delivery of health services. Examples of conditions selected as tracers are middle ear infection and associated hearing loss, vision disorders, iron deficiency anemia, hypertension, urinary tract infections, and cervical cancer. This program can be used to (1) compare health status among different population groups, (2) compare health status in relation to social, economic, medical care, and behavioral variables, and (3) compare various arrangements for health care delivery. The application of this method for the study of health care for children in Washington, D.C., has been reported by Kessner and Kalk (1973) and is discussed by Palmer (1976). Stevens (1975) has developed a method for evaluating nursing care that is similar to the tracer method (see Chapter 10).

Goal Attainment

Goal attainment refers to a process for assessing the efficacy of a program by examination or measurement of the predetermined goals (Kiresuk and Sander, 1979). LaPatra (1975) described the components of the goal attainment model as setting objectives, setting measures of objectives, collecting data, assessing the effect, and modifying the initial objective on the basis of the data analysis and interpretation. The following model by Shields is an example of a goal attainment model. Shields (1974) applies a process to each goal. For each goal the evaluator examines the categories of wherewithal, structure, operations, and outcomes.

Wherewithal refers to resources, materials, equipment, and physical facilities.

Structure consists of the organizational framework, that is, administrative structure, lines of authority, committee linkages, and patterns of communication.

Operations pertain to the processes and procedures for carrying out the program goals whether it is teaching, treating, or preventing and the performances of the workers doing the processes.

Outcomes refers to whether the goal was attained and to what degree as well as to other significant events related to the outcome.

The criteria applied to outcomes are: (1) effectiveness—whether the immediate purpose was attained; (2) efficiency—how cost efficient the program was; and (3) control—whether unexpected and potentially harmful events were associated with the program. If the program has more than one goal, the evaluation process is applied to each goal.

Systems Model

The systems model of evaluation focuses on the process as a working model or a social unit capable of achieving the goal (Schulberg et al., 1969). This model is concerned with objectives being achieved, subunits functioning in coordination, resources being maintained, and adaptation to the environment (LaPatra, 1975). The systems model examines aspects other than the goal; it recognizes that organizations have multiple goals and considers single goal attainment in relation to its effect on other goals in the system.

Three variables are described and evaluated in the systems model; the input, throughput, and output. *Input* consists of characteristics and conditions of people and the resources. *Throughput* refers to the human and nonhuman resources and process. *Output* refers to the products of the system (Baker and Northman, 1979). The systems model is more comprehensive, since it takes more elements into consideration for the evaluation.

Case Register

Systematic registration of contagious disease has been a practice for many years. Denmark began a national register of tuberculosis in 1921 (Horwitz, 1979). Its contribution to the reduction in the incidence of contagious diseases has been widely recognized (Clemmesen, 1979). Registers are also used for acute and chronic disease, for example, cancer and myocardial infarctions.

Registers collate information from such defined groups, and the information may be used for evaluation and planning of services, disease prevention, provision of care, and monitoring changes in patterns and care of diseases (Holland and Karhausen, 1979). The method is described here because of its use in evaluation of services. Information obtained by the community registers in Europe on myocardial infarction is a good example of the way a case register is used (Keil, 1979). The following are questions that were asked about cases of mycardial infarction for the community registers:

1. What is the incidence of disease? What differences in incidence are there between one community and another?
2. What percent recover? Or die?
3. Where does death occur?
4. How long do clients wait before calling a doctor?
5. How long is it before they see a doctor?
6. How many cases are associated with other major coronary heart disease risk factors?
7. How many are associated with environmental factors such as water hardness or air pollution?
8. What happens after clients leave the hospital and when they return to work? Is there a rehabilitation program?
9. How many had been seen by a physician shortly before the infarction?
10. What prevention measures are taken for persons considered susceptible?

The answers to these questions before and after implementation of a given program would give information about the impact of the program. A tuberculosis register indicates the degree to which infection is being controlled. Cancer registers make state, regional, national, and international comparisons possible and provide clues to etiological factors.

Evaluation Indexes

Doster (1979, p. 79) defines a health index as a "summary of the health features of a community that enable us to determine health care delivery needs." Doster (1979) further categorizes the health index into six headings: definition of community, people, environment, communication, health and illness indicators and health provider, resources, and services.

The founder of vital statistics, J. Graunt was interested in data on population, births, deaths, and other characteristics for the purpose of urban planning or redevelopment. The collection of vital statistics related to health problems is attributed to the public health movement in the middle of the nineteenth century (Ciocco, 1969).

Today the health and illness indicators such as mortality and morbidity data are probably cited more frequently than any other single indexes, not only for program planning but also for program evaluation.

The other categories identified by Doster can also be used for program evaluation.

SOURCES OF PROGRAM EVALUATION

Major sources of information for program evaluation are program participants, program records, and community indexes. The program participants or consumers of the service have a unique and valuable role in program evaluation. Whether the clients for whom the program was designed accept and use the service will determine to a large extent whether the program achieves its purpose. Thus their reactions, feelings and judgements about the program are very important to the evaluation.

The second major source of information for program evaluation is program records, especially clinical records. The most prominent example of the use of clinical records is the Donabedian (1966) model for evaluation. According to the Donabedian model, process and outcomes of care are often examined by review of clinical records. Most recently this has been done in the form of quality assurance (Chapter 10) and the audit (peer review). Although review of clinical records by professional peers was already being reported in the literature as early as the 1960s (Helbig et al. 1972), legislation in 1972 established the Professional Standards Review Organization to "promote effective, efficient and economical delivery of Medicare and Medicaid health services." For examples of outcome and process criteria the reader is referred to Haussman et al., 1977.

A third major source of evaluation is community indexes, previously described in evaluation indexes (p. 215). However, the evaluator must examine the community indexes in light of other variables or events in the community that may also facilitate or hinder achievement of the program's purpose.

TYPES OF MEASURES

To assess the response of participants in a program or consumers of a service, the evaluator may use a written survey in the form of a questionnaire or an attitude scale. Interviews, achievement tests, and observations are other ways of getting feedback about a program. Attitude scales are probably the most often used, and they are usually phrased in terms of whether the program met its objectives. The client satisfaction survey is an example of an attitude scale often used in the health care delivery system to evaluate the attainment of program objectives (refer to Chapter 10 for discussion of the pros and cons of the client satisfaction survey).

Morbidity and mortality have been used as indexes to evaluate a plan for community services and also to evaluate the effectiveness of community services. A decline in the morbidity or mortality from one particular cause may indicate the effectiveness of a program, particularly something that has the potential for a dramatic change such as an immunization program. Incidence and prevalence are also valuable indexes used to measure program effectiveness (refer to Chapter 7 for further discussion of rates and ratios).

SUMMARY

Planning programs and planning for the evaluation of programs are two of the most important activities for community health nurses to assure successful program implementation. Whether the program being planned is a national health insurance program like Medicare, a state health care program like early childhood developmental screening programs, or a local program like vision screening for elementary school children, the essential elements of planning are applicable.

Needs assessment is a key ingredient in the planning process. The target population for any program must be identified and involved in program development. If the target population does not recognize the need for a health services program, that program is designed to fail regardless of the commitment of health providers and the resources of the program.

A number of tools are available for assisting planners in needs assessment. Some of the major tools used for needs assessment are census data, key informants, community forums, surveys of existing community agencies, surveys of community residents, and statistical indicators.

Several procedural methods can be applied to plan program offerings. A few of these methods are the Planning, Programming and Budgeting System, Program Evaluation Review Techniques, the Critical Path Method, and the Multi-Attribute Utility Method.

The application of the planning process to program development is an indication that the planners wish to reduce the gap between program goals and the realities of program implementation and the likelihood of unanticipated occurrences during program implementation.

As one develops plans for program implementation, one should also develop the plan for program evaluation. All persons involved in program implementation should be a part of the plan for program evaluation. The major benefit of program evaluation is to determine whether the program is fulfilling its stated goals. Quality assurance programs are prime examples of program evaluation in health care delivery. Evaluation data are used to justify the continued existence of programs in community health.

Program evaluation focuses on goal attainment and the efficiency and effectiveness of program activities. Many methods of program evaluation are described in the literature. The primary method of evaluation used in health care today is Donabedian's Evaluative Framework. The Goal Attainment Method, Systems Model, Tracer Method, and Case Register are other methods applied to program evaluation.

Program records and community indexes serve as the major sources of information for program evaluation. Surveys, interviews, observations, and tests are measurements used to assess consumer and participant response to health programs.

Planning for the evaluative process is an integral part of program planning and should *not* be considered something begun after the program has been in operation for several months. As economic resources become scarce, nursing and the health care system must be able to justify their existence, prove the responsiveness of their services to consumer needs, and show their professional concern for accountability. Planning and evaluation will assist in meeting these objectives.

BIBLIOGRAPHY

American Public Health Association: Glossary of administrative terms in public health, Am. J. Public Health **50**(2):225-226, Feb. 1960.

Anderson, O.: Influence of social and economic research on public policy in the health field—a review, Milbank Mem. Fund Q. **44**:11-51, 1966.

Baker, F., and Northman, J.E.: Input-throughout-output evaluation of a school mental health clinic. In Schulberg, H.C., and Baker, F., editors: Program evaluation in the health fields, vol. 2, New York, 1979, Human Sciences Press.

Barentson, P.: *Critical path planning: present and future technique,* Princeton, 1970, Brendon Systems Press.

Beatty, W.H., editor: Improving educational assessment and inventory of measures of affective behavior, Washington, D.C., 1969, Association for Supervision and Curriculum Development, National Education Association.

Bice, T.: Health services planning and regulation. Williams, S., and Torrens, P., editors: Introduction to health services, New York, 1980, John Wiley & Sons, Inc.

Bloch, D.: Interrelated issues in evaluation and evaluation research, Nurs. Res. **29**(69):69-73, March-April, 1980.

Ciocco, A.: On indices for the appraisal of health department activities. In Schulberg, H. C., Sheldon, A., and Baker, F., editors: Program evaluation in the health fields, New York, 1969, Behavioral Publications, Inc.

Clemmesen, J.: Registration in the study of human cancer. In Holland, W.W., and Karhausen, L., editors: Health care and epidemiology, Boston, 1979, G.K. Hall & Co.

Commission on Hospital Care: Hospital care in the United States, New York, 1947, The Commonwealth Fund.

Committee on the Costs of Medical Care. Medical care for the American people, Chicago, 1932, University of Chicago Press. Reprinted, Washington, D.C., 1970, Department of Health, Education, and Welfare.

Cordes, S.: Assessing health care needs: Elements and processes. Fam. Community Health **1**:2, 1978.

Cronbach, L.J., et al.: Toward reform of program evaluation, San Francisco, 1980, Jossey-Bass Inc, Publishers.

Curren, W.: A national survey and analysis of state certificate of need laws for health facilities. In Havinghurst, C., editor: Regulating health facilities construction, Washington, D.C., 1974, American Institute for Public Policy Research.

Davidson, S.: Community nursing care evaluation, Fam. Community Health **1**(1):37, 1978.

Deniston, O.O.L., Rosenstock, I.M., and Getting, V.A.: Evaluating program effectiveness. In Schulberg, H.C., Sheldon, A., and Baker, F., editors: Program evaluation in the health fields, New York, 1969, Behavioral Publications, Inc.

Donabedian, A.: Evaluating the quality of medical care, Milbank Mem. Fund Q. **44**:164, 1966.

Donabedian, A.: The quality of medical care. In Abelson, P.H., editor: Health care: regulation, economics, ethics, and practice, Washington, D.C., 1978, American Association for the Advancement of Science.

Dorsey, J.L.: Certificate of need laws, Arch. Surg. **106**:765, 1973.

Doster, C.: Health index of a community. In Community health today and tomorrow, NLN Pub. No. 52-1768, New York, 1979, National League for Nursing.

Edwards, W., Guttentag, M., and Snapper, K.: A decision-theoretic approach to evaluation research. In Struening, E., and Guttentag, M., editors: Handbok of evaluation research, Beverly Hills, Calif., 1975, Sage Publications Inc.

Edwards, W.: Social utilities, The Engineering Economist, Summer Symposium Series 6, 1977.

Finger, K.: Certificate of need procedure under the national health planning and resources development act of 1974, N.Y. State Bar J. **49**(4):308-317, June 1977.

Fuerstein, M.T.: Community participation in evaluation: problems and potentials, Int. Nurs. Rev. **27**:187, Nov.-Dec. 1980.

Gordon, M.: Determining study topics, Nurs. Res. **29**(2):83, 1980.

Griffith, J.: Quantitative techniques for hospital planning and control, Lexington, Mass., 1972, Lexington Books.

Gronlund, N.E.: Stating behavioral objectives for classroom instruction, New York, 1970, Macmillan Publishing Co, Inc.

Hanlon, J., and Pickett, G.: Public health: administration and practice, St. Louis, 1979, The C. V. Mosby.

Havighurst, C.C.: Regulation in the health care system, Hospitals **48**:65, 1974.

Haussman, R.K.D., and Hegyvary, S.T.: Monitoring quality of nursing care. III. Professional review for nursing: an empirical investigation, Hyattsville, Md., Aug. 1977, DHEW Pub. No. HRA 77-70, Department of Health, Education, and Welfare.

Haussman, R.K.D., Hegyvary, S.T., and Newman, J.F.: Monitoring quality of nursing care. II. Assessment and study of correlates, Bethesda, Md. DHEW Pub. No. HRA 76-7, Department of Health, Education, and Welfare, Aug. 1977.

Hegyvary, S.T.: An evaluator's perspective, Nurs. Res. **29**:91, March-April 1980.

Helbig, D., O'Hare, D., and Smith, N.: The care component core—a new system for evaluating quality of inpatient care, Am. J. Pub. Health 62:540-546, 1972.

Holland, W. W., and Karhausen, L., editors: Health care and epidemiology, Boston, 1979, G. K. Hall & Co.

Horwitz, O.: Epidemiological parameters for the public health evaluation of a chronic disease. In Holland, W.W., and Karhausen, L., editors: Health care and epidemiology, Boston, 1979, G. K. Hall & Co.

Hyman, H.: Applications of methods of evaluation for studies of encampment for citizenship, Calif., 1962, University of California Press.

Institute for Health Planning: A glossary of health care delivery and planning terms, Madison, Wis., 1981, The Institute.

Jelinek, R., Hussmann, R.K.D., and Hegyvary, S.T., et al.: Methodology for monitoring quality of nursing care, Bethesda, Md. 1974, DHEW Pub. No. HRA 76-25, Department of Health, Education, and Welfare.

Keil, U.: Community registers of myocardial infarction as an example of epidemiological register studies. In Holland, W.W., and Karhausen, L., editors: Health care and epidemiology, Boston, 1979, G. K. Hall & Co.

Kessner, D.M., and Kalk, C.E.: Contrasts in health status: a strategy for evaluating health services, vol. 2, Washington, D.C., 1973, Institute of Medicine, National Academy of Sciences.

Kiresuk, T.J., and Sander, H.L.: Goal attainment scaling: research, evaluation, and utilization. In Schulberg, H. C., and Baker, F., editors: program evaluation in the health fields, vol. 2, New York, 1979, Human Science Press.

Knutson, S.L.: Evaluation for what. In Schulberg, H. C., Sheldon, A., and Baker, F., editors: Program evaluation in the health fields, New York, 1969, Behavioral Publications, Inc., pp. 42-50.

Krueger, J.C.: Establishing priorities for evaluation and evaluation research, Nurs. Res. 29:115, March-April 1980.

LaPatra, J.W.: Health care delivery systems: evaluation criteria, Springfield, Ill., 1975, Charles C Thomas, Publisher.

LeBreton, P.: Measuring a nursing services department's effectiveness designing the assessment instrument, Nurs. Health Care 1:3, 1980.

Mager, R.F.: Preparing objectives for programmed instruction, San Francisco, 1962, Fearon Publishers, Inc.

McCarthy, C.: Planning for health care. In Jonas, S., editor: Health care delivery in the United States, New York, 1977, Springer Publishing Co., Inc.

McCarthy, C., and Jonas, S.: Planning for health services. In Jonas, S.: Health care delivery in the United States, ed. 2, New York, 1981, Springer Publishing Co., Inc.

Mullen, P.D.: Qualitative methods for evaluative research in health education programs, Health Educ. 13:11, May-June 1982.

Palmer, R.H.: The present range of provider performance in the United States. In Greene, R., editor: Assuring quality in medical care, Cambridge, Mass., 1976, Ballinger Publishing Co.

Phaneuf, M.C.: Future direction for evaluation and evaluation research in health care, Nurs. Res. 29:123, March-April 1980.

Posavac, E.J., and Carey, R.G.: Program evaluation: methods and case studies, Englewood Cliffs, N.J., 1980, Prentice-Hall, Inc.

Program evaluation, NLN Pub. No. 15-1738, New York, 1978, National League for Nursing.

Public Law 89-749, Comprehensive health planning and public services amendments of 1966, Nov. 3, 1966.

Public Law 79-725, Hospital survey and constuction act, Aug. 13, 1946.

Public Law 93-641, National health planning and resources development act, Jan. 4, 1975.

Rakich, J., Longest, B., and O'Donovan, T.: Managing health care organizations, Philadelphia, 1977, W. B. Saunders Co.

Roman, D.: The PERT system: an appraisal of program evaluation review technique. In Schulberg, H., et al., editors: Program evaluation in the health fields, New York, 1969, Behavioral Publications, Inc.

Rossi, P., and Freeman, H.: Evaluation: a systematic approach, Beverly Hills, Calif., 1982, Sage Publications, Inc.

Ruybal, S.: Community health planning, Fam. Community Health 1:9, 1978.

Schulbert, H. C., and Baker, F., editors: Program evaluation in the health fields, vol. 2, New York, 1979, Human Sciences Press.

Schulbert, H. C., Sheldon, A., and Baker, F.: Program evaluation in the health fields, New York, 1969, Behavioral Publications, Inc.

Shields, M.: An evaluation model for service programs, Nurs. Outlook 22:448, July 1974.

Soumelis, C.G.: Project evaluation methodologies and techniques, Paris, 1977, UNESCO.

Stufflebeam, D.L.: Evaluation as enlightenment for decision making. In Educational evaluation and decision making, Itasca, Ill., 1971, Peacock Publishers, Inc.

Suchman, E.A.: Evaluative research, New York, 1967, Russell Sage Foundation.

Welch, L.B., et al.: Program evaluation: an overview, Nurs. Health Care 1:186, Nov. 1980.

Wiest, J., and Levy, F.: A management guide to PERT/CPM, Englewood Cliffs, N.J., 1969, Prentice-Hall, Inc.

Wholey, J.S.: Perspective on evaluation from the U.S. Department of Health, Education, and Welfare, Nurs. Res. 29(2):109, 1980.

Chapter
10

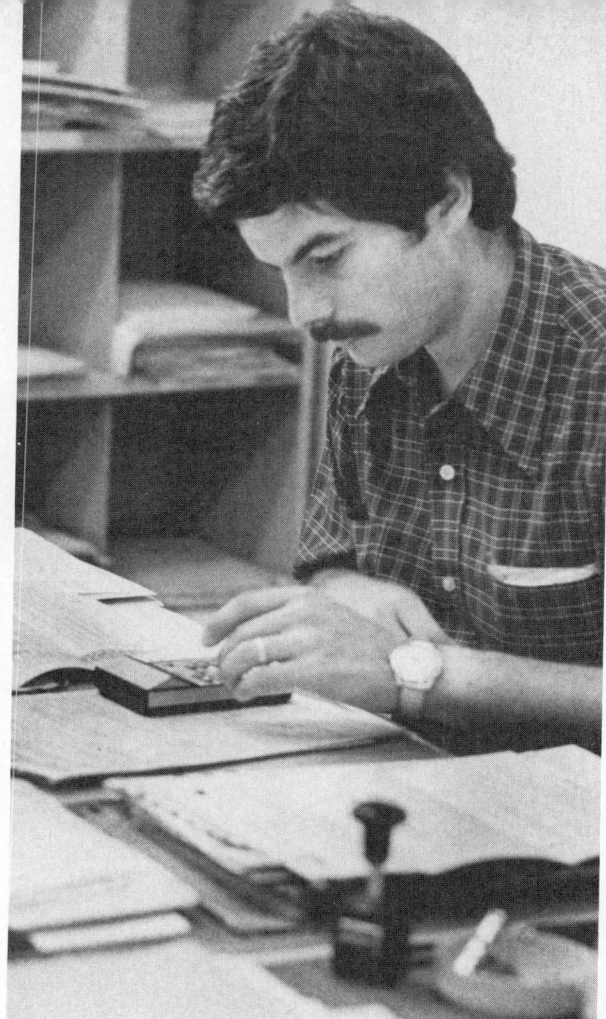

MARCIA STANHOPE

RECORD KEEPING AND QUALITY ASSURANCE IN COMMUNITY HEALTH NURSING

Because the health care delivery system has grown into the largest industry in the United States, resulting in considerable effect on the total population, society is demanding greater accountability and increased efficiency and effectiveness from the system. Quality assurance, or quality control, is the tool used in industry to assure the public that it is getting top value for money spent.

One may question why a system focused on the delivery of a service needs to be concerned with quality assurance. The major demand for quality assurance programs has resulted because of the vast changes that have occurred in the health care system over time. Some of these changes are increases in third-party in-

surance coverage, involvement of the federal government in the health care system, demand for service, technological advances, and numbers of health professionals providing care. Other changes include changing consumer expectations for cost, accessibility and equality, changing population demography, rising costs, and the monopolistic character of the system.

Both consumers and providers have a vested interest in the quality of the system. Jonas (1981) indicates that the health care provider has three basic reasons to be concerned about health care quality: (1) the principle of nonmaleficence—above all do no harm—has been a basic precept of the health care system since the writing of the Hippocratic Oath; (2) the principle of beneficience—do good work—is a basic precept of professionalism; and (3) the strong social work ethic in our culture which places a high value on "doing a good job in and of itself." Jonas says that in health care there is a direct link between doing a good job and individual survival.

Records are maintained on all clients of the health care system to provide complete information about the client and to show the extent and quality of care being given the client within the system. Records are an integral part of the system and of a quality assurance program. This chapter focuses on the development and implementation of a quality assurance program in community health nursing; on the components of a quality assurance program; on tools and methods for evaluating quality; and on the purposes, kinds, and documentation of records in community health nursing.

DEFINITIONS AND GOALS

Quality assurance is defined as the monitoring of the activities of client care to determine the degree of excellence attained in the implementation of the activities. The quality control process has been defined as "the comparison of actual results (performance) to expected results (desired outcomes) and the taking of corrective action when warranted and feasible" (Rakich et al., 1977, p. 322). An implicit factor in quality assurance is the accountability of the provider in the delivery of client services. *Accountability* means being responsible for activities of client care and being answerable to the client for the activities performed (Bergmen, 1980).

The goals of quality assurance are (1) to ensure the delivery of quality client care and (2) to demonstrate the health providers' efforts to fulfill their societal responsibility (Jonas, 1981; Rakich et al., 1977).

A variety of approaches and techniques are utilized in quality assurance programs. *Approaches* are methods used to ensure quality and *techniques* are tools for measuring quality (Jonas, 1981). This chapter describes several approaches and techniques used in quality assurance programs.

HISTORICAL DEVELOPMENT OF QUALITY ASSURANCE IN NURSING AND HEALTH CARE

Quality assurance approaches have been evident in nursing since Florence Nightingale in the 1860s called for a uniform format for the collection and presentation of hospital statistics to direct efforts to improve hospital treatment. One of the oldest quality assurance approaches, licensure, has been a major issue in nursing

since 1892. As mentioned in Chapter 1, by 1923 all states had permissive or mandatory laws directing nursing practice. Today revision of nurse practice acts is an ongoing process to assure the public that minimum competence in the expanding practice of nursing will be maintained (Bullough, 1975). From 1912 to 1939 the interest in quality nursing education led to the development of three nursing organizations involved in accrediting nursing programs: The National Organization for Public Health Nursing (1912) with accrediting programs in colleges and universities preparing public health nurses; the Association of Collegiate Schools of Nursing (1932), which required its member schools to meet certain educational standards; and the National League for Nursing Education (1939) with accrediting basic nursing programs (McCloskey, 1981).

The 1950s brought the development of tools to measure quality assurance. One of the first tools to be published was the Phaneuf Nursing Audit (1952), which has been used extensively in Community Health Nursing Practice.

In 1966 the American Nurses' Association (ANA) in its bylaws created the Divisions on Practice. From this came the charge in 1972 to the Congress for Nursing Practice to develop standards to be used in instituting quality assurance programs. The Standards for Community Health Nursing Practice were distributed to the ANA Community Health Nursing division members in 1973 and are listed in Appendix G (Blake, 1981).

In 1972, the year of the Congress for Nursing Practice, the Joint Commission on Accreditation of Hospitals (JCAH), already requiring hospitals to develop quality control systems, clearly delineated the responsibilities of nursing in its standards for nursing services. JCAH called upon nursing to clearly plan, document, and evaluate nursing care provided. During the same year the Social Security Act (Public Law 93-106) was amended to establish the Professional Standards Review Organization (PSRO) to mandate the review of the delivery of health care to recipients of Medicare, Medicaid, and maternal and child health benefits. Although PSRO was primarily designed for medical care evaluation, it has served to make quality assurance a primary issue for all professionals in health care delivery.

In nursing, efforts continue to be directed toward the development of approaches and techniques to assure quality nursing care. These efforts are evidenced in the quality assurance model developed by the ANA (1977), the study by Jacobs et al. (1978) to define critical requirements of safe practice, the ANA study of nurse credentials (1979), and the NLN study of accreditation (1979). Two efforts specifically directed toward strengthening community health nursing practice have been the development of frameworks for community health nursing practice by the ANA (1980) and the APHA (1980). A discussion of these two models can be found in Chapter 6.

APPROACHES FOR A QUALITY ASSURANCE PROGRAM

Two major categories of approaches exist in quality assurance—the general and the specific (Jonas, 1977). The general approach examines the person's or agency's ability to meet established criteria or standards at a given time. Examples of general quality assurance approaches used in the health care system are licensure, certification, and accreditation (Hinsvark, 1981; Jonas, 1981). *Credentialing* refers to the general quality control process indicating the attainment of minimum standards by the person or agency. Licensing, certification, and accreditation are all examples of approaches to credentialing.

According to Hinsvark (1981), the credentialing process has four functional components: (1) to produce a quality product; (2) to confer a unique identity, for example, registered nurse; (3) to protect the provider and the public; and (4) to control the profession. Credentialing has two basic components—mandatory and voluntary. *Mandatory credentialing* requires statutory law; state nurse practice acts are examples of mandatory credentialing. *Voluntary credentialing* is performed by an agency or institution. Certification examinations offered to nurses by the ANA are examples of voluntary credentialing.

Specific approaches to quality assurance are methods used to evaluate identified instances of provider and client interaction. Examples of specific approaches to quality control are agency staff review committees (peer review), utilization review committees, research studies, PSRO, client satisfaction surveys, and malpractice litigation. The overall goal of the specific quality assurance approaches is to monitor the events and outcomes of client care (LoGerfo and Brook, 1980). The functional components are (1) to identify problems between provider and client, (2) to intervene in problematical cases, (3) to provide feedback to the interaction participants, and (4) to provide documentation for interactions between provider and client.

The specific approaches are often voluntarily implemented by agencies and provider groups interested in the quality of interactions in their setting. However, the state and federal governments often call for a mandatory program to be established within public health agencies. For instance, through state departments of human resources and state health laws, regulations are set forth requiring periodic utilization review, peer reviews (audits), and other quality control measures within public health agencies that receive funds from state taxes, Medicaid, Medicare, and other public funding sources.

General Approaches
Licensure

Licensure is one of the oldest general quality assurance approaches in the United States. Licensure exists for both individuals and agencies. Approximately 35 professions and 17 types of agencies have mandatory licensure (Jonas, 1981).

Individual licensure is a contract between the profession and the state, in which the profession is granted control over entry into and exit from the profession and over quality of professional practice. Jonas (1981) cites several disadvantages to professional licensure: (1) professional self-interest, (2) questionable attention to regulating quality, (3) rigidity in job descriptions, (4) some limits on geographical mobility because of different state law requirements, and (5) discouraging of innovative and creative use of personnel.

When professionals are granted control over their own practice through licensure, questions arise about the professions's interest in safeguarding its own territory or protecting the consumer from unsafe practitioners. Will the profession be interested in regulating quality by setting standards of care and policing the profession to see that standards of care are upheld, or will the profession set standards and provide only a token sanction to those who do not uphold the practice standard?

The licensing process requires that regulations be written to define the scope and limits of the professional's practice. It is from these regulations that job descriptions evolve to set minimum and maximum limits on the functions and responsibilities of the practitioner. Some view the job descriptions as limiting practice to legally defined groups and as precluding people external to this defined group from being assigned duties normally practiced by the legally defined group. It is in this manner that employing agencies are restricted from hiring physical therapists, for example, for registered nurse positions.

Limited geographical mobility of professionals results because of differing licensure requirements from state to state. Although the nursing discipline enjoys *reciprocity,* or the recognition and acceptance of a professional's licensure between certain states, a nurse moving from one state to another could conceivably be required to meet a new set of criteria before receiving licensure in the new state. For example, state continuing education requirements or minimum licensure examination board scores may be different.

The issue over innovative and creative use of personnel led to a movement during the 70s in favor of *institutional licensure,* that is, allowing the employing agency to be responsible for the competence of the people they employ. This concept was not well received by the nursing and medical professions and to date has not been accepted as the answer to the disadvantages of professional licensure. The concern expressed is that poorly trained persons may be employed at minimum salaries to deliver a lower quality of health care to the consumer.

Licensure of nurses has been mandated by law *since 1903* when North Carolina, New York, New Jersey, and Virginia enacted laws on nurse registration. Today 49 of the 50 states have mandatory nurse licensure. *Mandatory nurse licensure* requires all who practice nursing for compensation to be licensed. One state has a *permissive licensure* law, meaning that a person can practice nursing without a license as long as the term *registered nurse* is not used and the practitioner does not purport to be licensed (Pinkerton, 1981).

Accreditation

Accreditation, a voluntary approach to quality control, is used for institutions whereas licensure is primarily used for individuals. From 1954 the National League for Nursing (NLN), a voluntary organization, has established standards for inspecting nursing education programs and community health–home health programs for the purpose of accrediting them. In addition, the state boards of nursing accredit basic nursing programs so their graduates may be eligible for the licensing examination. The accreditation function may be classified as *quasi-voluntary.* Although appearing to be a voluntary participatory program, accreditation is often linked to governmental regulation that encourages programs to participate in the accrediting process. Examples include the federal Medicare regulations restricting payments to accredited hospitals and home health care agencies and the federal program funding for nursing that is tied to the secretary of education's recognition of program accreditation by the NLN, by regional associations of colleges and secondary schools, or by designated state boards of nursing (Jonas, 1981; McCloskey, 1981).

Although accreditation of institutions assumes that certain standards of physical and organizational structure will assure quality health care or quality education at a given time, there are several arguments against the need for accreditation: (1) accreditation has not defined quality health care or education; (2) accreditation does not focus on health or educational outcomes; (3) review by colleagues is suspect, and self-interest may be promoted; (4) innovative and creative programs that deviate from established standards are discouraged; (5) institutional objectives are variable and not subject to standardization, thus making program comparisons meaningless; and (6) federal funding ties have caused accreditation to become quasi-voluntary (Jonas, 1981; McCloskey, 1981).

The advantages of accreditation are that it provides a means for effective peer review and an opportunity for an in-depth review of program strengths and limitations. However, since the accreditation process primarily evaluates physical structures, organizational structures, and personnel qualifications, serious consideration must be given to specific measures of the quality of health care delivery and to educational outcomes to provide more relevance to the accreditation process.

Certification

Certification, another general approach to quality, combines features of licensure and accreditation. Certification is usually a voluntary process within professions for looking at a person's educational achievements, experience, and achievements on examination to determine the person's qualifications for functioning in an identified specialty area, such as community health nursing.

In 1958 the ANA began to study implications for establishing a certification program in nursing. The reasons set forth for the need for such a program were to provide peer recognition to nurses involved in direct client care and to provide the health care consumer with further evidence of nursing's competence to accept increasing responsibilities in health care delivery. In 1966 five clinical units were established within the ANA to determine standards of nursing excellence: Medical-Surgical, Geriatric, Community Health, Psychiatric and Mental Health Nursing, and Maternal-Child Health. These units functioned to develop certification criteria, applicant eligibility, and certification mechanisms. In 1982 fifteen certification areas existed and 10,500 nurses had been certified by ANA since the programs inception (ANA, 1983). To become a certified community health nurse one must have a baccalaureate degree in nursing and 2 years of practice as a community health nurse immediately before application. In 1982 there were 217 certified community health nurses in the United States (ANA, 1983).

Certification has become a major issue in health care as evidenced by the proliferation of certification programs and the many organizations involved in the certification process. In 1971 the Department of Health, Education, and Welfare recommended that certification in health care be studied (ANA, 1979). In 1977 the

ANA study of credentialing in nursing was started. This study resulted in a proposal to establish an umbrella organization in nursing for credentialing so that "differences in certification could be eliminated and consistencies could be instituted for all nursing certification programs" (Jones, 1981).

Although usually a voluntary process, certification can be a quasi-voluntary process. For example, to function as a nurse practitioner in some states, one must show proof of educational credentials and take an examination in order to be "certified" to practice within the boundaries of the state.

The major concerns about certification as a quality assurance mechanism are that data are lacking about clinical competencies of the practitioner at the time of certification; data are lacking about the quality of the practitioner's output (competencies) following the certification process; and except for occupational health nurses, certification has not been recognized by employers as an achievement beyond basic preparation, so financial rewards have not occurred. Although the nursing profession has accepted the certification process as a mechanism for recognizing competence and excellence in nursing practice, certifiers must consider the utility and validity of the certification process as it is now set up and must be able to communicate to the public what it means to them to have certified nurses in health care delivery.

Other Approaches

Other general approaches to quality assurance defined in the ANA study of credentialing in nursing involve charter, recognition, and education degrees. *Charter* is the mechanism by which a state government agency, under state laws, grants corporate status to institutions with or without rights to award degrees. The ANA position is that a state government should charter not only university-based programs but nursing programs outside the university setting, such as hospital schools of nursing. *Recognition* is defined as a process whereby one agency accepts the credentialing status of and the credentials conferred by another. An example of *recognition* occurs when state boards of nursing accept the credentials of a nurse practitioner when the credentials are awarded by ANA or a specialty credentialing agency. *Academic degrees* are titles awarded individuals recognized by degree-granting institutions as having completed a predetermined plan in a branch of learning. At present there are four academic degrees awarded in nursing with some variations at each degree level: Associate of Arts/Science; Bachelor of Science in Nursing; the master's degrees—Master of Science in Nursing and Master of Nursing; and the doctorate in nursing—Doctor of Philosophy, Doctorate of Nursing

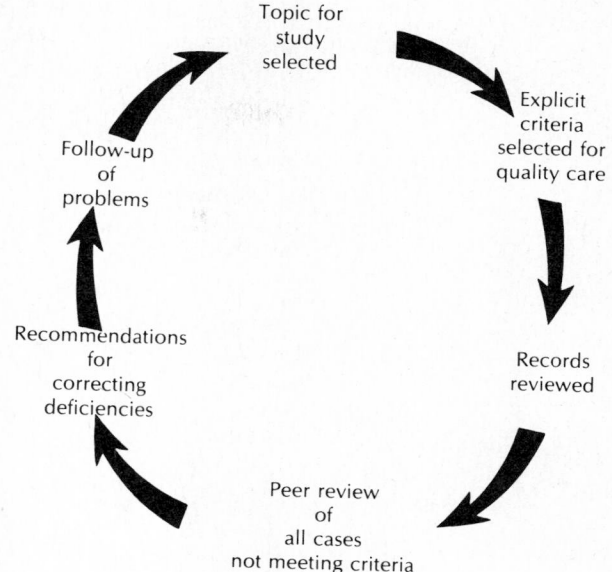

Fig. 10-1. The audit process.

Science, Doctorate of Science in Nursing, or Doctorate of Nursing.

Specific Approaches
Staff Review Committees

Staff review committees are the most common specific approach to quality assurance in the United States. Staff or peer review committees are designed to monitor client-specific aspects of care appropriate for certain levels of care. The audit has been the major tool used by peer review committees to ascertain quality of care. Specific kinds of audit instruments are presented later in this discussion. For explicit suggestions for the development of the peer review process, refer to the NLN administrator's handbook (CHHA/CHS, 1978).

The audit process (Fig. 10-1) consists of essentially six steps: (1) selection of a topic for study; (2) selection of explicit criteria for quality care; (3) review of records to see if criteria for quality care are met; (4) peer review of all cases that do not meet criteria for quality care; (5) specific recommendations to correct deficiencies, such as staff development programs, changes in procedures, or supervisor consultation with staff; and (6) follow-up of the topic to see that problems have been eliminated (LoGerfo and Brook, 1980).

Two types of audits are used in nursing peer review: concurrent and retrospective. The *concurrent audit* is a method of evaluating quality of ongoing care through appraisal of the nursing process. The advantages of the concurrent audit are (1) identification of deficiencies at the time care is given; (2) provision of a mechanism for identifying and meeting client needs during the caring process; (3) implementation of measures for fulfilling professional responsibilities to the consumer; and (4) provision of a mechanism for communicating on behalf of the client. The disadvantages of the concurrent audit are that (1) it is time consuming; (2) it is more costly to implement than the retrospective audit; and (3) since care is ongoing, it does not present the total picture of care the client will receive (Trussell and Strand, 1978).

The *retrospective audit* evaluates quality of care through appraisal of the nursing process following the client's discharge from the health care system. The advantages of the restrospective audit include that (1) it provides for comparison of actual practice to standards of care; (2) it provides for analysis of actual practice findings; (3) it provides a total picture of care given; and (4) it provides more accurate data on which to base corrective action. The retrospective audit has several disadvantages: (1) the focus of evaluation is directed away from ongoing care; (2) client problems are identified after discharge when there is no chance to assist that client with these problems; and (3) corrective action can only be used to improve practice for future clients. In 1972 the ANA published guidelines for peer review in nursing.

Utilization Review

Utilization review differs from peer review in that utilization review is directed toward assuring that care is actually needed and the cost is appropriate for the level of care provided. LoGerfo and Brook (1980) described three types of utilization review: (1) *prospective*—an assessment of the necessity of care before giving service; (2) *concurrent*—a review of the necessity of services while the care is being given; and (3) *retrospective*—an analysis of the services received by the client after the care has been given.

Utilization review grew in the mid twentieth century out of concern for increasing health care costs. The first committees were developed between insurance companies and professional groups and became mandatory under the 1965 Medicare Law as a cost control measure (Jonas, 1981; LoGerfo and Brook, 1980).

The utilization review process includes the development of explicit criteria that serve as indicators of the need for services and the length of service. Utilization review has been used primarily in hospitals to establish need for client admission and the length of hospital stay. In community health, especially home health care, utilization review establishes criteria for admission to agency service, the number of visits a client may receive, the eligibility for client services such as a nursing aide or physical therapist, and discharge. Chapter 35 discusses eligibility criteria for home health clients under federally regulated programs. If clients do not meet established criteria or if services are overutilized by the agency on the client's behalf, then the agency is sanctioned or denied reimbursement by third party payers for services provided the clients.

Utilization review has several advantages: (1) it is designed to assist clients to avoid unnecessary care; (2) it may serve to encourage the choice of care options by providers, such as home health care rather than hospitalization; (3) it can provide guidelines for staff and program development; and (4) it provides a measure of agency accountability to the consumer. The major disadvantage to utilization review is that not all clients fit the classic picture presented by the "explicit criteria" that serves as the basis for approval or denial of care. For example, an elderly female client is admitted to the home health care agency for management after hospital discharge. The client is paraplegic as result of CVA. After several weeks of physical therapy and speech therapy the client showed little sign of progress. The utilization review committee considered the client's condition to be stable and did not recognize the continued need for management to prevent future complications. Medicare payment was denied.

Within the utilization review process of Medicare and Medicaid, appeal mechanisms have been built in. The appeal allows providers and clients to present additional data that may help to reverse the original decision to deny payment.

For explicit suggestions on the development of utilization review process, refer to the NLN administrator's handbook (CHHA/CHS, 1978).

Professional Standards Review Organizations

Professional Standards Review Organizations (PSRO) program was established in 1972 in an amendment to the Social Security Act (Public Law 92-603) as a publicly mandated utilization and peer review program. This law provided that medical, hospital, and nursing home care under Medicare, Medicaid, and Title V Maternal and Child Health Programs would be reviewed for appropriateness and necessity and would be reimbursed accordingly.

The PSRO program was designed to have three components: (1) concurrent review to certify the necessity of client admission and continued hospital stay; (2) medical care evaluation studies (MCE) in which a topic for study is chosen and a retrospective analysis is used to determine quality of care and effective use of health care services (the MCE study process is the same as the audit process described in Fig. 10-1); and (3) a profile analysis in which aggregate statistical data are collected and which serves to identify utilization practices, to determine topics for MCE, to monitor effectiveness of review activities, and to establish local, regional, and national utilization norms (HCFA, 1979; Werner, 1981).

The PSRO programs have been administered by the Office of Professional Standards Review Organizations, Health Standards and Quality Bureau of Health Care Financing Administration (HCFA), since 1977. The PSRO regulations require that management applications be submitted to HCFA by an agency in order to be recognized as one of the 203 official PSROs designated under the law. State medical societies and nonprofit foundations for medical care were primarily awarded these management contracts. These designated agencies through their boards, which have a physician proportion of 51%, were to set local PSRO policies. The actual implementation and plan of utilization review could be controlled by the PSRO or could occur within the hospital. Within the hospital setting there was usually a nurse coordinator to conduct the concurrent medical review program (Werner, 1981).

Community health agencies and nursing services were omitted under the original PSRO guidelines, although the PSRO regulations established an option to include community health agencies at some future date. In 1974 PSRO contracted with the ANA to develop criteria for review of nursing care and guidelines for the participation of nurses in PSRO. Although the 1977 amendments to PSRO called for more nursing involvement in national policy making, to date, little evidence can be cited that this has occurred. With the introduction of "New Federalism" by President Reagan, there is doubt that publicly supported PSROs will continue. The 1982 Tax Equity and Fiscal Responsibilty Act abolished the PSRO program and established the Utilization and Quality Control Peer Review Program.

Evaluative Studies

Evaluative studies for quality health care have grown throughout the twentieth century. Three major models have been used to evaluate quality: Donabedian's structure-process-outcome model, the sentinel model, and the tracer model.

Donabedian (1966) introduced three major methods of evaluating quality care. These methods are *structure*—the evaluation of the setting and instrumentalities used to provide care, such as facilities, equipment, characteristics of the administrative organization, client mix, and the qualifications of the health providers; *process*—the evaluation of activities as they relate to standards and expectations of health providers in the management of client care; and *outcomes*—the net changes that occur as a result of health care or the net results of health care.

Data for structural evaluations can be obtained from the existing documents of an agency or from an inspection of a facility. For example, if one wants to do an evaluative study of structure in community health nursing, one might look at the ratio of nurses to clients, at the educational preparation of nurses and the ratio of nurses to clients with different disability levels, and at the defined responsibilities of nurses with different educational preparation in the organizational structure and their actual responsibilities. Two major assumptions relate to structurally oriented studies: (1) that if the organizational structure is optimal, better care will be provided; and (2) that quality of organization, physical structure, and staff can be described (Jonas, 1981; Williams, 1980).

Data for process evaluations can be collected through direct observation of provider encounters and review of records. Examples of process-oriented studies abound in the nursing literature. An audit instrument with established criteria for evaluating nursing performance is an example of a useful method for a process-oriented nursing study. The basis for a process-oriented study can be direct observation of client care using a client encounter protocol, which identifies the nurse's activities relative to history taking, nursing diagnosis, implementing appropriate nursing procedures, providing appropriate illness prevention and health promotion counseling, and record keeping.

The assumptions underlying process evaluative studies are that (1) health care is necessary to prevent illness and maintain or promote health; (2) good health care leads to good outcomes; and (3) good health care can be defined (Jonas, 1981).

Both the checklist approach and the criteria mapping approach are used to establish the client encounter protocol. The checklist approach is simply a "laundry list" of activities the nurse should perform to give good care. Table 10-1 illustrates a checklist approach to evaluate the community health nurse working with a hypertensive client. The criteria mapping approach is similar to clinical decision making. In criteria mapping an evaluation of good care depends on the presence or absence of certain signs, symptoms, or client needs in a specific situation. Table 10-1 also illustrates the criteria mapping approach to evaluation.

Data for outcome evaluative studies can be collected from vital statistics records, such as death certificates, in-person or telephone client interviews, mailed questionnaires, and client records. Nurses need to engage in more outcome-oriented studies to show nursing's efficacy in health care delivery. Community health nursing could study the outcome of various screening techniques used with clients. For example, when hearing and screening tests are performed on a group of school children, follow-up data could be collected from physi-

Table 10-1. Comparison of checklist approach and criteria mapping approach for assessing the process of care in a home visit to *selectively* assess client with diagnosed hypertension

Checklist	Criteria mapping
Observe and assess	**Observe and assess**
Temperature, pulse, and respiration	Temperature, pulse, and respiration
Blood pressure	Blood pressure — lying, sitting, and standing:
Intake and output	*If pressure variation between three readings is wide:*
Edema	Check side effects of medications
Instructions to client	Check medication compliance
Taking own blood pressure	Consult physician
Accurate measure of intake and output	*If orthostatic hypotension is evident:*
	Instruct client to stand up slowly and to sit or lie down if dizziness occurs
	Check known side effects of prescribed medications
	Edema
	If increase is noted:
	Check client's weight
	Check medication prescribed
	Check medication compliance
	Give client instructions:
	Avoid restrictive clothing
	Tie shoelaces loosely
	Never cross legs
	Elevate legs while sitting
	Avoid salt in foods
	Weigh self same time each day
	Intake and output
	If intake and output are inadequate:
	Instruct client on accurate measuring and recording
	Instruct client on amounts and kinds of fluids to drink for 24 hours

cians' records to determine the number of false positive cases identified by the nurses performing the tests. Such a study would provide data about community health nurses' abilities to perform effective screening tests.

Two categories of outcome measures are reflected in the literature: general health status indicators, or the physical, emotional, and social aspects of health; and disease specific indicators, which include morbidity and mortality, presence of symptoms, and behavioral disabilities known to occur with a specific disease. The basic assumption underlying outcome studies is that health care interventions will change the person's health status.

The tracer method described by Kessner and Kalk (1973) is a measure of both process and outcome of care. This method is more effective in evaluating health care of groups rather than of individual clients and in evaluating care delivered by an institution rather than by an individual provider.

To use the tracer method, one must identify a volume of clients with particular characteristics requiring specific health care management. Kessner and Kalk (1973) described the following essential characteristics for implementing the tracer method. A tracer, or a problem, should have a definite impact on the client's level of function; well-defined and easily diagnosed characteristics; population prevalence high enough to permit adequate data collection; a known variation resulting from utilization of effective medical care; well-defined management techniques in either prevention, diagnosis, treatment, or rehabilitation; and understood (documented) effects of nonmedical factors on the tracer. Stevens (1975) provided a taxonomy for selecting client groups for tracer outcome studies in nursing: (1) a particular disease; (2) similar treatment; (3) similar needs; (4) similar community; (5) similar life-style; and (6) similar illness stage.

The tracer method has been used by physicians and by nurse practitioners to identify persons with certain illnesses, such as hypertension, ulcers, and urinary tract infections, and to establish criteria for good medical and nursing management of the illnesses. The criteria has been used by peer review panels to evaluate the actual care given and to evaluate the changes in client status (Brook and Appel, 1973; Sibley et al., 1975). Except in the case of nurse practitioners, nursing has not used this evaluative method. The tracer method seemingly could provide nurses with data to show the differences in outcome as a result of nursing care standards.

In 1976 Rutstein described the sentinel method of quality evaluation based on the epidemiological method. This method is an outcome measure for examining specific instances of client care. The characteristics of this method are as follows: (1) cases of unnecessary disease, disability, complications, and untimely death are counted; (2) the circumstances surrounding the unnecessary event, or the *sentinel,* are examined in detail; (3) a review of morbidity and mortality is used as an index to determine a critical increase in the untimely event, which may reflect changes in quality of care; and (4) health status indicators such as changes in social, economic, political, and environmental factors are reviewed, which may have an effect on health outcomes. Changes in the sentinel indicate potential problems for others. For example, increases in mosquito populations may result in an increase in encephalitis in certain communities. Chapter 7 discusses the application of epidemiology in community health nursing.

Client Satisfaction

Client satisfaction is another specific approach to measuring quality of care. Client satisfaction can be assessed using in-person or telephone interviews and mailed questionnaires. Data from client satisfaction surveys are used to measure structure, process, and outcome of care given. In community health nursing, satisfaction surveys are used to assess care received during a specific agency admission, the clients personal nursing care, or the total care the client received from all services. Satisfaction surveys may measure the technical content of client care, attitudes about the care received and the providers of care, and perceptions of the situation (environment) in which the care was received. A study of client satisfaction conducted by Birch and Wolfe (1975) has indicated that clients are more critical of interpersonal and situational components of care than they are of the content of care. This may be true because consumers want to be treated as human beings and, given this treatment, trust the provider to have the ability to provide good care; consumers may not understand what is ideal care; or they may fear reprisal if they complain.

Satisfaction surveys are an essential aspect of quality assessment because the survey data give us clues to reasons for client compliance or noncompliance with plans of care. The surveys provide data about health-seeking behaviors, the likelihood of malpractice litigation, and the likelihood of continuing client-provider-agency relationships. The NLN (CHHA/CHS, 1978) provides an example of a client satisfaction survey (Discharged Patient Questionnaire) which can be used in a community health agency (Appendix A).

Malpractice Litigation

Malpractice litigation will only be mentioned here as a specific approach to quality assurance imposed on the health care delivery system by the legal system. Malpractice litigation typically results from client dissatis-

faction with the provider and with the content of care received. Medical literature abounds with examples of cases of malpractice that flourished through the 70s. Several reasons were given for the increase in malpractice suits: some provider care was of poor or doubtful quality and was recognized as such by the consumers; professions were not showing the capability to police their own ranks and reduce the risk of poor quality care to the consumers; and there was an apparent deterioration in provider and client relationships (Jonas, 1981). Nursing is not immune from malpractice litigation. A discussion of legal issues affecting community health nurses can be found in Chapter 5. If community health nursing establishes a sound quality assurance program, thereby policing its own client care quality, the risk of quality control measures being imposed by an external source such as the legal system can be reduced.

MODEL QUALITY ASSURANCE PROGRAM

The primary purpose of a quality assurance program is to ensure that the results of an organized activity are consistent with the expectations from the organized activity (Rakich, 1977). To evaluate the total picture of organized activity, the structure, process, and outcome components of health care delivery should be considered. All personnel affected by a quality assurance program should be involved in the development and implementation of the program components including administration, management, and staff. If personnel arrive at the agency after the quality assurance program has been developed, then adequate orientation to the program should be provided and personnel acceptance of the program should be assessed.

In 1977 the ANA introduced a schema for a model quality assurance program. The box on p. 228 depicts the model, which identifies these seven basic components of a quality assurance program: identifying values; identifying structure, process, and outcome standards and criteria; selecting measures (techniques) to assess the degree of attainment of the standards and criteria; making interpretations about the strengths and weaknesses of care given; identifying alternative courses of action; choosing courses of action; and taking action.

To use the ANA schema for quality assurance, an organization formulates objectives for the total agency. These objectives are used to form subobjectives, or level objectives, for each service provided by the agency and for each category of provider in each service, for example, nursing services and all personnel employed by nursing services in the public health department.

Once objectives are formulated, the required input

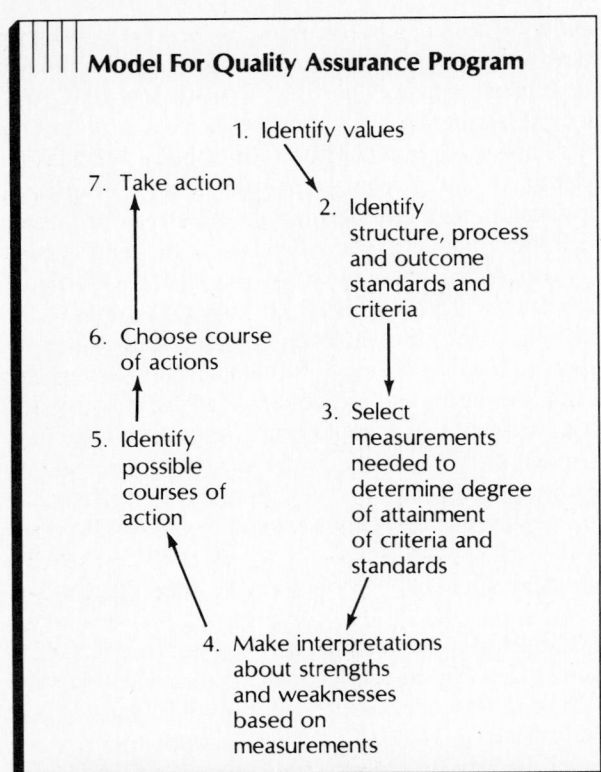

Model For Quality Assurance Program

1. Identify values

2. Identify structure, process and outcome standards and criteria

3. Select measurements needed to determine degree of attainment of criteria and standards

4. Make interpretations about strengths and weaknesses based on measurements

5. Identify possible courses of action

6. Choose course of actions

7. Take action

From American Nurses' Association: Quality model: a plan for implementation of the standards of nursing practice, Kansas City, Mo., 1977, The Association. Reprinted with permission of ANA.

resources are identified to accomplish the objectives. Need for the input resources of manpower, supplies and equipment, facilities, and finances are described. If the required input resources are not available to implement the identified objectives, an organization is restricted in the delivery of a quality service to the consumer. In determining necessary program input, community resources and consumer needs and wants must be examined to plan realistic programs for a community. Consider an example in which the Public Health Department has surveyed the community and identified consumer interest in a new family planning program. The objectives for the program have been written and the nursing services office has been directed to open the clinics by the beginning of the new year. However, the director of nurses has been unable to employ enough nurses for the clinic to begin. Therefore the administration decides that without nurse power the clinic cannot deliver quality services, and the opening of the clinic is postponed until all input resources are available to meet the program objectives.

Once input resources are determined, then policies, procedures, and job descriptions are formulated to serve as behavioral guides to the employees of the agency. These documents should reflect the essential

provider qualifications needed to implement the services of the agency.

Establishing organization objectives, identifying necessary input resources, and formulating policies, procedures, and job descriptions will lead to the development of standards, identification of efficient provider activity, delineation of program costs, and utilization of resources.

Values Identification

Values identification, the first step in a quality assurance program, serves to define the beliefs of the agency about humanity, nursing the community, and health. The development of an agency philosophy describes the nature and the scope of services to be provided by the agency; the clients to be served such as the individual (across the age span), families, groups, and communities; the services to be offered; and the available resources to provide services. The philosophy will also describe the goals of health care services to be offered by the agency, such as primary, secondary, and tertiary prevention goals. Once the philosophy and objectives are written, Donabedian's framework for evaluating health care programs can be actively used.

Identification of Standards and Criteria

Identification of standards and criteria for quality assurance begins with the writing of the philosophy and objectives of the organization. The philosophy and objectives of an agency serve to define the *structural standards* of the agency. Evaluation of structure is a specific approach to quality appraisal. In evaluating the *structure* of an organization, the evaluator ascertains whether the agency is adhering to the stated philosophy and objectives. Is the agency providing services to populations across the age span? Are primary, secondary, and/or tertiary preventive services offered? Other standards of structure are defined by the licensing or accrediting agency, such as the NLN standards for accrediting home health agencies (NLN, 1980). Other standards of structure include the organizational chart, which shows supervisory methods, communication patterns, staffing patterns, and sometimes staff assignments. How assignments are made, the client mix, and staff qualifications are also standards of structure used to evaluate the quality of an agency. These are several questions the evaluator can ask about the standards of structure: Does the agency use the methods of supervision described in the policies and procedures? Do the nurses function within the scope of their job descriptions? Do staff members have the qualifications required by this agency? *Review of agency documents* (audit), *self-studies*, and *utilization review* are the techniques employed for evaluating agency structure.

Standards of structure are evaluated internally by a committee composed of administration, management, and staff members for the purpose of issuing a self-study report quarterly, annually, or before an accreditation visit by a state or a voluntary agency. Standards of structure are also evaluated by a group external to the agency. Utilization review committees are often composed of an external advisory group with community representatives for all services offered through an agency, such as nurse, physical therapist, speech therapist, physician, board member, and administrator from a sister agency.

The evaluation of *process standards* is a more specific appraisal of the quality of care being given by agency providers. Criteria for evaluating the activities of all agency personnel need to be defined to make inferences about the quality of care received by the agencies' clients. Agencies use a variety of methods to determine criteria for evaluating provider activities. An agency can choose to develop process standards around one of the conceptual models described in Chapter 6 such as a developmental model. An agency can choose to use the standards of care set forth by the providers' professional organization, such as the ANA community health nursing standards; or in the case of nursing one can use the nursing process and apply it to the activities of the nurse as the activities correspond to the procedures of care defined by the agency.

The primary approaches used for process evaluation include the peer review committee and the client satisfaction survey. The techniques employed for process evaluation are direct observation, questionnaire, interview, written audit, and videotape of client and provider encounters.

Numerous *audit instruments* can be found in the nursing literature to evaluate the process of care. The instrument most often used in community health nursing is the Phaneuf Nursing Audit (Phaneuf, 1976). This 50-item instrument measures seven functions of professional nursing as they relate to the nursing process. This instrument is an example of a retrospective audit instrument that presents a picture of the total nursing care received by the discharged client. The instrument has been found to have a measure of internal validity and reliability (Stanhope, 1981; Stanhope and Murdock, 1981).

Two tools that have often been used in conjunction with the Phaneuf Nursing Audit are the Slater Nursing Competencies Rating Scale and the Quality Patient Care Scale (Felton, 1975). The Slater Nursing Competencies Scale is an 84-item scale intended to rate nurses' performances in the clinical setting after direct observation of an identified number of nurse and client encounters. The nurse's performance is judged against criterion variables representative of a gamut of nursing responsibilities for providing client care (Wandelt and Stewart, 1975). Ager reported a measure of validity and reliability for this instrument.

The Quality Patient Care Scale (QUALPACS) is a 68-item scale intended to measure the quality of care received by clients either by direct nurse-client encounters or from interventions with others on behalf of the client (Wandelt and Ager, 1975). Ager (1975) reported a measure of validity and reliability for QUALPACS.

Other nursing audit instruments or methodologies that may be used or adapted to evaluate process are the Rush-Presbyterian-St. Luke's Medical Center–Medicus Methodology for Monitoring Quality Patient Care (Jelinek et al., 1974), the Professional Practitioner's Performance Rating Scale (Dunn, 1970), the CASH Nursing Care Evaluation Instrument (Smith, 1975), the Critical Incident Performance Appraisal System (Brief, 1979), the Professional Nurse Performance Evaluation Method (Bernhardt and Schuette, 1975), or the Standards of Nursing Care by Carter (1976).

The client satisfaction survey may also be used to evaluate the process of ongoing care as documented in the literature (Trussell and Strand, 1978). The survey may be conducted by direct interview or by questionnaire.

Once data are collected to evaluate nursing process standards, the peer review committee reviews the data to identify strengths and weaknesses in the quality of care delivered. The peer review committee is usually an internal committee composed of representatives of the nursing staff who are trained to administer audit instruments and conduct client interviews.

The evaluation of outcome standards, or the end results of nursing care, is one of the more difficult tasks facing nursing today. To be able to identify net changes in the client's health status as a result of nursing care will give the nursing profession data to show the efficacy of nursing in the health care delivery system. Research studies using the tracer method or the sentinel method to identify client outcomes and client satisfaction surveys are approaches that may be used to evaluate outcome standards. Techniques that can be used to evaluate outcome standards are client classification systems that use admission data on the client's level of dependence or client's problems and discharge data that may show changes in levels of dependence (Daubert, 1977; Martin, 1982; Rosser and Watts, 1972), admission and discharge data, morbidity data, community agency readmission data, the community agency referral to hospital, and client satisfaction surveys.

Rissner (1975) developed a client satisfaction survey to evaluate client attitudes and the content of nursing care in a primary care setting. Decker et al. (1979) reported the development of criteria sets for evaluating outcome of community health nursing care, and Kline et al. (1980) reported the development of a process and outcome evaluation program for community health nursing in the state of Georgia. However, community health nursing has been primarily involved in evaluating program outcome to justify program expenditures rather than in evaluating client outcome. Outcome evaluation assumes that health care has a net positive effect on client status. The major problem with outcome evaluation is determining which nursing care variables are primarily responsible for causing changes in client status. In community health nursing there are multiple uncontrolled variables in the field which have an effect on client status, such as environment and family relationships, and it is often difficult to determine whether these extraneous variables are the cause of changes in client status or whether nursing interventions have the most effect.

Criteria and Standards Evaluative Measures

Selection of measures to determine the degree of attainment of criteria and standards has been discussed in the previous section. To summarize, the approaches and techniques used to evaluate structural standards and criteria are utilization reviews, review of agency documents, self-studies, and review of physical facilities. The approaches and techniques for the evaluation of process standards and criteria are peer review, client satisfaction surveys, direct observations, questionnaires, interviews, written audits, and videotapes. The evaluative approaches for outcome standards and criteria include research studies, client satisfaction surveys, client classification, admission, readmission and discharge data, and morbidity data.

The approaches and techniques an agency uses in a quality assurance program often depend on the state or federal guidelines that must be followed to satisfy credentialing requirements. Regardless of the scope of the governmental requirements, a model quality assurance program should include measures for evaluating structure, process, and outcome standards and criteria. Inferences made about the quality of services delivered by an agency are dependent on evaluating all aspects of the health care agency.

Health Provider Evaluation

Inherent in any quality assurance program should be the individual evaluation of health provider personnel. Although the overall agency structure, the process of care delivered by health provider groups, and client outcome may be evaluated, it is also essential to determine the individual provider's contribution to the overall picture of the quality of the agency to protect the

individual clients who are the recipients of the provider's care.

Past history of the evaluative process indicates that *personnel evaluation* has often been based on traditional trait ratings of personality and performance traits. Examples of trait rating measures are personal appearance, leadership, responsibility, accuracy, creativity, and ability to articulate. The problem with these measures is that they are not specific enough to measure concrete behavior and therefore are subject to broad interpretation by evaluators (Porter et al., 1974).

The present trend in personnel evaluation is to use appraisals based on specific performance objectives. Porter describes three methods used to evaluate performance: single global ratings, behaviorally anchored ratings, and objectives-oriented ratings.

The *single global ratings* scale includes a number of behaviors that are all-inclusive of the performance expected of a nurse in community health. Supervisors rate nurses on all the behaviors and assign a total score or single rating for overall job performance. One aspect of the Phaneuf Nursing Audit is the provision of a single global rating of a nurse in which the nurse may be rated as excellent, good, average, poor, or unsafe in the delivery of nursing care. The global rating for the Phaneuf audit is obtained by adding the score obtained by the nurse on 50 identified behaviors. Based on the total points received, the nurse is then assigned a quality rating of excellent to unsafe.

This type of performance evaluation technique allows for comparison of a nurse with peers and offers a mechanism for effectively attaining agreement among separate supervisor ratings. However, global ratings do not relate directly to specific behaviors of the nurse and do not contribute to motivation for change, planning for staff development, or the development of better job descriptions. For the nurse with a low level of trust in the organization, this type of rating may lead to defensiveness and rejection of the evaluation. This rating scale is often used to make decisions about raises and promotions because of the ease with which supervisors can compare employees and because the rating is seemingly reflective of a number of behaviors included in a total scale.

Behaviorally anchored ratings are evaluative tools that include direct observation of a list of behaviors the nurse should perform in delivering quality care. An example of a behaviorally anchored rating in nursing is the Slater Nursing Competencies Scale. Such a scale allows the supervisor to rate the nurse on a list of behaviors that can be generalized to all nurses. This type of scale provides a better rating method than the single global ratings scale because certain nurse behaviors can be assessed. Development of better job descriptions could result from the assessment of nurse

Table 10-2. Select advantages and disadvantages of health provider evaluation methods

Method	Advantages	Disadvantages
Trait ratings	Inexpensive Less time consuming	Permit subjective interpretation by evaluator Examine nonspecific behaviors
Objectives-oriented ratings	Pinpoint performance deficiencies Provide self-evaluation Collect data specific to evaluatee Motivate personnel	Expensive Time consuming Difficult to compare groups of providers Evaluation of merit difficult
Behaviorally anchored ratings	Collect data specific to group, such as nurses Give better overall performance rating Pinpoint deficiencies for staff development Provide comparative measures for groups Useful for evaluating merit	Expensive Require direct supervisor observation, therefore time consuming Ratings nonspecific to individual behavior
Single global ratings	Provide comparative measures for group Inexpensive Collect data from records Less time consuming	Unable to pinpoint behaviors specific to provider Nonmotivating Unable to pinpoint specific deficiencies Unable to use to develop job descriptions

behaviors in a specific setting, such as community health. The behaviorally anchored rating scale, however, will not give nurses a rating based on behaviors specific to the individual and may not enhance motivation to develop objectives for future job improvement. This scale may provide data about behaviors that are performed well, performed poorly, or are missing. The data can be used as a basis for staff development programs to improve care delivered by the agency nurses.

The *objectives-oriented ratings* tools are developed jointly between the supervisor and the nurse. These tools reflect agreement on specific performance objectives to be met by the nurse as well as on how these objectives are to be measured.

The development of objectives-oriented rating tools allows staff members to have input into their evaluation and also allows the supervisor to collect data specific to the individual about acceptable levels of performance and attainment of specific goals. This type of performance rating is said to be both more objective and explicit to the nurse; it allows the supervisor to pinpoint specific accomplishments of individuals and allows these persons to say how they have met their goals (self-evaluation). When evaluation focuses on individual accomplishments, the nurse becomes less defensive and is more motivated to attain future goals because of the personal feedback given about job performance (Porter et al., 1974).

The objectives-oriented rating is not always the evaluative method of choice; it is difficult to compare groups of nurses since evaluative objectives and measures are specific to each individual. Determining pay raises and promotions based on merit becomes more

difficult, since it is possible for several persons to meet their objectives but to function at different performance levels.

Instances occur when different ones of the performance evaluation measures discussed may be more appropriately used. The advantages and disadvantages of each method are outlined in Table 10-2. The objectives-oriented approach is the most costly to implement because of its individualized nature; the behaviorally anchored ratings are also costly because they require direct behavioral observations by supervisors; and the single global ratings are least costly because data can be collected from client records and do not require direct supervisor observations.

The behaviorally anchored and the objectives-oriented ratings are more useful in pinpointing behaviors specific to groups and individuals respectively and provide better performance ratings, better data for staff development, and better data for developing job descriptions. The behaviorally anchored and the single global ratings provide better comparative measures and are more useful for determining promotions and pay raises. The three behaviorally oriented evaluative approaches are preferable to the trait ratings because of the differences in subjectivity and specificity of the evaluation.

Interpreting Measurement Data

Interpreting measurement data is an essential component of the quality assurance process because it allows for the identification of discrepancies between the quality care standards of the agency and the actual practice of the health providers; data interpretation most importantly allows for the identification of strengths in the implementation of the standards of care.

Once the approaches and techniques to be used in the quality assurance program are determined, the program must be organized and implemented so that patterns of health care delivery can be established for the agency. These patterns must reflect the total agency functioning over time to generate valid data on which to base decisions about the strengths and limitations in meeting the agency's standards and criteria. The amounts of time and the effects on identifying substandard performance were discussed by Porter et al. (1974) as a factor to consider in the evaluation process. Problems with agency structure and client outcome may take a longer time to identify than process performance problems. In process evaluation the time spent may not be long enough when evaluating a process using concurrent audits or when using behaviorally anchored personnel evaluation ratings. The nurse may say that these ratings do not accurately reflect total performance in providing client care and may ignore the evaluation as irrelevant to actual performance. However, if all performance decisions are based on retrospective audit data, the interval between appraisals may be too long and the nurse may ignore the evaluation as irrelevant to present practice performance. Some combination of ongoing and retrospective evaluation may be essential to make process evaluation meaningful.

Selected regular intervals for evaluation should be established within the agency and periodic reports written so the combined results of the elements of structure, process, and outcome efforts can be analyzed and health care delivery patterns and problems can be identified. These reports should be collected and used for comparison to establish an ongoing picture of changes occurring within the agency.

Action Identification

Identification and choices of possible courses of action to correct the weaknesses within the agency should involve both the administration and the staff. The courses of action chosen should be based on their significance, economic benefit, and timeliness (Porter et al., 1974; Rakich et al., 1977). For example, if there is a nursing problem dealing with the recording of client health education, the agency administration and staff may analyze the problem to see why it is occurring. If the reasons given by the nurses include lack of time to do paperwork properly, case overloads that reduce the amount of time spent with clients, or lack of available resources for health education, it may not be significant to choose to provide a staff development program on the importance of recording and doing health education. It may be more important to assess how to provide the time and resources necessary for the nurses to offer health education to clients. Economically it may be more beneficial to provide dictating equipment and clerical assistance so nurses can dictate notes and other paperwork, thereby providing more client contact time, or it may be economically more beneficial to employ an additional nurse and reduce nurse caseloads.

The timeliness of the courses of action identified and chosen is also critical. If the recording problem has been a recurrent one and has not been shared with the staff and if administration decides to make unilateral decisions to reduce caseloads or introduce dictating equipment, the decisions may be viewed by the staff as negative and may result in reduced motivation and poorer job performance (Porter et al., 1974). However, when time is allowed for staff members to give input into decisions that directly affect their work, they will tend to be more committed to the decisions and more motivated to improve the standards of health care delivery.

Taking Action

Taking action is the final step in the quality assurance model. Once the alternative courses of action are chosen, actions must be implemented for change to occur in the overall operation of the agency. Follow-up and evaluation of actions taken must occur in order for improvement in quality of care to be assumed. Documentation is essential to the evaluation of quality care in any organization. The following section focuses on the kind of documentation that normally occurs in a community health agency.

RECORDS
Purposes of Records

Records are an integral part of the communication structure of the health care organization. Accurate and complete records are required by law and must be kept by all agencies, governmental and nongovernmental. In most states, the state departments of health stipulate the kind and content requirements of records for community health agencies.

Records serve the purposes of providing complete information about the client, indicating the extent and quality of services being rendered, resolving legal issues in malpractice suits, and providing information for education and research (Warren, 1978).

Community Health Agency Records

Within the community health agency many types of records are kept and used to predict population trends in a community, identify health needs and problems, analyze health trends, plan programs, evaluate programs, prepare and justify budgets, and make administrative decisions (Hanlon and Pickett, 1979). The kinds of records kept by the community health agency may include *reports* of accidents, births, census, chronic disease, communicable disease, mortality, life expectancy, and morbidity, reports of child and spouse abuse, reports of occupational illness and injury, and reports of environmental health.

Other types of records kept within the agency are *records* used to maintain administrative contact and control of the units (departments) of the organization. Three types of records make up this category: clinical, financial, and service. The *clinical record* is the client health record, or chart, used by all health care providers for the purpose of communicating observations, interventions, and prescribed regimens for client care. The clinical record consists of two major content sections: the client's history, including such information as client demography, admission data, primary provider's name, chief health problem, and financial information; and the clinical history, which includes diagnosis, progress notes, physical examination and health assessment, past history of health or illness problems, consultations and referrals, flow charts of medications, diagnostic studies and vital signs, and discharge summaries (Warren, 1978).

The *provider service records* include information about the numbers of home visits made daily, transportation and mileage, the providers' time spent with the client, and the amount and kinds of supplies used. The service record is completed on a daily basis by each provider, summarized weekly for a record of individual personnel service and payment, and summarized monthly and annually to indicate trends in health care activities and costs relative to personnel time, transportation, maintenance, and supplies. The provider service records are used to correlate with the agencies' *financial records* of salaries, overhead, and transportation costs and serve as the basis for the cost accounting system (Hanlon and Pickett, 1979).

Three additional kinds of service records seen in the community health agency are the *central index system,* the *annual implementation report,* and the *annual summary* of agency activities. The central index system is a data filing system that indicates the services requested, services offered, active and inactive clients of the agency, and a profile of the agency's clients. The central index system may be subdivided into a computer file for ready retrieval of the these data, and the actual chart files that are centrally located in a records office (library) for easy retrieval by health providers. The central index file serves to organize the ongoing activities of the agency and to summarize the history of the agency's services.

The annual implementation plan is developed at the beginning of each fiscal year to set forth the short- and long-term goals of the agency. The plan includes annual program objectives based on community health problems, methodology for meeting the objectives, the process to be used for evaluating the objectives, and the annual projected budgetary, personnel, and facilities requirements. The annual implementation plan usually reflects the plans for the total agency and for each unit of the agency.

The annual implementation plan serves as the basis for the agency's annual report. The annual report reflects the success of the agency in meeting the annual objectives, changes in population trends and health status during the year, the actual versus the projected budgetary requirements, the number of services offered, the number of clients served, and the plans and changes recommended for the future. The annual report, like other service records, is often required by funding agencies and state departments of health. The report is used to justify the continued existence of an agency, the budgetary requirements, the relationship of the agency to the community, and requests for funding from governmental and charitable organizations.

Documentation of Provider Care

Problem-oriented medical record keeping (POMR), the concept developed by Weed in 1969, is the most widely used method of documenting client care today. This method has been modified in nursing and is based on the problem-solving process (nursing process) of assessing client problems, developing a plan to resolve client problems, implementing the plan, and evaluating the client outcomes. The problem-oriented record (POR) system has four basic components: the data base—the assessment instrument, the problem list—the assessment outcome, the initial plan and treatment regimen, and progress notes—the implementation and evaluation tool.

The *data base* is the gathering of information about the client's history including psychological, sociocultural, economic, and physical history. The data base includes the health assessment completed by the nurse and a past family health history. Information sources for this assessment tool include the client, family, all other health providers, and diagnostic studies. The data base should be a standardized form accepted for use by all providers of services to the client. The information on the data base is used to make judgments about the client's problems.

The *problem list* reflects the inferences made by the health care team about the identification of the client's problems. This list has several basic components: a list of numbered problems, date of problem onset, and date problem became inactive or the date of problem solution. Nurses often find it difficult to "name" a client problem for the problem list and thus resort to using medical diagnoses or symptomatology to identify problems.

The POR system of recording fosters the development of the multidisciplinary record. The data base can provide for input about the client from data collected by each provider, such as the physical examination by the physician or nurse practitioner, the health assessment by the community health nurse, and the socioeconomic history by the social worker. This type of data base format reduces the need to duplicate observations, interviews, and questions of the client by various providers. Similarly, the problem list should reflect all client problems as identified by all providers responsible for the client's care—medical, nursing, social, and others. Such a format allows each provider to have a total clinical picture of the client and should provide the base for the development of a care plan that is multidisciplinary and thereby reduces the risk of overlap and duplication of provider services.

The POMR format designed by Weed called for the statement of a *plan of care* using three components: diagnostic considerations, therapeutic plans, and client education for each problem named on the problem list. The *plan of action* provides for establishing priorities for nursing interventions to assist the client toward problem resolution. As problems are resolved, nurses can focus on other identified problems of the client; or as nursing interventions seem ineffective, new courses of action are identified to move the client to problem resolution.

The fourth ingredient of the POR system is the *progress notes*. The format for the progress notes is the SOAP note, which is the acronym for subjective data, objective data, assessment, and plan written by each health provider for each client encounter. The *subjective data* for the SOAP note are facts obtained from the client, family, or caretaker about the client. The subjective data reflect information the nurse is given by someone else. *Objective data* reflect the direct observations of the nurse, information gathered from diagnostic studies, or vital signs. The *assessment* is the nurse's interpretation of the data gathered about the presenting problem, and the *plan* usually reflects what the nurse will do during the client encounter and what the nurse will do before or at the next visit to move the client toward problem resolution.

A problem that often arises in using the POR format is a lack of understanding about where to record the interventions during the visit and the planned follow-up interventions. This problem has led to modification of the SOAP format to a SOAAP format, which includes an *action statement* following the client assessment. The modified format seems to provide a clear picture of ongoing and follow-up activities planned for the client and provides an easier system for auditing all components of nursing care activities.

Another problem arising from the POR format is where to record data about client evaluation or expected outcomes. Another modification of SOAP has been an addition of an *evaluation statement* to the format, which becomes SOAPE. This format allows the nurse to list the changes expected in client status resulting from the nursing interventions. These expected outcomes (changes) serve as the foundation for evaluating the care the nurse has given to the client.

Several advantages to the use of POR in the community health setting have been described: the system allows for a multidisciplinary approach to client problem resolution; standardized problem identification enhances quality assurance programs; the system emphasizes client care by focusing attention on the the client problems; the system encourages brief, concise recording which is oriented to the client problems; continuity of care is enhanced by the problem list and the multidisciplinary approach; a new provider can review the chart and become fully acquainted with the client and the services delivered in a short time; and the system allows for easy evaluation and auditing of client care.

As an outgrowth of quality assurance efforts in the health care system, comprehensive methods are being designed to document and measure client progress and client outcome from agency admission through discharge. An example of such a method is the client classification system developed at the Visiting Nurses Association of Omaha, Nebraska (Martin, 1982). This comprehensive method of evaluating client care has several components: a classification system for assessing client problems and categorizing client problems; a data base; a nursing problem list; and anticipated outcome criteria for the classified problems. Such schemes are viewed as having the potential to improve the delivery of nursing care, documentation, and the descriptions of client care. Briefly, implementation of comprehensive documentation methods will enhance nursing assessment, planning, implementation and evaluation of client care and will allow for the organization of pertinent client information for more effective and efficient nurse productivity and communication.

SUMMARY

Quality assurance programs in health care delivery are the mechanisms for maintaining control over the system and for requesting accountability from the individual providers within the system. A quality assurance program consists of varying general and specific approaches and techniques utilized for the purpose of evaluating the structure, process, and outcomes of client care. The ANA has put forth a model quality assurance program that reflects the components of the nursing process in the evaluation of client care activities.

Records kept by community health agencies are instrumental in identifying elements of health care delivery which establish a total picture of the efficacy of the agency to the client community. The POR system of recording and comprehensive client classification and evaluation schemes are efficient methods for ready evaluation of direct client care delivered by the agency's health providers. A quality assurance program has the potential for enhancing health care delivery and reducing overlap, duplication, and costs of health care services.

BIBLIOGRAPHY

Ager, J.: Testing the quality patient care scale. In Wandelt, M., and Ager, J.W., editors: Quality patient care scale, New York, 1974, Appleton-Century-Crofts.

American Nurses' Association Committee for the Study of Credentialing in Nursing: The study of credentialing in nursing: a new approach, vols. 1 and 2, Kansas City, Mo., 1979, The Association.

American Nurses' Association: Quality model: a plan for implementation of the standards of nursing practice, Kansas City, Mo., 1977, The Association.

American Nurses' Association: A conceptual model of community health nursing, Kansas City, Mo., 1982, The Association.

American Nurses' Association: Take the extra step . . . become a certified nurse, Kansas City, Mo., 1983, The Association.

American Nurses' Association Congress on Nursing Practice: Standards of nursing practice, Kansas City, Mo., 1973, The Association.

American Public Health Association: The definition and role of public health nursing in the delivery of health care, Washington, D.C., 1980, The Association.

Bailit, H., et al.: Assessing the quality of care, Nurs. Outlook 23(3):153, March 1975.

Bergmen, R.: Accountability—definition and dimension, Keynote address at Second National Conference of Israeli Nurses, Tel Aviv, Oct. 1, 1980.

Bernhardt, I., and Schuette, L.: P.E.T.: a method of evaluating professional nurse performance, J. Nurs. Adm. 5:18, Oct. 1975.

Birch, I., and Wolfe, S.: Consumers assess alternative kinds of health service, Paper presented at annual meeting, American Public Health Association, Chicago, Nov. 1975.

Blake, B.: Quality assurance: an ethical responsibility, Supervisor Nurse, 12:32, Feb. 1981.

Brief, A.: Developing a usable performance appraisal system, J. Nurs . Adm. 9(10):7, Oct. 1979.

Brook, R., and Appel, F.: Quality-of-care assessment: choosing a method for peer review, N. Engl. J. Med. 288:1323, 1973.

Brook, R.H., Davies, A.R., and Kamberg, C.J.: Selected reflections on quality of medical care evaluation in the 1980s, Nurs. Res. 29(2):127, March-April 1980.

Bullough, B.: The first two phases in nursing licensure. In Bullough, B., editor: The law and the expanding nursing role, New York, 1975, Appleton-Century-Crofts.

Carter, J.: Standards of nursing care, New York, 1976, Springer Publishing Co., Inc.

Council of Home Health Agencies and Community Health Services: Accreditation of homes health agencies and community nursing services: criteria and guide for preparing reports, New York, 1976, National League for Nursing.

Council of Home Health Agencies and Community Health Services: Administrator's handbook for the structure, operation and expansion of home health agencies. New York, 1978, National League for Nursing.

Daubert, E.: A system to evaluate home health care services, Nurs. Outlook 25(3):168, March 1977.

Decker, F., et al.: Using patient outcomes to evaluate community health nursing, Nurs. Outlook 27(4):278, April 1979.

Donabedian, A.: Evaluating the quality of medical care, Milbank Mem. Fund Q. 44:166, 1966.

Dunn, M.: Development of an instrument to measure nursing performance, Nurs. Res. 19:502, Nov.-Dec. 1970.

Felton, G.: Increasing the quality of nursing care by introducing the concept of primary nursing: a model project, Nurs. Res. 24(1):27, Jan.-Feb. 1975.

Front, F.: Three methods of nursing audit, Dimen. Health Serv. 51:38, Sept. 1974.

Hanlon, J., and Pickett, G.: Public health administration and practice, St. Louis, 1979, The C.V. Mosby Co.

Health Care Financing Administration: HCF research report: P.S.R.O. program evaluation, Washington, D.C., 1979.

Hinsvark, I.: Credentialing in nursing. In McCloskey, J., and Grace, H., editors: Current issues in nursing, Oxford, England, 1981, Blackwell Scientific Publications, Inc.

Jacobs, A., et al.: Critical requirements for safe/effective nursing practice, Kansas City, Mo., 1978, Pub. No. 651, ANA Council of State Boards of Nursing.

Jelinek, A., et al.: A methodology for monitoring quality of nursing care, DHEW Pub. No. (HRA) 74-25, Bethesda, Md., 1974, Health Resources Administration.

Jonas, S.: Measurement and control of the quality of health care. In Jonas, S., editor: Health care delivery in the United States, New York, 1981, Springer Publishing Co., Inc.

Jones, F.: Certification for specialization. In McCloskey, J., and Grace, H., editors: Current issues in nursing, Boston, 1981, Blackwell Scientific Publications, Inc.

Kessner, D.M., and Kalk, C.E.: Assessing health quality—the case for tracers, N. Engl. J. Med. 288:189, 1973.

Kissinger, C.: Community nursing administration: Quantifying nursing utilization, J. Nurs. Adm. 3:43, Sept.-Oct. 1973.

Kline, M.: Quality assurance in public health, Nurs. Health Care 1(4):192, Nov. 1980.

Krumme, U.: The case for criterion-referenced measurement, Nurs. Outlook 23(12):764, Dec. 1975.

Lindeman, C.: Measuring quality of nursing care. Part I, J. Nurs. Adm. 6:7, June 1976.

Lindeman, C.: Measuring quality of nursing care. Part II, J. Nurs. Adm. 6:16, Sept. 1976.

LoGerfo, J., and Brook, R.: Evaluation of health services and quality of care. In Williams, S., and Torrens, P., editors: Introduction to health services, New York, 1980, John Wiley & Sons, Inc.

Martin, K.: A client classification system adaptable for computerization, Nurs. Outlook 30:515, Nov.-Dec. 1982.

McCloskey, J.: ANA's nursing accreditation. To what end? In McCloskey, J., and Grace, H., editors: Current issues in nursing, Oxford, England, 1981, Blackwell Scientific Publications, Inc.

McCloskey, J.: The state board test pool exam: entrance to professional nursing. In McCloskey, J., and Grace, H., editors: Current issues in nursing, Boston, 1981, Blackwell Scientific Publications, Inc.

Mullins, A.C., Colavecchio, R.E., and Tescher, B.E.: Peer review: a model for professional accountability, J. Nurs. Adm. 9(12):25, Dec. 1979.

National League for Nursing: Historical perspective of NLN's participation in the ANA credentialing study, NLN accreditation update, Report No. 1, New York, Oct. 1979, The League.

National League for Nursing: Criteria and standards manual of NLN/APHA accreditation of home health agencies and community nursing services, New York, 1982, The League.

Norman, J.: The clinical specialist as performance appraiser, Supervisor Nurse **9:**61, July 1978.

Office of Professional Standards Review: PSRO Program Manual, Washington, D.C., 1974, Department of Health, Education, and Welfare.

Osterweis, M., and Bryant, E.: Assessing technical performance at diverse ambulatory care sites, J. Community Health **4**(2):104, 1978.

Phaneuf, M.: A nursing audit method, Nurs. Outlook **5:**42-45, 1965.

Phaneuf, M.: The nursing audit: profile for excellence, New York, 1976, Appleton-Century-Crofts.

Phaneuf, M.C., and Wandelt, M.A.: Quality assurance in nursing, Nurs. Forum **13**(4):329, 1974.

Pinkerton, S.: Legislative issues in licensure of registered nurses. In McCloskey, J., and Grace, H., editors: Current issues in nursing, Oxford, England, 1981, Blackwell Scientific Publications, Inc.

Porter, L., Lawler, E.,, and Hackman, J.: Evaluating work effectiveness. In Bass, E., editor: Organizational practices and social processes, New York, 1974, McGraw-Hill Book Co. (Originally published in 1957.)

Public Law 97-248, Tax Equity and Fiscal Responsiblity Act of 1982.

Rakich, J., Longest, B., and O'Donovan, T.: Managing health care organization, Philadelphia, 1977, W.B. Saunders Co.

Rissner, N.: Development of an instrument to measure patient satisfaction with nurses and nursing care in primary care settings, Nurs. Res. **24**(1):45, Jan.-Feb. 1975.

Rosser, R., and Watts, V.: The measurement of hospital output, Int. J. Epidemiol. **1**(4):361-368, 1972.

Rutstein, D.D., et al.: Measuring the quality of medical care: a clinical method, N. Engl. J. Med. **294**(11):528, 1976.

Sibley, J., et al.: Quality-of-care appraisal in primary care: a quantitative method, Ann. Int. Med. **83:**46-52, 1975.

Smith, R.L.: Internal properties of the C.A.S.H. nursing care evaluation instrument, Health Serv. Res. **10**(2):136, 1975.

Stanhope, M.: A concurrent and retrospective evaluation of the effects of intrinsic and extrinsic motivating factors on nurse performance in home health care setting, unpublished doctoral dissertation, Birmingham, March 1981, University of Alabama.

Stanhope, M., and Murdock, M.: A psychometric measure of the Phaneuf Nursing Audit, Paper presented at the American Public Health Association Annual Meeting, Los Angeles, Nov. 1981.

Stevens, B.: The nurse as executive, 1975, Contemporary Publishing.

Trussell, P., and Strand, N.: A comparison of concurrent and retrospective audits on the same patients, J. Nurs. Adm. **8:**33, May 1978.

Waller, M., and Davids, D.: Performance profiles based on nursing activity records, J. Nurs. Adm. **2:**60, Sept.-Oct.1972.

Wandelt, M., and Ager, J.: Quality patient care scale, New York, 1975, Appleton-Century-Crofts.

Wandelt, M., and Stewart, D.: Slater nursing competencies rating scale, New York, 1975, Appleton-Century-Crofts.

Warren, D.: Problems in hospital law, Germantown, Md., 1978, Aspen Systems Corp.

Weed, L.: Medical records, medical education and patient care, Chicago, 1970, Year Book Medical Publishers, Inc.

Werner, J.: PSROs and hospital accreditation. In McCloskey, J., and Grace, H., Current issues in nursing, Oxford, England, 1981, Blackwell Scientific Publications, Inc.

Williamson, J.: Information management in quality assurance, Nurs. Res. **29**(2):78, March-April 1980.

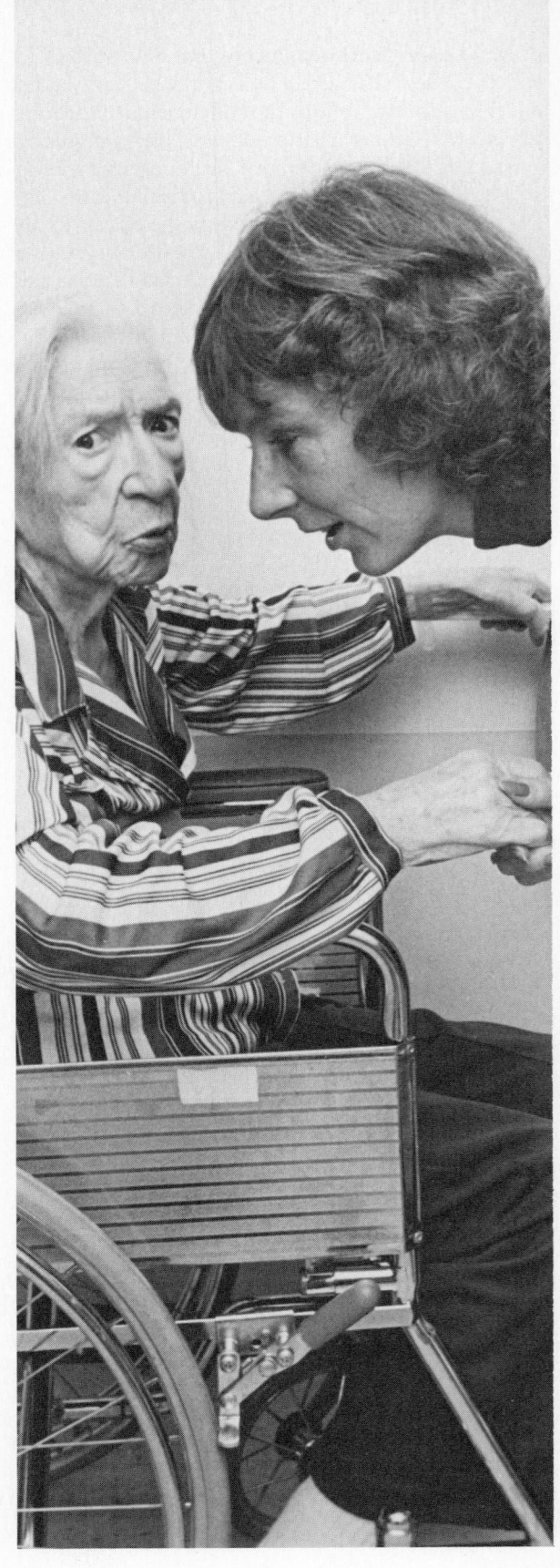

Part Three

THE PRACTICE OF COMMUNITY HEALTH NURSING

The primary orientation of health care delivery through the decades has been one of care and cure of the individual. Today with the reduction in the impact of communicable disease, there is evidence of life-style influences on health and consumer demands, illness prevention, and health promotion for individuals, families, groups, and communities. These changes in health care delivery have influenced changes and expansions in the practice of community health nursing.

As indicated in Chapter 11, if illness prevention and health promotion activities are to be effective and appropriate, the community health nurse must be aware of the sociocultural influences on the individual's and the family's health beliefs and practices. However the nurse should not overlook the possibilities of the new or resurgence of the old communicable and infectious disease that may be contracted in the greater community.

Concern currently exists about a return to environmental and social conditions that may lead to more infectious disease by the year 2000. As is pointed out in Chapters 12 and 13, the community health nurse must continually be concerned about prevention, control, case finding, reporting, and maintenance strategies as they relate to communicable and infectious processes and environmental, social, and occupational risks and related problems.

With the increasing emphasis on healthy life-styles, Americans are interested in factors of living that can result in health problems and in finding ways to reduce the risk of such problems. Chapter 14 discusses self-health care and health-risk appraisal and reduction and Chapter 21 deals with the nurse's role in promoting health through nutrition and exercise.

The community health nurse may work with the individual and family to promote health behaviors (Chapter 15). However, the nurse may find that strategies to introduce health behaviors directed at illness prevention and life-style changes lend themselves to working with groups in the community. Chapter 16 discusses basic group concepts that may be used for promoting health behaviors through groups, identifying community groups and their contributions to community life, and assisting groups to work toward community health goals.

Continued.

Part Three

Although it is necessary to identify health-risk factors among individuals and groups in the community, it is of paramount importance that community health nurses learn to identify and work with health problems of the total community. A healthier community life-style and quality of life for the residents can be promoted in this way. Chapter 17 provides conceptual clarity and guidelines for nursing practice with the client community.

While assessing a client community, the nurse will be struck by the data that show the increase in the number of mental health problems among the population. Although mental health problems can be caused by heredity, the populace is becoming more aware of problems related to living conditions and social and economic problems like violence, human abuse, and substance abuse. Chapters 18, 19, 20, and 22 address these issues and the nurse's role and functions relative to prevention, problem identification, and interventions, including those in both maturational and situational crises.

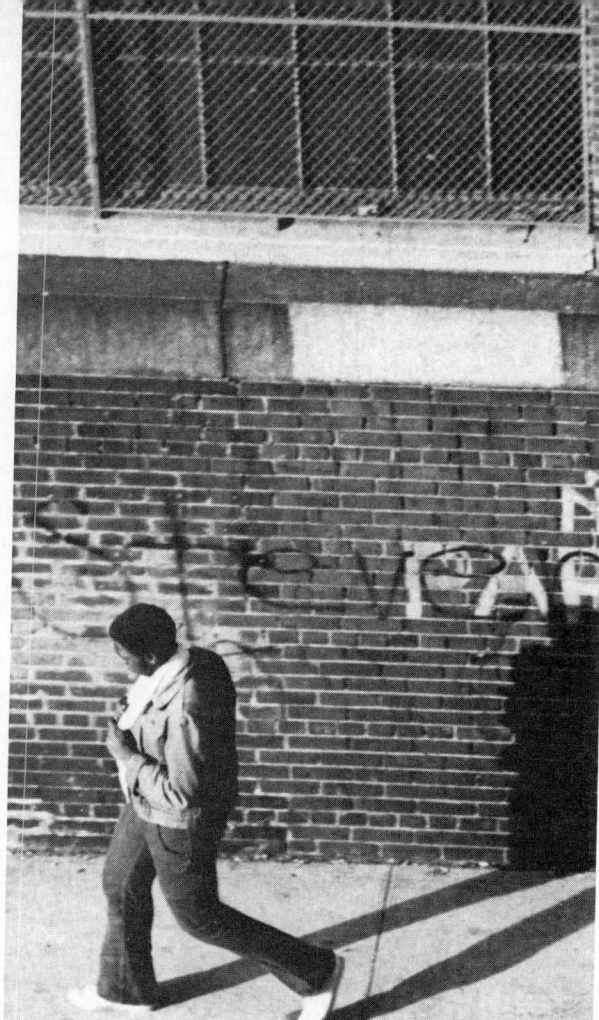

Chapter

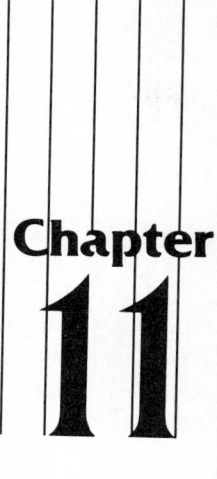

ELEANOR BAUWENS
SANDRA ANDERSON

SOCIAL AND CULTURAL INFLUENCES ON HEALTH CARE

The premise of this chapter is that health care is based not only on knowledge of the physical causes of disease but also on sociocultural influences. Often nurses must plan and give care to individuals and families whose health beliefs and practices differ from their own. If the care is to be effective and appropriate, the nurse must have knowledge of the importance of cultural influences as well as specific cultural values.

The purpose of this chapter is to help nurses deliver more personalized, culturally appropriate care to all clients. Ideally it will increase nurses' sensitivity to sociocultural influences on health care and thereby improve their ability in the assessment, intervention, and evaluation of health problems. We explore the meaning of culture, cultural differences, specific cultural groups in the United States, and poverty, and we provide guide-

lines for cultural assessment and cultural relevant health care.

MEANING OF CULTURE

Culture enables us to interpret our surroundings and the actions of people around us and to behave in ways that make sense. "Culture consists of standards for deciding what is, what can be, how one feels about it, and how to go about doing it" (Goodenough, 1966, pp.257-258). Some anthropologists conceive of culture as a set of rules. Each culture provides the individual with a set of rules for behaving and interpreting the behavior of others. This set of rules can be compared to a cultural grammar. Harrison and Ritenbaugh (1981) elaborate on the idea that "culture is to behavior" as "language is to speech." This definition implies that rules are not always in people's conscious awareness, but if they are broken, people become uncomfortable. For example, if greetings and farewells are not exchanged in an appropriate manner, either party may feel uncomfortable and the relationship may be awkward.

Viewing culture as a set of rules also implies that there are methods by which to learn explicit and implicit cultural rules. Explicit cultural rules are those in people's conscious awareness, those more easily learned than implicit rules, and those people do not consciously recognize. Nevertheless, there are ways to learn about the implicit rules through talking with people and observing their behavior. The rules can then be inferred from what people say they should do and from observations and descriptions of what people actually do.

One individual does not need to know all the rules of grammar to communicate by speech; neither does a person need to know all of the cultural rules to act appropriately and understand the behavior of others. In other words, individuality in behavior, perception, and feelings is taken into account. When enough grammar is known, individuals can create new sentences and make themselves understood in a variety of situations. Understanding cultural rules allows for the interpretation of behavior and helps a person act appropriately.

CONCEPTS RELEVANT TO CULTURE
Holism

Anthropologists believe that culture can best be viewed in the total social context. The concept of holism requires that human behavior not be isolated from the context in which it occurs and that the culture be viewed and analyzed as a totality. Culture is a functional, integrated whole with the parts interrelated and interdependent. The various components of a culture, such as the political, economic, religious, kinship, and health systems, perform separate functions and mesh to form an operating whole. To understand any one system, each must be viewed in relation to the others and to the culture as a whole. A whole culture is often said to be more than the sum of its parts (Benedict, 1934).

Culture Change

Any change in one or more systems affects the whole. Culture is never static but is in a constant process of adding or deleting elements. This process of change is a result of contact between groups and of forces within a group. Culture change usually creates new challenges and problems. Culture involves creative adaptation and retention of behavioral precedents that are passed on through language, customs, beliefs, attitudes, values, goals, laws, traditions, and moral codes. At times prece-

dents become outmoded or maladaptive and thus provide a potential source of conflict (Elling, 1977). This potential source of conflict may reflect the ability of a society to adapt to change whether it is introduced from within or without. The health status of a society is related to its ability to adapt to change.

In a society such as the United States, which has become increasingly technological as scientific medicine has steadily advanced, some individuals have become alienated from orthodox medicine. The search for treatment goes beyond allopathic methods of healing. For example, chiropractic contradicts the monolithic concept of scientific medicine, but it has gained status because of political, social, and legal changes.

Enculturation

Cultural behavior, or how to act appropriately, is socially acquired, not inherited. Patterns of cultural behavior are learned through the process of enculturation, sometimes called socialization. Enculturation is the process of acquiring knowledge and internalizing values. Through this process persons achieve competence in their own culture. Children acquire their culture by watching adults and making inferences about the rules for behavior. Cultural behavior patterns provide explanations for life events, which are important for nurses to understand. These events include such things as birth, death, puberty, childbearing, rearing of children, illness, and disease. As children grow in society, they learn certain beliefs, attitudes, and values about these life events, and this knowledge is carried throughout the life span, unless necessity or force compels them to learn different ways.

Culture-Bound

Whenever people learn a culture, they are to some extent imprisoned without knowing it. Anthropologists refer to this existence as being "culture-bound"; that is, living within a particular reality that is considered as *the* reality. All of us have learned ways to interpret our world based on our enculturation. Our interpretations are understandable and persuasive to those brought up to share the same frame of reference, but out interpretations may sometimes make little sense out of context. We are culture-bound within our own culture and profession, nursing. Being culture-bound within nursing means that we are likely to view our modern scientific approach to health and illness as the only way. Clients may view this modern scientific approach differently, judging that in some ways it meets their needs, and in other ways it does not. Dissatisfaction with medical treatment and practitioners, the movement toward self-care, and the striving for freedom of choice and individual responsibility have led to an increased interest in alternative health services. Western medicine is often practiced in unscientific ways. Desirable outcomes may occur independently of the physician's intervention, or the intervention may lead to iatrogenic consequences (Young, 1978).

Ethnocentrism

Because we look at the world from our own particular cultural viewpoint, we often believe our way is best, which is "ethnocentrism." It is important for nurses not to consider their own way the best and other people's ideas as ignorant or inferior. The ideas of lay individuals may be valid and certainly influence their health care behavior. The beginning of culturally appropriate health care lies in the awareness of the community health nurse that people may live by different rules and priorities from those of the health care provider, and these rules and priorities decisively influence health-related behavior. Health care providers tend to act on the assumption that their world view conforms to the way the world really is or ought to be. When people are judgmental of other cultures, they go beyond healthy cultural identification. Anthropologists refer to the term *cultural relativism* to denote that cultures are neither inferior nor superior to one another. Cultural relativists believe that there is no single scale for measuring the value of a culture; rather it must be understood as being relative to the total cultural context. The following comment by Jelliffe (1969, p. 61) refers to nutrition specifically, but it can be applied to any aspect of culture:

> . . . all different cultures, whether in a tropical village or in a highly urbanized and technologically sophisticated community, contain some practices and customs which are beneficial to the health and nutrition of the group, and some which are harmful. No culture has a monopoly on wisdom or absurdity.

For health professionals it is necessary to realize the existence of cultural relativism in regard to modern scientific medicine. Nurses must realize that not even their own beliefs and professional practice are immune to the universality of scientifically unsound behavior. Tripp-Reimer (1982) studied the concepts of ethnocentrism and cultural relativity in an Appalachian population served by Appalachian and non-Appalachian health professionals. She observed that it is not only the client who has a culture but the health care provider also enters the clinical situation with predetermined values, beliefs, and perceptions. She noted that "the provider's culture biases the interpretation and understanding of client behavior . . . (and) it will diminish the quality of care available for minority clients" (Tripp-Reimer, 1982, p. 188).

Stereotypes

Stereotypes are exaggerated beliefs and images that are popularly depicted in the mass media and folklore. Usually these images are false and serve to obscure important differences among members of a group and exaggerate those between groups. The perceived, exaggerated differences between two groups help to justify negative behavior of people in one group toward others. Individuals can be found to fit the stereotypes, but there are many more who do not. Stereotypes are commonly reflected by false and insensitive expressions such as "Indians are drunks," "blacks are lazy," "poor whites are trash," or "nurses are passive." Stereotyping can lead to inaccurate assessments and interventions based on preconceived notions rather than on unbiased, nonprejudicial observation and questioning. Health professionals must remain sensitive to individual variation within groups.

Cultural Values

The cultural system is composed of value orientations. A *value* is a type of belief about how one should or should not behave. *Beliefs* are "statements which the subject holds as true, but which may or not be based on empirical evidence: thus, the strength of a belief does not depend on its degree of correspondence with objective fact . . ." (Horn, 1979, p. 63). All belief systems are culture-bound because they are based on cultural factors and the meaning that individuals ascribe to these factors. Individuals assign meaning to health and illness based on their values and beliefs. Thus the behavior of clients in regard to health and illness can be more accurately understood by knowing something about their beliefs and values.

Cultural values are the prevailing and persistent guides influencing thinking and actions of people. Individuals' beliefs and values influence the kind of health care considered acceptable or desirable. Values provide powerful motivation and standards for behavior. For instance, if people value prevention, they will generally have their children immunized against disease. If prevention of illness is not valued, immunizations are likely to be ignored, even if provided free of charge.

There are two types of values: public and personal (Goodenough, 1966). Public values tend to be objectified by policies and laws; personal values are usually unverbalized and individualized. People may agree on public values but may vary greatly on personal values. Acceptance of rules requires that public values be reasonably compatible with personal values. When incompatibility exists, the society strives for agreement between public and personal values as is evidenced by the conflict over abortion in the United States.

One of the most important elements shared by a culture is its values. Shared values give a culture stability and security; they provide a standard for behavior. If two people share a similar culture and their experiences tend to be similar, their values will tend to be similar. However, no two people have exactly the same value pattern, but they are enough alike to recognize similarities and to identify the other as "one of my kind" (Goodenough, 1966).

The nurse should not expect to have an understanding of the value system of a family or cultural group after the first contact. The nurse should realize the importance of gathering data to help understand the values people have regarding health care because cultural values determine what people believe to be good or bad, adequate or inadequate health care (Leininger, 1976). Even in situations when the cultural backgrounds of the client and nurse are assumed to be similar, problems can arise if the nurse concentrates only on the disease and fails to recognize the sociocultural aspects influencing health and illness. Community health nurses have their own sets of values that influence their ways of thinking and behaving. Sometimes practitioners and clients can be torn between beliefs in two conflicting systems of viewing health care. Maintaining a sensitivity to the individual as a unique human being and to the culture as a whole can help nurses provide personalized and culturally appropriate care.

CULTURAL DIFFERENCES

All segments of the population in the United States share certain common elements in life patterns and basic beliefs. However, because of different cultural traditions and increasing mobility, a homogeneous culture is seldom found. In a homogeneous culture individuals tend to share the same attitudes, interests, and goals. Generally people are likely to do what is expected or to follow the norms, but discrepancies occur in all cultures. Society presents to individuals what they should do (ideal), but their actual behavior (real) only approximates the norm, especially if the norm is not highly valued. The actual behaviors tend to cluster toward a trend or mode. Individuals who grow up in the same society acquire certain standardized ways of dealing with objects and people. This means that even among total strangers in a completely unique situation there is some level of subjective understanding of what is normal and abnormal in overt behavior, what people actually do.

Ethnic Collectivity

People who have been reared in an "ethnic collectivity" (a group with common origins, a sense of identity, and shared standards for behavior) often acquire from

that experience cultural norms that determine the thought and behavior of individual members (Harwood, 1981). The effects of this enculturation carry over to health care and become an important influence for activities relative to health and illness behavior.

Social scientists speak about American culture as if it included a set of values shared by everyone. However, even within an ethnic collectivity intraethnic variations can be expected and are apparent in health behaviors. For example variations are seen in conceptions of mental illness (Guttmacher and Elinson, 1971), in definitions of health and illness, in skepticisms about medical care, in use of health care services (Berkanovic and Reeder, 1973), and in willingness to assume a dependent role when ill (Greenblum, 1974; Suchman, 1964).

The term *bicultural* implies that a person straddles two cultures, life-styles, and sets of values. To understand biculturalism it is necessary to discuss differences in the terms ethnicity, race, and minority. Ethnicity is frequently used to mean race, but it includes more than a biological identification. *Ethnicity* refers to groups whose members share a common social and cultural heritage passed on to each successive generation. Members of an ethnic group feel a sense of identity. *Race* is a biological term. Racial group members share distinguishing physical features like skin color, bone structure, and genetic traits such as blood grouping. Ethnic and racial groups may overlap. In such cases the biological and cultural similarities can reinforce one another. A *minority* may consist of a particular racial, religious, or occupational group that constitutes less than a numerical majority of the population. In this sense all of us belong to various kinds of minorities (Bullough and Bullough, 1982). Sometimes a minority group is designated because of its limited access to power or assumed inferior traits and undesirable characteristics. A numerical majority may be considered a minority because they lack the kind of power that usually accompanies majority status. Bicultural group members may share ethnic and racial characteristics of the larger group of which they are a part, but they also share a common culture different from that of the larger group.

Cultural Shock

"Cultural shock" is one of the effects of working with individuals from different cultural backgrounds. Leininger (1976, p. 7) describes cultural shock as "the feelings of helplessness and discomfort and the state of disorientation experienced by an outsider attempting to comprehend or effectively adapt to a different cultural group because of differences in cultural practices, values, and beliefs." Cultural shock sometimes makes health care providers feel uncomfortable or even angry. Kubricht and Clark (1982) surveyed nurses and foreign clients to identify areas in which needs were unmet and problems were encountered by nurses who were caring for these people. the survey revealed that foreign clients experienced feelings of boredom, anxiety, and fear; nurses experienced feelings of frustration and inadequacy; communication was either inadequate or nonexistent; the lack of culture-specific information was a significant problem; and resources to meet these needs were not consistently available.

Nurses can help reduce cultural shock by knowing about the different cultural groups with whom they are working. Ways of learning about culturally different clients include transcultural course work and experiences. Even with preknowledge, the nurse may regard clients as strange and have difficulty communicating; likewise, the client may perceive the health system and health care providers as unusual and incomprehensible. During a period of adaptation it is important for nurses to develop respect for others who are culturally different but at the same time maintain their own sense of worth. Community health nursing practice requires tolerance of beliefs that may be counter to those of the nurse.

Communication Patterns

Obvious barriers are present when two people speak different languages. Familiarity with the language of the client is one of the best ways to gain insight into a culture. Kluckhohn (1972) wrote that every language is also a special way of looking at the world and interpreting experiences. Each different language has a whole set of unconscious assumptions about the world and life. Kluckhohn believed that people see and hear what the grammatical system of their language makes them sensitive to. It is a high priority of the community health nurse working with clients who speak another language to comprehend at as many levels and with as many senses as possible.

However, barries to communications also may exist when individuals speak the same language. Nurses may have difficulty explaining things in simple jargon-free language that clients can understand. It is important to ascertain that the message is received and understood as the sender intended it. The nurse and the client can employ a feedback mechanism to facilitate communication. Much of the information we transmit to each other is conveyed by facial expression, posture, body movement, and voice tone. For example, the Anglo may value straightforward criticism to the person's face, but the Papago Indian finds that action impolite. As a result, Papago clients may be unwilling to criticize health personnel directly even if they are dissatisfied with their care.

Cultural differences are reflected in communication patterns. For instance, the actual terms used may vary according to to whom you speak, when you speak, acceptable and taboo topics, and the social situation. For example, Saunders (1954, p. 116) describes the effect that the inability to understand Spanish-speaking people's ways of looking at things may have on the English speaker's assessment of their "worth" " . . . in English a clock runs, while in Spanish, it walks (*el reloj anda*). Such a simple difference as this has enormous implications for appreciating differences in the behavior of English and Spanish-speaking persons. If time is moving rapidly, as Anglo usage declares, we must hurry. . . . If time walks, as the Spanish-speaking say, one can take a more leisurely attitude toward it. . . . " An attempt to understand a people's world view through their language can avert some major misunderstandings.

Personal Space and Contact

Personal space is a boundary that is invisible and flexible. Insel (1978) describes personal space as a "portable bubble" that continuously surrounds the individual. This invisible cushion of air provides a margin of safety and security. The bubble expands, shrinks, and changes in permeability according to the social situation, the physical area, the culture of the individual, and the relation to others present (Meisenhelder, 1982). Body or eye contact accepted or even expected in one culture may be taboo in another. Touching may be considered an intrusion of personal space in some cultures, but in others many forms of traditional healing require touching as part of the healing process or as a comfort measure.

Hall (1966) observed and interviewed northeastern Americans to learn about their use of personal space. He identified four zones: (1) intimate distance that extends up to 18 inches from the body, (2) personal distance as an area of 18 inches to 4 feet from the individual (3) social distance of 4 to 12 feet, and (4) public distance of 12 feet or more. People are usually not aware of the use of personal space according to zones; nevertheless, the use of personal space is certainly influenced by culture.

Watson (1970) studied cultural differences in the use of personal space. He compiled a range of space by nationality and found that Americans, Canadians, and British require the most personal space, whereas Latin Americans and Arabs need the least. He noted that within the same cultural group individuals interacted at a uniform distance according to the situation. Because people do not consciously recognize their use of personal space, they have difficulty understanding a different cultural pattern. As a result, acts of friendliness may be misinterpreted as threatening behavior if personal space has been invaded.

An understanding of personal space by the community health nurse can facilitate the nursing assessment process and has significance for nurse-client interaction. Health professionals often feel that they have access to any area of the client's body. The client may develop patterns of avoidance and withdrawal to protect personal space. Nevertheless, close contact is necessary when performing a physical assessment, for example. The nurse should attempt to reduce anxiety by recognizing the individual's need for personal space and taking the appropriate action to provide privacy. Clients should be allowed to direct the use of their personal space whether they are in their homes or in the hospital setting so that individual identity and integrity are preserved.

Cultural Views of Disease and Illness

In countries such as the United States there is an extremely complex system of health beliefs and practices. Variation in these beliefs and practices may be found across ethnic and social class boundaries and even within families. Currently the generally accepted approach is the biomedical model, which emphasizes biological concerns. These concerns are often considered more "real," significant, and interesting than psychological and sociocultural issues (Kleinman et al., 1978). Most health professionals in modern Western settings are primarily interested in the treatment of diseases and abnormalities in the structure and function of body systems. Kleinman et al. view the biomedical approach as culture-specific (culture-bound) and value-laden. The biomedical model represents one end of a continuum, the scientific pole. At the other pole is traditional content, the popular beliefs and practices that usually diverge from medical science (Chrisman, 1977). Health belief and practices of individuals vary along this continuum.

In the last decade anthropologists and sociologists have made a distinction between illness and disease. The human experience of illness is not necessarily identical to the biomedical interpretation of disease. Illness is the individual's perception of being sick. Disease is only diagnosed when the condition is a deviation from norms as established by Western biomedical science (Fabrega, 1971). Illness may occur in the absence of disease; for instance, 50% of the visits to a physician are for complaints without a definite biological basis. "Illness is culturally shaped in the sense that how we perceive, experience and cope with disease is based on our explanations of sickness" (Kleinman et al., 1978, p. 252.) Disease is described in medical-surgical nursing textbooks; however, nurses must also be familiar with the personal and cultural reactions to disease or discomfort.

Culture influences our expectations and perceptions of symptoms; the way we label sickness; when, how, and to whom we communicate our health problem; and how long we remain under care. Because health and illness are shaped by cultural factors, there is variation in health care behavior, health status, and patterns of sickness and care within and between different cultures. Health care behavior refers to social and biological activities of the individual based on maintaining an acceptable health status or on altering an unacceptable condition. Health status refers to the success with which a person had adapted to the total environment. Health care behavior influences health status, which influences health care behavior, and both are affected by sociocultural forces such as economics, politics, environmental influences, and the health system (Elling, 1977).

The model in Fig. 11-1 can be used to portray the relation of sociocultural patterns to the health care system, as well as many other factors that have a bearing on health. This model is broad in scope and is used to communicate that sociocultural influences impinge not only on the individual's health status but also on the entire health system. The many interrelations also indicate that a change in any one factor has an impact on the others.

If there is a discrepancy in the way health care providers and consumers view disease and illness, there may be a disagreement between what is important in health care to clients and to providers (Harwood, 1981). If the health provider and the client share the same beliefs and values, agree on appropriate treatment, and anticipate the same outcome, the client can be expected to comply with the provider's proposed health care. To the extent that the provider and client differ, the client's behavior can be expected to differ from what the provider desires, although the ways in which it may diverge cannot always be predicted. The community health nurse should not attempt to compete with or change clients' values but instead should try to help them maximize their health by adhering to their own values.

People who have been reared in a group with common origins and a sense of identity often share basic concepts and attitudes toward health and illness as well as styles of behavior and concerns about the world. The effects of enculturation influence health-seeking behaviors and activities to prevent and treat disease. Nevertheless, there is individual variation, and appreciation of this helps to prevent the common tendency of health professionals and others to stereotype ethnic group members, which can be dangerous. If health workers are conversant only in bits of isolated aspects of health beliefs and behaviors, holism is lost and intracultural variation obscured. An accurate description of the cul-

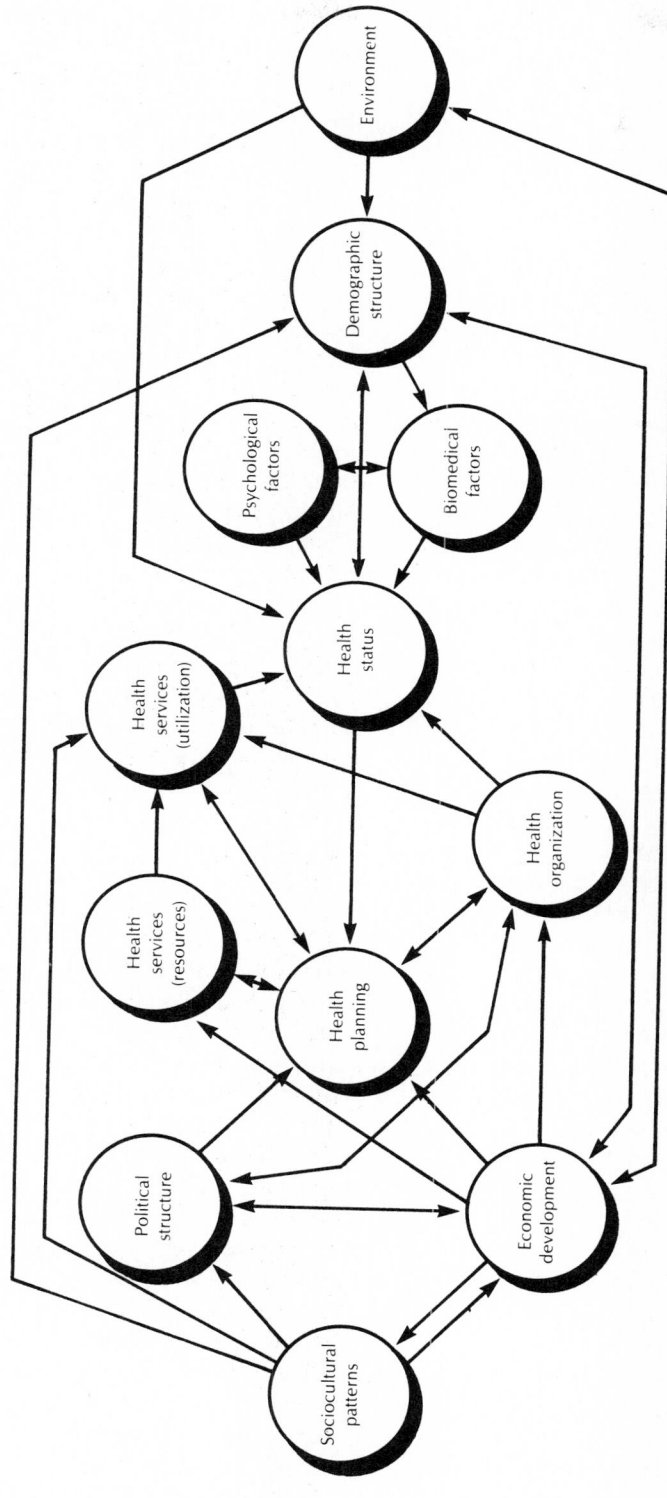

Fig. 11-1. Sociocultural patterns and the health system. (From De Miguel, J. M.: A framework for the study of national health systems, Fig. II., Inquiry 12(2):10-24, 1975. Reprinted with permission of the Blue Cross Association.)

ture and behavior of ethnic group members ideally provides an assessment of the range of behavior and the commonly held cultural beliefs and values. Without this knowledge, health professionals find themselves confronted with what appears to them to be strange and curious notions, and they feel the need to overgeneralize.

DIVERSE CULTURES OF THE UNITED STATES

Most people are aware of cultural diversity between their own country and another; however, cultural differences also exist within a country. The United States has many diverse cultures, since historically a variety of groups immigrated to this country. Although broad cultural values are shared by most people, a rich diversity of values and beliefs exists, including variation in health and illness beliefs. Nevertheless, nursing tends to be practiced in an ethnocentric manner. Generally, nursing has been taught and practiced as if all clients were members of the dominant American group, white, Christian, and of European ancestry (Ruiz, 1981). Because familiarity with this American group is widespread, it is not discussed in this chapter. (For information on low-income Anglos see Bauwens [1977], and for middle-income Anglos see Hautman and Harrison [1982].)

Information about the cultural backgrounds of Asian Americans, black Americans, Mexican Americans, Middle Eastern–Arab Americans, and Native Americans is presented as illustrative examples to help in understanding how cultural factors can and do influence client behavior and to highlight the importance of using cultural background data in providing nursing care. Factors that produce diversity between and within ethnic groups include historical factors, education, sex, place of birth, geographical location, socioeconomic status, and religious affiliation. The purpose of these examples of specific ethnic groups is not to present a detailed description of their culture and health behavior but to introduce to nurses and other health workers an appreciation of the multiple factors that influence health and illness beliefs.

Asian Americans

The likelihood of nurses having contact with Asians in the United States is greater than ever before. Historically the largest groups have been the Japanese, Chinese, Filipino, and Korean. A more recent influx of refugees from Viet Nam, Cambodia, and Laos has increased the Asian population, especially on the West Coast. A wide range of health beliefs and behaviors exists not only between the various groups but also within each group.

The Chinese Americans have been selected to serve as an example of Asian American groups. Early Chinese settlers in the United States were predominantly men who arrived in large numbers around 1850 to further their economic situation. They came with the idea of temporarily leaving their families to earn money and then returning to their homeland or eventually reuniting the family in the United States. Immigration laws intervened, and for those Chinese men who chose to stay, it means that their families were restricted from joining them (Spector, 1979).

The form of extended household associated with traditional China in which grandparents, parents, siblings, and even aunts, uncles, and cousins lived under one roof is rare in the United States today. However, often members of Chinese families still maintain strong emotional bonds and a sense of responsibility for mutual assistance as needed. Traditional customs and preferences that may or may not be present in Chinese American families include a male-dominated household, women viewed as liabilities because of the transfer of their loyalties to the husband's family at the time of marriage, preference and indulgence of boys, and respect for and deference to the elderly (Henderson and Primeaux, 1981).

If nurses are knowledgeable about the prescribed roles in the particular Chinese American families, they will be able to assess and intervene more appropriately. Special care is needed when dealing with individual's and family's expressions of feelings even though they may be nonverbal (Henderson and Primeaux, 1981). Most Asians strongly emphasize harmony and avoidance of conflict in groups. Direct confrontations are usually avoided even if one must accept the blame. It is important for all to maintain self-esteem and not lose face, and this is achieved at times by nonresponsiveness.

Recent examination by Yu (1982) of available vital statistics showed that Chinese Americans have a lower infant mortality (6.3 per 1000 live births under the age of 1 year in 1978) than white Americans (12.0 per 1000) (Fig. 11-2). What are some plausible explanations for this low infant mortality among Chinese Americans? One explanation may be the reporting errors of births and deaths. Misreporting of race, especially when interracial marriages are involved, may be a source of error. Some researchers suggest that the low death rates, if not the result of errors in reporting, might be accounted for by rarity of teenage pregnancies in Chinese Americans. However, it seems the Chinese advantage is evident in every age group. The larger proportion of educated women among Chinese Americans has been considered. Again, Chinese American women have the lowest death rate at every level of education. Cultural

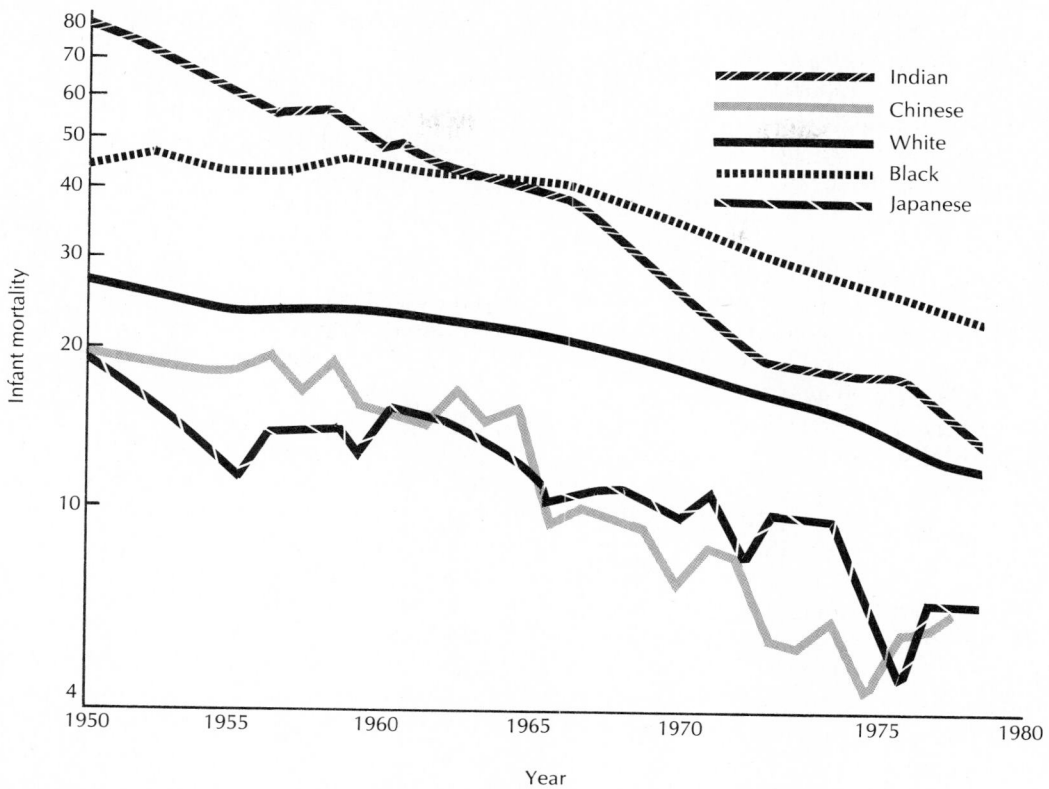

Fig. 11-2. Infant mortality per 1000 live births by race from 1950 to 1978. (From National Center for Health Statistics.)

influence on the health habits and life-style of Chinese Americans may be part of the explanation for differential statistics in infant mortality. Cultural influence on behaviors of women during pregnancy might include the following: (1) eating one or more types of Chinese herbs during pregnancy and just before delivery of the baby, (2) eating traditional foods, and (3) giving special herbs to the infants. At the present time all of these practices have been minimally studied to understand any possible association with infant mortality (Yu, 1982). Additional factors influencing the apparent differential in infant mortality among whites and Chinese might be found in other culturally determined health practices and life-styles, such as higher prevalence of smoking and substance abuse among white women as compared to Chinese American women. Precisely how the maternal intrauterine environment may be shaped by cultural health habits and practices is not clear but is worthy of attention and research.

Black Americans

Blacks are individuals who define themselves as belonging to an ethnic group or who are so defined and treated as such by their significant others. Members in an ethnic group exhibit behavior appropriate to the identity that is claimed. The best way to determine ethnic group membership is to ask individuals how they identify themselves. In the past various terms have been used to describe blacks: colored, negro, Afro-American, and black. Caution is advised in labeling clients because, depending on their age, they may prefer a term to which they attach dignity. Jackson (1981) notes that blacks constitute a highly heterogeneous group; in other words, no typical black individual exists. Because blacks have highly visible physical traits such as skin color, many health professionals have a tendency to treat blacks as if they were all alike. However, black Americans display considerable variation in their health attitudes and behaviors.

Most of the black Africans who came to this country during the seventeenth and eighteenth centuries were different from other immigrants because they came unwillingly on slave ships, primarily from West Africa. Emancipation did not end the problem of being black in this country. Segregation and discrimination are ongoing problems that have produced not only inadequate health care but also poverty, lack of education, and negative psychological responses.

Some of the differences in health problems are the result of varying genetic pools and hereditary immunity. However, many of these differences are more closely associated with economic status than with race. Poverty, discrimination, and social and psychological barriers tend to keep people from using services that are available. These three factors interact and reinforce each other, which partially explains the fact that mortality and morbidity are higher for blacks (Bullough and Bullough, 1982).

The black family is often oriented around women (matrifocal). Within the family the wife and/or mother is often charged with the responsibility for protecting the health of family members. She is expected to assist them in maintaining good health and in determining treatment if a family member is ill.

In general, black Americans have a strong religious orientation. Most belong to protestant faiths. The most common and frequently cited method of treating illness is prayer (Spector, 1979). Snow (1970) stated that many of her informants found it impossible to separate religious beliefs from medical ones. In some instances illnesses may be viewed as punishment for failure to abide by God's rules. Thus spiritual healers may be sought for curing illnesses; they generally have their own special curing techniques. Snow found that whether an individual comes from a rural or urban background is important in the selection of a health care provider. In general, those individuals who were reared in the rural South grew up being treated by folk practitioners. In many cases they did not encounter a physician until adulthood; thus they are most likely to turn to a neighborhood folk practitioner when ill. White (1977) claimed that folk medicine is still used within the black community because of humiliation in the mainstream health care system, lack of money, and lack of trust in health workers. Many go to physicians mainly because of the control of medicines and not because they feel the physician is superior in knowledge or training.

It is important for the community health nurse to recognize that black Americans are a heterogeneous group. Nevertheless, many are still influenced by ethnic group customs and traditions. Nurses have a responsibility to improve accessibility to health care, to provide culturally relevant health care, and to assist blacks to improve their own health status.

Mexican Americans

For this chapter the term *Mexican American* is used as a general designation for individuals of Mexican ancestry who live in only the southwestern states where studies were conducted. Given the regional encultura-

tion and socioeconomic variation existing within the Mexican American populations, it is difficult to formulate conclusions about an entire ethnic group with such diversity as rural villagers in New Mexico and Colorado (Saunders, 1954; Weaver, 1970), agricultural laborers in Texas (Rubel, 1966), low-income residents in Arizona (Kay, 1977), or urban lower-class individuals in California (Clark, 1970). Not only do studies represent different populations but also differing definitions of Mexican American are used (Quesada, 1973). Thus any discussion of Mexican Americans is complicated by the problem of defining this population.

Mexican Americans moved northward from Mexico into the southwestern section of the United States. Therefore unlike most other immigrants, they are close to their homeland. There is also geographical similarity between the southwestern United States and northern Mexico, so that the Mexicans who moved north were more or less at home. Because of the geographical closeness, there is considerable movement of Mexican Americans back and forth between the two countries, since many still have relatives in Mexico.

Traditionally the family maintains a position of prominence in Mexican-American culture and is characterized by a close-knit kin group. Ties beyond the nuclear family link grandparents, uncles, aunts, and cousins. A Mexican American is expected to turn to the family first to fulfill needs; seeking outside help often is done at the expense of pride and dignity of both the individual and the family. Practices are passed from generation to generation. If strong ties exist between the client and the family, the advice of the family may be followed rather than that of the community health nurse. The nurse may suggest that the client solicit the opinions of other family members regarding proposed actions. This demonstrates that the nurse understands the family's importance in health matters.

Language is also a cultural factor that influences health care practices. If a language barrier exists, it can be overcome by providing translators or Spanish-speaking health care providers. Mexican-American clients may be fairly fluent in English, yet when exposed to treatment plans in technical language, they may not comply with the regimen because of its unfamilarity or miscommunication.

Religion is often an important cultural factor affecting health beliefs and practices. Many Mexican Americans are members of Catholic churches and turn to religious practices to overcome illness. Folk cures today often include prayers before the treatment begins (Kay, 1977).

Health is viewed as harmonious relations within the social and spiritual realms. Disruptions in social relations or breaking cultural rules are believed to have a bad effect on an individual's mental and physical well-being (Madsen, 1964). Rubel (1966) noted that Mexican Americans structure folk illness concepts into two major categories: (1) *males naturales* (natural illnesses) and (2) *mal puesto* (bewitchment). The first category includes four promient folk syndromes: *molera caida* (fallen fontanel), *empacho* (indigestion infection), *mal ojo* (evil eye), and *susto* (fright); the second category includes such disorders as *brujeria* (witchcraft). Mal puesto is a declining belief and is generally used after several other diagnoses have been tried and treatment has been unsuccessful (Madsen, 1964; Rubel, 1966).

A wide variety of folk practitioners is used, including *curanderos* (folk healers), *sobadoras* (masseuses), and *parteras* (lay midwives). Generally an individual is referred to these folk practitioners by a family member, relative, or friend who has previously used their services or is aware of their reputations (Madsen, 1964).

Mexican Americans recognize a number of scientific disease categories and folk concepts of illness. However, recognition does not necessarily imply acceptance of scientific causes of disease. Causation may still be attributed to a lack of harmonious relations (Kay, 1977). Folk or scientific beliefs may be selectively chosen depending on such factors as the nature of the illness episode or the ability of folk or scientific treatment to produce a satisfactory outcome. Kay indicated that curanderos refer individuals to biomedical practitioners for serious illness and sometimes encourage treatment for folk illnesses by traditional and scientific means.

Nurses should elicit the client's view of the illness and recognize that Mexican Americans come with a culturally determined set of norms, and many have their own culturally derived concepts and interpretations about specific health problems. Denial of folk disorders by health professionals only reinforces the belief that these disorders lie outside scientific medicine's competence. Thus the client is encouraged to continue other forms of treatment. "The pervasiveness of folk medicine, its vitality, and self-sufficiency are noteworthy. It is not a question of a random collection of beliefs and superstitions. Folk medicine flourishes today because it is a functional part of the people's way of life" (Foster, 1952, p. 5).

Identifying cultural patterns is important in collecting data for planning nursing care. It is essential that the community health nurse be familiar with and understand the various cultural factors that may influence the health beliefs and practices of Mexican Americans and may determine their acceptance of health care services.

Middle Eastern–Arab Americans

Little attention has been given in the literature to the health care needs of Middle Eastern–Arab Americans. Only recently have Arabs immigrated to the United States in significant numbers. There are now between 2 and 3 million permanent and temporary residents in the United States, originally from the Middle East (Meleis and Sorrell, 1981). Most of the Arab Americans come from Palestine, Lebanon, Egypt, Iraq, and Yemen; some also come from Jordan, Syria, and other Arabian countries. In addition to geographical origination, Arabs are frequently characterized by the Arabic language and the Islam religion. They share the values, customs, and beliefs of the Arab culture.

Social properties of the Arab culture that are of interest to health care providers have been described by Meleis (1981) and Meleis and Sorrell (1981) and are listed as follows: (1) Affiliation with family is needed if an Arab is to cope satisfactorily with daily events and/or life crises. Arabs usually do not actively seek advice but feel help should be offered without a specific request. Visiting between family members is viewed as a social obligation during illness and other significant life events, which should be remembered in regard to hospital visitation. (2) Western medicine is usually highly valued even though the will of God, the "evil eye," and hot and cold shifts may be used to explain certain diseases. An effective cure and not personal care is expected of the health care system. They prefer to receive personal care from their families. Many Arab Americans believe that the more intrusive the procedure, the better the chance for recovery. (3) Arabs tend to give as little information as possible about themselves and their families to strangers. They may wonder about the personal nature of questions that may appear to others as routine. Arab clients frequently present a general description of their health status as any illness thought to affect the whole individual and the well-being of the entire family. Pain is also experienced in a generalized way. (4) Arab society is oriented to the present, as many believe that planning ahead has the potential of defying God's will. Arab American women tend not to plan ahead for labor, delivery, and a new baby. Lack of planning should not be interpreted as maternal disinterest in the infant. Their values concerning planning and prevention make it difficult for some Arab Americans to use contraceptives. When birth control is practiced, Arab American women are more likely to prefer intrauterine devices because of the value placed on intrusive treatment. (5) Arab American women usually dress conservatively. Since they value modesty, it is important to protect patients from unnecessary exposure. Topics related to sex and reproduction are discussed with female relatives and friends but not with men or strangers. "Extreme tact needs to be exercised when involving the wife in any discussion without the husband . . . he can be employed to enhance the compliance of the family in all areas of health care including contraception" (Meleis and Sorrell, 1981, p. 176).

This general profile of Arab Americans does not fit any individual exactly but fits most of them in some way. Meleis (1981, p. 1183) offers an important caveat: "The line between individualizing care based on cultural diversity and stereotyping is a very fine one."

Native Americans (American Indians)

Confusion over who is a Native American is compounded by the lack of an adequate definition. In 1954 the United States Bureau of Indian Affairs admitted that it could not determine an adequate definition of who an Indian is or was (Josephy, 1969). Thus the term *Indian* in government reports can refer to a cultural group, a racial group, or a legal concept. As defined by the 1979 census, the largest concentrations of Indian populations in the United States were in Arizona and Oklahoma with 95,000 Indians each and New Mexico with approximately 72,000. Alaska, California, North Carolina, South Dakota, New York, Montana, Washington, and Minnesota are other states with large numbers of persons classified as Native Americans.

Among the Navajo, a southwestern Indian tribe, infant mortality has been reduced dramatically in recent years, although it is still higher than in the general United States population. In 1955 there were approximately 139 Navajo infant deaths per 1000 live births (Kunitz and Levy 1981). The infant mortality for Native Americans fell from 62.5 per 1000 in 1955, to 32.2 in 1967, to 20.1 in 1971 (Fig. 11-2). In 1977 the infant mortality was 18.8 for Native American boys and 12.3 for Native American girls (Vital Statistics of the United States, 1981). Infant mortality is influenced by the use of prenatal care, birth weight of the infant, feeding patterns, nutritional status of the infant and mother, and complicated pregnancies. Improvements in the future will probably be associated with improved living conditions and increased socioeconomic status rather than improved medical care (Oakland and Kane, 1973).

Providing effective health care to Native Americans is complicated by the fact that each nation or tribe has its own language, religion, and belief system regarding health and illness and its treatment. There are also variations in geography, distribution of wealth, and social organization. What is effective among one group may not be among another group (Vogel, 1970). The problem for the community health nurse is to fit traditional customs into effective preventive health care. The nurse must be aware that all Native Americans are not the same; they are not even members of the same tribe.

Individuals range from those uneducated in Anglo ways to those well-educated in their own and Anglo cultures. The nurse has to determine where the client is located on the continuum (Kniep-Hardy and Burkhardt, 1977).

The Native American family is frequently an extended family that includes several households. In addition, other individuals, formalized through a religious ceremony, can become the same as parents in the family network. Grandparents are family leaders, and respect for individuals increases with age. The family is important during periods of crises when family members serve as sources of support and security. The family structure has implications for the community health nurse, since family members need to be included in actively caring for the client (Primeaux and Henderson, 1981).

Religion is integrated into a distinct way of living and interpretation of life and is constantly present, whereas in the Western world religion generally is viewed as a discrete body of knowledge practiced in a specific place. Traditional healing ceremonies are ritualistic ways to handle illnesses and deaths. Some rituals may be performed by the family, or a traditional specialist may be sought to perform the ceremonies (Primeaux and Henderson, 1981). It is important for the community health nurse to recognize that Native Americans' health beliefs and practices today are a combination of Western medicine and traditional religious practices. Even though Anglo physicians and hospitals have been made available to Native Americans on reservations, old ways to treat illnesses continue to exist and are incorporated into the modern referral system in some places. As Ackerknecht (1942, p. 508) noted,". . . the strong connection between these (healing) rites and the whole religion and tradition of the tribe produce certain psychotherapeutic advantages for the medicine man which the modern physician lacks." For example, a Navajo nursing student related an incident about her mother-in-law who lives on the Navajo reservation. A physician diagnosed the woman as having breast cancer, based on positive mammography and a biopsy. Surgery was recommended (radical mastectomy), but her mother-in-law refused. Instead she went to a medicine man who sucked out the inflicting cause. The mother-in-law still returns to the physician for periodic checks that include mammography. The student stated that she is thankful that her mother-in-law is well, but the physician remains appalled by this outcome, which included no further problems.

The knowledge of health beliefs and practices can assist the community health nurse in the management of the individual client and in the planning of health care delivery to specific cultural groups. Knowledge of the culture enhance the ability of the nurse to understand clients' problems, since cultural beliefs and values affect the way in which individuals recognize illness, select a health care provider, and determine their expectations of the provider. There may be the simultaneous use of various health services by clients and the switching serially from traditional to Western scientific medicine or other forms of practice. As illustrated in the example about the student nurse's mother-in-law, there is a strong ideological tendency to accept orthodox medicine, but at the same time there are pragmatic reasons to use unorthodox practitioners.

POVERTY

There is no agreement about how poverty should be defined or measured; in fact, no one really knows the extent of poverty in the United States. Any attempt at defining and measuring poverty must consider numerous variables. The federal government's poverty standards are defined and measured strictly in terms of income; that is, an absolute standard is used. Some have agreed that poverty should be defined by relative standards, accepted standards of what human life requires.

Absolute and Relative Standards

Poverty may be defined in absolute or relative terms. An absolute standard attempts to define some basic set of resources necessary for adequate existence. The federal government defines poverty in absolute terms using the Social Security Administration standards as the official measure. This standard varies by place of residence, family size, and sex of the family head. The basis for the standard is the cost of food. Farm families are presumed to need 85% of the cash income required by nonfarm families because they can grow crops and thus not spend as much money for food. In 1980 the poverty income for a nonfarm family of four was $8414 and for a farm family of four, $7152. Increases in the SSA poverty standard are based on the consumer price index. The consumer price index reflects current market prices for food as determined by the United States Department of Agriculture.

A relative standard attempts to define poverty in terms of the median standard of living in a society. Townsend (1974, p. 15) stated the "Individuals, families and groups . . . can be said to be in poverty when they lack the resources to obtain the type of diets, participate in activities, and have the living conditions and amenities which are customary, or are at least widely encouraged or approved, in the societies to which they belong." If a relative standard were to be used, the poor might be defined as those who earn 50% of the median income for their family size. For example, in 1980 the

median income for four-person families was $21,023. Any four-person family with an income of less than $10,511 would be considered poor. This would raise the poverty level for a four-person family in 1980 by $2097 over the estimated 1980 SSA standard of $8414, which would increase the poverty count significantly. A major attraction of the relative standard is that it more clearly delineates the overall distribution of wealth in the United States.

Health and welfare programs for the poor are based on absolute standards, which are misleading because they do not consider all of the dimensions, such as access to basic services, regional variations, and assets. As a result, many of the deserving poor do not receive assistance. The working poor have incomes too high to be considered eligible for public assistance programs, yet because of inflation, common needs such as food and health care are inaccessible.

Other Definitions of Poverty

The word *poverty* has assumed numerous other meanings at different times and places. Definitions of poverty are in large measure historically conditioned and are based on standards and aspirations of society set in terms of what is considered technically possible. As standards and potentials change, so must the definitions of poverty. In 1914 Hollander defined the poor as lacking the necessary clothing, food, shelter, and education. Today in the United States people are perceived as poor even if they have the minimum required for subsistence.

Poverty also has been defined in terms of values. Valentine (1968, p. 13) stated that the primary meaning of poverty is, "A condition of being in want of something that is needed, desired, or generally recognized as having a value." Thus poverty is a relative term meaning a lack of necessary things, such as goods and services sufficient to meet minimum needs. The essence of poverty is inequality; that is , poverty is relative deprivation—too little money, food, housing, health care, and educational opportunity.

Psychologically, poverty can be defined in terms of deprivation and helplessness. The poor are deprived not only of the minimum adequate provisions for physical life but also of adequate sensory, social, and emotional stimuli for normal development. This definition is frequently criticized because it implies that the poor are "culturally deprived" and therefore lacking in experience or in culture (i.e., middle-class values). It is not that the poor are deprived of culture; it is that the culture with which they are associated is derogated because they are impoverished and powerless.

Research studies (Dohrenwend and Dohrenwend, 1969 and 1974; Dunham, 1965; Hollingshead and Redlich, 1958) investigating the relation of socioeconomic status and psychological disorders have been done. Most of these studies report that psychological disorders are more common among poor people than middle- or upper-class individuals. Usually it is the lowest class that has the largest number of mentally ill individuals. Poverty seems to be a factor in mental illness; however, it is not clear whether poverty is a cause or a consequence. Carefully controlled research is still needed.

Whether the poor are defined economically or psychologically, they can be described from the perspective of alienation. That is, they are outside the mainstream of the dominant society. Individuals with power are drawn mostly from upper- socioeconomic groups, and the poor typically do not have any great influence over decision made by these individuals.

Culture of Poverty

Oscar Lewis was an early formulator of the concept, "culture of poverty" in his works, *The Children of Sanchez* (1961) and *La Vida* (1966). Essential to this concept is the idea that poverty is not merely economic deprivation but also entails personality traits, some of which are psychologically compensatory and rewarding. Like other aspects of culture, such elements are passed from generation to generation through enculturation. Many of the poor have beliefs, values, and life-styles that are not an adjustment to low income but an ingrained way of life that is self-perpetuating and reinforced by each new generation. Lewis (1966) noted that the socioeconomic interests and values of the larger society are causal factors in the development and perpetuation of poverty. He contended that to eliminate poverty, these life-styles and ways of perceiving the world and one's place in it must be abolished if poverty is to be eradicated.

Numerous critics have disagreed with Lewis' rationale. Valentine (1968) disagrees with the causes of behavior, the reasons for the deprivation of the poor, and the directions that social policies should take. He and other critics (Kahn, 1969; Leacock, 1971) of the concept fear that those unsympathetic to the poor will use the concept to withdraw aid or institute programs in line with the protestant ethic.

There are dangers associated with the use of the culture of poverty concept. For example, if the existence of a distinct and self-perpetuating culture of poverty were widely accepted, public funds might be diverted from programs to create more jobs, more housing, and better schools to those for more social work and reeducation of a psychiatric nature. Moreover, the culture of poverty concept serves to sustain the complacency of the more affluent by shifting the onus away from themselves and onto the shoulders of the poor, referred to by Ryan (1971) as "blaming the victim." Another danger that may be associated with the concept is that if the poor can be characterized as disorganized, deviant, or even sick, it would be foolhardy to permit them to share in decisions about the allocation of funds or to give them any control over their lives.

However, the culture of poverty concept may be handy if carefully used. For example, the controversy and research about the concept may help us understand the range of values of the poor, the function of their specific values, and in what situations they emerge. Attention to life-styles can tell us how and why certain groups are excluded from the mainstream and are unable to obtain adequate services. The insight gained can guide health care planners and others to restructure health care so that it is equally available to the poor.

Poverty and Health

There is a reciprocal relation between poverty and health. It has long been recognized that economic deprivation and health status are intertwined. For example, in 1828 Villerme showed that mortality in France was closely linked to the living conditions of different social classes (Rosen, 1963).

In the early twentieth century the health of the poor was still deplorable. In the United States industrial expansion, urban growth, and immigration coincided to produce congested areas with inadequate housing. Poverty, malnutrition, and disease were widespread. Campaigns demanded governmental action to eliminate or ameliorate the consequences of poverty with respect to health. Between 1910 and 1920 American social policy was formulated, and legislation in relation to health was passed. The depression of the 1930s forced on the United States an urgent need to reconsider and to change established patterns of federal and state aid. Through these measures there was a recognition of the health hazards and poor health to which people were subjected because of economic instability.

By the 1960s it was evident that poverty and its attendant ills had not disappeared. With the passage of the Economic Opportunity Act in 1964, the United States declared war on poverty and rediscovered the poor. Congress passed antipoverty legislation to coordinate federal agencies with services and resources related to poverty and to enable the poor to become the recipients. In 1965 Congress enacted the Medicare and Medicaid programs. Medicare is financed through the Social Security system. Medicaid, the state-run program to purchase medical care for low-income persons, is financed by the federal government and each state. Arizona is the only state that has not participated in Medicaid; however, in October 1982 the Arizona Health

Care Cost Containment System (AHCCCS), an experimental health care financing and delivery system, began operation. This marks the first time substantial federal health care funds have come into Arizona. The federal portion is on a capitated basis and is in the form of a 3-year research and demonstration grant (Arizona Department of Health Services, 1982).

From the standpoint of most indicators, the health status of rural people is poor, particularly when contrasted with the health of the total population. The death rates of infants and mothers are significantly higher in rural areas than in urban areas. Additionally, work-related disability rates are high because of accidents resulting from hazardous work environments (Health Status in Rural America, 1977). Most sparsely settled rural areas lack medical personnel and resources as well as strong lobbies in special interest areas. The poor are unlikely to use preventive health care because of more pressing priorities (Bauwens, 1977; Koos, 1954).

Although the health problems of the general rural populations are severe, they are even more critical for migrant farm workers. Migrants generally are more frequently ill, acutely and chronically, than the majority of Americans (Skenhin, 1974). Bissell (1976) noted that "the infant mortality rate is 125 percent above the national average." The accident rate among children of migrants is high because there is little supervision while the mother is working in the fields. Lack of sanitary facilities and overcrowding contribute to the spread of infectious diseases. Housing is frequently improvised and inadequate. The migratory conditions and poverty render the migrants less able to seek health care and these conditions account for the greater probability of their acquiring diseases. In general, poor people get sick more and stay sick longer because of inadequate health maintenance, lack of prevention, poor nutrition, and limited access to adequate personal health services.

The poor are more vulnerable to disease and less able to cope with it than the nonpoverty population. Because of this vulnerability, community health programs should ideally focus attention on populations in which there are high incidences of chronic and communicable diseases, high infant death rates, high birth rates, environmental hazards, and multiple social problems. The community health nurse needs to be involved in the planning and implementing of such programs. The programs ideally take into account social and cultural factors, respect values, mobilize local resources, and concentrate on meeting the needs of the poor. To meet these needs, health programs may encounter difficulties for at least four reasons:

1. The methods used may have to be adapted or especially designed to reach the individuals.

2. Geographically the individuals may be remote from the health centers, adding to problems of transport.
3. Politically the individuals may have little access to power and therefore little influence on the allocation of resources.
4. The values held by the individuals may be different from those of the program planners and administators, and the setting of objectives and appraising of results of the programs may have to follow criteria that differ from those adopted by the rest of the population.

When working with the poor, nurses need to be able to identify the strengths and weaknesses of poor clients without imposing their own values. Facts regarding poverty life-styles need to be distinguished from myth and prejudice. The following questions should be considered by the nurse: Do I perceive the values of the poor client as different from my own? If yes, how do the values differ? Do I expect the poor client to conform to my values? What does the client expect of me as a health professional? This value clarification is necessary for nurses to examine their own attitudes with respect to poor clients.

CULTURAL ASSESSMENT

The material in this section is meant to assist nurses to be aware of and sensitive to sociocultural factors that affect health and the health care system. Awareness of sociocultural factors is necessary when assessing a community, family, and individual. Several relevant areas to guide the nurse in the assessment of these factors are found in *Community, Culture and Care* by Brownlee (1978).

Community Sociocultural Factors

The following is a list of pertinent sociocultural factors to be assessed in the community:

1. Existing influences that divide people into groups within the community, such as ethnicity, religion, social class, occupation, place of residence, language, education, sex, race, and age
2. Conditions that lead to social conflict and/or social cohesion
3. Attitudes toward minority groups, youth and the elderly, and males and females
4. Division of the community into neighborhoods or districts and the characteristics of these
5. Formal and informal channels of communication between health programs and the community
6. Barriers that may be the result of differences in cultural beliefs and practices

7. Political orientation in the community (attitudes toward authority and its use in health problems)
8. Patterns of migration either in or out of a community and their effect on health care services
9. Relation of religion and medicine within the community (who and what causes various illnesses and how they can be prevented)
10. Types of diseases or illnesses thought by various members of the community to exist (culture-specific conditions, such as illnesses caused by hot and cold imbalances and diseases of magical origin)

Family and/or Individual Sociocultural Factors

When assessing families or individuals, the community health nurse needs to be aware of the following:

1. Typical family households, roles played by family members and kinship groups, and patterns of residence
2. Events, rituals, and ceremonies considered important within the life cycle, such as birth, baptism, puberty, marriage, and death
3. The health beliefs and values of the family members and the social meaning attached to wellness and illness
   a. Beliefs concerning body organs and or systems and how they function
   b. Particular methods used to help maintain health, such as hygienic and self-care practices
   c. Attitudes toward immunizations, screening tests, and other preventive health measures
   d. Beliefs and practices surrounding conception, pregnancy, childbirth, lactation, and rearing of children
   e. Attitudes toward mental illness, deformities, and death and dying
4. The person(s) in a family responsible for various health-related decisions, such as what to do when ill, where to go, who to see, and what advice to follow
5. Health topics that may be sensitive or taboo to the client
6. Possible conflicts between family health beliefs and practices and the teachings and practices of an established health program
7. Beliefs, rules, and preferences or prejudices concerning food, such as those believed to cause or cure illness
8. Culturally appropriate ways to enter and leave situations, including greetings, farewells, and convenient hours to make a home visit

Cultural assessment of the community, family or individual includes all of the preceding factors. The community health nurse needs to spend time to learn the culture before beginning any efforts at intervention or change. Specific families and individuals do not always reflect the "typical" cultural pattern. The nurse must remain sensitive to individual variations.

GUIDELINES FOR CULTURALLY APPROPRIATE HEALTH CARE

Modern Western medicine considers the biomedical model to be the best if not the only view of disease. This cultural conditioning of health professionals leads to depreciation or even denial of the client's view. To compensate for this inherent bias it is suggested that nurses elicit clients' interpretations of their health problems.

Client's Explanatory Model

Kleinman (1980) developed the concept of a client explanatory model by which an individual pulls together various beliefs and applies them to an illness to provide a meaningful explanation of the events surrounding the illness and to choose an appropriate course of action. The client's model deals with one or more of the same five questions for illness as used in the medical model: (1) etiology, (2) onset of symptoms, (3) pathophysiology, (4) course of illness, and (5) treatment. Usually the client's model is more concrete, is not completely articulated, and may be inconsistent and based on erroneous evaluation of evidence. "Nonetheless, they (clients' models) are comparable to clinical models . . . as attempts to explain to clinical phenomena" (Kleinman et al., 1978, p. 256). The client's model reflects cultural beliefs, social class, education, occupation, religious affiliation, and past experience with illness and health care.

Clients often hesitate to disclose their models to health professionals. Once the client is assured that the health care provider is genuinely interested, his model can usually be elicited by the nurse with a few simple, direct questions. The following set of questions will help to elicit the client's explanation of the illness (Kleinman et al., 1978, p. 256):

1. What do you think caused your problem?
2. Why do you think it started when it did?
3. What do you think your sickness does to you? How does it work?
4. How severe is your sickness? Will it have a short or long course?
5. What kind of treatment do you think you should receive?

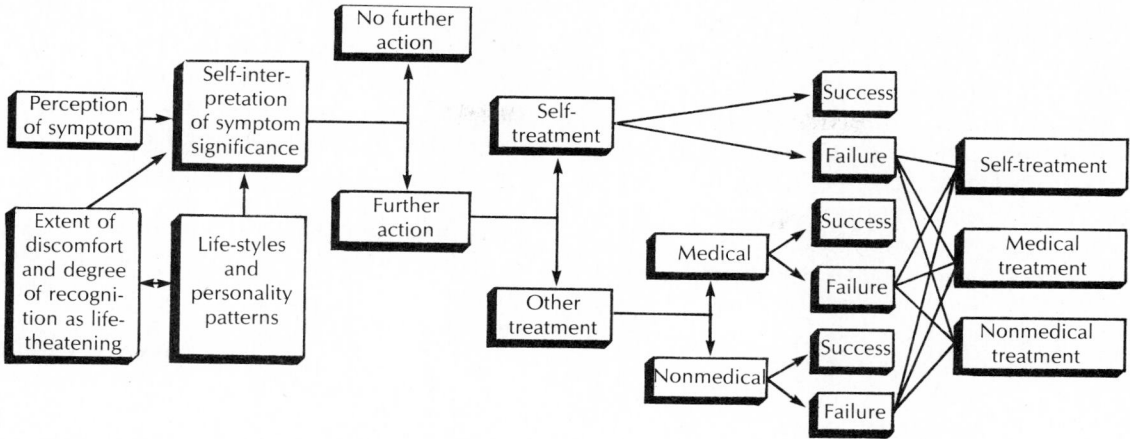

Fig. 11-3. Process of symptom management. (From Jackson, J. J.: Urban black Americans. In Harwood, A. K., editor: Ethnicity and medical care, Cambridge, Mass., 1981, Harvard University Press, p. 83. Reprinted by permission.)

Client's Perception of Symptoms

A model developed by Jackson (1981) illustrates the process that a client might use from the initial self-perception of illness symptoms to treatment, whether that treatment is self-care, medical, or nonmedical (Fig. 11-3). The model begins with the perception of a symptom, which implies that the individual has identified that something is wrong. The individual then evaluates the significance of the symptom. Many factors influence the interpretative process, such as cultural beliefs and values, extent of discomfort, and previous experience with illness. Jackson (1981) believes that the level of income, social class, education, and disruption of activity are major variables that determine the client's process of symptom management. Based on the interpretation, the client may or may not initiate further action. If further action is considered necessary, the person can choose self-treatment or treatment by others, medical or nonmedical. The client then makes a decision about the success or failure of the selected treatment. If the treatment is deemed a failure, vacillation among alternative sources of health care or simultaneous use of two or more alternatives is likely to occur. Mechanic (1969) believes that the major goal of treatment is symptom abatement.

Cultural Health Practices

Cultural health practices can be considered as efficacious, neutral, or dysfunctional (Pillsbury, 1982). Efficacious practices are recognized by Western medicine as being beneficial to health even though they may be very different from scientific practices. Beneficial prac-

tices should be actively encouraged by community health nurses, although they may seem foreign to mainstream health professionals. A treatment strategy congruent with the client's own beliefs has a better chance of being successful. For example, cultural beliefs about the efficacy of herbal teas must be considered by the community health nurse, since some are therapeutic (dehydration can be treated with tea). Treatment with tea may be as efficacious as water. Another example is the use of the traditional birthing position of kneeling, which seems to be more beneficial for women than the horizontal position advocated by Western medical practice (Cominsky, 1977).

Neutral (harmless) practices are of no significance one way or another to the health of the individual. They may be considered unimportant by the health professional, but for the individual the health practices may be linked with beliefs that are closely integrated into everyday behaviors. Examples of practices that are neutral include "the ritual disposal of the placenta and cord, interpretation of signs in the cord, avoidance of sexual activity during various stages of pregnancy, culturally prescribed hygiene practices and avoidance of exposure during a lunar eclipse" (Johnston, 1980, p. 13). Even though these practices do not require intervention by the practitioner, the nurse should respect their significance and meaning to the individual.

In all cultures there are practices that are dysfunctional or harmful from a health point of view. In Western countries the excessive use of sugar and overrefined flour is partially responsible for the high incidence of dental caries and obesity. Health education should be focused on dysfunctional or harmful health practices. Efforts should be made to assist clients to modify harmful practices.

Williams and Jelliffe (1972) included a category of uncertain practices in their cultural assessment system. This category includes practices with unknown effects, such as swaddling newborns and the use of abdominal binders for mothers and infants. In most instances practices do not perfectly fit into one category or another. "Health practices are relatively more or less beneficial or harmful when compared to alternative practices" (Greene and Johnston, 1980, p. 13).

In addition to culturally specific health care practices, individuals may turn to alternative health practitioners for a variety of reasons. Harwood (1981) listed the following general reasons why individuals might use alternative healers: (1) lack of availability and accessibility of mainstream health services, (2) lack of satisfaction with treatment, (3) lack of trust in the ability of Western medical practitioners to effectively treat psychosocial problems, and (4) lack of knowledge of Western medical practitioners in the treatment of culture-bound syndromes.

In many cases alternative healers complement the delivery of mainstream health care services. Often they are more available and accessible than Western health care providers. They are familiar with culture-bound syndromes and cultural traditions. In addition, they often establish warm relations with clients and their families.

Principles for Nursing Practice

Based on the discussion of culture and cultural differences, principles for nursing practice can be identified.

The nurse should be aware of the client's cultural interpretation of health, illness, and health care. A client's perception and definition of an experience as an illness is partially the result of culturally learned beliefs and the amount and kind of exposure to mainstream health culture. Clarification of the variety of client interpretations by different cultural groups is important. The objective is to be aware of and sensitive to the fact that there are multiple factors underlying client behaviors. The nurse should question clients concerning their ideas about health and illness in a nonjudgmental way that elicits the client's concepts and communicates genuine interest.

The nurse should identify sources of discrepancy between clients' and health providers' concepts of health or illness. A frequent source of poor communication between clients and nurses is when one party uses a term to label an illness or a symptom and that term is unfamiliar to the other person. Another source of miscom-

munication occurs when the client and the nurse use the same term but mean different things. For example, the term *family* has a variety of meanings for different segments of the community. Lack of communication may go undetected because the client and the nurse are using the same term. The nurse should check with the client as to the meaning for the unknown term, and the client should be encouraged to request clarification from the nurse. Discrepancies will then become apparent and should be discussed. Methods of handling discrepancies include educating the client; adapting the nursing care plan to the client's system (i.e., agreeing to a therapeutic plan that accommodates the client and the nurse to some degree); or working within the client's system by using a therapeutic care plan that is considered effective by the nurse and appropriate for the client's culture.

The nurse should be aware of the cultural values that affect client's use of the health care system. Cultural values shape human health behaviors and determine what individuals will do to maintain their health status, how they will care for themselves and others who become ill, and where and from whom they will seek health care. Cultural preferences for certain modes of treatment suggest that nursing interventions may be more effective if they include culturally perferred treatment modes. For example, the nurse might mention the use of herbal teas in addition to the usual use of water or juice when caring for Mexican American clients.

The nurse should evaluate the effectiveness of nursing actions with clients from diverse cultural groups. One way to evaluate the effectiveness of nursing actions is by monitoring the client's adherence to treatment regimens. Clients judge regimens not only on a medical basis but also on a social and cultural basis. Whether the regimen is adhered to or not may depend on such conditions as explaining the regimen using vocabulary that the client can understand; accommodating the client's life-style, dietary patterns, and health beliefs; and enlisting the client's family in reinforcing treatment regimens. The specific family members enlisted for support may differ according to the client's ethnic affiliation.

Knowledge of cultural patterns enhances the ability of the nurse to assess and understand the client's health beliefs and practices. Assessment of sociocultural factors enables the nurse to identify ways in which individuals and families may differ from the typical cultural pattern. Sensitivity to individual variations makes it possible to plan culturally appropriate interpretation of health problems. It is important to be aware of the process that clients use from the initial self-perception of their illness symptoms to treatment. The nurse must be aware of how clients evaluate the success or failure of the treatment. Cultural health practices are described as being beneficial, neutral, or harmful.

The overall purpose of this chapter has been to help nurses deliver more personalized, culturally appropriate care to all clients. If clients are to be treated in a holistic manner, the nurse must constantly be aware of their attributes and health beliefs and practices.

SUMMARY

Sociocultural variables related to health care have been discussed. The premise that health care is based not only on knowledge of the physical causes of a disease but also on sociocultural influences has been introduced. Culture has been defined as a set of rules that help people act appropriately. The following cultural concepts that have relevance for nurses have been discussed: holism, culture change, enculturation, culture-bound, ethnocentrism, stereotypes, and cultural values.

The mobility of people and their cultural diversity increase the likelihood that nurses will come in contact with a variety of cultural life-styles and traditions. Often nurses must provide care for individuals from different cultural groups. This chapter has explored cultural trend items in the following areas: ethnic collectivity, cultural shock, communication patterns, personal space and contact, and cultural views of disease and illness. Diverse cultures of the United States, namely, Asian, black, Mexican, Arab, and Native American, have been presented as examples to provide cultural background data to assist nurses in providing culturally relevant nursing care. Poverty has been addressed from the economic, psychological, and cultural perspective, and the reciprocal relation between poverty and health has been discussed.

BIBLIOGRAPHY

Ackerknecht, E.H.: Problems of primitive medicine, Bull. Hist. Med. **11**:508-509, 1942.

Arizona Department of Health Services: AHCCCS (Arizona Health Care Cost Containment System) Bulletin, Phoenix, Dec. 14, 1982, AHCCCS Public Information Office.

Bauwens, E. E.: Medical beliefs and practices among lower-income Anglos. In Spicer, E.H., editor: Ethnic medicine in the Southwest, Tucson, 1977, University of Arizona Press.

Benedict, R.: Patterns of culture, Boston, 1934, Houghton Mifflin Co.

Berkanovic, E., and Reeder, L.G.: Ethnic, economic and social psychological factors in the source of medical care, Soc. Prob. **21**:246-259, 1973.

Bissell, K.A.: The migrant farmworker, Washington, D.C., 1976, The Catholic University of America.

Brownlee, A. T.: Community, culture and care, St. Louis, 1978, The C.V. Mosby Co.

Bullough, V.L., and Bullough, B.: Health care for the other Americans, New York, 1982, Appleton-Century-Crofts.

Chrisman, N.J.: The health seeking process, Cult. Med. Psychiatry **1**:351-377, 1977.

Clark, M.: Health in the Mexican-American culture, Berkeley, 1970, University of California Press.

Cominsky, S.: Childbirth and midwifery on a Guatemalan finca, Med. Anthropol. **1**:94, 1977.

De Migul, J.M.: A framework for the study of national health systems, Inquiry **12**(2):10-24, June 1975.

Dohrenwend, B.P.: Sociocultural and social-psychologist factors in the genesis of mental disorders, J. Health Soc. Behav. **16**:365-392, 1975.

Dohrenwend, B.P., and Dohrenwend, B.S.: Social status and psychological disorder: a causal inquiry, New York, 1969, John Wiley & Sons, Inc.

Dohrenwend, B.S., and Dohrenwend, B.P.: Stressful life events: their nature and effects, New York, 1974, John Wiley & Sons, Inc.

Dunham, H.W.: Community and schizophrenia: an epidemiological analysis, Detroit, 1965, Wayne State University.

Elling, R.H.: Socio-cultural influences on health and health care, New York, 1977, Springer Publishing Co., Inc.

Fabrega, H.: Medical anthropology. In Siegel, B.J., editor: Biennial review of anthropology, Stanford, Calif., 1971, Stanford University Press.

Foster, G.M.: Relationships between theoretical and applied anthropology: a public health analysis, Hum. Organization **11**:5-16, 1952.

Goodenough, W.H.: Cooperation in change, New York, 1966, Russell Sage Foundation.

Greenblum, J.: Medical and health orientations of American Jews: a case of diminishing distinctiveness, Soc. Sci. Med. **8**:127-134, 1974.

Greene, L., and Johnston, F.: Social and biological predictors of nutritional status, growth, and development, New York, 1980. Academic Press.

Guttmacher, S., and Elinson, J.: Ethno-religious variation in perceptions of illness: the use of illness as an explanation for deviant behavior, Soc. Sci. Med. **5**:117-125, 1971.

Hall, E.T.: The silent language, New York, 1959, Doubleday & Co., Inc.

Harrison, G., and Ritenbaugh, C.: Anthropology and nutrition: a perspective on two scientific subcultures, Fed. Proc. **4**:(11):2595-2600, Sept. 1981.

Harwood, A., editor: Ethnicity and medical care, Cambridge, Mass., 1981, Harvard University Press.

Hautman, M.A., and Harrison, J.K.: Health beliefs and practices in a middle-income Anglo-American neighborhood, Adv. Nurs. Sci. **4** (3):49-64, 1982.

Health status in rural America, Rural Health Report no. 1, Washington, D.C., 1977, Rural America.

Henderson, G., and Primeaux, M.: Transcultural health care, Reading, Mass., 1981, Addison-Wesley Publishing Co., Inc.

Hollander, J.: The abolition of poverty, Boston, 1914, Houghton Mifflin Co.

Hollingshead, A.B., and Redlich, F.C.: Social class and medical illness, New York, 1958, John Wiley & Sons, Inc.

Horn, B.M.: Transcultural nursing and child-rearing of the Muckleshoot people. In Leininger, M., editor: Transcultural nursing, New York, 1979, Masson International Nursing Publications.

Insel, P.M.: Too close for comfort, Englewood Cliffs, N.J., 1978, Prentice-Hall, Inc.

Jackson, J.J.: Urban black Americans. In Harwood, A., editor: Ethnicity and medical care, Cambridge, Mass., 1981, Harvard University Press.

Jelliffe, D.B.: Child nutrition in developing countries, Washington, D.C., 1969, U.S. Department of Health, Education, and Welfare.

Josephy, A.M., Jr.: The Indian heritage of America. New York, 1969, Alfred A. Knopf, Inc.

Kahn, A.O.: Studies in social policy and planning, New York, 1969, Russell Sage Foundation.

Kay, M.A.: Health in the Mexican-American barrio. In Spicer, E.H., editor: Ethnic medicine in the southwest, Tucson, 1977, University of Arizona Press.

Kleinman, A.: Patients and healers in the context of culture, Berkeley, 1980, University of California Press.

Kleinman, A., Eisenberg, L., and Good, B.: Culture, illness and care, Ann. Intern. Med. **88**:251-258, 1978.

Kluckhohn, C.: The gifts of tongues. In Samover, L.A., and Porter, R.E., editors: Intercultural communication: a reader, Belmont, Calif., 1972, Wadsworth, Inc.

Kniep-Hardy, M., and Burkhardt, M.: Nursing the Navajo, Am. J. Nurs. **77**:95-96, 1977.

Koos, E.: Health in Regionville, New York, 1954, Columbia University Press.

Kubricht, D.W., and Clark, J.A.: Foreign patients: a system for providing care, Nurs. Outlook **30**(1):55-57, Jan. 1982.

Kunitz, I.J., and Levy, J.E.: Navajos, In Harwood, A., editor: Ethnicity and medical care, Cambridge, Mass., 1981, Harvard University Press.

Leacock, E.: The culture of poverty: a critique, New York, 1971, Simon & Schuster.

Leininger, M.: Transcultural health care issues and conditions, Philadelphia, 1976, F.A. Davis Co.

Lewis, O.: The children of Sanchez, New York, 1961, Random House, Inc.

Lewis, O.: La Vida, New York, 1966, Random House, Inc.

Madsen, M.: The Mexican-Americans of south Texas, New York, 1964, Holt, Rinehart & Winston General Book.

Mechanic, D.: Illness and cure. In Kosa, J., Antonovsky, A., and Zola, I., editors: Poverty and health: a sociological analysis, Cambridge, Mass., 1969, Harvard University Press.

Meisenhelder, J.B.: Boundaries of personal space, Image **14**(1):16-19, Feb.-March 1982.

Meleis, A.I.: The Arab American in the health care system, Am. J. Nurs. **81**:1180-1183, 1981.

Meleis, A.I., and Sorrell, L.: Arab American women and their birth experiences, Am. J. Mat. Child Nurs. **6**:171-176, 1981.

National Center for Health Statistics: Vital statistics of the United States, 1977, vol. II, Mortality, Part A, Hyattsville, MD., 1981, U.S. Government Printing Office.

Oakland, L., and Kane, R.L.: The working mother and child neglect on the Navajo reservation, Pediatics **51**:849-853, 1973.

Pillsbury, B.: Doing the month: confinement and convalescence of Chinese women after childbirth. In Kay, M., editor: Anthropology of human birth, Philadelphia, 1982, F.A. Davis Co.

Primeaux, M., and Henderson, G.: American Indian patient care. In Henderson, S., and Primeaux, M., editors: Transcultural health care, Philadelphia, 1981, F.A. Davis Co.

Quesada, G.M.: Mexican Americans: Mexicans or Americans? Lubbock, Tex., 1973, Southwestern Council of Latin-American Studies.

Rosen, G.: The evaluation of social medicine. In Freeman, H.E., Levin, S., and Reeder, L.B., editors: Handbook of medical sociology, Englewood Cliffs, N.J., 1963, Prentice-Hall, Inc.

Rubel, A.: Across the tracks: Mexican Americans in a Texas city, Austin, 1966, University of Texas Press.

Ruiz, M.C.J.: Open-closed mindedness, intolerance of ambiguity and nursing faculty attitudes toward culturally different patients, Nurs. Res. **30**(3):177-181, 1981.

Ryan, W.: Blaming the victim, New York, 1971, Pantheon Books.

Samora, J.: Conceptions of health and disease among Spanish-Americans, Am. Cath. Sociol. Rev. **22**:314-323, 1961.

Saunders, L.: Cultural difference and medical care, New York, 1954, Russell Sage Foundation.

Shenkin, B.N.: Health care for migrant workers, Cambridge, Mass., 1974, Ballinger Publishing Co.

Snow, L.F.: Popular medicine in a black neighborhood. In Spicer, E.H., editor: Ethnic medicine in the southwest, Tucson, 1977, University of Arizona Press.

Spector, R.E.: Cultural diversity in health and illness, New York, 1979, Appleton-Century-Crofts.

Suchman, E.A.: Sociomedical variations among ethnic groups, Am. J. Sociol. **70**:319-331, 1964.

Townsend, P.: Poverty as relative deprivation: resources and style of living. In Weaderburn, D., editor: Poverty inequality and class structure, London, 1974, Cambridge University Press.

Tripp-Reimer, T.: Barriers to health care: variations in interpretation of Appalachian client behavior by Appalachian and non-Appalachinan health professionals, West. J. Nurs. Res. **4**(2):179-191, 1982.

U.S. Bureau of the Census: Statistical abstracts of the United States, 1979, Washington, D.C., 1979, U.S. Government Printing Office.

Valentine, C.A.: Culture and poverty, Chicago, 1968, University of Chicago Press.

Vogel, V.J.: American Indian medicine, Norman, Okla., 1970, University of Oklahoma Press.

Watson, O.M.: Proxemic behavior: a cross-cultural study, The Hague, Netherlands, 1970, Monitor & Co.

Weaver, T.: Use of hypothetical situations in a study of Spanish-American illness referral systems, Hum. Org. **29**:140, 1970.

White, E.H.: Giving health care to minority patients, Nurs. Clin. North Am. **12**:27-40, 1977.

Williams, C., and Jelliffe, D.: Mother and child health: delivering the services, London, 1972, Oxford University Press.

Young, A.A.: Rethinking the Western health enterprise, Med. Anthropol. **2**(2):1-9, 1978.

Yu, E.: The low mortality rates of Chinese infants: some plausible explanatory factors, Soc. Sci. Med. **16**(3):253-265, 1982.

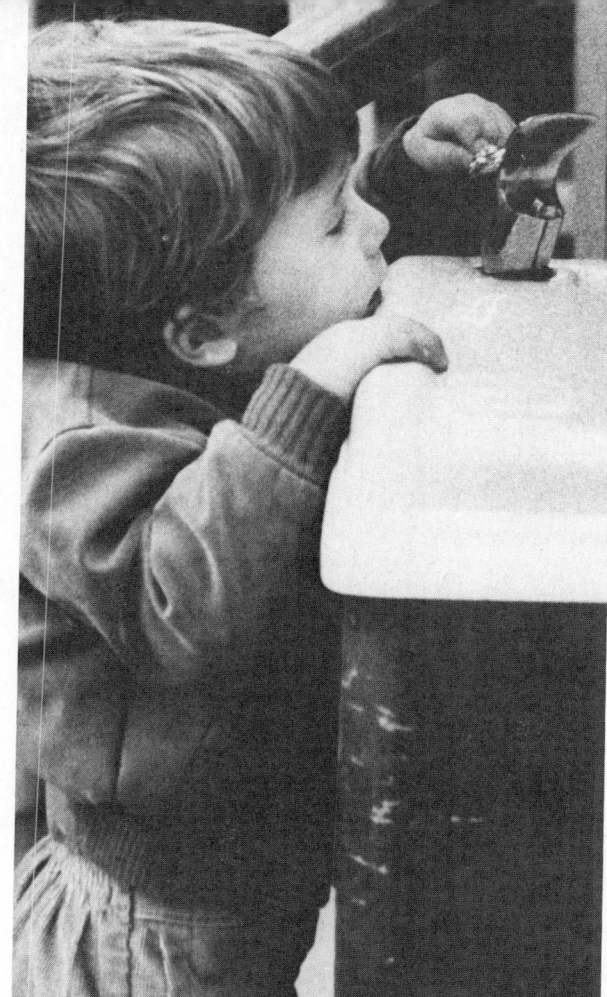

Chapter
12

JOAN TURNER

COMMUNICABLE DISEASES AND INFECTION CONTROL PRACTICES IN COMMUNITY HEALTH

In recent decades the impact of communicable diseases on contemporary society has been drastically reduced and altered by the combined efforts of such disciplines as medicine, nursing, microbiology, pharmacology, and sanitary engineering. Table 12-1 illustrates the declining mortality associated with heretofore common communicable diseases. The table shows only one aspect of the communicable disease problem, namely death. Other aspects that the community health nurse must be familiar with, are discussed in this chapter, and include surveillance mechanisms, temporal and geographical patterns, realized and potential effects of current and past immunization programs, the emergence of new communicable and/or infectious processes, and the increasing appearance of antibiotic-resistant organ-

isms. Incidence, mortality, and morbidity data are used to explore these phenomena.

The vast majority of persons who succumb to communicable diseases contract them in the larger community and are cared for at home. This chapter discusses the role of the community health nurse in prevention, control, finding cases, reporting, and maintenance strategies as they relate to communicable and infectious processes.

HISTORICAL PERSPECTIVE

Communicable diseases have helped to shape human destiny since earliest times. In fact, since humans are the only reservoir for many of these diseases, micro-

Table 12-1. Death attributed to common communicable diseases in the United States in 1900, 1935, and 1978

	1900	1935	1978
Influenza and pneumonia	202.2*	103.9	30.9
Tuberculosis	194.2	55.1	2.6
Diphtheria	40.3	3.1	†
Typhoid	12.0	2.7	†
Meningococcal infections	12.0	2.1	0.3

* All statistics represent rates per 100,000 persons.
† Some death rates for 1978 are not available.

biologists ponder such questions as, "which came first, human beings or infectious organisms?" It is supposed that humans who lived in the Paleolithic period (18,000 to 6000 BC) were susceptible to tapeworms and round-worms as well as tetanus and gas gangrene. However, the occurrences of epidemics or outbreaks involving large numbers of people were not evident until approximately 5000 to 4000 BC). Before that period of time, family groups were largely nomadic and isolated from similar social groups. As the first large cities came into existence and great numbers of persons lived in close proximity, the stage was set for innumerable epidemics of communicable diseases. Occasionally these epidemics came close to exterminating organized society.

Diseases such as tuberculosis, mumps, hepatitis, and influenza were present in Egypt as early as 3000 BC. Diseases that are now thought to be malaria and small-pox were documented in China around 400 BC. As discussed in Chapter 1, epidemics of measles, mumps, diphtheria, cholera, plague, and smallpox swept through Europe in the Middle Ages. More than half of all causes of death were related to communicable diseases during that time.

Examples of some of history's most notorious and lethal epidemics are the Black Death in Europe in 1345 AD, smallpox in the North American Indians in 1633, dysentery during the Crusades, and influenza pandemics of 1889 and 1918. In a few days, an epidemic of yellow fever left Napoleon with 3000 survivors out of 25,000 troops. Such mortality figured heavily in his ultimate defeat at Waterloo (Hare, 1955).

Communicable diseases continued to play a significant role in the death and illness of people through the colonial period in the United States, and they were still leading causes of death in 1900. In fact, the need to control the spread of communicable diseases rather than the concern for infected individuals stimulated the first health legislation in the United States including the establishment of health departments in colonial America. Nevertheless, the antibiotics of the 1940s, the vaccines of the 1950s, 1960s, and 1970s, and the general improvement in nutrition and sanitation gradually brought many of the killing and crippling communicable diseases under control.

CURRENT PERSPECTIVE

Some infectious diseases, such as smallpox, have been completely exterminated; the severity of attack has been lessened in others, and often death can be prevented. For instance, the dramatic decrease in death from pneumonia can be seen in Table 12-1. However, community health nurses cannot discount the real and potential impact that communicable and infectious processes have on society for at least five reasons (see box on next page).

First of all, failure to enforce the recommended schedule for communicable disease control (see Tables 12-5 and 12-6) or a break in community sanitation or water purification can result in an epidemic at any given point in time. An epidemic is not the only threat; communicable diseases also result in chronic disability and irreversible disease processes every year. For instance, it is estimated that the occurrence of rubeola, a disease that is 95% preventable by immunization, resulted in 600 cases of mental retardation in 1975 in the United States alone (Brown, 1975).

Second, community health nurses must be knowledgeable about communicable diseases to effectively counsel parents or family members in the care of potentially exposed or frankly infected persons. Often community health nurses are also in positions to recognize signs and symptoms of actual or impending disease and thus make appropriate referrals for diagnosis, treatment, and control.

Third, communicable disease plays a tremendous role in the economic viability of any given community and of the nation as a whole. Roger Ezeberg of the U.S. Department of Health, Education and Welfare estimated that the total economic loss from the 1968-1969 pandemic of Hong Kong influenza in the United States alone was $46 million (Beveridge, 1978). In addition, acute respiratory disease (i.e., the "flu" or a "cold") is the most common human illness and the principal reason for people to consult a physician. Approximately 156 million workdays are lost annually at a cost of $24 billion as a result of communicable and infectious diseases (Healthy People, 1979).

Fourth, community health nurses must recognize the changing trends underlying communicable and infectious disease processes. Although trends in specific diseases are discussed in some detail later in this chapter, one of the most important aspects of the changing pattern of communicable diseases lies in the resistance to usual treatment protocols now found in organisms that were once completely sensitive to a given antibiotic. Over the last 25 years, infection-causing bacteria have evolved that are literally impervious to antibiotics. The genesis of drug-resistant bacteria is thought to be the abuse or overuse of antibiotics. Lappe (1981, p. 225) said that if practitioners do not stop the misuse of antibiotics, "we may soon face a generation of germs that will not die." Abuse of antibiotics is not perpetuated by prescription alone but also by their use as additives to crop sprays, food preservatives, and animal feed.

Finally, considering only causes of mortality provides the community health nurse with a fragment of the view needed to deal effectively with the problem of communicable and infectious processes (Table 12–1). Gradually, attempts to deal with communicable and infectious processes of contemporary society on a larger scale are being mobilized, and the community health nurse continues to play an important role in those attempts. For instance, there is an international thrust behind judicious use of antibiotics, and much of the community health nursing role that corresponds with this movement involves professional and lay health education relating to the dangers of antibiotic misuse and guidelines for intelligent and therapeutic administration of these substances.

Infectious and/or Communicable Diseases

For purposes of this discussion, infection is a complex interaction of a host and parasite; the characteristics of both affect the interaction (Ramsay and Emond, 1979).

Communicable diseases are transmitted from one host to another by a variety of methods and are caused by specific agents that may be found in the environment. As discussed in Chapter 8, the minimum requirements for a communicable disease to occur are (1) a host that provides sufficient living conditions for the organism or parasite, (2) an agent that is capable of causing disease, and (3) a reservoir or environment where living conditions are sufficient for the maintenance and occasionally the growth and reproduction of the agent. Any communicable disease requires an interaction among these three components, host, agent, and environment. Interaction is the key word, since these three components may coexist without it, and the result might not be disease (see box on p. 262).

The great epidemics of the past create a picture of vast armies of microbiological invaders that have competed with humans throughout the ages for survival. However, such a picture is far from descriptive of the usual relationship of peaceful coexistence between the host and the microbiological parasite. Actually, many microbes live in symbiosis-producing metabolites essential for the nutrition of the host, whereas others appear to protect their host against invasion by more virulent organisms. A few parasites and hosts are poorly matched, and the result of that disequilibrium is frequently disease.

Occasionally, disease agents undergo a stage of development in another host; for example, *Trichinella spiralis* matures in swine, bear, and aquatic mammals and is excreted as live larvae.

Epizootic disease denotes a phenomenon in which an epidemic, similar to one in humans, strikes animals. Examples of such epizootic disease are yellow fever in monkeys, plague in rodents, and salmonella enteritis in farm animals. Under these circumstances, the host-parasite relationship is complex and easily disturbed.

Arthropod vectors also play an important part in the spread of many infectious diseases, particularly in the southeastern United States and other tropical and subtropical regions. In some infections, like malaria, the parasite must undergo development within arthropod vectors before it can be transmitted.

Factors Influencing Infection
Agent Factors

The following discussion describes various agent characteristics that are influential in disease causation (Ramsey and Emond, 1979).

Pathogenicity refers to the agent's relative ability to produce disease. The aspect of pathogenicity varies widely from one species to another and frequently de-

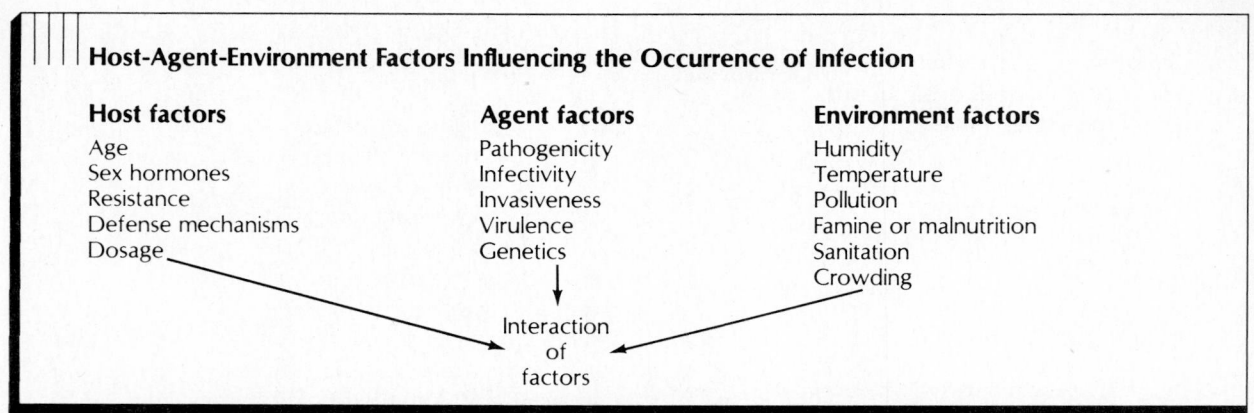

Host-Agent-Environment Factors Influencing the Occurrence of Infection

Host factors	Agent factors	Environment factors
Age	Pathogenicity	Humidity
Sex hormones	Infectivity	Temperature
Resistance	Invasiveness	Pollution
Defense mechanisms	Virulence	Famine or malnutrition
Dosage	Genetics	Sanitation
		Crowding

Interaction of factors

pends on various microbiological characteristics such as the presence of capsules or enzymes. One contemporary example of an enzyme produced by organisms is penicillinase, which results in the organism's ability to survive in the presence of penicillin.

Infectivity is the ability of the organism to spread rapidly from one host to another. High infectivity is not necessarily associated with the severity of disease. For example, chickenpox virus is believed to be one of the most infectious agents in contemporary times, but the disease is generally self-limited in that there are usually no permanent effects from it.

Invasiveness refers to the agent's ability to spread within the host. An example of this characteristic is the organism *Treponema pallidum,* which is capable of spreading throughout the body.

Virulence is the ability to produce severe disease. An example of this agent characteristic is the influenza-A virus, which is capable of producing more severe disease than the influenza-C strains.

Dosage refers to the fact that multiple organisms invading the host are more apt to overwhelm host defenses, whereas small numbers of the same organisms are frequently suppressed or tolerated without disease actually occurring. For instance, a host eating a hearty portion of salmonella-infected food would be more likely to get food poisoning than one who ate sparingly of the same food. Also, a mixed or multiple-agent infection often produces more serious effects than separate invasion by the components. For example, the onset of bacterial pneumonia in addition to a generalized influenza syndrome greatly increases the threat to the affected host.

Host Factors

In general, most disease processes produce the greatest morbidity and mortality in the very young and the very old in any given population, but there are some important exceptions. Many viral diseases produce much less disturbance (are less virulent) in the young. For instance, mumps are generally tolerated better by young children than middle-aged adults. However, chicken-pox in a newborn, although rare, is frequently life-threatening.

Males and females react differently to infection. Sex hormones influence the reaction of the tissues to infection. For instance, estrogens render the vaginal epithelium resistant to bacterial invasion whereas testosterone sensitizes the testes to mumps virus. Also, because of the slight physiological depression of the autoimmune system in pregnant women, they are particularly vulnerable to infectious disease and may suffer a high mortality during communicable disease outbreaks. Finally, cortisone and its derivatives lower host resistance to infection.

In humans, resistance to malaria and tuberculosis may differ among generations. For instance, the death rate of one generation during initial epidemic may be as high as 99%. However, with the subsequent destruction of most of the susceptible individuals in successive generations, the survivors of such epidemics and their descendents have a higher rate of immunity.

Both the host's local and systemic responses (defense mechanisms) to potential infection have a bearing on whether or not infection ultimately occurs. The quality and effectiveness of the host's defense mechanisms are in turn influenced by the wide range of factors related to the general well-being of the host. Chronically ill people and those with immunosuppression are more susceptible to infection. Conversely, those with a high level of health are generally less susceptible to infection. In addition, many facets of the host's ability to ward off infection are interdependent on environmental factors such as humidity, temperature, and crowding.

Environmental Factors

Environmental factors play a role in the infectious process. Because of the effect they have on the host and the agent, atmospheric factors such as humidity and temperature of the air play a significant role in the spread of infection. For instance, there is a temporal or seasonal pattern to many communicable diseases. Changes in humidity and temperature may alter the habits of the host and the state of the respiratory mucosa. In addition, air pollution and smoke tend to reduce the resistance of the respiratory tract to infection, and statistically these factors increase the incidence of pneumonia.

The so-called scourges of humanity, famine, pestilence, and war, occur together. Infection in the undernourished host generally results in disease that is virulent and often deadly. Lack of protein in the diet is believed to interfere with the development of cell-mediated immunity, and deficiencies of vitamin A lower the resistance of epithelial cells (Ramsay and Emond, 1979).

Contamination of food or water supplies with sewage may result in diseases ranging from cholera and hepatitis to salmonella and schistosomiasis. In fact, endemic (or those diseases particular to a given geographical area) strongholds for these and other communicable diseases exist in parts of the world where sanitation is poor or water is not purified. For instance, enteric diseases such as cholera are endemic to Asia and the Middle East.

Efficient transmission of most of the communicable diseases requires that large numbers of people interact. In addition, when people come into contact with animals or their by-products, the risk of contracting certain communicable diseases is increased. For instance, veterinarians are particularly susceptible to brucellosis and rabies, hunters who prepare animal hides are susceptible to anthrax, and bird fanciers are susceptible to psittacosis or parrot fever.

Summary

An infectious agent is necessary but not sufficient to produce disease. Although some of the complexities of the interaction that produces disease cannot always be fully understood, consideration of all factors is essential when constructing preventive or management strategies for communicable diseases.

Impact of the Contemporary Problem

Because communicable phenomena change over time, it is important to examine what diseases occur in contemporary times and how their occurrence is monitored.

Surveillance

Surveillance, a basic skill in communicable disease control, requires four sets of activities. Community health nurses may play a role in any or all four of these activities:

1. Identifying active cases and persons exposed to disease
2. Reporting suspected or confirmed cases to health authorities
3. Analyzing and interpreting reported information
4. Synthesizing information to implement control measures

The first step in surveillance is identifying the probable cases of active disease and additional individuals exposed to disease. Accomplishment of this activity requires that health personnel who see people in clinic or home settings be alert to objective and subjective signs and symptoms of various common communicable diseases. Individuals with fever, rash, swollen lymph nodes, nausea, vomiting, or diarrhea must be further evaluated to rule out communicable disease.

The second step in surveillance is reporting suspected or confirmed cases to a responsible health authority who is generally either the physician or nurse in charge of the communicable disease section of the county health department. In some instances, formal mechanisms exist for reporting suspected or confirmed cases, such as specific surveillance forms that may be completed and forwarded to the communicable disease branch of the county health department. More frequently, reporting observed or assumed cases is done by telephone. The community health nurse who reports by telephone or in written form must collect all information that may be requested, such as signs and symptoms exhibited by cases, date of onset, duration of symptoms, and any number of pertinent environmental and host factors.

The third step in surveillance is analyzing and interpreting reported information to determine the implications of a given disease manifestation. This step requires that current information be analyzed in light of past and present disease trends. These specialized activities are often carried out by an intradisciplinary team of people who function to prevent and control communicable and infectious processes. Although this team is typically headed by a physician with special interest and training in communicable diseases, nurses play a significant part in the ongoing activities of the team. Such nurses typically have considerable interest in communicable and infectious processes and advanced preparation in both community health nursing and epidemiology.

The final step in surveillance requires synthesizing

information so that an appropriate response to the disease outbreak can be made. At this point, measures are instituted to control the source of the problem. Controlling any given outbreak may require immunization, health education, quarantine, or rigorous screening programs.

Thus surveillance begins with the identification of a real or potential problem and is complete only after the problem is resolved and is therefore no longer a public threat. By examining the four sets of activities associated with surveillance, it can be seen that this is a multi-faceted process with many ramifications for community health nursing practice. It is through surveillance activities that the morbidity and mortality of a given disease over a period of months or years is known. It is also through surveillance that disease phenomena are monitored and ultimately controlled.

Surveillance System. Since 1961, the Centers for Disease Control (CDC) in Atlanta, Georgia, have been responsible for the collection of data on nationally notifiable communicable diseases on a number of other disease phenomena. In 1970 the Communicable Disease Center was renamed the Centers for Disease Control to reflect a broader mandate in preventive services. Over the last two decades, surveillance systems maintained by the CDC have expanded, and emphasis has shifted as incidence rates and disease characteristics have changed. Examples of the interest of the CDC in noncommunicable phenomena include family planning, childhood lead poisoning prevention, congenital birth defects, and chronic diseases.

In 1981 the CDC was officially reorganized and renamed the Centers for Disease Control. In that reorganization the department of Consolidated Surveillance and Communications Activity and the responsibility for publishing the Morbidity and Mortality Weekly Report (MMWR) were subsumed by the CDC.

Each week the CDC publishes the MMWR. These reports include weekly and cumulative totals of reported communicable diseases by geographical region and individual state. Although the format of the MMWR remains constant, various topics of public health interest such as unusual cases of disease, communicable disease outbreaks, and environmental hazards are discussed. Even though the MMWR is the best single source of information on the incidence of communicable and infectious diseases, the statistics cannot always be interpreted as totally accurate because of the phenomenon of "underreporting." Underreporting occurs when cases of a given disease are either not detected or the information is not forwarded to the CDC. Some diseases are more likely to be underreported than others. For example, mild communicable diseases such as chickenpox and rubella are frequently not reported to or detected by health officials. Also, the CDC estimates that only 1% of all salmonella infections are reported (CDC, Annual Summary, 1979).

On the other hand, diseases associated with serious consequences, such as encephalitis and rabies are probably reported quite accurately. Communicable disease requiring laboratory or clinical verification or one treated in the hospital is likely to be accurately reported.

Aside from a slight limitation in the reporting mechanism, the MMWR provides enlightening, authoritative and up-to-date information on many facets of communicable disease occurrence, prevention, and control. At this time the MMWR weekly and annual reports and a plethora of other government documents relative to specific communicable disease phenomenon may be obtained at minimal cost by writing:

Centers for Disease Control
Public Health Service
U.S. Department of Health and Human Services
Atlanta, Georgia 30333

Notifiable and Nonnotifiable Conditions

A disease classified as "nationally notifiable" is one that all states are legally responsible for reporting on a weekly, monthly, and annual basis to CDC. Other diseases may be classified as "optionally reported," and these are diseases that states may choose to report based on their statewide health regulations. Appendix I lists those communicable disease conditions reportable in most states.

In addition to the nationally notifiable communicable diseases, the MMWR and the national surveillance program also monitor the occurrence of other conditions of interest to community health nurses and others. Such communicable disease phenomena are optionally reported by given state health departments and include conditions such as giardiasis, histoplasmosis, infectious mononucleosis, meningitis, Reye's syndrome, strep throat, scarlet fever, toxoplasmosis, and influenza. In some instances, these diseases are reported only when they are believed to be occurring in epidemic proportion (in excess of expectations). At other times, a given disease is reported in a particular state because it is believed to be endemic and therefore an ongoing public health problem. For instance, histoplasmosis is believed to be endemic to the Ohio Valley region.

It is worth noting that it may be difficult to view weekly totals of various communicable diseases literally. For example, the statistics on influenza and pneumonia are "undercounts." To see the real impact of influenza, it is helpful to look at annual summaries (also published by CDC), which examine attributable or cause-specific deaths and the total number of cases reported. In 1978 there were 54,267 deaths attributed to influenza in the United States. That same year influenza and pneumonia ranked as the fifth leading cause of death, accounting for 3% of all deaths (CDC, Annual Summary, 1979).

Morbidity and Mortality Associated with Communicable Disease

As noted before, the only communicable diseases that ranked in the top five causes of death in 1978 were pneumonia and influenza. In 1979 chronic obstructive pulmonary disease replaced pneumonia and influenza as the fifth leading cause of death in the United States. Depending on how the data are viewed and how inclusive the topic is, a different picture can be obtained.

> Three million people in the United States, and over 150 million people around the world are still admitted to hospitals each year with infections. In the United States, the death rate from all infectious diseases is 123 per 100,000 persons, making them the Number 3 killer after heart disease and cancer (Lappe, 1981, p. 225).

In the preceding excerpt, Lappe is counting not only the deaths that occur from infectious or communicable diseases in the community but also the deaths that occur during the course of hospitalization in short- and long-term care facilities. These infections that occur during hospitalization but were not present or incubating on admission are termed *nosocomial*. It is variously estimated that at least 5% of all patients admitted to hospitals will die of nosocomial infections during their hospitalization. The rate is much higher among long-term care facilities such as nursing homes and rehabilitation centers. Nosocomial infections may occur at any body site ranging from the urinary tract to a surgical wound. The invading organism (agent) implicated in such infections is endogenous or part of the host's own microbiological flora in about 50% of the cases. The other 50% of invading organisms are classified as exogenous or external to the host's usual microbiological flora.

The outcome of nosocomial infections is that individuals who are so affected contribute to the overall impact of morbidity and mortality of communicable and infectious processes. (The role of the infection control practitioner, created to deal with the phenomenon of nosocomial infection, is discussed later in this chapter.)

Mortality from tuberculosis, hepatitis, encephalitis, syphilis, and rheumatic fever has decreased considerably. Deaths attributable to meningococcal infections slightly increased in recent years.

As seen in Table 12-2, the total number of deaths attributed to communicable diseases in the representative year of 1978 is 121,639. This figure is an under-

Table 12-2. Number of deaths in the United States in 1978 from various infectious and/or communicable diseases

Cause	Number of deaths
Specific notifiable diseases	4,680
Fungal infections	635
Respiratory infections	59,396
Miscellaneous infectious processes*	1,728
Nosocomial infections†	55,200‡
TOTAL	121,639

Data compiled from Centers for Disease Control: Annual summary, MMWR, 1979.
*Miscellaneous infectious processes include herpes zoster, meningitis (excluding meningococcal and tuberculosis), mononucleosis, streptococcal sore throat, scarlet fever, and toxoplasmosis.
†Based on Bennett's and Brachman's estimate that "3% of all nosocomial infection probably results directly in the death of the patient," (1979, p. xv).
‡Represents gross underestimates, since the number of deaths caused by nosocomial infections is given for acute (short-term) care facilities only.

count because some deaths were attributed to other causes and because the figures do not include nosocomial infection deaths for care facilities such as nursing homes and institutions for the mentally or physically disabled. The greatest impact of communicable diseases can be viewed by considering the effects of all communicable and or infectious phenomena under one category. (See Tables 12-3 and 12-4 for further information.)

Actually, when the impact from all communicable processes in one category is visualized, it is quite possible that, as Lappe asserted, communicable and infectious diseases rank as this nation's number three killer. In 1978 cancer was the second leading cause of death in the United States and accounted for 365,693 deaths. If all communicable and infectious diseases were considered a category or entity as cancer is and if accurate statistics were available, communicable and infectious diseases would rate much higher as a national killer than statistics on separate communicable processes now indicate.

Tables 12-3 and 12-4 also help to visualize the impact of communicable disease. It should be noted that the seven communicable diseases with the highest incidence are those diseases for which there is no active immunization except for hepatitis B for which vaccine was not developed in time to have impact on 1980 data and tuberculosis for which vaccine (BCG) is rarely used in the general U.S. population.

Table 12-3. Incidence of notifiable communicable diseases, United States, 1980*

Diseases	Number of cases reported
Gonorrhea	1,004,029
Chickenpox	190,894
Syphilis (all stages)	68,832
Hepatitis (all types)	59,996
Salmonellosis (excluding typhoid fever)	33,715
Tuberculosis	27,749
Shigellosis	19,041
Measles (rubeola)	13,506
Mumps	8,576
Aseptic meningitis	8,028
TOTAL	1,434,366

Compiled from Centers for Disease Control: Annual summary, MMWR, 1980.

* These data do not include estimates of the common cold or pneumonia and influenza, which are not mandatorily notifiable diseases.

Table 12-4. Deaths from specified notifiable diseases, United States, 1978

Cause of death	Number of deaths reported in 1978
Tuberculosis (all forms)	2,914
Hepatitis (all types)	508
Meningococcal infections	403
Encephalitis	185
Syphilis	169

Table 12-5. Temporal patterns in communicable or infectious diseases

Type of disease	Season of peak occurrence
Polio	Spring
Roseola infantum	Spring
Rubella	Late winter and spring
Meningococcal infections	Winter and spring
Rubeola (measles)	Late winter and early spring
Diphtheria	Autumn and winter
Rocky Mountain spotted fever	Summer
Legionellosis	July through October
Reye's syndrome	December through March

Temporal Patterns. Surveillance over many years has shown that several well-known communicable diseases show identifiable temporal patterns (Table 12-5). That is, certain communicable and/or infectious disease processes occur more frequently during one season of the year. Awareness of these seasonal fluctuations can alert the community health nurse to what disease phenomenon might be expected at any given time of year.

Pandemics. The term *pandemic* refers to a worldwide outbreak of the same epidemic disease phenomenon. Contemporary pandemics of communicable diseases have been essentially limited to the type-A influenzas. In this century there has been the Spanish or swine influenza pandemic 1918-1919, the Asian influenza pandemic of 1958-1959, and the Hong Kong influenza pandemic of 1968-1969. In the case of influenza, virologists restrict the definition of pandemic to mean a worldwide epidemic caused by a new subtype of influenza type A. It is believed that the characteristic of being a new subtype is important in that people are far more susceptible to a subtype that has not been demonstrated in the population previously than they are to those subtypes that are present at frequent intervals.

IMMUNIZATION PRACTICES

Although immunizing agents or vaccines are available for about 25 disorders (see box) only 7 are recommended for routine use (Tables 12-6 to 12-8). The remaining 18 vaccines are not recommended for routine use because the diseases are sufficiently rare to preclude routine immunization except to special-risk people, such as those at risk for Rocky Mountain spotted fever. In fact, the provision of protection against measles, mumps, rubella, polio, diphtheria, pertussis and tetanus has become a national priority. Because it was recognized in 1976 that a third of all children in the United States under the age of 15 were not properly immunized, President Carter began a major Childhood Immunization Initiative in 1977. Though the relative success of this initiative can be demonstrated by a decreased incidence of the 7 "childhood diseases," continued emphasis on proper immunization is essential.

Usually vaccines are recommended for either gener-

Diseases for which Active Immunization is Available

Adenovirus (types 4 and 7)
Anthrax
Botulism
Cholera (vaccine has only limited value)
Cytomegalovirus (experimental attenuated CMV vaccines are under evaluation)
Diptheria
Haemophilus influenza
Hepatitis B
Influenza
Measles (rubeola)
Meningitis (caused by *Neisseria meningitidis*)
Mumps
Pertussis
Plague
Pneumococcal infections
Polio
Rabies
Rocky Mountain spotted fever
Rubella
Salmonellosis (typhoid immunization affords protection in approximately 70% to 90% of subjects)
Smallpox
Tetanus
Trachoma conjunctivitis (temporary and limited protection study)
Tuberculosis (BCG effectiveness discussed later in this chapter)
Tularemia
Typhus
Yellow fever

Diseases for Which There is Passive Immunization

Botulism (but administration carries with it a great danger of sensitivity reaction)
Hepatitis type A (ISG)*
Measles (rubeola) (ISG)
Mumps
Rubella (ISG)
Smallpox
Tetanus
Varicella-zoster virus infection

*ISG, Immune serum globulin

al or specific use. Table 12-8 illustrates those vaccines that are recommended by the American Academy of Pediatrics for general use. Table 12-9 shows immunization procedures to be followed for children not immunized in early infancy.

Communicable Diseases for Which There is no Active or Passive Immunization Available

Actinomycosis
All arboviruses except Yellow Fever
Amebiasis caused by *Escherichia histolytica*
Ascariasis (roundworm infection)
Aspergillosis
Balantidiasis
Blastomycosis
Brucellosis (undulant fever)
Candidiasis (moniliasis, thrush)
Cat-bite fever
Cat scratch disease
Chlamydial infections
Coccidioidomycosis
Clostridium perfringens food poisoning
Coxsackie virus
Cryptococcosis
Echoviruses
Enterobiasis (pinworm infection)
Erythema infectiosum
Escherichia coli diarrhea
Gas gangrene
Genital herpes
Giardiasis
Gonococcal infections
Hemorrhagic fever
Herpes virus hominis (simplex infections)
Histoplasmosis
Impetigo
Larva migrans
Leprosy
Leptospirosis
Listeriosis
Lymphocytic choriomeningitis
Lymphocytosis
Malaria
Molluscum contagiosum
Mononucleosis
Mycoplasma pneumoniae infections
Otitis media
Parainfluenza virus infections
Pediculosis
Psittacosis
Primary amebic meningoencephalitis
Rhinovirus infections
Rickettsialpox
Roseola infantum
Scabies
Schistosomiasis
Shingellosis
Staphylococcal infections
Streptococcal infections (including pharyngitis, scarlet fever, and erysipelas)
Syphilis
Tapeworm disease
Tinea capiti, corporis, cruris, pedis
Toxoplasmosis
Trichinosis
Viral gastroenteritis

Table 12-6. Recommended schedule for active immunization of normal infants and children (routine diphtheria, tetanus, and pertussis immunization schedule summary for children less than 7 years old, 1981)*

Dose	Age or interval	Product
Primary 1	6 weeks old or older	DTP†
Primary 2‡	4 to 8 weeks after first dose	DTP
Primary 3‡	4 to 8 weeks after second dose	DTP
Primary 4‡	Approximately 1 year after third dose	DTP
Booster	4 to 6 years old, before entering kindergarten or elementary school (not necessary if fourth primary immunizing dose is administered after fourth birthday)	DTP
Additional boosters	Every 10 years after last dose	Td

* See text for important details.
† Prolonging the interval does not require restarting series.
‡ DT, if pertussis vaccine is contraindicated.

Table 12-7. Routine diphtheria and tetanus immunization schedule summary for persons 7 years old and older, 1981*

Dose	Age or inverval	Product
Primary 1	First visit	Td
Primary 2†	4 to 8 weeks after first dose	Td
Primary 3†	6 months to 1 year after second dose	Td
Boosters	Every 10 years after last dose	Td

Centers for Disease Control: MMWR, Aug. 21, 1981.
* See text for important details.
† Prolonging the interval does not require restarting series.

Table 12-8. Recommended schedule of vaccines[a] for active immunization of normal infants and children

2 months	DTP[b]	TOPV[c]
4 months	DTP	TOPV
6 months	DTP	[d]
1 year		Tuberculin test[e]
15 months	Measles,[f] Rubella[f]	Mumps[f]
1½ years	DTP	TOPV
4-6 years	DTP	TOPV
14-16 years	Td[g] — repeat every 10 years	

Report of the Committee on Infectious Diseases, ed. 19, Evanston, Ill., 1982. Copyright American Academy of Pediatrics, 1982.
[a] Concentration and Storage of Vaccines
Because the concentration of antigen varies in different products, the manufacturer's package insert should be consulted regarding the volume of individual doses of immunizing agents.

Because biologics are of varying stability, the manufacturer's recommendations for optimal storage conditions (e.g., temperature, light) should be carefully followed. Failure to observe these precautions may significantly reduce the potency and effectiveness of the vaccines.
[b] DTP, diphtheria and tetanus toxoids combined with pertussis vaccine.
[c] TOPV, Trivalent oral poliovirus vaccine. This recommendation is suitable for breast-fed as well as bottle-fed infants.
[d] A third dose of TOPV is optional but may be given in areas of high endemicity of poliomyelitis.
[e] Frequency of repeated tuberculin tests depends on risk of exposure of the child and on the prevalence of tuberculosis in the population group. For the pediatrician's office or outpatient clinic, an annual or biennial tuberculin test, unless local circumstances clearly indicate otherwise, is appropriate. The initial test should be done at the time of, or preceding, the measles immunization.
[f] May be given at 15 months as measles-rubella or measles-mumps-rubella combined vaccines (see Rubella, section 9, and Mumps, section 9, for further discussion of age of administration).
[g] Td, Combined tetanus and diphtheria toxoids (adult type) for those more than 6 years of age, in contrast to diphtheria and tetanus (DT) toxoids which contain a larger amount of diphtheria antigen. *Tetanus toxoid at time of injury:* For clean, minor wounds, no booster dose is needed by a fully immunized child unless more than 10 years have elapsed since the last dose. For contaminated wounds, a booster dose should be given if more than 5 years have elapsed since the last dose.

Table 12-9. Primary immunization for
children not immunized in early infancy*

Under 6 years of age

First visit	DTP, TOPV, tuberculin test
Interval after first visit	
1 month	Measles,† mumps, rubella
2 months	DTP, TOPV‡
4 months	DTP, TOPV
10-16 months or pre-school	DTP, TOPV
14-16 years	Td, repeat every 10 years

6 years of age and over

First visit	Td, TOPV, tuberculin test
Interval after first visit	
1 month	Measles, mumps, rubella
2 months	Td, TOPV
8-14 months	Td, TOPV
14-16 years	Td, repeat every 10 years

Report of the Committee on Infectious Diseases, ed. 19, Evanston, Ill., 1982. Copyright American Academy of Pediatrics, 1982.
* Physicians may choose to alter the sequence of these schedules if specific infections are prevalent at the time. For example, measles vaccine might be given on the first visit if an epidemic is under way in the community.
† Measles vaccine is not routinely given before 15 months of age.
‡ Optional.

Active Immunization

Active immunization requires that the host's autoimmune system be actively involved in forming specific antibodies against particular diseases, as opposed to passive immunization, in which protection is derived from inoculation with antibodies from a foreign host. The two general types of active immunity are (1) natural active immunity resulting from either a subclinical or symptomatic bout with the given disease and (2) artificial acquired immunity. The latter occurs when the host is injected with a disease-specific vaccine. This permits the duplication of the immune state that follows recovery from a specific communicable disease without exposing the host to the full consequences of the disease in question.

Artificial acquired immunity or vaccination is not without some risks to the host. Risks or side effects associated with vaccination depend on the nature of the specific vaccine; that is, whether it has bacterial or viral antigens and if the antigens are killed, whole organisms or live attenuated organisms. In general, the vaccine label explains its composition Table 12-10 describes some side effects of administering recommended childhood immunizations and corresponding nursing actions. There are several contraindications and special

circumstances for which the routine immunization administration schedule may be temporarily interrupted (Table 12-11).

Special Considerations for DTP Immunization*

At one time respiratory diphtheria was common and occurred primarily in children. Currently, the disease is rare and occurs mainly in unimmunized or inadequately immunized people. The ages of hosts infected with diphtheria recently in the United States suggest that many American adults are not protected. Adequate immunization is thought to protect the individual for at least 10 years. Even though such immunization reduces the risk of developing diphtheria and the severity of the clinical illness, it does not eliminate the possibility of an immunized host carrying *Corynebacterium diphtheriae* in the pharynx or on the skin (CDC, Aug. 21, 1981).

Even though the incidence of tetanus has decreased as a result of routine use of tetanus toxoid, the number of reported cases has remained relatively constant in the last decade (approximately 100 cases annually). For instance, in 1980, 95 cases of tetanus were reported in 33 states nationwide. Not only do two thirds of all cases occur in individuals 50 years old or more but the disease has occurred almost exclusively in people who are unimmunized, are inadequately immunized, or have an immunization history that is unknown. Although puncture-type wounds are often associated with tetanus, 5% to 10% of recent cases occurred in individuals who reported only superficial wounds or chronic skin lesions, such as decubitus ulcers. In general, tetanus toxoid is highly effective and is thought to produce protective levels of serum antitoxin that persist for at least 10 years after full immunization (CDC, Aug. 21, 1981).

Even though the routine use of pertussis vaccine has resulted in a substantial reduction in the incidence of and mortality from pertussis, the number of reported cases has changed relatively little in the past 10 years. Pertussis is a good example of a disease that may be underreported, since many cases are not accurately diagnosed. Most reported illnesses caused from host responses to *Bordetella pertussis* occur in infants and young children; two thirds of reported deaths occur in children less than 1 year old. However, older children and adults may serve as reservoirs of infection while they suffer nonspecific symptoms such as a severe respiratory infection. Pertussis is highly communicable and is frequently associated with severe sequelae and death. Vaccination early in life is essential. Because the incidence and severity of pertussis decrease with age and the vaccine may cause side effects and adverse re-

*The term *DTP* refers to a vaccine that provides immunization against diphtheria, tetanus, and pertussis.

Table 12-10. Possible side effects and nursing responsibilities of recommended childhood immunizations

Immunization	Reaction	Nursing responsibilities
Diphtheria	Fever usually within 24-48 hours Soreness, redness, and swelling at site of injection	Instructions for DTP: Advise parents of possible side effects; may recommend prophylactic use of aspirin or acetaminophen if fever occurred following previous DTP immunization; recommend its use if fever occurs following present immunization; advise parents to notify physician immediately of any unusual side effects, such as those listed under pertussis
Tetanus	Same as for diphtheria but may include urticaria and malaise All may have delayed onset and last several days Lump at injection site may last for weeks, even months but gradually disappears	
Pertussis	Same as for tetanus but may include loss of consciousness, convulsions, and thrombocytopenia	
Poliovirus (TOPV)	Essentially no side effects Vaccine-associated paralysis usually occurs within 2 months of immunization	See general comment to parents*
Measles	Anorexia, malaise, rash, and fever may occur 7 to 10 days after immunization Rarely (estimated risk 1 in 1 million doses) encephalitis may occur	Advise parents of more common side effects and use of antibyretics for fever; if a persistent high fever with other obvious signs of illness occurs, have them notify physician immediately
Mumps	Essentially no side effects other than a brief, mild fever	See general comment to parents
Rubella	Mild rash that lasts 1 or 2 days within a few days after immunization Arthralgia, arthritis, and/or paresthesia of the hands and fingers may occur about 2 weeks after vaccination and is more frequent in older children and adults	Advise parents of side effects, especially of time delay before joint swelling and pain; assure them that these symptoms will disappear; may recommend use of mild analgesics for pain

Whaley, L.F., and Wong, D.L.: Nursing care of infants and children, St. Louis, 1979, The C.V. Mosby Co.
* General comment to parents regarding each immunization: The benefit of being protected by the immunization is believed to greatly outweigh the risk from the disease.

actions, routine pertussis immunization is neither needed nor recommended for persons 7 years or older, except under unusual circumstances (CDC, Aug. 21,1981).

Side Effects and Adverse Reactions from DTP Immunization. Local reactions, generally erythema and induration with or without tenderness, are common after the administration of vaccines containing diphtheria, tetanus, or pertussis antigens. These reactions occur in approximately 40% to 70% of all DTP doses, are usually self-limited, and require no therapy. A nodule may be palpable at the injection site of absorbed products for several weeks. Abscesses at the injection site have been reported to be 6 to 10 per million doses. Mild to moderate fever (38.0° to 40.4° C [or 100.4° to 104.7° F]) occurs frequently in infants, and in about 50% of all doses administered, it shows up generally within several hours of administration and persists for 1 to 2 days. Fever and other systemic symptoms are much less

common following administration of preparations that do not contain pertussis vaccine.

Because severe systemic reactions such as generalized urticaria or anaphylaxis have been reported, epinephrine should be accessible during the immunization process. The exact frequency of severe events following pertussis vaccination is unknown, but reported ranges for some of these phenomena are shown in the following list.

1. Collapse or shocklike state (60 to 300 per million doses).
2. Persistent screaming episodes—prolonged periods of peculiar crying or screaming that cannot be controlled by comforting the infant (70 to 2000 per million doses).
3. Isolated convulsions with or without fever (40 to 700 per million doses).
4. Encephalopathy, with or without convulsions and manifested by a bulging fontanel with changes in

Table 12-11. Contraindications to routine immunizations

Contraindication	Immunization	Rationale	Nursing considerations
Acute febrile illness or chronic debilitating diseases	All	Masks febrile reactions from the immunization, decreases body's natural defense mechanisms	Explain reason for postponing immunization to parent and reschedule it at earliest return visit For chronic diseases, check with physician before administering any immunization
Gastroenteritis	Live poliovirus vaccine	May interfere with colonization of the viruses in the intestines, which is essential for the immune response to occur	Explain reason for postponing immunization and reschedule it as soon as possible
Altered immune system Immunologic disease Generalized malignancy (leukemia, lymphoma) Immunosuppressive therapy (steroids, antimetabolitics, radiation)	All live viral vaccines (measles, mumps, rubella, and polio)	Depressed immune defenses may result in extreme reactions to the immunizations	Emphasize to parents the need to prevent their children from exposure to any of these childhood diseases, since they cannot be artificially protected from them
Recently acquired passive immunity Blood transfusion or immune serum globulin within last 6 weeks Maternal antibodies during first year	Measles, mumps, and rubella vaccines	Presence of passive immunity prevents formation of antibodies to the vaccine	Inquire during the history concerning recent blood transfusions or injections of immune serum globulin; wait recommended 6 weeks before administering the immunization; follow suggested schedule for measles, mumps, and rubella (15 months)
Allergy to substances in vaccine, for example, egg protein, neomycin	Live virus vaccines grown on chick embryos, treated with neomycin	Known hypersensitivity to substance will also result in reaction to substance in vaccine	Check manufacturer's product information for specific contraindications and screen child for known allergies to potential foreign substances
History of nervous system disorders Reaction of high fever, somnolence, or convulsions following a DTP immunization	Pertussis vaccine	Danger of serious reaction to pertussis vaccination is greatly increased	Take a detailed neurologic history, including past convulsions, fainting spells, tremors, or twitching and specific reactions to DTP; report any such findings to a physician before administering the pertussis vaccine
Pregnancy	All live virus vaccines except for poliovirus	Potential risk to fetus, especially from rubella	Take a careful history of all women of childbearing age regarding the possibility of pregnancy or conception within the next 2 months

Whaley, L.F., and Wong, D.L.: Nursing care of infants and children. St. Louis, 1979, The C.V. Mosby Co.

the level of consciousness or focal neurological signs; the encephalopathy may lead to permanent neurological deficit (1.3 to 30.0 per million doses), (CDC, Aug. 21, 1981).

It is important for community health nurses to be aware of these and subsequent findings so they may intelligently counsel health consumers. Such findings sometimes cause generalized panic when presented to lay people in a biased fashion in the media. The community health nurse should encourage reporting of adverse reactions by parents and clients. Reports of severe or unusual reactions that seem to temporally correspond with immunization procedures should be forwarded to local and/or state health departments. Consulting CDC is recommended to obtain treatment protocols related to managing individuals who may have been in close contact with known diphtheria or pertussis infections to prevent potential spread.

Tuberculosis Immunization and Testing Practices

In 1980, 27,983 tuberculosis cases were reported to CDC. These data represent an increase of 0.6% (166 cases) from 1979 data. Before 1980 the number of reported cases of tuberculosis had decreased approximately 4% per year. One of the primary reasons associated with this increase was the large number of cases of tuberculosis among the Indo-Chinese refugees who were entering the United States during this reporting period (CDC, Feb. 13, 1981).

However, methods used in reporting and actual phenomena influence rates and their interpretation. For instance, for the first time in 1980 information about the Hispanic ethnicity of people with tuberculosis was collected. As a result of the analysis of those data, the indication is that tuberculosis does and will have higher rates in people of Hispanic origin that most other groups in the United States (CDC, May 14, 1982).

Efforts to control tuberculosis in the United States are directed toward early diagnosis and treatment (secondary prevention), which include therapy with isoniazid for infected individuals. In this country vaccine prepared from the bacillus of Calmette and Guerin (BCG) has been used mainly for selected groups of uninfected people who live or work where they have an unavoidable risk of exposure to tuberculosis (CDC, June 1, 1979).

BCG Vaccine. BCG vaccine has been in use for over 60 years. There are many different types of BCG vaccine available today, but each type varies in its ability to produce immunity in humans. For example, studies conducted before 1955 demonstrated liquid vaccines prepared from different BCG strains showed protection (immunization) rates ranging from 0 to 80% (CDC, June 1, 1979).

Production standards for BCG vaccines in the United States specify that the strain must demonstrate various characteristics of safety and potency and be capable of inducing tuberculin sensitivity in humans. However, the relation between sensitivity (the point at which a person shows a physiological antigenic response) and immunity (resistance to a given disease) is one which has not been proven. Just because an individual shows a sensitivity to tuberculosis by reacting to an intradermal skin test does not necessarily guarantee that immunity to tuberculosis is assured. In the United States BCG is manufactured as a freeze-dried vaccine that must be reconstituted, protected from exposure to light, and used within 8 hours of reconstitution.

Currently, CDC recommends that BCG be considered for the following high-risk hosts: (1) infants in a household who are tuberculin skin-test negative but who have repeated exposure to persistently untreated or ineffectively treated clients with sputum-positive pulmonary tuberculosis; (2) groups in which an excessive rate of new infection can be demonstrated, and the usual surveillance and treatment programs have failed or are not feasible (such groups might exist among those without a regular source of health care); and (3) some health workers who may be at increased risk of repeated exposure (CDC, June 1, 1979).

BCG should be reserved for persons who are skin-test negative (less than 10 mm induration [see next section on tuberculin skin testing]). Those who receive BCG should have a tuberculin skin test 2 to 3 months later. Since standards for BCG vaccines require that the strain must be capable of inducing tuberculin sensitivity, if the subsequent skin test is negative and the indications for BCG remain, a second dose of vaccine should be given. The dose is indicated by the manufacturer in the package labeling; one half of the usual dose should be given to infants under 28 days old. If the indications for immunization persist, these children should receive a full dose of BCG after 1 year of age (CDC, June 1, 1979).

Even though the World Health Organization recommends that BCG be given by the intradermal route, vaccines manufactured in the United States may be administered either intradermally or by percutaneous technique. Vaccination should be accomplished by the method recommended on individual package labeling.

Worldwide, BCG vaccine has been associated with many severe adverse reactions ranging from ulceration at the vaccination site to death. However, the frequency of complications pertaining to BCG vaccine made in the United States may be different. For instance, CDC reports that the frequency of ulceration ranges from 1% to 10%, and disseminated BCG infection and deaths are rare (1 to 10 per 10 million vaccinations) and occur almost exclusively in children with impaired immune responses (CDC, June 1, 1979).

BCG for prevention of tuberculosis should not be given to those with impaired immune responses or when immunological responses have been suppressed with steroids, alkylating agents, antimetabolites, or radiation. Pregnant women should not be vaccinated unless they are at high risk of infective tuberculosis. As is true of all adverse reactions to immunizations, all suspected reactions to BCG should be carefully investigated and reported to county or state health authorities. Such adverse reactions to BCG may occur as long as one year or more after vaccination.

Administration of Tuberculin Skin Test. Even though skin testing for tuberculosis is essentially a screening technique and not an immunization procedure, it is important for the community health nurse to be thoroughly conversant with tuberculin skin testing in relation to routine immunization procedures. For example, the reactivity to tuberculin skin testing may be depressed or suppressed for as long as 4 weeks by viral infections, or live virus vaccines, such as measles, polio, rubella, and mumps. A reactive or positive tuberculin skin test merely indicates that the individual has probably been exposed to and has formed some sensitivity to the causative agent of tuberculosis. Further diagnostic procedures should be carried out before a diagnosis of active disease is made.

To conduct a tuberculin skin test such as the Purified Protein Derivative (PPD) test, a sterile injection unit should be used to inject 0.1 ml of prepared solution intradermally. The substance should not be injected subcutaneously, but if subcutaneous injection should occur, no local skin reaction will develop, though highly susceptible persons may develop a general febrile reaction and/or acute inflammation around old tuberculosis lesions (PDR, 1981).

The result is read in 48 to 72 hours after the intradermal injection, and only induration is considered in interpreting a test; redness is not a criterion for interpretation. "Erythema of less than 10 mm should be disregarded. If the area of erythemia is greater than 10 mm and induration is absent, the injection may have been made too deeply and retesting is indicated" (PDR, 1981, p. 2010). Reactions 48 to 72 hours subsequent to intradermal injection, which show induration, are interpreted as follows: (1) negative reading—less than 5 mm induration; (2) doubtful reading—induration measuring 5 to 9 mm; (3) positive reading—induration at injection site, which measures 10 mm or greater. Doubtful readings may indicate retesting at a different injection site. A child who is known to have been exposed to an adult client with tuberculosis must not be adjudged free of infection until a negative skin re-

action is obtained at least 10 weeks after no longer being in contact with the infected individual (PDR, 1981).

Tuberculin skin testing should not be performed on known tuberculin-positive reactors because of the severity of reaction that occurs at the test site in very highly sensitive individuals. As with any biological agent, epinephrine should be immediately available in cases of hypersensitivity or acute reaction.

Measles, Mumps, and Rubella Virus Vaccine

The measles, mumps, and rubella vaccine (MMR) is recommended for general use beginning at 15 months of age. Before that age, children may fail to respond to one or all three components as a result of the presence of residual antibodies of maternal origin (transplacental immunity). In some geographical areas, where measles infection is highly likely to occur before 15 months of age, the decision may be made to immunize such infants. However, the younger the infant, the greater the possibility that seroconversion (the process whereby the body produces an immune state) will not occur. In any event, children who are immunized before 15 months of age should be revaccinated on the recommended schedule after they reach 15 months of age (PDR, 1981).

Often health professionals become complacent after immunizations are administered, but it should be remembered that vaccines have varying degrees of effectiveness under optimal conditions. For instance, a single injection of MMR may produce specific antibodies for protection against measles in 95% of the people immunized, against mumps in 96% of those immunized, and against rubella in 99% of those immunized. The small percentage of individuals who do not form specific antibodies in response to the vaccine remain at risk for the disease.

MMR should not be given to pregnant women, those who may be hypersensitive to neomycin (each dose of MMR contains 25 mg of neomycin), individuals diagnosed as active untreated tuberculosis cases, persons receiving corticosteroids or radiation therapy, or those with blood dyscrasias. MMR should not be given less than 1 month before or after immunization with other live viruses, and vaccination should be deferred for at least 3 months following blood or plasma transfusions or administration of human immune serum globulin. Thus it is important that careful histories are obtained on all individuals before immunization.

Just as the community health nurse should be well versed in all adverse reactions from immunization, it is important to note that administration of MMR has been associated with a corresponding incidence of encephalitis. However, the risk of such neurological disorders following live vaccine administration remains far less than that for such occurrences following actual infection with natural measles (PDR, 1981).

Passive Immunization

In passive immunity, protection is given to the host by inoculation with antibodies derived from another host. The immunity is effective almost immediately and persists for a few weeks before it disappears. There are three types of passive immunity: transplacental immunity, natural passive immunity, and artificial passive immunity. In transplacental immunity, IgG antibodies are transferred from the mother. Since the baby plays no active part in the process, its range of immunity is dependent on the variety of antibodies in the mother's blood. This is an important point because even though transplacental immunity against measles, for example, is possible, if the mother lacks antibodies against measles, the child will be born susceptible. To carry the point further, there are still instances of congenital tetanus in infants who are born to mothers not immunized against tetanus. Such phenomena occur with some frequency in underdeveloped nations.

Communicable diseases to which infants often receive *natural passive immunity* are mumps and diphtheria. Infants receive questionable amounts of immunity to pertussis; 40% of all fatalities in the United States attributable to pertussis occur in the first year of life. Natural passive immunity to chickenpox is not thought to occur at all; in fact, infection with chickenpox virus is frequently devastating during the first year of life.

In addition to acquiring natural passive immunity, infants may also acquire disease at birth from the mother through (1) infected amniotic fluid, (2) the maternal bloodstream, or (3) direct contact with infected maternal tissue in the birth canal. Specifically, syphilis, occasionally *Listeria monocytogenes,* and less frequently tuberculosis are acquired through the placenta (Korones, 1976).

In *artificial passive immunity,* protection is prompted by administering antibodies obtained from the same or a different species. Antibodies obtained from an immune member of the same species seldom cause severe reactions. An example of antibodies obtained from the same species is immune serum globulin (human), or ISG.

Animal Serums

The risk of serum sickness or severe reaction is increased when human hosts receive antibodies produced by active immunization in a different species. Tetanus and rabies serums, formerly produced in animals, are now produced in humans, making them much safer to administer. In four types of immunization animal serum continues to be used: (1) diphtheria, botulism, and gas gangrene; (2) tetanus and rabies exposure when special human gamma globulin is unavailable; (3) snake and spider bites; and (4) disorders in which immunosuppression with antilymphocyte serum is indicated (AAP, 1982).

Animal serums are avoided unless definitely indicated. Hence a careful history must be taken before sensitivity testing relative to asthma, hay fever, urticaria, and previous injections of animal serums. This history is followed by sensitivity tests that are administered with necessary equipment and personnel present to recognize and treat adverse reactions. For further information relative to sensitivity testing for serum reactions, the pharmacological information packaged along with these substances should be checked.

Immune Serum Globulins

ISG produces passive immunity and is an antibody-rich fraction of pooled plasma from normal donors. The advantages of ISG over plasma administration include (1) freedom from hepatitis viruses, (2) concentration of the antibodies into a small volume for intermuscular use, and (3) stable antibody content if properly stored (AAP, 1982).

ISG has occasional side effects, and for this reason its use is generally limited to disorders in which its efficacy has been established. Currently, there are only four disorders in which the value of ISG is clearly recommended: (1) measles prophylaxis or modification, (2) viral hepatitis type A (HAV) prophylaxis or modification, (3) viral hepatitis type B (HBV) prophylaxis when hepatitis B virus immune globulin is indicated but not available, and (4) antibody deficiency disease (AAP, 1982).

There are several other disorders in which the use of ISG may be helpful, but the benefit is not clearly established. One instance in which the value of ISG is highly debatable is related to its use in preventing rubella in the first trimester of pregnancy. It is important to remember that ISG does not actually prevent the occurrence of disease but rather alters or modifies its clinical course.

Special human ISGs are derived from the blood of individuals hyperimmunized or convalescing from specific infections. Because these preparations contain a higher concentration of antibodies to specific microbial agents than do ordinary ISGs, they are helpful in several disorders in which ISG is of no value (Table 12-12).

Table 12-12. Uses of special human immune serum globulins (ISG)	

Disease and special ISG	Comments
Tetanus immune globulin (human)	Used in prevention and treatment of tetanus, especially in nonimmunized subjects
Vaccinia immune globulin (human)	Used in prevention and treatment of vaccinia complications and for prevention of smallpox
Rabies immune globulin (human) (RIG)	Used when there is no vaccination before exposure*; valuable in prevention of rabies after exposure; given concurrently with human diploid cell rabies vaccine (HDCV), which induces an active response that takes 7-10 days to develop and persists about 1 year
Zoster immune globulin (human)	May be used in prophylaxis or modification of high-risk susceptible children exposed to varicella or herpes zoster; includes children with leukemia, disseminated malignancies, cellular immunodeficiencies, and those receiving high doses of immunosuppressives
Pertussis immune globulin (human)	Is of unproven value
Mumps immune globulin (human)	Is of unproven value

* People previously immunized or those vaccinated before exposure should receive HDCV (1.0 ml each dose) on days 0 and 3; it is not necessary to give these individuals RIG (CDC, 1980).

Foreign Travel Immunization Requirements

Nurses whose clients are traveling abroad may wish to request the publication entitled *Health Information for International Travel* (HEW Pub. No. 76-8280) from:

Centers for Disease Control
Overseas Travel
Atlanta, Georgia 30333

No further discussion is offered, since these guidelines change frequently; current guidelines should be checked when needed.

Immunization under Special Circumstances
Pneumococcal Polysaccharide Vaccine

Streptococcus pneumoniae is one agent that causes bacteremia and meningitis in infants and children. Death is the outcome in 5% to 15% of the cases, and a large number of survivors are permanently handicapped (Pelton, 1978).

The *S. pneumoniae* vaccine was licensed by the Food and Drug Administration in 1978, and it is recommended for high-risk youngsters over two years old and for adults with chronic illness or those who are at increased risk of pneumococcal disease or its complications. An example of a child who would probably require this vaccine is one with sickle-cell anemia. An example of an adult requiring vaccination might be one who is elderly and suffers from chronic obstructive pulmonary disease.

The community health nurse may have occasion to administer the vaccine to children. It should be given subcutaneously, and the parents should be informed that the child may suffer mild side effects such as low-grade fever, mild erythema, and induration at the injection site about four hours after administration. This reaction may last up to four days but usually subsides within 24 hours.

The safety of the pneumococcal vaccine in pregnant women has not been fully evaluated at this point. In addition, because of the marked increase in adverse reactions with reinjection of pneumococcal vaccine, second or booster doses are not recommended by the CDC (CDC, Aug. 28, 1981).

Meningococcal Vaccine

Sepsis and/or meningitis caused by *Neisseria meningitidis* poses a serious threat to children under 4 years of age because they have not yet developed protective antibodies. Furthermore, the prognosis of *N. meningitidis* infection is grave. About 10% of those infected die, and another 30% are left deaf or with brain damage (Pelton, 1978).

Two vaccines licensed in 1972 protect against the two types (A and C) or meningococci that most often cause epidemics of meningitis. Work is under way to develop a type B vaccine, since type B meningitis is the cause of most of the sporadic cases in this country. These vaccines are recommended for use in epidemic situations only. The type A vaccine is currently recommended only for children over 5 years of age, and the type C is only for administration to adults. The use of types A and C in younger age groups is under investigation. Side effects are similar to those seen after DTP administration (Table 12-10).

Impact of Current Immunization Programs

Before measles vaccine became available in the 1960s, epidemics occurred every two or three years with nearly 500 deaths caused by that disease in the United States annually. At that time it was an accepted but unhappy fact of life that nearly every child would get measles, and the same was true of rubella and mumps. As a direct result of the measles vaccine, which was introduced in 1963, the national incidence of measles has dropped 90%. Accompanying that decline has been a dramatic decrease in encephalitis following measles. In fact, complete elimination of measles is thought by some to be within reach in the United States, and eradication of measles has been set as a national goal.

Increased national emphasis, such as the Childhood Immunization Initiative in 1977, has resulted in a comparatively high immunization rate for measles and for other diseases among preschool and school-aged children. (See Table 12-13 for individual state requirements for immunization.) In a survey conducted by the Center for Preventive Services at CDC in 1980, most states showed their preschoolers to be 80% to 90% immunized with few exceptions.

TRENDS IN INFECTIOUS AND/OR COMMUNICABLE DISEASES

The following discussion explores the role and impact of selected communicable diseases or their phenomena on contemporary society. In some instances these phenomena are relatively new and therefore less understood than more familiar communicable diseases. In other instances the communicable phenomena discussed have significant impact on community health nursing practice and therefore warrant exploration.

Antibiotic Resistance

Microorganisms, like all living things, occasionally undergo genetic mutations as a result of alterations in the enzyme production of mutant cells. For example, when mutation occurs in a few cells of a given species of a microorganism that is multiplying in a host being treated with penicillin, the subsequent change occasionally alters a few cells in such a way that they are no longer susceptible to the action of penicillin. These microorganisms are then said to be *antibiotic resistant* or *drug fast.* This process is also referred to as *transfer of R-factor,* since it is the RNA of the cell that relays the genetic change. A similar resistance pattern may develop in any number of microorganisms in response to any chemotherapeutic drug. The resistant cells grow and ultimately replace sensitive cells.

In the preceding description, resistance occurred ostensibly in a person taking a therapeutic dose of penicillin, but that is usually not the case. The situation that is most often credited for the phenomena of resistant organisms is overuse or abuse of antibiotics. This abuse by physicians includes prescribing excessive doses, prescribing antibiotics prophylactically in preoperative or post-operative situations or in the presence of *presumed* viral infections, and prescribing antibiotics without the aid of culture and sensitivity reports.

Antibiotic resistance has been of great concern to infection control practitioners in episodic settings for over two decades, but resistance patterns are increasingly affecting a broader range of microbiological agents, including common communicable diseases. Perhaps one of the best known and most notorious communicable disease with an agent that has developed resistance to penicillin is gonorrhea.

The first evidence of penicillin resistance by *Neisseria gonorrhoeae* was demonstrated as early as the 1950s. Such strains have subsequently been reported in all parts of the world, but some still respond to higher doses of penicillin, which are given in combination with probenecid. Resistance to other antibiotics, including erythromycin, streptomycin, tetracycline, and chloramphenicol, has also been reported. By 1976 strains of higher resistance to penicillin were documented in the United States and traced to the Far East. Since 1976 these same highly resistant strains have been reported in numerous parts of the world (Reeves and Geddes, 1979).

Staphylococcus aureus is also frequently penicillin resistant. In recent years, reports of infections with methicillin-resistant *aureus* have increased. When methicillin, a member of the penicillin family was first developed, all strains of staphylococcus were believed to be sensitive to this antibiotic. Although that is no longer true, most of these methicillin-resistant strains seem to be occurring in large, medical school–affiliated hospitals. It is unknown whether or not this may represent a reporting bias in that such institutions tend to report nosocomial infections with high reliability. If such infections are truly more common in large medical school–affiliated hospitals, it may be because such institutions usually include burn and trauma units, which provide a source of periodic reintroduction of these organisms. For this reason, CDC recommends that people who are known to be colonized or infected with this particular strain of staphylococcus not be transferred to other medical facilities whenever possible. At this point, the potential risk of spread to healthy family contacts is not known but is probably small.

Table 12-13. Statewide immunization requirements*

State	School: To whom does the law or regulation apply?	Diphtheria	Pertussis	Tetanus	Measles	Mumps	Polio	Rubella	Day care: Are licensed day care facilities covered by the school law or other law or regulation?	Medical	Religious	Philosophical
Alabama	All enrolled—K through 12	X	X	X	X	X	X	X	Yes	X	X	
Alaska	All enrolled—K through 12	X	X	X	X		X	X	Yes	X	X	
Arizona	All enrolled—Public system— < 18	X			X		X	X	No	X	X	
Arkansas	All enrolled—K through 12	X	X	X	X		X	X	Yes	X	X	
California	All enrolled—K through 13	X	X	X	X	X	X	X	Yes	X	X	X
Colorado	All enrolled—K through 12	X	X	X	X	X¹	X	X	Yes	X	X	X
Connecticut	All enrolled—K through 12	X	X	X	X		X	X	Yes	X	X	
Delaware	All enrolled—K through 12	X	X	X	X		X	X	No	X	X	
Distr. of Col.	All enrolled—K through Age 25	X		X	X	X	X	X	Yes	X	X	
Florida	New enterers—any grade	X	X	X	X	X	X	X	Yes	X	X	
Georgia	All enrolled—K through 12	X	X	X	X	X	X	X	Yes	X	X	
Hawaii	New enterers—any grade	X	X	X	X	X	X	X	Yes	X	X	X
Idaho	All enrolled—K through 5	X	X	X	X	X	X	X	No	X	X	X
Illinois	All enrolled—K through 12	X	X	X	X		X	X	Yes	X	X	
Indiana	All enrolled—K through 12	X	X	X	X		X	X	Yes	X	X	X
Iowa	All enrolled—K through 12	X	X	X	X		X	X	Yes	X	X	
Kansas	New enterers—any grade	X	X	X	X	X	X	X	Yes	X	X	
Kentucky	New enterers—K and 1st	X		X	X		X	X	No	X	X	
Louisiana	New enterers—any grade	X	X	X	X		X	X	Yes	X	X	X
Maine	All enrolled—K through 6	X	X	X	X		X	X	Yes	X	X	X
Maryland²	All enrolled—K through 6	X	X	X	X		X	X	Yes	X	X	
Massachusetts	All enrolled—K through 12	X	X	X	X	X	X	X	Yes	X	X	
Michigan	New enterers—any grade	X	X	X	X		X	X	Yes	X	X	X
Minnesota	All enrolled—K through 12	X	X	X	X	X³	X	X	Yes	X		X
Mississippi	All enrolled—K through 12	X	X	X	X		X	X	Yes	X		
Missouri	All enrolled—K through 12	X		X	X		X	X	No	X		
Montana	All enrolled—K through 12	X	X	X	X	X	X	X	Yes	X	X	X
Nebraska	All enrolled—K through 12	X	X	X	X	X	X	X	Yes	X	X	
Nevada	All enrolled—K through 12	X	X	X	X		X	X	Yes	X	X	
New Hampshire	New enterers—K, 1, and transfers	X	X	X	X	X	X	X	Yes	X	X	
New Jersey	All enrolled—K through 12	X	X	X	X	X	X	X	Yes	X	X	
New Mexico	All enrolled—K through 12	X	X	X	X		X	X	Yes	X	X	
New York	All enrolled—K through 12	X		X	X	X	X	X	Yes	X	X	
North Carolina	All enrolled—K through 12	X	X	X	X		X	X	Yes	X	X	
North Dakota	All enrolled—K through 12	X	X	X	X	X	X	X	Yes	X	X	
Ohio	All enrolled—K through 12	X	X	X	X		X	X	Yes	X	X	X
Oklahoma	All enrolled—K through 12	X	X	X	X		X	X	No	X	X	X
Oregon	New enterers—5 through 14 yr	X	X	X	X		X	X	Yes	X	X	
Pennsylvania	New enterers	X		X	X	X	X	X	Yes	X	X	X
Rhode Island	All enrolled—K through 12, college	X	X	X	X		X	X	Yes	X	X	X
South Carolina	All enrolled—K through 12	X	X	X	X		X	X	Yes	X	X	
South Dakota	All enrolled—K through 12	X	X	X	X	X¹	X	X	No	X	X	X
Tennessee	All enrolled—K through 12	X	X	X	X		X	X	Yes	X	X	
Texas	All enrolled—K through 12, college	X	X	X	X	X	X	X	Yes	X	X	
Utah	New enterers—any grade	X	X	X	X	X	X	X	Yes	X	X	X
Vermont	New enterers—K, 1, and transfers	X	X	X	X		X	X	Yes	X	X	X
Virginia	New enterers—any grade	X	X	X	X		X	X	Yes	X	X	
Washington⁴	All enrolled—K through 12	X	X	X	X	X³	X	X	Yes	X	X	X
West Virginia	New enterers—any grade	X	X	X	X		X	X	Yes	X	X	
Wisconsin	All enrolled—K through 12	X	X	X	X		X	X	Yes	X	X	X
Wyoming	New enterers—under 11 years	X	X	X	X	X	X	X	Yes	X	X	
Subtotal: States and D.C. only		51	45	48	51	23	51	51		51	48	19
American Samoa	No statewide law regulation											
Guam	New enterers—any grade	X	X	X	X	X	X	X	Yes	X	X	
Puerto Rico	New enterers—K and 1	X	X	X	X		X	X	Yes			
Virgin Islands	New enterers—any grade	X	X	X	X		X	X	No			
TOTAL United States territories		51	48	51	54	24	54	54		52	49	19

¹ K only.
² 7-12 grades for measles only.
³ Through grade 1 only.
⁴ Requires immunity or course of immunization as recommended by the health department.
*This information provided by the state health departments.

According to CDC, all forms of tuberculosis were lower in 1979 than for any of the preceding 10 years, but in 1980 there was a 0.6% increase (CDC, Feb. 13, 1981). Regardless of the exact number of cases, pulmonary tuberculosis is still common in the world, reaching an incidence of 200 to 250 cases per 100,000 population in some areas of Africa, India, and the Far East (Reeves and Geddes, 1979). In 1980 region 10 in the United States (Alaska, Idaho, Oregon, and Washington) showed the greatest increase in the number of tuberculosis cases over preceding years. Region 3 (Delaware, District of Columbia, Maryland, Pennsylvania, Virginia, and West Virginia) showed the greatest decrease in the number of tuberculosis cases in 1980 as compared to preceding years (CDC, Feb. 13, 1981).

Initial resistance to the commonly used drugs for the treatment of tuberculosis has not shown any major changes in recent years in most economically advanced countries. However, resistance patterns are thought to be much higher in some countries, such as China. It is believed that the main reason for treatment failure in tuberculosis is incomplete or ineffective methods rather than the emergence of resistant strains per se (Reeves and Geddes, 1979).

Haemophilus influenzae type B is a common cause of meningitis in children. Although this agent was initially sensitive to ampicillin and chloramphenicol, strains that are resistant to one or both of these antibiotics have been demonstrated in the United States and other countries since 1974.

In addition to those agents already cited, there have been reports of resistant strains of the causative agents of syphilis, malaria, shigellosis, salmonellosis and typhoid (Reeves and Geddes, 1979).

It is difficult to accurately predict where resistance patterns will end or what the full ramifications of resistant strains are for the future. Some predictions are frightening at best, but at present it would seem that our chemopharmacopedic sophistication is such that treatment alternatives stay just a little ahead of the microorganism's amazing ability to form resistant patterns. It could be argued though that current treatment modalities stay more than a little behind the development of resistant strains of microorganisms.

What can be done? First, it is important to appropriately isolate and effectively treat people known to be infected with resistant strains. It is also important to detect carriers or those with subclinical infections with resistant strains. Meticulous initial case finding and then follow-up are essential when infectious people are found. Unfortunately, in many countries of the world antibiotics may be obtained without a prescription, and this is believed to account for the high rate of chloram-phenicol resistance in populations of such countries. It would be helpful if worldwide agreement could be reached on the principles of antibiotic usage. For instance, antibiotics important for treating human infections should be excluded from animal feeds. Also, no disease should be treated with antibiotics unless positively indicated by clinical and laboratory data. Even topical gentamicin should be avoided if possible because pathogens such as *Pseudomonas aeruginosa* may acquire resistance in its presence.

Finally, the principles of control of spread of resistant organisms, which are similar to those of any communicable disease, must be followed (i.e., good surveillance, rapid detection, isolation of infected patients, good hygiene, treatment of carrier and possibly contacts of cases and carriers), and some day a worldwide antibiotic policy.

Sexually Transmissible Diseases

In 1977 some 10 million cases of sexually transmissible diseases occurred in the United States; 86% were in the 15- to 29-year-old age groups. According to the CDC (1980), *venereal disease* is no longer an adequate term because it is too limited. Hence the terminology *sexually transmissible diseases* includes the following:

- trichomoniasis—3.0 million cases annually
- gonorrhea—2.5 million cases annually
- nongonoccocal urethritis (NGU, caused by organisms such as chlamydia and mycoplasma)—2.5 million cases annually)
- genital herpes—500,000 cases annually
- syphilis—80,000 new cases annually

Although these diseases vary widely in cause and effect on the host, the element they have in common is that they are all sexually transmissible.

Most of these diseases cause burning, itching, and discharge, but they may occur with few recognizable symptoms. They may recur because there is no evidence that one infection confers active immunity. Some of these diseases are capable of causing disability in the host, such as infertility, sterility, arthritis, pelvic inflammatory disease in females, and neurological damage and death. The presence of these diseases in pregnant women may have serious consequences for the unborn child as well.

No vaccines are currently available, but efforts are under way to develop a vaccine against gonorrhea. All persons who have frequent sexual contact with different partners should be examined periodically regardless of symptoms or the lack of them. Certain groups, including homosexuals, migrant workers, and the poor, are at higher risk for all the sexually transmissible diseases than the population at large (Healthy People, 1979).

Some of the essential elements for controlling these diseases include (1) educating the public, particularly high risk groups and adolescents, so that they understand early signs of disease and the kinds of sexual behavior that increases risk; (2) encouraging condom use among males with multiple partners; (3) screening high risk groups; (4) treating with antibiotics when appropriate in those found infected; and (5) identifying and treating sexual contacts (Healthy People, 1979).

Two sexually transmitted diseases are discussed in more detail, since they are comparatively new and are thought to have wide-ranging public health effects now and in the future.

Chlamydial Infections

Chlamydial infections are probably more widespread than is currently documented and are comparatively recently recognized clinical phenomena that are not well known to many health professionals. The agent, *Chlamydia trachomatis,* is a bacteria-like organism that is responsible for many animal and human diseases that community health nurses have occasion to assess and manage. Two species of chlamydia exist: *C. psittaci* and *C. trachomatis.* The former is responsible for the human disease psittacosis or parrot fever. *C. trachomatis* causes a number of clinical entities such as lymphogranuloma venereum, hyperendemic blinding trachoma, inclusion conjunctivitis, pneumonia of the newborn, nongonococcal urethritis, cervicitis, salpingitis, and epididymitis.

The signs and symptoms of chlamydial infections are similar to any nonspecific genitourinary infection in either males or females. In the male the disease is frequently asymptomatic with the exception of a slight uretheral discharge and transient burning on urination. In the female the symptoms vary from vaginal discharge and low abdominal pain to signs that are so mild that they may go undetected.

Like any other sexually transmissible disease, any sexually active host is a candidate for developing a chlamydial infection. Factors that increase a woman's susceptibility include multiple sex partners and contacts with men having nonspecific urethritis (NSU). Though chlamydial infections may be relatively asymptomatic, they are nonetheless capable of causing salpingitis and pelvic inflammatory disease. In addition, infants born to women colonized with chlamydia are susceptible to chlamydial pneumonitis.

Even though a specific laboratory culture can be taken from the cervix or penis to detect the presence of chlamydia, this is often not routinely done because of the expense involved (chlamydia-specific cultures cost at least $50). Currently, chlamydia is sensitive to tetracycline, making this drug the treatment of choice. Chlamydia-specific cultures are typically used when the clinical picture fails to respond to tetracycline and the specific organism must be identified to further treat the person. Control measures for genital chlamydial infections are generally the same as for all sexually transmissible diseases.

Genital Herpes Infection

Data compiled by CDC support the notion that an epidemic of genital herpes infection occurred in the United States from 1966 to 1979 and that the disease continues to occur in epidemic proportions. For instance, the number of consultations with physicians for genital herpes infection increased from a reported 29,560 visits in 1966 to 260,890 in 1979. Thus the rate at which people consulted fee-for-service, office-based physicians for genital herpes infection increased almost ninefold in the 13-year interval. In contrast, the same survey showed less than a twofold increase in the rate of consultation for oral herpes infections (CDC March 26, 1981).

The increased incidence of genital herpes infection is particularly noteworthy for community health nurses for several reasons. (1) There is an association between genital herpes infection and the development of cervical cancer. (2) Infections acquired during passage through the birth canal are often life-threatening to the newborn. (3) While a new drug, Acyclovir, is available for treatment of *initial* genital herpes infection, there is no specific treatment for *recurrent* or chronic genital herpes. These recurrences are common and are physically painful and emotionally distressing to affected individuals.

Acyclovir does have limitations. First, its effectiveness seems directly proportional to the disease stage in which it is employed. The earlier the drug is used, the more effective it is in halting the progression of the disease. Acyclovir is also effective for use in immunosuppressed individuals who suffer from genital herpes. The drug is not currently thought to be effective for chronic or recurrent genital herpes. As yet, there is insufficient data relative to its use in pregnant or lactating females.

Acyclovir is a cream that is applied topically to the affected region six times per day for 7 consecutive days. Clients should be instructed to wear a finger cot or rubber glove to apply the cream to avoid autoinoculation of other body sites.

According to CDC, social, demographic, and behavioral changes within the U.S. population during the past decade have placed an increased proportion of the people at risk for sexually transmitted diseases such as genital herpes (March 26, 1982). It is difficult to know whether or not this trend will continue well into the 1980s. The most important role for the community health nurse in relation to bringing genital herpes under control continues to be public education aimed at prevention when feasible and early diagnosis and treatment when the disease does occur.

Other Diseases of Special Concern
Pediculosis

Occurrences of pediculosis or lice infestation are worldwide, and outbreaks are common among schoolchildren and other groups. *Pediculosis* refers to infestations of the head or hairy parts of the body or clothing with adult lice, larvae, or nits (eggs) leading to severe itching and excoriation of the scalp or scratch marks on the body (Benenson, 1980).

From a public health standpoint, the louse is not only a human nuisance but also transmits epidemic typhus, trench fever, and louse-borne relapsing fever (Benenson, 1980). The mode of transmission is direct contact with an infected person and indirect contact with the personal belongings of an infected person, especially clothing and headgear. Pediculosis is communicable as long as lice remain alive on the infected person, on the clothing of an infected person, and until eggs in the hair and clothing have been destroyed. Diagnosis of pediculosis is accomplished by finding either lice or nits on hairy surfaces of the body.

Pediculosis is treated with lindane (Kwell). Kwell comes as a lotion and a shampoo and contains lindane 1% as its active ingredient. The client should be instructed to apply a sufficient quantity to cover only the affected and adjacent hairy areas. The lotion should be rubbed into the scalp and hair and left in place for 12 hours, after which a shower should be taken.

For head lice, the shampoo is used. The client should be instructed to use enough to thoroughly wet dry hair and skin of the affected and adjacent hairy areas. When the hair and skin are thoroughly wet with shampoo, small quantities of water are added, working the shampoo into the hair and skin until a good lather forms. Shampooing is continued for 4 minutes, and then the hair is rinsed thoroughly. When the hair is dry, any remaining nits or nit shells (debris) may be removed with a fine-toothed comb. One application is usually curative. Some people do suffer persistent pruritus after treatment; however, retreatment should not be instituted unless living mites are seen.

Measures that can be instituted to prevent spread, aside from specific treatment, include (1) avoiding physical contact with infected persons or their belongings or clothing and (2) educating the public on the val-ue of laundering clothing and bedding in hot water (55°C or 131°F for 20 minutes) or dry cleaning to destroy nits and lice.

Helminth Infections

There are many different varieties of parasites, or helminths, which infect humans. Though it is known that some of these infections are quite common in the United States, exact data are unavailable because helminth infections are not mandatorily reported to CDC. For instance, though most people have heard the expression, "You eat so much, you must have a tapeworm," both beef and pork tapeworm infections are thought to be quite rare in the United States yet occur frequently in parts of Africa, Asia, Mexico, Peru, and eastern Europe (Benenson, 1980). In the absence of data pertinent to the United States, it is reasonable to assume that tapeworm infections would be prevalent wherever infected beef or pork is eaten raw or very rare.

Ascariasis (Roundworm Infection). Roundworm infection is essentially a helminthic infection of the small intestine. Its occurrence is worldwide with the greatest incidence in tropical countries. In the United States the disease is more prevalent in the South where it affects children of preschool and early school age more than older children and adults.

Symptoms of roundworm infection vary, but often the first recognizable sign is when the parasites are regurgitated or passed in the stool. The sudden appearance of a brownish parasite the size of a fishing worm is alarming to the child, the parent, and the health professional alike. Should this occur, adults should gently grasp the parasite with gauze or tissue until it passes. It should then be flushed down the toilet and the child referred for treatment.

Treatment of roundworm, pinworm, and hookworm is considered together after a brief discussion of pinworm and hookworm infections.

Enterobiasis (Pinworm Infection). In enterobiasis the causative agent is *Enterobius vermicularis*. Symptoms include anal itching, disturbed sleep, local irritation, and often secondary infections resulting from scratching. The occurrence of pinworms is worldwide. Benenson (1980) said pinworm infection is the most common helminth infection in the United States. Prevalence is highest in children of school age and lowest in adults.

Diagnosis of pinworm infection is made by finding adult worms in feces or in the anal region, or by applying transparent adhesive tape to the perianal region on awakening and before the person bathes or uses the toilet. The adhesive tape may then be examined microscopically for the presence of pinworms or their ova.

Pinworms are transmissible by direct transfer of infective eggs to mouth or indirectly through clothing, bedding, food, or other articles contaminated with the eggs of the parasite. In heavily infested houses, pinworms can be inhaled via dust. It is noteworthy that pinworm infections of animals are not transmissible to humans.

The following are general methods for prevention of spread of pinworms: (1) remove sources of infection by treating infected persons with medication described below; (2) encourage daily changing of clean underclothing, night clothing, and bedsheets; (3) launder clothing and bedsheets from infected persons in temperatures at least 55°C or 132°F; (4) educate infected and susceptible persons in good personal hygiene, particularly in thorough washing of hands before eating or preparing food; (5) discourage nail biting and scratching the bare anal area; and (6) reduce overcrowded areas whenever possible.

Ancylostomiasis (Hookworm Infection). Hookworm infection refers to chronic debilitating disease with vague symptoms that vary in proportion to the degree of anemia and hypoproteinemia present in the host. The anemia and hypoproteinemia seen in hookworm disease is produced by the blood-letting activity of the adult nematode in the intestine. Also, the severity of symptoms varies with the degree of infestation in that every light infections produce few or no clinical effects (Benenson, 1980).

Hookworms are not transmitted from person to person, but infected persons can contaminate soil by defecation as long as they remain infected and untreated. Under favorable conditions, hookworm larvae remain infective in soil for several weeks. Hookworms hatch in soil, and these hatched larvae are capable of penetrating bare skin (usually the foot) whereon they migrate to the bloodstream and ultimately attach to the intestinal wall where they continuously repeat their life cycle. Diagnosis of infection is confirmed by finding hookworm ova in the stool by microscopic examination.

The only control measures pertinent to hookworm infection are education of the public about the danger of going barefoot outdoors and specific treatment of confirmed cases.

Treatment of Roundworm, Pinworm, and Hookworm Infections. There are several medications available with varying effectiveness for treating these three common helminth infections. The two medications that are discussed here are used to some degree for all three types of infections.

Mebendazole (Vermox) can be used for single and mixed infections of roundworm, pinworm, and hookworm. The tablet may be chewed, swallowed, or crushed and mixed with food. For the control of pinworms a single tablet is given orally one time. For the control of roundworm and hookworm infections one tablet is given twice a day for 3 days.

Mebendazole should not be used for pregnant women or children under 2 years of age. Its ultimate effectiveness is said to depend on a number of host characteristics. For instance, the drug is believed to be less effective if given in the presence of diarrhea. If the patient is not cured in 3 weeks, a second course of treatment is advised.

A second antihelminthic drug is pyrantel pamoate (Antiminth). Again, this substance is used to treat roundworms, pinworms, and hookworms. Pyrantel pamoate may be administered without regard to ingestion of food or time of day. No laxative is necessary, and the drug may be taken with milk or fruit juices. The recommended dose is 1.0 g (PDR, 1981).

Adverse reactions encountered with pyrantel pamoate are most often related to the gastrointestinal system, such as anorexia, nausea, vomiting, abdominal cramps, and diarrhea. Its use in pregnancy is not fully tested nor has this substance been proven safe for children under 2 years of age.

Kawasaki Disease

Kawasaki disease, (KD, formerly know as mucocutaneous lymph node syndrome) an acute febrile illness of unknown etiology, occurring predominately in children under 5 years of age, is increasingly detected in the United States. In the 2 years between 1976 and 1978, 261 cases were reported to CDC. As in Japan, where KD is endemic, the disease in the United States does appear to be associated with geographical area, time of the year, socioeconomic status, and environmental factors (CDC, Feb. 15, 1980). Most cases of KD reported to CDC over the last few years have occurred sporadically, although clusters have been reported in the United States, Japan, and Greece.

Diagnosis of KD is made on the basis of distinctive clinical findings. Since the most severe sequela of this disease is development of coronary artery aneurysms, prevention and/or early detection is important.

Treatment of KD, aside from being supportive in nature, is directed toward minimizing the incidence of cardiac complications. Even though one study used aspirin to reduce the incidence of coronary aneurysm formation (Kato et al., 1979), no drug or combination of drugs has been conclusively proven effective in reducing the severity of cardiac complications to date (CDC, Feb. 15, 1980). Additionally, it is not known how KD is transmitted nor has a specific infectious agent been isolated. For these reasons nursing management aimed at containing the infection or identifying contacts is obscure in that it is difficult to contain what cannot be identified.

Legionellosis

Legionaires' disease (later called LD or legionellosis) received considerable publicity during its outbreak in Philadelphia at the 58th annual convention of the American Legion in July 1976. Initially and for several subsequent weeks it was difficult to pick up a newspaper or listen to a newscast that did not address LD. This outbreak is an excellent example documenting the need of community health nurses to be well-informed on topics of local, regional, and national concern. Even though no one knew the answers surrounding the epidemic in Philadelphia, much misinformation circulated, and it was frequently the responsibility of health care personnel to clarify the facts. For instance, there were daily rumors among lay and professionals alike that there was a new outbreak of LD in a given part of town or neighborhood. Nothing was known about the mode of transmission, and the fear was that the disease would break out in an uncontrolled form.

During that epidemic in 1976, an estimated 182 cases including 29 deaths occurred in a 3-week span of time (CDC, Nov. 10, 1978). Initially, little was known about the causative agent or the mode of transmission, but more than $1.5 million dollars were spent by CDC in the ensuing year, to unravel this mystery (CDC, 1977). In 1978, as laboratory protocol for serum testing came into wider use, a group of epidemiologists agreed that LD would be a reportable disease for a 3-year period. One of the major results of increased surveillance was that sporadic cases of LD were reported in several states in the United States and in several other countries of the world over the next 12 months.

Gradually panic subsided, but the exact nature of the epidemic outbreak of LD in Philadelphia was never completely explained. For example, the mode of transmission appeared to be airborne, but there were some indications that the organism was transiently present in the water coils of the air conditioning system. The causative organism was subsequently named *Legionella pneumophila.* Shortly after the outbreak in Philadelphia, laboratory analysis of the serum from victims compared to serum on file at CDC from similar previous outbreaks demonstrated that LD was not a new disease entity. Only the causative organism was newly discovered, since the investigation of previous outbreaks had failed to identify a causative organism for any number of reasons, including the lack of sophistication of serological and microbiological processing of samples.

The biggest unanswered question surrounding the LD outbreak in Philadelphia relates to the elements of pathogenicity and virulence of *L. pneumophila.* Continued surveillance has revealed that *L. pneumophilia* is not a particularly pathogenic or invasive organism in

that hosts most usually affected are elderly or generally debilitated. The question of why 182 relatively healthy persons were affected in such a short time span in Philadelphia remains unanswered.

Legionellosis continues to be typified by sporadic (not epidemic) outbreaks and to exhibit seasonality with 51% of all cases for 1979-80 having a beginning in July through October. Approximately the same number of cases was reported for 1978 and 1979 with a slight decrease in 1980. The case fatality ratio for 1980 was about the same as for preceding years or about 16% (CDC, Annual Summary, 1980).

CARING FOR A CHILD WITH A COMMUNICABLE DISEASE AT HOME

The majority of communicable diseases occur in children who are usually cared for at home. For this reason community health nurses need to teach parents proper care of infected children. Although the discussion is geared toward infants and children, many of the general principles such as those related to adequate hydration and general comfort measures are readily applicable to the adolescent and adult.

Adequate management of the individual suffering from a communicable disease can result in earlier treatment of untoward effects such as high fever, sepsis, or pulmonary infiltration. Generally it is helpful to advise the parents of the expected course of the illness, including possible high fevers. If parents are aware of usual symptoms, when unexpected signs such as unconsciousness or seizure occur, they will be more likely to seek immediate medical attention. It is helpful to go over various treatment settings that are available to the parent for emergency treatment before the need arises.

The incubation period is of particular concern to parents who have other children at home or who have not had the disease in question themselves. Frequently it is necessary to counsel parents about preventive measures such as their own children being exposed to children who subsequently become ill. Most communicable diseases are transmissible before the onset of rash or other definitive symptoms occur. The boxed material on p. 267, and Tables 12-6 to 12-8 assist in making decisions about when to advise immunization and when to defer such intervention. Helpful too is a personal or office copy of a standard reference on communicable diseases, such as the *Report of the Committee on Infectious Diseases* (frequently called simply, *The Red Book*), which is updated every 4 years by the American Academy of Pediatrics.

When antibiotics are prescribed, the community health nurse should emphasize the importance of taking the recommended dosage for the entire time prescribed, regardless of signs of improvement. Taking antibiotics any less than the amount prescribed may not only result in a recurrence of infection but the recurrence may be caused by an organism that has become resistant to the original antibiotic. Antibiotics prescribed for one member of the family should never be saved and then administered to another family member or friend, no matter how similar the symptoms. Antibiotics should be purchased in amounts sufficient to complete a prescribed regimen of treatment and the remainder disposed of safely. Though nurses may understand this concept quite well, lay people tend to save unused medications for any number of reasons including their cost.

Some general tips to share with parents include the following. (1) Fever can usually be relieved by antipyretics, liberal fluids, and tepid water baths. The choice of antipyretics should be left up to family preference assuming no allergies exist. The child should be dressed lightly and kept well sheltered from the elements while febrile. (2) Itching associated with chickenpox and measles can be relieved by oral antihistamines (if the physician does not object), which can be purchased over the counter. The pharmacist can advise as to appropriate dosage when the drug is purchased. The parent should be told that antihistamines may cause drowsiness. Baths with 2 to 4 tablespoons of bicarbonate of soda may be helpful in relieving itching too. (3) Although a cough may be controlled with an over-the-counter cough suppressant, parents should be warned about the potential for "double-dosing" children with a cough mixture containing antipyretics and antihistamines.

Adequate hydration and nutrition during the acute and convalescent periods are essential. Often there are mouth or throat lesions in addition to a generally poor appetite. Some of the more acidic fruit juices may be poorly tolerated for this reason. The parent should be encouraged to offer small feedings at frequent intervals rather than two or three large meals a day. Also, the parent needs to be alerted to the dehydration effects of diarrhea that may accompany influenza syndromes.

As children begin to feel subjectively improved, there is a tendency to become too active. Bed rest is important throughout the acute and convalescent stages but may be mixed with other quiet activities consistent with the child's developmental level and tolerance. The child suffering from a communicable disease should not be isolated from family contact any more than is absolutely necessary.

Conjunctivitis from Measles

Measles may be accompanied by conjunctivitis, which causes some degree of photophobia. This condi-

tion generally passes with little ill effect. A warm washcloth over the eyes in the morning on arising helps to clear the mucus that may mat the eyelids and eyelashes. The "sickroom" should be lighted dimly with blinds or drapes closed against bright sunlight while photophobic symptoms are paramount. The germicidal effect of sunlight should not be discounted, and aside from the presence of unusual symptoms such as photophobia, the sick-room should be exposed to as much sunlight as comfort permits.

THE INFECTION CONTROL PRACTITIONER

It seems negligent to complete a chapter on communicable diseases without specifically delineating the emerging role of the infection control practitioner (ICP). This role was created in response to the episodic phenomenon of nosocomial infections in the middle 1950s. Since then, the role has proliferated so that about 80% of all hospitals in the United States with a bed capacity of 300 or greater employ at least one such practitioner full time (Emori et al., 1980). Further, the role is becoming increasingly visible in distributive care facilities such as health departments, home health care agencies, and extended care facilities.

Surveys have shown that the vast majority (approximately 94%) of ICP positions are filled by registered nurses (Emori et al., 1980; Turner, 1977). The role functions of this position are the prevention, surveillance, and control of nosocomial infections. In 1972 ICPs and physicians formed a multidisciplinary infection control organization called the Association for Practitioners in Infection Control (APIC). This organization has grown rapidly and currently has national, regional, and local chapters. The interested reader is encouraged to contact APIC for further information on infection control activities in any given geographical area.

APIC National Office
Rte. 21359 Milwaukee Ave.
Half Day, Illinois 60069

The biggest area of contention relative to the ICP role in the 1980s is the question of academic and clinical preparation of practitioners. APIC describes the bachelor's level practitioner as the desired level of entry into infection control practice. However, these roles frequently require a basic command of disciplines such as elementary statistics, research, epidemiology, microbiology, teaching-learning, and an ability to use change and communication theory. Because of such requirements, some educators are recommending that these individuals have master's degrees (Turner, 1978). Since the ICP role may be readily comparable to a type of clinical specialist role, master's preparation would seem most appropriate, especially when the role is performed in a large or complex agency setting.

SUMMARY

A serious effort has been made to portray the impact that communicable and infectious processes have on contemporary society and therefore on community health nursing practice. Even though communicable diseases are no longer the most frequent cause of morbidity and mortality, they still represent a major health problem. The nature and sometimes the name of communicable processes change over time, but they nonetheless retain a sinister ability to weaken, to disable, and to kill.

A good deal of irony surrounds humanity's relationship with the microorganism. Any student of microbiology understands our reliance on this basic life form. At the same time clinical microbiologists and infectious disease experts struggle to retain some margin of control over these rudimentary organisms.

The effort to monitor and control communicable disease phenomena is world-wide. However, the effectiveness of larger surveillance systems is dependent on astute individuals on the local level who must find cases and implement preventive, control, and maintenance strategies. Because of the practice arena involved, the community health nurse occupies a position of responsibility for all these functions. There are few other instances in which the opportunity to contribute in an intradisciplinary fashion for the common good is so operative.

BIBLIOGRAPHY

American Academy of Pediatrics: Report of the committee on infectious diseases, ed. 19, Evanston, Ill., 1982, AAP.

American Hospital Association: Infection control in the hospital, ed. 4, Chicago, Ill., 1979, The Association.

Benenson, A.S., editor: Control of communicable diseases in man, ed. 13, Washington, D.C., 1980, American Public Health Association.

Bennett, J.V., and Brachman, D.S., editors: Hospital infections, Boston, 1979, Little, Brown & Co.

Beveridge, W.I.: Influenza: the last great plague, New York, 1978, Prodist.

Brown, M.S.: What you should know about communicable diseases and their immunizations: a guide for nurses in ambulatory settings, Nursing 9(5):72, 1975.

Centers for Disease Control: BCG vaccines, MMWR, Atlanta, Ga., June 1, 1979, pp. 241-244.

Centers for Disease Control: Diphtheria, tetanus and pertussis: guidelines for vaccine prophylaxis and other preventative measures, MMWR, Atlanta, Ga., Aug. 21, 1981, pp. 392-407.

Centers for Disease Control: Genital herpes infections—United States, 1966-1979, MMWR, Atlanta, Ga., March 26, 1982, pp. 137-138.

Centers for Disease Control: Legionnaire's disease, Morbidity & Mortality Weekly Report (MMWR), Atlanta, Ga., Nov. 10, 1978, pp. 439-441.

Centers for Disease Control: Legionnaire's disease—Australia, MMWR, Atlanta, Ga., Jan. 5, 1979, p. 523.

Centers for Disease Control: Kawaski disease—New York, MMWR, Atlanta, Ga., Feb. 15, 1980, pp. 61-63.

Centers for Disease Control: Pneumococcal polysaccharide vaccine, MMWR, Atlanta, Ga., Aug. 28, 1981, pp. 410-411.

Centers for Disease Control: Methicillin—resistant *Staphylococcus aureus*—United States, MMWR, Atlanta, Ga., Nov. 20, 1981, pp. 557-559.

Centers for Disease Control: Tuberculosis—United States, 1980, MMWR, Atlanta, Ga., Feb. 13, 1981, pp. 55-56.

Centers for Disease Control: Tuberculosis among hispanics in the United States—1980, MMWR, Atlanta, Ga., May 14, 1982, pp. 237-239.

Centers for Disease Control: Annual summary, MMWR, Atlanta, Ga., 1979.

Centers for Disease Control: Annual summary, MMWR, Atlanta, Ga., 1980.

Centers for Disease Control: CDC updates senators on Legionnaire's disease—hospital infection control, Atlanta, Ga., 1977, pp. 144-145.

Dowling, H.G.: Fighting infection:conquests of the twentieth century, Cambridge, Mass., 1977, Harvard University Press.

Dubos, R.: Man adapting, New Haven, 1965, Yale University Press.

Emori, T.G., Haley, R.W., and Stanley, R.C.: The infection control nurse in U.S. hospitals, 1976-1977, Am. J. Epidemiol. 111(5):592-607, May 1980.

Fuerst, R.: Microbiology in health and disease, ed. 14, Philadelphia, 1978, W. B. Saunders Co.

Hare, R.: Pomp and pestilence, New York, 1955, Philosophical Library, Inc.

Healthy people: the Surgeon General's report on health promotion and disease prevention, DHEW Pub. No. (PHS) 79-55071, Washington, D.C., 1979, Department of Health, Education and Welfare.

Kato, H., Hoike, S., and Yokoyama, T.: Kawaski disease: effect of treatment on coronary artery involvement, Pediatrics 63(1):175-179, 1979.

Korones, S.B., and Lancaster, J.: High-risk newborn infants:the basis for intensive nursing care, St. Louis, 1976, The C. V. Mosby Co.

Lappe, M.: Antibiotic roulette, Reader's Digest, Oct. 1981, pp. 225-230.

Pelton, S.: Trends in immunization, Pediatr. Nurs. 5(4):45-52, 1978.

Physician's Desk Reference, ed. 35, Oradell, N.J., 1981, Medical Economics Books.

Ramsay, A.M., and Emond, R.T.: Infectious diseases, London, 1979, William Heinemann Medical Books, Ltd.

Reeves, D., and Geddes, A.: Recent advances in infection, New York, 1979, Churchill Livingstone, Inc.

Richards, N.M.: Infectious diseases. In Jarvis, L.L., editor: Community health nursing; keeping the public healthy, Philadelphia, 1981, F. A. Davis Co.

Turner, J.G.: Survey of infection control practitioners in Florida, Gainesville, Fla., 1977, University of Florida, Board of Regeants.

Turner, J.G.: The nurse epidemiologist:selection and preparation, Sup. Nurse 9(4):33-41, 1978.

Whaley, L.F., and Wong, D.L.: Nursing care of infants and children, St. Louis, 1979, The C. V. Mosby Co.

Youmans, G.P., Paterson, P.Y., and Sommers, H.M.: The biologic and clinical basis of infectious diseases, Philadelphia, 1975, W. B. Saunders Co.

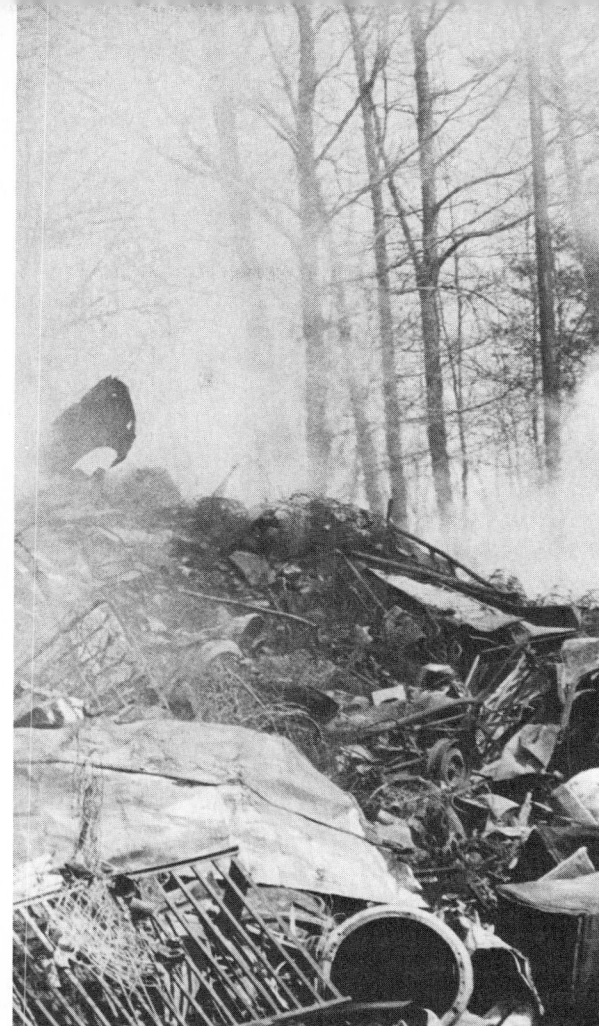

Chapter 13

JEANETTE LANCASTER
VIVIENNE BROWN

ENVIRONMENTAL AND OCCUPATIONAL HEALTH AND SAFETY

Despite achievements emerging with the advancement of society, problems of pollution, pestilence, and deterioration remain. Issues identified decades ago have not been solved. Today the problems have increased and the issues remain, although in increasingly complicated forms. Some are merely eyesores, others are serious enough to make the simple act of breathing a difficult task. Environmental problems are as old as history itself; over the centuries some have increased in severity, although others have diminished, but discouraging new problems have emerged. Nurses play a key role in detecting environmental and occupational health hazards as well as in developing and implementing health promotion and treatment programs.

Environmental degradation and deterioration have been concerns of environmentalists for many years; however, public awareness remained at low levels until the 1960s when it began to increase dramatically. Since the 1960s environmental groups have become more active. During 1982 several leading U.S. environmental groups criticized the Reagan administration's environmental policies. Criticism was aimed at the weakening of the Clean Air Act, failure to act on acid rain and toxic air pollutants, loosening of controls on hazardous wastes, and subsidizing of nuclear energy.

In 1970 the United States Environmental Protection Agency (EPA) was formed and given primary responsibility for controlling pollution and dealing with threats to life and the environment. The EPA has been accused of being lax in meeting deadlines, and some programs have never been initiated. Under the Reagan administration the agency encountered large reductions in personnel, authority, and budget. Many environmentalists believe the 1980s will see the demise of the EPA.

Even with EPA regulations and achievements, some environmental hazards have reached critical levels, posing a threat not only to health but also to the general quality and fabric of life. Newspaper, radio, and television repeatedly offer horror stories of chemical spills and exposures, acid rain, asbestos in city water, contaminated fish, and deterioration of the ozone level. Acid rain caused by ozone pollution is responsible for billions of dollars of damage to crops annually. Ozone depletion will result in increased susceptibility to skin cancer.

Dioxin is increasingly becoming a major contaminant. Dioxin is an ingredient in the defoliant Agent Orange. Agent Orange was widely used as a defoliant by U.S. forces in Vietnam, and it is one of the most deadly known chemicals. In 1976 a cloud of dioxin was accidently released into the air in Seveso, Italy, killing thousands of animals and causing hundreds of children to become ill. Birth defects in that area tripled. It is estimated that between one and 11 pounds of dioxin were responsible for this environmental mishap. The EPA has confirmed that dioxin is present in significant levels in many sites in Missouri. In humans dioxin has been linked to cancer, birth defects, and problems of the liver, kidneys, nervous system, and skin.

Air pollution continues as a threat to human health, affecting reactions to prescription drugs; altering an individual's susceptibility to infectious disease such as colds, influenza, and pneumonia; serving as a catalyst for heart disease; and contributing to chronic, often irreversible lung problems.

No discussion of environmental health and safety would be complete without a brief review of several classic disasters that have shaped many contemporary environmental health practices. Between December 3 and 5, 1930, several thousand people in the densely populated Meuse River Valley west of Liege, Belgium, were stricken, and 60 died as a result of industrial air pollution. In this narrow strip of land, barometric pressures were high, temperatures at or below freezing, and no wind was blowing. Factory smoke combined with fog to create a "soupy" mixture that settled on the grounded. Victims became hoarse, short of breath, and nauseated. Deaths were the result of heart failure in the elderly or others already weakened by other causes (Waldbott, 1978).

The Belgian disaster did not motivate other countries to take precautions against air pollution. The greatest air pollution disaster occurred in the United States in October, 1948, at Donora, Pennsylvania. Circumstances similar to those in the Meuse Valley led to the Donora disaster. Many factories, including zinc smelters and producers of wire, steel, and sulfuric acid, lined the river front, and freight trains emitted great clouds of smoke that rose to 350 feet. When a high pressure front moved in, rainfall added fog and moisture to the air. On October 26, an inversion began in cold weather with a wind velocity near zero. A constant smog blanket produced a virtually air-tight chamber, day and night, for more than five days, during which the air was permeated by an odor of sulfur (Waldbott, 1978). Twenty people died and 5,910 or 42% of the population, suffered from irritation of the eyes, nose, and throat, pain and chest constriction, cough, labored breathing, severe headaches, nausea, and vomiting.

A different type of disaster occurred in London, England, on December 4, 1952. As a high-pressure mass of cold air moved across the English Channel toward the Thames Valley, people used fireplaces extensively. With practically no wind, the city became engulfed in a heavy cloud of smoke that condensed in the moisture of London's fog. The greatly reduced visibility for trains and automobiles and for boats on the waterways led to many accidents. Although impossible to assess the death toll caused by respiratory and heart problems from the fog, 2,851 persons over the usual death rate for 1 week (between December 4 and 13, 1952) died and during the following week another 1,224 deaths were attributed to the presence of the fog. London suffered a second fatal fog in 1956 which claimed 1000 lives (Waldbott, 1978).

Similarly, water pollution poses a serious threat to life. No longer is safe drinking water assured. In Chesapeake, Virginia, homeowners have refused to drink city water. In the early 1970s the city purchased and installed miles of asbestos cement pipe. The EPA found asbestos fibers in the water flowing through the pipes. Residents quickly installed their own wells and refused to drink city water. The residents faced criminal charges for failing to comply with a city ordinance. Most of the charges have been dropped, but some residents filed suit against the city complaining of personal injury resulting from ingesting water containing a known carcinogen, asbestos. The residents may have justifiable grounds for their refusal to drink the water (Environment, 1982).

The EPA reported 192 outbreaks of disease attributed to drinking water, causing 36,800 acute illnesses between 1971 and 1977 (Your Guide, 1980). Recently suspected carcinogens called trihalomethanes have been discovered in water systems. Trihalomethanes are formed when chlorine reacts with natural substances in water. The EPA has proposed a rule that will regulate the trihalomethane concentration in drinking water.

The current ruling is being challenged by the American Water Works Association because of economic, technical, and procedural issues. Litigation by concerned groups opposed to EPA regulations is not uncommon.

Beaches that were once ideal vacation sites have deteriorated. Onshore and offshore oil spills at the Atlantic, Pacific, and Gulf shores have killed fish and birds and made beaches undesirable recreation areas. Lakes are polluted also; almost all fish species in Lake Ontario have been found to be contaminated. Fish have been tainted with DDT, mercury, toxaphene, and other chemicals dumped by industries. Chlorinated hydrocarbons that remain poisonous for years have accumulated. The lake itself, once pleasing to look at, now poses an eyesore. Waterways leading to the lake often serve as dumps containing radioactive debris (Brown, 1982).

Annually in the United States millions of tons of hazardous wastes are generated, often forcing residents to abandon homes built near chemical dump sites. Thousands of improper disposal sites remain scattered throughout the country. Another chemical hazard is pesticides, which are used increasingly. More than a billion pounds of pesticides are used annually in the United States. People suffering from the adverse effects of pesticides include farm workers, pesticide applicators, pesticide production employees, consumers of seafoods, and unsuspecting residents in communities affected by aerial spraying. Symptoms of pesticide poisoning may include dizziness, nausea, and abdominal pain in mild cases but convulsive seizures, coma, and death can occur in more severe cases.

A herbicide called Tordon contains picloram, the same ingredient found in a defoliant that was used in Vietnam. Timber companies in North Carolina have used picloram for 20 years, leading to a 90% increase in cancer death in that area (Deadly Chemical, 1982).

Even more threatening is the increased use of toxic substances such as chemicals. Chemicals that permeate and virtually characterize modern life have become a serious source of environmental contamination, and they are now thought to be a significant negative determinant of health and longevity. Each year thousands of new chemicals are discovered by the chemical industry, with hundreds introduced commercially. The immediate cause for concern arises from the sheer numbers of the chemical compounds, the diversity of their use, and the adverse resultant effect already attributed to some.

There has been a growing list of diseases, either known or suspected, caused by or associated with chemicals introduced into the environment. Emphysema and other lung disorders are linked to air pollution, lead poisoning to lead-based interior house paint and to the lead additives of gasoline, heart diseases to carbon monoxide, and permanent nerve disorders to mercury. A connection has been found between one type of lung cancer (mesothelioma) and the fibers produced in the manufacturing of asbestos. A form of liver cancer has been found in workers engaged in turning vinyl chloride into polyvinyl chloride. In spite of this growing list, the full magnitude of the problem of chemicals in the environment has not been determined.

The production and maintenance of a healthy, stimulating, and enjoyable environment will require a combination of increased litigation, vigorous enforcement of existing laws, increased cooperation by business, and greater public awareness and education. Community health nurses can make significant contributions to this process.

HISTORICAL PERSPECTIVE

The environment played a key role in early community health measures. In biblical times many customs, taboos, and religious practices were derived from interactions between people and environmental conditions. Moses' Law satisfied both religious and sanitary conditions. As people became aggregated or urbanized, problems such as an adequate supply of water and the removal of wastes were apparent. As early as 3000 to 1500 BC, the Minoans and Egyptians built flood dikes, drainage, and irrigation systems and had public water systems (Hanlon and Pickett, 1979). The Romans built impressive aqueducts, drainage systems, gutters, and public baths and paved the streets. As cities developed in the Middle Ages, communicable diseases came into existence. Pandemics of cholera associated with polluted water and bubonic plague carried by rats reduced the population of Europe. Leprosy probably started in Egypt and was spread by the Crusaders. Also, around 1440 AD bubonic plague or black death began in China and was carried to India and then to Egypt. During this time bacteria carried by the rat flea could be traced to points of origin at seaports.

During the Renaissance the microscope was developed, which enabled scientists such as Pasteur and Koch to establish the role of bacteria as a cause of disease.

In the United States the development of the colonies led to textile and paper mills. The demand for an endless number of products increased, and the nation's transition from a farm economy to early industry was under way.

Another historical change was the replacement of flatboats with railroads as a means of transportation. Railroads pushed their way across the frontier, linking two oceans. Hastily constructed steel mills with their numerous emissions provided the tracks on which the trains ran and newly dug coal mines provided their fuel. Factories still depended on workers' skills; as technology increased, so did the demand for workers.

Environmental health in the United States was seriously questioned after 1850 following publication of the *Report of the Sanitary Commission of Massachusetts* (Rosen, 1957). This report, while largely ignored at the time of publication, is regarded today as a landmark document because of the implications for environmental health. Recommendations specific to environmental health included the development of a systematic plan for observing atmospheric phenomena, smoke prevention, measures to ensure pure air and water, adequate drainage, sewage, and pest control. Other recommendations dealt with occupational health, housing, pest control, food, drugs, and schools. Ironically, many of the problems addressed in the report exist today.

The Industrial Revolution brought new hazards to people and the environment. The use of machinery and suboptimal work methods led to stress, physical injuries, and chemical exposures. Cities doubled in size. Knowledge of sanitation and personal hygiene was unavailable for the poor and the hundreds of immigrants who flocked to this country in search of jobs.

Conditions in the mines and the steel mills were deplorable in the early twentieth century. In the large cities sweatshops were a constant threat to life and health for many workers. Men, women, and children put in 70- and 80-hour work weeks in factories. Tuberculosis and other diseases were common among workers. The early 1930s brought badly needed legislation that changed working hours for children and adults. New automated machines and techniques replaced the old. Sophisticated mechanization led to mass production, and cities became increasingly overcrowded. Emissions from industries and automobiles polluted the air. Factories discharged industrial wastes into the air and waterways.

World War II brought an increasing number of women into the labor forces. Women worked with chemicals and gases, such as benzidine and vinyl chloride, both of which are now considered to be carcinogenic. After the war men replaced a large majority of women in the work force and continued to work with these and other carcinogenic substances. The use of amines such as benzidine has now been banned in foreign countries; they are not used in the United States either but were until the 1970s. Many of the women workers during World War II have since developed bladder cancer.

As the demand for supplies and products increased, so did the pressures to keep costs down and production

up. The results were increased accidents, injuries, and deaths. Legislation regulating workplace hazards was passed in 1970 with the enactment of the Occupational Safety and Health Act (OSHA). The law requires employers to comply with specific standards promulgated by the Department of Labor. In addition to OSHA, the act created the National Institute for Occupational Safety and Health (NIOSH) within the Department of Health and Human Services (DHHS) to conduct research on occupational hazards and recommend new standards to OSHA. Both agencies have tended to be understaffed and underfunded. The effectiveness of OSHA and NIOSH has also been diminished by the lengthy process involved in setting standards. The true picture of occupational injuries is frequently difficult to assess because workers often change jobs and in doing so are exposed to a variety of substances over a period of time. This complicates attempts to identify a specific substance as the cause of a disease. Many diseases result from the cumulative effects of exposure to substances both on and off the job.

People are currently experiencing the most varied and intense life stressors in the history of humanity. Tremendous advances in science, technology, education as well as the social and behavioral sciences are altering the ability of individuals, families, groups, and communities to maintain balance and stability. Not all of these changes are positive. Despite considerable knowledge about the relationship between health and the environment, waterways are increasingly polluted, the air is filled with noxious substances and pesticides, and radiation and nuclear power threaten livelihood. Each attempt to make life more comfortable and pleasant leads to new sources of pollution and stress.

Past models of looking at environmental influences on health are no longer effective for the complex problems of the twentieth century. Although some water, air, or noise pollution in isolation may not disrupt homeostasis, when all three are present in combination with factors such as crowding, interpersonal stress, and chemical or biological hazards, the cumulative impact can disrupt the ability to cope successfully with environmental stimuli.

ECOLOGY AND ENVIRONMENTAL HEALTH

Ecology, the age-old study of living organisms in interaction with the environment, provides a model for looking at environmental health. Ecology is concerned with the broad conceptualization of the interrelationships between living and nonliving things. The term *ecology* was first proposed by German biologist Ernst Haeckel in 1869; the word is derived from the Greek root *oikos,* meaning house. Ecology literally means the study of organisms at home. Ecology is concerned with both the structure and functioning of the organism; it attends to the surroundings as well as that which is surrounded.

Ecology, in order to study the interrelationships within an environment, is action oriented and focuses on what can be rather than ending its conceptualization of the human/environment relationship with either what has been or what is. The term *biosphere* refers to the world of living things and is made up of numerous ecosystems. Each *ecosystem* represents all living and nonliving parts that support a chain of life within a selected area (Wilner et al., 1978) and is the sum total of all existing subsystems.

In each ecosystem, nature provides specific conditions essential for supporting plant and animal life. Each ecosystem is a "circle of life" comprising four principal types of components: (1) sunlight, water, oxygen, carbon dioxide, organic compounds, and other nutrients for plant growth; (2) plants, which convert carbon dioxide and water into carbohydrates through photosynthesis; (3) consumers of the products of plants: herbivores (for example, cows and sheep) and carnivores (man and other meat-eating animals); (4) decomposed organisms such as bacteria, fungi, and insects.

Barry Commoner's "laws of ecology" help to explain the scope of environmental health. Commoner (1971) organized an informal series of laws of ecology, with the first one holding that "everything is connected to everything else" and stating that sunlight, water, oxygen, carbon dioxide, organic compounds, and all organisms are interconnected. The second law, "everything must go somewhere," stipulates that one organism's excretion or waste is taken up by another organism as food. The third law, "nature knows best," holds that human changes within a natural system do not always improve that system and may prove to be detrimental. The fourth law, "there is no such thing as a free lunch," stipulates that anything removed from the natural environment by human effort must be replaced and anything added to the natural environment must be removed if the environment is to be preserved. The extent to which these laws are violated or obeyed determines the status of the environment. These laws call attention to the interrelated nature of the human environment and support the need for using an ecological perspective in viewing environmental health.

In studying ecosystems it is also necessary to consider people as part of, not separate from, a life support system composed of the atmosphere, water, soil, plants, and animals that function together to keep the system viable. When people are considered a part of their environment, it is essential to consider attitudes, values, and perceptions. The behavior of people is influenced by their values and attitudes about themselves, others, and the world around them. Similarly, one's perception of reality is usually more influential in determining behavior than the reality itself. People act in accordance with what they perceive, think, feel, and cherish.

From an ecological perspective the environment is a multifaceted system made up of biophysical and sociocultural components. The interrelationships between the total person and the total environment are dynamic. Each makes demands on the other, as people try to adapt to the environment or adapt their needs and desires to meet the current state of the environment. Adaptation is a process, not an event. For any organism to survive, it must learn to adapt. Nothing remains fixed or constant in a living system; rather, living systems are in a constant state of adaptation as organisms continually accommodate to new stressors. Not all adaptations are smooth or positive in outcome. A system can be overloaded so that it cannot adapt to the stimuli. For example, people can be temporarily placed in a noisy situation that is intolerable but over time they may adjust, for example, to the sound of large airplanes landing near their homes, or the sound may decrease. However, if the noise overload is too great or is constant, a person can experience psychotic symptoms caused by continuous sensory overload.

People often overlook the multiple interactions required to maintain a stable relationship among living and nonliving parts of the environment. A classic example of the lack of an orientation to planning occurred in Borneo with a World Health Organization mosquito control program (Harrison et al., 1969). After a community was heavily sprayed with DDT, the mosquitoes were controlled, but roofs began to be eaten by caterpillars, which were unaffected by the DDT. The spray also killed wasps that previously ate the caterpillars. The problem was complicated following indoor spraying to control houseflies. Previously, a small harmless gecko lizard ate the houseflies. However, when the lizards ate the diseased flies, the lizards became debilitated and were easily captured by their predators, the cats. As cats disappeared, the rat population boomed, invading houses and threatening Borneo with the plague (Hanlon and Pickett, 1979). This example shows how easily, with the help of people, an ecosystem can be thrown out of balance. Throughout the remainder of the chapter consider how each of the environmental hazards could ultimately lead to an equally undesirable outcome.

Not only do people contribute to the status of their environment, but they are products of that environment; therefore, the environment is a determinate of health and well-being. *Environmental health* may therefore be defined as that aspect of community health which is concerned with these forms of life, substances, forces, and conditions in the surroundings of people that may exert an influence on their health and well-being. Environmental health embodies the absence or presence of illness, health maintenance, human efficiency, and the enjoyment of life.

Many parts of the environment can produce health hazards: biological organisms, toxic chemicals, radioactivity, ineffective waste disposal, noise, and other physical and psychosocial forces.

IDENTIFICATION OF ENVIRONMENTAL HAZARDS

Many contemporary changes disrupt the circle of life. Hanlon and Pickett (1979) propose two contexts for describing the human and environment relationship. The first includes elements of the natural environment hazardous to health such as biological agents of disease or injury, including microorganisms, plants, and animals; weather; radiation; naturally occurring chemicals; and geological perturbations such as earthquakes and volcanoes. The second context consists of health hazards brought on by the actions and maladaptations of people to their environment and includes suicide, accidents, genetic damage, poisoning, and health threats from pollution. Chapters 20, 22, 26, 27, and 38 discuss some of these environment hazards.

The modern environment is hazardous in at least two ways: it contains noxious and stressful events and it changes so quickly that people are unable to adapt. As discussed in Chapter 38, the rate of change offers phenomenal stress caused by rapid and often novel requirements for human adaptation. Even small doses of a contaminant over a long period of time can disrupt health. Factors within the environment often work together to reinforce one another (synergism) or act in opposition (antagonism). Problems, because of their interactive nature, cannot be considered in isolation but rather must be viewed from an ecological perspective. Community health nurses are called on to provide information to consumers and agencies about the effect of the environment on health as well as to carefully assess for environmental hazards and plan appropriate interventions. To do this, an understanding of contemporary environmental contaminants is needed.

Biological Hazards

Biological hazards include disease-producing agents that can enter the human body. They consist largely of bacteria, viruses, and other microorganisms and parasites (Hanlon and Pickett, 1979). As discussed in Chapters 7 and 12, for a disease to be transmitted, a host source, causative agent, and means of transmission must be present. The following outline depicts selected environmental aspects of the host-agent-transmission model.

Environmental Impact Analysis Areas.*

Potential impacts to the physical environment
  Air
    Climate
    Air emissions
    Air quality
  Water
    Water requirements
    Water availability
    Water quality
  Physiography
    Soils
    Geology
    Topography
    Drainage modifications
  Solid wastes
    Quantity
    Disposal
  Mineral resources
    Consumption
    Depletion
Potential impacts to the biological environment
  Flora
    Terrestrial
    Aquatic
    Endangered species
  Fauna
    Terrestrial
    Aquatic
    Endangered species
  Ecological relationships
    Ecological balance
    Critical species in food chain
    Productivity
    Diversity
Potential impacts to human environment
  Socioeconomic impacts
    Population and demographic changes
    Economic conditions
    Employment
    Wages
    Tax base
  Social conditions
    Noise
    Pressure on services such as police, fire, schools, and
      hospitals and on utilities and transportation

*From Golden, J., et al.: Environmental impact data book, Ann Arbor, Mich., 1979, Ann Arbor Science Publishers, Inc.

Changes in daily living patterns
Land use
Water use
Aesthetics
Special interest points
    Archaeological
    Paleontological
    Historical
    Recreational
Human health effects
    Air emissions
    Water residuals
    Solid wastes

Biological hazards are primarily concerned with bodily entry of disease-producing infectious agents (Purdom, 1980). Many biological hazards are described in detail in Chapter 12. In general, biological hazards are transmitted either through the escape of an agent from a source or reservoir to a susceptible host.

Some people are more seriously affected by communicable disease than others, depending on their state of health, level of immunity, heredity, and environmental and other prevailing conditions at the time of exposure (Purdom, 1980). Common forms of invading pathogens are bacteria, fungi, and mold.

Water

As discussed in Chapter 1, water has served as a waste disposal mechanism since early recorded history. Rome channeled its sewage into the Tiber River through aqueducts. Epidemics of typhoid fever, cholera, and dysentery occurred during the Middle Ages when the same bodies of water were used for waste disposal and for drinking. In the last century oceans, lakes, and rivers have become dumping sites for sewage and industrial wastes. Health hazards come from ingesting polluted water from one of the following sources: waterborne viruses and bacteria, waste heat, radioactivity, industrial pollutants, oil spills, and underground pollution from dumping.

Waterborne viruses and bacteria require moisture, a food medium, and proper temperature and pH to survive any length of time; therefore, water is an excellent medium for cultivating bacteria. Bacteria is normally filtered out of water as it moves through soil; waste that follows passageways along fissures in rocks, coarse gravel, or limestone conveys bacteria. Shallow wells may become contaminated when the distance the water travels through the soil is insufficient to filter out bacteria. Most communities have wells 450 to 1400 feet deep.

Bacteria or viruses may enter wells through surface water, by the use of contaminated water to prime pumps, through contamination of ropes, by buckets handled with unclean hands, or by cross connectors between water pipes and waste piping. Most outbreaks of waterborne diseases occur in private supplies, but contaminated public supplies affect more people.

Waterborne bacteria diseases include typhoid and parathyphoid fevers, dysentery, and cholera. Waterborne viral diseases include infectious hepatitis and poliomyelitis. The pathogens responsible for these diseases are found in the intestinal and urinary tracts of infected people.

The *temperature of water* directly influences the toxicity of many pollutants and the growth of bacteria and viruses. Aquatic life is damaged when industry dissipates heat in circulating water. As aquatic life is harmed, the circle of life or food chain is disrupted. Many factories use cooling towers to lower water heat; however, only a fourth to two thirds of the heat can be dissipated by this method.

Small amounts of toxic chemicals in water threaten all forms of life. For example, mercury has for many years been discharged from both industrial and agricultural sources. As it increases in concentration in the food chain, mercury can result in serious or even fatal poisoning, neurological disorders, or birth defects (Spath and Crook, 1981). Not only are food sources poisoned by chemicals in water, but recreation is also affected. Swimming in contaminated waters can increase the incidence of gastrointestinal disease.

Radioactivity has been introduced into water in areas such as mining or milling, which use radioactive substances. In addition, industries making and testing atomic bombs release radioactive substances.

Water pollution can be broadly defined as the addition of something that changes the natural qualities of water. Industry has altered water quality for years by dumping industrial waste into rivers and seas. Industrial wastes primarily consisting of paper, chemicals, primary metal, or petroleum are derived from the manufacturing process. These pollutants deplete the dissolved oxygen, causing fish to die and odors to develop. Contaminants, although not lethal to fish and shellfish, do render them inedible to humans.

Certain pollutants, such as phosphates, promote excess growth of nutrients in lakes. The nutrient, in a process called *eutrophication*, promotes the growth of algae, which cause cloudy, odorous water and produce deposits. These deposits are incompatible with most forms of aquatic life.

Oil spills and discharge from onshore and offshore facilities threaten marine life. Oil spills kill fish and certain birds and make beaches unusable for recreation. Moreover, oil-laden sediment can move with bottom currents and contaminate unpolluted offshore areas. As a result, the sea floor near an oil spill remains toxic to animals for long periods following the initial spill.

Food

An estimated 2 to 10 million people in the United States contract a foodborne disease annually. These diseases rank second only to the common cold as the most frequent cause of illness (Wilner et al., 1978). Environmental hazards related to food are of three main kinds. The first consists of *microbiological contamination* and usually occurs as a result of deposits of toxins on food. Contaminated foods may cause salmonellosis and shigellosis, illness from *Clostridium perfingens, Vibrio,* and viruses, and food poisonings from *Staphylococcus* and *Clostridium botulinus* toxins. Food poisoning from microbiological contamination is caused by the transfer of an organism through food to a human victim after which internal growth of the organism occurs.

A second environmental problem related to food is *chemical additive contamination.* Most Americans consume 5 pounds of chemical additives in food each year (Wilner et al., 1978). Chemical food additives fall into two categories: intentional additives and incidental additives. Intentional additives are deliberately used in food processing to enhance or conserve nutritional value or to improve or maintain flavor, color, texture, or consistency. The use of these additives is sanctioned by the Food and Drug Administration under the GRAS list (Generally Recognized As Safe). Typical GRAS additives include vitamins A_1, D_2, D_3, carotene, ascorbic acid, riboflavin, and others. A complete listing of such additives may be found in the *Federal Register.*

Incidental additives enter and remain in food as a result of their use as pesticides or herbicides, after addition to animal food, from packaging material, or through chemical changes brought about by processing methods. In these cases the levels in food must not exceed the tolerances set by the FDA.

A third environmental hazard relates to *suboptimal food handling.* Careless food handling, inadequate pretreatment, a contaminated environment, a high bacterial count, and poor food storage have negative influences on food safety and quality. A major community health nursing role in regard to food is that of education. Both consumers and other health care providers need to be well informed about the potential adverse effects of food contamination, additives, and improper handling. Education can be conveyed in a variety of ways including direct provision of facts to individual clients or groups, classes on the effects of environmental hazards, and a variety of public service announcements.

Air Pollution

The toxic action of a pollutant is rarely the same for any two individuals because of varying human factors (Purdom, 1980). Pollutants occur either as gases or fine particles referred to as particulate matter. Although both forms are present in the atmosphere simultaneously, gases constitute about 90% of all pollutants. A pollutant exerts its effect by either depressing or stimulating normal functioning within an organ (see Fig. 13-1).

Virtually all human activities bring people into contact with some form of air pollution. Indoors, people are exposed to vapors in the kitchen, fumes from cleaning detergents, particulates in cosmetics, aerosols in spray cans, tobacco smoke, fibrous particles from rugs, draperies, blankets, and clothes. In homes and commercial establishments, central heating and air conditioning circulate dust continuously (Purdom, 1980).

Outside, people are exposed to particles from insects, animal and human excretion, odors, gases from marshes, and dust from fields and streets. During spring and summer, pollen adds to the burden of particles to be inhaled, while spores, constitutents of decaying plants and animals, bacteria, and viruses permeate the air throughout the year. The terrain affects air pollution. For example, fumes are more easily concentrated in one area in hilly sites, particularly when people settle in a valley.

Five main classes of human-generated air pollution are: (1) carbon monoxide, a significant element in motor vehicle exhaust; (2) sulfur oxides, produced mostly by the combustion of coal, fuel oil, and natural gas; (3) hydrocarbons, a family of compounds containing carbon and hydrogen; (4) nitrogen oxides, mainly emitted by power plants and in transportation vehicle exhausts; and (5) particulate matter such a dust, soot, or ash.

At present, limited information is available concerning the possible health effects of many chemical compounds. The immediate cause for concern arises from the number of chemical compounds available, their versatile use, and the adverse effects associated with some chemicals (see Table 13-1).

The chemical industry is the major source of hazardous wastes. Since 1958 the 53 largest chemical manufacturers have disposed of over 750 million tons of unwanted by-products. Industry, transportation, and agriculture are also major contributors of hazardous chemical wastes. Many chemicals in liquid waste effluents make their way to water supplies, industrial and transportation vehicle exhausts permeate the air, pesticides are often found concentrated in humans and animals, with many containing high levels of residues from agricultural pesticides.

Air pollution emissions from transportation vehicles are the pollutants from the burning of fuel for automo-

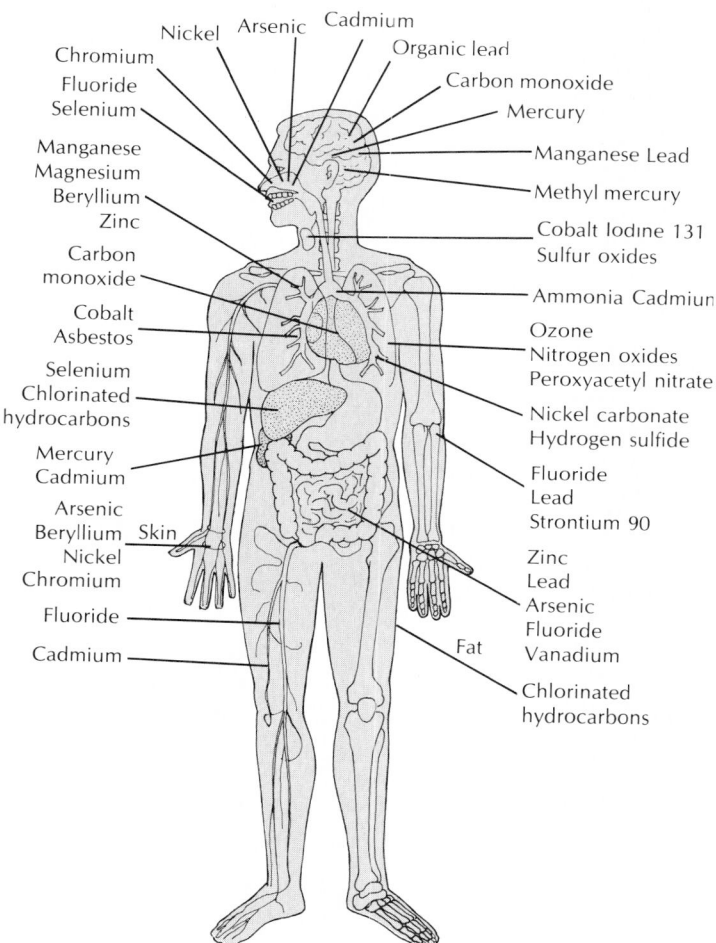

Fig. 13-1. Main targets of major air pollutants. (From Waldbott, G. L.: Health effects of environmental pollutants, ed. 2, St. Louis, 1978, The C. V. Mosby Co.)

Table 13-1. Examples of specific effects of pollutants

Groups	Agent	Principal affected organs
Respiratory pollutants		
Pulmonary irritants	Sulfur oxides	Lining of the respiratory tract
	Nitrogen oxides	
	Ozone	
	Chlorine	
	Ammonia	
Dusts	Quartz	Pulmonary interstitial tissue
	Silica	
	Carbon	
	Asbestos	
	Cobalt	
	Iron oxides	
Granuloma-producing agents	Beryllium	Lungs
Fever-causing agents	Zinc	Alveoli
	Manganese	
	Hemp, cotton	
Asphyxiating pollutants	Carbon monoxide	Hemoglobin
	Hydrogen sulfide	Respiratory center
Systemic pollutants	Lead	Nerve tissue
	Mercury	Brain, bowels
	Fluoride	Bones, teeth
	Cadmium	Blood vessels, kidneys
	Chlorinated hydrocarbons	Fat tissue, liver
	Organophosphates	Nerve-muscle synapsis
Host-specific agents		
Allergenics	Thiocyanate	Respiratory tract
	Formaldehyde	Skin, lungs
Carcinogenics	Strontium 90	Bones
	Iodine 121	Thyroid
	Nickel carbonate	Lungs, sinuses
	Chromium	Nose
	Asbestos	Pleura
	Selenium	Testicular tissue
	Arsenic	Skin
Mutagens	Most systemic pollutants; organic mercury, lead, chlorinated hydrocarbons, arsenic, fluoride, cadmium	

From Waldbott, G.L.: Health effects of environmental pollutants, ed. 2, St. Louis, 1978, The C.V. Mosby Co.

biles, trucks, buses, ships, railroads, and airplanes. Such emissions are 25 times greater in cities than in rural areas. Exhausts from transportation vehicles produce about 60% of the total air pollutants and as much as 90% in certain urban areas. These emissions result from the burning of gasoline as well as diesel fuel, distillates, and residual oils.

Emissions from transportation vehicles may be calculated from the total gallons of fuel consumed for each source. Standard emission factors and fuel consumption data are used to obtain the weight of pollutants discharged. Standard emission factors are determined from a statistically valued sample and are established by the Department of Health and Human Services. Adjustments are calculated and are made to account for pollution-reduction devices.

Burning of coal, gas, and oil constitutes the principal source of sulfur oxides and nitrogen oxide. Coal is burned in power plants, in many industrial processes, as well as for domestic and commercial heating purposes. Coal, oil, and gas are used for space heating and gas and oil for heating of water; gas is used for cooking. Public utilities are a major source of sulfur oxide, nitrogen oxides, and particulate matter.

Industrial processes produce 56% of particulates. Certain kinds of industry produce more particulates than others. These types of industry include power plants that emit carbon, silica, aluminum, and iron oxide; the construction industry, which emits various kinds of dust; cotton ginning industry, a major source of trash, dust, and lint; and the feed and grain industry, a source of dirt (silicates), grain dust, and chaff.

Just as with the detection of potential health problems resulting from food sources, community health nurses often assess the presence of air pollution. Frequently the community health nurse is the one individual who recognizes the total type and amount of pollution with which clients come in contact. For example, a person working in an industry that emits noxious fumes and living in an area polluted by a different type of substance is particularly at risk for developing a pollution-related health problem. Also, nurses have many opportunities to assess the hazards of air pollution in the home and instruct families in proper ventilation, cleaning techniques, and use of pollutants.

Physical Hazards

Physical hazards can cause death, disease, or disability (Purdom, 1980). Historically, the effects of earthquakes, volcanic eruptions, floods, and tidal waves have been dramatic. In recent years, synthetic physical hazards have joined the ranks of naturally occurring hazards. Among the more widespread physical hazards are radiation, noise, solid waste, insects and rodents, and accidents.

Radiation

People have been exposed to radiation from the sun and minerals since the origin of our species. The extent and effect of *natural radiation* are unknown. However, currently, natural radiation accounts for about 55% of the total radiation for the average American. Of the natural sources, cosmic radiation emanates from the sun and other parts of earth and consists of many types of particulate and electromagnetic radiation. It increases during solar flares and is greatest at high altitudes. Cosmic radiation accounts for about 30 millirem (0.03 rem) per year (Silberstein and Silberstein, 1981).

Natural radiation also comes from the soil and certain rocks. Although radioactivity is low in most sedentary rocks, it is high in volcanic rocks. Some natural materials release small amounts of radiation. Living in a brick or stone house adds about 30 millirems of exposure annually compared to living in a wooden house (Silberstein and Silberstein, 1981). "One millirem is one one-thousandth of a rem; rem stands for 'roentgen equivalent man' and reflects the amount of radiation absorbed in human tissues" (Wilner et al., 1978, p. 255). The radioactivity in residential dwellings depends on the composition of the dwelling as well as local geological formation.

A third source of natural radiation comes from normal body potassium. A radioisotope known as potassium 40 constitutes about 0.01% of the potassium in the body. People receive between 15 and 20 millirems per year from potassium 40 and about 0.7 from carbon 14, which is formed within the atmosphere by the action of cosmic radiation and then incorporates in body tissues.

An additional natural form of radiation involves the possible loss of protection from ultraviolet rays of the sun. Released gases may be destroying the stratospheric protective layer of ozone, thereby permitting more of the sun's ultraviolet radiation to reach earth. An increased dose of ultraviolet radiation is linked to skin cancer in light-skinned people. The hazardous gases are fluorocarbons known by the trademark Freon. This gas is often used in spray can repellants and in refrigerators, freezers, and air conditioners. Fluorocarbons are highly stable, and instead of breaking down over time, they accumulate and move upward into the stratosphere, interrupting the ozone layer (Wilner et al., 1978).

Radioactive minerals also present serious hazards for miners. According to Hanlon and Pickett (1979) a group of 907 uranium miners with 3 years of underground experience has 17.8 times the normal death rate for heart disease, 5 times the rate for respiratory cancer, and 4.5 times the rate for nonautomotive accidents.

Uses of *synthetic radiation* include x-rays and radioisotopes in clinical diagnosis and treatment; radioisotopes in industry for measuring, testing, and processing; electric power generation; lasers in science, industry, and medicine; and electronic devices at home (Wilner et al., 1978). At present, between one third and one half of all critical medical decisions are based on radiology (Hanlon and Pickett, 1979). Medical uses account for about 94% of all exposure to synthetic sources of radiation, or about 40% of the total radiation exposure for a person (Wilner et al., 1978). Numerous devices serve to decrease the amount of radiation in medicine. The size of the x-ray beam has been reduced to limit exposure to only the required areas. Lead-containing aprons shield the gonadal region, and a variety of techniques are used to filter the beam.

The effects of radiation depend on the dose, type of radiation, and the sensitivity of various organs to the particular radiation. Some side effects of high levels of radiation are disruption of bone marrow, ulcers of the skin, diminished kidney function, pumonary edema, and a diminished concentration of red and white blood cells and platelets. Other side effects have been linked to genetic damage to cells, causing mutations that may be passed on to subsequent generations. Unborn fetuses are at risk from radiation exposure. Irradiation of the mother immediately before conception or at the time of conception results in a high incidence of prenatal deaths. Nurses must caution clients about the possible effects of radiation and instruct them to inform all other health care providers treating them if they have undergone radiography.

The interest in nuclear energy as a source to generate

electric power has increased because of declining oil reserves. The dilemma that arises in nuclear power production is how to dispose of the reactor wastes. Waste is produced as a result of activation of extraneous products found in coolants and as a result of nuclear fission.

The most outstanding potential source of radioactive pollution is the testing of nuclear weapons. The product of instantaneous and delayed fallout may be carried around the world several times with a number of years required before the bulk of the radioactive material is deposited on the ground. A community's proximity to a source of fissionable material such as a nuclear reactor or its importance as a military target should be known to community health nurses. A nuclear reactor accident could leave an area larger than Louisville, Kentucky, uninhabitable for a year. Unprepared citizens exposed to radioactive fallout may die or develop radiation sickness or cancer years after exposure.

A 1-megaton nuclear warhead exploding with the force of one million tons of TNT could kill from a few hundred to several million people, depending on the target's population density. Fallout radiation would leave 8,000 square miles unfit for human habitation for at least a year (Fetter, 1981).

A growing industry is based on the production and use of artificial radionuclides and compounds in research establishments and in hospitals. Through injection of radioisotopes into the body, organs have been scanned to determine the presence or absence of certain diseases. Industry, biology, and agriculture make use of radioisotopes as tracers. These procedures become hazardous to the environment as radioactive materials are discharged with the sewage into the waterways, thus affecting aquatic life and humans through drinking water and the food chain.

A relatively new potential source of environmental pollution is the use of nuclear energy as a power source for rocket propulsion and satellites. The hazard in this use of nuclear energy stems from the possibility of a satellite failing to go into orbit at the point of launching. At this point, isotopic power devices have the potential to liberate radioactive substances into the atmosphere.

Noise

Noise is defined as any unwanted sound within the environment. Noise pollution is concentrated in cities, with urban areas becoming steadily noisier. The sources of noise include construction activity, aerospace vehicles, diesel trucks, power mowers, radio and television sets, and people. Noise is particularly difficult to deal with because it is highly subjective.

Noise is a health hazard according to its level, frequency, and length of exposure. Depending on these three factors, noise reaction falls into the categories of annoyance, disruption of activity, loss of hearing, and physical or mental deterioration (Hanlon and Pickett, 1979).

The magnitude or level of noise is measured in decibels (dB). One dB represents the weakest sound level audible to the healthy human ear. The dynamic range of the ear or the difference between the loudest and the faintest sound is about 12 dB (Bruce, 1981). Generally, the danger level for hearing loss for most people is about 80 dB, and the current standard for workplace exposure is 90 dB averaged over 8 hours. The Environmental Protection Agency (EPA) defines 75 dBs as a long-range goal for workplace exposure (UAW Sound Security Department, 1979). The dB scale is based on powers of 10. Each increase in 10 dB is equivalent to multiplying the intensity by 10; in other words, 30 dB is 10 times as intense as 20 dB and 40 dB is 10 times as intense as 30 dB.*

Noise can affect a person's psychological and physical well-being. Communication is disrupted by increasing noise, particularly in industries where people must shout to communicate. The quality of work is diminished in the presence of noise. Physiological responses to noise include vasoconstriction of the peripheral blood vessels, slow and deep breathing, skeletal muscle tension, and galvanic skin responses. People exposed to loud noises of long duration have an increase in urinary output, an increase in urinary catecholamines, and an increase in blood pressure.

Various forms of wildlife are also effected by noise pollution. Generally animals adapt to a predictable, regular noise or to continuous noise. A grizzly bear will run when disturbed by the noise level of 81 dB. When sound reaches a level of 165 dB, it can kill small animals; the energy of the sound wave is converted to heat within the animal's body (Wilner et al., 1978).

An individual's length of exposure to noise is largely determined by socioeconomic status, life style, and occupation. Essentially how people spend time determines their exposure to noise. How people react to noise is largely determined by their perception of the noise. Some people are more sensitive to noise than others. Several specific ways in which noises either annoy or disrupt health are described in the following section.

Noise as an Annoyance. Annoyance is the most widespread reaction to noise. The noise level, frequency, and length of exposure influence how annoying a noise is. A major characteristic of environmental noise is unpredictability; noise often startles people,

---

*Sound frequencies are measured in hertz (Hz), or units of frequency representing cycles per second. The audible range of frequencies for the human ear is between 16,000 and 20,000 Hz.

disrupting their physiological and psychological stability. An annoying noise can aggravate existing physical disorders, disrupt sleep, lower the body's resistance to disease or physical stress, interrupt concentration, and generally disturb feelings of well-being. As noted, noise interferes with communication because people instinctively speak louder when the noise level increases (Bruce, 1981). Noise from machinery can interfere with instructions or the hearing of safety signals. Workers continuously exposed to high-intensity noises show an increased incidence of nervous complaints, nausea, headaches, instability, argumentativeness, sexual impotence, mood changes, and anxiety (Cohen, 1981).

The greatest physiological effect of noise is temporary or permanent hearing loss. Temporary impairment, or auditory fatigue, occurs after a short exposure to an intense noise. Exposure to a continuous high sound level with no recovery time between exposures can cause permanent hearing damage (Hanlon and Pickett, 1979).

In 1972 Congress passed the Noise Control Act, which is based on the following premises: uncontrolled noise can pose health hazards; major sources of noise are construction and transportation equipment, motors, engines or electrical equipment; and primary responsibility for noise control remains with state and local governments, although on occasion federal intervention may be required. The act includes provisions for the identification of major sources of noise, the establishment of noise emission standards, and for individuals to institute civil action in their own behalf against any person or governmental agency violating the noise Control Act (Wilner et al., 1978, p. 261).

Methods of Noise Control. The Noise Control Act provides one method of regulation to monitor and reduce noise. Bruce (1981) proposed the source-path-receiver concept of noise control. For example, the source may be a machine, the highway, neighborhood children, or pets. The receiver is the recipient of the unwanted sound, and the path is the route the noise takes between the source and the receiver. Control of the source includes use of quieter equipment, relocation of source, or better maintenance of equipment.

Interference in the path can take the form of a barrier such as trees between houses and a highway or an enclosure such as a shed for noisy equipment. Wrapping or muffling the sound, acoustical absorption materials, surface damping, or application of a coating to lightweight panels can reduce noise radiations.

Receiver controls include such tactics as use of earplugs or relocation of the receiver. Each form of control should fit the situation and the people involved. Nurses can assess noise sources and help clients plan suitable methods of interruption of noise pollution.

Waste Disposal

Solid Wastes. Of the 4.3 billion tons of solid wastes produced annually, an estimated 360 million tons come from household, municipal, and industrial sources; 2.3 billion tons are agricultural wastes; and 1.7 billion tons are mineral wastes (Wilner et al., 1978). The traditional methods of disposing of these wastes included the open burning dump or the poorly designed smoking incinerator. Incinerators and dumps violated air pollution regulations and were breeding grounds for rats, flies, and other rodents. The most commonly used solid waste disposal methods today are sanitary landfills and incineration.

In sanitary landfills, waste is disposed of in canyons, swamps, and ravines and then compacted by heavy machinery and covered with earth before rodent infestation can occur. By filling the undesirable plot, the site can be integrated into the surrounding lands for public or private use.

Even though it is the best known method of waste disposal, landfilling is not without fault. When rainfall infiltrates the landfill surface or when the groundwater table saturates a part of the landfill, matter can be leached by the water moving through the system. As the water drains from the landfill, it carries debris or dissolvent matter with it. As a result, the possibility exists for contamination of underground waters and surface water supplies.

Unlike a sanitary landfill, incineration of solid wastes can be located on the premises of apartments, department stores, hospital and similar establishments. On-site incineration reduces the volume and weight of wastes, which must be removed for final disposal. Incinerators are used in hospitals for destruction of pathological waste because heat destroys most pathogens.

Incineration of solid wastes yields a high percentage of volume reduction; however, the total weight reduction achieved depends on the amount of glass, metal, and other noncombustible materials. The volume reduction is generally between 70% and 85% and the weight reduction is between 50% and 80%. It is this volume and weight reduction that gives incineration its appeal as a method of solid waste disposal. The hazards of incineration result from the environmental nuisances of noise, dust, and air pollution.

Disposal of wastes is both costly and difficult. Each of the methods just described have advantages and disadvantages. New methods of waste disposal are being tried. One method grinds waste and subjects it to jets of air to separate paper from metals and plastics. Iron and steel can be removed by magnets. In two other methods, once the material is ground, it is incinerated and produces a glasslike slag used in bottles, building materials, or highway aggregate. The second method suspends and centrifuges the ground waste into various components (Hanlon and Pickett, 1979).

Approximately two thirds of the cost of solid waste disposal comes form pickup and transfer to a collection site. Compactors can reduce cost by providing a smaller mass for collection. There are at least five reasons for more effective management of solid wastes (Chanlett, 1981):

1. Decrease pathogen transmission
2. Reduce discarded toxic and infectious materials
3. Increase esthetic effect of areas previously used for waste disposal
4. Recover materials and energy
5. Maintain costs

Solid waste provides fertile areas for pathogen transmission resulting from its attraction for flies and rodents. Mosquitoes breed on water accumulated in bottles, cans, and other containers in open dumps. Mosquitoes are associated with the transmission of yellow fever, dengue, or hemorrhagic fever.

Other wastes. Other wastes include toxic materials such as poisons, inflammables, infectious contaminants, explosives, and radionuclides (Chanlett, 1981). Hazardous materials make up about 10% of industrial waste output. Disposal of such wastes is difficult. Some can be neutralized, others burned, and still others buried or distilled. Although few cases of human injury are documented, the example of Love Canal has caused concern about the potential for disaster. A rising water level at Love Canal at Niagara Falls, New York, caused by excessive rainfall, brought chemical wastes to the water surface. The site was about a mile long, following an old canal previously used as a chemical dump. Later the area was filled and used for a school and 100 homes. Problems became apparent in 1978. Alleged health hazards included a high miscarriage rate, increased birth defects, children being burned on contact with the oozing liquid, and several cancer deaths. Tests demonstrated the presence of 82 chemicals, 11 of which are on the suspected carcinogenic list. The economic loss in depreciation of homes and the emotional loss from fear are quite high (Chanlett, 1981), but the actual human injury at Love Canal has yet to be established.

Nuclear shipments are an area of concern because of the risks posed from transporting the wastes from power plants to disposal sites. People opposed to transporting the wastes cite leaky casks or the possibility of a truck accident. To date there have not been any accidents, but some near accidents have occurred. If an accident occurred in New York City and just 1% of leaking radiation found its way into the city, the predicted results would be 1300 deaths immediately or within days or weeks, followed by 170,000 delayed cancer

deaths (Holzer, 1982). Currently New York City is leading the nation's opposition to ban nuclear shipments.

Methods of Waste Disposal. The esthetic offenses of irresponsible waste discard must be emphasized. Dumping of refuse along streets and on vacant land is a tribute to the lack of value some Americans place on the cleanliness and beauty of their homeland. Many counties have effectively dealt with unsightly dumping by installing the "green box." The green box is a large metal box with a capacity of 4 to 12 cubic yards and is placed at road intersections near service stations and grocery stores (Chanlett, 1981). Conveniently located, these boxes serve residents and travelers alike. The contents are collected regularly and transported to a sanitary landfill. This disposal method has reduced open dumping by 70% to 75% in southeastern United States.

In recent years it has become increasingly apparent that natural resources, if used at the present rates, will not sustain the same quality of life for an indefinite period. Recycling is thriving, and 25% of the 200 million tons of major metals, rubber, glass, and textiles processed annually are recycled materials. Copper, stainless steel, nickel, aluminum, lead, steel, and zinc are particularly valued. Currently the federal government supports several recycling efforts, and both states and private enterprise are active participants in this process. As an example, private efforts have established 1300 recycling centers that process 1 million of the 4 million cans produced annually. Recycling these cans saves $300 per ton, since the electricity required to reprocess the cans is only 5% of that needed to refine bauxite ore.

Solid wastes as sources of energy yield mixed reviews. The best method equips incinerators with heat recovery equipment to generate steam that can heat or produce electricity.

As mentioned, the largest costs associated with waste disposal come from collection. The cost for public or private disposal efforts runs about $25 per person per ton of solid waste a year (Chanlett, 1981). Management skills are being applied to the business of solid waste collection, since costs for the United States approach $4 billion annually. Collection routes, hauling times, and methods of containing waste (bag or can) are being evaluated to improve cost effectiveness.

Essentially, two choices exist for the disposal of waste; "burn it" or "bury it." Both methods are currently in use; however, the latter will become more difficult as population increases and less land is available for waste disposal purposes.

An increasingly popular goal is "transform it" and this includes composting. However, in the United States composting has been less successful than in other countries. Basically, composting is an aerobic process whereby bacteria, especially fungi, feed on organic material. A carbon/nitrogen ratio of 30:1 is needed to provide the nitrogen for forming new protoplasm. If the pile is stirred regularly to renew its oxygen supply, it becomes an excellent soil conditioner, but it is not a complete source of fertilizer, since compost is low in phosphorous and potassium. Composting has been effective in many countries including Switzerland, Japan, Thailand, South Africa, Israel, West Germany, The Netherlands, England, Scotland, France, and Mexico (Chanlett, 1981).

The future will witness new methods of solid waste disposal. Poor burial sites of the past have later posed far-reaching dangers. Sites used in the past are yet to be identified. Subsequently, in later years homes, schools, industry, and recreational areas were built on these sites. It is not known how the contents of solid waste affect people. It can be anticipated that refillable bottles will be used more extensively, new packaging efforts will reduce the volume of discardable paper and plastics, and more materials will be repaired rather than discarded.

Vector Control

Insect and rodent control is commonly referred to as *vector control* because of the disease transmission potential. "The rodent is the host for the flea, which is the vector, or carrier, of plague and endemic typhus; anopheles mosquitoes transmit malaria" (Wilner et al., 1978, p. 264).* Vector control is most effectively carried out by modifying and regulating the environment to reduce or prevent propagation. Vectors of community health concern are rodents and arthropods. Among rodent vectors, rats, ground squirrels, and prairie dogs are most important, since they spread the plague. Of the arthropods certain mosquitoes, flies, fleas, roaches, lice, mites, and ticks are important sources of disease. In the United States insects exact a far greater toll on health and life than anything else (Hanlon and Pickett, 1979).

Vector control has become a reality in recent decades, since the life cycles of many organisms have become known. However, control requires the cooperation of many groups, organizations, and the public. Buildings must be constructed to keep rodents from entering, kept in good repair, and maintained free of food wastes. Pest control measures must be carefully carried out so that unsuspecting people and animals are safe. Nurses must consistently assess for the presence of vectors as they make home visits and see clients in clinics,

schools, work sites, and other community health settings. Once the presence of vectors are noted, nurses can provide relief measures through education of clients or referral to agencies that might provide vector control services.

Trapping is often used in rodent control, although it is a slow and difficult process. Poisons, while effective for rodents, do pose new hazards for people, especially children. One material, red squill, kills rodents because they cannot regurgitate but only acts as an enteric for humans, poultry, and other animals (Wilner et al., 1978). The problem of rodent control is complex, since an estimated 14,000 people are bitten by rats annually. In the United States, plague-infected wild rodents have spread eastward from the West Coast at a rapid rate. The ecological distribution of plague is not clearly understood. However, murine typhus is endemic in several southeastern and some western states where rats and mice infest households. Many health departments are launching programs to tackle the rodent problem but challenges still exist.

Since *mosquito* "eggs hatch and the larvae and pupae develop only in quiet water and under certain conditions, mosquito control is most effectively accomplished by eliminating or modifying these waters" (Wilner et al., 1978, p. 265). Each species prefers one type of water. Anopheles mosquitoes prefer clean, shallow water, whereas *Aedes aegypti,* which transmits yellow fever and dengue, prefers water near people, including rainwater. *Culex tarsalie,* the vector for encephalitis, breeds in a variety of nonsalty waters such as surplus irrigation waters. *Aedes,* a vicious daytime biting mosquito, prefers salt marshy areas, whereas *Culex fatigans,* the cause of urban filariasis, prefers water heavily contaminated with human wastes (Wilner et al., 1978).

Mosquito control includes draining and filling marshes and low areas, stocking larvae-eating fish, varying water level to cause larvae and pupae to be exposed to waves and currents, spraying, improving irrigation practices, providing better drainage systems, and conducting public education on control methods.

Accidents

Annually 75 million Americans are injured severely enough to need medical attention or restriction of their activity (Healthy People, 1979). In 1978 in the United States the age-adjusted death rate for all accidents was 44.3 per 100,000 population. Motor vehicle accidents accounted for 23.4 per 100,000, suicides 12.0 per 100,000, and homicides 9.6 per 100,000 (Health: United States, 1981). Table 13-2 further displays the rates for and sources of accidents to demonstrate male/female and black/white variations. In addition, Table 15-2 shows death rates by age group from 1950 to 1978 for

---

*A vector is an agent that actively carries a germ to a susceptible host. Vectors are considered animate vehicles for the transmission of pathogenic organisms and include birds, beasts, bugs, or people.

Table 13-2. Age-adjusted death rates for accidents

Race, sex, and cause of death	Year				
	1950	1960	1970	1975	1978
All persons					
All causes	841.5*	760.9	714.3	638.3	606.1
All accidents	57.5	49.9	53.7	44.8	44.3
Motor vehicle accidents	23.3	26.5	27.4	21.3	23.4
White male					
All causes	963.1	917.7	893.4	812.7	773.1
All accidents	80.9	70.5	76.2	64.8	64.5
Motor vehicle accidents	35.9	34.0	40.1	31.7	35.2
White female					
All causes	645.0	555.0	501.7	445.3	425.5
All accidents	30.6	25.5	27.2	22.4	22.9
Motor vehicle accidents	10.6	11.1	14.4	10.9	12.6
Black male					
All causes	1373.1	1246.1	1318.6	1174.3	1113.1
All accidents	105.7	100.0	119.5	92.4	84.0
Motor vehicle accidents	39.8	38.2	50.1	35.8	35.0
Black female					
All causes	1106.7	916.9	814.4	688.4	650.5
All accidents	38.5	35.9	35.3	27.6	26.1
Motor vehicle accidents	10.3	12.7	13.8	9.4	9.8
All accidents					

From Health: United States, 1981, Pub. NO. 82-1232, Hyattsville, Md., 1981, Department of Health and Human Services.

*Deaths are calculated per 100,000 resident population.

motor vehicle accidents. These figures indicate that accidents pose a major health problem. Community health nurses are involved in prevention and rehabilitation of injuries sustained in these accidents.

Accidents can occur at any time and in any setting; most result from carelessness or ignorance and could have been prevented (Jarvis, 1981). The focus of nurses in community health must be on reinforcement of safe living, working, and recreational settings. To do so requires careful environmental assessment. Chapter 17 provides guidelines for completing an assessment of the entire community. However, a later section of this chapter provides a discussion of ways to assess the quality of the environment.

Motor vehicle crashes account for almost half of all deaths from unintentional injuries. Nonfatal injuries among men often occur at work, and for women the home presents a high-risk environment. Some occupations such as construction work, farming, firefighting and mining are especially high in risk.

Age. For all injuries combined, population-based death rates are highest for the elderly: 164 per 100,000

people aged 75 to 84 compared to 86 per 100,000 for people aged 15 to 24. (All statistics in this section come from Healthy People, 1979, pp. 55-71.)

It is often difficult to assess the full scope of the problem of accidents, since many are not reported. However, several statistics are provided to emphasize the scope of the problem. Certain population groups are at greater risk because of either greater exposure to hazards, decreased ability to avoid hazards, decreased resistance to injury, or less likelihood of survival once injured (Healthy People, 1979).

Fig. 13-2 shows the injury death rate by age per 100,000 population of the United States. In children under five, falls constitute the leading cause of nonfatal injuries, but the largest number of fatalities involve automobiles, drownings, and fires. Table 13-3 presents the leading categories of unintentional injury deaths. Teenagers and young adults because of their activities and behavior are exposed to more high-risk activities than other groups. Contact sports, motorcycling, high-speed driving, and the use of firearms increase the accident potential for this age group. In the 15- to 24-year-

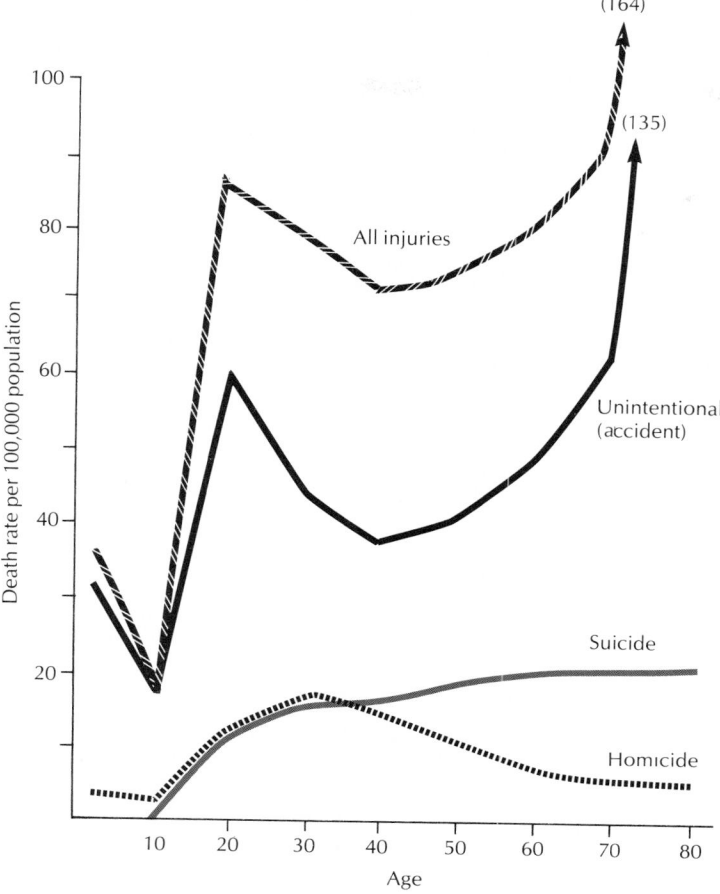

Fig. 13-2. Injury death rates by age per 100,000 population in the United States. (From Healthy people: the Surgeon General's report on health promotion and disease prevention, background papers, Pub. No. 79-55071A, Hyattsville, Md., 1979, Department of Health, Education, and Welfare.)

old group, about three fourths of all deaths result from injuries: 24,000 accidental 5,000 homicidal, and 4,800 suicidal.

The high death rates of the elderly reflect their poor clinical experience and their susceptibility to complications following injury. Although comprising only one tenth of the population, people over 65 suffer one fifth of all injury deaths. They are especially susceptible to falls and burns.

Sex. Men are twice as likely as women to suffer a fatal injury, and they have a 50% greater likelihood of a nonfatal injury associated with transportation, recreation, work, and assaults. Following menopause, women become more susceptible to injury because of the onset of osteoporosis (Healthy People, 1979).

Motor Vehicle Crashes. Roughly 1 death in 40 in the United States involves a motor vehicle. Factors affecting the risk of occupant death or injury from motor vehicle accidents include the amount of highway travel, road characteristics, speed, vehicle crashworthiness, and restraint use. Better designed and repaired roads are reflected in lower accidents. Specific factors to consider in assessment of road quality include illumination, the presence or quality of structures separating opposing lanes of traffic, signs, and range of visibility.

High speeds increase the risk of motor vehicle accidents. The size of vehicles also influences the likelihood of death or injury. Small cars have more crashes per mile and injuries per crash than larger cars. There are, however, many ways in which vehicles can be made safer, including energy-absorbing steering wheels, windshields and instrument panels that dissipate some of the energy by deforming when struck by a head or knee, padding of surfaces that project into the passenger compartment, restraint systems, and door locks. In the United States, although seat belts have been standard equipment in cars for more than a decade, only 20% of front seat occupants use them (Healthy People, 1979).

||| **Table 13-3.** Leading causes of accidental deaths by age groups

Under 5 years	15 to 24 years	Over 75 years	All ages*
Motor vehicle accidents	Motor vehicle accidents	Falls	Motor vehicle accidents
Fire, burns	Drowning	Motor vehicle accidents	Falls
Drowning	Firearms	Pedestrian accidents	Pedestrian accidents
Pedestrian accidents	Pedestrian accidents	Fire, burns	Drowning
Falls	Poisoning	Poisoning	Fire, burns
Poisoning	Fire, burns	Drowning	Poisoning

From Healthy People: The Surgeon General's report on health promotion and disease prevention, background papers, Pub. No. 79-55071A, Hyattsville, Md., 1979, Department of Health, Education, and Welfare.

*If homicides and suicides were included, firearms (which cause about 31,000 deaths annually) would be the second leading category for all ages combined.

Usage increases with educational level; however, many people fail to use them even though they know about their effectiveness.

Children are at special risk, since they may be unable to secure a restraint system and must rely on their parents or other caretaker to protect them. Only 7% of children wear seat belts or ride in adequate infant or car seats (Healthy People, 1979). Placing children in the back seat reduces the risk of injury but is still less effective than seat belts.

Other vehicular accidents involve motorcycles, mopeds, bicycles, and pedestrians. About 4000 motorcyclists and 1000 bicyclists were killed in 1977. The rapid increase in moped use indicates that they may pose an additional hazard to health. Injuries can be reduced in many of the same ways as with automobiles. However, helmets are particularly useful as a safety measure. Increased injuries followed the 1976 repeal of the mandatory helmet use regulation (Healthy People, 1979).

Accidents at Home, Work, and Play. The kitchen is the most frequent site of home accidents, whereas the bedroom is the most frequent site of fatal ones (Hanlon and Pickett, 1979). Females in lower-income groups have the highest female home accident rate, and males in high-income groups have the highest male accident rate.

As will be discussed in greater detail later in the chapter, the work site should be safe and free of hazards. Carelessness, such as spilling water or other liquids on the floor or improperly positioning extension cords and objects in walkways, poses accident hazards. Equipment needs to be in good repair, protected according to need, used properly, and equipped with appropriate safety devices. Stairs should have railings, and steps should have safety treads.

Many accidents occur in the recreational area when people play, relax, or engage in sports. Participants may overestimate their ability and become exhausted during a recreational activity. They may fail to observe safety rules, use faulty equipment, or use equipment for purposes for which it was not intended. Playgrounds should be free of glass, tin cans, and other debris (Jarvis, 1981).

Sports-related injuries total more than two million annually. Although injuries leading to permanent damage are uncommon, their severity does warrant mentioning. Permanent spinal cord injury results most frequently from gymnastics and football. The use of protective equipment should be encouraged. Water sports pose health hazards, with drowning being the largest cause of fatalities. Death rates because of drowning are highest for males and for people between the ages of 1 and 24. Community health nurses must actively assess the multiple environments in which they see clients to detect the presence of unsafe activities, equipment, and so forth. Active assessment should be followed by vigorous educational efforts and enforcement of safety regulation and laws.

Chemical Hazards

Chemical hazards, while by no means new, are increasing annually. In addition to chemicals occurring in nature, an estimated two million other chemicals are currently known. Of these 30,000 are synthetic; approximately 1000 new synthetic chemicals are introduced annually (Hanlon and Pickett, 1979). At present limited information is available concerning the possible health effects of many chemical compounds. One problem with chemicals is that they abound in the workplace, existing in the form of gases, dusts, mists, and vapors. Industrial gases affect the body directly or indirectly; some cause an acute effect, whereas others can be linked to chronic effects occurring from repeated low-level exposures. Nitrogen dioxide, sulfur dioxide, and hydrogen sulfide are extremely irritating to the eyes and upper respiratory tract. Cyanide presents itself in various forms in industry. One form, hydrogen cyanide, a side product from blast furnaces, coke ovens, and gas works interferes with the body's utilization of oxygen. Some mild symptoms of cyanide poisoning include headache, weakness, nausea, and vomiting. Higher doses result in cessation of breathing and death. Repeated insults from exposure to gases may result in chronic cough or bronchitis in mild cases. In more severe cases the result may be emphysema or pulmonary edema.

Dusts

Dusts, extremely common in the work place, involve many different kinds of substances. The lung disease associated with dusts is called *pneumoconiosis.* One problem with dusts results from the size of the particles. Some are so small (visible only by means of a microscope) that they can easily enter the nasal passages and remain in the lungs. The classic example of exposure to a certain type of dust particle that has been linked to cancer is exposure to asbestos. Asbestos, a fibrous mineral, has been used widely for insulation and fireproofing, in textiles, drywall compounds, cement, and thousands of other products. For years scientists knew that exposure to asbestos caused asbestosis, a severe and sometimes fatal scarring of the lungs, but it was not until the 1960s that asbestos was recognized as the cause of mesothelioma. This type of cancer is associated with the membranes that surround the lungs and line the abdominal cavity. Asbestos has also been linked with cancer of the larynx and the gastrointestinal tract. It is difficult to estimate the number of workers and consumers who have been exposed to asbestos. Recently in North Carolina asbestos was found in the insulation material in school buildings. Steve McQueen, the actor, died from mesothelioma.

In the past many employees working with asbestos brought the fibers home on their clothes, thus exposing their families. A worker exposed to asbestos for 1 day may develop cancer in later life as a result of the exposure. The asbestos entering the nasal passages remain deposited in the lungs. It is estimated that hundreds of thousands of asbestos workers will die as a result of exposure. This estimate does not include family members or consumers who have been exposed.

Other types of dusts affecting workers are coal, silica, and wood. Sandblasters and tunnel workers exposed to silica dust have contracted silicosis, which results in massive fibrosis of lung tissue with increased susceptibility to tuberculosis and infection. Silicosis is also associated with pulmonary hypertension and cor pulmonale.

Coal miners, exposed to coal dust, may develop large, solid, black lung masses as a result of black dust deposited in the lungs. This disease is referred to as simple pneumoconiosis, or more appropriately as "black lung." Carpenters, foresters, loggers, and pulp, paper mill, and plywood mill workers are among those exposed to wood dusts. Some of these workers are showing an abnormally high rate of cancer of the stomach, lymph, and blood-forming tissues.

Byssinosis, another type of lung disease, has been identified among workers in cotton mills. The disease is similar to nonoccupational bronchitis and has been confused with emphysema.

Organic Chemicals

Organic chemicals are substances containing carbon. Thousands are used in industrial processes as solvents, intermediates, and starting materials. Carbon tetrachloride, a common solvent, is used as a drying agent for spark plugs, a dry cleaning agent, a fire extinguishing agent, a fumigant, and an anthelminthic agent. Excessive exposure may result in depression of the central nervous system whereas acute exposure causes kidney damage. The vapors from perchlorothylene, another organic chemical, have toxic effects on the liver.

Exposure to various forms of ether may cause dermatitis, lung disease, eye irritation, or kidney or liver damage. For years, hospitals used ethyl ether as a general anesthetic. Most hospitals have discontinued using it, preferring other anesthetics, but women working in operating rooms where ethyl ether is still used have an increased risk of miscarriage, birth defects in their children, liver and kidney disease, and cancer.

Aromatic hydrocarbons such as benzene, toluene, xylene and northalone irritate the skin, eyes, and upper respiratory tract. Benzene, once the most commonly used solvent in the industry, has been linked to leukemia. Aldehydes and ketones, organic compounds containing carbon, are widely used in industry and chemical synthesis. Excessive exposure to ketones may result in coma, respiratory depression, or death in severe cases.

Naturally Occurring Chemicals

Many naturally occurring chemicals are hazardous to humans. For some of these, trace or small amounts are beneficial, whereas excesses or deficiencies cause health problems. For example, excesses or deficiencies of metals such as cadmium, selenium, chromium, lead, copper, zinc, and lithium may be related to major degenerative diseases such as heart disease, muscular dystrophy, diabetes, multiple sclerosis, cancer, mental illness, or congenital malformations (Hanlon and Pickett, 1979). Previously mentioned, asbestos has carcinogenic properties because of its composition of trace metals and chemical compounds such as benzpyrene. *Benzpyrene* is also found in tobacco smoke, and asbestos workers who smoke have up to 30 times greater risk of lung cancer than their nonsmoking counterparts. In addition, trace metals such as Ni, Cr, and Fe, are associated with certain types of asbestos fiber. Cancer may be activated by a reaction among benzpyrene compounds, an enzyme, and the particular trace metals (Hanlon and Pickett, 1979).

The trace element *cadmium* has been found in the kidneys of people dying from hypertensive complications. The chief sources of cadmium are foods grown in soils containing cadmium from fertilizers, beverages in containers coated with galvanized zinc, and vegetables, drinking water, coffee, and tea (Hanlon and Pickett, 1979).

Chromium is associated with cardiovascular disease, and *lead* has many harmful properties. In addition to numerous industrial uses, lead is found in the environment. Occupational safeguards have limited many of lead's harmful effects; however, tetraethyl lead used as an antiknock and power-increasing gasoline additive continues to present health problems. Not only does this compound pollute the environment, but it also is highly toxic when inhaled or absorbed through the skin, largely leading to cerebral or central nervous systems symptoms (Hanlon and Pickett, 1979).

Inorganic *nitrites* and *nitrates* contaminate drinking water and are especially dangerous for infants up to 6 weeks who have not yet developed certain metabolic enzymes. Infants also have a more readily reactive hemoglobin level and a small blood volume relative to fluid intake.

Molds

Another group of toxic chemicals, often classified as a biological hazard, includes fungi called *molds*. Mold deteriorates food fiber, induces plant disease, and can cause pulmonary and invasive diseases in people. Some food molds produce toxic metabolites known as mycotoxins. The oldest mycotoxin, ergot, infects cereal grasses, especially rye, and can cause serious epidemics. The last outbreak of ergotism was reported in 1951 in southern France. Many victims showed central nervous system symptoms such as hallucinations, depression, and self-destructive manias (Hanlon and Pickett, 1979).

Other mycotoxins include the aflatoxins, produced by mold on peanuts and other agricultural products. Even in low doses, aflatoxins can cause acute intoxication, liver damage, and cancer of the liver in animals. The entire effect on humans is not known. Reaction to chemicals depends on the toxicity and concentration of the chemical, individual susceptibility, and the duration of exposure. The effect is often related to the body weight of the person as well as the chemical's state (solid, liquid, gas) at the time of exposure.

Pulmonary Irritants

Some substances pass rapidly through the respiratory system whereas others remain in the lungs for extended periods of time. Prolonged or continuous exposure to certain gases, vapors, and fumes can lead to chronic inflammatory or neoplastic changes as well as lung fibrosis. Gases and vapors of low water but high fat solubility pass through the lung to the blood and are carried to organ sites for which they have affinity.

The principal respiratory diseases induced by pollutants are bronchiectasis, emphysema, pulmonary fibrosis, pulmonary edema, and partial collapse of lung tissue. Although the range and list of pulmonary irritants is endless, some are particularly common and exhibit diverse effects.

Sulfur oxide has been extensively researched; its presence serves as an indicator of pollution because it gives off bluish-white plumes and reduces visibility. This substance is generated by burning wood, coal, and petroleum products. The degree of irritation depends on the concentration in the atmosphere and the size of the particles (Waldbott, 1978). Sulfur oxide interacts with a variety of other pollutants. For example, January 22, 1970, in Detroit, salt was used to melt snow and ice on the streets. Droplets of sulfuric acid coalesced with the sodium chloride (salt) to form the highly irritating hydrochloric acid, leaving a residue of sodium sulfate (Kellogg, W.W., et al., 1972).

Nitrogen oxide (N_2O) comes primarily from automobile exhaust and almost all forms of combustion; it is a by-product of many industries and is used in making explosives. In high concentration nitrogen oxide reduces the oxygen-carrying capacity of blood by increasing the blood level of methemoglobin. In contrast, nitrogen dioxide is about four times as toxic as nitrogen oxide. Insoluble in water, nitrogen dioxide passes through the trachea and bronchi into the alveoli of the lungs where it forms nitrous and nitric acid. Both are highly irritating to the mucous lining of the lungs. Both short- and long-term exposure to nitrogen dioxide increases susceptibility to infection by decreasing the ability of the lungs to clear inhaled infectious organisms.

Acute nitrogen dioxide poisoning can occur in farmers filling silos. During the early weeks when a silo is being filled, nitrogen dioxide is generated from moldy silage. Similar incidents occur in power plants as people work with boilers and industrial gases. Symptoms of chronic poisoning range from slight irritation, burning and pain in the throat and chest, to violent coughing and shortness of breath. Nitrogen oxide reacts with alkali in lung tissue, causing edema. Nitrogen dioxide interacts with tobacco smoke, causing smokers to be at higher risk for developing health problems. This gas has poor warning qualities because it smells good.

Ozone (O₃) is an unstable colorless gas with an oxidizing power surpassed only by fluorine. Originally viewed as beneficial because it was believed to have bacterial action and to assist in the oxygenation of blood, ozone is now recognized as one of the most dangerous irritants to eyes, throats, and lungs (Waldbott, 1978). It is found in smog created by the interaction of hydrocarbons, nitrogen oxides, and sunlight. In the air it can be a threat to aviation personnel at altitudes over 30,000 feet (Werthamer et al., 1970).

Synthetic sources of ozone include high-voltage electrical equipment such as electrical insulators, x-ray and ultraviolet ray equipment, quartz lamps, and electrostatic air cleaners. Ozone is used as a commercial bleaching compound and sterilant. Ozone impairs the functioning of pulmonary macrophages by thickening the walls of small pulmonary arteries, resulting in chronic pulmonary disease, emphysema, and right heart failure (P'an, A.Y.S. et al., 1972). Because it depresses respiration and causes lung edema, ozone interferes with normal lung ventilation.

Chlorine, a common toxic gas, is frequently used in the chemical industry for preparation of organic and inorganic agents such as trichlorethylene, vinyl chloride plastics, pesticides, herbicides such as DDT, refrigerants and propellants such as Freons, detergents, and pharmaceuticals (Stahl, 1969). It is also used in the paper industry.

Acute epidemics have occurred repeatedly from accidents associated with the handling or emptying of liquid chlorine cylinders. In March, 1961, while supposedly empty chlorine cylinders were being handled, the main valve of one slipped off, causing 156 people to be immediately stricken. Some had lung hemorrhages; others experienced asthmalike wheezing and pneumonia-like lung infiltration for as long as 35 months (Kowitz et al., 1967). Other episodes of chlorine spillage have led to congestive heart failure, pulmonary edema, and pneumonia.

Only one other gas, *carbon monoxide,* will be discussed, although many more affect health. Carbon monoxide (CO), because it deprives the hemoglobin of its oxygen-carrying ability, is a common asphyxiant (Waldbott, 1978). It is a poisonous gas produced by incomplete combustion and is particularly dangerous since it cannot be seen, smelled, or tasted by potential victims. Carbon monoxide is considered the greatest single, nonindustrial hazard. It is responsible for half of all fatal poisoning in the United States; often the engine of a running car or an open, unlighted gas burner is used in suicide. Oceans are a major source of CO (Coburn, 1970), as are automobile exhausts, cigarette smoke, and gas and coal heating systems.

When CO replaces oxygen in the blood, the functioning of lungs, brain, and heart is impaired. Initial symptoms range from dizziness, headaches, nausea, and general fatigue to impairment of memory and loss of muscular control (Waldbott, 1978). It is a deceptive gas because of its poor warning characteristics and because people affected by it may appear drunk and act belligerent. Smokers are affected at lower concentrations, although less seriously.

Chemical Pesticides

Chemical pesticides vary considerably and include insecticides, fungicides, herbicides, rodenticides, arachnicides (spider killers, and nematocides (worm killers). Over the past 20 years the use of these chemical substances to destroy unwanted insect, animal, or vegetable life has increased tremendously. Spraying, dusting, baiting, drenching, dipping, and painting are used to eliminate pests. In an attempt to avoid one hazard to health, other hazards are often invited—air pollution, water pollution, and consumption of these chemicals through food products. Not all noxious material acts on the desired target. A portion of the applied chemical contaminates the air, water, soil, plant life, wildlife, and humans.

Pesticides remaining in the air are quickly diluted in large masses of air to what would appear to be harmless concentrations. The "harmless concentration" in air must be questioned, however, when concentrations of chemicals are found in migrating animals thousands of miles from its use. Pesticides settling on soil may be carried into larger bodies of water by runoff. Pesticides in water are concentrated in fish, which in turn are consumed by humans. Pesticides falling on plant surfaces may be consumed by animals or harvested with crops, or leaves may be carried away by wind or waters. In any event, the pesticide is eventually consumed by people either by consumption of the crop or of animals grazing on the crop.

Chlorinated hydrocarbons and organophosphorus compounds (Parathion) are the most dangerous environmental chemicals. The chlorinated hydrocarbons include DDT, benzene hexachloride, lindane, dieldrin, endrin, aldrin, chlordane, isodrin, toxophene, and similar compounds designed to kill insects. The second group of pesticides, the organophosphates, includes insecticides and herbicides such as parathion, malathion, azodrin, diazonion, TEPP, and phosdrin.

DDT, the most widely used and best known chlorinated hydrocarbon, is a matter for great environmental concern. Most uses of DDT have been barred since 1972 (Wilner et al., 1978). Three properties render DDT one of the most dangerous chemical pollutants: (1) it is extraordinarily stable with the half-life of the residues ranging up to 20 years (Woodwell et al., 1971); (2) its high solubility in fat and low solubility in water enable it to penetrate into animal food products; and (3) the high vapor pressure of DDT causes it to evaporate from soils and plants and to circulate widely in the atmosphere.

Unlike the chlorinated hydrocarbons, the organophosphates produce no chronic effects on the ecosystems. In fact, some organophosphates, such as malathion, which are extremely poisonous to insects, have relatively little effect on mammals. However, other organophosphates such as parathion, have caused serious illness among humans.

Pesticides can and do present a problem. In Florida, specifically Dade County, roughly 2 million pounds of pesticides are spread over that county each year. That averages out to be more than 1 pound of pesticide per person. Questions arise based on the fact that only three quarters of an ounce is needed to spray an entire acre for mosquito control. Migrant farmworkers are especially at risk and are frequently sprayed while working in fields. A large number of farm workers have not been adequately trained to work with pesticides. Problems have occurred because restricted-use pesticides have been applied by inexperienced applicators. The EPA requires that certain information be included on every pesticide label, including directions for use, first aid instructions, storage and disposal guidelines, and rules for general or restricted use. Ironically, many migrant workers are unable to read. Pesticide poisonings have resulted from workers entering fields recently sprayed or from pesticide drift. Working conditions in the fields are often intolerable. Because of the lack of toilets, washing facilities, and drinking water, migrant workers have a high rate of infectious diseases and kidney and bladder problems. Very few pesticide poisonings are reported.

The EPA is responsible under the Federal Insecticide, Fungicide, and Rodenticide Act (FIFRA) for protecting human health and the environment from unreasonable harm from pesticides. The agency has been accused of being extremely lax regarding its responsibility to protect workers. OSHA has recently developed standards for migrant farm workers.

Chemical Effects on Fetus

Another area of concern is the effect of a chemical on the unborn fetus. Environmental hazards enter the body through inhalation, skin contact, and ingestion. These three routes will be presented in more detail later in this chapter. Important questions can be raised regarding the potential health effect a toxic substance may have on the fetus. The primary way a chemical or other hazardous substance reaches the unborn child is through the placenta. Most chemicals or toxins cross the placental barrier and enter the circulatory system of the developing fetus. After these chemicals enter the expectant mother's body through one or more of the routes mentioned earlier, they eventually find their way into the mother's circulation and then into the child's. Some chemicals are rapidly transported across the placenta. The mother's liver will detoxify some substances, and the kidneys will excrete others. Because the tissues of the fetus are developing rapidly, they are more susceptible to adverse effects than are adult tissues.

The question pertaining to the potential health effects of toxic substances may be receiving an answer in the form of birth defects associated with the mother's exposure. For example, there is a possible correlation between dioxin and birth defects in Vietnamese children. To date, scientists cannot accurately predict exactly how much of a toxic substance will reach the fetus, or at what concentration the fetus can be exposed without resultant adverse effects.

Areas of Concern

The immediate cause for concern arises from the number of chemical compounds available, their widespread use, and the adverse effects associated with some. Exposure to low levels of these chemicals may produce or aggravate chronic disease. These chronic diseases are not associated with the workers' environment. Identifying the specific cause of a disease is sometimes difficult. Many workers change jobs frequently. They are exposed to various chemicals at different times. The onset of a chronic disease may not appear for several years, thereby making it difficult to determine the source. Other diseases may result from cumulative exposures.

Threshold limit values (TLVs) are the maximum concentration to which workers can be exposed for 8 hours a day without developing disease. Because they are based on average exposure, workers may conceivably be exposed to higher levels at certain times. Although TLVs have been established for many chemicals, it is virtually impossible for the government to establish TLVs for all chemicals because of the vast numbers of the chemicals in use. Problems arise because monitoring of TLVs is left up to industry. Often industries do not have the necessary monitoring equipment. OSHA has the broad responsibility for monitoring chemical exposure in the workplace, but because of understaffing, they cannot do the work that is necessary. The existing TLVs have been established without regard to individual susceptibility or the cumulative effects of chemicals.

The three primary routes of entry of environmental

hazards are inhalation, skin contact, and ingestion. The adult human being has a large gas-tissue interchange (90 square meters of total surface, 70 square meters of alveolar surface). This large surface combined with the blood capillary network (surface of 140 square meters) with its continuous blood flow allows for a rapid absorption of many substances from the air into the alveolar portion of the lungs and on into the blood stream. Chapter 12 in the discussion of communicable disease presents additional information on entry and modes of action.

Chemical Effects on Body Systems

The inhalation of pollutants affects not only the respiratory and cardiovascular systems and the brain, but the gastrointestinal tract, kidneys, and many other target organs are affected. Fig. 13-2 illustrates the health effects of several environmental pollutants on target organs. Table 13-1 presents examples of specific effects of several pollutants.

Hazardous substances affect people not only through inhalation but also through skin contact. A major purpose of the skin is to serve as a barrier against the entry of foreign substances; however, substances do penetrate the skin or react with substances on the skin surface to cause a primary irritation (dermatitis). The main routes of skin absorption are through epidermal cells, hair follicles, and sebaceous glands. Toxic substances are absorbed more rapidly when the person is sweating or wearing wet clothes as well as when the skin is abraded.

Ingestion of environmental hazards is easier to monitor and control than inhalation and skin contact. Toxicity by mouth is generally of a lower order than that by inhalation because of poor absorption into the blood stream, the high acidity as the substance goes through the stomach, as well as subjection to the alkaline medium of the pancreatic juice on passing through the small intestine. Exceptions to these characteristics are arsenic, cadmium, lead, and mercury (Waldbott, 1978).

Psychosocial Hazards

Sociological and psychological variables in the environment are more difficult to define than are biological, chemical, and physical hazards. However, any consideration of the environment must take into account psychosocial influences that are hazards. Many of these hazards are described in Chapters 18, 20, and 38, which deal respectively with community mental health, violence and human abuse, and the recognition and management of stress. So that redundancy will be avoided, this section is somewhat briefer than preceding ones, but this should not be interpreted as a minimization of the health hazards associated with the psychosocial components of the environment.

Dubos (1969) contends that mental characteristics are shaped by the environment, and genes only determine responses to stimuli. Environmental stimuli affect people from the time of conception. Survival depends on a variety of environmental stimuli, but often it is the amount and rapidity of stimuli that determine a person's ability to adapt. Although people can adapt to psychosocial stressors, they often experience stress that ultimately leads to disorders of the body or mind.

Noise, overcrowding, lack of privacy, lack of opportunity for social interaction, lack of space, boredom, excessive leisure, tedium, traffic, crowds, and feelings of estrangement from the mainstream of life can be psychosocial hazards.

Change constitutes a psychosocial hazard for nearly everyone. Both positive and negative changes require human energy for adaptation. Chapter 38 elaborates on change as a stressor. Change, inevitable for most people, is more tolerable if it occurs at a reasonable rate and does not conflict with previously held values or beliefs.

Many societal changes result in potential psychosocial hazards such as increasing mechanization and automation, mobility, and dehumanization of societal institutions. People must adapt to new jobs, new homes, and new social groups, often without assistance from friends, family, or social support networks. Other psychosocial stressors and potential health hazards come from changing female and ultimately family roles as described in Chapter 18.

The United States has increasingly becoming a country of many cultures. When people holding highly divergent beliefs and attitudes live in close proximity, the potential for stress and often conflict arises. Chapter 11 describes key social and cultural variables affecting community health nursing.

COMMUNITY HEALTH NURSING AND ENVIRONMENTAL AND OCCUPATIONAL HEALTH

Community health nurses must have an understanding of the biological, physical, chemical, and psychosocial hazards affecting both male and female workers, the general public, the elderly, and children as well as potential health effects on the unborn fetus. Community health nurses may be actively involved in the control of communicable diseases. Therefore nurses must be aware of the many factors that influence the spread of disease. Nurses who work in the community should be aware of the types of environmental hazards. They must also know where to locate sources of information identifying the specific effects a hazard may have on an individual or an entire community. Currently there are many occupational and environmental health resources available. These might include programs offered by universities, public health departments, medical centers, community health centers, or information obtained from federal agencies such as the EPA, OSHA, NIOSH, Centers for Disease Control (CDC), and the National Institutes of Health (NIH).

Voluntary agencies are excellent sources, because they are involved in health maintenance and disease prevention. The American Heart Association, the American Lung Association, the National Association for Mental Health, and the Arthritis Foundation are some of the voluntary agencies. These organizations have pamphlets that are excellent resource material both for the nurse and the consumer.

Newspapers are excellent resources. In some cities articles that discuss the effects of environmental degradation and deterioration appear daily or weekly. Some articles address current research, while others discuss the role of the federal government.

It is important that community health nurses understand the role others play in the workplace and in the community. In the work setting large companies employ part- or full-time physicians who are trained in occupational medicine. The physician is responsible for advising management concerning health conditions of the workers, health hazards that may exist in the plant, and safeguards to protect the health of workers. Occupational medicine is a relatively new subspecialty of medicine. A few years ago, only a small number of physicians were trained in this field, but advances have been made. Some medical schools now incorporate occupational medicine into their general curriculum.

On-the-job accidents or extreme exposures to toxic substances or physical hazards may produce acute effects that are easily recognized or identified. Low-level insults occurring over a long period of time are the culprits of chronic disease. People are exposed to these insults daily both at work and in the environment. Generally speaking, the person who visits a physician is not asked about work exposures to toxic substances, consequently the causal relationship between work and health may be overlooked. This is an area in which community health nurses should become more involved. Many small industries do not have the services of an occupational health specialist. Therefore, the nurse in the clinic or outpatient department may be the first person to come in contact with the worker. It is important that nurses take a complete work history to determine what the worker has been exposed to on the job.

The nurse should advise the worker to keep a written record of all job exposures to chemical, biological, and physical hazards. Such a record may assist in helping identify the specific cause or causes of a chronic disease.

The role of occupational health nurses has expanded considerably in recent years. The nurse is involved in planning, organizing, and developing occupational health programs, sometimes in conjunction with a full-time physician or in consultation with a physician. The nurse is responsible for record keeping, health assessment, health screening, and acute illness intervention. Many nurses are involved in the rehabilitation of the worker, in counseling and in health education.

Because of their close relationships with workers and since both management and labor view nurses as neutral, nurses are in a strong position to work toward promoting occupational health programs. Since World War II tremendous gains have been made in implementing occupational health programs in manufacturing, service, and commercial establishments. Industry is concerned with maintaining maximal levels of production and healthy workers are a key resource for meeting this goal. The industrial community needs the same careful assessment as would be provided for the general community, and nurses often carry out health assessments of industry as well as design and implement health programs.

The nature of health programs in industry varies from a one-nurse first aid station to a comprehensive, multidisciplinary health program for workers and their families. The health of workers is a vital public health concern since one third of a worker's day is generally spent on the job. Workers are entitled to a safe environment that promotes their physical and emotional health. Essentially, occupational health nursing is the blending of nursing and community health philosophy and skills to prevent disease and injury and promote optimal health, productivity, and social adjustment.

Occupational health nurses tend to have functions that fall into three general categories: administration, direct nursing care, and health education and promotion. Administratively they are responsible for establishing, maintaining, and evaluating a program for employee health. This includes maintenance of worker occupational health records, development and maintenance of an occupational health nursing manual, training of other health personnel, coordination of the occupational health team, cooperation with federal and state occupational health regulatory groups, and participation in educational programs of students.

Direct nursing care includes health assessment, screening, monitoring, counseling, and the provision of services when occupational injuries or injuries occur. Health assessment includes preemployment, periodic, and terminal evaluation of employees and includes many of the primary care skills described in Chapter 33. The nurse frequently screens for recognized health problems affecting workers, including hypertension, cardiovascular disease, or diabetes. Although most employees have another source of health care, the nurse can monitor their adaptation to chronic illness and can often provide guidance and assistance when such intervention is needed.

A major nursing activity is that of health education. As with all types of health education, the first step is assessment of environmental hazards and worker or occupational team member educational needs, which includes both employee and health team in-service programs on health and safety as well as one-to-one counseling of workers. The Occupational Safety and Health Act of 1970 requires that workers be told about any possible hazards in the workplace, and the nurse is often given this responsibility.

Health education includes both formal and informal teaching. During each encounter with a worker nurses can provide health education related to the worker's needs. For example, hypertensive employees often benefit from diet counseling, especially with regard to preparing foods with low salt content. Group as well as individual teaching is used to provide information needed to maximize employee health. Health education also includes interpreting health and welfare benefits to workers so they know what is available both through the employer and the community. The nurse can make appropriate referrals and procure a variety of services unavailable within the occupational health unit.

Employee health educational programs can include a wide range of topics. Possible topics might deal with alcoholism, cancer, obesity, exercise, nutrition, stress management, coping effectively with retirement, and so forth. Programs can also be developed around safety measures, avoidance of hazards in the workplace, and other topics specific to a work setting.

Another responsibility of the occupational health nurse is to act as a resource person with respect to the community. The nurse should have current knowledge pertaining to community health resources. Community health nurses working in clinics or public health departments should have an understanding of the occupational health nurse's role and strive to work together in complimentary ways. The community health nurse may be involved in the establishment of a disaster plan for a hospital, a plant, or a factory. The establishment of such a plan will require coordinated efforts.

The industrial hygienist is the professional who is most often identified with the recognition and control of toxic substances in the workplace. If the company does not have an industrial hygienist, the safety specialist may be charged with this responsibility in addition to establishing and maintaining a safety program. The nurse working in the clinic may be the first to detect a potential health problem stemming from the work setting. The community health nurse has the responsibility for notifying the industrial hygienist, the occupational nurse, the physician, or the safety specialist so the appropriate methods for identifying and controlling the toxic substance can be undertaken.

Community health nurses come in contact with many workers who do not benefit from the services of these occupational health specialists. Therefore, the nurse must be able to advise the worker on the recognition of health hazards. Workers should be advised that any abnormal eye irritation, especially on entering the workplace, may be a warning that exposures or TLVs are too high. Some chemicals produce mild eye irritations, whereas others can be more damaging. Therefore, early detection is important. If irritation occurs, the worker should report it to the appropriate authorities in the workplace as this may be an indication of a potential health hazard. Detecting an odor may indicate exposure to a dangerous chemical. many chemicals have a distinctive odor. Sulfur dioxide has a strong suffocating odor, hydrogen sulfide has a characteristic rotten egg odor, and chlorine has a distinct odor similar to that of household bleach.

An excess of dusts or fumes may indicate a nonexistent or a poorly functioning ventilation system. For noise exposure, the general rule is that if a worker must yell to be heard at a normal conversation distance, then the noise levels may be too high and permanent damage may result over a period of prolonged exposure. The other health effects resulting from noise have been discussed. Careful handling of chemicals and the proper handling of chemical spills are important in the workplace.

Recurring symptoms or prolonged illness may indicate a potential problem and workers should be advised to consult a physician. Since symptoms may occur gradually, workers sometimes assume that frequent headaches or a constant cough are nothing to be alarmed about; however, those symptoms may be the initial indicators of a chronic progressive disease, which if detected early, may be preventable.

For the most part, physicians and nurses are involved in the practice of curative medicine, the "hands on" healing practice. However, preventive medicine is gaining interest, and it has practical application with regard to environmental health. The mechanisms responsible for the degenerative disease process (for example, cancer, heart disease, and diabetes) remain somewhat obscure, but the causes of some environmentally induced diseases are relatively accessible.

The causes must be identified, and then approaches toward reducing the long-term effect can be instituted. Preventive measures may include identifying blood lead levels to determine a worker's exposure to lead, pulmonary function testing, audiometric testing, or periodic medical examinations. In some cities if the air becomes extremely polluted, an alarm will sound. This serves as a warning to children or the elderly with chronic respiratory problems that they should be extremely cautious. This is an example of a preventive environmental practice.

A key community health nursing role is assessment of the environment: home, school, recreational area, work site, or community as a whole. Community health nurses, especially those involved with home health care, must do a careful assessment of the safety of the home. Electrical cords should not be hidden under throw rugs. This is especially true in situations where elderly people might trip. Cleaning agents contain chemicals, and if not used and stored properly, these agents may be hazardous. Elderly people with poor eyesight are at risk. One example involved an elderly woman who mixed several cleaning agents, which lead to unconsciousness and severe respiratory irritation. Improper food storage in the home has resulted in many cases of food poisoning. Children who have ingested cleaning agents or plant fertilizers are regularly taken to emergency departments. For some, ingestion has been fatal.

Schools present many hazards. Accidents occur with regularity on playgrounds, gyms, grandstands, and bleachers. High schools have laboratories with chemicals that may result in burns to individuals or fires from explosions. Machinery in shops pose a threat. Poor lighting, littered floors, and narrow or broken stairs are other areas of concern. Improper playground equipment has caused numerous injuries to children.

A few selected chemical hazards of the work site have been discussed. Other hazards are machinery, equipment, undesirable working habits, such as poor lighting and poor ventilation systems. Many accidents occur because employees have not been adequately trained to operate machinery. Improper selection of employees is another hazard. Diabetics, epileptics, and people with hypotension, allergies, heart conditions, or respiratory problems such as asthma or chronic bronchitis should be carefully screened before job placement. Continuous monitoring after job placement should also take place. The manual handling of materials is found in almost every business and industry and is a leading source of serious injury resulting in need for worker's compensation. Environmental assessment is an ongoing process regardless of site. Accurate assessment can detect environmental risks before they become health hazards.

In assessing the environment, community health nurses should consider the degree of potential toxicity present or proposed through an introduction of some substance or activity and should determine whether a health hazard will be likely. From the perspective of physical, chemical, and biological hazards *toxicity* refers to the ability of a substance to cause injury to biological tissues. The *hazard* associated with the substance is the likelihood that it will cause injury in a given environment or situation.

Both recognition and interaction are important. The person who drove to work in heavy traffic or walked down a busy street is exposed to carbon monoxide. This exposure may be greater than carbon monoxide exposure in the workplace. The person who smokes a pack of cigarettes a day may be exposed to higher levels of carbon monoxide than those associated with the workplace. People who consume excess amounts of alcohol are more susceptible to the effects of carbon tetrachloride. Similarly, exposure to silica increases the susceptibility of tuberculosis. People with asthmatic conditions should not be placed in dusty work areas. Consequently, both an assessment of the individual and the environment is necessary.

Community health nurses must be aware of what hazards exist in the community. This information is gained by careful observation as the nurse travels through the community. Observations might include the presence and characteristics of trash collection sites, standing water, the quality of the air as determined by sight and smell, the level and type of noise, and the conditions of housing including their closeness to one another. The outline on p. 290-291 presents many areas for assessment.

Community health nurses use the nursing process to assess the quality and safety of the environment and to plan and implement interventions. Because other health and safety providers often have greater designated responsibility for environmental control, the nursing role in many areas includes assessment and reporting to the appropriate agency as well as being health educator and advocate or catalyst for environmental change.

Upon observing a potential or actual environmental hazard, nurses report them to the appropriate regulatory or intervening authority or citizen action groups. In some cities, the health department, county commission, housing authority, or other agency maintains responsibility for some aspect of environmental safety. It is important to know which local agencies handle specific environmental problems so quick and accurate referrals can be made. Frequently, citizen action groups are vital forces in instigating environmental change. The nurse alerts such groups to health hazards and works with them as they establish an intervention plan.

Another nursing action is education of environmental health and safety to school children, health providers, fire and police personnel, and the general public. These groups must be informed about environmental issues such as pollution, vehicular safety, product safety, and the presence or potential for additional physical, chemical, biological, and psychosocial hazards.

Nurses must often serve as catalysts to see that actions are taken. Often it is easy to persuade individuals and groups that an occupational or environmental health factor is potential. Interventions may be designed but may never get implemented. The nurse serves as a vital force to see that people follow through on the plans and commitments they make.

ROLE OF GOVERNMENT IN ENVIRONMENTAL HEALTH AND SAFETY

The decades of the 1960s and 70s, especially the last half of the latter 70s, will be known in environmental history as the Age of Realization. People finally recognized how badly they had fouled up their own nests with multiple forms of pollution. Enforcement actions started in 1899 with the Refuse Act (Banks, 1971). Over the years standards for control of emission of air pollutants were established and the Environmental Protection Agency (EPA) was created.

Early local governmental efforts dealt with services such as water supply, sewage collection and deposit, refuse collection and disposal, control of rodents and pests, and regulation of housing and recreation. Some of the earliest efforts at environmental control were performed by the official health departments in Philadelphia, New York, Baltimore, and Charleston. They directed activities toward community sanitation and the prevention of filth and oral disease. Often separate departments tended to specialize in specific entities such as food sanitation and housing sanitation. In some instances, the specialization was extreme, with food sanitation divided into milk, meat, and food divisions. The state health department and other statewide environmental health and safety agencies are responsible for ensuring that all people within the state receive comprehensive services. Few, if any, direct services are performed at the state level, and the pattern of organization among states varies.

The national level is primarily charged with establishing regulations. The initiative to clear up the environment began slowly in the 1960s with the passage of five pieces of environmental legislation dealing with air and water pollution (Sandhu, 1981). By 1981, 42 major federal legislative acts served to control the hazardous or toxic substances released into the environment.

The trend over many years has been to look carefully at the way people influence the environment and vice versa. In 1967, a task force was established by the Secretary of Health, Education, and Welfare to assure that all Americans could live in a healthy environment "by controlling pollution at its source, reducing hazards, converting waste to use, and improving the esthetic value of man's surroundings" (Hanlon and Pickett, 1979, p. 628). Since that time, the Task Force on Environmental Health and Related Problems has struggled for a coordinated environmental health protection system. The struggle bore fruit with the National Environmental Policy act of 1969, which declared a national environmental policy, established a Council on Environmental Quality and paved the way for the formation of the EPA in 1970. Creation of the EPA consolidated the federal environmental efforts into one agency and gave it far-reaching authority to control air and water pollution, including noise, radiation, and toxic substances (Sandhu, 1981). One of the highest priorities of the EPA is the identification and assessment of toxic substances.

Other agencies besides the EPA involved in controlling hazardous materials include the Food and Drug Administration (FDA), OSHA, NIOSH, the Consumer Product Safety Commission, and the Food Safety and Quality Service. In addition, the Toxic Substances Strategy Committee Group (1977) and the Regulatory Council (1978) promote and improve coordination of regulatory activities.

The focus of the government's role in toxic substances is to reduce exposure.

Legislative Acts

The federal government has been involved in environmental legislation since the 1800s. The first federal legislation to regulate pollution of waters was the Rivers and Harbors Act of 1899.

In 1960 the passage of five pieces of environmental legislation spurred the regulatory initiative to make the environment more livable. Early environmental legislation addressed air and water pollution. Later Congress looked at food additives. The FDA believed that food additives containing any carcinogenic hazard should be banned. The EPA has been responsible since 1970 for controlling and abating pollution in the areas of air, water, noise, pesticides, solid waste, toxic substances, and radiation. The agency has regulatory authority in all matters pertaining to air, water, noise, and pesticides under specific federal laws (Your Guide, 1980). The major legislative acts pertaining to these subjects have been summarized (see Table 13-4).

Water Quality Legislation

The EPA's current water regulation program is built on the federal Water Pollution Control Act Amendments of 1972, known as the Clean Water Act. As men-

Table 13-4. Selected examples of major environmental legislative acts involving the Environmental Protection Agency

Subject	Legislative act	Purpose
Air pollution	Air Quality Control Act, 1970; amended, 1977	The act grants EPA authority to establish national air quality standards to protect community health and welfare. The act also calls for states to examine air quality more closely and, if standards are not being met, to revise state plans.
Water quality	Water Pollution Control Act Amendments, 1972	The act imposes on EPA the task of restoring and maintaining the chemical, physical, and biological integrity of the nation's waters.
Water quality	Safe Drinking Water Act, 1974; amended, 1977	The act requires that EPA issue regulations that set national standards to protect drinking water.
Ocean dumping	Marine Protection Research and Sanctuaries Act, 1972	The act authorizes EPA to establish a dumping permit program and site for dumping. The Army Corps is authorized to control dredged material.
Noise	Noise Control Act, 1972; amended, 1978	The act calls for EPA to establish standards and promulgate regulations concerning major sources of noise. The act further requires EPA to conduct research into the effects and control of noise and to help states and local assistance programs.
Solid waste	Solid Waste Disposal Act, 1965; Resource Conservation and Recovery Act, 1976	The acts provide for the establishment of regulations and devise EPA programs to ensure safe disposal of wastes, i.e., toxic substances, pesticides, explosives. They also require states to look at existing waste disposal sites and develop plans.
Toxic substances	Toxic Substances Control Act, 1976	The act compels industry to develop adequate data on the effect of chemical substances on health and the environments and to regulate and ban substances when necessary.

tioned in Table 13-4, the basic purpose of the act is to restore and maintain chemical, physical, and biological integrity of waters (Your Guide, 1980). The act requires states to establish water quality standards for all significant bodies of surface waters. To achieve these goals, states must control sources of discharges of water pollutants. The major provisions of the act call for Municipal Pollution Control by allocating federal funds to be used for sewer rehabilitation, construction, or the modification of existing facilities. Other provisions call for limitations on the amount and types of effluent material released into the nation's waters. Any industry intending to discharge pollution must first secure a permit, and EPA has the responsibility for reviewing and approving state permit programs. The agency also monitors the quality of water, with special emphasis on temperature, microbiological content and oxygen supply.

In some instances the United States Army Corps of Engineers and EPA have a mutual interest in protecting the water. This protection applies to some marshes, bogs, and swamps. Any filling of wetlands or dumping of dredged materials requires a permit from the Army Corps of Engineers, which must first be approved by EPA.

The Safe Drinking Water Act was amended in 1977 so that EPA must issue regulations that set national standards to protect drinking water (Your Guide, 1980). These standards are necessary since organic and inorganic chemicals as well as pesticides still filter into our water supply.

Air Pollution Legislation

Federal air pollution programs seek to protect public health and welfare from harmful effects of air pollution (Your Guide, 1980). To achieve this goal, EPA issues two kinds of ambient air quality standards, or maximum acceptable levels of pollution for the outdoor air surrounding the general population. Primary ambient air quality standards deal with particulates, sulfur oxides, carbon monoxide, nitrogen oxides, ozone, and lead. Secondary standards protect plants, animals, and materials from harmful pollution.

EPA also sets nationwide emission standards for air pollution sources, such as emissions from motor vehicles. The automobile industry, as required by law, must work on controls to reduce emissions from automobiles. States must establish controls for attaining standards for vehicles already in use by mandatory inspection and maintenance programs. State and local governments are encouraged to upgrade public transportation systems. One means of reducing emissions is to reduce the use of private automobiles by making public transportation more desirable.

The agency sets source performance standards or emission standards with which industries and smaller plants must comply. Finally, EPA establishes national standards for hazardous air pollutants or toxic pollutants that endanger human health even in small amounts. These are currently in effect for asbestos, beryllium, mercury, and vinyl chloride. One of the most important provisions of the law gives EPA the authority to get a federal court to impose a fine as high as $25,000 per day for violators of the clean air regulations.

Noise Legislation

The authority for noise abatement and control is administered under the Noise Control Act of 1972, which was amended through the Quiet Communities Act of 1978 (see Table 13-4). The EPA sets noise emission standards for some products, railroads, trucks and buses, airports, and aircraft. The agency is researching the physiological and psychological effects of noise on people. Through this legislation, EPA is charged with (1) establishing standards and promulgating regulations concerning major sources of noise, (2) conducting research into the cause, effects, and control of noise, and (3) helping state and local assistance programs. The agency with primary responsibility for regulating noise in the workplace is the Occupational Safety and Health Administration.

Pesticide Legislation

Congress passed the original Federal Insecticide, Fungicide, and Rodenticide Act in 1947. This bill was subsequently strengthened and amended in 1972, 1975, and 1978. The regulation of pesticides is handled by EPA's Office of Pesticides and Toxic Substances. The pesticide control program registers pesticides, trains people to apply pesticides, and conducts monitoring and research (Your Guide, 1980).

Waste Legislation

Federal support of methods for safe solid waste disposal began in 1965 with the Solid Waste Disposal Act (Table 13-4). In an effort to limit the improper disposal of waste, the Resource Conservation and Recovery Act of 1976 was enacted. Under the act EPA establishes regulations and devises programs to ensure safe disposal of waste. The act requires states to look at existing waste disposal sites and to develop and implement plans for solid waste disposal.

Toxic Substances Legislation

The Toxic Substances Control Act (TSCA), or Public Law 94-469, was passed by Congress and signed into law on October 11, 1976, and became effective January 1, 1977. The general purpose of this act is described in Table 13-4. Under the TSCA, the EPA has authority to compile and publish an inventory of chemical substances either manufactured or imported for commercial purposes.

The TSCA requires testing of some chemical substances if there is evidence of unreasonable risk to health or the environment. EPA may also prohibit the sale, use, or disposal of new or existing chemicals if these are found to present an unreasonable risk to health or the environment. The agency also researches and monitors the effects of toxic chemicals.

Radiation Legislation

Several federal agencies are responsible for protecting the public from radiation. The agencies' major responsibilities are to set radiation standards, assess new technology, and monitor radiation in the environment.

Criticism of EPA

The EPA conducts extensive research in an effort to control and abate the nation's pollution problems. EPA's Office of Research and Development has 15 laboratories throughout the nation for the purpose of conducting such research.

In recent years there has been much criticism and controversy regarding the federal regulatory attempts. The EPA, accused by some of being understaffed, recently saw additional personnel losses. Attempts to reduce inflation by tightening economic controls forced the agency to operate under much tighter budget constraints.

Environmentalists criticize EPA standards as being lax. They cite polluted rivers and streams, dead water birds, and fish kills as examples of environmental degradation. However, state and local governments blame EPA standards for keeping new business from entering their states. Throughout the years some state legislators, in an effort to appease industry, have attempted to weaken environmental enforcement. Chemical manufacturers have criticized EPA efforts for more stringent control, although chemicals found to be extremely dangerous have been banned. Workers suffering from chronic diseases, attributed to the use of such chemicals, are calling for stricter controls. EPA is not the only agency concerned with the control of toxic substances. Five agencies have formed the Interagency Regulation Liason Group (IRLG). The IRLG comprises the EPA, the Occupational Safety and Health Administration, the Food and Drug Administration, the Consumer Product Safety Commission, and the Food Safety and Quality Service of the Department of Agriculture.

ROLE OF PRIVATE SECTOR IN ENVIRONMENTAL HEALTH AND SAFETY

Some manufacturers of pesticides, farmers, and citrus growers question the approach the government has taken to regulate pesticide use and want less stringent controls. Migrant farm workers and advocate groups point to the lack of federal involvement regarding personal protective equipment. They cite unsanitary field conditions, lack of drinking water, and an increasing number of unreported pesticide poisonings each year.

Environmentalists and some scientists have expressed concern about pollutants such as trihalomethanes in water, whereas other researchers and scientists point out that a direct causal link between drinking water quality and cancer incidence has not been established. The controversy goes on and on. As health care professionals, nurses must objectively assess the effect of the environment on health. As new legislation is passed and old legislation amended, they must continue to ask questions, attempt to remain objective, and weigh the evidence of both sides. They must be able to comprehend the complexity of each problem as well as the ramifications involved in possible alternatives, bearing in mind that the best approach toward solving any environmental problem is an informed one.

SUMMARY

The challenge of maintaining environmental health and safety is tremendous. Each innovation seems to exact a price in terms of destruction or threat of pollution to the environment. This chapter has discussed significant biological, chemical, physical, and psychosocial hazards and has pointed out the governmental role in maintaining and regulating environmental health and safety.

Community health nurses are in key positions to detect environmental hazards. Although nurses do not al-

ways directly combat these hazards, they monitor, report, and serve as action-oriented catalysts. Community health nurses must recognize potential hazards in the communities they serve and aid clients in protecting themselves against these health risks. Water, air, soil, and food are only a few possible health hazards. To implement an ecological approach to community health, nurses must be constantly aware of the interaction among people and the environments in which they live. This human and environment interaction and its effect on health have been sources of concern since early recorded history. Many problems have been solved, but new and often more challenging and resistant ones continually arise.

BIBLIOGRAPHY

Banks, H.O.: Comprehensive health planning in relation to environmental problems, Am. J. Public Health **61**:1972-1979, 1971.

Brown, M.: The forgotten great lake, Audubon **84**(6):88-95, Nov. 1982.

Bruce, R.D.: Noise pollution. In Jarvis, L.L., editor: Community health nursing: keeping the public healthy, Philadelphia, 1981, F.A. Davis Co., pp.647-658.

Cahill, C.: Citizens challenge asbestos pipe use, Environment **24**(4):43-44, May 1982.

Chanlett, E.T.: Solid waste management. In Jarvis, L.L., editor: Community health nursing: keeping the public healthy, Philadelphia, 1981, F.A. Davis Co., pp.667-680.

Coburn, R.F.: Biologic effects of carbon monoxide, Ann. NY Acad. Sci. **174**:1-43, 1970.

Cohen, S.: Sound effects on behavior, Psychology Today **15**:38-46, Oct. 1981.

Commoner, B.: The closing circle: nature, man and technology, New York, 1971, Alfred A. Knopf, Inc.

Deadly chemical, deadly fear, Charlotte Observer, Nov. 7, 1982, p. 2A.

Dubos, R.: The crisis of man in his environment, Proceedings of Symposium on Human Ecology, Pub. No. 1929, 1968, Department of Health, Education and Welfare, pp.12-23.

Fetter, S., and Tsipis, K.: Catastrophic releases of radioactivity, Sci. Am. **4**:41-47, 1981.

Golden, J., et al.: Environmental impact data book, Ann Arbor, Mich., 1979, Ann Arbor Science Publishers, Inc.

Hanlon, J.J., and Pickett, G.E.: Public health: administration and practice, ed. 7, St. Louis, 1979, The C.V. Mosby Co.

Harrison, G., Gates, D., and Halling, C.S.: Ecology: the great chain of being, Ekistics **27**:161, March 1969.

Health:United States, 1981, DHHS Pub. No. (PHS) 82-1232, Hyattsville, Md., 1981, Department of Health and Human Services.

Healthy people: the Surgeon General's report on health promotion and disease prevention, DHEW Pub. No. (PHS) 79-55071A, Hyattsville, Md., 1979, Department of Health, Education, and Welfare.

Holzer, H.: A doomsday scenario on 59th street, New York **15**:21, May 24, 1982.

Jarvis, L.L.: Community health nursing: keeping the public healthy, Philadelphia, 1981, F.A. Davis Co.

Kellogg, W.W., et al.: The sulfur cycle, Science **175**:587-596, 1972.

Kowitz, R.A., et al.: Effects of chlorine gas upon respiratory function, Arch. Environ. Health **14**:545, 1967.

Lancaster, J.: Community mental health nursing: An ecological perspective, St. Louis, 1980, The C.V. Mosby Co.

Nelson, K.W.: Government regulations—environmental and occupational health, Am. Ind. Hyg. J. **42**:633-636, Sept. 1981.

P'an, A.Y.S., Beland, J., and Zygmunt, J.: Ozone-induced arterial lesions, Arch. Environ. Health 24:229-232, 1972.

Purdom, P.W., editor: Environmental health, New York, 1980, Academic Press, Inc.

Rosen, G.: A history of public health, New York, 1957, M.D. Publications.

Sandhu, S.S.: Regulation of environmental pollutants: introductory remarks **37**:1-3, Jan. 1981.

Silberstein, C.A., and Silberstein, E.B.: Ionizing radiation and community health. In Jarvis, L.L., editor: Community health nursing: keeping the public healthy, Philadelphia, 1981, F.A. Davis Co., pp.681-691.

Spath, D.P., and Crook, J.: Water pollution. In Jarvis, L.L., editor: Community health nursing: keeping the public healthy, Philadelphia, 1981, F.A. Davis Co., pp.659-666.

Stahl, Q.R.: Air pollution aspects of chlorine and hydrogen gas, Litton Systems, Inc., Bethesda, Md. 1969, Pub. No. 188087, Department of Commerce, National Bureau of Standards.

United Auto Workers Sound Security Department: What every representative should know about health and safety, Pub. No. 449, Detroit, 1979, UAW, p. 6.

Waldbott, G.L.: Health effects of environmental pollutants, ed., St. Louis, 1978, The C.V. Mosby Co.

Werthamer, S, et al.: Ozone-induced pulmonary lesions, Arch. Environ. Health **20**:16-21, 1970.

Wilner, D.M., Walkley, R.P., and O'Neill, E.J.: Introduction to public health, ed. 7, New York, 1978, MacMillan Publishing Co., Inc.

Woodwell, G.W., Graig, P.P., and Johnson, H.A.: DDT in the biosphere: where does it go? Science **174**:1101-1107, 1971.

Your guide to the Environmental Protection Agency, Washington, D.C., Dec. 1980, Office of Public Awareness, EPA.

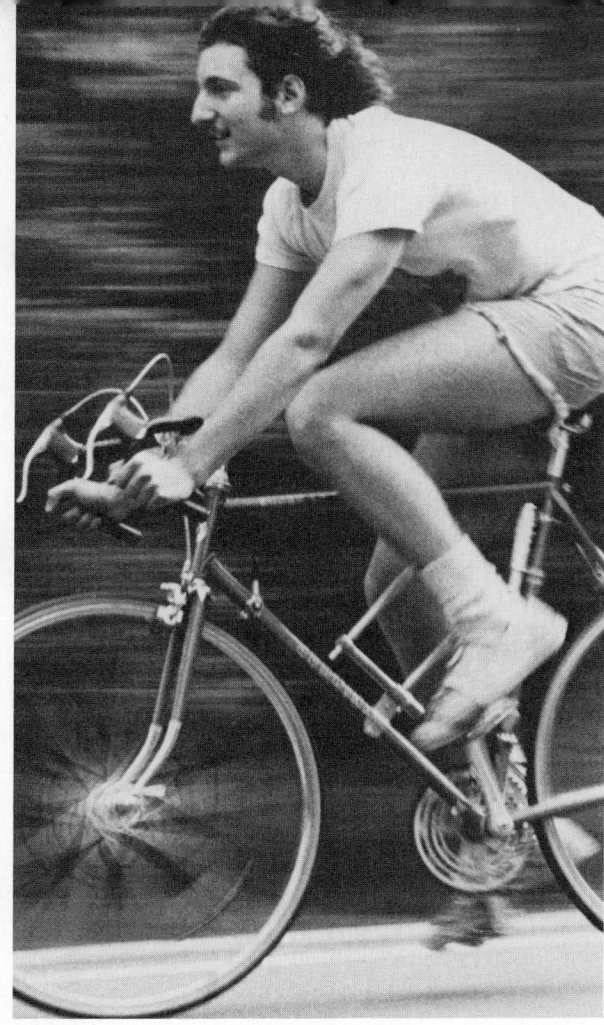

14

JEAN GOEPPINGER

SELF-HEALTH CARE THROUGH RISK APPRAISAL AND REDUCTION: IMPLICATIONS FOR COMMUNITY HEALTH NURSING

A marked resurgence of interest in self-health care is readily apparent today. Many Americans exercise regularly (even enthusiastically), maintain their weight at recommended levels, and deliberately attempt to manage their stress. Some drive at reduced speeds, drink fewer alcoholic beverages than in the past, and no longer smoke. Other are jogging on country lanes and in city parks, joining structured physical fitness programs, patronizing natural food stores, gardening organically, and engaging in a variety of relaxation techniques at home and at work.

Newspaper articles and radio and television programs provide additional evidence of the growing interest in self-health care, as does the rapid proliferation of commercial weight-reduction programs, smoking cessation plans, and health spas. The private sector has also been active in other ways. The San Francisco–based National Center for Health Education, a private institution, was founded in the middle of the 1970s. About the same time the health and life insurance industry began to support the Advisory Committee on Education for Health, and the American Hospital Association developed its Center for Health Promotion. These centers and the Advisory Committee have published reviews of relevant literature and programs and have developed recommendations for the insurance and health care industries.

The federal government has been involved also. During the past decade the Office of Health Information and Health Promotion (now the Office of Health Information, Health Promotion, Physical Fitness, and Sports Medicine) was established in the Office of the Assistant Secretary for Health, as was the Bureau of Health Education (now the Center for Health Promotion and Education) in the Centers for Disease Control. *Healthy People: The Surgeon General's Report on Health Promotion and Disease Prevention* and the subsequent volume, *Promoting Health/Preventing Disease: Objectives for the Nation,* were published. The National Heart, Lung, and Blood Institute sponsored such seminal research as the Multiple Risk Factor Intervention Trials (MRFIT) and the Stanford Heart Disease Prevention Program.

Naturally, critics exist who find as much to impugn in the renewed commitment to self-health care as advocates have to commend. Critics argue that social change, not simply individual change, is prerequisite to health (Kronenfeld, 1979); professional interest in self-health care has subverted the basic consumer orientation (Fonaroff, 1977; Levin, 1976); the efficacy of self-health care has not been systematically and convincingly demonstrated, and consequently it has been adopted for faddish, not scientific reasons (Breslow, 1978b); the cost effectiveness of self-health care has been assumed, not established (Gori and Richter, 1978; Veatch, 1980); and fostering individual healthful changes requires unethical manipulation of human behavior (Warwick and Kelman, 1973).

The debate between critics and proponents of self-health care is important. It suggests that despite the rhetoric of support and recent progress, important barriers to the full adoption of self-health care remain. The criticisms just presented require careful attention. Health professionals in particular can direct their efforts to resolving questions of efficacy.

This chapter focuses on health risk appraisal and reduction, areas of self-health care in which questions of efficacy are already being addressed. The context within which health risk appraisal and reduction have developed is described first. The scientific basis for health risk appraisal and reduction, data related to the issue of efficacy, are then presented. Methods of appraising and reducing health risk at individual and community levels are reviewed, and the community health nurse's roles in assessment and intervention are emphasized.

SELF-HEALTH CARE

The concept of people helping themselves in health matters is not unique. Very likely the practice of self-health care antedates recorded history. Early writings appear in ancient Chinese, classical Greek, and the Bible. Americans have been involved since colonial times. For example, Thomas Jefferson required a medical self-help course for students entering the University of Virginia during the early years of the nineteenth century (Weiss, 1977). Self-health care as engaged in today has a variety of meanings.

History

Self-health care has always included mystical and pragmatic components. For instance, in classical Greek literature the goddess Hygeia represented the belief that humans could remain healthy if they lived rationally. Certain activities of daily living, like exercise, were essential to the maintenance of health, and tributes to Hygeia were important. Similarly, in biblical times various food laws were promulgated to please Yahweh and ensure health.

Eventually, as knowledge of the human body and the mechanisms of disease was acquired, the emphasis of self-health care shifted. The original goal of health protection was balanced by a second goal of disease treatment; lay responsibility was offset by a growing confidence in persons with specialized training (health care professionals).

The nurturance of health and the provision of care to the ill remained lay functions to a limited extent, however. Many health-related activities continued to occur in the family environment and to be directed or performed by wives and mothers, even though dependence on professional health care increased.

Currently, self-health care is again assuming a dominant position. It is competing with, if not supplanting, professional health care. For instance, some versions of self-health care emphasize lay diagnosis and self-treatment as opposed to professional diagnosis and collaborative management. Other more conservative versions focus on teaching people how to work with their health care providers. The effects of either version on the professional health care system are similar. Professional roles in health care are undergoing renegotiation, and the economic security of the existing health care system is threatened. The self-health care system is also endangered, for increased cooperation with its professional counterpart also increases the likelihood of formalization, bureaucratization, and professionalization. In this scenario the lay resource may become an extension of the professional system.

The revitalization and perhaps the assimilation of

self-health care occurring now is a phase in the cyclical rediscoveries of professional health care and self-health care. The recurrent popularity of self-health care may be partially attributed to U.S. history. For example, frontier American society is well remembered for its reliance on self-help. Americans on the frontier survived without the benefit of expert advice. In the true spirit of Jacksonian democracy, they not only depended on self-help but also scorned advice from outsiders. In health as in other areas of life, the older, wiser, and more experienced family members provided the nursing care. If these family members were literate and financially secure, they probably consulted the medical encyclopedia on the parlor bookshelf. If they were illiterate and impoverished, they undoubtedly used folk remedies that were part of the culture's oral tradition. In either case self-health care on the frontier also retained its original religious links. Early popular self-care books, like *Primitive Physic* by John Wesley (1747), the founder of Methodism, were regularly recommended at prairie revivals.

The current renaissance of interest in self-health care may be related to today's political climate. Authority in general has been challenged; racial minorities demanded their rights in the 1960s, and women and patients made their demands in the 1970s. The challenge to a professional health care system, which many believe exemplifies elite rather than democratic control, is clearly illustrated in the ideology of self-care. In the opening sentences of *Medical Nemesis, the Expropriation of Health*, Illich stated, "The medical establishment has become a major threat to health. The disabling impact of professional control over medicine has reached the proportions of an epidemic" (1976a, p. 3).

Illich considered the epidemic iatrogenic or medically induced. Two types of iatrogenesis, social and cultural, are relevant to self-health care. Social iatrogenesis fosters people becoming "consumers of doubtful nostrums rather than changing the morbid social and political conditions that are the major causes of ill-health" (Illich, 1976b, p. 69). Cultural iatrogenesis, on the other hand, turns "patients into passive consumers, objects to be repaired, voyeurs of their own treatment . . . It destroys our autonomous ability to cope with our bodies and heal ourselves" (Illich, 1976b, p. 73). Changes occur at the level of the individual and are instituted not *by* but *for* the person by a professional.

Illich chastised American health professionals and society for robbing persons of self-health care abilities and skills. Politicians and legislators promote self-care because of their interest in cost containment rather than a belief in the individual's ability to preserve his own health.

In fact, medical advances are only minimally related to increases in life expectancy. McKinlay and McKinlay (1977), among others, have been articulate and convincing advocates of the position that medical measures contributed minimally to the decline in mortality in the United States since the turn of the century. Their secondary analysis of data on mortality from 10 major infectious diseases since 1900 suggested that chemotherapeutic and prophylactic medical measures were in many instances introduced decades after the marked decline in mortality began.

If medical measures were not principally responsible for the modern decline in mortality, another explanation is necessary. The main contributors to the decline seem to have been better standards of living, including improvements in sanitation, personal hygiene, and diet, thereby leading to a newly favorable balance in the host-agent relationship (McKeown et al., 1975).

This conclusion has been drawn for chronic illnesses as well as for communicable diseases. Wildavsky (1977) noted that the medical system affects only 10% of the variability in common health indexes, that is, infant mortality, disability days, and adult mortality. He attributed the remainder of the variability to factors over which physicians lack control, "from individual lifestyle (smoking, exercise, worry), to social conditions (income, eating habits, physiological inheritance), to the physical environment (air and water quality)" (1977, p. 105).

In the public arena these conclusions were first supported by LaLonde. In *A New Perspective on the Health of Canadians* (1974), the then Canadian Minister of National Health and Welfare categorized the determinants of health as fourfold: human biology, environment, life-style, and health care (Fig. 14-1). The document was extraordinarily influential among policymakers in this country. For example, *Healthy People: The Surgeon General's Report on Health Promotion and Disease Prevention*, adopted three of LaLonde's four categories as risks to health. The major risk categories delineated were inherited biological, environmental, and behavioral (Healthy People, 1979a). Illich would have added health care as the fourth risk.

These research findings and governmental statements give credence to the principle that health has multiple determinants and indirectly to the concept of self-health care. Three of the four determinants of risks to health, human biology, environment, and life-style, are more under lay than professional control.

Self-health care, despite its renewed popularity, lacks consistency of definition. Definitions vary according to the following attributes: instigator, target, goal, and knowledge base. In turn, labels for the definitions vary

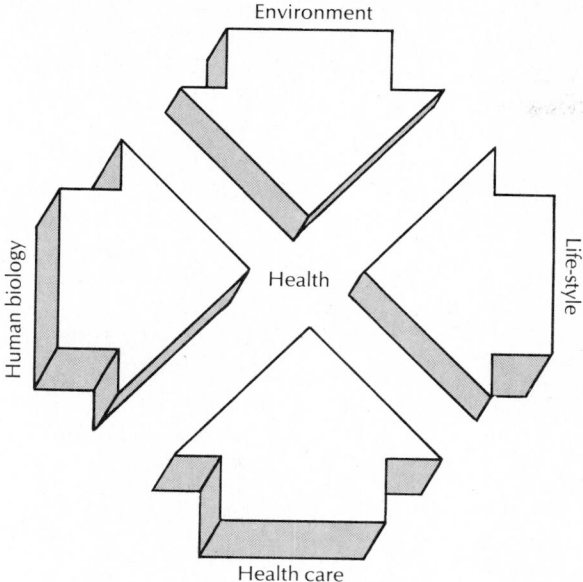

Fig. 14-1. Determinants of health. (Adapted from Lalonde,
M.: A new perspective on the health of Canadians, Ottawa,
1974, Government of Canada.)

from life-style management to self-help, self-care, or
self-health care. In the following subsection the various
meanings of self-health care are analyzed.

Meaning

A comprehensive paradigm of self-health care that
includes the four attributes previously delineated has
been developed by Lorig (1980). The instigator of care
refers to the party responsible for initiating health care,
the lay person or the professional. The target of care
denotes the intended beneficiary of care, the individual
or the social system. The goal is the purpose or function
of care, either health promotion or disease prevention.
The types of knowledge on which health care is based
are categorized as philosophical, cultural, or scientific.
So defined, these dimensions are used as a framework
to analyze the various meanings of self-health care that
are widespread today.

Most commonly, self-health care is conceptualized
as lay-initiated. Individuals are believed able to carry
out health care on their own. However, sometimes self-
health care is defined as compliance, the ability of individuals to carry out only prescribed health care. (The
prescriptions are matters of professional judgment.)
Less frequently, self-health care is seen neither as an alternative nor as an extension of professional health care
but as a supplement.

The second dimension is the target of self-health

care. Self-health care may aim for change at the personal or social system level. Approached from a clinical
model, it emphasizes changes in the individual's health
beliefs and practices. Critics (e.g., Ryan, 1976) often
suggest this represents victim-blaming because individuals alone are not responsible for the choices of health-
compromising behaviors or for the consequences.
These responsibilities are shared with society. Self-
health care approached from a public health perspective emphasizes social responsibility and societal
change rather than individual reform.

The goal of self-health care is variable. Self-health
care has been advocated for health promotion or protection and primary prevention, early detection, and
treatment of disease. The goal of risk appraisal and reduction is generally more circumscribed and involves
either primary prevention or early detection.

The final dimension is the knowledge base for self-
health care. Early proponents often based their self-
health care practices on religious or philosophical tenets. This rationale has persisted but is of diminished
importance. Cultural or folk–medical beliefs and popu-
larized scientific medicine have come to be as important.

Contemporary literature about self-health care emphasizes varying aspects of this paradigm. For instance,
Levin, one of the most prolific writers on self-care, subsumed self-health care under the professional health
care delivery system, based it therefore on scientific
medicine, and targeted it to individual change. However, he construed the goal very broadly and defined self-
health care as a process in which a "layperson can function effectively on his or her own behalf in health promotion and decision-making, in disease prevention,
detection, and treatment" as "the primary health resource in the health care system" (1977, p. 115).

Another health educator, Green, defined self-care
differently but just as restrictively. His definition included only diagnostic and treatment activities that
were formerly the responsibility of professional health
care providers and excluded "basic prevention activities which consumers may and should take which providers have not themselves traditionally provided or
controlled" (Green et al., 1977, p. 168). Self-health care
is an alternative to professional health care, directed to
the individual, aimed at diagnosis and treatment, and
based on scientific medicine.

Nurses have always emphasized people's natural
self-care capacities. Orem, a contemporary nursing
theorist, described self-care as "the practice of activities
that individuals personally initiate and perform on
their own behalf in maintaining life, health, and well-
being . . . an adult's personal continuous contribution

to his own health and well-being" (1971, p. 13). The nursing profession is essential, according to Orem, because individuals are not always self-sufficient. Nursing is necessitated by self-care deficits. Consequently, though self-health care is a lay responsibility, professional contributions are periodically required to sustain or enhance its discharge. Like Levin and Green, Orem's focus is on the individual, and the basis of at least that portion of self-care provided by professionals is scientific.

From Lorig's perspective each of these definitions is restrictive. A more complete definition of self-health care must include the full range of possibilities when all four dimensions are considered. Self-health care "encompasses those activities, continuous and episodic, volitional and unintentional, which people can do for themselves, individually or collectively, in a variety of health and illness matters. These activities complement professional health care services" (Goeppinger, 1982, p. 380).

Relation to Risk Appraisal and Reduction

Within the global approach to self-health care, risk appraisal and reduction can be understood as ways in which professionals can assist individuals and groups develop a portion of their self-health care agendas. The goal of risk appraisal and reduction is the primary prevention or early detection of disease; the knowledge base is the growing body of research findings regarding the relation between certain risk factors and mortality and the effectiveness of intervention in inducing and sustaining risk-factor modification.

It is the cumulation of scientific evidence that makes health risk appraisal and reduction such an attractive aspect of self-health care for the health professional. The findings from the Human Population Laboratory's study of Alameda County lend considerable support to the hypothesis that the presence of selected health risk factors is directly related to excess mortality. The study design is prospective, and the original probability sample included 6928 Alameda County residents; hence the findings can be generalized with some confidence (Breslow, 1972).

After the original health practices survey (5½ years later), mortality was determined to be inversely related to the following health habits: eating three meals daily at regular intervals, eating breakfast, sleeping 7 to 8 hours a night, using alcohol moderately, exercising regularly, not smoking, and maintaining a desirable height/weight ratio (Belloc, 1973). A 45-year-old man engaging in six or seven of these habits could expect to live 11 years longer than a man engaging in three or fewer habits. A 45-year-old woman who engaged in six or seven of these habits could expect to live 7 years longer than a woman engaging in fewer than four habits.

Nine years subsequent to the original survey, analyses have confirmed and extended the original findings. The inverse relationship between health practices and mortality persisted (with mortality decreased as the number of health practices increased), but dietary practices were no longer found to be significant. Using only the 3892 white adult members of the sample on whom mortality data were available, Wiley and Camacho (1980) found cigarette smoking, alcohol consumption, physical exercise, hours of sleep per night, and weight in relation to height significant predictors of mortality. Berkman (1977) also found that mortality was negatively correlated with the strength of the respondent's social networks, such as marriage, contacts with close friends and relatives, church membership, and ties with formal and informal groups.

Additional data continue to verify the relation of health risk factors to mortality. Concurrently, other research has concentrated on the efficacy of intervention in modifying known health risks. The findings of three studies, although they must be qualified, suggest health education can foster behavioral changes in clients, and these changes decrease health risks and possibly even lower the incidence of related diseases.

The Stanford Heart Disease Prevention Program is in essence a field trial of the relative effects of a mass media campaign and those of such a campaign plus intensive face-to-face instruction on three cardiovascular disease risk factors: cigarette smoking, systolic blood pressure, and serum cholesterol (Maccoby et al., 1977). After 2 years there was a substantial increase in knowledge about cardiovascular disease and its risk factors and a decrease in all health risk behaviors in the two experimental communities. A comparable increase in knowledge and decline in risk were not noted in the control community. On the contrary, the differences in knowledge were statistically significant ($p < .05$), and the risk of cardiovascular disease, although not statistically significant, did increase about 7% in the predicted direction. Intensive face-to-face counseling was found especially effective in inducing behavioral change.

These findings have to be accepted with caution. High-risk subjects in the media-only community showed almost no reduction in cardiovascular risk. Furthermore, the lack of a face-to-face instruction only experimental condition makes it impossible to evaluate completely the relative efficacy of media-based intervention (Leventhal et al., 1980). Finally, the persistence of change after 2 years was not examined; nevertheless, the findings were encouraging.

Similar results are emerging from a study in North

Karelia, Finland, a largely rural area with extraordinarily high rates of cardiovascular disease (Puska, 1978). In the early 1970s more than half of North Karelian males smoked. They also ingested large amounts of animal fats and had grossly elevated serum cholesterol levels. Many suffered from untreated hypertension. Excess mortality from cardiovascular disease, particularly among middle-aged men, was high.

Concerned about these risks, North Karelians asked the government for help. A risk-management program involving retraining of health professionals, reorganization of public health services, production of low-fat dairy products and low-fat and low-salt sausages, development of patient information services, and organization of public health education evolved to help residents control blood pressure, stop smoking, and decrease cholesterol intake. These interventions began in 1972 and concluded in 1977.

Subsequent evaluations revealed that the prevalence of the three risk factors decreased more in North Karelia than in the comparison county (Bauer, 1981). Cigarette smoking declined, more low-fat milk was consumed, and an increased proportion of hypertension was controlled.

The findings regarding behavioral change have been considered "sounder and more convincing" (Wagner, 1982, p. 51) than those regarding cardiovascular disease and mortality. Although the incidence of myocardial infarction and stroke has dropped, whether or not changes among health-related behaviors, risk-factor levels, morbidity, and mortality are truly "biologically significant" (Wagner, 1982, p. 52) remains to be seen after further monitoring. Fortunately, data collection is continuing.

The Multiple Risk Factor Intervention Trial (MRFIT) program is also directed at lowering risks from smoking, high serum cholesterol levels, and hypertension. Unlike the Stanford and North Karelia studies, it is a controlled clinical trial. The purpose is to determine whether or not counseling can yield an appreciable decrease in cardiovascular disease and mortality of high-risk males. Although the final results are not available, preliminary analyses suggest that participants in the experimental condition have reduced their cholesterol levels, controlled their hypertension, and stopped smoking. The first two changes averaged slightly over half the expected changes, and cigarette smoking cessation exceeded predictions (Neaton et al., 1981).

Each of these studies illustrates that rather simple, often community-based health education can contribute to risk-factor reduction. However, it has not been established that even statistically significant reductions in risk produce comparable reductions in morbidity and premature mortality. Yet many believe we cannot wait patiently and passively to establish these relationships. "The best we can seek is to avoid action based on imprudent interpretation of available data and to promote action against risk factors based on prudent interpretation of available data, at the same time striving for better and more pertinent evidence" (Breslow, 1978a, p. 456).

Overviews of several methods for assessing and managing health risks are presented in the next two sections. As Breslow requested, their claims are carefully evaluated against available data.

METHODS OF HEALTH RISK APPRAISAL

The goal of health risk appraisal is to collect and analyze data about health risks experienced by an individual or group and to provide that individual or group with the information necessary to reduce the identified risks. Health risk appraisal may be carried out on an individual or a personal level and on a community or a collective level. It may involve epidemiological and/or clinical approaches. An epidemiological approach to health risk appraisal is required to establish the presence or absence of health risks at the community or collective level. These approaches are discussed more fully later in the chapter. A clinical approach to health risk appraisal is required to establish the presence or absence of health risks at the individual or personal level. Both approaches are important to community health nurses and are consequently considered here.

Appraising Individual Health Risks

At least three types of individual health risk appraisals are common today. They include the Health Hazard Appraisal in any of its many versions, the Lifetime Health Monitoring Program, and the Wellness Appraisals or Inventories.

Although each type of appraisal is rather complex, the basic concepts and procedures are described. A full exposition of each type can be found in the references cited. Examples are displayed in Appendix D.

Health Hazard Appraisal (HHA)

Among the earliest proponents of individual health risk appraisal were two family physicians who called their approach *prospective medicine* (Robbins and Hall, 1970). Unlike physicians in conventional curative medicine, they wanted to deal with an individual's health, not disease, from the perspective of what was likely to occur and not what had already happened. They realized that most chronic diseases do not happen instantaneously but have a predictable sequence. They knew that the characteristic precursors of many diseases can also be monitored and controlled. The natu-

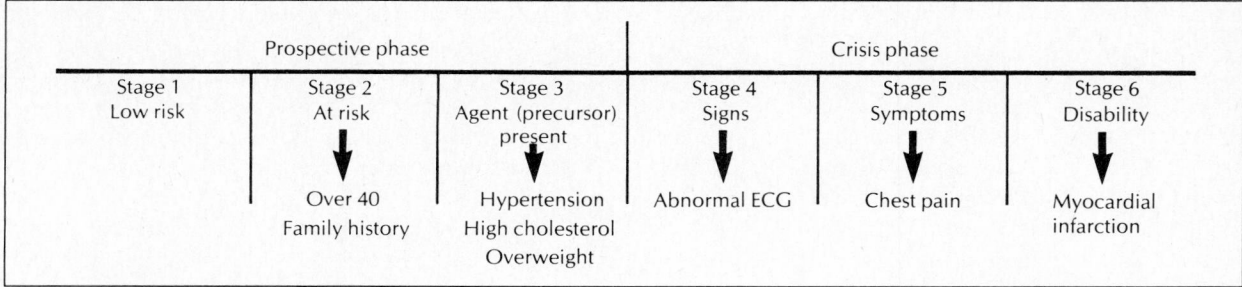

Fig. 14-2. Natural history of arteriosclerotic heart disease.

ral history of one such illness, arteriosclerotic disease, is diagrammed in Fig. 14-2.

Robbins and Hall operationalized the concept of prospective medicine by developing a method of profiling risk termed the *Health Hazard Appraisal.* The objectives of the Health Hazard Appraisal are to (1) assess the total risks to a client's health based on knowledge of the client, the natural history of certain diseases, and the major causes of mortality for aggregates of the client's age, sex, and race; (2) initiate lifestyle changes in the client to avoid disease precursors and minimize their pathogenic influence; and (3) institute medical therapy as early in the course of a disease as possible.

To accomplish these objectives data are collected by a self-administered questionnaire, basic laboratory tests, and a miniclinical examination. The questionnaire (see Appendix D) elicits data about certain common personal habits that are known to compromise health, such as cigarette smoking, family health history, and use of certain medical services like cervical cancer screening. The laboratory testing is limited to obtaining the serum cholesterol level. The physical examination consists of height, weight, and blood pressure measurements.

These personal data are then compared with data compiled from the 10 major causes of death for an aggregate of the client's age, sex, and race, the average probability of dying, and the precursors and risk intensities associated with each cause. An appraisal and achievable age are computed. The appraisal age is that of the average person in the same racial, sex, and age group with a total 10-year risk similar to that of the individual being assessed. For example, a 20-year-old white woman might have an appraisal age of 15 if she has good health habits and is fortunate genetically. Another 20-year-old white woman may have an appraisal age of 25 if she smokes, fails to use a seat belt, and does not have regular breast examinations. This person's achievable age, the age she might achieve by modifying certain health hazards, would be considerably lower.

The achievable age represents the lower 10-year risk projected if the individual complies with the prescribed changes.

In the decade subsequent to Robbins and Hall's initial work, health hazard appraisal instruments proliferated rapidly. At least 12 health risk appraisals are in current usage (Doerr and Hutchins, 1981), and some are medically focused, like Robbins and Hall's Health Hazard Appraisal. Many others are expanded versions that include issues related to mental health, social health, and even the environment. Two instruments that illustrate the difference are the Health Risk Index and Hettler's Lifestyle Assessment Questionnaire (see Appendix D).

The Health Risk Index is compiled from data on illnesses; family medical history; and life-style factors related to specific diseases, selected physiological areas, and to a lesser extent emotions and feelings. These data are compared to mortality data. The Lifestyle Assessment Questionnaire, on the other hand, includes (1) a wellness inventory requesting data on personal habits, feelings and emotions, community, automobile safety, rest and relaxation, and fitness; (2) a life-style assessment with separate sections on personal growth and risk of death; and (3) a medical alert. Only data from the risk of death portion of the life-style assessment are compared to mortality data. Other health hazard appraisal instruments range between these two extremes.

Versions of health hazard appraisal instruments have also been developed specifically for children, such as the Know Your Body program, developed by the American Health Foundation in New York City (Williams et al. 1980). It was designed to identify chronic disease risk factors in schoolchildren 11 to 14 years of age and to return findings and health prescriptions to the children in a "Health Passport."

Lifetime Health Monitoring Program (LHMP)

As a substantial portion of physician time is spent evaluating the health of apparently well people (often considered the "worried well"), Breslow and Somers

(1977) proposed a Lifetime Health Monitoring Program (see Appendix D) suitable to medical practice. Like the Health Hazard Appraisal, it uses clinical and epidemiological data to identify specific needs for health care, but unlike its counterpart, it focuses on needs appropriate to particular stages of the life cycle. It also does not require the collection of data in a standardized fashion.

The objective is to focus health evaluation and counseling on the health problems apt to occur in each of 10 different age groups. To illustrate, it is recommended that the age group 40 to 59 be tested for hypertension, breast, cervical, and gastrointestinal cancer, and counseled on changing nutritional needs, physical activity, and the use of cigarettes, alcohol, and drugs. An ad hoc advisory committee of the Institute of Medicine developed drafts for all 10 age groups. A set of criteria to guide the choice of procedures appropriate to each age group was also developed (Bauer, 1981).

Wellness Inventories

The various wellness inventories are slightly different than the generic Health Hazard Appraisal (Robbins and Hall, 1970) or the Lifetime Health Monitoring Program. They customarily define health risks more broadly and emphasize lay control. Like the Lifetime Health Monitoring Program, they focus on health promotion as well as disease prevention.

Typically, wellness inventories are concerned with a wide range of personal habits. For example, Clark's Wellness Assessment (1981) has six categories: eating well, being fit, feeling good, caring for self and/or others, fitting in, and being responsible. Ardell (1977) includes in his index inventories related to self-responsibility, nutritional awareness, physical fitness, stress management, and environmental sensitivity. Travis' Wellness Self-Evaluation (1977) includes a Life Change Index, Eating Habits Survey, Wellness Inventory Symptom Checklist, Medical History, Purpose in Life Test, Stress Assessment, and Creativity Index. In contrast, Robbins and Hall's Health Hazard Appraisal includes only those health habits whose relationships to disease have been clearly documented.

The health habits with which wellness inventories are concerned are seldom amenable to professional control. The lay individual is assumed to be the locus of control. Equally obvious is that the philosophical posture of the wellness appraisal is proactive, not reactive. The Health Hazard Appraisal is designed to avert disease and premature death; wellness appraisals may foster disease prevention, but they do so by advocating health enhancement or promotion. "One holds the line, the other moves forward" (Ardell, 1977, p. 56). The Lifetime Health Monitoring Program reflects a balanced commitment to disease prevention and health promotion. Irrespective of the type of individual health risk appraisal and the breadth of the its goal, certain limitations exist.

Adequacy of Appraisal Methods

Methodologies to help identify individual health risks are inadequate. Limitations abound, although only certain ones are salient to practice. The practice-related limitations are (1) the inconsistency with which various health characteristics and behaviors are measured and analyzed, (2) the assumption that health risk appraisal alone is successful in changing behaviors or improving health, and (3) the likelihood that emphasis on personal responsibility and individual health habits may foster an oversimplified understanding of the determinants of health and disease.

First, although there is a growing consensus that health (and disease) has three if not four determinants (Fig. 14-3), the relative attention each appraisal method devotes to human biology, environment, and life-style varies. Some appraisals include only the risk indicators identified from a large and carefully controlled data base. These generally fall within the category of human biology, less frequently life-style, and even more infrequently environment. Others like the wellness inventories include "behaviors for which the scientific evidence of their predictive importance remains controversial; characteristics for which scientific evidence that intervention is efficacious remain controversial; and characteristics about which the client can do nothing" (Wagner et al., 1982, p. 349). None of the appraisal methods includes assessments of health care, a fourth likely determinant of health and disease. This set of limitations means that interpretations and recommendations vary widely depending on the appraisal method used, and therefore comparisons have to be made cautiously.

The second practice-related problem is that definitive evidence is lacking to support the success of health risk appraisal in stimulating behavior change. Early advocates mistakenly assumed that appraisal was synonymous with intervention. Of the three randomized controlled studies reported by Wagner et al. (1982), only one found behavioral changes, and even these statistically significant results had dubious clinical importance. Unfortunately, despite this evidence, health risk appraisal programs have continued to be misrepresented as interventions.

The third problem is the danger that appraisals emphasizing only those factors for which the scientific evidence is compelling may delude proponents of self-health care into believing that environmental and social factors are unimportant. By focusing on human bi-

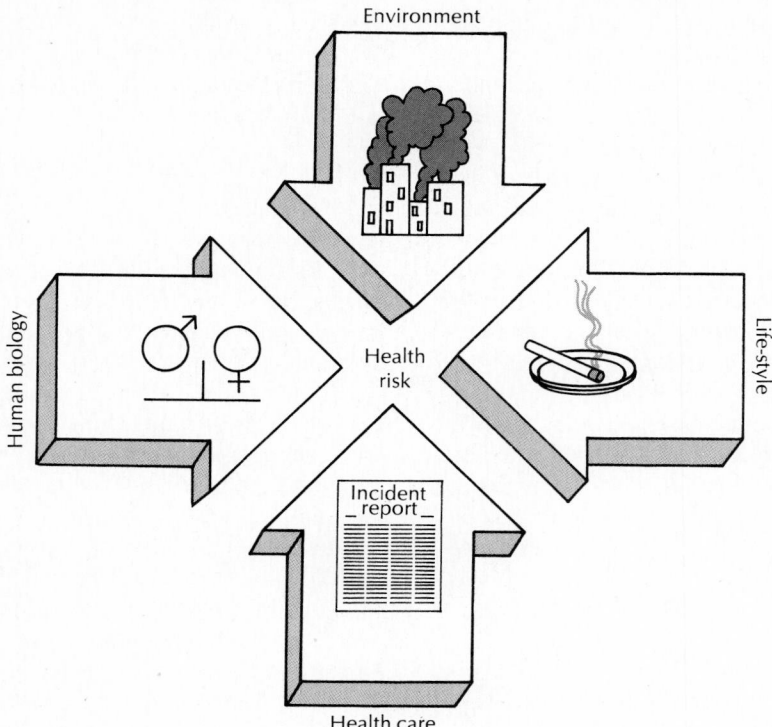

Fig. 14-3. Areas of health risk appraisal.

ology and life-style, health professionals and lay persons alike may unintentionally "blame the victim" (Ryan, 1976). Identifying risks that the individual cannot of his own volition ameliorate may simply generate excessive anxiety and guilt.

Despite these limitations, health risk appraisal provides the individual with a permanent record containing epidemiologically derived but personalized information that can be taken home, mulled over with family and friends, and used to gauge progress in mitigating health risks over time. It also provides the nurse with information necessary to design disease prevention and health promotion strategies for patients. Such tangible evidence for "silent" risks like hypertension may be extremely beneficial.

Appraising Public Health Risks

Health risk appraisals can be used to estimate the risks to a defined population from a number of chronic, and to some extent, preventable diseases. Three approaches to establishing public or aggregate health risks exist. They are (1) epidemiological measures, including the well-established mortality and morbidity data and health risk appraisals; (2) vital statistics, the demographic correlates of health and illness; and (3) community competence levels.

The use of mortality data and to a lesser extent morbidity figures to establish health risk is undoubtedly the most accepted approach. These techniques are thoroughly discussed in Chapter 7. Similarly, the results of health risk appraisals for a given aggregate may be compiled to form a composite picture of risk. This has been done with industrial employees (Durfee and DeGrassi, 1979).

The use of certain demographic data in which the relation to health and illness, although contextual or indirect rather than direct, has been thoroughly documented and is also appropriate. Dependency ratios, socioeconomic status, race, sex, and education provide a second tool for estimating public health risks.

The third approach, the use of community competence levels, has been proposed but not tested. The potential use is thoroughly described in Chapter 17, where community competence is presented as a potential correlate if not a measure of community health. Like certain demographic measurements community competence levels may be an important contextual variable, but this would occur at the level of community process, not structure. The possible use to health risk appraisal of certain demographic measurements and the concept of community competence needs further study. Just as critical is the need to integrate health risk appraisal into

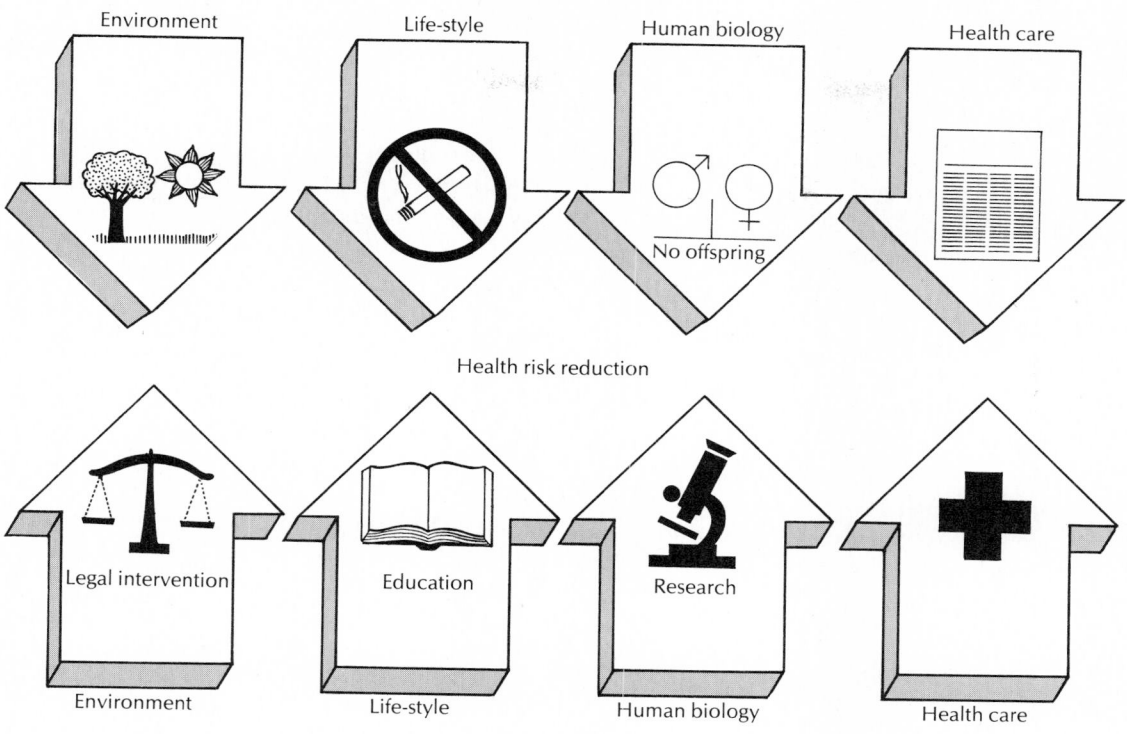

Fig. 14-4. Aims of health risk reduction.

high quality risk reduction programs, which are discussed in the next section.

METHODS OF HEALTH RISK REDUCTION

Health risk reduction can focus on minimizing risk and/or maximizing opportunity in any or all of the four determinants of health/disease—environment, lifestyle, human biology, and health care (Fig. 14-4). It may also originate at individual and societal levels. Microlevel interventions, those performed at the individual level, may be most feasible in the areas of human biology and life-style. Macrolevel interventions, those carried out at the societal level, may be essential in the areas of environment and health care. Both microlevel and macrolevel interventions may be required to sustain changes in the areas of life-style and health care. The individual may be able to initiate change in these areas, but individual change without corresponding system change in unlikely to be maintained.

Individual, societal, and composite (individual and societal) changes are discussed in this section. Examples are drawn from the four major categories of health

determinants, and the community health nurse's roles are emphasized.

Individual Change

Individual approaches are the most popular among the proposed interventions. They require behavioral changes by individuals on their own behalf. The common characteristic of changes at the individual level is that people "use their own personal interest, know-how, ingenuity, and resources to achieve the risk reduction" (Blum, 1982, p. 23). Others may be involved, but the locus of control for change rests with the individual.

Microlevel changes in the area of life-style are the most celebrated. Intervention directed to exercise and physical fitness, smoking cessation, nutrition and weight control, and stress management are commonplace. The presentation of a comprehensive overview of behavioral intervention strategies in any of these areas is beyond the scope of this chapter. The reader is encouraged to consult the wide variety of readily available sources for a more thorough understanding of each strategy.

One typology of behavior change strategies, proposed by Pender (1982, p. 210), seems especially useful. She clustered strategies for "self-modifications" as (1) self-confrontation, (2) cognitive restructuring, (3) modeling, (4) operant conditioning, (5) counterconditioning, and (6) stimulus control. Further, she suggested that nurse and client be "mutually involved" in the selection of specific strategies. The behavioral contract was recommended as a mechanism for the joint establishment of health goals and strategies for change.

Self-confrontation, one intervention strategy, is based on the premise that change ensues when the individual recognizes inconsistencies within his values, beliefs, and behaviors or between his and those of others he emulates. As Pender (1982) noted, this strategy has been used successfully as an approach to smoking cessation. However, the use of feedback from health risk appraisals as an inducement to behavior change, which is predicated on the efficacy of self-confrontation (appraisal age versus achievable age), is unconvincing.

An intervention using *cognitive restructuring* aims to "teach clients to think more rationally and thus gain greater control over their own lives and health" (Pender, 1982, p. 215). For example, rational thinking about obesity and the necessity of weight loss is reflected in the following statement, "I have difficulty controlling my between meal snacking." In the same situation, "I'll never be slender. I've always been chubby," exemplifies irrational thinking. The procedures for applying the principles of cognitive restructuring to clinical intervention have been outlined by Goldfried and Sobocinski (1975); however, research to determine the impact on health behavior has not been done.

Systematic, controlled research on the effects of *modeling,* a more common intervention strategy among nurses than cognitive restructuring, has also not been done. Modeling consists of providing the client with opportunities to observe the behavior of others. For example, alcoholics who have successfully achieved the client's own health goal of abstinence may well serve as models. This strategy is thought to be especially helpful when the client is unsure of the behaviors that are required to achieve the goal. Modeling of risk-averting behavior is inherent in the professional obligations of nurses.

Perhaps the most effective self-modification strategies for healthful change are those using *conditioning.* They are based on the principle that behavior is determined by its consequences. As a result, health-generating behaviors must be identified and rewards provided. The nurse who uses conditioning strategies with clients needs to be well informed about ways of sensitizing individuals to their health-generating and health-damaging behaviors, the appropriate use of rewards, and the gradual shaping of healthy behaviors. The nurse could,

for example, reward a client who had maintained a regular exercise program with praise and by noting increased muscle tone. The relative merits of each strategy must be assessed. Two books have been written to provide information about these topics, one by LeBow (1973) and the other by Berni and Fordyce (1977).

Counterconditioning is a special type of conditioning in which the aim is to replace an undesirable link between a stimulus and a response with a more desirable one. For instance, the nurse might aim to help a client replace tension with relaxation in a stressful situation.

Stimulus control, the final strategy identified by Pender, is also used by nurses. Its theoretical underpinnings are especially appropriate to risk reduction, since they emphasize the antecedents or precursors and not the consequences of behavior. So far, however, sets of antecedents such as the Health Belief Model and Personal Health Behavior (Becker, 1974) and Health Locus of Control/Health Value (Wallston and Wallston, 1978) have not been demonstrated to be strong predictors. Additional research is needed before effective risk reduction interventions can be based on these concepts.

Other microlevel interventions may be targeted to the area of human biology. The application of new knowledge in genetics is one example in which only individual change would be considered ethically acceptable. Two individuals with recessive genes for sickle-cell anemia, for instance, may be counseled about the risks to their future offspring but not proscribed from reproducing.

Societal Change

Interventions at the societal level or macrolevel interventions are less popular than those directed to individual change, probably because it is easier scientifically and politically to assume that the individual is responsible for his own health. The individual may indeed be responsible but only to a limited extent. For example, how can the individual be held solely responsible for driving recklessly when Detroit continues to manufacture large and powerful automobiles with government subsidies? Many changes in life-style, like driving habits, undoubtedly require concurrent changes at the societal level.

In areas like the environment, societal change may be most essential. Only legislation to control environmental hazards from chemical and physical agents will lower the excess mortality from occupationally induced cancers. The need to earn enough to purchase basic necessities precludes many from quitting jobs with well-established health risks, like coal mining. The fulfillment of basic needs constrains the freedom to choose jobs where personal health is not at risk. As a result, the risks themselves, and not the individual's exposure to them, must be altered.

Clean air and water, as well as safe jobs, require group action. State legislation mandating the inspection of wells and the laboratory examination of well water is a traditional example of risk-reducing surveillance. Negotiations between the United States and Canada on the pollution of the Great Lakes are another creative example of group action for environmental health at the international level.

Societal level change is also deemed by many to be a prerequisite to health system reform. Some advocate political revolution as a means to health system reform; more support legislation at the national level to ensure minimal health care for all. A typology of societal change strategies might include both.

Composite Change

It is clear that effective multidimensional risk reduction involves health-generating changes at the individual and societal levels. It is equally clear that the community health nurse acting alone cannot be considered an intervention mechanism. Change requires the nurse to use multiple mechanisms, such as behavioral contract, the establishment of coalitions, the use of small interacting groups, cooperation with lay advisors, the mass media, public policy, and legislation (state, federal, and international). These are more fully discussed in Chapters 5 and 17; therefore in the next and final section only the rationale for involving community health nurses in risk appraisal and reduction and an example of one nurse's roles are presented.

ROLES OF THE COMMUNITY HEALTH NURSE

Risk appraisal and reduction are integral aspects of self-health care. They are equally important aspects of community health nursing. Disease prevention and health promotion have been integral to public health since its earliest days. They are just as important today, perhaps even more so as the disease picture shifts from infectious to chronic disease, and our abilities to discern and influence the determinants of chronic disease improve.

Community health nursing is a part of this tradition. Although intensive care following a head injury and postoperative care following mutilating surgery occupy some professional nurses, disease prevention activities have in the past and continue to occupy much of the community health nurse's time. The renewed emphasis from lay persons and professionals on disease prevention, health promotion, and self-health care simply provides new challenges for established skills. Health risk

appraisal serves as a way of responding to the challenges.

Though the philosophy of public health provides the orientation to risk appraisal and reduction, community health nursing's unique synthesis of clinical and aggregate skills provides the practice guidelines. Community health nurses commonly provide services to individuals, families, and other groups, as do nurses in other areas, but the knowledge base of community health nursing practice has been broadened to include epidemiology. Community health nurses give care, for instance, to individuals when self-health care demands exceed their capabilities. These nurses do so because the clients' needs for health reflect aggregate needs. Consequently, community health nurses are ably prepared to assist with risk appraisal and reduction. They have the wide range of skills necessary to work with individuals, families, and groups and the knowledge to understand the epidemiological and behavioral evidence for health risk assessment and management.

Community health nurses working in a preschool immunization clinic, for example, have an excellent opportunity to introduce parents and children to the concepts of disease prevention and health promotion. In addition to providing the usual information about immunization schedules, school-induced separation anxiety, and possible side effects of the immunizations, the nurse could elicit information about the status of the parents' health. One enterprising nurse did this and as a result was able to broaden considerably the care that was offered.

The nurse, using a simplified version of the Health Hazard Appraisal, discovered the following. One child's father, a white 30-year-old truck driver, had an appraisal age of 43 years and achievable age of 25. He was at greater risk than his contemporaries for motor vehicle accidents, arteriosclerotic heart disease, suicide, cirrhosis of the liver, stroke, and cancer of the lungs. He had a sedentary job that kept him apart from his family for long periods, drank 25 to 40 bottles of beer a week, never wore a seat belt, was hypertensive (blood pressure 200/106), smoked two packs of cigarettes a day when he was "on the road," carried 200 pounds on a 5½-foot frame, was "tense," and drove 198,000 miles annually. The nurse ascertained which of these risks he considered modifiable; worked with the man, his entire family, and his driving partner to develop an intervention plan that would bring his appraisal age down to 35 years; and referred him and his family to several community agencies for additional assistance with specific risk reduction actions.

The nurse's efforts were so successful and the client was so satisfied that soon other drivers and their wives began calling for advice Eventually, the drivers' labor union was approached, and it gave support to a small health risk identification and reduction program for all interested drivers belonging to the local union. This was conducted by the nurse and agency colleagues. Similar programs, run by nurses, have been reported in the professional literature (e.g., Grove et al., 1979).

SUMMARY

In this chapter risk appraisal and reduction have been presented as important ways for community health nurses to assist individuals, families, aggregates, and other community groups in achieving improved self-health care. The four areas in which self-health care could be targeted, human biology, environment, lifestyle, and professional health care, were reviewed. The environment and life-style were emphasized as especially important to risk appraisal and reduction because of the growing body of data on our abilities to successfully modify risk in these areas. Methods of appraising individual and aggregate health risks were reviewed and evaluated, as were selected intervention strategies. The chapter concluded with an illustration of community health nursing action to appraise and reduce risks at the individual and group levels.

BIBLIOGRAPHY

Ardell, D.B.: High level wellness: an alternative to doctors, drugs, and disease, Emmaus, Pa., 1977, Rodale Press, Inc.

Bauer, K.G.: Improving the chances for health: lifestyle change and health evaluation, San Francisco, 1981, National Center for Health Education.

Becker, M.H., editor: The health belief model and personal health behavior, Thorofare, N.J., 1974, Charles B. Slack, Inc.

Belloc, N.B.: Relationship of health practices and mortality, Prev. Med. **2**:67, 1973.

Berkman, L.F.: Psychosocial resources, health, behavior and mortality: a nine-year follow-up study. Paper presented at the annual meeting of the American Public Health Association, Washington, D.C., Oct. 1977.

Berni, R., and Fordyce, W.E.: Behavior modification and the nursing process, St. Louis, 1977, the C.V. Mosby Co.

Blum, H.J.: Social perspective on risk reduction. In Faber, M.M., and Reinhardt, A.M., editors: Promoting health through risk reduction, New York, 1982, Macmillan Publishing Co., Inc.

Breslow, L.: A quantitative approach to the World Health Organization's definition of health: physical, mental, and social well-being, Int. J. Epidemiol. **1**:347, 1972.

Breslow, L.: Prospects for improving health through reducing risk factors, Prev. Med. **7**:449, 1978a.

Breslow, L.: Risk factor intervention for health maintenance, Science **200**:908, July 1978b.

Breslow, L., and Somers, A.R.: The lifetime health monitoring program: a practical approach to preventive medicine, N. Engl. J. Med. **296**:601, 1977.

Clark, C.C.: Enhancing wellness: a guide for self-care, New York, 1981, Springer Publishing Co., Inc.

Doerr, B.T., and Hutchins, E.B.: Health risk appraisal: process, problems, and prospects for nursing practice and research, Nurs. Res. **30**:299, 1981.

Durfee, J.H., and De Grassi, A.: Health hazard appraisal in the workplace. Proceedings of the fifthteenth annual meeting on Prospective Medicine and Health Hazard Appraisal, Bethesda, Md., 1979, Health and Education Resources, p. 71.

Faber, M.M., and Reinhardt, A.M.: Promoting health through risk reduction, New York, 1982, Macmillan Publishing Co., Inc.

Fielding, J.E.: Appraising the health of health risk appraisal, Am. J. Public Health **72**:337, 1982.

Fonaroff, A.: Issues in self-care: preface, Health Educ. Monogr. **5**(2):108, 1977.

Goeppinger, J.: Changing health behaviors and outcomes through self-care. In Lancaster, J., and Lancaster, W., editors: Concepts for advanced nursing practice: the nurse as a change agent, St. Louis, 1982, The C.V. Mosby Co.

Goetz, A.A., and McTyre, R.B.: Health risk appraisal: some methodologic considerations, Nurs. Res. **30**:307, 1981.

Goldfried, M.R., and Sobocinski, D.: Effect of irrational beliefs on emotional arousal, J. Consult. Clin. Psychol. **43**:504, 1975.

Gori, G.B., and Richter, B.J.: Macroeconomics of disease prevention in the United States, Science **200**:1124, 1978.

Green, L.W., et al.: Research and development issues in self-care: measuring the decline in medicocentrism, Health Educ. Monogr. **5**:161, 1977.

Grove, D.A., et al.: Application of a risk-factor identification and reduction program in a corporate setting. Proceedings of the fourteenth annual meeting on Prospective Medicine and Health Hazard Appraisal, Bethesda, Md., 1979, Health and Education Resources.

Healthy people: the Surgeon General's report on health promotion and disease prevention, DHEW Pub. No. (PHS) 79-55071, Washington, D.C., 1979, Department of Health, Education and Welfare.

Healthy people: the Surgeon General's report on health promotion and disease prevention, Background papers, DHEW Pub. No. (PHS) 79-55071A, Washington, D.C., 1979b, Department of Health, Education and Welfare.

Hettler, B.: Lifestyle assessment questionnaire, Stevens Point, 1978, University of Wisconsin, Stevens Point Foundation.

Illich, I.: Medical nemesis, the expropriation of health, New York, 1976a, Random House, Inc.

Illich, I.: Medicine is a major threat to health, Psychology Today **9**:66, May 1976b.

Kasl, S.V.: Cardiovascular risk reduction in a community setting: some comments, J. Consult. Clin. Psychol. **48**:143, 1980.

Kronenfeld, J.J.: Self care as a panacea for the ills of the health care system: an assessment, Soc. Sci. Med. **13**(A):263, 1979.

Kuller, L., et al.: Primary prevention of heart attacks: the multiple risk factor intervention trial, Am. J. Epidemiol. **112**:185, 1980.

LaLonde, M.: A new perspective on the health of Canadians, Ottawa, 1974, Government of Canada.

LeBow, M.D.: Behavior modification: a significant method in nursing practice, Englewood Cliffs, N.J., 1973, Prentice-Hall, Inc.

Leventhal, H., et al.: Cardiovascular risk modification by community-based programs for life-style change: comments on the Stanford study, J. Consult. Clin. Psychol. **48**:150, 1980.

Levin, L.S.: Self-care: an international perspective, Soc. Policy **6**:70, 1976.

Levin, L.S.: Forces and issues in the revival of interest in self-care: impetus for redirection in health, Health Educ. Monogr. **5**:115, 1977.

Lorig, K.: Arthritis self-management: a joint venture. A multiple outcome patient education evaluation, doctoral dissertation, Berkeley, 1980, University of California at Berkeley, 1980.

Maccoby, N., et al.: Reducing the risk of cardiovascular disease, J. Community Health **3**:100, April-June 1977.

McKeown, T., Record, R.G., and Turner, R.D.: An interpretation of the decline in mortality in England and Wales during the twentieth century, Popul. Studies **29**:391, 1975.

McKinlay, J.B., and McKinlay, S.M.: The questionable contribution of medical measures to the decline of mortality in the United States in the twentieth century, Milbank Mem. Fund Q. **55**:405, Summer 1977.

Medical datamation: health risk index, Bellevue, Ohio, 1980.

Mooney, H., and Rives, N.W.: Measures of community health status for health planning, Health Serv. Res. **2**:124-145, 1978.

Multiple risk factors intervention trial group: Statistical design considerations in the NHLI multiple risk factor intervention trial, J. Chronic Dis. **30**:261, 1977.

Neaton, J.D., et al.: The multiple risk factor intervention trial (MRFIT). VII. A comparison of risk factor changes between the two study groups, Prev. Med. **10**:519, 1981.

Orem, D.: Nursing: concepts of practice, New York, 1971, McGraw-Hill Book Co.

Pender, N.J.: Health promotion in nursing practice, New York, 1982, Appleton-Century-Crofts.

Promoting health/preventing disease: objectives for the nation, DHHS Pub. No. (PHS) 0-349-256, Washington, D.C., 1981, Department of Health and Human Services.

Puska, P.: North Karelia project: a community program for the control of cardiovascular disease (abstract), Conference on Prevention, Institute of Medicine, Washington, D.C., Feb., 1978.

Robbins, L.C., and Hall, J.N.: How to practice prospective medicine, Indianapolis, 1970, Methodist Hospital of Indiana.

Ryan, W.: Blaming the victim, New York, 1976, Random House, Inc.

Travis, J.W.: Wellness workbook for health professionals, Mill Valley, Calif., 1977, Wellness Resource Center.

Veatch, R.M.: Voluntary risks to health: the ethical issues, J. Am. Med. Assoc. **243**:50, Jan. 4, 1980.

Wagner, E.H.: The North Karelia project: what it tells us about the prevention of cardiovascular disease, Am. J. Public Health **72**:51, 1982.

Wagner, E.H., et al.: An assessment of health hazard/health risk appraisal, Am. J. Public Health **72**:347, 1982.

Wallston, K.A., and Wallston, B.S., and DeVellis, R.: Development of the multidimensional health locus of control (MHLC) scales, Health Educ. Monogr. 6(2):160, 1978.

Warwick, D.P., and Kelman, H.C.: Ethical issues in social intervention. In Zaltman, G., editor: Processes and phenomena of social change, New York, 1973, John Wiley & Sons, Inc.

Weiss, D.: Who has been responsible for our health in the past? Paper presented at a workshop of the Kentucky Bureau of Health Services, Lexington, March 22, 1977.

Wesley, J.: Primitive physic: or, an easy and natural method for curing most diseases, London, 1747, Thomas Trye.

Wildavsky, A.: Doing better and feeling worse: the political pathology of health policy, Daedalus **106**:105, 1977.

Wiley, J.A., and Camacho, T.C.: Life-style and future health: evidence from the Alameda county study, Prev. Med. **9**:1, 1980.

Williams, C.A.: Community health nursing—what is it? Nurs. Outlook **25**:250, 1977.

Williams, C.L., Carter, B.J., and Eng, A.: The know your body program: a developmental approach to health education and disease prevention, Prev. Med. **9**:371, 1980.

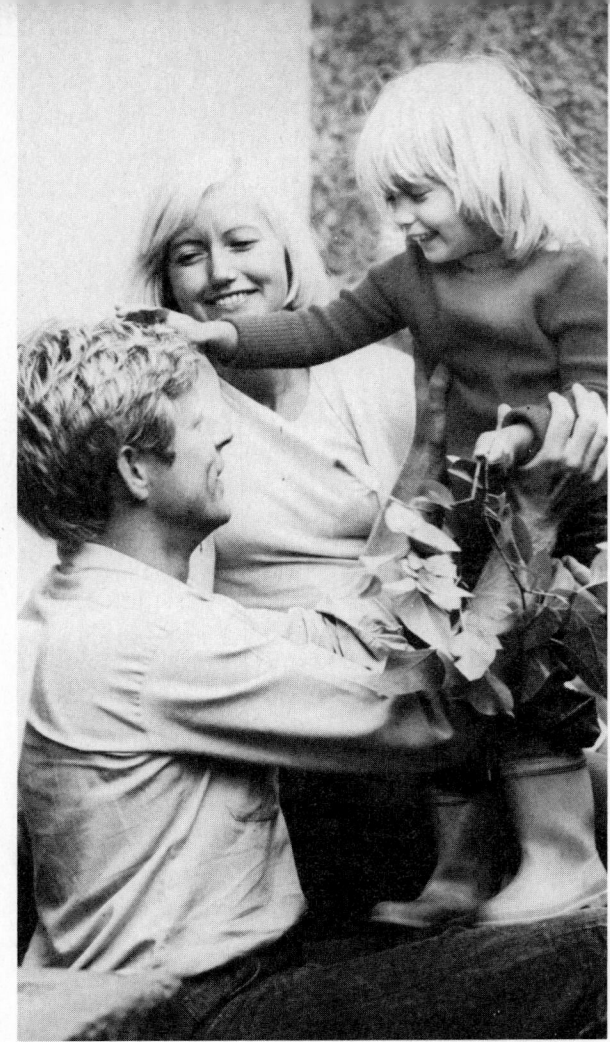

Chapter 15

ROSEMARY JOHNSON

PROMOTING THE HEALTH OF FAMILIES IN THE COMMUNITY

The family is considered the natural and fundamental social unit of society and as such occupies a unique position between individual family members and the community. The family as a mitigating force between individuals and the larger society influences the health and illness behavior of family members, affects the health of the community, and effects health-related changes in the community. Traditionally, the family has been conceptualized as an essential unit of service in community health nursing, and the goal of improving the health of families has endured over time.

The family, as society's most significant unit of social behavior, has been undergoing considerable changes that have affected the family's structure, functions, and interactions, both within the family and in the community. Concomitant with these changes have been changes occurring in other areas related to the health of

families, such as approaches to the delivery of health-illness care, economic and political priorities for health-illness care, and the education and socialization of health care professionals such as community health nurses. All of these changes, as well as those addressed elsewhere in this text, have implications for promoting the health of families in the community.

This chapter discusses selected areas related to family health promotion, with an emphasis on the community health nursing process. It is not possible within the scope of a single chapter to examine all the content areas related to the family; thus the reader is encouraged to draw from the many chapters in the text which have direct application to the study of family health promotion. Chapters 11, 14, 19, and 23 to 28 have content with direct implications for family health.

The concept of the family as a unit of community

health nursing care has been evolving over time, especially during the twentieth century. It is important to briefly review the events that have influenced the evolution of this concept. Throughout much of history the management of physical and emotional illness has been a responsibility assumed by the traditional family within the home environment. By 1850 families started to share the task of caring for ill family members with others, such as physicians (Farrell and Schmitt, 1979). During the 1880s visiting nursing associations began to develop, and visiting nurses, initially called district nurses, started to provide short-term client care in homes. The nurses' home visits included instruction to families about how to care for the ill family members and, in addition, emphasized a healthy life-style for all family members. Through contact with the family and individual family members in the home setting, the visiting nurse became increasingly aware of the influence that the family had on the individual's health.

During the first decade of the 1900s there also was a growing awareness of the relationship between the health of the family and the health of the community. The identified interaction between the health of the individual, family, and community led to the development of new ideas about the scope of practice of the community health nurse. By the middle of that same decade the community health nurse was providing total nursing services for individuals and families.

Since the 1920s numerous official publications and position papers have included statements addressing the concept of the family as a unit of community health nursing service. One of the earliest statements was published in 1932 by the National Organization for Public Health Nursing. Several decades later the Community Health Nursing WHO Expert Committee (1974, p.11), expressed concern over the diminishing importance of family health nursing in community health nursing and made the following statement in a position paper: "Family health nursing is based on the concept of the family as a unit and is directed towards meeting the health needs and concerns of the family by encouraging it to use its own resources . . . [as well as] . . . available health services."

Recent statements by the American Public Health Association Public Health Nursing Section (1980) and the American Nurses' Association Division on Community Health Nursing (1980) describe the family unit, and family members, as the focal units of care for community health nurses. Thus for over half a century the concept of the family as a unit of community health nursing service has been operationalized through the published statements of these two professional groups.

Although there has been a past and present emphasis on health care for the family unit, a close examination of community health nurses' practice reveals that the focus of health care to families has been on individual family members rather than directed toward and provided for the family as a social unit. Community health nurses directing and continuing to direct their services to the health and illness behaviors of individual family members, rather than focusing on the family as the unit of health and illness behavior, has been examined by community health nurses both in education and in practice. There is a general consensus that conceptualization and implementation of family health care are very difficult. One factor contributing to the difficulty in conceptualizing family health care is that the concept of the family itself is changing. In addition, family functions and interaction processes for varying family structures are not clearly defined. This has important implications for the community health nurse, who must be knowledgeable about the relationship between family functions and processes and family health behavior. In addition, the criteria for judging family health are not well formulated.

Numerous factors mitigate against the implementation of the family unit approach in community health nursing. One contributing factor is the financial reimbursement policies of insurance companies and government programs, which make payments for services for individuals rather than families. In addition, many third party payer programs cover illness care and exclude wellness care. Also, there are health care systems (including health departments) that foster an individual client approach.

Service factors that may contribute to inhibiting a family unit approach are the size of the community health nurses' case loads and the health care delivery patterns that influence community health nurses' working hours and accessibility to the total family. In addition to service factors, nursing education must be considered as a negative influence on the professional socialization of students to practice family health care. Many nursing education programs continue to emphasize nursing care of individuals, whether sick or healthy, with less emphasis on the health of the family unit.

Promoting the health of families in the community is difficult, but the perceived difficulties must be tempered with a firm professional conviction that the family unit is a legitimate client of the community health nurse. The challenge for community health nurses is to learn how to assist families to stay well; to value physical, psychological, social, and environmental well-being over morbidity; and to promote healthful family lifestyles. A further challenge for community health nurses is the integration of family health promotion and prevention activities into existing health service delivery systems.

Thus the community health nurse needs to be knowledgeable about how families protect their health, improve their health status, prevent illness, and generate health-protective behaviors in family members. In addition, the community health nurse needs to be knowledgeable about the relationship between community health, family health, and individual health, and how these in turn are influenced by social, cultural, political, and environmental factors. These knowledge areas provide a framework for directing community health nursing care in relation to family health promotion.

THE FAMILY UNIT

The social significance of the family has been founded in its mediating function within the larger society where it "links" the individual family member to societal structures. This linking process serves a society's needs through motivating individuals' participation in the production and distribution of food; protection of the young, old, and sick; socialization of the young; and so forth (Goode, 1964; Leslie, 1973). Although all family units do not fit the traditional definition (i.e., nuclear family) each family, regardless of its structure, has the potential for serving societal needs in one way or another. In addition, families tend to be similar in relation to needs such as affectional interchange; reasonable stability; financial resources for food, clothing, and shelter; educational opportunities; and the availability and accessibility of health services.

Families with which the community health nurse works will represent a variety of structures and living arrangements. The community health nurse is responsible for assisting the family to promote its health, to meet family health needs, and to cope with health problems within the context of the existing family structure and life-style. Thus community health nurses must be knowledgeable about family structures, functions, processes, and roles; in addition, they must be aware of and understand their own values and attitudes pertaining to the family and varying family-life-styles.

The Family in Historical Perspective

Historically the family unit operated as a functional system for mutual protection and survival, which required the combined efforts of all family members. Functions such as health and illness care were performed essentially in the home and usually by the mother. Generally there tended to be a close, supportive relationship with extended family members, and frequently extended family members shared resources

(e.g., food) and services (e.g., care of the sick) with each other. With the advent of industrialization and the growth of bureaucracy, families relinquished to other institutions in society many of the functions once considered the responsibility of the family. Changes having relevance for the family units could be summarized as follows:

1. Families and individual family members became more geographically mobile.
2. Women began to experience increased social opportunities such as moving into higher education and careers.
3. Emphasis on emotional health for the family and individual family members increased.
4. Importance was being accorded to personal enrichment.
5. The divorce rate increased.
6. Acceptance of singlehood in some societies increased.
7. Unemployment rates increased, especially as related to adult children and adult males.
8. Blurring of sex roles occurred.
9. Children became more involved in guiding their own development.
10. New birth technologies and alternatives to childbearing surfaced.
11. People were living longer, and thus, for many, an increased amount of time was being spent in the marital role.
12. More emphasis was placed on leisure time.
13. Experimentation with family forms occurred in response to these social changes and the changing needs of the family unit and individual family members.

Goode (1964) made an interesting observation about the study of family change. He stated that examination of family changes is influenced by prevalent myths from the past. It cannot be shown that family life has changed much through the centuries, but societies tend to develop myths indicating that families of the past lived in greater harmony than do the families of the present.

A consequence of family changes and the emergence of variant family forms has been the increased difficulty associated with defining the family concept. The importance of defining the family rests in the fact that the way one defines the family will determine to some extent how one operationalizes the family's functions and role in society.

Defining the Family

Definitions of the family abound in the literature and frequently are conceptualized in relation to the discipline represented by the definer. For example, a biological approach may conceptualize the family as a unit with the biological function of perpetuating the species. A psychological approach will emphasize the family as a basic unit for personality development and the development of subgroup relationships, such as the parent-child relationship. The discipline of economics views the family from the perspective of how the unit works together to meet material needs. Sociology emphasizes the family's characteristics as a social unit interacting with the larger society. Many definitions of the family include aspects of all these disciplines.

A definition of the nuclear family will be presented first, since this family system is still predominant in the United States. The *nuclear family* has been defined "as a small group consisting of parents and their non-adult children living in a single household" (Farber, 1973, p. 2). Another definition, which is similar to the definition of the nuclear family, views the *family* as "a cluster of people, whose relationship is stipulated by law in terms of marriage and descent, and whose precise membership varies according to the circumstances" (Farber, 1973, p. 2).

In contrast to Farber's definitions, the following two definitions represent broader conceptualizations of the family. Jordheim (1980, p. 61) views the *family* as a "relationship community of two or more persons," in which individuals may come from the same or differ-

ent kinship groups. In a somewhat similar approach Mauksch (1974, p. 522) views the *family* as a basic human unit with "generic properties," namely, "the coexistence of more than one human being involving continuous, presumably permanent sharing of living facilities, a perception of reciprocal obligations, a sense of commonness, and sharing of certain obligations toward each other and towards others." I perceive Mauksch's definition of the family to be congruent with my philosophy about family. This definition encompasses family forms previously excluded by nuclear family definitions.

Thus definitions of the family range from viewing the family as having one structure exclusively to perceiving the family as a household unit representative of various types of family structures. A broad definition or conceptualization of the family is needed in community health nursing, since community health nurses work with families representative of all the aforementioned definitions, that is, families that represent both traditional and nontraditional structures.

Traditional and Nontraditional Families

There is an increasing pluralism in family forms. In addition, the same individual may participate in a number of family life-styles over a lifetime.

The varieties of family forms are numerous, and

Traditional Families
1. Nuclear family—husband, wife, and offspring living in a common household
   a. Single career [husband only working]
   b. Dual career
      1) Wife's career continuous
      2) Wife's career interrupted
2. Nuclear dyad—husband and wife alone: childless, or no children living at home
   a. Single career
   b. Dual career
      1) Wife's career continuous
      2) Wife's career interrupted
3. Single parent family—one head, as a consequence of divorce, abandonment, or separation (with financial aid rarely coming from the second parent), and usually including pre-school and/or school-age children
   a. Career
   b. Non-career
4. Single adult living alone
5. Three generation family—may characterize any variant of family forms 1, 2, or 3 living in a common household
6. Middle aged or elderly couple—husband as provider, wife at home (children have been "launched" into college, career, or marriage)
7. Kin network—nuclear households or unmarried members living in close geographical proximity and operating within a reciprocal system of exchange of goods and services
8. "Second career" family—the wife enters the work force when the children are in school or have left the parental home

these forms overlap and are too subtle for adequate categorization. One attempt at developing a typology of family structures is reflected in the work of Sussman and Cogswell. Sussman's classification (1971) of traditional family structures is outlined in the box on the preceding page.

Cogswell and Sussman's examination (1972) of the increasing variants of the traditional family resulted in the further development of a typology that included experiments with traditional marriages, experimental family forms, and experimental marriages (unions). This typology essentially focuses on the positions or roles present in each family type and identifies the most salient and predominant patterns of relationships and activities.

A taxonomy of experimental families and marriages is found in the box below. The group marriage families are considered to be "experimental" families, since procreation and child rearing are involved. The procreation of children and their socialization may be involved in some of the experimental marriages (unions), but for the most part the alliances focus on adult members' needs for identity, intimacy, and interaction (Cogswell and Sussman, 1972).

Macklin (1980) identified additional nontraditional family alternatives that complement those of Cogswell and Sussman. These additional alternatives are as follows:

1. Never-married singlehood
2. Voluntary childlessness
3. Binuclear family (joint child custody and coparenting)
4. Reconstituted or blended family (stepfamily)

The increased proportion of elderly persons in American society and a growing concern for their welfare has resulted in more attention focused on alternative relationship options for that age group. Some of the alternatives discussed are as follows (Macklin, 1980, p. 915):

1. Polygyny (more than one female mate at one time)
2. Various communal arrangements, e.g., "share-a-home": a quasi-family of nonrelated aged persons share a common household and expenses
3. "Affiliated family": older nonkin are integrated into a younger family unit
4. Nonresidential affiliations: maintenance of relationships with relatives, e.g., intimate family networks, new extended families, expanded families

Working with and serving the needs of families with varying family structures and functions have many implications for health professionals and health-illness care agencies. Pluralism in family forms requires a variety of approaches to meet family health needs.

Community health nurses should continue to devel-

Experimental Forms of Families and Marriages

Group marriage families

Form A: Common residence or compound of households
1. Composed usually of three or more monogamous couples
2. Practice sexual exclusivity
3. Members have ready access to one another for social interactions
4. Share resources, common facilities, and socialization of children
5. Some communes take this form

Form B: Similar to Form A
Sexual swapping within group is practiced

Form C: Mixture of formerly married couples and singles
1. May be composed of all singles
2. With or without sexual swapping

Form D: Multilateral marriage similar to Form B
1. Usually involving fewer than six members
2. Most frequently two-family monogamous couples
3. Sometimes only three persons

Experimental "marriages"

Form A: Nonrelated adults sharing a common household
1. Involving a division of labor
2. With or without sexual accessibility

Form B: Heterosexual cohabitation where there is a de facto marriage with recourse to legal requirements

Form C: Homosexual unions involving same sex pairings in a single household
1. Sharing roles, intimacies, experiences, and resources
2. In some instances more than two members may form a colony or commune

Form D: Affiliated family usually involving unrelated members of different generations
1. For example, aged woman and a single parent and offspring
2. A division of labor appropriate to needs and capabilities of participants

Adapted from Cogswell, B. E., and Sussman, M. B.: Fam. Coord. **21**:506-507, 1972. Copyrighted 1972 by the National Council on Family Relations. Reprinted by permission.

op their knowledge about and understanding of different family structures. This helps the nurse to intervene more effectively with each family on an individual basis to promote and protect the family's health. Furthermore, community health nurses should question whether health care services, social support systems, and their own services are available and accessible to all types of families. Presently most health care services are geared to the traditional, single-career, nuclear family. These services may be inadequate for meeting the needs of other families. For example, the time of the day and week when agency and community health nursing services are available may be incongruent with the schedule of working parents. Action directed at the evaluation and redesigning of health care services may be necessary.

Family Roles and Functions

Working with families necessitates a fundamental knowledge base about family structures and family roles and functions. Knowledge in these areas is essential to adequately *assess* the family and to effectively plan, intervene, and evaluate care *with* the family. There is a vast amount of literature available on family theory and family research. The reader with further interest in this topic is directed to scholarly works in the field of family sociology.

Family Roles

Family roles are related to the organizational structure of the family, the division of labor in the family, and family processes. Part or most of one's lifetime is spent in some type of family in which there are defined role relations, as well as the rights and obligations of each member of the family unit (Goode, 1964). Before examining various family roles and the obligations associated with those roles, it is important to define the terms *role* and *position.*

1. *Role*—a set of characteristic behaviors, prescribed and proscribed, expected of people occupying a given position
2. *Position*—an identity given to two or more persons who share specific attributes or behaviors that set them apart from other people

In a family, an individual will occupy a position of spouse, parent, or sibling, and certain roles are associated with each position. An example of a set of behaviors related to the spouse position would be the sexual role. Positions and roles within the context of any family can change over time. There are societal as well as family expectations for behaviors associated with certain family roles and these expectations may not be congruent. Similarly, differences may exist within families. Each

family tends to modify family roles in relation to the family structure and to forces internal and external to the family unit.

Adult Role. The work of Nye (1976) has been selected as an example of family adult roles. The enactment of these roles (described here), as well as the behaviors associated with the roles, will vary in relation to the family form, that is, traditional or nontraditional family form.

1. *Child socialization:* encompasses processes and activities in the family which contribute to the development of the child's social and mental capacities
2. *Child care:* involves provision of physical and emotional care to the child for the purpose of developing a healthy individual
3. *Provider role:* includes the production of goods and services needed by the family or the obtaining of them through the exchange of goods and services
4. *Housekeeper role:* involves preparing and maintaining the goods and services for the family's use. This role also includes services in the home that contribute to family members' pleasure and comfort
5. *Kinship role:* includes the maintenance of contact with kin and, in addition, implies assistance during periods of crisis
6. *Sexual role:* requires mutual participation of both partners, with the implicit assumption that both partners enjoy the sexual relations
7. *Therapeutic role:* entails assisting the family member to cope with problems and providing emotional support, as well as handling interfamilial problems
8. *Recreational role:* implies family recreation and possesses aspects of relaxation, entertainment, and personal development

Sibling Role. As noted previously, one of the positions that may exist within a family is that of sibling. Sibling roles may include involvement in the household division of labor such as child care tasks. Siblings are also instigators of socialization in the family as well as recipients of the socialization process.

A *sibling relationship* refers to the nature of interaction between brothers and sisters. Schvaneveldt and Thinger (1979, pp. 459-460) listed functions performed on a day-to-day basis within the sibling (sib) interactional system:

1. *Identification:* process by which a sib experiences life vicariously through the behavior of the other sib(s) and learns through the other sib's experiences

2. *Differentiation:* process of a sib defining one's own identity and space in the family rather than fusing with a sib
3. *Mutual regulation:* process whereby sibs serve as "mirrors, sounding boards, and testing grounds" for each other
4. *Direct services:* sibs teach each other skills, "manipulate powerful friendship rewards for each other," control resources, act as buffers for each other, and so forth
5. *Negotiate with parents:* sibs negotiate with parents for one another, form coalitions against adult power, and serve as translators between a sib and parents
6. *Pioneering:* one sib initiates a process, thereby giving permission to other sibs to follow accordingly

Linking Role. One final family role that requires attention is the linking role (Sussman, 1974, p. 233). This involves "competencies in handling the normative demands of bureaucracies while sustaining a modicum of humanness and family identification." The socialization process for the linking role includes representing the family or kin, such as the elderly, in dealing with bureaucratic organizations. The family's objectives and needs for physical maintenance, specifically the need for health care, requires a linking role. For example, to meet a specific need the family may have identified that it must have contact with the health care agency, a bureaucratic organization. The linking relationship between the family and the health care agency is facilitated by a selected family member who contacts the agency to negotiate for needed services. An alternative approach might be to contact a linking group in the community who assumes responsibility for reducing social distance between a family and an agency. The community health nurse, assuming an advocacy position, might assume this linking responsibility, thereby reducing the family-agency social distance.

■   ■   ■

The preceding discussion of family roles has included references to various family-related functions associated with specific roles. The following section will continue the discussion of family functions, but from a more general perspective.

Family Functions

A *function* may be defined as an expected action of someone in a given role. It is through the enactment of family roles that family functions are fulfilled.

All families have certain functions that are performed to maintain the integrity of the family unit and to meet the family unit's needs, individual family member's needs, and society's expectations. Family members in systems with two or more individuals have functional responsibilities in relation to their social position. Depending on the position one occupies, the member may function as provider, homemaker, companion, health motivator, and/or sexual partner. These roles are important for the maintenance of the family system. The family unit also fulfills its responsibilities toward the larger community through constructive participation in appropriate organizations and through the exchange of services with various other social systems.

One approach to examining family functions is in relation to the family's physical, affectional, and social properties (Murray et al., 1975). Examples of these three types of functions are as follows:

1. *Physical functions:* provision of food, clothing, and shelter; protection against danger; provision for health and illness care
2. *Affectional functions:* meeting emotional needs
3. *Social functions;* provision for social togetherness; fostering self-esteem; supporting creativity and initiative

Another approach to the examination of family functions is from a task-oriented perspective. A *task* is defined as a "function, but with work or labor overtones assigned to or demanded of the person" (Murray et al., 1975). Sussman (1971) delineates the main tasks of families as being the following:

1. The socialization of children
2. Strengthening the competency of family members in relation to their adjustments within organizations (e.g., school, place of occupation)
3. Appropriate use of social organizations
4. Providing an environment that fosters the development of identities and affectional behavior
5. Creating a satisfying, emotionally healthy environment essential to the family's well-being

Implicit in many of the aforementioned functions and tasks is the function of *adaptation,* both within the family and in relation to society. The adaptation function is vital to the family in a society experiencing rapid and pervasive social changes. By adapting its structure and functions, the family meets the changing needs of society and other social systems. The following example illustrates a family's adaptation to a larger social system:

The American economic system requires a mobile labor force. Thus when an employing company dictates that an adult family member move to another city to further the company's objectives, either the entire family moves, the respective family member makes the move alone and commutes periodically to see the family, or the individual may resign from the job. Regardless of the final decision, family members and the family as a whole experience changes.

> ### Criteria for Assessing Family's Strengths
>
> - The ability to provide for the physical, emotional, and spiritual needs of a family.
> - The ability to be sensitive to the needs of the family members.
> - The ability to communicate effectively.
> - The ability to provide support, security, and encouragement.
> - The ability to initiate and maintain growth-producing relationships and experiences within and without the family.
> - The capacity to maintain and create constructive and responsible community relationships in the neighborhood, the school, town, local and state governments.
> - The ability to grow with and through children.
> - The ability to perform family roles flexibly.
> - An ability for self help and the ability to accept help when appropriate.
> - Mutual respect for the individuality of family members.
> - The ability to use a crisis experience or seemingly injurious experience as a means of growth.
> - A concern for family unity, loyalty, and interfamily cooperation.

Adapted from Otto, H. E.: Fam. Process **2**:333, Sept. 1963.

Vincent (1967) states that the family's adaptive function may have "spongelike" characteristics. That is, the family may absorb much of the blame for social problems such as delinquency and alcoholism. Another form of family adaptiveness to the larger society is families' compliant behavior in the political and health-illness systems. Compliant behavior as adaptation may be interpreted as appropriate if the consequences are in the family's best interest. On the other hand, compliant behavior may be inappropriate if it places the family in a passive recipient position and the family's power and authority are relinquished.

Otto's criteria (1963) for assessing family strengths address both family functions and family processes (see box above). *Family strengths* are defined as "those factors or forces that contribute to family unity and solidarity and that foster the development of the potentials inherent within the family" (Otto, 1973, p. 88). Family strengths are considered to be interrelated and vary according to the family life cycle stages.

The family strengths' framework has proved to be valuable for community health nurses in psychosocial assessment and in planning health care programs with families. The community health nurse can assist the family in identifying and developing its strengths and in using these strengths for family problem solving (Otto, 1973).

FAMILY HEALTH

Family health as a concept is based on the premise that health of the family unit is more than the sum of the individual family members' health-illness behaviors. The family as a social unit develops a system of values, beliefs, and attitudes about health and illness that are imparted to and demonstrated through the health-illness behaviors of the family members. The family also functions as the primary intermediary for transmitting health-related cultural traits to the next generation. It is through the family that family members learn the beliefs and practices concerning health and illness of the larger society.

The general concept of family health as presently used is ambiguous, sometimes referring to the health of family members and at other times meaning the state of the family itself. The World Health Organization (1976, p. 17) proposes using the term *familial health*, which "connotes the relative functioning of the family as the primary social agent in the promotion of health and well-being." An interesting observation has been pointed out by the WHO Study Group on Statistical Indices of Family Health (1970, p. 13) in relation to defining family health. The group states that health in relation to the family should not be defined in terms of "absence or presence of disease," since only individuals, per se, have diseases. Furthermore, "physical or mental health can be measured only in respect to the individual family members." Thus if the family is regarded as a unit in relation to health behavior, with family patterns of illness, responses to symptoms, and use of health and illness facilities, it should be recognized that these behaviors are representative of individuals acting in the name of, or through the influence of, the family (World Health Organization, 1976, p. 20). This perspective on family and individual health should be viewed within the context of the interrelationship between family structure and functioning and family members' health.

Family health is frequently described in terms of the family's or family members' interpersonal relationships, developmental tasks, family processes, coping behaviors, functioning, and family organization and integration. For example, family health and illness have been conceptualized as family processes and as products of continuously interacting forces within the family, among family members, and within each family

---

Interrelationship Between Family Health and Family Members' Health

Family factors affecting family members

- Sociodemographic characteristics
- Organization (size, composition, etc.)
- Developmental stage
- Roles/role relationships
- Division of labor functions
- Processes (communication, decision making, etc.)
- Socialization processes
- Developmental (physical, psychosocial) support
- Level of functioning
- Attitudes toward individual family members
- Health standards
- Health values, beliefs, attitudes
- Health goals

Family members' factors affecting family and other family members

- Transmission of congenital defect
- Transmission of disease
- Developmental disability
- Long-term health problem
- Terminal illness
- Health risk behaviors
- Decision maker
- Problem solver
- Health care provider
- Experiences in community
- Experiences with health-illness
- Care providers
- Family role (mother, father, etc.)

Reciprocal factors

- Health practices
- Initiator of health behavior
- Priority placed on health
- Conceptualization of health-illness
- Source/cause of illness
- Source/cause of health problems
- Definer of sick role
- Coping behaviors
- Resources

---

member (Mauksch, 1974). Smilkstein (1980, p. 224) states that "a *family in health* is one whose members perceive it as cohesive and offering the nurturement and resources that are necessary for personal growth and sustenance in the face of life's challenges."

In the last analysis, each family unit must be viewed from an individual family perspective which includes that family's unique biological, physical, and social-psychological characteristics. The uniqueness of the family will be further influenced by its sociodemographic characteristics (socioeconomic status, ethnicity, etc.), and its relationship with the broader society in which the family is situated. Finally, and most importantly, the family unit will define continuously and systematically for itself the parameters of health and illness, as well as what constitutes appropriate health promotion and maintenance behavior.

Relationship Between Family Health and Individual Health

The family is the primary social system within which the individual develops, is nurtured, and becomes socialized and where personal growth and autonomy are fostered. The family contributes to individual family members' health through supporting their (members')

biophysical and psychosocial development. Within the family system individual members learn to interact with others and develop social skills. The members learn how to cope with personal, family, and societal problems, and they learn methods for developing external family linkages with community groups and organizations. It is also within the family unit that members develop their concept of health and establish their health habits.

The health-illness behaviors of the family as a whole and of family members as individuals are dynamically interrelated and are continuously interacting with and influencing each other. Health problems in one family member affect the other family members and impact on the family as a whole. The level of the family's functioning and state of organization influence the behavior of individual members. The family, rationally or irrationally, establishes health standards and practices that are imparted to the members. Many of the conceptions about health and illness and healthful and unhealthful actions acquired by the child are learned in unplanned, unintentional, accidental ways in the family (Hochbaum, 1970).

Another important factor associated with the interrelationship between family health and individual health is that family members possess individual characteristics, personality, and behavioral style. Individual members are perceived and responded to differently by other family members, thereby influencing individual health and illness behavior. The individuals themselves through their interactional experiences in the family and in society develop their own perceptions about health, illness, and health practices. Thus the individual's concept of health is the result of experiences inside and outside the family and may be modified in relation to new experiences and developmental transitions. Changes in health behaviors of individual family members may contribute to modifications in the general health behavior of the family unit. The box on the opposite page summarizes some of the factors associated with the interrelationship between individual and family health. The lists are not considered to be comprehensive, and the reader is encouraged to include additional factors.

Family Health Estate Concept of Mauksch

A family health concept that focuses on the interdependence of the health of the family and the health of individual family members has been developed by Mauksch (1974). This conceptualization, referred to as the *family health estate,* views each family (a primary human unit) as a unique and distinct health behavior unit. The family health estate concept can serve as an "organizing principle for knowledge" about the family's health that is not attainable by inquiring into the health behavior of individual family members only (Fig. 15-1). The family as a unit represents a fusion or combination of the properties that the "family members contribute within the context of their culture, their awareness of health relevant knowledge, and their unique individual ways of introducing these factors into the emerging family" (Mauksch, 1974, p. 524). The emerging family, consisting of the founding individuals and any additional members who join the unit, develops health values, health habits, and health risk perceptions characteristic of that individual family. The family health estate also involves health-related roles and task allocations within the family system.

Fig. 15-1 depicts the family (A) as founded by unit members (B) who infuse their biological and psychosocial properties, cultural norms, values, beliefs, attitudes, etc. into the family system. Each individual's properties interact with and are modified by the properties of the other individual. This interactional process (linking) continues during the inclusion of other members (C) into the family system (A) and/or through social interactions (linking) outside of the family. The linking processes within the family may be positive (pleasurable, stress reducing, etc.) or negative (uncomfortable,

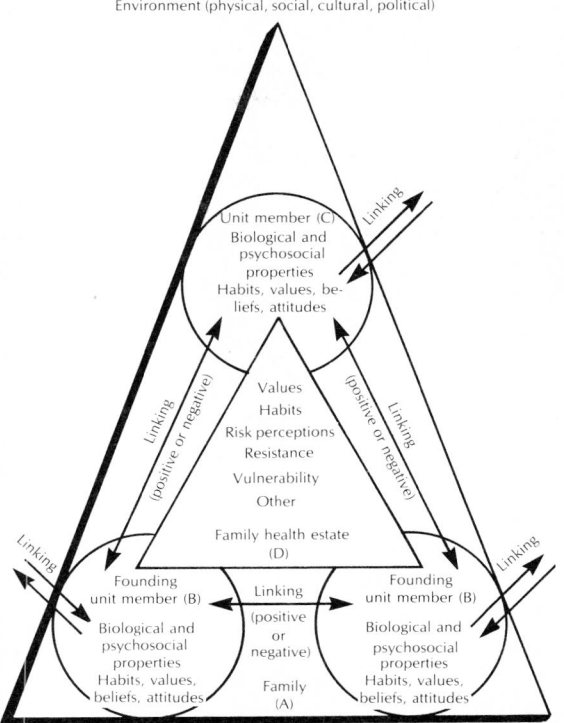

Fig. 15-1. Schematic portrayal of the family health estate as described by Mauksch. (From Mauksch, H.: Soc. Sci. Med. 8:521, 1974.)

stress producing, etc.). Threats to the family's health may be a consequence of the weakening of the family linking system (disorganization), with resulting implications for the health status of the individual family members. Conversely, any dysfunction that affects a family member may affect the family unit. The health of the family as a functioning unit can and should be distinguished from the health of the family members who possess individual health status and are subject to individual illness risks. The family's health values, perceptions, beliefs, and attitudes; health habits; and so forth—the family health estate—influence the family unit and individual behavior in relation to health promotion, "disease prevention, illness susceptibility, illness management, recuperation and reintegration, and illness consequences" (Mauksch, 1974, p. 525). In turn, individual experiences in social systems outside the family, such as school and occupational health programs, can influence the family health estate (D) through the modification or changing of habits. Similarly, family experiences with health and life-threatening situations can alter the family health estate. In the final analysis, health and illness are viewed as products of continuously interacting forces within the family, among its members, and within each family member.

Family Health Tasks

A basic family function is to protect the health of its members and to provide supportive, nurturing care during periods of illness. One of the premises inherent in health promotion and illness/disease/disability prevention is that the primary responsibility for health belongs to the individual and the family. The manner in which the family carries out its health-illness care responsibilities, and the ability to do so, will be influenced by factors such as the family's structure, division of labor, socioeconomic status, and ethnicity. The list of health-related functions and tasks in the adjoining box is applicable to most families, but the extent to which these functions and tasks will be observed for every family will vary in accordance with the aforementioned family characteristics.

The community health nurse supports the family in its ability to perform health-related functions and tasks, contributes through assisting the family in strengthening its resources for carrying out these responsibilities, and intervenes more directly as necessitated by the family situation. Effective intervention with the family will be based on an adequate family assessment, which includes data about the family's health status (organization, functioning, etc.); individual family member's health status; health standards and practices in the family; family conceptions about health and illness; family perceptions about its responsibility for health-illness care; health-illness care resources; and family values, attitudes, and beliefs related to health and illness.

FAMILY HEALTH AND COMMUNITY HEALTH

The health of families and the family's health-illness activities are intrinsically related to the health of the larger community. As stated in the American Public Health Association's definition (1980) of public health nursing, public health nurses work with families in accomplishing the goal of "improving the health of the entire community." The American Nurses' Association's definition (1980) makes it explicit that nursing directed to families "contributes to the health of the total population." The health-illness behaviors of families influence the health status and health-illness care resources in the community. Similarly, the health status of the community and the availability, accessibility, and attractiveness of health-illness care resources in the community can affect the health status and health-illness behaviors of families.

Levels of Wellness

Dunn (1967, p. 167) states that " . . . the family stands in between individual wellness and social well-

---

Family Health Functions and Tasks

- Provision of adequate food, shelter, and clothing
- Maintenance of health-supporting physical home environment
- Maintenance of health-supporting psychosocial home environment
- Provision of resources for maintenance of personal hygiene
- Provision for meeting spiritual needs
- Health education
- Health promotion (nutrition, exercise, etc.)
- Health-illness decision making
- Recognition of developmental disruptions
- Recognition of health disruptions
- Seeking health care
- Seeking illness care
- Seeking dental care
- First aid
- Supervision of medications (prescribed and over-the-counter)
- Illness care (short-term and long-term)
- Rehabilitation care
- Involvement with the community's health

---

ness. You can't really have high-level wellness for either individuals or social groups unless you have well families." To achieve wellness the family must be an integrated unit striving to develop its fullest potential physically, mentally, spiritually, and socially. Family health then includes the promotion and maintenance of physical, mental, spiritual, and social health for the family unit and for individual family members. The individual-family-social wellness relationship addressed by Dunn could be depicted as shown in Fig. 15-2.

The levels of wellness of the individual family members, the family, and the larger society are all interrelated either directly or indirectly. For example, the impact of the level of wellness of the individual family member on the community, as well as the impact of the community's level of wellness on the individual, may be indirectly mediated by the family. And as noted by Dunn, the family's wellness level influences the wellness status of both the community (society) and the individuals in the family. For example, the healthy family serves as a resource for the community through preparing and providing healthy family members who are capable of adequately functioning in designated social roles, such as parental, student, and occupational roles. Families experiencing nonhealth states can collectively influence the health status of the community in which they reside, are less capable of participating adequately in their socially designated roles, and can place excessive de-

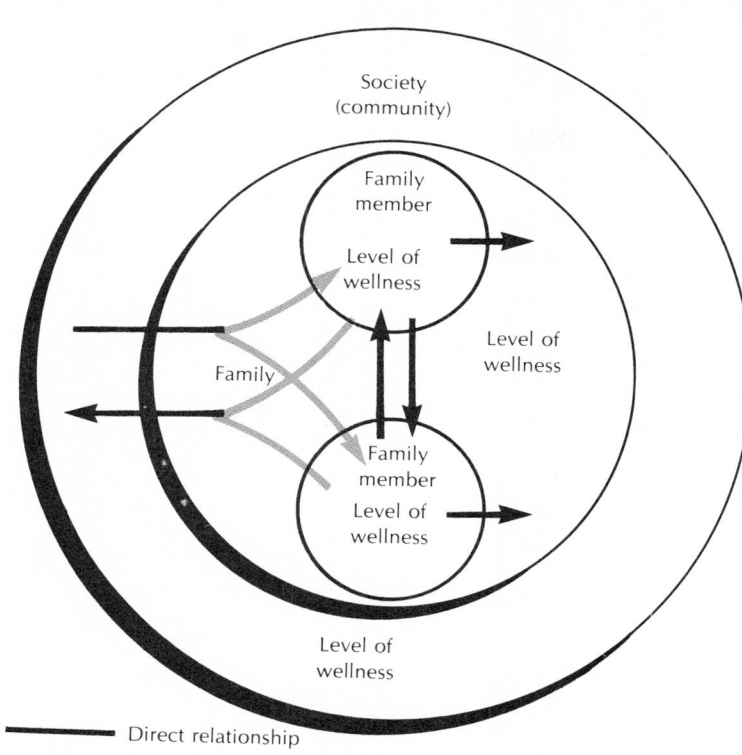

Fig. 15-2. Relationships of individual, family, and social wellness.

——————— Direct relationship

——————— Indirect relationship

mands on the illness care systems as well as other human service systems in the community.

Indirect Influences

Families are capable of influencing or contributing to the health of the community through other means also. Families may politically influence the enactment of health-related legislation such as the availability of family planning resources and more stringent drunken driving laws. Additionally, family members contribute directly to health-supporting and illness care agencies through financial contributions, volunteer work, and blood donations (Pratt, 1976). Thus by promoting and maintaining the health of family members and by participating in the successful functioning of the larger community, the family is also contributing to the promotion and maintenance of the health of the community.

Systems Perspective

Another approach to examining the relationship between family health and community health is from a systems perspective. Blum (1976), building on Brody's hierarchy (1973) of systems for homo sapiens, demonstrated the relationship between systems as relevant to illness and disability. Brody's hierarchy of systems started with subatomic particles, the smallest system, and progressed to the biosphere level. The systems in

the hierarchy most relevant for this discussion (in ascending order) are cells, tissues, organs, body systems, persons, families, communities and organizations, nations (societies), and cultures.

A system in the hierarchy interacts with the systems directly above it and the systems directly below it: the system's homeostasis is dependent on these interactions (Blum, 1976). If some force(s) overcomes the homeostatic mechanisms of the initially affected system, this system may in turn act as a disrupting force on the systems directly above and below it. The resulting impact could have both a domino and ping-pong effect. That is, there could be sequential disruptions throughout all systems (domino effect), as well as the resulting disruptions in the systems above and below (ping-pong effect). As depicted in Fig. 15-3, a force (health situation) may originate within the individual and affect only the family (e.g., a temporary illness), or it may affect both the family and community (e.g., alcoholism and drunken driving). Similarly, misuse of alcohol could be a family behavior having innumerable implications for the health of individual family members and the community.

Blum (1976) exemplified one instance of the spread of disequilibrium downward through the hierarchy of systems as a consequence of cultural values and change in relation to war and peace values:

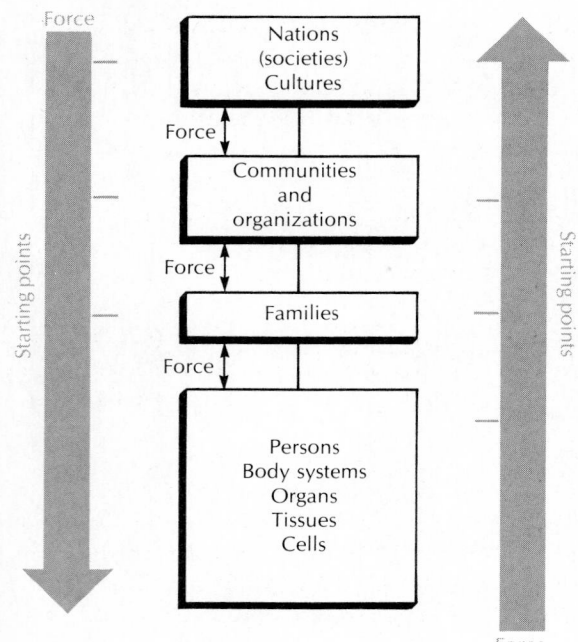

Force

Starting points

Nations
(societies)
Cultures

Force

Communities
and
organizations

Force

Families

Force

Persons
Body systems
Organs
Tissues
Cells

Starting points

Force

Fig. 15-3. Family health and community health: a systems perspective.

Hypothetically, assume that numerous cultural systems decide that the values of peace and general human welfare take priority over war and full domestic employment, and there is a resulting national policy that the manufacturing of armed services aircraft will cease. Some communities would experience a loss of income, and possible out-migration of engineers and skilled workers. Concomitantly, the families of aerospace engineers previously employed by such aircraft industries would experience economic and emotional stress, and possible role realignment or changes if, for example, the spouse had to seek employment, or an adult child had to drop out of college. Additional changes might be the loss of health insurance and other benefits. Consequences for the individual engineer could be the loss of self esteem, and the need to learn new skills as well as adjusting to changing life styles. The final outcome for one or more of the family members could be the development of digressive social behaviors, or other stress related illnesses. At this point one might begin to observe the spread of disequilibrium upward through the hierarchy of systems, as the behaviors of individual family members begin to impact on the health status and coping behavior of the family. The family's ability or inability to cope adequately, and to adjust with or without consequential family disorganization has obvious consequences for the community. Family disorganization places demands on the community's health and human services' resources, as well as reducing the availability of productive, contributing family mem-

bers in the community. Multiple families experiencing states of disorganization would eventually affect the general health status of the community.*

Conclusions

In some health-related situations the family functions as the dependent variable and the community as the independent variable in the illness/disease/disability prevention and health promotion causal relationships. That is, the community as the independent variable influences or affects families' health status and health promotion behavior. In other situations, the family serves as the independent variable and affects the health status, health promotion, and illness/disease/disability prevention functions of the community.

FAMILY HEALTH PROMOTION AND ILLNESS PREVENTION

Health promotion and illness/disease/disabilty prevention are the essence of community health nursing practice and comprise a major goal in working with families. The expected outcomes of health promotion with the family are the continuation of the family's adequate level of functioning and coping or improvement in one or both of these behaviors; the maintenance of or improvement in the family's general overall health status; and the family's continued assumption or increased assumption of self-responsibility (family) for promoting and protecting the family's health.

There are numerous definitions of health promotion, the majority of which are similar to Leavell and Clark's definition (1955) of *health promotion* as a primary level of prevention. Leavell and Clark delineated three levels of prevention: *primary prevention* includes health promotion and specific protection; *secondary prevention* involves early diagnosis and prompt, adequate treatment; and *tertiary prevention* focuses on rehabilitation. The three levels of prevention are not necessarily discrete categories of behaviors and activities; some activities related to one level of prevention may be appropriate activities for another level of prevention. For example, a health promotion activity such as health education may be viewed as a specific protection activity also, with the difference being in the educational content.

Generally, health promotion involves behaviors and procedures, such as good nutrition, exercise, and adequate rest and relaxation, directed at supporting or im-

*Modified from Blum, H. L.: Expanding health care horizons: from a general systems concept of health to a national health policy, Oakland, Calif., Third Party Associates, Inc.

proving health and well-being of a nonspecific nature. Specific protection involves measures directed toward a particular health problem risk factor, or disease. The application of the prevention measure, such as immunizations, is for the purpose of preventing the disease or problem from ever occurring in the individual. Health promotion may involve the support of existing health life-styles, the modification or change of existing lifestyle behaviors, or the addition of new behaviors and practices.

In addition to the aforementioned outcomes of health promotion with the family, Pender (1982) identified the following expected outcomes (for the family) of health promotive nursing care: competence in minimizing barriers that prevent personal or family growth and development, improved ability to make rational health-related decisions, ability to assess correctly the needs for professional health care, judicious use of health care services, and greater availability and accessibility of health-promoting rather than health-damaging options.

For most of the health promotion outcomes addressed, the family is an active participant. Thus the family can be perceived as motivated and responsible for adopting, adapting, and using active strategies for health promotion or as being a passive recipient of health promotion and prevention. There is the risk that if the family assumes the passive role to any great extent and for long periods of time, the family's motivation for self-responsibility may decrease considerably. Examples of a family's *passive position* are found in situations in which health care providers tend to assume the family's decision-making and problem-solving functions. Among *active strategies* are activities related to basic health habits such as eating three regularly scheduled meals a day; no snacking; moderate exercise, at least two or three times a week; 7 or 8 hours of sleep each night; no smoking; maintenance of moderate weight; and no consumption of alcohol or only in moderation (Belloc and Breslow, 1973).

Health Models

Family health promotion must be examined within the context of the family as a sociocultural system as well as within the broader sociocultural system external to the family. Five variables directly related to the family's sociocultural orientation are motivation, perception, values, attitudes, and beliefs. These five factors are interrelated and intrinsically influence health promotion behavior.

Motivation involves a conscious or unconscious need or desire to act. Assuming that health behavior is caused behavior, then motivation factors such as

needs, concerns, wants, and expectations are involved in governing health promotion behavior. Furthermore, the manner in which the motives are expressed in relation to any situation, such as health promotion will depend on the way health promotion is perceived and interpreted and judged, as well as on the individual's concerns associated with health promotion. For example, in one family, some family members may be motivated to exercise because of a desire to improve their physical appearance while other family members may perceive exercise as a means of avoiding high blood pressure. Although there are various reasons why family members exercise, the entire family is motivated to exercise.

Perception is the process of acquiring knowledge about oneself and the surrounding environment. This information results in a personal definition of the world in which the individual resides. Perception is associated with assumptions developed from personal experiences such as health-illness situations. How the family or individual family member responds to a proposed health promotion activity, such as dietary changes, will be influenced by the perceptions associated with the changes, as well as perceptions about alternative actions.

Values, attitudes, and beliefs are interrelated and have both direct and indirect influence on health behavior. These three variables are associated with tendencies to respond to the environment and people in distinctive positive or negative ways. The family's personal and social values; beliefs about itself and the external sociocultural world; and attitudes toward others and itself guide family health behaviors.

1. *Values* refer to the felt importance, desirability, or worth of phenomena or actions.
2. *Attitudes* are opinions held about tangible and intangible phenomena that affect one's actions.
3. *Beliefs* are judgments or the acceptance of phenomena as real or true.

Family planning exemplifies the interrelatedness of values, attitudes, and beliefs. A family's religious and cultural value orientations may strongly influence their values regarding the interference with natural reproductive processes. These values in turn influence the family's tendency to respond favorably or unfavorably toward family planning measures and will influence the family's judgment about family planning as right or wrong.

Perceptions, beliefs, attitudes, and values are formed and changed throughout developmental and situational experiences. Beliefs are considered to be easier to change than attitudes, and attitudes are easier to change or modify than values (Rokeach, 1968).

Health Belief Model

The aforementioned variables in combination with other variables, particularly sociodemographic factors, have been studied in relation to their function as determinants of health behavior. Several such studies culminated in the health belief model (Rosenstock, 1974). The model was formulated to explain health-related behavior at the level of individual (i.e., family member) decision making. Although the formulation focuses on individual perceptions, many of the variables are relevant to the family unit.

The major components of the health belief model are *beliefs* (perceived susceptibility, perceived seriousness, perceived benefits of taking action and barriers to action), *cues to action,* (advice from others, newspaper articles), and *modifying factors* (demographic variables such as age or sex, sociopsychological variables such as personality or reference group, structural variables such as knowledge about and experience with health situations). All of these factors function together in relation to the likelihood of engaging in health-promotive or health-preventive behavior. Decision making related to engaging or not engaging in a particular health-promotive or health-preventive behavior involves perceptions about susceptibility and serves as a stimulus for appropriate action.

Although not identified as such in the health belief model, a relationship should be noted between the demographic, sociopsychological, and structural variables and cues to action. For example, the kind of materials read may be associated with age, sex, and social classes and advice from others may tend to be from peer groups. In addition, the relationship between cues to action and perceived action benefits/action barriers should be viewed as important. For instance, advice from others can influence perceptions about the benefits or negative aspects of certain health behaviors.

The health belief model can be applied to the case of a middle-aged couple with below average income (one family member recently unemployed). Both family members are at high risk for hypertension and in need of changing some of their health habits, such as engaging in moderate exercise and reducing their weight, salt intake, alcohol consumption, and stress. In assisting this family to change or modify some of their life-style behaviors and add new practices, the community health nurse would need to know the family's perceptions about hypertension as well as perceptions about engaging in health practices that could contribute to reducing the risk (susceptibility) of becoming hypertensive. Do the family members perceive that they are at risk for hypertension? What are their perceptions about the seriousness of hypertension, such as the physical threat, the implications regarding work, and so forth?

What factors are associated with their perceptions of the threat of hypertension, for example, knowledge about hypertension? What are their perceptions about the benefits and barriers to changing health practices? This particular family may perceive that the family members are at risk for hypertension because of their age, may view hypertension as serious because of their present family situation as well as what they know about the condition, and see some benefits in starting to modify one or more of their health practices. At the same time, they may believe that there are some health practices that they cannot change. Knowing about the family's perceptions in relation to hypertension provides the community health nurse with important information (data) essential to planning and working with this family.

Preventive Behavior Model

Suchman (1967) proposed a model of preventive behavior that has relevance for both the individual member and the family. The model proposes that individuals and groups such as the family be assessed according to personal readiness factors, social control factors, and situational or action factors (Fig. 15-4).

The *personal readiness factors* include recognition of the seriousness of the health problem, acceptance of personal vulnerability, predisposition to take health-preventive or health-protective action, motivation to act, ability to act (physically and psychologically), knowledge about the desired health action (knowing how to act), and belief in the desired action.

The *social control factors* exemplify the interrelationship between the individual member's and family's health-related behaviors. One of these factors is social pressure to act; the individual must feel that the family approves of the desired health action and that the family will take action also. The health behavior act must be incorporated into the individual's role performance and be appropriate for fulfilling role obligations, such as those expected of the parent role. Finally, the health action must be congruent with the values and usual behavior patterns of the individual and family (Suchman, 1967).

The *situational or action factors* tend to be associated with the implementation phase of the health action. The health behavior must offer the individual and family more benefits (rewards) than discomforts (giving up pleasurable habit). The family environment must be favorable for the use and completion of the action, the action should not demand too much effort or be too disruptive, and it should produce the effect desired by the individual and family. Finally, the health action to be taken must be attractive, and the individual and family must not have had previous negative experi-

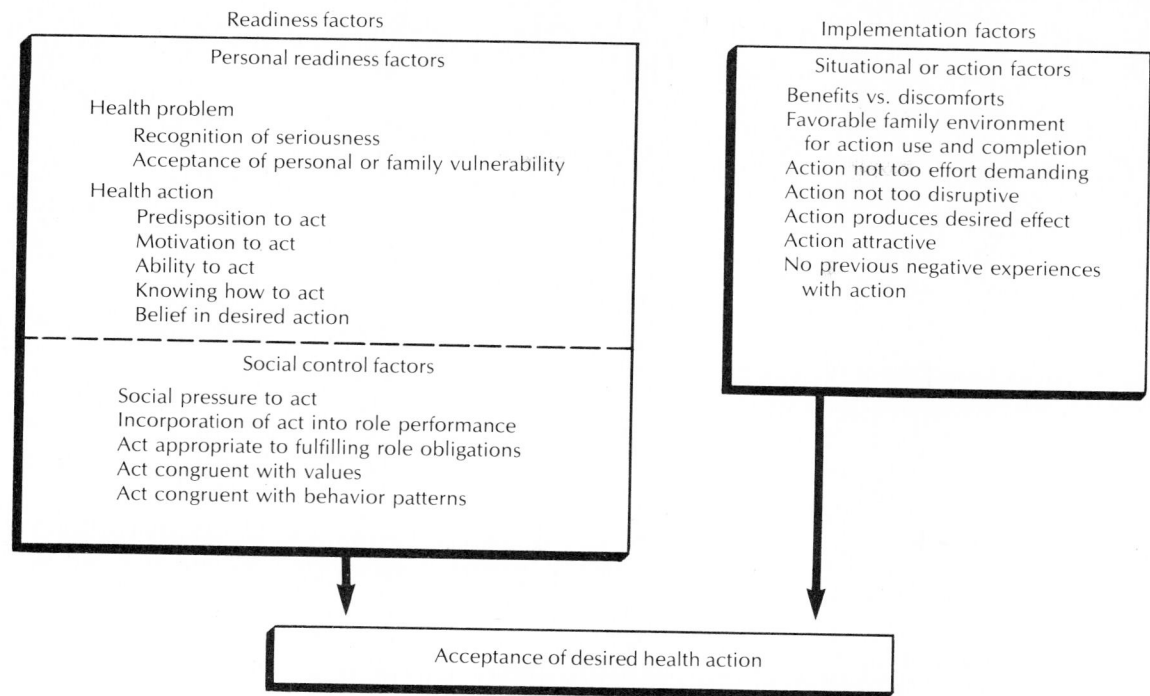

Fig. 15-4. Schematic portrayal of Suchman's preventive behavior model.

ences with the desired action. The degree of acceptance of the desired health action will be dependent on the extent to which the conditions of all of the aforementioned factors are met (Suchman, 1967).

The Suchman model introduces more variables for the family health assessment process, such as personal readiness factors related to the desired health action (e.g., ability and knowing how to act) and social control factors related to family and social roles, in addition to those included in the health belief model.

Social-Ecological Perspectives Health Model

Another approach to assessing health promotion and prevention behavior has been formulated by Moos (1979). The conceptual framework, referred to as a social-ecological perspective, examines the relationship between environmental and personal variables and health status. The framework derives its name from the inclusion of social-environmental and physical-environmental (ecological) variables (Fig. 15-5). The framework depicts a unidirectional causal flow for purposes of simplicity, but it should be acknowledged that there is an interrelationship between the different sets of factors based on feedback mechanisms.

The *environmental factors,* not to be considered inclusive, are grouped into four sets of variables that influence family health directly or indirectly. The *physi-*

cal setting variables include such factors as topography, temperature, rainfall, and architectural and design characteristics. In addition to directly affecting health status, physical environmental factors may influence health indirectly through its effect on the social environment. *Organizational factors* refer to industrial sites, educational institutions, health and illness care facilities, etc., that are related to functional effectiveness and use of health care services. The *human aggregate factors* refer to sociodemographic characteristics such as age, education, and socioeconomic background. The *social climate* (environment) has three basic dimensions. The relationship dimension examines the degree of the family's involvement in the environment and the extent of the mutual support and open communication between the family and societal components. The personal growth (goal orientation) dimension assesses family development in a specific setting. The dimensions of system maintenance and system change refer to the degree of orderliness in the environment as well as its response to change (Moos, 1979).

The *personal system* variables explicate the individuality of responses to varying environments. The personal system factors influence a family's perception of the environment or situation and affect the psychological and intellectual resources available to that family for managing the situation. The variables identified for

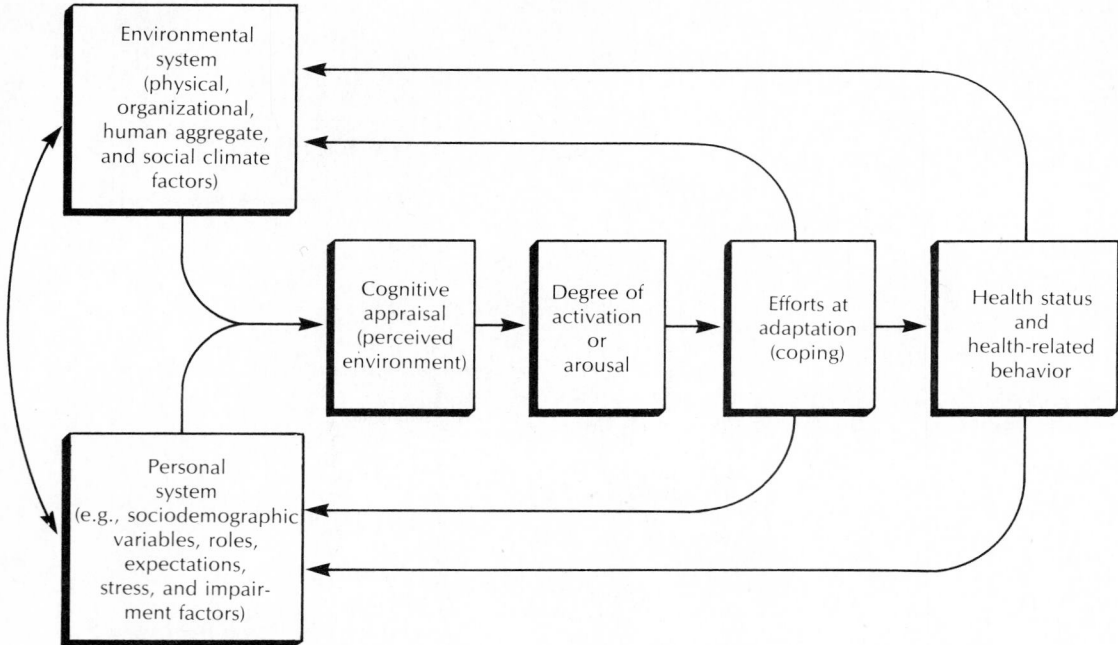

Fig. 15-5. A simplified model of the relationship between environmental and personal variables and health. (From Moos, R. H.: Social-ecological perspectives in health. In Stone, G. C., Cohen, F., and Adler, N. E., editors: Health psychology—a handbook: theories, applications, and challenges of a psychological approach to the health care system, San Francisco, 1979, Jossey-Bass, Inc., Publishers. p. 529.)

the personal system in the model are representative of the many factors (values, attitudes) that influence family responses.

Three mediating factors intervene between the environmental and personal systems and health status and health-related behavior. The first of these, *cognitive appraisal* (perception of the environment) is usually, although not always, an essential intervening factor. *Activation or arousal* usually occurs in response to the way the environment is perceived, and this in turn may result in *adaptation and coping efforts* directed at changing some aspect of the environmental or personal system.

Health status and health-related behavior are dependent variables and are influenced by the environmental and personal systems, as well as the mediating factors of cognitive appraisal, activation or arousal, and efforts at adaptation. Moos (1979, p. 532) categorized the health-related variables into five indexes related to "the onset and development of illness, course of illness and outcome of treatment, utilization of health services and compliance with treatment, functional effectiveness, and satisfaction and well being."

Examples of the application of the social-ecological framework can be found in studies of the relationship

between health, population density, and crowding. A major implication of the social-ecological model for community health nursing is that it introduces another important set of variables (environmental factors) for use in the family health assessment process. The community health nurse should collect data not only about the family's personal system, but about the family's environmental system as well. Equally important is an assessment of the family's perceptions about its environment and the ways with which it copes with the environment. Finally, in addition to obtaining objective data about the family's perceptions about the relationship between its environment, health status, and health-related behavior. It is significant to note that the family's perceptions about the environment (home, neighborhood, social) and the relationship of the environment to health status and health related behavior may differ from the nurse's perceptions.

Factors Supporting or Impeding Family Health Promotion

Numerous factors may support a family's attempts at protecting and improving its health status, as well as impede or block the family's efforts in this direction. Examples of these variables are the family's structure,

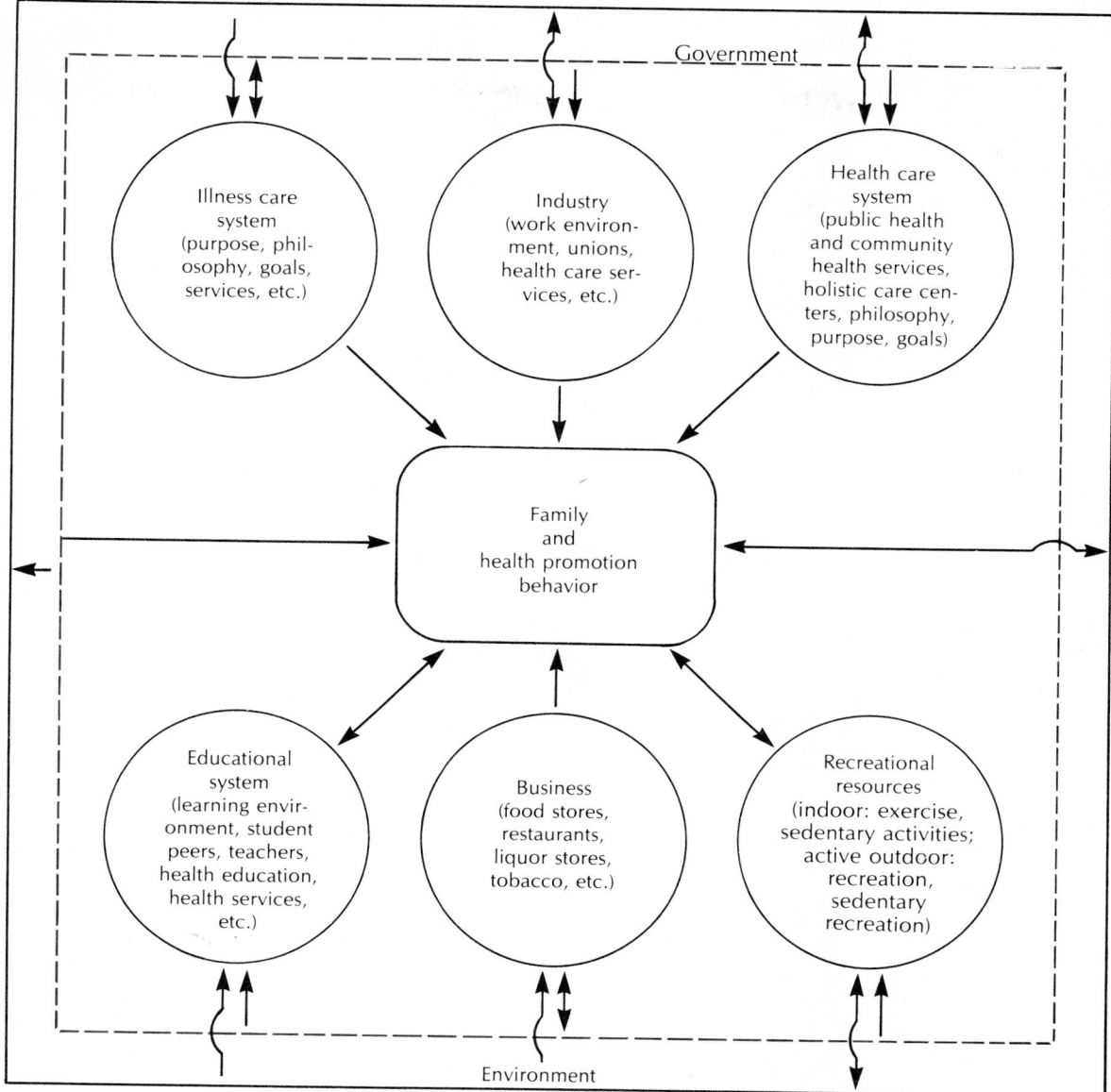

Fig. 15-6. Family health promotion and the ecological system.

values and beliefs, sociodemographic characteristics, and extent to which necessary internal and external supports are available.

An additional factor that must be considered is the family's attitude toward health actions that result in long-range gratification, given the long-range nature of health promotion activities. An important goal may be to stimulate families to act in the absence of any perceived immediate threat to health. Since a goal of health promotion is supporting or improving health, it is important to know the value assigned to health by different families, as well as to know about their perceptions of the short- and long-range rewards.

In summary, the family must be predisposed to assuming responsibility for practicing health promotion; there must be enabling conditions (family and community resources) allowing and supporting family responsibility for health promotion; and the family must perceive a need and benefit related to health promotion (Andersen, 1974).

In addition to working with families and assisting them in their efforts to maintain and improve health, the community health nurse has an obligation to become knowledgeable about and involved with the forces in the macroenvironment that may or may not be supportive of the family's endeavors. These forces are inherent in various societal systems such as the government, education, industry, business, and health-illness care systems. Examples of macroenvironmental forces are political decisions that may govern the availability and accessibility of needed resources supportive of family health, the philosophy and goals of health-illness care systems that emphasize illness care for the individual, and the easy access to and availability of over-the-counter drugs and alcoholic beverages. While all social systems have a direct influence on the family, the family's influence on the external systems may or may not be reciprocal.

Fig. 15-6 depicts the relationship between the family (and its health behavior) and various systems, or factors, in the macroenvironment. Although some of the relationships do not depict a symmetrical effect, the family has some influence on the other systems, such as the illness care agency, but to a much lesser degree than the systems have on the family. The two systems with which the family probably has the strongest reciprocal relationship are the educational system and the recreational system. The educational system provides health services and health education opportunities directed at health promotion for the school-aged individual. In addition, the school environment includes a school-aged peer system that may or may not be supportive of the individual's health promotion activities. The family in turn has considerable influence in determining the nature and content of health education programs in the school, which may or may not be in the child's best interests.

The family's influence on the recreational system tends to be one of supply and demand. Recreational facilities such as jogging tracks for physical exercise and video games (a sedentary recreation) are examples of diverse types of recreation resources that have developed at different rates in response to public demands and interests.

Other systems have an asymmetrical relationship with the family. Large industries may have health education and exercise programs for employees, as well as health care services. On the other hand, industries may serve as repositories for stress situations related to the job and be a prime source of environmental pollution. It would be inappropriate to examine the family-industry relationship without considering the contributions unions have made to improving environmental working conditions for employees and improving the family health and dental insurance benefits.

Health-illness care systems may or may not be supportive of families' health promotion activities by virtue of the services offered, the accessibility of the services, and the families' willingness or ability to pay for health protective services. In addition, most third party payer plans do not include reimbursement to health care providers for health promotion services.

Businesses, such as food, clothing and liquor stores, through their advertising procedures contribute to making many products attractive that may be detrimental to one's health. Some of these products, such as alcohol, are major contributors to serious long-term health problems. Thus it becomes imperative that health promotion activities extend beyond the boundaries of individual and family life-styles to the physical and social environment. Health promotion must be integrated into the other sources of influence on health such as the physical environment and the economic, social, governmental, and legal systems. "The concept of health promotion has yet to mature as a national institution . . . as the success of self-responsibility for personal health becomes more evident, public appreciation of and demand for the concept of health promotion will rapidly further its maturation" (Watkin, 1980, p. 35).

COMMUNITY HEALTH NURSING PROCESS WITH FAMILIES

The goal for the community health nurse is to promote the health of the family unit and family members through support and assistance in their health promotion and illness/disease/disability prevention efforts. This goal is put into practice through the nursing process, which, in community health nursing, is based on theories, concepts, and principles of nursing and the public health sciences. Nursing process can be described as an organized, systematic, deliberate act of moving through a series of developmental stages toward goal achievement (Yura and Walsh, 1978). The stages, or phases, are dependent on each other and consist of assessing, planning, implementing, and evaluating. The nursing process can be conceptualized as a dynamic phenomenon that involves analyzing data, making decisions, solving problems, and setting goals in collaboration with the family.

An integral part of the community health nursing process is the establishment and maintenance of an effective working relationship with the family. Inherent in this working relationship is the ability to analyze and understand one's own values, attitudes, and perceptions about different family structures, varying family life-styles, and diverse family health practices. Self-awareness on the part of the community health nurse can contribute to the development of an accepting, trusting nurse-family relationship in which both nurse and family respect each other's basic integrity.

The environments in which the community health nurse and the family or family members interface vary.

The setting may be the family's home, a clinic, the school, or some other community site. The physical setting in which the family and nurse interact may influence the family's and nurse's response to the immediate situation. The family may perceive itself as more in control in the home setting, with the community health nurse being a "guest," while other community settings (e.g., clinics) are viewed as being the nurse's territory with the nurse in control. The community health nurse also has feelings and perceptions about the appropriateness and comfort of one setting over another. For example, the nurse may experience a sense of discomfort associated with an initial home visit to a family. This may be caused by such factors as the nurse experiencing a sense of decreased control in the nurse-client situation, feeling uncomfortable about the family's lifestyle, and having unclear goals for the visit.

The community health nurse will tend to use two approaches in working with the family. One approach will emphasize working with the family as a unit, while in other instances the emphasis is on individual family members. The two approaches are interrelated and used interchangeably. For instance, the community health nurse may initiate the nursing process with the total family unit, shift the approach to a single family member or dyad (such as parents), and then refocus the nursing intervention toward the entire family unit.

The community health nurse, when working with the family unit, may experience feelings of inadequacy about interacting with the family as a small group. Such concerns about simultaneously working with a number of individuals are quite common considering that most of the nurse's experiences involve working with people on a one-to-one basis. Working with the family through group action requires knowledge about group behavior, appropriate physical settings for group functioning, and the leadership process. The development of group skills and the experience of working with groups should contribute to the community health nurse's ability and competency in working with the family group (Chapter 18).

Conceptual Frameworks for Study of the Family

Conceptual (or theoretical) frameworks provide a guiding structure for studying family interaction and development. A single conceptual framework, or a framework developed from several conceptual approaches, serves the purpose of directing the nursing process in relation to family assessment, development of the family health care plan, selection of the implementation strategies, and formulation of an evaluation plan. Numerous conceptual frameworks can be used for studying families, such as anthropological, struc-

ture-functional, institutional, interactional, situational, psychoanalytical, sociopsychological, and developmental. Some of these frameworks may be discussed within theoretical categories such as systems theory and role theory. This section will briefly address a sampling of the conceptual frameworks for purposes of explicating the relevance of a framework for the nursing process.

Interactional Framework

The interactional approach focuses on the family as a unit of interacting personalities and examines the symbolic communication processes by which family members relate to one another. Within the family each member occupies a position or positions to which a number of roles are assigned. Family members define their role expectations in each situation in relation to the reference group and through their perceptions of the role demands. Family members judge their own behavior by assessing and interpreting the actions of others toward them. The responses of others in the family serve to challenge or reinforce the family members' perceptions of the norms or role expectations.

Central to the interactional approach is the process of role taking. Every role exists in relation to some other role, and interaction represents a dynamic process of testing conceptions about each other's roles. Through family interaction the result of the testing process is stabilization or modification of roles. The ability to predict other family members' expectations for one's role enables each member to have some knowledge of how to react in the role and how other members will react to the performance in the role.

Assessment of the family within an interactional framework would emphasize (1) family functioning relative to interaction between and among family members, for example, the messages communicated about family role expectations, such as the socialization of children in relation to role development, and (2) family communication patterns relative to messages sent about health and illness behaviors appropriate for different roles, such as differing behaviors appropriate for the child versus the father.

Structural-Functional Framework

Within the structural-functional framework the family is viewed as a social system with members who have specific roles and functions. The structure and function of the family can be analyzed (1) relative to social systems external to the family (i.e., socialization of family members for social roles); (2) from the perspective of internal relationships within the family and between family subsystems (i.e., division of labor between family members); and (3) with respect to the reciprocal relationship between the family and the personality development of family members (i.e., development of personalities needed to carry out family functions) (McIntyre, 1967). General assumptions in the structural-functional approach include the following (Eshelman, 1974):

1. The family is a social system with functional requirements.
2. The family is a small group possessing certain generic features common to all small groups.
3. The family as a social system accomplishes functions that serve both the individual and society.

Studying the family from a structural-functional perspective also includes analyzing the family as a system with boundaries that regulate input from and output to the environment. The boundaries facilitate or interfere with adaptation. The family as a social system consists of individuals organized into a single unit so that change in any family member inevitably results in changes in the entire family system (Friedman, 1981).

The structural-functional approach provides a framework for assessing family structure and functions such as the socialization process of family members for roles and behaviors necessary for living and interacting in society; the socialization process for family members in relation to cultural and social norms; values, rights, and privileges assigned family roles; enactment of family roles; locus of authority and decision making in the family; development of coping behaviors; family subsystems; and communication patterns. Other examples of the structural-functional approach include the family health estate, the interrelationship between family and individual health, and the relationship between family health and community health, all discussed previously.

Developmental Framework

The last conceptual approach to be discussed will be the developmental framework, which incorporates aspects of social systems theory, the structural-functional approach, and the sociopsychological approach. The major focus of the developmental framework is the nuclear family. The developmental framework identifies the developmental stages of a family from the beginning of marriage to the death of the surviving spouse. The family is viewed as a system that changes through time as a result of the following:

1. Changes in the age composition of the family members (e.g., family members aging through time)
2. Plurality patterns (e.g., expanding and contracting family)
3. School placement of the children (e.g., first child entering school to last child leaving school)

4. Functions and status of the family within the larger social system (e.g., starting a career or exiting from the work role and moving into the retirement role)

Application of the developmental framework to the family divides the family into different chronological stages. Duvall (1977) categorized family development into eight stages referred to as the "family life cycle": beginning family (establishing a marriage), early childbearing family (oldest child is infant through 30 months), family with preschool children (oldest child is 2½ to 5 years of age), family with school-aged children (oldest child is 6 to 13 years of age), family with teenager(s) (oldest child is 13 or 20 years of age), launching family (period from first child leaving home to last child leaving home), middle-aged family (middle-aged marital dyad up to retirement), and aging family (retirement to death of both spouses).

Family developmental tasks, defined as "a growth responsibility that arises at a certain state in the life of a family, successful achievement of which leads to satisfaction and success with later tasks, while failure leads to . . . difficulty with later family developmental tasks" (Duvall, 1971, p. 149), have been delineated for each of the family stages. Examples of family developmental tasks appear in Table 15-1.

Many of the family developmental tasks in Table 15-1 are more relevant for the nuclear family than for variant family structures. Duvall (1971) delineated eight family developmental tasks that are more universal in their family application. These eight tasks are as follows: "physical maintenance; allocation of resources; division of labor; socialization of family members; reproduction, recruitment, and (or) release of family members; maintenance of order; placement of members in the larger society; and maintenance of motivation and morale." This listing still precludes some of the variant family structures addressed previously, such as childless families.

The achievement of family developmental tasks at each family stage is interrelated with the accomplishment of developmental tasks by individual family members. In working with the family it is important for the community health nurse to be knowledgeable about both family development and individual human development, since both are occurring simultaneously and are in a reciprocal relationship. Assessment of the family and family members' developmental stages and performance of associated tasks provide the community health nurse with essential data for family health care planning and anticipatory guidance. (The reader should refer to Chapters 25 through 28 for a discussion of individual developmental tasks across the life span.)

Table 15-1. Family developmental tasks

Family stages	Developmental tasks
Beginning family	Establishing a marriage
	Relating to kin network
	Family planning
Early childbearing family	Stabilizing the family unit
	Reconciling family members' conflicting developmental tasks
	Facilitating developmental needs of mother, father, and infant
Family with pre-school children	Nurturing and socializing children
	Maintaining a stable marriage
Family with school-aged children	Socializing children
	Promoting school achievement
	Maintaining satisfactory marital relationship
Family with teen-ager(s)	Balancing teenage freedom and responsibility
	Maintaining open parent-child communication
	Maintaining a stable marital relationship
	Building a foundation for future family stages
Launching family	Releasing children as young adults
	Readjusting the marriage
	Assisting aging parents
Middle-aged family	Strengthening the marital relationship
	Sustaining relationships with parents and children
	Providing a healthy environment
	Cultivating leisure-time activities
Aging family	Adjusting to retirement
	Maintaining satisfactory living arrangement
	Adjusting to reduced income
	Adjusting to health problems
	Adjusting to death of spouse

Adapted from Friedman, M.: Family nursing: theory and assessment, New York, 1981, Appleton-Century-Crofts, p. 50-64.

Conclusions

In concluding this section on frameworks for the study of the family, it can be stated that each framework offers a particular focus for assessing the family, and adopting a single framework may preclude the assessment of other relevant areas of family life. Also, the three frameworks have overlapping concepts. Given the increasing variation in family structures, the family must be assessed from many perspectives so that all dimensions of a particular family are evident.

Preprocess Goals

Initiating the community health nursing process requires careful consideration of the approach to be used with the family for developing an effective, productive nurse-family relationship. There are *preprocess goals* that the community health nurse and family will work toward either before or during the assessment phase of the nursing process. The preprocess goals involve establishing a mutual nurse-family trust relationship, defining the nurse's role in the family's health care, assisting the family to feel comfortable in the client role, and

developing a positive environment in which to implement successfully the nursing process (Yura and Walsh, 1978). Implicit in these goals is mutual decision making (involving the family and nurse), which will determine the parameters of the nurse-family working relationship.

The receptivity of the family to the community health nurse will vary from one situation to another. For example, a family who has had numerous debasing experiences with human services workers may be very suspicious of the nurse and the intent of the visit and may reject the nurse's presence. The community health nurse will need to cope as objectively as possible with feelings of rejection and at the same time explore with the family their perceptions about the purpose of the visit and their feelings about past experiences with other professionals. The nurse and family together should discuss and define what the nurse's role should be in this particular family situation: What are the family's expectations of the nurse? How can the nurse be assistive? In addition, the nurse and family should discuss the family's role in the situation, with emphasis on the family's autonomy and participation in the decision-making process relevant to the health situation. The community health nurse may find that working with the family on the preprocess goals takes more than one contact in view of the family's past experiences. Working with the family in this manner can result in the development of a reciprocal relationship between professional and family, can develop a positive environment in which to implement the nursing process, and can serve to reinforce past positive relationships families may have had with other professionals.

The Assessment Process

Assessment is the systematic collection, classification, and analysis of data for the purpose of identifying the family's, and family members', health-related strengths and problems. Generally, information is obtained about family processes and interaction patterns that help define the family's health-illness behavior; personal, social, cultural, and environmental factors that influence a family's perceptions, values, attitudes, and beliefs about health and illness; the family's utilization practices of formal and informal health care resources; the family's self-care health practices and resources; and the general level of health of the family and its members. The assessment phase is critical to the total nursing process, since the identification of family strengths and problems provides direction for planning, selection of implementation strategies, and evaluation.

The *total assessment process* consists of a series of phases: collecting subjective and objective data related to the family's health and illness behaviors; analyzing the initial data for accuracy and completeness; collecting more data if necessary; and analyzing the data for identification of family health risks, health problems, and potential family stressors, as well as family strengths, resources, and coping ability. The data are analyzed, also, for the interrelationship between family, environmental factors, and the family's health status and health practices.

Data Collection

Several approaches are possible in collecting family data, such as use of a questionnaire, interviewing, and the participant observer method. Sources of family data, other than the family, are agency records and other human services workers who have been associated with the family.

The questionnaire, though least desirable of all the methods, can be given to the family to complete essential family household data and selected factual data about family health and illness. The questionnaire

method can be an effective and efficient adjunct to the interview. For example, if the community health nurse is meeting with the total family, each family member (as appropriate) can be requested to complete a brief questionnaire asking for objective information relevant to that family member. The use of the questionnaire can be preceded or followed by a family interview for the collection of additional data.

The interview has long been considered the most effective data-gathering process. Two approaches to interviewing are the direct method, or the structured interview, and the indirect method. The structured interview can be used with the family for the purpose of collecting considerable factual information in a short time. The interview guide consists of a previously ordered set of questions of a direct nature.

The indirect method of interviewing, like the direct method, has a purpose; the questions used in the indirect interview process are less structured and allow the family or family member to express thoughts and feelings more freely (e.g., "Would you please share with me the things the family does to protect its health?" as opposed to "Does anyone in your family smoke?"). While the indirect method of interviewing can elicit considerable information from the family, it is important for the community health nurse to direct the discussion, as necessary, to keep the interview purposeful. Effective interviewing requires knowledge about the interview process (verbal communication, nonverbal communication, listening) and involves practice in the application of this knowledge.

Another approach that can be used in the assessment process is the participant observer method. Considerable data can be collected by observing family patterns of decision making, relationships between family members, communication patterns, patterns of family activities, health practices, the physical environment of the home and neighborhood, and so forth.

The amount and type of data to be collected from the family, the setting in which the data collection occurs, the data collection method(s) selected, and the length of time or number of family contacts required in this assessment phase will be determined by factors related to the family, the community health nurse, and the health care agency. Each agency will have specified forms for collecting family data. In addition, the community health nurse will want to develop an assessment guide and/or form that directs the collection of data essential for family health care. An example of a family health assessment guide is in Appendix B. This guide identifies general data areas that can be adapted for use in a variety of community health nursing settings.

Data Analysis

The initial family data collected by the community health nurse should be examined for accuracy and completeness. This process may result in the identified need to collect additional data, such as the need to obtain more information about a specific health situation. Any questionable data should be validated with the family. Missing data may be forthcoming if the family is asked to submit additional information the nurse may need for planning purposes. Once data collection has been completed, the data are collated, similar data are grouped together and arranged in some sequence for the purpose of formulating conclusions, and finally the data are examined for relationships. For example, the data may be examined for the relationship between identified health problems and family sociodemographic characteristics.

Data analysis is most effective if the family is involved in the analysis process. General uses of data analysis based on both subjective and objective data include identification of the following:

1. Family's sociodemographic profile (age, sex, education, ethnicity, religion, occupations, etc.)
2. Environmental factors supportive of or inhibiting health practices (home, neighborhood, school, occupational setting, etc.)
3. Perceptions, values, attitudes, and beliefs about health and illness (folk medicine orientation, value placed on health, etc.)
4. Family processes and interaction patterns related to health-illness behavior (decision making, group problem solving, etc.)
5. Coping behavior (family's practices in dealing with stress and health problems, intrafamily resources for coping, external resources for coping, potential resources for coping with stress and health problems, etc.)
6. Family and family members' health practices and risk behaviors (smoking, alcohol use, stress, nutrition, exercise, dental care, accident prevention, family planning, immunizations, etc.)
7. Utilization practices related to formal and informal health care resources (use of faith healer, nurse practitioner, physician, etc.)
8. Ability and potential for self-care (abilities regarding maintaining health and preventing illness)
9. Health status of family and family members (general level of functioning in physical, emotional, developmental, social areas)
10. Potential health problems/high risk potential (hypertension, accidents, etc.)
11. Strengths and barriers that support or interfere with needed family and community health nursing actions (value conflicts, etc.)

Yura and Walsh (1978) have developed a typology of judgments that the nurse must make about the family data. The nurse may determine that (1) problems are not in evidence and the family is presently maintaining its health; (2) no problem exists but there is a potential problem; (3) a problem exists but is being handled successfully by the family; (4) a problem exists with which the family needs some form of assistance; (5) a problem exists that requires health care intervention; (6) a problem is present and requires further study and diagnosis for purposes of resolution or management; or (7) a problem exists in a family member which is not limiting the individual but the appropriate intervention (e.g., surgery) will place the person in a temporary state of dependency.

Three other types of problems about which the nurse makes judgments are of a more serious nature: (1) A problem may exist which necessitates immediate and continuous intervention by the health care team. (2) A crisis may suddenly be imposed on the family, with which the family may or may not be able to cope. (3) A long-term and permanent problem may require supplemental care over an extended period of time. The aforementioned problems may exist singularly or in combination for the family.

Many family health problems in community health tend to fall in the first five judgment categories of the Yura-Walsh typology. The family health problems usually are of a nonacute, or episodic nature, and tend to be less urgent. Many of the problems can be managed by the family with or without community health nursing support. In addition, numerous family health problems are of an anticipatory nature rather than of a nature requiring immediate intervention.

A list of the family's strengths, resources, and problems should be developed jointly by the family and community health nurse. Since family health care involves change in some area of the family's behavior, the family must see a need for change. The family's involvement in the data analysis process and in problem identification assists the family in perceiving the extent of the problems. The family's or family members' health problems will be categorized according to the immediacy of needed action. The crucial nature of the problem, availability of resources, family readiness to cope with the situation, among others, are criteria that can be helpful in assisting the family and nurse to decide which problems should be given priority for intervention and which problems can be handled in the future. In determining family problems it is important to identify the problems for which nursing action will make a difference, such as assisting the family to act on or cope with its situation.

The capacity of the family to cope with health and health-related situations is an important data area for analysis and for planning. The coping behavior involves decision making relevant to a course of action to be taken or not taken. Janis and Mann (1977) delineate five basic coping patterns a family or family member might use to handle realistic health threats:

1. The family may decide to continue its health risk behavior, ignoring information about the risks and potential outcomes. This type of behavior is termed *unconflicted persistence*.

2. *Unconflicted change* consists of the family uncritically adopting the most salient and strongly recommended new course of protective or preventive action.

3. During *defensive avoidance* the family decides to evade the conflict by procrastinating, shifting the responsibility to others, or rationalizing the least objectionable alternative, remaining selectively inattentive to important information about risk reduction.

4. The family, for a variety of reasons such as emotional excitement or panic, may decide on a hasty solution thought to provide quick relief to the threat, while ignoring the possible undesirable consequences. This type of behavior is called *hypervigilance*.

5. Unless a threat is immediately serious, *vigilance* behavior tends to result in decisions that are most beneficial for the family. The vigilance pattern involves the family in seeking essential information about the situation, assimilating the information as objectively as possible, evaluating the alternatives, and then making a decision about how to handle the situation.

Identification of the family's coping pattern has important implications for the next phase of the nursing process—planning.

Planning

The planning process involves the determination of appropriate community health nursing actions for assisting the family to achieve specified outcomes (see Appendix B for a sample of a family health care plan). Planning involves the family and community health nurse jointly in determining goals, setting priorities, and identifying alternate courses of action for resolving problems. In addition to assigning priority to the diagnosed or identified problems, problems are differentiated in relation to those which can be managed by the family, those which can be resolved by nursing intervention, and those which should be referred. The operational plan includes immediate, intermediate, and long-range goals; objectives; designated family and nursing actions; and expected outcomes. If no problems exist, the community health nurse verifies the family's state of wellness and plans with the family to periodically meet for assessment purposes (Yura and Walsh, 1978).

Goals and objectives serve as criteria for selecting appropriate courses of nursing actions and provide the means for continuous and summative evaluation of the nursing interventions. A *goal* is a statement of purpose that provides direction for the overall plan, including the objectives and evaluation. *Objectives* are behavioral statements that are more specific than goals and are stated in terms of achieving a measurable amount of progress toward a goal. According to Reinke (1972) specifications for an objective include *what* (nature of what is to be attained); *extent* (amount of whatever is to be attained); *when* (time when determined outcome will exist); *who* (individual or family in whom attainment or change is desired); and *where* (location, e.g., home, where condition will be acted on). The goals and objectives should be congruent with the family's general goals, philosophy, and values. They should also be realistic, achievable, and challenging for the family. The family health care plan will include goals and objectives for the family unit and may also include subobjectives for family members.

Implicit in the planning phase of the nursing process are problem solving and decision making. Family involvement in planning provides problem-solving and decision-making experiences for the family. For example, families can participate in decisions about self-care, choosing among courses of action, and establishing priorities. In addition, they can be involved in problem solving regarding how to best use resources economically, to strengthen existing family resources, to anticipate future health needs, and to handle other similar situations. Observation of the family problem-solving and decision-making experiences provides the community health nurse with additional information about the family's verbal and nonverbal communication patterns, creativity, intrafamily support, communications conflict, centralization or distribution of power, and type of leadership (Klein and Hill, 1979).

Holistic Approach

The holistic approach to planning addresses the physical, mental, and spiritual aspects of the family; emphasizes the family's uniqueness; approaches the family within the context of its cultural and social context; emphasizes the family's responsibility for its own health, self-care, and health education; focuses on health promotion and prevention of illness/disease/disability; and plans in relation to the family's developmental stage and tasks, as well as individual family members' stages of development and accompanying developmental tasks. Other considerations, from a holistic perspective, are the emphasis on appropriate nutritional behaviors as well as exercise and stress-reduction and the assistance given to the family to view illness problems as opportunities for understanding risk behaviors and psychosocial stresses that may have contributed to the problems (Hastings et al., 1981).

Contracting Approach

Another approach that involves the family in problem solving and decision making is the process of contracting. The contract is a verbal or written agreement between the nurse and the family which specifies the goals of the family's health care and the relationship-between the nurse and the family. The underlying philosophy in contracting involves belief in the dignity, worth, and autonomy of the person and the family and affirmation that the family's health is its responsibility. The contracting process encourages both the family and the community health nurse to examine their values and beliefs about health and to consider alternatives to the family's risk behaviors that will improve the quality of life for the family (Hayes and Davis, 1980).

Contracting has a problem-solving format in which the community health nurse and the family share perceptions about the identified family health problems and strengths and share their rationale for the ranking of or priorities given to the problems. Once the problems have been assigned priorities, the family and nurse establish mutually agreed on goals, objectives, and target activities, or steps for achieving the goals and implementing the objectives, and develop the evaluation plan. The contract (written or verbal) includes a description of the responsibilities and expected activities for both the family and nurse; the implementation plan, including the time limits for accomplishment of specified activities or changes; and the evaluation measures. Various aspects of the contract, such as time, are renegotiable. See Appendix B for a sample of a family–community health nurse contract.

Review

Before implementing the nursing plan, the community health nurse and family should conduct a critical review of the completed planning process. This review should include the following:

1. A reassessment of the identified family health needs and concerns to ensure completeness
2. An assessment of the degree to which the family was involved in developing the care plan objectives
3. An assessment of the extent to which the objectives can be achieved realistically by the family and nurse

4. Verification that the recommended actions or interventions are physically, psychologically, and socially possible for the family to accomplish

The community health nurse should review the care plan also to ensure that the objectives are specifically defined and written, stated in terms of specific changes in behavior to be achieved, broken down into intermediate steps or subobjectives for periodic evaluation, and stated as a baseline from which progress toward achievement of the goal(s) and objectives can be measured (Knutson, 1969).

Implementation

Strategies for health care implementation involve *change.* A common goal of helping efforts is to effect some kind of change, and the nature of the problem or situation will determine when and where change must occur. Change is a goal for intervention with the family to strengthen the family's opportunities for improved general functioning, enhanced quality of life, increased self-awareness and autonomy, and development of a stronger sense of self-responsibility for health promotion and illness/disease/disability prevention (Eriksen, 1977).

Implementation is defined as the initiation and completion of actions necessary to accomplish defined goals (Yura and Walsh, 1978). *Strategy* is conceptualized as a method by which nursing action improves the health of families. Examples of implementation strategies are anticipatory guidance, health counseling, health education, modification of the family's physical environment, strengthening family resources, health care guidance, direct care provision, stress reduction, assistance to the family in identifying and using social supports, facilitation of family processes (decision making, problem solving), self-care monitoring, and referrals. Strategies may be implemented and carried out by the community health nurse, by the family, or by others (e.g., health aides or extended family members). Of utmost importance throughout the implementation phase of the nursing process is a continued awareness (by the nurse) of the family's attitude toward and perceptions about the strategies being used. An effective evaluation plan, as well as the nurse-family contract, should facilitate the ongoing assessment of the family's attitudes and the family's progress toward goal achievement.

Self-responsibility is inherent in health promotion and illness/disease/disability prevention. Families vary in ability and readiness to assume responsibility for health promotion and illness prevention activities without the assistance of resources outside the family. The reasons for this wide variation are numerous, including sociodemographic factors and limited socializing experiences. The community health nurse must be prepared to assist some families to have a learning experience that is almost developmental in nature. That is, some family members will need to have the opportunity to have a socializing experience in which they can learn the health protection behavior. This beginning learning experience must be reinforced, rewarded, and supported through continued learning opportunities until the behavior is incorporated into the family's value system.

The socialization process is much more complex than the simplified process just outlined and may require additional outside resources to support its implementation, such as adequate income and available dental services.

Tapia's schema (1975) of families' level of functioning exemplifies the preceding discussion and can be compared to developmental stages of the individual through the life span. The levels of family functioning range from infancy to maturity, with the intermediate levels being childhood, adolescence, and adulthood. Since the families differ in their ability to accomplish certain tasks, and their responses to health services vary, the community health nurse's working relationship with the family should be appropriate to the family's level of functioning. For example, if a family is functioning at the "infancy" level, the nurse functions as a "good mother" to the family, and the nursing activities emphasize assisting the family to develop trust and to progress to another level of functioning. The family functioning at the maturity level is able to operate independently in relation to health promotion activities without need for community health nursing intervention. Thus if nursing efforts are concentrated on nursing activities appropriate to the family's level of functioning, the nursing measures should be more meaningful to the family and more economical in relation to both the family and the community health nurse's time and efforts.

Community Health Nursing Strategies for Family Health Care

Family Self-Care. *Self-care* implies self-responsibility and is viewed as a family strategy for improving or maintaining health; it can become a nursing strategy when the community health nurse provides support to the family for self-care. Thus the concept of *family self-care* subsumes the family functioning on its own behalf in health promotion, illness/disease/disability prevention, illness/disease/disability detection, and treatment. This level of functioning takes place both in the home and in the primary health care setting. Preconditions for self-care are the family's understanding of its health status, health problems, and health behaviors and of the implications these factors have for the

family's future. An understanding of family self-care necessitates knowledge about the family's customs and life-styles and their influence on episodic actions, such as self-diagnosis and self-treatment. Family self-assessment tends to be based on criteria personally perceived as relevant. It can be assumed that there will be considerable variation in self-care behaviors among families because of differences in family structure, stages of individual and family development, and the family's sociodemographic characteristics. (The reader should refer to Chapter 14 for a discussion of self-care and risk factor analysis.)

Counseling. Anticipatory guidance, anticipatory problem solving, and health counseling comprise strategies appropriate for the community health nurse who is assisting families develop the ability to assume increased responsibility for self-care and to cope more effectively with potentially stressful events or situations. Actually, there are overlapping areas in all three approaches.

Anticipatory guidance assists the family to "identify potentially stressful situations and prepares (it) either by lessening the impact of the situation through appropriate planning or by developing support systems such as family and friends that serve as buffers against the undesirable effects of the impending stress situation" (Pender, 1980, p. 10). The community health nurse using anticipatory guidance is actually assisting the family in developing resistance to situational or developmental stress events. Anticipatory guidance is a form of family education that is future oriented in terms of discussing how a situation is likely to be, how the family may behave in the anticipated situation, and what type of family behavior should be appropriate for the situation. The purposes of anticipatory guidance are to prepare the family for life changes and to strengthen the family resources for effective coping with changes (Pender, 1980).

Anticipatory problem solving tends to be oriented toward health promotion more generally and starts where the family currently is in relation to identifying perceived or anticipated problems. The family is helped to estimate risks and stresses likely to occur in relation to the anticipated problem. The phases in clinical problem solving start with scanning and formulating (exploration of issue of concern) and then progress through appraising (assessment), developing readiness to solve the problem, planning, implementing, and evaluating. An important aspect of the implementation stage is its focus on how to solve the future problem. To develop and test skills the family actually practices the steps in the plan of action. Goals in this process are to assist the family in identifying problems more precisely and to help the family arrive at generalized approaches to problem solving (Pridham et al., 1979). See Appendix B for a family problem-solving guide.

Health counseling is defined as a helping process used to facilitate the client's development of independence, ability in decision making, and ability to take action related to the family's health. There are aspects of both anticipatory guidance and anticipatory problem solving in health counseling.

Through counseling the nurse is able to assist the family in clarifying beliefs, values, and feelings associated with various problems. For example, the nurse may help the family explore perceptions about a health-damaging behavior and feelings about changing the-behavior. The nurse may guide the family toward answers to questions such as the following (Pender, 1982): What are the perceived positive and negative consequences of alternative choices regarding the health problem? How can the negative consequences by attenuated and the positive consequences strengthened? What does the family perceive as potential sources of immediate and long-range gratification from the alternative actions? Additional areas for clarification are the family's interpretation of health and health-related events, its philosophy of life, its rituals, its methods of identifying and accomplishing goals, and its perceptions about family roles, functions, and processes.

Throughout the counseling process the community health nurse provides the family with facts and information important to making informed decisions for actions to be taken. This information must be accurate, complete, appropriate for the respective family (e.g., at the appropriate level of functioning), and presented in an objective, nonjudgmental way. Through health counseling the community health nurse can assist the family in its ability to act judiciously in relation to family health.

Referral Process. Another community health nursing strategy related to family health is the *referral process*. The purpose of the referral is to introduce the family to community resources, and the goal is to enhance family self-care capabilities in using resources. The referral may be initiated by the family, community health nurse, or another human services workers; it may be written or verbal. An example of the referral process can be found in the community health nurse's and family nurse practitioner's working relationship. The community health nurse functions as a case finder in the community and can refer family members to the family nurse practitioner as appropriate. The family nurse practitioner can, in turn, refer family members and families to the community health nurse for follow-up for family health counseling, environmental assessment, and so forth.

Although families' levels of handling referrals vary, it is essential that the family is involved in and, oriented to the process. Generally the basic steps in the community health nursing referral process are as follows, with the family's and nurse's responsibilities varying:

1. Establish a working relationship (joint responsibility)
2. Establish the need for a referral (joint responsibility)
3. Set objectives for the referral (joint responsibility)
4. Explore resource availability (family and nurse involved, but nurse may take lead)
5. Client decides to use or not use referral (a family right, but joint responsibility regarding exploring reasons and alternatives as necessary)
6. Make referral to resource (family or nurse)
7. Facilitate referral (nurse in assistive role)
8. Evaluate and perform follow-up (family and nurse evaluate together, and family or nurse follows up)

One of the resources the family may be encouraged to use is its social network or support system. *Social network* refers to the set of contacts with relatives, friends, neighbors, etc. through which the family "maintains a social identity and receives emotional support, material aid, services and information, and develops new social contacts" (McKinlay, 1981, p. 78). According to Hogue (1977) a *support system* is the same as a social network and may be a spontaneous or natural network (e.g., friends), an organized support system not directed by professional workers (eg., parents coping with adolescents' group), or an organized support system directed by a professional worker (e.g., a stress reduction group). The referral process used in relation to the social network/support system may be from the family, professional sources, or a lay referral system (friends, neighbors, etc.).

In summary, the referral process is a means whereby the community health nurse assists the family to use necessary resources and ensures coordination of family health care. The coordination process, in turn, involves the community health nurse in mediating between the family and fragmented services for the purpose of integrating the services for the family and providing for continuity of care. (Refer to Chapter 35 for the referral and coordination roles of the community health nurse.)

The Health Team. Throughout the family health care process the community health nurse may be working directly (intervenes directly) or indirectly (delegates intervention) with the family and working individually or as a health team member. Health services and other human services are interdependent, and no single professional is capable of meeting the family's needs alone. The family *health team* consists of the family, the community health nurse, and others such as extended family members, health care professionals (family nurse practitioner, physician, nutritionist), human service workers (social worker, etc.), health aides, and members of the clergy. The composition of a health team varies, but the process remains the same—an organized group effort for the purpose of providing integrated services to the family. An integral part of the health team process is the *health team conference*, which provides an opportunity for intrateam communications, problem solving, and decision making. An essential participant in the conference should be the family or a family member. The community health nurse should be aware of the need for the family's participation in the team conference and, in addition, should be aware of the possibility that the family members may need assistance and support in being active participants and feeling that their ideas are important.

Competency for collaboration, such as that needed for effective team functioning, requires a knowledge base in group process, conflict resolution, problem solving, and evaluation. In addition, the community health nurse needs to be knowledgeable about public health and nursing and the nature of the other professions represented on the team. It is not unusual to find some overlap in interests and functions among the various professionals. Therefore attributes important for all the professional team members are professional confidence, respect for own ability, flexibility, trust in colleagues, sensitivity to different approaches to problem solving, sensitivity to colleagues' need for self-esteem, and acceptance of professional conflicts. The interprofessional team member needs to be adept in interpersonal communication and relationship skills (Kane, 1977).

Evaluation

Evaluation is the process of measuring the extent to which the predetermined objectives are met. The community health nurse's intervention with the family may actually involve three elements of evaluation: effectiveness of the family's involvement in their health care, degree to which the objectives were achieved and effectiveness of intervention strategies employed by the nurse and the family.

There are two types of evaluation: formative and summative. *Formative evaluation* is a continuing process that measures progress toward goal achievement throughout the implementation phase of the nursing process. There may be identified checkpoints during the implementation phase which serve as markers for the formative evaluation. The results of the formative evaluation will indicate whether or not changes are needed in the nursing plan or intervention strategy. For example, weekly home visits for family health counsel-

ing were planned by the community health nurse and family. After a 3-week period the nurse and family evaluated the effectiveness of the health counseling visits through demonstrated family progress in self-care. The family's progress indicated that the nursing visits should be changed to every other week.

The *summative evaluation* is conducted at the conclusion of the nursing process and determines the extent to which the overall objectives were met. The evaluation outcomes determine what type of community health nursing action is still needed. The family may have responded as expected, and the problem is considered resolved. Since no further community health nursing intervention is indicated, the family and nurse formulate a plan for the family's continued self-care.

A second type of outcome is one in which the family's problem may not have been resolved, although the immediate goals for care were met. The family's situation is reassessed, the plan of care modified accordingly, and the community health nurse's involvement continued. An example of the second type of summative evaluation outcome is the hypertension situation discussed previously in which the family members felt there were some life-style behaviors that could be modified or changed in the near future and others that they could not work on presently. Since they did modify some of their health habits, the present care plan is revised, a new contract developed, and the working relationship continued.

A third type of summative evaluation outcome may provide evidence that the health behavior manifestations of the family are similar to what they were during the initial assessment phase and little or no progress has been made in relation to problem resolution. At this point the family's situation and intervention strategies require evaluation to determine the most appropriate course of action to pursue. For example, in the hypertension situation the family may be unable to modify any of the health habits written into the care plan. At this point the nurse and family reassess the situation and attempt to determine the factors contributing to the lack of progress toward meeting the health care plan objectives. Were the objectives unrealistic for the family to achieve in the designated time? Had the family's attitudes or motivation changed? The future course of action planned by the nurse and family will depend on the assessment outcomes.

A fourth type of summative evaluation outcome indicates that new problems have developed. The new or emerging problems are assessed, and the original plan is modified to accommodate planning for additional strategies appropriate to the new problems. A new problem that developed for the high-risk hypertensive couple was that the family member who had been working was no longer employed. As a consequence, the family is now experiencing additional stress and life-style changes, necessitating a reassessment of the situation and the development of a health care plan congruent with the family's present situation.

■   ■   ■

The nursing process consists of stages that are continuous and dynamically interrelated. For the nursing process to be most effective, the community health nurse and the family need to function collaboratively in all of the stages—assessing, planning, implementing, and evaluating.

SUMMARY

Community health nurses' work with families is becoming increasingly complex because of the variations in family structures, the intricate relationship between family and individual health, the multiplicity of factors that influence the family's health behavior, and the changing nature of social-environmental forces, which are constantly impinging on the family. Implementing health promotion for families within the context of changing family and social environments requires community health nursing competencies based on theory and research. Working with families necessitates the continuing pursuit of knowledge derived from nursing, family theory, theories about health promotion, and the public health sciences.

The community health nurse should perceive family health–related responsibilities as encompassing more than competency in working directly with families. Community health nurses' commitment to family health promotion includes involvement in epidemiological studies that focus on the family (Chapter 8), conduction of clinical research directed toward community health nursing intervention for family health promotion (Chapter 9), participation in health programs development for families (Chapter 12), and involvement in political issues supporting or mitigating against health promotion.

BIBLIOGRAPHY

American Nurses' Association: A conceptual model of community health nursing, Kansas City, Mo., 1980, The Association.

American Public Health Association: The definition and role of public health nursing in the delivery of health care, Washington, D.C., 1980, The Association.

Andersen, R.: A behavioral model of families' use of health services, ed. 2, Research Series 25, Chicago, 1974, Center for Health Administration Studies, University of Chicago Press.

Ball, D.W.: The family as a sociological problem: conceptualization of the taken-for-granted as prologue to social problems analysis, Soc. Probl. **19:**295, 1972.

Belloc, N.B., and Breslow, L.: The relation of physical health status and health practices, Prev. Med. **1:**67, 1973.

Blum, H.L.: Expanding health care horizons: from a general systems concept of health to a national health policy, Oakland, Calif., 1976, Third Party Associates, Inc.

Brody, H.: The systems view of man: implications for medicine, science, and ethics, Perspect. Biol. Med. **17:**71-92, 1973.

Cassell, J.: Planning for public health: the case for prevention. Paper presented at Conference on Redesigning Nursing Education for Public Health, Washington, D.C., 1973, Division of Nursing, Department of Health, Education, and Welfare.

Cogswell, B.E., and Sussman, M.B.: Changing family and marriage forms: complications for human service systems, Fam. Coord. **21:**505, 1972.

Dillehay, R.C.: Attitudes and beliefs. In Knutson, A.L., editor: The individual, society, and health behavior, New York, 1965, Russell Sage Foundation.

Dunn, H.L.: High-level wellness, Va., 1967, R.W. Beatty, Ltd.

Duvall, E.M.: Family development, ed. 4, Philadelphia, 1971, J.B. Lippincott Co.

Duvall, E.M.: Marriage and family development, ed. 5, Philadelphia, 1977, J.B. Lippincott Co.

Eriksen, K.: Human services today, Reston, Va., 1977, Reston Publishing Co., Inc.

Eshleman, J.R.: The family: an introduction, Boston, 1974, Allyn & Bacon, Inc.

Farber, B.: Family and kinship in modern society, Glenview, Ill., 1973, Scott, Foresman & Co.

Farrell, M.P., and Schmitt, M.H.: The American family: an historical perspective. In Hymovich, D.P., and Barnard, M.U., editors: Family health care: vol. 1, ed. 2, New York, 1979, McGraw-Hill Book Co.

Friedman, M.M.: Family nursing: theory and assessment, New York, 1981, Appleton-Century-Crofts.

Goode, W.J.: The family, Englewood Cliffs, N.J., 1964, Prentice-Hall, Inc.

Green, L.W.: Health promotion policy and the placement of responsibility for personal health care, Fam. Community Health **2:**51, Nov. 1979.

Hardy, M.E.: Role stress and role strain. In Hardy, M.E., and Conway, M.E., editors: Role theory: perspectives for health professionals, New York, 1978, Appleton-Century-Crofts.

Hastings, A.C., Fadiman, J., and Gordon, J.S., editors: Health for the whole person, Boulder, Colo., 1981, Westview Press, Inc.

Hayes, W.S., and Davis, L.L.: What is a health care contract? Health Values: Achieving High Level Wellness **4:**82, March/Apr. 1980.

Helvie, C.O.: Community health nursing: theory and process, New York, 1981, Harper & Row, Publishers, Inc.

Hochbaum, G.M.: Health behavior, Belmont, Calif., 1970, Wadsworth, Inc.

Hogue, C.C.: Support systems for health promotion. In Hall, J.E., and Weaver, B.R., editors: Distributive nursing practice: a systems approach to community health, Philadelphia, 1977, J.B. Lippincott Co.

Henkel, B.O.: Solving health problems though small group action. In Spradly, B.W., editor: Contemporary community nursing, Boston, 1975, Little, Brown & Co.

Janis, I.L., and Mann, L.: Decision making: a psychological analysis of conflict, choice, and commitment, New York, 1977, The Free Press.

Jordheim, A.E.: Alternate life-styles and the family. In Reinhardt, A. M., and Quinn, M.D., editors: Family-centered community nursing: a sociocultural framework, vol. 2, St. Louis, 1980, The C.V. Mosby Co.

Kane, R.A.: Competency for collaboration. In Reinhardt, A.M., and Quinn, M.D., editors: Current practice in family-centered community nursing, St. Louis, 1977, The C.V. Mosby Co.

Keller, M.J.: Toward a definition of health, Adv. Nurs. Sci. **4**(1):43, Oct. 1981.

Klein, D.M., and Hill, R.: Determinants of family problem solving effectiveness. In Burr, W.R., et al., editors: Contemporary theories about the family: research based theories, New York, 1979, The Free Press.

Knutson, A.L.: The individual, society, and health behavior, New York, 1965, Russell Sage Foundation.

Knutson, A.L.: Evaluation for what? In Schulberg, G.C., Sheldon, A., and Baker, F., editors: Program evaluation in the health fields, New York, 1969, Behavioral Publications.

Leavell, H.R., and Clark, E.G.: Preventive medicine for the doctor in his community: an epidemilogic apporach, ed. 3, New York, 1965, McGraw-Hill Book Co.

Leslie, G.R.: The family in social context, ed. 2, New York, 1973, Oxford University Press.

Levin, S.L., Katz, A.H., and Holst, E.: Self-care: lay intitiatives in health, New York, 2976, Prodist.

Macklin, E.D.: Nontraditional family forms: a decade of research, J. Marr. Fam. **42**:905, 1980.

Mauksch, H.: A social science basis for conceptualizing family health, Soc. Sci. Med. **8**:521, 1974.

McIntyre, J.: The structure-functional apporach to family study. In Nye, F.E., and Berardo, F.M., editors: Emerging conceptual frameworks in family analysis, New York, 1967, Macmillan, Publishing Co. Inc.

McKinlay, J.B.: Social network influences on morbid episodes and the career of help seeking. In Eisenberg, L., and Kleinman, A., editors: The relevance of social science for medicine, Boston, 1981, D. Reidel Publishing Co., Inc.

Milsum, J.H.: Health, risk factor reduction and life-style change, Fam. Community Health **3**:1, May 1980.

Moos, R.H.: Social-ecological perspectives on health. In Stone, G.C., Cohen, R., and Adler, N.E., editors: Health psychology—a handbook, San Francisco, 1979, Jossey-Bass, Inc., Publishers.

Murray, R., Meili, P., and Zentner, J.: The family—basic unit for the developing person. In Murray, R., and Zentner, J., editors: Nursing concepts for health promotion, Englewood Cliffs, N.J., 1975, Prentice-Hall, Inc.

Nye, F.I.: Role structure and analysis of the family, Beverly Hills, Calif, 1976, Sage Publications, Inc.

Nye, F.I., and Berardo, F.M., editors: Emerging conceptual frameworks in family analysis, New York, 1967, Macmillan Publishing Co., Inc.

Otto, H.E.: Criteria for assessing family strengths, Fam. Process **2**:329, Sept. 1963.

Otto, H.E.: A framework for assessing family strengths. In Reinhardt, A.M., and Quinn, M.D., editors: Family-centered community nursing: a sociocultural framework, vol. 1, St. Louis, 1972, The C. V. Mosby Co.

Pender, N.J.: Health promotion: challenge of the 1980s, nursing lecture, Muncie, Ind., Apr., 1980, Ball State University.

Pender, N.J.: Health promotion in nursing practice, New York, 1982, Appleton-Century-Crofts.

Pesznecker, B., Drayr, M.A., and McNeil, J.: Collaborative practice models in community health nursing, Nurs. Outlook **30**:298, 1982.

Pratt, L.: Family structure and effective health behavior: the energized family, Boston, 1976, Houghton Mifflin Co.

Pridham, K.F., Hansen, M.F., and Conrad, H.H.: Anticipatory problem solving, Sociol. Health Ill. **1**:177, Sept. 1979.

Reinke, W.A., editor: Health planning: qualitative aspects and quantitative techniques, Baltimore, Md., 1972, The Johns Hopkins University Press.

Rokeach, M.R.: Beliefs, attitudes, and values, San Francisco, 1968, Jossey-Bass, Inc., Publishers.

Rosenstock, I.M.: Historical origins of the health belief model. In Becker, M.H., editor: The health belief model and personal health behavior, Thorofare, N.J., 1974, Charles B. Slack, Inc.

Rowe, G.P.: The developmental conceptual framework to the study of the family. In Nye, F.I., and Berardo, F.M., editors: Emerging conceptual frameworks in family analysis, New York, 1967, Macmillan Publishing Co., Inc.

Schvaneveldt, J.D. The interactional framework in the study of the family. In Nye, F.I., and Berardo, F.M., editors: Emerging conceptual frameworks in family analysis, New York, 1967, Macmillan Publishing Co., Inc.

Schvaneveldt, J.D., and Thinger, M.: Sibling relationships in the family. In Burr W.R., et al., editors: Contemporary theories about the family: research based theories, New York, 1979, The Free Press.

Smilkstein, G.: The cyle of family function: a conceptual model for family medicine, Fam. Pract. **11**:223, 1980.

Suchman E.A.: Preventive health behavior: a model for research on community health campaigns, J. Health Soc. Behav. **8**:197, Sept. 1967.

Sussman, M.B.: Family systems in the 1970s: analysis, policies, and programs, Ann. Am. Acad. Pol. Soc. Sci. **396**:40, July 1971.

Sussman, M.B.: Family, kinship, and bureaucracy. In Sussman, M.B., editor: Sourcebook in marriage and the family, ed. 4, Boston, 1974, Houghton Mifflin Co.

Tapia, J.A.: The nursing process in family health. In Spradley, B.W., editor: Contemporary community nursing, Boston, 1975, Little, Brown & Co.

Vincent, C.E.: Mental health and the family, J. Marr. Fam. **29**:18, 1967.

Watkin, D.M.: Maintenance, prevention, and promotion: changing public and private sector views of individuals' responsibility for personal health. In Reinhardt, A.M., and Quinn, M.D. editors: Family-centered community nursing: a sociocultural framework, vol. 2, St. Louis, 1980, The C.V. Mosby Co.

World Health Organization: Community health nursing: report of a WHO expert committee, Technical Report Series No. 558, Geneva, 1974, The Organization.

World Health Organization: Statistical indices of family health, Technical Report Series No. 587, Geneva, 1976, The Organization.

Yura, H., and Walsh, M.B.: The nursing process: assessing, planning, implementing evaluating, ed. 3, New York, 1978, Appleton-Century-Crofts.

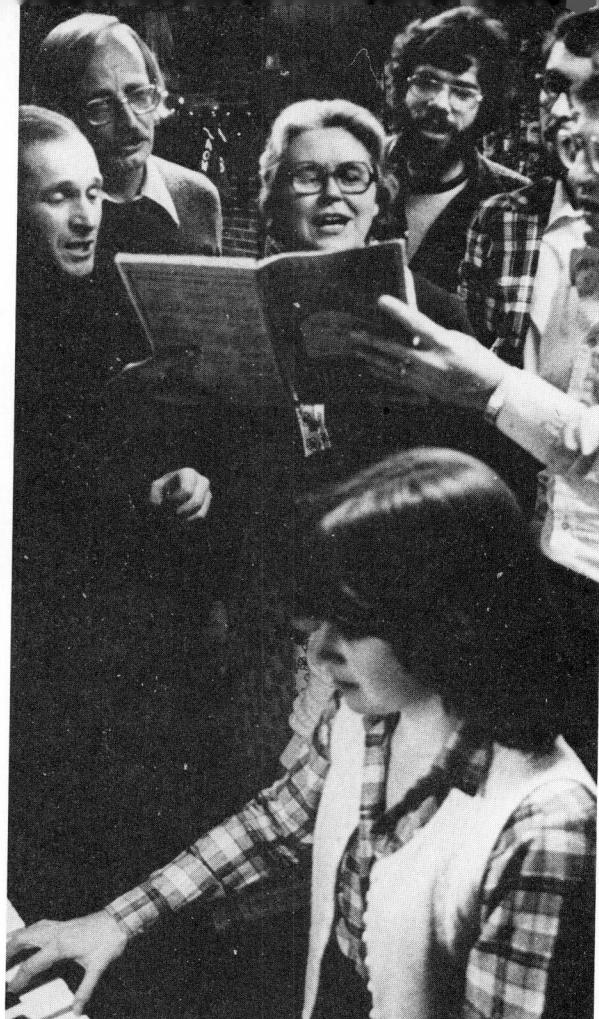

Chapter 16

PEGGYE GUESS LASSITER

WORKING WITH GROUPS IN THE COMMUNITY

Working with groups is an important skill for community health nursing. In daily practice nurses routinely plan and implement health-focused action with clients, other nurses, and other health care workers. Nurses often participate in groups in which they are encouraged to observe their own responses to the membership and leadership. Such study and experience enrich a person's knowledge of group concepts and application to groups of clients, work groups, and community groups. Working with clients through group approaches is helpful in most health care settings and is especially important for community health nursing, since group methods are often effective for work toward community health goals.

Additionally, groups are often an inexpensive mode by which information can be communicated, decisions made, and issues and concerns handled. As discussed in Chapter 8, community health nurses often use groups to communicate health information to a group of clients who can come together once or on a regular basis to receive the same type of assistance, rather than repeating the information several times to separate individuals. In an era of decreasing resources, groups are becoming an increasingly popular format for community health nursing intervention.

Groups hold power for individuals and communities, and this power lies in the ability to bring about change. Changes are often needed to improve health and well-being for individuals and communities. Groups are crucial for the development of individuals, and some individual changes for health are possible to achieve with group support and encouragement; these changes would be difficult to attain without that support. The attitudes that individuals have are developed in kin and friendship groups; continued membership throughout life in other groups influences thoughts, choices, behaviors, and values. People tend to find their social needs met through association with others, and groups are a natural vehicle for these needs.

Groups form for varied reasons; they may form to address a clearly stated purpose or goal, or the purpose may seem somewhat vague. They may form naturally as individuals are attracted to each other by shared values, interests, activities, or personal characteristics. On the other hand, people may come together to accomplish a task and become a group even when personal attraction is low.

Community groups represent the collective interests, needs, and values of individuals; they provide a link between the individual and the larger social system. Through groups people may express personal views and relate them to those of others. Groups serve the whole community as communication networks and may be viewed as an organization of community parts. Identifying groups, their goals, member characteristics, and their place in the community structure is an important first step toward understanding the community and assessing its health. Through community groups nurses may assist people to identify priority health needs and capabilities. Group methods may be used to implement community changes.

GROUP CONCEPTS

Basic group concepts are presented in this chapter. These concepts may be used in nursing practice to promote individual health through group work, to identify community groups and their contributions to community life, and to assist groups in working toward community health goals.

Group Definition

A *group* is a collection of interacting individuals who have a common purpose or purposes. Each member influences and is in turn influenced by every other member to some extent. The members' characteristics bring a composition to the group that in part determines the degree and kind of influence among them. Key elements in this group definition are *member interaction* and *group purpose,* both of which are necessary to the definition (Fig. 16-1).

Bertcher stated, ". . . a successful group is composed of two or more individuals who *do* interact over time in relation to one or more goals that are valued by each of these individuals; further, their interaction occurs in such a way that each must be dependent on the other to some degree as they try to achieve their common

goal(s); and each feels that they have been able to influence the others to some degree" (1979, p. 15).

The following four examples illustrate member interaction and group purposes. First, families are a unique example of community groups and the most familiar group form. Family purposes are numerous, including psychological support and socialization of their members. Usually families share kinship bonds, common living space, and economic resources. Interactions are diverse and frequent because of the multiple ties between members and the particular functions delegated to families by society. Group concepts offer one study approach to family groups.

A second example is groups formed in response to particular community needs. The purpose of such community groups is clearly to address specific problems or opportunities. For example, in one community residents banded together to form a neighborhood association to protect their health and welfare. This neighborhood of upper middle-class homes was located in an unincorporated area. Over a period of 3 years the residents were threatened with multiple environmental hazards, including forest fires (fire hydrants had been overlooked in developing part of the area), establishment of a small airport near the homes, and construction of an interstate highway adjacent to the homes. To protect their interests residents formed a neighborhood association and elected officers to represent their interests in a constructive manner.

Member interactions in this group focused on work toward the stated purpose. If these adults are also attracted to each other because of compatible interpersonal styles and shared beliefs, the influence of members on each other is strengthened. Interactions between members are influenced by the group purpose and the interpersonal dimensions of attraction.

Third, groups in the community often occur spontaneously because of mutual attraction between individuals and obvious and keenly felt personal needs. Young and single adults sharing similar desires for socialization and recreation are likely to form loosely structured groups. Through parties and other social meetings the young adults establish themselves in new ways of behaving and relating. They select partners, test ideas and attitudes, and establish their identity within a group of people with similar developmental needs. The unstated purpose is to test and become familiar in adult roles. Interactions between members serve to establish relationships appropriate to developing adult needs.

A fourth example is health promoting groups, which are formed as individuals meet in the community and health care settings and discover common challenges to their physical and emotional well-being. The purposes

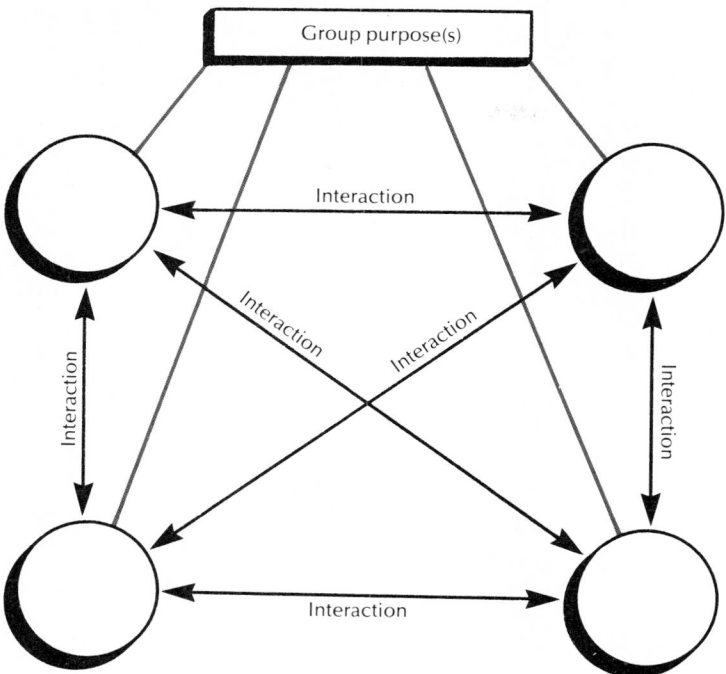

Fig. 16-1. A group is a collection of interacting individuals who have a common purpose or purposes.

of health promoting groups are to improve health for the members and to master specific threats to health. Chapters of Alcoholics Anonymous, Parents without Partners, and La Leche League illustrate such health promoting groups. Interactions between members are personally supportive and include group problem solving and education. Health promoting groups usually organize around particular purposes, and member interactions facilitate work toward those purposes. These groups may be either of two types: established groups or selected membership groups, both of which are discussed.

How do purpose and interaction vary in these four examples? For some groups purpose is obvious and may be easily stated by members. This is true for groups organized to address specific community needs or health challenges. For families, social groupings, and many spontaneously formed groups the purposes are unstated. However, the purpose for the groups can be determined by studying their activities as a group over a period of time. Highly personal and multipurpose groupings serve individual and collective needs in concrete, function-oriented ways and in subtle, less obvious manners.

Purpose and member interaction are important components of all groups, but the expression of purpose, the manner of member interaction, and the intensity of the interaction vary. Group purposes and member interactions help distinguish the group's function for its members and the community.

Established Groups

There are advantages to using established groups for individual health change when membership ties are made and the people can use the structure already in place. Some beginning work of selection and making the group attractive has already been done. Membership ties in established groups influence individuals, and even in newly formed groups people bring emotional and social ties from previous and parallel group memberships. People are influenced by the interaction in one particular group and by their alliance with other important groups to which they belong. Memory serves to keep the norms and role expectations from one group present in a person as he moves from group to group. Individual behavior is then influenced not only by the membership, purpose, attraction, norms, leadership, and structure of the established health group but also by those processes remembered from other valued group memberships. Consideration of the multiple influences on members helps to determine an appropriate grouping for each situation and its peculiar dimensions.

Before deciding to work with established groups, the nurse must judge whether or not introducing a new focus is compatible with existing group purposes. In some cases individual health goals enhance existing group purposes, and the nurse may be seen as an important resource for bringing information for health, behavior, and group process. Nurses observe collective needs based on client contacts and assessment of other community data. Just as other nursing interventions are based on assessment of need and knowledge of effective treatment, groups are similarly formed from assessment of priority community needs for individual health change and consideration of group effectiveness in working toward those changes.

How can the community nurse enter existing groups and direct their attention to individual health needs? One nurse employed by an industrial firm noted the deleterious effect of managerial stress on several individuals. They had elevated blood pressure, stomach pain, and emotional tension. The nurse learned that the stressed adults were members of a jogging team that met weekly for conversation in addition to regular parallel workouts. The joggers readily accepted the offer to work together on individual stress management, seeing the need of their fellow members caught in high stress circumstances and the accompanying danger to health. High level health had been a shared value by all team members, and though jogging was seen as an enjoyable and health promoting activity, they had never articulated a shared purpose for improved health. In this circumstance the nurse observed a need for stress reduction, felt that the individuals at risk would be best able to achieve stress reduction when supported through a group process from valued friends, and proposed a new purpose be added to the jogging team's activities.

Selected Membership Groups

Nurses are familiar with group work in which members are selected because of the nature of their individual health needs. For instance, individuals with diabetes are brought together to consider diet management and physical care and to share in problem-solving remedies; community residents are brought together for social support and rehabilitation following treatment for mental illness; or the isolated elderly are brought together for socialization and hot meals.

Members' attributes are an important consideration in composing a new group. As noted earlier, members are attracted to others from similar backgrounds, with like experiences, and with common interests and abilities. This suggests selecting members so that common ties or interests balance out dissimilar traits. When the nurse is able to arrange it, the membership for selected groups should contain one or more individuals with expressive and problem-solving skills and some who are comfortable in supportive roles. Many people show ability in task and maintenance functions, and others have undeveloped potential for such functions. Support and training for group effectiveness within the unit build cohesion. As members perform increasingly valuable functions for the group, they become more attracted to it and more attractive to others.

The size of the group influences effectiveness; generally 8 to 12 people are considered a good number for small group work focused on individual health changes. Groups of up to 25 members may be effective when their focus is on community needs such as the group discussed previously that formed a neighborhood association. Large groups often divide and assign tasks to the smaller subgroups, with the original large groups meeting less frequently for reporting and evaluation.

Recruitment and selection among candidates for optimum group membership require judgment based on knowledge of group concepts. Selection can be facilitated by setting member criteria for specific groups. The criteria usually suggest a mixture of member traits, allowing balance for the process of decision making and growth.

Group Purpose

When the need for particular health changes is established and group work is selected as the most effective intervention, a purpose or goal for a proposed group must be stated. Clear statement and presentation of this purpose are essential in establishing criteria for member selection. A group purpose clearly stated facilitates recruitment of prospective members to the group.

Such a clear statement of purpose facilitated new group formation in one housing development in Xeona. There were numerous reports of child abuse and neglect according to the local department of social services. Routine home visits for well-child care documented high stress between parents and their offspring, and some parents requested guidance from the community health nurse in child discipline. The community health nurse felt that a parent group would address that community need. Nurses who were involved selected the following purpose for the group: "Dealing with kids for child and parent satisfaction." The purpose showed process, to help parents deal with kids, and the desirable outcome, satisfaction for parents and children. As potential members were approached, this statement of purpose for the group helped the individuals decide whether or not they wanted to join.

Appeals for membership may be public with all who elect to join accepted. In such situations the membership is self-selected, based on the stated group purpose. In this type of recruitment adequate publicity must be available to those in need of particular health changes. Prospective members often wish to discuss the purpose with leaders or clarify questions concerning the purpose at the first group meeting. Their commitment to the health group is partly based on individual goals and how well the group goal satisfies their personal objectives.

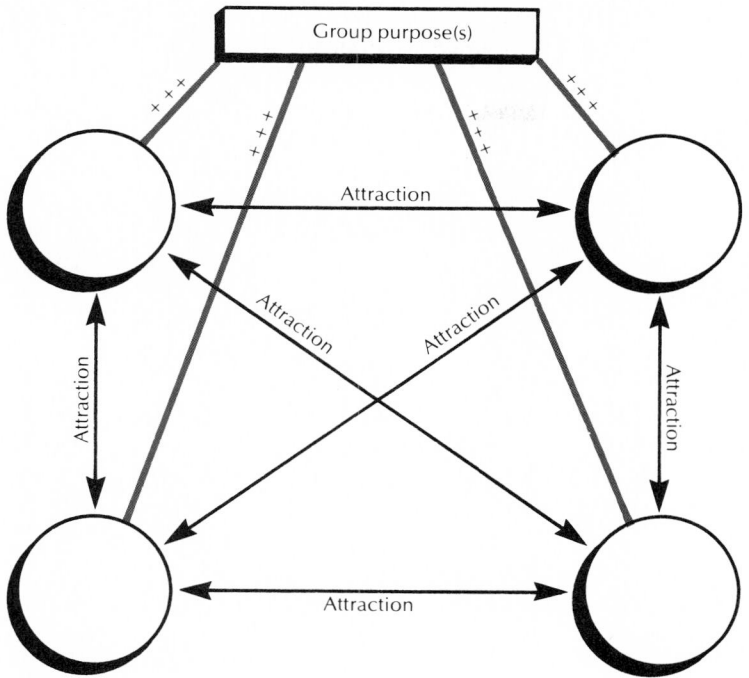

Fig. 16-2 Cohesion is the measure of attraction between members and member attraction to group purpose(s).

Cohesion

The measure of attraction between members and to the group is called *cohesion*. This pull to each other, to the group, and to its purposes operates for an overall group valence or attraction measurement. Individuals in a highly cohesive group identify themselves as a unit, work toward common goals, are willing to endure frustration for the sake of the group, and defend the group against outside criticism. Attraction is increased when members feel accepted by others, see like qualities in each other, perceive that others like them, and believe they share similar attitudes and values (Fig. 16-2). Some individual attributes that influence attraction between members include physical and interpersonal characteristics, behaviors, skills, knowledge, beliefs, and values. Members' traits that increase group cohesion and productivity include (1) congruence between personal goals and those of the group, (2) attraction to group goals, (3) attraction to other selected members, (4) distribution of leading and following skills, and (5) existence of problem-solving skills.

Functions of members that facilitate movement toward the group purpose are termed *task functions*. These task-directed abilities of any member improve his attractiveness. These traits include cognitive ability in problem solving, access to material resources, and skills in directing. Of equal importance are abilities to provide affirmation and support for individuals in the group; these functions that help members to stay with the group and feel accepted are termed *maintenance*

functions. Ability to help people resolve conflicts and ensure social and environmental comfort is also a maintenance function. Task and maintenance functions are necessary to group progress. Naturally those members who supply such group requirements are attractive, and an abundance of such traits within the membership tends to increase group cohesion.

Members' attributes held in low regard or judged as personally repulsive or threatening decrease attraction toward those members and the group as well. Behaviors and attitudes that are poorly understood by others in the group also tend to decrease group cohesion.

Commonly shared characteristics usually contribute to group attraction for members, whereas differences tend to decrease attractiveness. Members' perceptions of differences can create marked competition and jealousy. However, differences in members' characteristics increase group cohesion if they support complementary functioning or provide contrasting viewpoints necessary for decision making. Cohesion factors are complex; multiple influences affect member attraction to each other and to the group goal. Group productivity and member satisfaction are positively affected by high group cohesion. Two group examples illustrate factors that influence group cohesion and result in effectiveness.

A community health nurse initiated and provided beginning leadership for a group of clients who had been treated for burns. Ten residents, all from one town, had been discharged in 3 months from the local burn unit. The stated purpose for the group was to assist members in the difficult transition from hospital to home. Each person had been treated for extensive burns in an intensive care treatment center; had relied heavily on health workers for physical, social, and emotional rehabilitation; and had faced the challenge of resuming work and family roles. Individuals shared some similar experiences and hopes for the future. The individuals varied in the amount of trauma and stress experienced, and they differed widely in psychological readiness for return to ordinary daily routines. One woman was able to return quickly to her job as cashier in a large supermarket. The strength of her determination to overcome public reaction to her scars, coupled with an ability for words and empathy for others, were marked differences from others in the group. These differences proved very attractive to other members, inspiring them to work toward a return to their own roles in life. Her differences were perceived as attainable by other members. The cohesion for this group was in the member attraction to the common purpose of returning, after hospitalization, to successful life patterns, including work, and managing relations with others. Each member also felt that others with similar burn experiences could facilitate goal attainment. This example shows that certain member experiences, such as crises or traumas, although they are not highly valued by group members, may help individuals define their life situations as similar to each other and may increase member attraction.

Being different from the general population and like the other group members is for some a compelling force for the group. (For others, conversely, it repels them from the group, as they cannot tolerate the thought of their own likeness to some aversive characteristic such as disfigurement.) Empathy for another's pain, learned only through mutual experience, may provide each individual with a required perspective for problem solving or validation of reality. The nurse in the previous example helped members use common experiences and learn from their differences.

Differences created tension in one self-help group for victims of spouse abuse. Nurses met a severe challenge stemming from the differences they presented as non-victims. The community health nurses had been invited by professional staff members to assist the group in its process and to provide health information as needed. Victim members of the group felt that the nurses could not truly understand the intensely personal and devastating injury each had experienced, and they spoke directly to this point. They initially isolated the nurses from membership but tolerated their presence. Attraction of the group diminished, and attendance at meetings fell. Discussion of superficial issues occupied group time as the victim members avoided topics of member safety and violence in general. The nurses encouraged all the members to describe experiences seen as threatening to self-respect in their family and work

roles. The nurses revealed some of their own struggles for responsible self-direction and control. Such redefinition of self and variations in respect to abuse status supported a focus on similar individual goals rather than differences in life experiences. Group members supported one another to assert individual rights for safety, to locate employment, to make living arrangements necessary for independence from the abuser, and to identify needs for personal interactional changes. Cohesive forces for responsible status and the clear purpose of maintaining member safety contributed to successful group work. Thus member traits and the way they are perceived are shown to influence group cohesion and effectiveness.

Members' attraction to the group depends also on the nature of the group itself. The group programs, size, type of organization, and position in the community are influencing factors. When goals are perceived clearly by individuals and group programs or activities are believed to be effective, attraction to the group is increased.

The concept of cohesion helps to explain group productivity. Some cohesion is necessary for people to remain with a group and accomplish the set goals. Attractiveness positively influences member motivation and commitment to work on the group task. Cohesion for groups may be increased as members better understand the experiences of others and are able to identify common ideas and reactions to various issues. Nurses facilitate this process by pointing out similarities, contrasting supportive differences, or helping members redefine differences in ways that make those dissimilarities compatible.

Norms

Norms are standards that guide, control, and regulate individuals and communities. All members of a group understand and acknowledge the unwritten and frequently unspoken rules for that group, known as norms. The *group norms* represent the standards for group members' behaviors, attitudes, and even perceptions. All groups have norms and mechanisms whereby conformity is accomplished. Group pressures are brought to bear on members to bring about conformity to norms (Sampson and Marthas, 1981). Group norms serve three functions: (1) to ensure movement toward the group purpose or tasks, (2) to maintain the group through various supports to members, and (3) to influence members' perceptions and interpretations of reality.

The first function means that certain norms keep the group focused on its task or direct movement toward the end on which members have agreed. Diversion from a steady focus is permitted only as members respect central goals and feel committed to return to them. This compelling force to return to agreed on work is the *task norm,* the strength of which determines the intensity that the group has in keeping to its work.

In the second function *maintenance norms* create group pressures to ensure affirming actions for members and to help in maintaining comfort. Individuals in groups seem most productive and at ease when their psychological and social well-being is nurtured. Attention to social and psychological tension of members and the resulting steps to support them at high stress points are maintenance behaviors. Healthy maintenance norms may lead a group to pay attention to conditions like temperature, space, and seating, which ensure the physical comfort of the group during meeting times. The group is maintained by those arrangements that minimize physical tension for members, and this attention to arrangements may include meeting in places that are easily accessible and comfortable to the participants, providing refreshments, and scheduling meetings at convenient times.

A third function of group norms relates to members' perceptions of reality and is of equal importance to group performance. Daily behavior is largely based on the way each aspect of life is understood. Through socialization individuals learn how to gather information, assign meaning to that information, and react to situations in such a way that satisfies needs. Decision-making and action-taking processes are influenced by the meanings ascribed to reality. Individuals need validation of these interpretations of reality and look to others to reinforce or to challenge and correct their ideas of what is real. Groups serve to examine the life situations confronting individuals. As individuals gather information, attempt to understand that information, make decisions, and consider the facts and their implications, they can take responsible action not only in relation to self and group but also for the community.

A group culture or composite of the norms develop, and though norms dictate behaviors and perceptions, it is important to know that the nurse cannot dictate them. The nurse can implicitly and explicitly support rules, attitudes, and behaviors, which in turn can lead to certain norms. Only when the rules, attitudes, and behaviors become part of the life of the group, independent of the nurse, are they norms.

Fig. 16-3 shows that group norms affect members, tending to pressure them to see relevant situations in the same way that others view them. Strong normative pressure may develop to provide support for members considering change. Benne, describing the function of small groups for planned change, pointed out that individuals develop their value orientations through internalizing the norms of small groups on which they de-

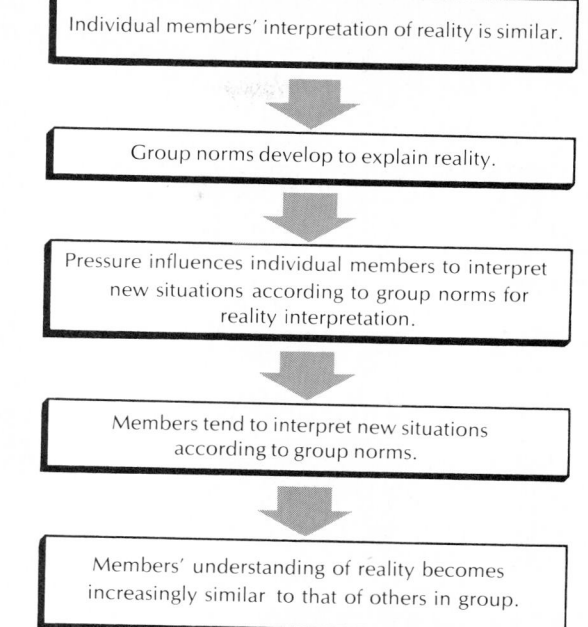

Fig. 16-3. Influence of group reality norms on individual members.

pend, notably families. "Changes in value orientations of individuals may be accomplished by seeking and finding significant membership in a small group with norms that are different in some respects from the normative orientation these individuals bring to a group" (1976, p. 76).

To illustrate, if a group of people who have diabetes defines uncontrollable diet as harmful, they will direct their efforts toward influencing each other to maintain diet control. The role of the nurse in such a group would involve providing accurate information about diet and the disease process, including cause and effect relationships between food intake and disease, and continually displaying a belief that health through diet control is attainable and desirable.

When members of any group have similar backgrounds, their scope of knowledge may be limited. For example, female members in a spouse abuse group may believe that men are exploitive and harmful based on common childhood and marriage experiences. Such a stereotyped view of men could be reinforced by members' similar perceptions and might lead to continuing anger, fear of interactions with men, and a hostile or helpless approach to family affairs. Nurses or group members who have known men in loving, helpful, and collaborative ways can describe their different and positive perceptions of men, thereby adding information and challenging beliefs based on more limited experiences. The group functions to influence members' perceptions and interpretations of reality. The health and condition of the individual improves as members' perceptions of reality become based on a full range of data, and cause and effect factors are understood. Nurses bring an important perspective to groups in which similar backgrounds limit the understanding and interpretation of personal concerns.

Leadership

Leadership in groups is an important and complex concept that involves guiding or directing a course. In a group the members' behaviors that lead include all of those actions that determine and influence the group movement. Leadership behaviors and definitions are shown in the box on the opposite page. Members who have a strong influence over others are identified as leaders.

Sources of leader influence are knowledge, ability, access to needed resources, personal attractiveness, status or position in the community or organization, and ability to control sanctions for others. Leadership behaviors may be concentrated in one or a few persons, or they may be dispersed and shared by many. Effective leadership is necessary for positive group functioning. Leadership is often described as patriarchal, paternal, or democratic, and each of these has a particular effect on members' interaction, satisfaction, and productivity. Some groups reflect a combination of leadership styles.

When the final authority for group direction and movement is vested in one person, the leadership style is *patriarchal* or *paternal.* Patriarchal leadership may control members through rewards and threats, often keeping them in the dark about the goals and rationale behind prescribed actions. Paternal leadership wins respect and dependence from followers by parentlike devotion to members' needs at the leader's own expense yet controls group movement and progress through interpersonal power vested in singular leadership. Patriarchal and paternal styles of leadership are authoritarian. For groups in which immediate task accomplishment or high productivity is the goal, these styles are effective. This is especially true for efforts that are technical rather than interpersonal in nature. However, group morale and cohesiveness are typically low under these styles of leadership; members may fail to learn how to function independently, and issues of authority and control disrupt productivity whenever the followers tire of submission to the one leader.

A paternal style was effective in the following situation. Mary Jones, a community health nurse, called her neighbors together to alert them to the threat of undesirable drug traffic in the neighborhood. The residents agreed with Mary that several recent drug-related arrests in the area signaled a need for community concern. No one knew what to do, but all felt quick action was desirable. Mary had experience in organizing people to work quickly, knew local resources, and thought that information, education, and residents' collaboration with police could substantially control the drug traffic problem locally. She organized the neighborhood group, assigned and monitored their tasks, and praised them highly as progress was made toward the goal of keeping the area free of drug sales. This leadership approach was effective for several weeks but required Mary to maintain a high level of activity.

A different style of leadership, *democratic,* is characterized by a cooperative structure that promotes and supports members' functioning in all aspects of decision making and planning. Members influence each other as they explore goals, plan steps toward the goals, implement those steps, and evaluate progress.

The previous situation also serves to illustrate the democratic style of leadership. As Mary Jones' neighbors became knowledgeable about controlling drug use and working with educators and police, they began to share the daily responsibilities to keep the project going and to generate new ideas and activities. Bob Smith realized that control of drug sales in one neighborhood failed to address the problem for the larger community. He organized a larger task force to look into the problem in other neighborhoods. Various members served in leadership roles as the project evolved. The change in leadership styles broadened the effectiveness of this community group as the members brought their collectively greater resources to bear.

A more common experience for nurses is illustrated in this example. A committee of nurses for a small community health organization met weekly to improve nursing services. Tom initiated a revision of written standards. Several members of the group felt threatened that their daily work would change and that a resulting evaluation by new standards would find them inferior or somehow needing to alter familiar procedures. Jane supported the work toward updated standards. She also was sensitive to the necessity of continuing support and affirmation of each nurse's worth on the committee. She often interrupted Tom's drive toward stating and refining standards by asking members to respond to suggestions, noting to the group the excellent contributions. Sara provided a touch of humor whenever group tension became high. Amber provided a critical, questioning support to the decision-making process and led the members to evaluate each step. In these and other ways group members shared leadership tasks. Some served predominately to push the group toward its objective, whereas others facilitat-

Examples of Leadership Behaviors

- Advising — introducing direction based on knowledgeable opinion
- Clarifying — checking out meanings of interaction and communication through questions and restatement
- Confronting — presenting behavior and its effects to the individual and group to challenge existing perceptions
- Evaluating — analyzing the effect or outcome of action or the worth of an idea, according to some standard
- Initiating — introducing topics, beginning work, or changing the focus of a group
- Questioning — bringing about analysis of views by questions that support examination
- Suggesting — proposing or bringing an idea to a group
- Summarizing — restating discussion or group action in brief form, highlighting important points
- Supporting — giving the kind of emotionally comforting feedback that helps a person or group continue ongoing actions

ed that movement forward by maintaining member involvement through support. For this group the chairperson served as convener but did not dominate in leader activities. The members accomplished the work of writing and implementing an audit for new nursing standards in a democratic leadership style.

Generally speaking, shared leadership in groups increases productivity and cohesion, resulting in friendly interactions between members. It builds appreciation for the work of leadership and inhibits power seekers. Shared leadership supports an idea of group wholeness, flexibility, and freedom. It might be hypothesized that a group in which the leadership is established in one effective and knowledgeable member would benefit from stability in its structure, predictability in its movement, and efficiency in its expenditure of energy. Follower roles would be clear and expectations explicit. Such an arrangement is efficient for groups of short duration, for those with a clearly defined purpose, and for those for which quick action is urgent. Such a leadership arrangement would be efficient for a disaster team but not for a planning committee.

Group Structure

Structure describes the particular arrangement of group parts that help to describe the group as a whole. Communication structure and role structure are two such descriptive frameworks. A *communication structure* identifies the parts according to message pathways and member participation in sending and receiving messages. Such communication structures can be mapped from observation of groups in action. People who are very active in receiving and sending messages and who serve as channels for messages because of their verbal skills, personal attractiveness, or spatial position are central in the structure. These central individuals derive influence in the group from their access to and interpretive control over communication flow.

Role structure for a group describes the expected behaviors of members relative to each other as the group interacts over time (see box on the next page). The role assumed by each group member has certain functions or behaviors that are displayed in the group and serve a purpose in the life of that group. Examples of roles are leader, follower, task specialist, maintenance specialist, evaluator, peacemaker, and gatekeeper. Members' roles in the group may be described by their predominate actions. Identification of a group's role structure can be accomplished by observation of members' behavior as the group operates. Communication and role structures are interrelated. Identification of communication patterns helps also to determine roles, since people occupying particular roles are characterized by certain kinds of communication.

In the earlier example of nurses working on standards of nursing service, Tom served a role as task specialist, Jane as maintenance specialist, and Amber as evaluator. These members occupied particular roles repeatedly and were expected by others to maintain their behavior to serve the purposes of the group.

A person occupying a gatekeeper's role controls outsiders' access to the group. Since gatekeepers are active in deciding issues of outsider entry, they use influence to either facilitate or block communication between outsiders and group members. Identification of those in gatekeepers' roles is crucial in community work when established groups are used for community health. The gatekeeper usually comes forward to confront the nurse after beginning contacts are attempted. An invitation to communicate further with group members is extended only after the nurse and gatekeeper determine mutual benefits and possible risks from continued contact between the nurse and the group.

Conflicts in groups may develop from competition for roles or member disagreement about the role ascribed to them. Struggles between members often result more from disagreement over dominance or out of competition for a favored position than from a conflict

---

Expected Behaviors Defining Group Roles

- Leader — guides and directs group activity
- Follower — seeks and accepts the authority or direction of others
- Task specialist — focuses or directs movement toward the main work of the group
- Maintenance specialist — provides physical and psychological support for group members, thereby holding the group together
- Evaluator — analyzes the effect or outcome of action or the worth of ideas according to some standard
- Peacemaker — attempts to reconcile conflict between members or takes action in response to influences that disrupt the group process, threatening its existence
- Gatekeeper — controls outsiders' access to the group

---

regarding group goals or steps in decision making. When group structures are considered from role and communication perspectives, the nurse and members of the group can more clearly understand the pressures affecting conflicting behavior and can work to resolve matters productively.

The following is an illustration of structure analysis leading to conflict resolution.

A small church in the rural town of Cookville initiated a project for youth recreation. The teens of Cookville had little opportunity for recreation, aside from driving around the countryside; the roadway was frequently used as a speedway by the restless youths. The church enlisted the high school principal and the community health nurse to work with a project group, and it was dynamic. All supported the development of a local youth center and worked energetically toward that goal.

After 2 months of smooth work together, many arguments erupted at meetings. Conflicts about the supervision of the proposed center, the site for the physical plant, and numerous smaller concerns seemed to dominate planning time. The group had active, aggressive members; four of these individuals seemed to talk the most and to resist argument resolution. After several frustrating meetings, the nurse asked the group to consider their roles in decision making. She suspected that the disagreements were related to members' functions in the group rather than their ideas. The nurse was supportive to each person as the roles and expectations of each member of the project group were explored. The four most talkative individuals expressed personal wishes to direct the planning and displayed aggravation when these attempts were thwarted. Other members described supportive and task functions but did not seek dominance in leadership functions. The open analysis of role structure made clear to the members that arguments grew out of competition for directing roles rather than from true disagreements about the recreation project. The open discussion in this situation also resulted in an agreement to divide the project work into several task areas to be led by separate area directors. Members expressed relief that basic agreement about the purpose remained intact, and they were able to modify their role expectations to accommodate all members. They joked together about being a collection of bosses and renewed their productive work.

PROMOTING INDIVIDUALS' HEALTH THROUGH GROUP WORK

Health behavior is influenced greatly by the groups to which people belong and for which they value membership. Individuals live within a social structure of significant others such as family, friends, workers, and acquaintances. The patterns and directions of everyday activities are learned in a family, and these are later reinforced or challenged by new sets of important others. These groups form the context in which values, beliefs, and attitudes are formed; individuals usually consider the responses of others in all types of decisions regarding personal welfare.

The following example illustrates the effects of a person's social network on health behavior.

Mary Berton worried about a lump recently discovered in her breast. She first asked her husband, Lew, to confirm its presence, which he did. He agreed that she should arrange for a diagnostic evaluation, and an appointment was arranged. Mary talked with Lew about the possible consequences of malignancy, and she noted Lew's concern for her safety. She was fearful of radical surgery and its impact on her relationship to Lew, but she did not discuss that with him. Mary telephoned two close friends from her work place and asked them to meet her for coffee. Even though they felt it was premature to fret about the lump being malignant, they discussed all they knew about treatment for breast cancer, including the trials, defeats, and successes of three mutual friends who had had surgery for breast cancer. Each of the experienced friends had reacted differently to her own situation, and Mary's friends retold familiar details. The retelling seemed important in grasping the current situation and helping Mary sort out her feelings. She was assisted in facing the reality of risk, recognizing the need to follow through with diagnostic procedures, selecting able medical sources, and managing her emotional stress.

Mary's friends' and husband's responses to her situation influenced her assessment, decision making, and subsequent behavior. The work done by Mary and her friends in response to her health need is important business. It illustrates a common mechanism among individuals and the groups to which they belong. The groups described in this example are Mary's family group, which includes Mary and Lew, and Mary's friendship group, of which those who met for coffee are a subset.

Groups supportive of individual health changes are unavailable to some people because of their social or emotional isolation. Also, existing groups sometimes work contrary to health goals. Individuals isolated from supportive groups or hindered by their group connections may find movement toward health very difficult, and they may benefit greatly through newly organized groups established for specific purposes. Isolated individuals may have low self-esteem, be mentally ill, be socially stigmatized, and be interpersonally abused. They may be disadvantaged, gifted, or deviant, or they may simply live a rural existence or be engaged in solitary work.

As community nurses enlarge their knowledge of group concepts, develop skills in working with varied groups, and become aware of the power in groups for individual changes, they will become available, visible, and sought for group work. At times community health nurses work with existing groups, and at other times they select members for new groups. A decision about whether to work in established groups or to begin new ones is based on the clients' needs, the nature of existing groups, the purpose of the groups, and the membership ties in existing groups.

Beginning Interactions

Once a group forms, work begins on the stated purpose. Early meetings require further clarification of both individual and group goals. Members with varying degrees of openness present themselves and their backgrounds. They begin to interact with each other by seeking and giving information about themselves and their circumstances and at the same time demonstrating their capabilities in problem solving and group participation. The nurse assists by supporting ideas and feelings, inviting participation, giving information, clarifying thoughts, and suggesting structure. The method for proceeding toward the purpose varies according to the nurse's skill and preference but also to group composition and the multitude of skills brought by members.

Nurses in beginning groups should place priority on helping members interact with a degree of satisfaction. This requires close attention to maintenance tasks of attending, eliciting information, clarifying communication when needed, and recognizing contributions of members. Attending includes simple responses to people, such as listening carefully to their speech and not-

ing their mood, dress, and informal conversation as they enter the meeting. Attending behavior communicates recognition and acceptance of the person and his presentations to the group.

A beginning format that focuses on whatever brought each member to the group provides recognition and helps the individual acknowledge similar and different perspectives. Members may be asked to describe what each hopes to accomplish in the group and what experiences each has previously had in groups. Member to member exchanges are encouraged; individuals are recognized and supported as they take on leadership functions.

Even in beginning sessions of groups, some patterns of work are formulated. Members try out familiar roles and test their individual abilities. Those approaches to member support, leadership, and decision making, which are comfortable and productive for the members, become normative ways for the group to work. The nurse enters into such models creatively, evaluating style and productivity according to appropriateness for the members and nurse. The work of the group is begun even as the goals for health change are examined carefully and are realistically accepted. During this early period, members' attractions to each other and to the group begin to develop.

Conflict

Groups at work experience conflict. Members come with unique personalities and often disagree about many aspects of the group's work and the part that each member plays. Open discussion of differences and disagreements can promote individual and group growth. The nurse should promote such openness, though making it clear that respect for each person and point of view is necessary. This lays the groundwork for a group norm that supports member esteem during conflict and resolution. Conflict in groups may grow from unspoken or generally unrecognized issues. These conflicts are sometimes communicated subtly in themes such as control and dependence.

Often the conflict regarding status in the health group represents concerns brought in by members who experienced similar problems in other important groups like their families (e.g., one person's struggle for leadership and dominance is mirrored from a similar struggle at home). Persons in victim roles, for example, may have integrated low esteem and self-accusation into their views of themselves. The replay of problematic interpersonal transactions in the group allows critical examination by supportive members and leads to healing, understanding, and rejection of low self-evaluation and to the practice of presenting a healthier self.

Problem Solving for Health Change

Work toward established health goals is facilitated by community health nurses through their considerable knowledge of health and health risks for individuals, groups, and communities. Problem-solving and decision-making skills and strategies for change are part of the nurse's resources for such group work.

Basic teaching is sometimes used as an early method. Members benefit from understanding facts and cause and effect links, the known associations between environment, body response, wellness, and pathology that are pertinent to the health change goal. Participation in formal learning may help people focus on the reality of the problems faced and ways to understand them. The potential of a group for effecting individual change is only addressed fully when members work actively and directly through discussion and other approaches to problem solving. Expectant parent groups illustrate a type of community group in which teaching is a highly appropriate method. Participants need to understand facts concerning pregnancy, labor and delivery, self- and infant care, parenting, and adjusting to change. Along with factual understanding, they need an opportunity to practice the skills required in anticipated tasks and to explore their attitudes and emotional responses to the anticipated family changes. Specific learning activities in the group would likely include practice for baby baths and situation enactment of family activity after the baby comes home. Such experiential learning activities, which require interaction between members and use of materials highly relevant to the change goal, are useful.

One way to consider change for health is through analysis of motivating and restraining forces for individuals and groups. For this analysis the group considers major factors that influence the particular change proposed for health. Included are the encouraging and supportive forces for change and the interfering and resistive influences that each person experiences from all sources, including important individuals within the family, work, and community groups. These forces are identified during group meetings, where others help to plan action steps for overcoming interferences and promoting facilitative factors. The group members learn from each other and the nurse to deal effectively with multiple outside influences as they relate to the individuals' desired health goals.

Relationships within the group become increasingly important because of the shared understanding of the what, how, when, and where of health needs and changes. Normative pressures within the group keep members engaged in the agreed-on work and support the progress made by each individual. A group worksheet is presented on the opposite page. This worksheet helps to organize influences for and against goal attainment. Describing and listing the supportive forces and resistive influences for change help people clarify the multiple factors operating in any change. The study of factor sources, whether they arise within the individual, the work group, other valued groups, or the community at large, reveals areas requiring action. Such an analysis encourages consideration of diverse influences.

For the Xeona group at high risk for abusive parenting, eight parents showed up for the first meeting. Some came because they knew the nurse calling the meeting and thought she could help them with discipline problems. Two came only because it was strongly advised by their spouses, and others came because of the stated and publicized purpose of dealing with kids for parent and child satisfaction. Offering child care during meetings permitted parent attendance.

During the first two group meetings they described their children and some of the satisfying and frustrating experiences of parenting. Frustrations in work and family relations also surfaced, along with stress regarding finances and housing. Central to the concern of each was an expressed wish to be a better and happier parent. Neglect and violence were not mentioned in early group sessions.

As parents became acquainted, they noticed that they had similar frustrations about discipline. They described their anger, which sometimes erupted in slaps and beatings. They also expressed shame and confusion about these angry expressions of frustrations. After about 3 months, they felt strength from their mutual support and were able to face some changes that were expressed as "finding and using better ways to discipline kids."

What happened in the group to enable recognition of needs and plans to change abusive behavior? The people felt care and respect first from the nurse and later from each other. They recognized comparable frustration in parenting and failure to deal well with anger. Empathy for others in similar circumstances and with shared needs motivated them to work together on their parenting problems. They were encouraged by the nurse's and other group members' belief in each one's ability to change to a healthier parenting position with accompanying responsible behavior. The group helped each parent plan action steps toward individual goals. Progress on individual steps was reported each week with resulting support and reinforcement. The result was a reduction of the abuse and neglect of children by group members.

Evaluation of Group Progress

Evaluation of individual and group progress toward health goals is important. Action steps toward the goal are specified from the earliest planning. These small steps may be suggested in response to learning objectives, from listed action steps designed to support facili-

Group Worksheet: Influences For/Against Attainment of Goal

Group goal: _____

Related individual goals: _____

Influences within individuals

        For: 1 _____

              2 _____

              3 _____

  Against: 1 _____

              2 _____

              3 _____

Influences within work group

        For: 1 _____

              2 _____

              3 _____

  Against: 1 _____

              2 _____

              3 _____

Influences from other valued groups

        For: 1 _____

              2 _____

              3 _____

  Against: 1 _____

              2 _____

              3 _____

Community influences

        For: 1 _____

              2 _____

              3 _____

  Against: 1 _____

              2 _____

              3 _____

tative forces and deal with resistance forces, or from whatever problem-solving plan the group designs. These action steps and the indicators of achievement are articulated in discussion and written in a group record. Celebration is built into the group's evaluation system to help individuals recognize and reinforce each step toward the health goal. Celebration may include concrete rewards such as special foods and drinks, or it may be personal expression of joy and member-to-member approval. Celebration for group accomplishments marks progress, rewards members, and motivates each person for continuing work.

Summary of Health Promotion Through Group Work

Groups are a powerful mechanism for promoting individual health change. Community health nurses may effectively use small group methods to promote individuals' health through existing groups and those established for individual health changes. This section addressed initiating the group, working toward group goals, and evaluating group effectiveness.

COMMUNITY GROUPS AND THEIR CONTRIBUTION TO COMMUNITY LIFE

In a broad context community health nurses focus on the community and its health which may be viewed according to health outcomes experienced by the people or to the structure of services and resources available and used. Community health may also be defined as community competence, a comprehensive state of physical, emotional, and social well-being of the people that results from interactive processes between the community parts. Nurses are interested in the whole of the community and its component parts.

Identifying Community Groups

An understanding of group concepts provides a beginning basis for identifying community groups, their goals, member characteristics, and group norms. Nurses may begin community assessment by identifying community subsystems and the formal groups within them. This formal community structure is mapped from data in public documents, such as a community comprehensive plan, and from local media. Community residents, especially those in leadership positions, may provide additional information about the various formal groups, their functions, and their position in the community. It is important to note the harmony among the goals of various formal groups; the overlap, cooperation, or competition in function; the differences and similarities between member character-

istics; and the congruence or lack thereof between formal group standards.

The membership in formal groups can be determined by noting member rolls. The demarcation between subsystems and for formal groupings within them is determined by the statements of community residents about who belongs, works with, or affiliates with particular groupings.

Informal groups are usually identified through interviews with key spokespersons. Informal groups also become distinguished by action or service in the community that is recognized in the news media. Informal groups include friendship, neighborhood, and social network groupings.

Groups are ranked in the community on the basis of such characteristics as social prestige or power. Power in turn is associated with the hierarchies of position in the community subsystems of economics, government, education, religion, health, and welfare. Those in high level positions have greater capacity for influencing community-wide matters than those in relatively lower positions. The nurse should consider the extent to which formal and/or informal groups are linked through family and friendship ties.

After the community subsystems, formal groups, and representative informal groups are identified and links between them are mapped, the nurse may further study the community group structure through observation of each group's goals and their appropriateness to overall community goals. Both stated and unstated goals are identified in this process.

Goals for the community and for various groups are studied through media sources and community informants. In community health assessment the nurse documents needs, resources, and vision for change as perceived by the people living and working in the community. The data may be organized according to the opinions of and behaviors from the groups identified. Since individuals develop, refine, and change their ideas within the context of the groups to which they belong, the matrix of community health needs and desires for change may also be understood according to the group structure of the community. An illustration of community need assessment from a group perspective is diagrammed in Fig. 16-4. Analysis of groups, their health needs, and their desire for change suggests collaborative links and a willingness to change.

Interlinking Subsystems

Edwards and Jones (1976) described the community according to differentiated and interlinking subsystems such as family, economy, government, religion, education, health, and welfare. These community subsystems

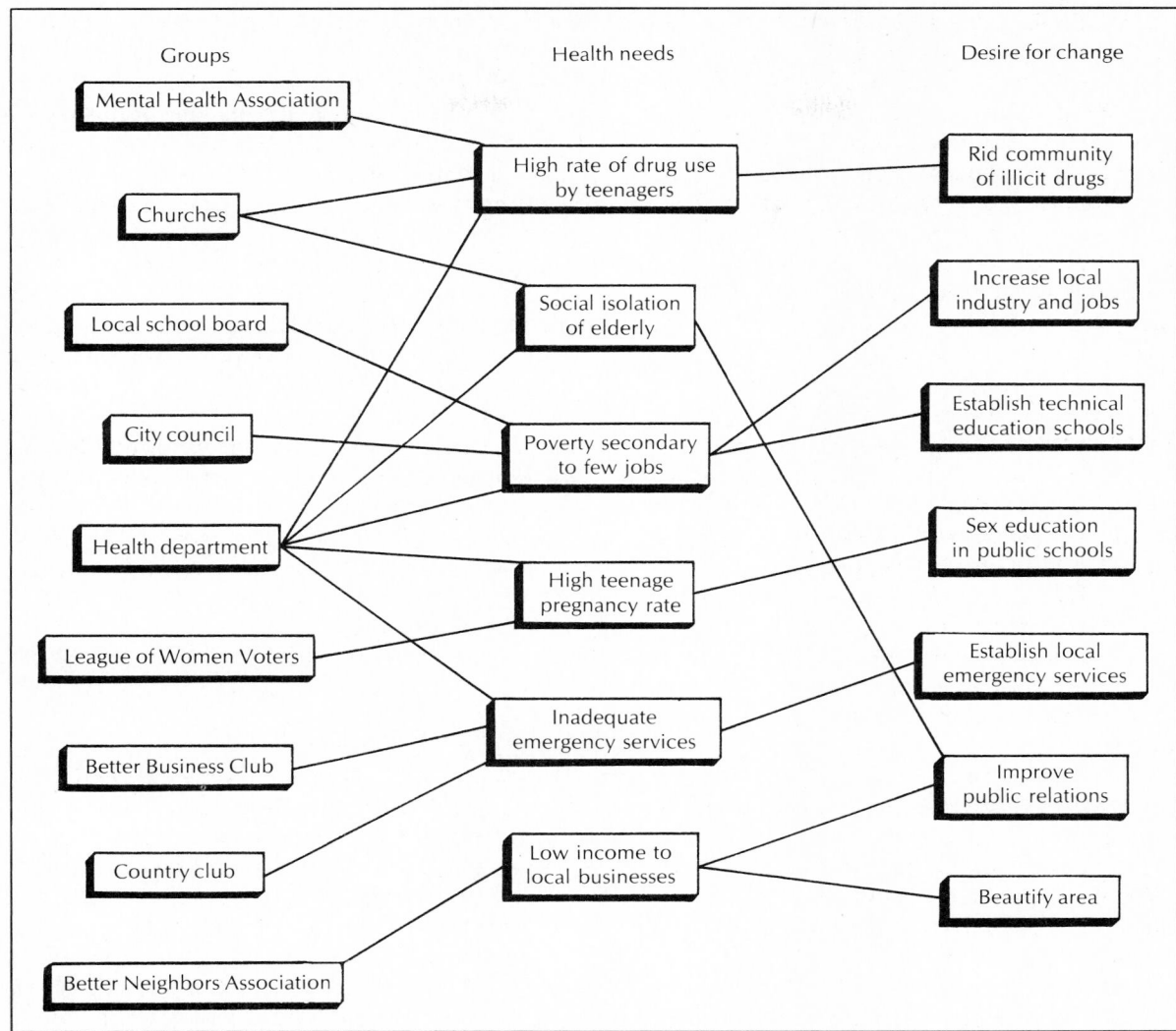

Fig. 16-4. Community identifies health needs and desire for change.

are linked vertically to the larger society and horizontally to each other through various communication and cooperative exchanges. Functioning within and between subsystems of the community are individual persons, informal groups such as friendship and other spontaneous groups, and formal groups such as schools, churches, and businesses.

The interrelatedness among individuals is built partly on the network of roles and status levels that exist in the various formal and informal groups in the community's social structure (Edwards and Jones, 1976). Informal groups are linked to the extent that their members have connections with formal groups that are in turn part of the community subsystems. The informal and unofficial channels of interaction that develop between

status levels (formal and informal groups) serve to link groups, thus contributing to the community integration. For example, the relationships and patterns of influence existing in local extended family groups are likely to influence the many other groups to which those family members belong. Members of a family in Goff county actively participate in the board of county directors, the school board, the protestant mission council, the youth advisory commission, and the county rescue squad. This family's conservative political views, especially those related to local management of financial affairs, are reflected in the conservative fiscal posture of these five separate community groups.

The various group norms regarding member communication and interaction with others and the degree of harmony between group goals influence the overall harmony and free exchange between individuals and groups in the community. Links between formal groups depend on the degree of coordination, cooperation, and competition between community subsystems. Many communities sanction various cooperative links by means of coordinating groups, such as interagency councils. Links to county, state, and national subsystems exist to a large extent as local groups are increasingly controlled by special community organizations and events.

The small group is potentially able to influence and change the larger social community of which it is a part. The social system depends on groups for governing, making policy, determining community needs, taking steps to alleviate those needs, and evaluating program outcomes. The small group is a mechanism for interrelatedness between community subsystems, certain subsystems and their counterparts in the larger social structure, and factions within subsystems. Change in the composition and function of strategic small groups may produce change also for the wider social system that depends on small groups for direction and guidance (Benne, 1976).

WORKING WITH GROUPS TOWARD COMMUNITY HEALTH GOALS

Community health nurses may use their understanding of group principles to work with community groups toward needed health changes. The groupings appropriate for this work include both established, community-sanctioned groups and groups for which nurses select members representing diverse community sectors.

Existing community groups formed for community-wide purposes such as elected executive groups, health planning groups, better business clubs, womens' action groups, school boards, and neighborhood councils are excellent resources for community health assessment, since part of their ongoing purpose is to determine and respond to community needs. These types of groups are powerful actors for community health because they are already established as part of the community structure. When a group representing a community sector is selected for community health intervention, the total community structure is studied. Data about family ties, experiences with resource centers, and lifelong contacts to other sector groups are obtained. Groups are subject to existing community values, strengths, and normative forces.

How might community health nurses assist established groups work toward community goals? The same interventions recommended for groups formed for individual health change are beneficial to community health–focused groups. Such facilitative interventions include building cohesion through goal clarity and individual attraction to groups, building member commitment and participation, keeping the group focused on the goal, maintaining members through recognition and encouragement, maintaining member self-esteem during conflict and confrontation, analyzing forces effecting movement toward the goal, and evaluating progress. On entering established groups, nurses seek to assess the leadership, communications, and normative structures. Knowledge and activity resources of the nurse facilitate involvement in the group planning, problem solving, action, and evaluation steps. The steps for community health change parallel those of decision making and problem solving in other methodologies.

One community health nurse joined the Oswald neighborhood group after several client families recounted stories of multiple gunshot injuries to youths in the neighboring homes. Seven young males aged 14 to 21 had been injured in separate shoot-outs during recent months. The neighbors, mostly parents, formed a concerned parent group to discuss the dangers for all residents and especially for their sons. The clients knew that Ms. Brown, the nurse, knew how to help groups "get their act together" and take action on problems. They had worked with Ms. Brown for the neighborhood health fair. Her assessment was that the Oswald neighborhood could improve their relations if the adults and youths recognized and redirected some emerging problems.

Ms. Brown attended the first few group meetings, taking a back seat as Mrs. Knight, a local resident and parent, recounted the recent violent occurrences, and others added details about the shootings. Feelings ran high and everyone wanted to speak out about the threats to themselves and their families. Urgency for action kept people task directed. Soon they focused on two action goals: (1) to limit youths' access to firearms by getting the weapons out of neighborhood homes and (2) to establish a supervised youth recreation center to provide alternative activities for youth. Both goals were reasonable, partial solutions to the problem of teenage violence in Oswald; they required commitment and high-energy expenditure from the majority of the neighborhood residents. Ms. Brown offered to help the group consider action steps toward the goals that were possible, economical, efficient, and productive. She helped the group identify factors that facilitated their work toward goals and other factors that hindered progress. To accomplish the first goal, limiting youths' access to firearms, the group analyzed facilitative and hindering forces. This analysis led to action steps that would increase residents' awareness of danger from firearms, identify homes where firearms were kept, determine household regulations over these firearms, and launch a person-to-person communication that supported strict control for all guns. Commitment to this community intervention was heightened by the group's fear of violence, and they spent many hours within a 2-week period of time to implement steps toward the goal. Their action produced a dramatic effect in the community, culminating in a neighborhood rally, during which most residents spoke on record for strict gun control.

The second goal for a supervised youth center took longer for accomplishment. Although shoot-outs no longer occurred in the community and Oswald became a safer place to live, the youths previously involved in the neighborhood violence remained dissatisfied and conflicts between them and outside gangs continued. Plans to address the continuing needs of local youths included a support group for management of conflict, vocational training classes for young people, service activity projects in a local church, and youth representation on the newly formed neighborhood council. Since adults and youths in Oswald realized that gang action and violence were problems in adjoining neighborhoods, they began linking with citizens in those neighboring areas to promote concern about guns and violence. They recognized that safety in Oswald depended on wider community exchanges and continued work.

Community groupings, because of their interactive roles, seem to be logical and natural action clusters for community health change. As the decision-making and problem-solving capabilities of community groups are strengthened, the groups become more able representatives of the whole community as well as its sectors. Community health nurses improve the community's health through work with groups toward that goal.

SUMMARY

Group concepts are clusters of statements that describe the phenomena of groups. The concepts presented in this chapter—member interaction, group purpose, cohesion, norms, leadership, and structure—provide a basic framework for understanding group behavior. The concepts appear deceptively simple, but application to live groups reveals their complexity for individuals wishing to influence group behavior. Though each group concept is initially considered in isolation, the combination of concepts provides a multidimensional structure for group analysis. Group behavior is complex because of the many factors influencing individual members, member interaction within the group, and the group's community environment.

A serious student will want to study different groups, analyzing the various dimensions presented by these group concepts. Such study illustrates the interplay of influences on groups and their members. It allows an orientation to what works and does not work in groups. Since the interactions are multiple and complex, per-

ception of contributing factors is necessarily limited. Accuracy is improved through experience, and students can widen their understandings and validate their observations through discussions with participants. Discussion and analysis of observed groups in conjunction with experienced teachers enrich the student's study of groups. The learning activities for this chapter are designed to support the student's growth in understanding groups.

Considered study of all kinds of groups enriches the nurse's sensitivity to group dynamics and helps distinguish the interplay of factors operating to enable or hinder group effectiveness. A group concept framework is like using one lens for looking at changing behavior for all clients and health systems delivering care. The group is both a natural phenomenon affecting everyday life and a deliberate methodology for influencing change for health, which is the essence of nursing practice.

The illustrations in the chapter describe real group situations. However, it is impossible to describe every feasible combination of elements in a cookbook fashion. The nurse must use creativity in the application of knowledge in unique situations. A series of questions to guide the implementation of concepts should be asked. What is the problem? Who are the people involved? Is group methodology the best route to accomplish the objectives with these particular people? If so, at what level—individual member focused or community focused? Will the problem be best addressed by an established group, or should members be selected for forming a new group? What is the nursing role in establishing the new group? What strategy is suitable for entering an existing group?

It should be remembered that interventions are products of established knowledge, techniques, and personal attributes such as life experience, personality, and personal style. Ability to work in a group context may vary according to all of these factors along with group members' attributes and needs.

Supervision or consultation assists in self-evaluation and development of group strategies. Such feedback is essential to developing self-awareness in group practice. Literature describing specific interventions with particular problems and/or types of groups is available, and a bibliography is listed for this purpose.

Through knowledge of group behavior, skill in group practice, and appreciation of the power that groups have, community health nurses may substantially enlarge the scope of their impact on health for individuals and communities. Community health nurses are challenged to use the opportunities for change through work with groups.

BIBLIOGRAPHY

Alinsky, S.D.: Rules for radicals, New York, 1971, Vintage Books.

Benne, K.D.: The current state of planned changing in persons, groups, communities, and societies. In Bennis, W. G., et al., editors: The planning of change, ed. 3, New York, 1976, Holt, Rinehart, & Winston General Book.

Bennis, W.G., et al., editors: The planning of change, ed. 3, New York, 1976, Holt, Rinehart, & Wiston General Book.

Bertcher, J.H.: Group participation: techniques for leaders and members, Beverly Hills, 1979, Sage Publications, Inc.

Bertcher, H.J., and Maple, F.: Creating groups, Beverly Hills, 1977, Sage Publications, Inc.

Callahan, J., et al.: Processing a task group: a continuing education committee at work planning a conference, J. Cont. Educ. Nurs. **11**:8, Sept. 1980.

Cartwright, D., and Zander, A., editors: Group dynamics, ed. 3, New York, 1968, Harper & Row Publishers, Inc.

Cottrell, L.S.: The competent community. In Kaplan, B.H., et al., editors: Further explorations in social psychiatry, New York, 1976, Basic Books, Inc., Publishers.

Edwards, A.D., and Jones, D.: Community and community development. The Hague, Netherlands, 1976, Mouton Publishers.

Forsyth, D.M., et al.: Preventing and alleviating staff burnout through a group, Psychosoc. Nurs. Ment. Health Serv. **35**:8, Sept. 1981.

Henkel, B.O.: Solving health problems through small group action. In Spradley, B.W., editor: Contemporary community nursing, Boston, 1975, Little, Brown & Co.

Kagey, J.R., et al.: Mental health primary prevention: the role of parent mutual support groups, Am. J. Public Health **71**:166, Feb. 1981.

Krawczyk, R.M.: Peer participation conferences: a dynamic method of nursing instruction, Nrs. Ed. **17**:5, Oct. 1978.

Lipson, J.G.: Consumer activism in two women's self-help groups, West. J. Nurs. Res. **2**:393, 1980.

Michael, M.M., et al.: Symposium on the self-care concept of nursing: use of the adolescent peer group to increase the self-care agency of adolescent alcohol abusers, Nurs. Clin. North Am. **15**:157, March 1980.

Nix, H.: Why Parents Anonymous? J. Psychiat. Nurs. **18**:23, Oct. 1980.

Politser, P.E., et al.: Social climates in community groups: toward a taxonomy, Community Ment. Health J. **16**:187, 1980.

Sampson, E.E., and Marthas, M.: Group process for the health professions, ed. 2, New York, 1981, John Wiley & Sons, Inc.

Shamansky, S.L., and Pesznecker, B.: A community is . . . , Nurs. Outlook **29**:182. March 1981.

Smith, L.L.: Finding your leadership style in groups, Am. J. Nurs. **80**:1301, 1980.

Spradley, B.W., editor: Community health nursing concepts and practice, Boston, 1981, Little, Brown & Co.

Veninga, R.: Are you a successful communicator? Can. Nurse **74**:34, Nov. 1978.

Walsh, S.: Parents of Asthmatic Kids (PAK): a successful parent support group, Pediat. Nurs. **7**:28, May/June 1981.

Yalom, I.D.: The theory and practice of group psychotherapy, New York, 1975, Basic Books, Inc., Publishers.

Chapter
17

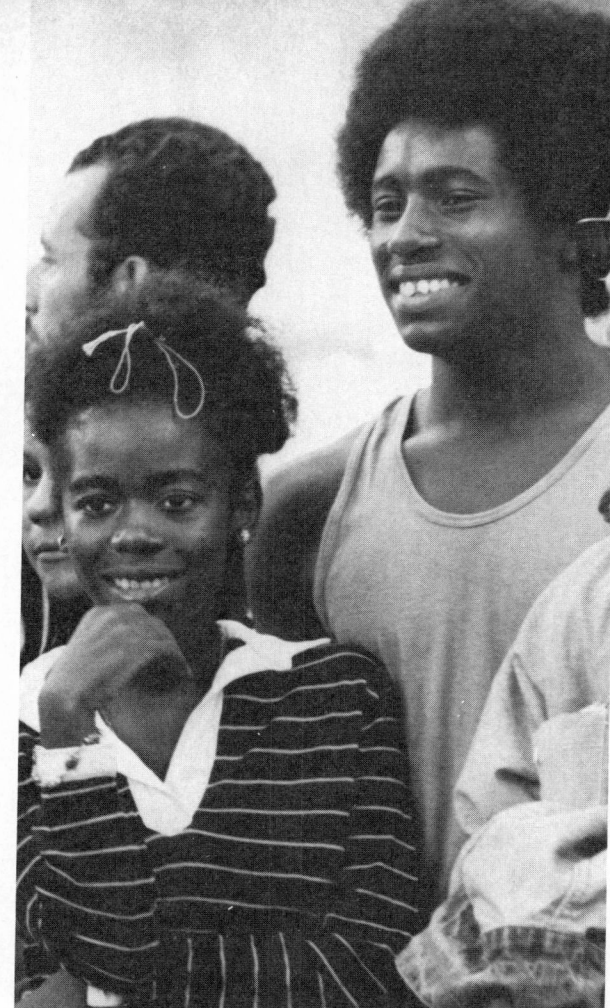

JEAN GOEPPINGER

COMMUNITY AS CLIENT: USING THE NURSING PROCESS TO PROMOTE HEALTH

Nurses have traditionally considered the community as one of their clients. Some nurses, especially community health nurses, have even viewed the community as their most important client. Irrespective of the relative emphasis given to the community, the concept of "community as client" has never been adequately defined. Consequently, nursing practice directed to the community as client has been neglected. The proportion of nursing practice devoted to the community has been minimal, and the effects of that practice, to the limited extent that they have been documented, have been disappointing.

This chapter provides both conceptual clarity and guidelines for nursing practice with the community client. Use of the nursing process to promote community health is emphasized. Initially the various meanings attributed to the concept of community as client are delineated and analyzed. One definition is adopted for use throughout the chapter. Next the reasons for considering the community as an appropriate nursing client are considered. The three concepts that are basic to nursing practice with the community client are examined in the subsequent section. They are (1) community, the target of change; (2) community health, the goal of change; and (3) partnership for community health, the means of change. Guidelines for nursing practice with the community client follow. Principles and tools to assist in the nursing assessment of community health and nursing intervention for community health are presented. Examples are included to illustrate the use of the nursing process in promoting the health of the community.

COMMUNITY AS CLIENT

A wealth of issues exists today in community health nursing. Paramount among them are the concern and confusion surrounding the nature of our clients. The fundamental questions are (1) whether a community *practice setting* ensures that the community is the client, (2) whether the community itself or certain segments of the community such as individuals, families, and aggregate groups are the clients; and (3) whether the community client is both the *unit* and the *target of service.*

The community has simultaneously been discussed as the setting of service (Archer and Fleshman, 1979), the unit of service (Goeppinger, 1980; Skrovan et al., 1974), and the target of service (Freeman, 1973; Williams, 1977; Wood and Ohlson, 1977). Typologies encompassing all three meanings have been created (Archer, 1976; Archer and Fleshman, 1975; Spero, 1977). They suggest that such diverse interpretations are not mutually exclusive. The lack of unanimity about the nature of our clients is, however, confusing.

This section critically reviews the most common meanings ascribed to the concept of community as client.

Summary of Definitions

The uniqueness of community health nursing has customarily been attributed to its practice setting. The community has been conceptualized as the client simply because community health nursing care did not occur in the hospital.

At the turn of the century, for instance , the practice environments of community health nurses were homes rather than hospitals. Nurses wore blue rather than white uniforms, worked as diligently to promote health as to treat illness, and most importantly, were guests in clients' homes. Community health nurses practiced in clients' natural environments, their homes, and not in the hospital. Early community health nursing textbooks included lengthy descriptions of the home environment and tools for assessing the extent to which that environment was conducive to family members' health. Health education about the home environment was frequently a major part of nursing care. The community environment was treated similarly with attention focused on the extent to which the community supported or impeded health.

Gradually more nurses began to move out of the hospital. School and industry as well as home became legitimate practice sites for nurses. The exodus from the hospital continued with the creation and institutionalization of the nurse practitioner role in community settings.

As the sites of practice broadened, the uniqueness of community health nursing which had been attributed to the practice setting—home, school, industry, and health center—became less convincing. Many of the nurses who were now community based did not even take into account the environments in which they practiced. Instead, practice was oriented to the individual patient and family. The *Conceptual Model of Community Health Nursing* of the American Nurses' Association (1980, p. 4, Assumption 5) represents just such a position. Consequently, the location of practice became an inadequate reason for identifying the care occurring there as oriented to the community as client, for the actual clients are the individual and family, not the community.

A more recent perspective identifies the community as client when the community itself is the unit of service. The community—not the individual, family, or aggregate—is defined as the unit of nursing service. Nursing practice is aimed at assisting communities to identify, articulate, and successfully manage their health concerns. Similar orientations to community practice are held by some social workers and community organizers. The communities in such practices are generally neighborhood or locality based.

This approach to specification of the community has not been readily accepted by community health nurses. Nursing care delivered to individuals or families, that is, direct clinical care, has been and remains a more popular concept.

Direct clinical care can, however, be oriented to the community client when the unit of service is not equated with the target of service. Many community health nurses have long espoused just such a notion.

Both Freeman (1973) and Williams (1977), for example, write that personal clinical care delivered to individuals and families residing in community settings is community health nursing care when it is focused on the health of a population group such as the community. This notion is consistent with the central emphasis of community health practice on the health of population groups, with nursing's emphasis on direct clinical care, and with current thinking about the importance of synthesizing personal clinical care with care directed to the health of specific population groups (Kark, 1974). This chapter is built on the perspective of the community as the target of service.

The Community Client

The community is considered the client or target of service when nursing practice, regardless of setting or unit of service, is community oriented. Community-oriented practice means that healthful change is sought for the community's benefit. The focus is on the collec-

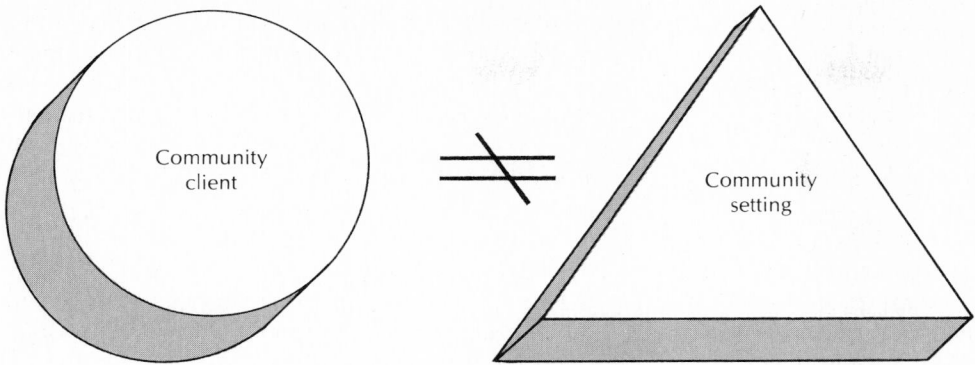

Fig. 17-1. Is community client determined by the practice setting?

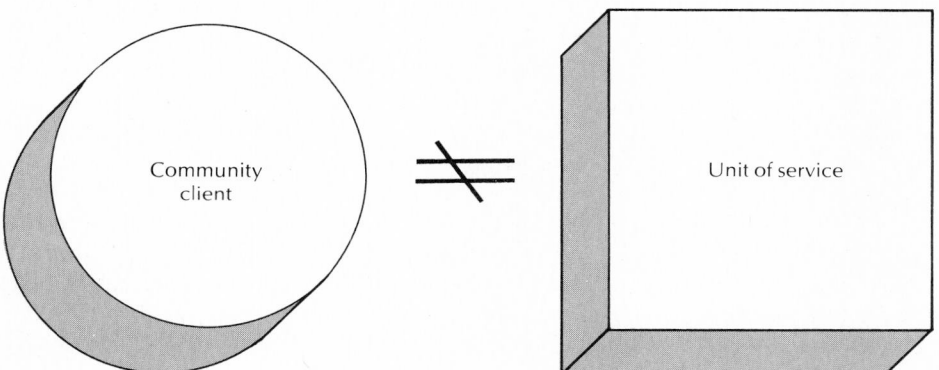

Fig. 17-2. Is community client synonymous with unit of service?

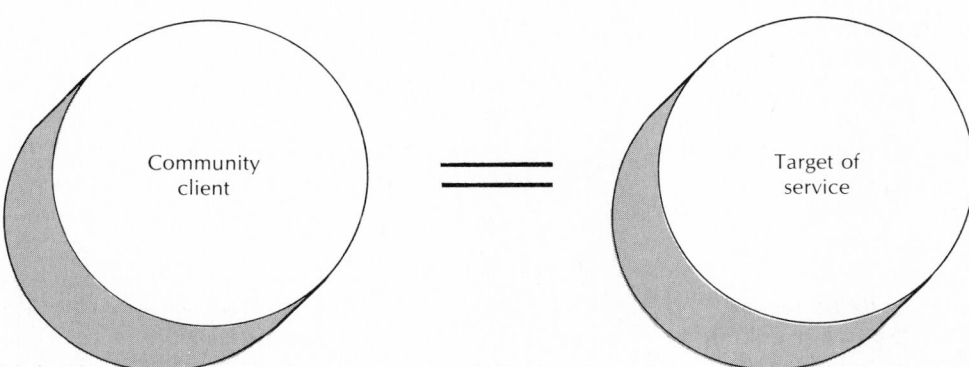

Fig. 17-3. Is community client the target of service?

tive or common good instead of individual health. The units of service may be individuals, families or other interacting groups, aggregates, institutions, and communities. Although change may be sought from these various units, change is intended to impact on the whole that comprises these units, not merely on the units themselves. When the target of change is the community, the client is the community. A visiting nurse's target might be, for example, an entire work force and not the single disabled worker in her case load. In this instance the nurse would provide service with the goals of returning the worker to the job and maintaining a productive work force. The nurse would not intend merely to help the individual achieve independence in personal hygiene.

Relevance of the Community Client to Nursing Practice

As defined earlier, the *community client* is salient, if not essential, to nursing practice for several reasons. One, this definition recognizes the potential power of a merger between nursing practice that is oriented to the individual and community health practice that is oriented to the collective. Two, it respects the complexity of the change process. Three, it provides a framework within which multiple nursing roles can be organized in a complementary fashion. And four, it reinforces nursing's particular strengths in working with interacting groups such as families and special interest groups such as dieters or new parents.

The concept of community client casts direct care services within the essence of community health practice. Direct nursing care can be offered to the individual person or family members, for instance, because their needs for health represent a common rather than a unique problem. Therefore, changes in their health will impact on the health of their communities. Decisions are made at the individual level in the light of their effect on the collective. The health of the collective is the goal. Community health nursing intervention to avert family abuse, for instance, would be undertaken primarily because of the social, not the individual, costs of abuse.

The concept of community client also highlights the complexity of the change process. Change for the benefit of the community client often must occur at several levels, ranging from the individual to the societal. As Ryan (1976), points out the victim cannot always be blamed and expected to correct the deficit without concurrent changes in the "helping" professions and public policy. The solutions to life-style–induced health problems such as smoking, overeating, and speeding, for instance, involve not merely the individual's choice of health-promoting habits but also societal facilitation of healthful choices. Most individuals cannot alter their habits alone. They require the support of family members, friends, and community health care systems that include professional nurses and relevant social policies.

A commitment to healthful change for the community client requires a process of change at each of these levels. As a result, nursing roles with multiple units of service are required. One nursing role would emphasize the individual and direct personal care skills. Another nursing role would focus on the family as the unit of service. A third nursing role would focus on the community, especially constituent community groups.

Although the concept of community client encompasses nursing practice with multiple units of service, community health nursing's special affinity for interacting groups can be emphasized. Interacting groups such as the family and voluntary associations have long been the clients and partners of community health nurses. These groups have recently been characterized as *mediating structures,* and their strength as buffers between the individual and society recognized (Berger and Neuhaus, 1977). This comes as no surprise to community health nurses. However, we can use this "new" information to strengthen arguments for the relationship between traditional modes of practice and community-oriented practice.

The definition of community client as the target of service requires that three additional concepts (namely, community, community health, and partnership for community health) be understood.

BASIC CONCEPTS FOR COMMUNITY-ORIENTED PRACTICE

Community-oriented practice is targeted to the community, the population group for whom healthful change is sought. The goal is community health, more appropriately considered health-promoting change rather than a fixed state. The most important mechanism of facilitating change for health is one of partnership between the lay public and health professionals and among health professionals.

Community

The concept of community has even more meanings than does the concept of community client just discussed. Each discipline concerned with the community —sociology, demography, community psychology, urban planning, and architecture, to name a few—has its own perspective and definition. These have been adopted, often without much thought, by those of us engaged in community-oriented practice. In this subsection some current definitions and typologies of *community* are discussed, a classification system that categorizes the plethora of definitions by their common characteristics is presented, and definitional issues are noted. My definition, used to guide my own and the community-oriented practice of nursing students, is presented last.

Community Defined

Some authors define community very simply. Hanchett (1979, p. 7), for example, defines the term as "people in relationship with others." Others define it more elaborately. Edwards and Jones (1976, p. 12) use the following definition. The community is a "grouping of people who reside in a specific locality and who exercise some degree of local autonomy in organizing their social life in such a way that they can, from that locality base, satisfy the full range of their daily needs." The report on community health nursing of the expert committee of the World Health Organization (1974, p. 7) includes this definition: "A community is a social group determined by geographic boundaries and/or common values and interests. Its members know and interact with one another. It functions within a particular social structure and exhibits and creates norms, values and social institutions."

Still other theorists and writers present typologies rather than single definitions. Two of these typologies are particularly well known to community-oriented practitioners.

Blum, a health planner, describes 11 kinds of community in the typology in the 1974 edition of his classic text, *Planning for Health*. They are listed in the box on this page.

As may be seen, this typology encompasses a wide range of characteristics, as does the one provided by Archer and Fleshman (1979). Unlike Blum, however, these well-known community health nurses cluster the many types of communities into only three categories. Communities are (1) emotional, that is, dependent on a "sense or feeling of community" (Archer and Fleshman, 1979, p. 23); (2) structural or involving "time and space relationships among people" (Archer and Fleshman, 1979, p. 24); and (3) functional, dependent on some achievement or the fulfilment of some common need.

These definitions and typologies suggest that no one approach can be expected to account for the diversity of meanings attributed to the concept of community. Like Archer and Fleshman, several authors (Hanchett, 1979; Shamansky and Pesznecker, 1981; Wellman and Leighton, 1979) have reduced the diversity to manageable proportions by identifying dimensions common to most definitions. These dimensions are presented next, together with a summary of the remaining issues.

┃┃┃ The Types of Community

Face-to-face community
Neighborhood
Community of identifiable need
Community of problem ecology
Community of concern
Community of special interest
Community of viability
Community of action capability
Community of political jurisdiction
Resource community
Community of solution

From Blum, H.L.: Planning for health, New York, 1974, Human Sciences Press, pp. 498-510.

Community Analyzed

Wellman and Leighton (1979, p. 365) note that most definitions of *community* include three dimensions: (1) networks of interpersonal relationships that provide friendship and support to members, (2) residence in a common locality, and (3) "solidarity sentiments and activities." The basic elements of community identified by Hanchett (1979, p. 10) and Shamansky and Pesznecker (1981, p. 183) are similar. Hanchett includes people, place, resources and services, and relationships among the people and among the people, place, and resources. Shamansky and Pesznecker phrase the elements as interrogative pronouns: who, where and when, and how and why.

Hanchett as well as Shamansky and Pesznecker consider people and interaction among the people as basic. These elements are similar to the first dimension identified by Wellman and Leighton.

With respect to the second dimension, that of common locality, Hanchett mentions place and Shamansky and Pesznecker identify a time and space dimension. Like Wellman and Leighton, they agree that people coexist within a particular space and, in Shamansky and Pesznecker's case, within a given space and time.

Finally all three sets of authors mention a functional dimension, although different characteristics are emphasized. Wellman and Leighton and Hanchett accentuate the function of social support. Wellman and Leighton label the notion of bond or ties as solidarity. Hanchett (1979, p. 10) notes, "People in relationship to one another are the essential elements of community." Shamansky and Pesznecker recognize the importance of social participation and mutual support functions but add three others, those of production-distribution-consumption, socialization, and social control. The interrelationships among the authors' dimensions are depicted in Table 17-1.

Table 17-1. A comparison of selected definitions of community

Authors	Dimension		
	Personal	Structural	Functional
Wellman and Leighton	Interpersonal networks	Residence in a common locality	Social support
Hanchett	People; relationships among people	Place	Resources and services; relationships among people, place, resources, and services
Shamansky and Pesznecker	Who? People	Where and When? Space and time	How and why? Social participation, support, production-distribution-consumption, socialization, and social control

Adapted from Wellman, B., and Leighton, B.: Networks, neighborhoods, and communities: approaches to the study of the community question, Urban Affairs Q. **14:**353-390, 1979; Hanchett, E. S.: Community health assessment: a conceptual tool kit, New York, 1979, John Wiley & Sons, Inc.; and Shamansky, S. L., and Pesznecker, B.: A community is, Nurs. Outlook **29:**182-185, 1981.

Even if the dimensions of people, location, and function are common to many definitions of community, the difficulties of conceptualization are not resolved. At least three problems remain.

One, definitions of community and community health are often repetitive. Definitions of community that include shared sentiments and actions often overlap with definitions of community health that focus on the process dimension of effective functioning or community competence. When this happens, only healthy communities can be considered communities at all.

Two, even the briefest exposure to community-oriented practice reveals the frequent absence of definitive geographical or political boundaries to demarcate the community, the lack of correspondence between the catchment or receiving areas of health and welfare institutions and the boundaries of the communities, and the extension of social relationships beyond a single community. These issues have led to intense and prolonged arguments about whether the community, especially the modern urban community, has been "lost" (Hunter, 1975; Luloff and Wilkinson, 1977; Suttles, 1972). These arguments remain unresolved.

Three, one can question whether continued emphasis on the locality-based community is warranted, given the shift in funding priorities to categorical aid programs and block grants. The frequent disparity between local needs and federally determined services is obvious to any community worker. As a result, community may be more meaningful as an analytical rather than a service term.

I believe that community-oriented nurses need to recognize these problems and to develop their own responses to them. I have, however, continued to find the concept of community helpful and have used the following definitions to shape my practice.

Community Specified

The *community* is a locality-based entity, composed of systems of formal organizations reflecting societal institutions, informal groups, and aggregates, which are interdependent, and whose function or expressed intent is to meet a wide variety of collective needs.

The definition includes the spatial, personal, and functional dimensions delineated earlier. It uses "locality-based," the spatial dimension; "an entity composed of systems of . . . organizations . . . groups, and aggregates," the personal dimension; and working "to meet a wide variety of collective needs," the functional dimension. Interdependence, or interaction among the systems, is also recognized. Unless noted otherwise, this interpretation is the one meant whenever the term community is used subsequently.

Community Health

The concept of community health has three common characteristics or dimensions: status, structure, and process. They specify community health and the goal of community-oriented practice in different ways.

The Status Dimension

Community health defined in status or outcome terms is certainly the most well-known and accepted approach. The physical, emotional, and social components of community health are frequently measured by traditional morbidity and mortality, life expectancy indexes, risk factor profiles (physical), consumer satisfaction and mental health indexes (emotional), and crime rates and functional levels (social). Other status measures such as worker absenteeism and infant mortality reflect the impact of all three components.

When community health is understood as being measured by status, the most appropriate strategy for improving community health is one of disease prevention. For if disease—physical, emotional, and social—can be averted or treated in its presymptomatic stages, status measures of community health will improve.

The Structural Dimension

Community health viewed from a structural perspective can refer both to community health services and resources and to attributes of the community structure itself, commonly identified as social indicators or correlates of health. Utilization patterns, treatment data from various health institutions, and provider/population ratios represent the first meaning.

The problems in using these measures are serious. Inequities in access to care and quality of care are well known. The erroneous assumption of a direct causal relationship between the provision of service and improved health is mentioned less frequently (Miller and Stokes, 1978; Mooney and Rives, 1978). Such problems necessitate cautious use of these measures.

Demographic characteristics such as dependency ratios, socioeconomic and racial distributions, and median educational levels represent the second meaning. Their relationships to health status have been thoroughly documented. For instance, health status is inversely related to age and directly related to socioeconomic levels.

Strategies to alter the structural dimension, either health services or demographic characteristics, and thereby improve community health are less well understood than is disease prevention. They include program planning and community development, respectively.

The Process Dimension

Community health defined as the process of effective community functioning or problem-solving is the least well established definition. It is, however, as appropriate to community-oriented nursing as the status and structural definitions because it directs the study of community health toward health promotion through effective community action (Wilson, 1976), an important aim of community-oriented nurses.

My colleagues and I have expanded on this approach. We have put into operation the notion of community health as process by refining the construct of community competence. Defined originally by Cottrell (1976, p. 197), community competence is a process whereby the components of a community—the organizations, groups, and aggregates identified in the defini-

Table 17-2. The conditions of community competence

Condition	Definition
Commitment	The affective and cognitive attachment to a community "that is worthy of substantial effort to sustain and enhance" (Cottrell, 1976, p. 198)
Self-other awareness and clarity of situational definitions	The lucid and realistic perception of one's own and the other community components' identities and positions on issues
Articulateness	The technical aspects of formulating and stating one's views in relation to the other's views
Effective communication	The accurate transmission of information based on the development of common meaning among the communicators
Conflict containment and accommodation	The inventive, effective assimilation and management of true, that is, realistically perceived differences
Participation	Active, community-oriented involvement
Management of relations with larger society	Adeptness at recognizing, obtaining, and utilizing external resources and supports and, when necessary, stimulating the creation and use of alternative or supplementary resources

From Goeppinger, J., et al.: Community Health is community competence, *Nurs. Outlook*, **30**(8):467, 1982.

tion on p. 384—are able to "collaborate effectively in identifying the problems and needs of the community; . . . achieve a working consensus on goals and priorities; . . . agree on ways and means to implement the agreed-upon goals; and . . . collaborate effectively in the required actions."

Eight essential conditions of competence were also proposed (Cottrell, 1976). They are commitment, self-other awareness and clarity of situational definitions, articulateness, effective communication, conflict containment and accommodation, participation, management of relations with the larger society, and machinery for facilitating participant interaction and decision making. The conditions have been defined (see Table 17-2), and indicators of each condition and procedures to gather and generate data about them have been developed (University of Virginia, 1981).

Although the process dimension of community health has only begun to be elaborated and the tools for assessing community processes remain incomplete, the approach can be defended for these reasons. First, measuring the impact of community-oriented nursing services on community health status is difficult because there is often a chronological distance between nursing service and changes in status. For example, interventions to improve the nutritional status of mothers and infants require weeks not days for healthful changes in hematocrit levels to be observed. However, the impact of intervention on process measures like grocery shopping patterns is more immediate.

Second, although the ratio of community health nurses to population is inversely correlated with mortality (Miller and Stokes, 1978), we do not understand why. Because our present health care services generally have less influence on health status than assumed, the critical factor may be process rather than structure. Community-oriented nurses in a local rural community, for instance, worked with the residents' council and the area health department to improve communication about possible solutions to a long-standing problem of water contamination. Although state monies were unavailable, cooperation between the residents and health department personnel did result in the private funding of a single, safe communal well.

Third, nurses are especially well prepared to work with interacting groups. Consequently, it is probably that nursing interventions to strengthen interactions within and/or among community groups, organizations, and aggregates impact favorably on community health understood as process. This is also clearly exemplified in the vignette given in the preceding paragraph. As a result of the preceding considerations, my definition of community health emphasizes process, although status and structural dimensions are included.

Community Health, a Synthesis

Community health is the meeting of collective needs through problem identifying and managing interactions within the community and between the community and the larger society. This requires commitment, self-other awareness and clarity of situational definitions, articulateness, effective communication, conflict containment and accommodation, participation, management of relations with the larger society, and machinery for facilitating participant interaction and decision making.

The status dimension of community health is covered by the phrase, "collective needs," which includes needs for health. Activities to meet these needs involve interactions at formal and informal levels, the structural and process dimensions. The process dimension is central. This is clearly reflected in the last sentence of the definition, which delineates the eight essential conditions of competence.

Strategies to improve community health depend, to some extent, on the dimension of community health that is emphasized. If the emphasis is on the status dimension, the most appropriate strategy is usually disease prevention. When, for instance, the problem is infant mortality, one strategy is to prevent pregnancies among the very young and the very old. On the other hand, if the emphasis is on process, the better strategy is health promotion. For example, if family life education is precluded because of ineffective communication among families, children, school board members, religious leaders, and health professionals, the most effective strategy is to open discussion and negotiate a mutually satisfactory resolution. The strategy that benefits the structural dimension is dependent on the interpretation. A focus on health service suggests a program planning orientation whereas a focus on community demography suggests community development, a form of health promotion. All strategies must include a component of partnership, the basic means to improve community health.

Partnership for Community Health

Most changes aimed at improving community health involve, of necessity, partnerships among community residents and health workers from a variety of disciplines. Quite commonly the community is passively involved in activities conceived and carried out by the health sector. Community residents, for example, are viewed as data sources and recipients of intervention. This form of partnership could be labeled passive participation. In contrast, the type of lay-professional partnership with which this chapter is concerned is active participation. Here power at all stages of the community health assessment-planning-implementation-evaluation process is shared among lay and professional persons.

Historically nurses' participation in community change has also been passive. The power, the method of inducing significant changes, has rested with other community workers, usually the physician health officer and the health planner. Community health nurses, like the communities they serve, have frequently been informed of desired changes with no input regarding the selection of these changes. Unlike communities, however, nurses have generally been actively involved in the implementation phase. Intervention *by* the nurse, albeit *for* the community's benefit, has been a predominant practice mode.

The monopoly of the change process previously held by health care providers is now being challenged—appropriately—by an increasingly enlightened public, some assertive community health nurses, and a few health care institutions. The World Health Organization, for instance, has made partnership, defined as community involvement, a basic tenet of its campaign, "Health for all by the year 2000" (Mahler, 1981, pp. 8-9).

Partnership Defined

Partnership is often equated with participation and involvement of the community or its representatives in healthful change. The meanings of participation and involvement range from manipulation or engineered support to consultation (the invitation of community members' opinions) to control (the decisive exercise of power by community members). The definition of partnership advocated here encompasses that portion of the range extending from consultation to control, that is, active participation or involvement. *Partnership* is the informed, flexible, and negotiated distribution (and redistribution) of power among all participants in the process of change for improved community health.

The three main characteristics of partnership are denote by the adjectives "informed, flexible, and negotiated." Partnership is *informed*. This is probably the most basic characteristic. Lay and professional partners must be informed, that is, cognizant of their own and the other's perceptions, rights, and responsibilities. Partnership is also *flexible*. Lay and professional partners must recognize the different as well as similar contributions each can make to a given situation. Professionals often contribute, for example, substantive expertise lacked by lay persons. On the other hand, lay persons' definitions of community health problems are often more appropriate than those of professionals. Because contributions vary and each situation demands different contributions, the distribution of power must be *negotiated* at every stage of the change process. Partnership, so defined, is as essential a concept for community health nurses as the concepts of community and community health.

Partnership Justified

Partnership is important because health is not given but generated and because new and more efficacious forms of lay-professional partnership are gradually being identified. Although health services may be given, health itself cannot be given. Health is created, optimally from the interactions among health service providers, recipients, and their environments. Consequently, community health and partnership are intricately related. Maternal-child health in our own and underdeveloped countries, for example, is affected more by wise grocery shopping and improvements in home gardening than by the provision and compliant ingestion of vitamin and mineral supplements. Changes in consumer behavior and horticultural practices require active participation by both lay and professional people. Partnership in problem identification and goal setting is especially important because it engenders the commitment essential to successful change.

The salience of partnership to improved community health is supported by the growing body of literature establishing its effectiveness. Studies have documented, for example, the utility of partnership models involving village health workers (Kingma, 1975), Latina opinion leaders (Lorig and Walters, 1980-1981), health facilitators (Salber, 1981), lay advisors (Salber, 1979; Salber et al., 1976), and health guides (Warnecke et al., 1976). The roles of these partners-in-health have included offering advice, making referrals, sympathetic listening, and instituting programs.

Despite the data, professional health workers, including community health nurses, often have challenged the notion of partnership. In community and clinical practices, compliance is preferred rather than collaboration. And in the literature are questions such as the following: Is "evaluation of health care quality by consumers" an illegal intrusion into professional prerogatives (Kelman, 1976)? Is it possible for the ordinary health professional to be a partner in change rather than a change agent (Bodenstein, 1974)? Can the health care consumer determine the "right" goals?

Conclusions

The meaning of partnership, like the meanings of community and community health, is not fully understood; neither is any single meaning universally accepted. Sufficient clarity and agreement do exist, however, to consider them as elements of a conceptual framework for community-oriented nursing practice.

In the following sections three concepts form the framework within which the nursing process, understood as guidelines for community-oriented nursing practice, is presented; the concepts are (1) community, the target of change; (2) community health, the goal of change; and (3) partnership for community health, the means of change. Using the nursing process to promote community health includes assessment, planning, implementation, and evaluation.

NURSING ASSESSMENT OF COMMUNITY HEALTH

The nursing assessment of community health requires that relevant existing data be gathered, that additional data be generated, and that the data base be interpreted. These concepts are considered first. Then methods of assessment are reviewed, assessment guides are presented, and issues are delineated.

Key Concepts

The systematic collection of data about community health necessitates gathering or compiling existing data, frequently statistical in nature, and generating missing data, often by participant observation in the community and its constituent groups and by interaction with key community members. These data are then interpreted and community health problems and capabilities identified.

Data Collection

The primary goal of data collection is to acquire usable information about the community and its health. Consequently data have to be gathered and generated. The acquisition of existing, readily available data is labeled *data gathering.* These data usually describe the demography of a community, age, sex, socioeconomic, and racial distributions, for example; its vital statistics, including selected mortality and morbidity data; its institutions, including health care organizations, and the services they provide; and health manpower characteristics.

Other data, generally not statistical in nature, are less easily acquired. Often such data must be developed by the nurse data collector. The development of data is labeled *data generation.* Data that frequently require generation include information about a community's knowledge and beliefs; values and sentiments; goals and perceived needs; norms; power, leadership, and influence structures; and problem-solving processes.

The first type of data covers numerical information obtained from reports and studies, data that have been collected by others via structured interviews and questionnaires. The second type of information may include numerical data and data collected by others. Generally, however, these data are collected by the nurse as a result of interaction with community members and groups. The data are therefore more apt to be collected via informant interviewing and participant observation. Also the data are more likely to be related to the process dimension of community health than to status or structural dimensions. They are often less readily quantified.

The composite data set or data base, including data that are both gathered and generated, forms the factual base for the diagnosis of need. Community health problems and community health capabilities are identified from the data by a process of data interpretation.

Data Interpretation

The primary goal of data interpretation is the attribution of meaning to the data. Data are analyzed and synthesized; themes are noted; and *community health problems,* needs for action, and *community health capabilities,* the resources available to meet the needs, are identified. Problems are indicated by discrepancies between both the nurse's and the community's concepts of community health and the available data. Capabilities, on the other hand, are suggested by congruence between the nurse's and the community's concepts of community health and the data. The notions of problem and capability and therefore the impetus for change originate in human values, in this instance, values about health. And often the values of the nurse and the community differ.

The nurse's values about community health are revealed in the definition itself. For example, I obviously value the problem-solving process, a wide range of needs, and the collective or community perspective. Yet the community's values may result in a somewhat different understanding of community health, and consequently different problems and capabilities may emerge. For that reason data interpretation should not simply be approached from a conceptual framework. The framework may blind the nurse to the community's perceptions. Problem and capability identification is optimally the result of a process of interaction between the nurse and the community, that is, partnership.

One widely accepted technique for encouraging lay participation in problem identification is the Program Planning Model proposed by Delbecq and Van de Ven (1971). This model can be used in problem identification and program planning. It maximizes the contributions of a variety of groups with diverse interests and varying expertise such as one encounters in community practice. It depends heavily on nominal groups, "groups in which individuals work in the presence of one another but do not interact" (Delbecq and Van de Ven, 1971, p. 467), the separation of personal from collective problems, and a round-robin procedure for listing problems without concurrently evaluating or elaborating on them.

The Program Planning Model, popularly referred to as the nominal group process, was compared in one study with three other approaches to identifying and "prioritizing" health needs (Scutchfield, 1975). These approaches were community diagnosis, random consumer survey, and comprehensive health planning ratings. The nominal group process, which involved consumers as well as health care providers, resulted in a greater emphasis on lack of services and facilities and on financing problems than did the community diagnosis. The community diagnosis method, involving only health professionals, yielded a greater emphasis on particular diseases. Missing in the community diagnosis, Flexner and Littlefield note (1977, p. 246), is the understanding that "what the consumer feels is important may in fact be important, . . . , even though this perspective may be alien to the 'objective information' orientation" of the data gatherer.

Consequently a variety of methods to collect and interpret data is essential. Methods that encourage the nurse to attend to the community's perception of its health problems and capabilities are as important as those that are structured to yield knowledge the nurse considers essential. Several of these methods are discussed in the next subsection.

Methods of Assessment

At least five methods of collecting and interpreting data are useful to the community health nurse. They are informant interviewing, participant observation, secondary analyses of existing data, surveys, and windshield surveys. They can be clustered into two distinct but complementary categories: those methods that rely on what is observed by the data collector and those methods that rely on what is reported to the data collector. Informant interviewing, participant observation, and windshield surveys are examples of the former; secondary data analyses and surveys represent the latter.

In the following paragraphs, the methods are described, the appropriate use of each method considered, and the importance of multiple assessment methods, that is, *triangulation,* stressed. Excellent references exist for each method; the reader is referred to them for comprehensive discussions.

Observational methods are essential to community health nursing. *Informant interviewing,* that is, directed conversation with selected members of a community about community members or groups and events, is basic. So is *participant observation,* the "conscious and systematic sharing, in so far as circumstances permit, in the life activities, and on occasion, in the interests and affects of a group of persons" (Kluckhohn, 1940, p. 331).

Informant interviewing and participant observation methodologies are particularly suitable techniques for obtaining information about community beliefs, norms, values, power and influence structures, and problem-solving processes. Such data are seldom reducible to enumeration, and as a result, they are often not collected. Even worse, impressions—intuitive and unverified—are sometimes substituted for data. Yet these data are as important to understanding a community and community health as the data that are more readily quantified.

A *windshield survey* is the motorized equivalent of simple observation. Through an automobile windshield many dimensions of a community's life and environment are carefully observed. Common characteristics of street people, neighborhood gathering places, the rhythm of community life, housing quality, and geographic boundaries are some of the dimensions that can be readily observed.

All of these methods require sensitivity, openness, curiosity, and the abilities to listen, taste, touch, smell, and see "life" as lived in a community at levels far beyond that required to understand and cope with one's own daily routines. Thorough discussions of observational methods are beyond the scope of this text. The interested reader is referred to Filstead (1972), Glazer (1972), Polit and Hungler (1978), Seaman, (1982), and Weick (1968).

Secondary analyses of existing data, for example, content analyses of minutes from community meetings and surveys, are also important. *Secondary analysis,* in which the community health nurse utilizes previously gathered data, is extremely valuable because it is efficient and economical. Many secondary sources—public documents, minutes from meetings, statistical data, and health records—are readily available. Major disadvantages of working with existing data (missing, inaccurate, or erroneous information) are often not as critical in community health because demographic and vital statistics are collected in standardized ways so that opportunities for error are minimized.

Surveys, in which data from a sample of persons are reported to the data collector, are equally useful but somewhat less efficient and economical than observational methods and secondary analyses. They require time-consuming and costly investments in the data collection stage and are not easily incorporated into much community nursing practice. They are, however, necessary for certain community problems. A lack of accessible personal health services, for example, cannot be readily and reliably documented in any other fashion.

Both survey and secondary analysis methodologies are well described in *Nursing Research: Principles and Methods* (Polit and Hungler, 1978). In addition, several manuals exist to assist community workers in developing, conducting, and analyzing a survey. A good example, informative and pragmatic, is *Needs Assessment: A Model for Community Planning* (Neuber, 1980).

As no way of collecting data is without bias, it is advantageous to use the most appropriate methodologies for the type of data sought and to use several methods with different methodological weaknesses. Triangulation, the use of multiple complementary methodologies, is essential and quite consistent with community health nursing practice. Except for perhaps the survey, all of the preceding methodologies are commonly used by the nurse.

The nursing assessment of community health—data collection and interpretation—is not random but focused. Focus or perspective can be provided by a conceptual framework such as the one presented here and by detailed assessment guides. Examples of both are discussed next.

Assessment Guides

Concepts specified at an operational level, that is, stated in behavioral or observable terms, can serve as assessment guides. The concepts of community and community health, as defined earlier, have been made operational for just such a purpose.

The concept of community, for instance, has been specified as presented in Table 17-3. The original definition (see p. 383) includes three dimensions: (1) place or space, (2) people or person, and (3) function. Each of these dimensions is specified by several indicators. The spatial dimension is represented by indicators like geopolitical boundaries and size and by characteristics of the physical environment such as land usage patterns.

When combined, the indicators for each of these three dimensions constitute a portion of the Assessment Guide in Appendix F. The specification of community health—its status, structure, and process dimensions—is presented in Table 17-4. In this way the concepts of community and community health provide the framework for the Assessment Guide. Together the concepts and Assessment Guide constitute the Community Health Assessment Model, the basis of the Community Oriented Health Record (see Appendix F). Data, problems, and capabilities are all organized by the model.

To assist the community health nurse collect and interpret data about the process dimension of community health, I have developed a companion assessment guide, The Community Competence Assessment Manual (University of Virginia, 1981).* This manual, like the Assessment Guide of the Community Oriented Health Record, has been useful in orienting community health nurses to community practice.

Other assessment guides have been constructed which might also be useful. The Community Nursing Survey Guide is one such example (see Tinkham and Voorhies, 1977, Chapter 11, and University of Virginia, 1981). The kinds of information Tinkham and Voor-

*Further information can be obtained from the author of this chapter.

Table 17-3. The concept of community made operational

Dimensions	Indicators
Place or space	Geopolitical boundaries
	Local or folk name for area
	Size in square miles, acres, blocks, census tracts
	Transportation avenues — rivers, highways, railroads, sidewalks
	Physical environment — land usage patterns, condition of housing, etc.
People or person	Number and density of population
	Demographic structure of population — age, sex, socioeconomic, and racial distributions; rural/urban character; dependency ratio; etc.
	Informal groups — block clubs, service clubs, friendship networks, etc.
	Formal groups — schools, churches, businesses, industries, governmental bodies, unions, health and welfare agencies, etc.
	Linking structures
Function	Production, distribution, consumption of goods and services
	Socialization of new members
	Maintenance of social control
	Adapting to ongoing and expected change
	Provision of mutual aid

hies consider important—data about the community itself, demographic and epidemiological information about the people, data about the environment, knowledge about communication channels, data about health facilities and personnel, and knowledge about community health nursing services and programs—are similar to those specified in the Assessment Guide. They do not, however, cover the process dimension of community health as thoroughly as the Assessment Guide and the Community Competence Assessment Manual.

Another guide, in the form of a handbook for community-level personnel, has been developed by Connor (1969). The handbook provides a simple and comprehensive yet flexible approach to understanding the community. The community worker's attention is focused on 12 elements of the community social system, such as resources, history, values and sentiments, and goals and felt needs, and 11 patterns of social relationships within the community, such as the family, government, health, and communication networks. To-

|||| **Table 17-4.** The concept of community health made operational

Dimensions	Indicators
Status	Vital statistics — live births, neonatal deaths, infant deaths, maternal deaths, deaths
	Disease incidence and prevalence for leading causes of mortality and morbidity
	Health risk profiles of selected aggregates
	Functional ability levels
Structure	Health facilities — hospitals; nursing homes; other — industrial and school health services, health departments, voluntary health associations, categorical grant programs, prepaid health plans, etc.
	Health-related planning groups
	Health work force — physician, dentist, nurse, environmental sanitarian, social worker, significant others
	Health resource utilization patterns — bed occupancy days, patient/provider visits, etc.
Process	Commitment
	Self-other awareness and clarity of situational definitions
	Articulateness
	Effective communication
	Conflict containment and accommodation
	Participation
	Management of relationships with the larger society
	Machinery for facilitating participant interaction and decision making

gether these constitute "the social compass applied to the community" (Connor, 1969, p. 25). The social compass provides a systematic, conceptually based approach to gathering information about the community.

All of these guides provide a perspective on data collection. They ensure that the data collected are comprehensive and consistent with the community health nurse's conceptual framework. But they also determine whether the data are collected at all and how they are interpreted. Consequently it is essential to remember that the community's perception of its health may vary markedly from that of the nurse. It is critical to remain open to any data and data interpretations, despite the comfort of a highly structured assessment guide. The most salient data and the most appropriate interpretations may not fit every assessment guide. They should

not be discarded but rather treated as the highly significant information they are. The community's presentation of data is basic.

Assessment Issues

Gaining entry is perhaps the biggest challenge in assessment. The community health nurse is usually an outsider and often represents an established health care system that is not trusted or even known by community members. The possibility of indifference or even active hostility exists. In addition, the community health nurse may feel insecure about her skills as a community worker, and the community itself may refuse to acknowledge its need for these skills.

Since the nurse's success in collecting and interpreting data and later in planning, initiating, and evaluating intervention depends, in large part, on the way she is viewed, entry is critical. Successful entry can often be facilitated by participating in community events, looking and listening attentively, visiting persons in formal leadership positions rather than attempting immediately to discern and contact informal leaders, employing some sort of assessment guide as a framework, and using a peer group for support.

Once entry at an initial level has been accomplished, *role negotiation* often becomes an issue. The nurse must decide how long to segregate the two roles as collector of reliable data and as intervenor. The dangers of overinvolvement and premature response to health needs and social injustice are compelling.

Role negotiation can be aided by a thoughtful and consistent presentation of the reasons for one's presence in the community; by sincere demonstrations of one's commitment to the community, for example, keeping appointments and verbally stating the importance of getting the community members' perceptions of collective health needs; and by respecting persons' rights to choose whether or not they work with the nurse.

Maintaining *confidentiality* is also important. Nurses must take scrupulous care to preserve the identity of community members who provide sensitive or controversial data. In some cases the nurse may have to consider withholding data; in other situations she may be legally required to disclose data.

The issues of attending to community as well as professional perceptions of problems, entry, role negotiation, and confidentiality are of a different order than the issue of *small area analysis*. The concern here is with the lack of statistical data on small communities and the inappropriateness of making conclusions about data gathered for small areas, for example, about mortality rates calculated when the denominator is as small as 5000. This issue frequently compromises the validity of many identified health problems. It reinforces the usefulness of triangulation, because if similar health problems are identified irrespective of the assessment method, increased confidence can be placed in their validity.

Recognition of these issues reinforces the importance of data collection and interpretation in partnership with the community.

■   ■   ■

Nursing intervention to assist communities in healthful change is dependent on understanding the community and its health, that is, on a deliberate, systematic, and informed nursing assessment. Nursing intervention for community health includes planning, implementation, and evaluation phases, just as it does at individual and familial levels. Though the intervention process is similar at the various levels, intervention strategies differ. The planning, implementation, and evaluation phases are presented in this section. Nursing roles, activities, and issues that are particularly pertinent to community-oriented practice are highlighted.

PLANNING FOR COMMUNITY HEALTH

The planning phase includes analyzing and "prioritizing" the community health problems identified earlier, establishing goals and objectives, and identifying intervention activities to accomplish the objectives.

Problem Analysis and Prioritization

The aim of *problem analysis* is to clarify the nature of the problem. The analyst can identify the origins and impact of the problem, the points at which intervention might be undertaken, and the parties that have an interest in the problem and its solution. Analysis often requires the development of a problem matrix in which the direct and indirect precursors and consequences are identified and interrelationships among problems and their precursors and consequences are mapped. This is important because one can anticipate that several of the same precursors and consequences underlie many of the problems. The common precursor(s) may be the problem of highest priority.

Problem analysis should be undertaken for each identified problem. It often requires the organization of a special group composed of the nurse, persons whose areas of expertise relate to the problem, persons whose organizations have the capabilities to intervene, and representatives of the "community of identifiable need" (Blum, 1974, p. 499), the community experiencing the problem. Both substantive and process specialists must participate. Together they can identify the

problem correlates and explicate the relationships between each correlate and the problem.

In the Problem Analysis Sheet of the Community Oriented Health Record (see Appendix F) the user is directed to just such a process. Problem correlates, precursors and consequences, are listed in the first column. Correlates are sought from all facets of community life. In the second column the relationships between each correlate and the problem are noted. And in the third column data from the community and the literature which support the relationship are presented in capsule fashion.

An example of one community health problem, suspected infant malnutrition, and a few of its correlates are sketched in the box on the next page. This example illustrates a linear form of problem analysis. Other forms of problem analysis—circular, feedback, and branching—are found in the excellent workbook by Koberg and Bagnall (1981).

After problems have been submitted to a cursory review, they should be put through a ranking process to determine their relative priority. This ranking process, in which problems are evaluated and priorities are established according to predetermined criteria, is called *problem prioritization*. It should involve the contributions of community members, substantive experts, and administrators and resource controllers.

Problem prioritization can be facilitated by the use of predetermined criteria. Criteria I have found helpful include (1) community awareness of the problem, (2) community motivation to resolve or better manage the problem, (3) nurse's ability to influence problem solution, (4) availability of expertise relevant to problem solution, (5) severity of the consequences if the problem is unresolved, and (6) quickness with which resolution can be achieved. These criteria are listed in the first column of the Problem Prioritization sheet of the Community Oriented Health Record (see Appendix F).

Blum clusters 54 such criteria into four classes: technological aspects, health aspects, general social concerns, and planning concerns (1981, pp. 155-156). In my criteria the last two, severity of consequences and quickness of resolution, represent health aspects; the first two, community awareness and community motivation, exemplify general social concerns; and the remaining criteria; nurse's ability and availability of relevant expertise, are examples of planning concerns.

Other sets of criteria may be used (for an example, see Dever, 1980, p. 361) or developed by the nurse. The criteria do need to be agreed on before intervention and by a variety of reference groups.

Given an acceptable and comprehensive set of criteria and a list of problems, the process of assigning priorities itself is rather simple. The criteria are weighted (see

PROBLEM ANALYSIS: SUSPECTED INFANT MALNUTRITION IN JEFFERSON COUNTY

Name of community: _Jefferson County_

Problem/statement: _Suspected infant malnutrition in Jefferson County_

Problem analysis

Problem correlates	Relationship of correlates to problem	Data supportive to relationships (refer to appropriate sections of Data Base _and_ relevant research findings in current literature)
1. _Improper diets_	_Diets lacking in required nutrients contribute to malnutrition._	
2. _Ignorance_	_The norm is to bottle feed rather than breast feed._	
3. _Lack of money_	_Infant formulas are expensive._	

Appendix F, for more details).* Then each problem is rated according to the criteria (column 4), the rationale for the rating is noted (column 5), the significance of the problem is computed (column 6), the significance scores of the problems are contrasted, and priorities are established. The most significant problems, those with the highest priority, are selected as the focus for inter-

*This is a judgmental process that, ideally, precedes problem analysis and is engaged in by community members, substantive experts, and resource controllers.

vention. The process of establishing a significance score for the problem of suspected infant malnutrition is diagrammed in the box on the next page.

Establishing Goals and Objectives

Once high-priority problems are identified, relevant goals and objectives are developed. The _goal,_ generally a rather global statement of the desired outcome, and _objectives,_ the precise statements of the desired outcome, are carefully selected.

PROBLEM PRIORITIZATION: SUSPECTED INFANT

MALNUTRITION IN JEFFERSON COUNTY

Problem prioritization

Criteria	Criteria weights (1-10)	Problem	Problem rating (1-10)	Rationale for rating	Problem significance (weight X rate)
1. Community awareness of the problem	5	Suspected infant malnutrition in Jefferson County	10	Health service providers, teachers, and a variety of parents have mentioned problem.	50
2. Community motivation to resolve the problem	10		3	Most feel this problem is irresolvable as majority of those affected are indigent.	30
3. Nurse's ability to influence problem resolution	5		8	Nurse skilled at consciousness raising and mobilizing support.	40
4. Ready availability of expertise relevant to problem resolution	7		10	WIC program, nutritionists available. County extension agent interested.	70
5. Severity of consequences if problem is left unresolved	8		5	Effects of marginal malnutrition not too well documented.	40
6. Quickness with which problem resolution can be achieved	3		3	Time to mobilize rural community with no history of social action lengthy.	9
					Total = 239

```
                    GOALS AND OBJECTIVES:
          SUSPECTED INFANT MALNUTRITION IN JEFFERSON COUNTY

Name of community: ___Jefferson County_____

Problem/concern: ___Suspected infant malnutrition_____

                         Goals and objectives

Goal statement: _____To document and, if appropriate, reduce the incidence
                      and prevalence of infant malnutrition
```

Present date	Objectives (number and statement)	Completion date
1-80	No. 1 80% of infants seen by health department, neighborhood health center, and private physicians will have their developmental levels assessed.	6-80
1-80	No. 2 WIC program eligibility will be ascertained for 80% of infants seen by health department, neighborhood health center, and private physicians.	6-80
1-80	No. 3 An outreach program will be implemented to identify at-risk infants not now known to health care providers.	6-80
1-80	No. 4 WIC program eligibility will be ascertained for 75% of at-risk infants.	1-81
1-80	No. 5 75% of all infants eligible for WIC food supplements will be enrolled in the program.	12-81
1-80	No. 6 50% of the mothers of infants enrolled in WIC will demonstrate 3 ways of incorporating WIC supplements into their infants' diets.	6-81

An example of a goal and objectives relevant to the problem of suspected infant malnutrition is depicted in the box above. The goal is simply to reverse the problem, that is, to document and, if appropriate, reduce the incidence and prevalence of infant malnutrition. The objectives are more precise. In addition, they are behaviorally stated and incremental.

It is usual for a group rather than an individual to be responsible for establishing goals and objectives. Such a group should include persons who have participated in the assessment and problem analysis and prioritization, because goal achievement is more likely to occur when the goal is a mutual one.

Plan: ASSESS INFANT'S DEVELOPMENTAL LEVELS

Name of community: _Jefferson County_

Objective number and statement

1. _80% of infants seen by health department, neighborhood health center, and private physicians will have their developmental levels assessed._

Date	Intervenor activities/means	Plan Value (1–10)	Plan Probability (1–10)	Activity/means selected for implementation
1-80	1. WIC program supplies personnel to assess infant developmental levels.	1	10	Insufficient personnel and time. Existing community resources (potential)
			Total 10	ignored.
1-80	2. WIC program provides in-service education to staff on assessment of infant development.	5	5	Antipathy between WIC personnel and other health workers high. Need for education must be assessed first and enthusiasm for
			Total 25	objectives created.
1-80	3. CNP provides in-service education to staff in assessment of infant development.	3	10	CNP can't do it alone!
			Total 30	
1-80	4. CNP assists WIC personnel to identify in-service educational needs of area health care providers about assessment of infant development.	8	8	Most likely to build on existing community strengths. CNP skilled in needs assessment and interpersonal techniques needed
			*Total 64	to decrease antipathy.
1-80	5. CNP assists WIC personnel to identify driving and restraining forces relative to implementation of objective.	10	8	Without this, change effort likely to fail.
			*Total 80	

*Means selected.

PLAN: IMPLEMENT AN OUTREACH PROGRAM

Name of community: _____ *Jefferson County* _____

Objective number   3. *An outreach program is implemented to identify at*
and statement   *risk infants not now known to health care providers*

Plan

Date	Intervenor activities/means	Value (1-10)	Probability (1-10)	Activity/means selected for implementation
1-80	1. *CNP identifies and trains lay advisors in community as case finders.*	*8*	*6*	*Lay leaders already known, proven to be effective change agents; can't however, be paid.*
			Total 48	
1-80	2. *Local hospital administrators alter job descriptions of nurses in maternity and pediatrics to include case finding and referral.*	*8*	*5*	*All babies in Jefferson County born in hospital since 1978. Administrator interested in community. Administration powerful can alter nurses' job descriptions. Nurses hate*
			Total 40	*student nurses.*
1-80	3. *CNP encourages public health nurses to do better job of case finding.*	*8*	*2*	*Public health nurses have historic role in case finding. CNP not well known by PHNs. PHNs reported to be overworked.*
			Total 16	
1-80	4. *WIC personnel devote 1 evening/week to case finding.*	*1*	*10*	*One nurse (nonresident) eager to do this. Doesn't develop exiting community*
			Total 110	*resources.*

*Means selected.

Once goals and objectives are established, intervention activities to accomplish the objectives can be identified.

Identifying Intervention Activities

Intervention activities are the means by which the objectives are realized. They are the strategies that spell out what must be done to achieve the objectives, the ways in which change is affected and the problem cycle is interrupted.

Because alternative intervention activities do exist, they must be identified and evaluated. The process of sketching out possible interventions and selecting the best set of activities for each objective is often unconscious and intuitive. To make the process deliberate, the Plan sheet of the Community Oriented Health Record (see Appendix F) was developed. Examples of identifying and evaluating alternative activities related to the goals of documenting and reducing infant malnutrition are depicted on pp. 396 and 397.

In the box on p. 396 five intervenor activities are listed in the second column, each of which is relevant to the first objective. The first two activities involve Women, Infants and Children (WIC) program personnel as the principal change agents. The last three involve the writer (community nurse practitioner, or CNP), WIC program personnel, and the staff of the health department, neighborhood health center, and private physicians' offices.

The likely effectiveness of each of the activities is considered in the third and fourth columns. The *value,** the likelihood that the activity will foster achievement of the objective and eventual resolution of the problem, is noted first. Clearly it is more valuable to educate others in the assessment of infant development (activity 4) than to do it for them (activity 1). It is also valuable to analyze the change process necessary to accomplish the objective (activity 5). Consequently, activities 4 and 5 have higher value scores than activity 1.

On the other hand, the *probability,** the likelihood that the means can be implemented, is highest when only the CNP is involved, because she has more control over her behavior than over the behavior of others. Therefore activities 1 and 3 have a higher probability than activities 2, 4, and 5.

The reasons for the numerical scores are noted briefly in the fifth column. The activities with the highest scores, computed by multiplying the value times the probability, are selected, since it is important both to

---

*The value and probability scores of intervenor activities may range from 1 (low) to 10 (high). The range of 1 to 10 was arbitrarily determined.

impact on the objective (value) and to be able to carry out the means (probability).

A second example of plan development is depicted in the box on p. 397. The activities relate to Objective 3 in the box on p. 395, implementation of an outreach program.

IMPLEMENTING INTERVENTION FOR COMMUNITY HEALTH

The work of transforming a plan for improved community health into progress towards the achievement of goals and objectives constitutes the third phase of the nursing process, *implementation.* Implementation efforts may rest primarily with the person or group who established the goals and objectives or they may be shared with or even delegated to others. The issue of centralization of implementation efforts is salient. The community health nurse's position on the issue can be influenced by a variety of factors. Several of the factors, as well as four important implementation mechanisms, are considered next.

Factors Influencing Implementation

Implementation efforts are shaped by the nurse's preferred mode of practice, the type of health problem that has been selected as the focus for intervention, the community's readiness to participate in problem resolution, and the characteristics of the social change process. The nurse who participates in community-oriented intervention has a key position and brings to the effort knowledge and skills not possessed by other intervenors. The question is one of how the nurse uses the position, knowledge, and skills.

Nurse's Preferred Mode of Practice

Nurses can act as content experts, helping communities to select and attain task-related goals. In the instance where infant malnutrition was suspected, the nurse used her epidemiological skills to help ascertain the incidence and prevalence of malnutrition. The nurse in this situation also served as a process expert by acting to increase the community's own capabilities in documenting the problem rather than by merely contributing her substantive expertise.

The roles of fact gatherer, analyst, and program implementor have been distinguished from those of enabler-catalyst, teacher of problem-solving skills, and activist-advocate (Rothman, 1974b). Bodenstein (1974) considers the former as change agent roles and the latter as change partner roles. Community health nurses, like other health professionals, have been socialized to impose change, to act as change agents rather than as change partners. We can, however, respond more flexibly.

Type of Health Problem

The nurse's choice of role can be dependent on the nature of the health problem and the community's history in decision making as well as on professional and personal preferences. Some health problems clearly suggest that certain intervention roles are appropriate. A problem in community health process, for instance, the lack of democratic problem-solving capacities, requires the nurse to select teacher, facilitator, and even advocate roles. Problem-solving skills must be explained and modeled. A community health status problem, on the other hand, frequently requires fact-gatherer and analyst roles. Some problems require multiple roles. The example of suspected infant malnutrition is such a problem. Managing conflict among the involved health care providers demanded process skills; collecting and interpreting the data necessary to document the problem required both interpersonal and analytical skills.

Community's History of Participation

The community's history of participation in decision making is critical. If a community is skilled in identifying and managing its problems and has a history of success in doing so, the nurse may appropriately play the role of technical expert or advisor. If the community is lacking problem-solving skills or a history of successful change efforts, quite different roles may be required. The nurse may have to focus on developing problem-solving capabilities or achieving one successful change so that the community becomes empowered to assume responsibility for promoting change on its own behalf.

The Social Change Process

The nurse's role depends on the social change process. Not all communities are receptive to innovation. Innovation has been found to be inversely related to the extent to which a community adheres to traditional norms and directly related to high socioeconomic status, a perceived need for change, the presence of liberal, scientific, and democratic values, and a high level of social participation by community residents (Rothman, 1974a, pp. 422-436).

The innovation itself also indicates how well it will be accepted. Innovations with the highest adoption rates are those perceived as relatively more advantageous than the other alternatives, compatible with existing values, amenable to a limited trial before full-scale adoption, easily explained or demonstrated, geographically accessible, and simple (Rothman, 1974a).

For example, community residents might go to an immunization clinic rather than a private physician if the clinic is nearby and less expensive and if the physician is not available when needed.

The final variable in the social change process is the diffusion and adoption process. Innovations are accepted more readily when the diffusion process is compatible with the community's norms, values, and customs, information is relayed through the appropriate communication mode (the mass media for early adopters and face-to-face for late adopters), other communities support the community's change efforts, opinion leaders are identified and used, and communication about the innovation is clear and unambiguous (Rothman, 1974a).

Conclusion

Since the factors that shape implementation are multiple and their impact on the change process complex and varying, the community health nurse must be adaptable. The roles used to initiate change may differ from those used to maintain or stabilize it. And the roles required to initiate, maintain, and stabilize change may vary from community to community and from one intervention to another within the same community. Irrespective of the community health nurse's specific role, several mechanisms of implementing intervention for improved community health are important. The mechanisms are (1) the small group, (2) lay advisors, (3) the mass media, and (4) public policy.

Implementation Mechanisms

Implementation mechanisms are the vehicles or modes by which innovations are transferred from the planners to the units of service. The community health nurse *alone* is never considered an implementation mechanism, for change on behalf of the community client requires *multiple* implementation mechanisms. Instead, the nurse must identify and use appropriately all relevant aids to intervention. In this subsection small interacting groups, lay advisors, the mass media, and public policy are emphasized as implementation mechanisms or aids.

Small interacting groups, formal and informal, are essential implementation mechanisms. Many of the formal groups in the community—families, legislative bodies, health care recipients, and service providers, for example—are fully considered elsewhere in the text. Some of the informal groups, such as neighborhoods and social action groups, have also been discussed. The commonality among these diverse groups is their location between the community and the individual levels. Because of their intermediate position, they can and do act to support and constrain change efforts at the community and individual levels. They are potentially powerful simply because they are mediating structures (Berger and Neuhaus, 1977).

Consequently the community health nurse needs to ascertain which groups view the proposed change as beneficial and which do not. New small groups may need to be formed to facilitate the change, and accommodations may have to be made in the innovation or diffusion process to increase receptivity. Initially the innovation may have to be directed to groups with a majority of *early adopters,* those with broad perspectives and abilities to adopt new ideas from mass media information sources, and to groups whose own goals are like those of the intervention plan (Rothman, 1974a).

Lay advisors often perform a similar function to early adopters. They are individuals who are influential in approving or disapproving new ideas and from whom others seek advice and information about new ideas (Rothman, 1974a). Lay advisors or opinion leaders are characterized by conformity to community norms, heavy involvement in formal service organizations and informal social groups, specific areas of expertise, and a slightly higher social status than their followers (Rogers, 1962; Warnecke et al., 1976). In community health literature they are frequently referred to as health facilitators (Salber, 1981; Salber et al., 1976), village health workers (Kingma, 1975), and health guides (Warnecke et al., 1976) as well as opinion leaders (Lorig and Walters, 1980-81) and lay advisors (Salber, 1979; Service and Salber, 1977). These persons are also labeled gatekeepers and key informants.

Irrespective of their title, lay advisors have been found to be helpful in community-oriented intervention. In one study, for example, they increased breast self-examination practices among Latina women by about 40% (Lorig and Walters, 1980-81). In another study, rural blacks in North Carolina were provided with a higher percentage of arthritis care by lay advisors than by physicians (Salber, 1981).

Both small interacting groups and lay advisors are particularly useful in instituting change among late adopters. Groups dominated by early adopters and lay advisors can be reached through the mass media.

Mass media is typically an impersonal and formal type of communication and is useful in community-oriented intervention to provide information quickly to large numbers of people. Use of mass media is efficient because the proportion of resources to population covered is low and populations can be targeted. Information about venereal disease can, for example, be more effectively disseminated through rock than through classical music stations.

In addition to being efficient, use of the mass media is effective. The Stanford Heart Disease Three Community Program showed that residents of the community receiving media-only intervention did increase their knowledge about cardiovascular risk factors and improve their dietary patterns. Residents of the community receiving the mass media campaign combined with face-to-face intervention also reduced their cardiovascular risk (Maccoby et al., 1977). Similar findings have been reported from the North Karelia Study in Finland (McAlister et al., 1982).

Public policy can also play a critical part in the adoption of healthful community-oriented change. An intent of public policy in the field of health is to address collective human needs. It frequently serves to constrain individual choice for the public good. Drivers have been urged for several years, for instance, to wear automobile seatbelts. The incidence of automobile fatalities was not reduced, however, until recently when drivers were required to observe lowered speed limits. Obviously public policy can facilitate choices that promote community health.

If public policy that will encourage or even allow health-generating choices is to be enacted, the community health nurse must actively lobby for it. The nurse must also eagerly seek out small groups and lay advisors and use the mass media as aids to implementation. Working with naturally occurring small groups like the family and with lay advisors is familiar to most community health nurses. Working with legislators and using the mass media are less familiar. Yet all resources must be used in efforts to achieve healthful change in the community client.

The use of a small group to initiate community-oriented change is illustrated in the Progress Notes of the Community Oriented Health Record (see box on next page). A plan requiring the use of lay advisors is sketched on the Plan sheet of the Community Oriented Health Record (see box, p. 397).

Any implementation efforts, no matter what mechanisms are used, must not only be documented but evaluated. Evaluation is important to determine and improve the effectiveness of community-oriented nursing practice and thereby to increase our knowledge base and ability to compete for funds.

EVALUATING INTERVENTION FOR COMMUNITY HEALTH

Simply defined, *evaluation* is the appraisal of the effects of some organized activity or program. It may involve the design and conduct of evaluation research, in which the methods of social science research are used to determine program effectiveness, efficiency, adequacy, appropriateness, and unintended consequences (Kane

Progress notes

PROGRESS NOTES

Name of community: _Jefferson County_

Goal: _To document and, if appropriate, reduce the incidence_

and prevalence of infant malnutrition

Date	Narrative, Assessment, Plan (NAP)	Budget, Time
	(Record both objective and subjective data. Interpret these data in terms of whether the objectives were achieved and whether the intervenor activities utilized were effective. The plan is dependent on the assessment and may include both new or revised objectives and activities.)	
2-14-80	Objective 1, Means 4	
	Narrative: Meeting to develop needs assessment was attended by CNP, 2 WIC personnel, and physicians from health department, neighborhood health center, and local medical society. Consensus rapidly achieved among 5 of 6 participants that goal, objectives, and means (especially Objective 1, Means 4) were appropriate. Physician representing medical society consistently objected, stating vehemently that private sector had long provided adequate medical care for area youngsters. One WIC staff member angrily questioned how physician could document "adequacy." Physician responded that federal aid created more need than disease did. He would not recommend that medical society support the effort. CNP cowered, afraid that this confrontation would jeopardize entire effort. Eventually, however, physician left, and plans were made to develop and conduct needs assessment, with or without the medical society's help.	
	Agenda: CNP to develop needs assessment tool with WIC personnel and health systems agency planner. Physicians to develop list of providers to be contacted. Neighborhood health center physician to get a place on medical society agenda and attempt to clarify our plans. WIC personnel to contact nonphysician health workers to introduce plan and develop provider list.	

Continued.

PROGRESS NOTES—Cont'd

Assessment: *Plans made to proceed with needs assessment*	*$100 2 hours meeting*
and garner support essential to accomplishment of objective.	*and 2 hours preparation*
Group process problematical, and CNP ineffective due to dis-	
comfort with conflict between physician and WIC staff member.	
Plans: *Meeting scheduled for 2-28-80 to deal with agreed-on*	
agenda.	
Before 2-28 meeting, CNP will discuss ways of better	
handling conflict with consultation group, collaborate in	
drafting needs assessment, and telephone others by 2-21 to	
determine their progress.	
J. Goeppinger, RN, CNP	

et al., Deniston, 1974). It may also involve the more rudimentary process of assessing progress by comparing the objectives and the results. Since an entire chapter is devoted to program planning and evaluation in community health (Chapter 12) and comprehensive references are readily available,* this section deals with the comparison of objectives and results.

Evaluation has already begun in the planning phase with the establishment of goals and measurable objectives and the identification of goal-attaining activities. After implementation of intervention, only the accomplishment of the objectives and the effects of the intervention activities have to be appraised. The Progress Notes of the Community Oriented Health Record (see Appendix F) direct the nurse to perform such appraisals concurrently with implementation. In assessing the data recorded there, the nurse is requested to evaluate whether the objectives were achieved and whether the intervenor activities used were effective and to decide whether the costs in money and time were commensurate with the benefits. This process is depicted in the box on the preceding page. Here the nurse has noted progress toward the needs assessment and the difficulties encountered in dealing with conflict among the group members.

Such an evaluation process is oriented to community health, since the intervention goals and objectives are derived from the nurse's and the community's concep-

tions of health. Simplistic as it appears, it is not without problems. The lack of a control community or even adequate baseline information makes it questionable to attribute success, or failure, to the intervention. Nursing interventions may also have such diffuse and therefore weak effects that our crude measures do not discern them. Basic models for the practitioner to use in determining cost benefit estimates and cost effectiveness are not commonplace. And finally, the lay role in evaluation has never been fully accepted. Professionals have adopted partnership in assessment and implementation more readily than in evaluation. The issue of who has the power to define, judge, and institute change in professional activities is by no means resolved.

SUMMARY

Using the definition of community client as the target of service and the key concepts of community, community health, and partnership for health, the nursing process of assessment, planning, implementation, and evaluation to promote community health has been described and illustrated.

BIBLIOGRAPHY

American Nurses' Association: Issues in evaluation research, Pub. Code. G-124 2M 9/76, Kansas City, Mo., 1976, The Association.

American Nurses' Association: A conceptual model of community health nursing, Pub. Code. CH-10 3M 12/80R, Kansas City, Mo., 1980, The Association.

Archer, S.E.: Community nurse practitioners: another assessment, Nurs. Outlook **24**:499-503, 1976.

*See American Nurses' Association, 1976; Ciarlo, 1981; Fink and Kosecoff, 1978a; Fink and Kosecoff, 1978b; Fitz-Gibbon and Morris, 1978; and Morris and Fitz-Gibbon, 1978.

Archer, S.E., and Fleshman, R.P.: Community health nursing: a typol-ogy of practice, Nurs. Outlook **23**:358-364, 1975.

Archer, S.E., and Fleshman, R.P.: Community health nursing patterns and practice, North Scituate, Mass., 1979, Duxbury Press.

Arnstein, S.R.: Eight rungs on the ladder of citizen participation. In Cahn, E.S., and Cahn, J.C., editors: Citizen participation: a case-book in democracy, Trenton, N.J., 1970, Community Action Train-ing Institute.

Berger, P.L., and Neuhaus, R.J.: To empower people: the role of medi-ating structures in public policy, Washington, D.C., 1977, American Enterprise Institute for Public Policy Research.

Blum, H.L.: Planning for health, New York, 1974, Human Sciences Press.

Blum, H.L.: Planning for health: generics for the eighties, New York, 1981, Human Sciences Press.

Bodenstein, J.W.: The role of health professionals—Africanization in mission hospitals, Contact **21**:3-10, 1974.

Ciarlo, J.A.: Utilizing evaluation, concepts and measurement tech-niques, Beverly Hills, Calif., 1981, Sage Publications, Inc.

Connor, D.M.: Understanding your community, Oakville, Ontario, 1969, Development Press.

Cottrell, L.S.: The competent community. In Kaplan, B.H., Wilson, R.N., and Leighton, A.H., editors: Further explorations in social psychiatry, New York, 1976, Basic Books Inc., Publishers.

Delbecq, A.L., and Van de Ven, A.H.: A group process model for problem identification and program planning, J. Appl. Behav. Sci. **4**:466-492, 1971.

Dever, G.E.A.: Community health analysis: a holistic approach, Ger-mantown, Md., 1980, Aspen Systems Corp.

Edwards, A.D., and Jones, D.G.: Community and community devel-opment, The Hague, Netherlands, 1976, Mouton Publishers.

Feuerstein, M.T.: Participatory evaluation—an appropriate technol-ogy for community health programmes, Contact **55**:1-8, 1980.

Filstead, W.J.: Qualitative methodology: firsthand involvement with the social world, Chicago, 1972, Markham Publishing Co.

Fink, A. and Kosecoff, J.: An evaluation primer, Beverly Hills, Calif., 1978a, Sage Publications, Inc.

Fink, A., and Kosecoff, J.: An evaluation primer workbook: practical exercises for health professionals, Beverly Hills, Calif., 1978b, Sage Publications, Inc.

Fitz-Gibbon, C.T., and Morris, L.L.: How to design a program imple-mentation, Beverly Hills, Calif., 1978, Sage Publications, Inc.

Flexner, W.A., and Littlefield, J.E.: Comment on alternative methods for health priority assessment, J. Community Health **2**:245-246, 1977.

Freeman, R.B.: The dilemma of public health nursing today: redesign-ing nursing education for public health, DHEW Pub. No. (HRA) 75-75, Bethesda, Md., 1973, Department of Health, Education and Welfare, Division of Nursing.

Glazer, M.: The research adventure, promise and problems of field-work, New York, 1972, Random House, Inc.

Goeppinger, J.: Community health nursing is primary nursing care in society. In Flynn, B.C., and Miller, M.H., editors: Current perspec-tives in nursing: social issues and trends, St. Louis, 1980, The C.V. Mosby Co.

Goeppinger, J., Lassiter, P.G., and Wilcox, B.: A process definition of community health, Unpublished materials, Charlottesville, 1981, University of Virginia.

Goeppinger, J., Lassiter, P.G., and Wilcox, B.: Community health is community competence, Nurs. Outlook **30**:464, 1982.

Hanchett, E.S.: Community health assessment: a conceptual tool kit, New York, 1979, John Wiley & Sons, Inc.

Hunter, A.: The loss of community: an empirical test through replica-tion, Am. Sociol. Rev. **40**:537-552, 1975.

Hyman, H.H.: Health planning, a systematic approach, Rockville, Md., 1982, Aspen Systems Corp.

Kane, R.L., Herson, R., and Deniston, O.L.: Program evaluation: is it worth it? In Kane, R.L., editor: The challenges of community medi-cine, New York, 1974, Springer Publishing Co., Inc.

Kark, S.: Epidemiology and community medicine, New York, 1974, Appleton-Century-Crofts.

Kelman, H.R.: Evaluation of health care quality by consumers, Int. J. Health Serv. **6**:431-442, 1976.

Kingma, S.J., editor: Primary health care and the village health work-er, Contact **25**:4-12, 1975.

Kluckhohn, F.: The participant-observer technique in small commu-nities, Am. J. Sociol. **46**:331-343, 1940.

Koberg, D., and Bagnall, J.: The all new universal traveller: a soft-systems guide to creativity, problem-solving and the process of reaching goals, Los Altos, Calif., 1981, William Kaufman, Inc.

Lorig, K., and Walters, E.G.: Cuidaremos: the HECO approach to breast self-examination, Int. Q. Community Health Educ. **1**:25-134, 1980-1981.

Luloff, A.E., and Wilkinson, K.P.: Is the community alive and well in the inner city? Am. Sociol. **42**:827-828, 1977.

Maccoby, N., et al.: Reducing the risk of cardiovascular disease: effects of a community-based campaign on knowledge and behavior, J. Community Health **3**:100-114, 1977.

Mahler, H.: The meaning of "health for all by the year 2000," World Health Forum **2**:5-22 1981.

McAlister, A., et al.: Theory and action for health promotion: illustra-tions from the North Karelia project, Am. J. Public Health **72**:43-50, 1982.

Milio, N.: Promoting health through public policy, Philadelphia, 1981, F.A. Davis Co.

Miller, M.K., and Stokes, C.S.: Health status, health resources, and consolidated structural parameters. Implications for public health care policy, J. Health and Soc. Behav. **19**:263-279, 1978.

Mooney, A., and Rives, N.W., Jr: Measures of community health sta-tus for health planning, Health Serv. Res. **2**:129-145, 1978.

Morris, L.L., and Fitz-Gibbon, C.T.: How to measure program imple-mentation, Beverly Hills, Calif., 1978, Sage Publications, Inc.

Neuber, K.A.: Needs assessment: a model for community planning, Beverly Hills, Calif., 1980, Sage Publications, Inc.

Polit, D.F., and Hungler, B.P.: Observational methods. In Nursing re-search, principles and methods, Philadelphia, 1978, J.B. Lippincott Co.

Rogers, E.: Diffusion of innovations, New York, 1962, The Free Press.

Rothman, J.: Planning and organizing for social change, action princi-ples from social science research, New York, 1974a, Columbia Uni-versity Press.

Rothman, J.: Three models of community organization practice. In Cox, F., et al., editors: Strategies in community organization: a book of readings, Itasca, Ill., 1974b, F.E. Peacock Publishers, Inc.

Ryan, W.: Blaming the victim, New York, 1976, Vintage Books.

Salber, E.J.: The lay advisor as community health resource, J. Health Polit. Policy Law **3**:469-478, 1979.

Salber, E.J.: Where does primary health care begin? The health facilita-tor as a central figure in primary care, Isr. J. Med. Sci. **17**:100-111, 1981.

Salber, E.J., Beery, W.L., and Jackson, E.J.R.: The role of the health facilitator in community health education, J. Community Health **2**:5-20, 1976.

Scutchfield, F.D.: Alternative methods for health priority assessment, J. Community Health **1**:29-38, 1975.

Seaman, C.C., and Verhonick, P.J.: Research methods for undergrad-uate students in nursing, New York, 1982, Appleton-Century-Crofts.

Service, C., and Salber, E.J., editors: Community health education: the lay advisor approach, Durham, N.C. 1977, Community Health Education Program, Department of Community and Family Medicine, Duke University.

Shamansky, S.L., and Pesznecker, B.: A community is . . . , Nurs. Outlook **29**:182-185, 1981.

Skrovan, C., Anderson, E.T., and Gottschalk, J.: Community nurse practitioner: an emerging role, Am. J. Public Health **64**:847-853, 1974.

Spero, J.: Issues and concerns in graduate education in public health nursing, Unpublished paper presented at American Public Health Association convention, Washington, D.C., 1977.

Suttles, G.D.: The social construction of communities, Chicago, 1972, University of Chicago Press.

Tinkham, C.W., and Voorhies, E.F.: Community health nursing, evolution and process, New York, 1977, Appleton-Century-Crofts.

University of Virginia School of Nursing: Community competence assessment manual, Unpublished, Oct. 1981.

Warnecke, R.B., et al.: Health guides as influentials in central Buffalo, J. Health Soc. Behav. **17**:22-34, 1976.

Warren, R.L., editor: New perspectives on the American community, Chicago, 1977, Rand McNally & Co.

Weick, K.E.: Systematic observational methods. In Lindzey, G., and Aronson, E., editors: The handbook of social psychology, ed. 2, Reading, Mass. 1968, Addison-Wesley Publishing Co.

Wellman, B., and Leighton, B.: Networks, neighborhoods, and communities: approaches to the study of the community question, Urban Affairs Q. **14**:363-390, 1979.

Williams, C.A.: Community health nursing—what is it? Nurs. Outlook **25**:250-254, 1977.

Wilson, R.N.: Editorial note to the competent community. In Kaplan, B.H., Wilson, R.N., and Leighton, A.H., editors: Further explorations in social psychiatry, New York, 1976, Basic Books, Inc., Publishers.

Wood, J., and Ohlson, V.: Graduate preparation for community health nursing practice. In Miller, M.H., and Flynn, B.C., editors: Current perspectives in nursing; social issues and trends, St. Louis, 1977, The C.V. Mosby Co.

World Health Organization: Community health nursing: report of a WHO expert committee, Technical Report Series No. 558, Geneva, 1974, WHO.

Chapter 18

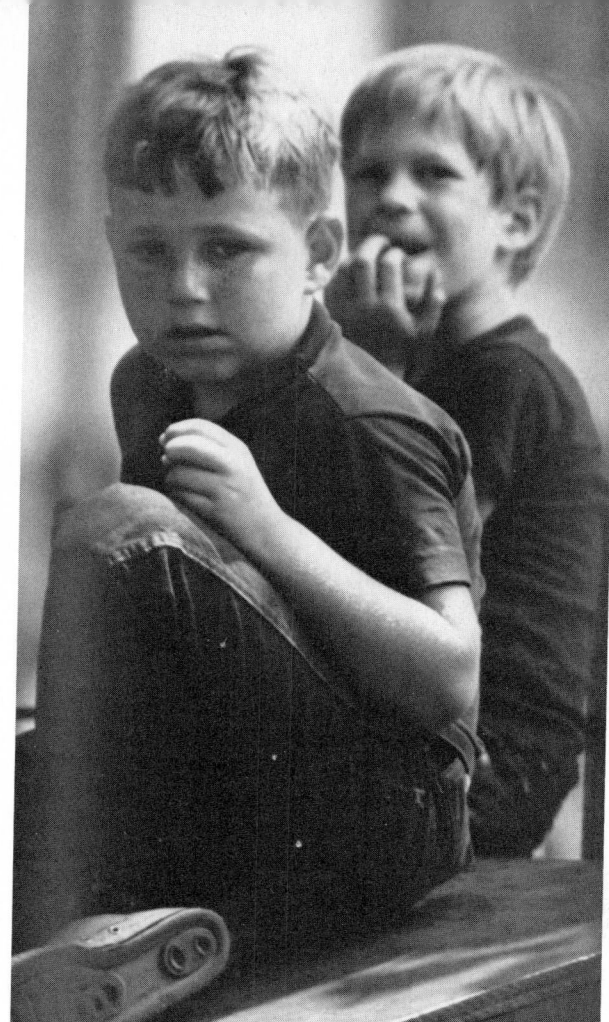

DAVID KERSCHNER
JEANETTE LANCASTER

COMMUNITY MENTAL HEALTH: PROBLEM IDENTIFICATION, PREVENTION, AND INTERVENTION

Mental health problems annually affect an increasing number of American families. According to the President's Commission on Mental Health (1978) nearly 15% of the population of the United States need some type of mental health service at any given time. It is also estimated that as many as 25% of the population suffer from what are considered to be mild forms of emotional disorder such as depression or anxiety. Mental health problems and needs frequently confront community health nurses. These problems are often complex and tend to result from the interaction of many factors, including heredity, family relationships, living conditions, and social and economic constraints. Since people suffering from psychological maladies often re-

main in or return to the community following treatment, community health nurses must be able to assess the presence of mental health problems and plan and implement interventions within the confines of the resources available in the community. To do this, it is necessary to understand how mental health services are typically organized, including the history of their development. Other sections of this chapter discuss current challenges to the maintenance of mental health, creation of a preventive framework, major risk factors working against maintenance of mental health, major mental health problems, and selected methods of intervention. Particular attention is given to medication management of mentally ill persons in the community.

CONCEPTS OF MENTAL HEALTH AND ILLNESS

Mental health and illness represent an area filled with unknowns. Definitions of mental health vary considerably, and the cause of most forms of mental illness remains elusive or highly debatable. Since no universally accepted definition of mental health exists, program planning in community health for this population group is complex. Definitions of mental health range from the absence of mental disease to the attainment of one's maximal capabilities.

Concepts of mental health and illness have changed dramatically in the last two centuries. In the fifteenth century the mentally ill were considered to be "possessed," and witch-hunting and exorcism of demons were ways in which communities responded to this health disruption (Wilner et al., 1978). A book published in 1489 entitled *Malleus Maleficarum (Hammer Against Witches)* contained instructions for identifying a witch. This book served as a guide for "handling" mentally afflicted people for nearly 300 years; many of the criteria used in 1489 to detect witches are symptoms currently associated with mental illness (Wilner et al., 1978).

Following the era of demon possession it was next thought that disease resulted from organic defect or injury. If no lesion was found, people demonstrating aberrant behavior were considered immoral or criminal, and suitable punishment was leveled against them.

In recent times efforts have been directed toward differentiating mental health from illness. Anthropologists, however, point out that what seems like illness in one culture may be viewed as acceptable behavior elsewhere. Chapter 11 describes social and cultural aspects of community health nursing. Considering social, cultural, and individual differences affecting and evidenced in people, it can be seen that mental health is always relative—to time, place, and situation (Taylor, 1982). However, several characteristics of mental health are generally accepted. These are the ability to cope with maturational and situational stressors, to cope with reality, to love and be loved in return, to accept oneself, and to think and act independently (Taylor, 1982). Marmor and Pumpian-Mindlin (1950, p. 30) defined mental health as "that state in the interrelationships of the individual and his environment in which the personality structure is relatively stable, and the environmental stresses are within its absorptive capacity."

Like mental health, mental illness is usually determined in terms of an individual's relationship to the environment. According to Taylor (1982), p. 115) "mental illness is a complex problem that is thought to be a unique response involving an individual's personality as it interacts with his environment at a time when he is particularly vulnerable to stress."

Although these definitions are by no means universally accepted, their breadth allows their adaptation to specific situations. Mental health, viewed from a community health perspective, is a complex process whereby people maintain at least a moderate degree of adaptation to the environment and are able to function in everyday activities and cope with daily stressors. Illness ensues when the person is unable to maintain a state of equilibrium with the environment and thereby becomes incapable of acceptable functioning with daily activities. The next section briefly traces the development of community mental health as a system of care. Historical antecedents serve as determinants of many of today's beliefs and forms of care in community mental health.

DEVELOPMENT OF COMMUNITY MENTAL HEALTH AS A SYSTEM OF CARE

The methods of treating mental illness have changed dramatically in the past century. This section highlights several significant changes in mental health in order to explain current attitudes and stereotypes about mental illness. Community mental health, as a treatment philosophy, was mandated by the Community Mental Health Centers Act of 1963 and will be discussed in detail in a later section of this chapter.

Community mental health, a treatment approach implemented through comprehensive community mental health centers, is considered the fourth revolutionary development in the field of psychiatry. The first revolution occurred in 1793 when Pinel removed the chains from mentally ill patients confined in Bicêtre, a hospital outside Paris. The second revolution was ushered in with the inception of Freudian psychoanalytic treatment about 100 years after the work of Pinel. The advent of psychotropic drugs commenced the third revolution and in many ways made it possible to treat mentally ill persons from a community mental health approach (Taylor, 1982).

The basic philosophy underlying community mental health is that behavior is determined by two sets of variables: the person and the situation. As such, this philosophy is consistent with public health thinking. To implement this philosophy, community mental health requires a different orientation from the medical model that prevailed in psychiatry for many years. Treatment is more encompassing than merely removing an emotionally disturbed person from the stressful setting, making the necessary psychological repairs, and returning the person to the same setting. Community mental health focuses on helping the individual, the family, and also the community to interact in more adaptive ways so that mental health is maintained.

Humanitarian Reforms in Mental Health

Prior to 1840 people deemed to be mentally ill were sent to jails, asylums, or county homes. These forms of shelter and removal of the afflicted person from society protected the afflicted people from being harmed, and from harming others and provided them with food and shelter. Treatment, as such, was unheard of for the mentally ill person. At this time, mental illness was viewed as an incurable affliction, and the only logical goal seemed to be to remove the sick person from the community so no harm would come to anyone. During this era a few private hospitals were available for patients who could afford this luxury.

Benjamin Rush, often called the "father of American psychiatry," led the movement for humane treatment of mentally ill people. Although instrumental in introducing a humanitarian way of thinking into psychiatry, he continued to use remedies such as blood-letting, purgatives, and a torturelike device known as the "tranquilizer."

The work begun by Rush was carried on enthusiastically by a former schoolteacher, Dorothea Dix, who in 1841 appointed herself inspector of institutions for the mentally ill. Traveling the land, she crusaded for enlightened treatment for patients. Dix insisted that each state should assume the financial and caretaking responsibility for its own residents. Her exhaustive efforts on behalf of mental health led to the establishment of 32 mental hospitals in the United States. At this time most of the hospitals were built in rural areas both for the patients to benefit from fresh air and also to keep them isolated from the mainstream, since they were feared by others.

As the population of the United States grew, the number of hospitals did also, until 1900. At this time the completion of new hospitals virtually came to a halt, which meant that existing facilities soon became overcrowded and deplorable conditions became the standard. The care of mentally ill people in the United States continued to deteriorate until Adolf Meyer took up the crusade that had been carried on by Dix. Meyer, the first person to describe and campaign for community mental health, proposed that a clinic for the mentally ill be established in communities so certain population groups could be studied and treated. The mental health movement received a major impetus in 1908 from the publication of Clifford Beers' book *A Mind That Found Itself.* In this book Beers graphically recounted his experiences as a psychiatric patient and urged reform and public education for mental health

(Hanlon and Pickett, 1979). He is credited with the establishment of the Connecticut Society for Mental Hygiene, whose purpose was to combat ignorance about the cause and nature of mental illness. In 1909 the National Committee for Mental Hygiene was organized. This organization was a forerunner of the National Association for Mental Health.

In the following decade, 19 state mental hygiene societies and 16 societies in other nations were organized. The International Congress for Mental Hygiene was established in 1922, and in 1930 the first International Mental Hygiene Congress was held in Washington, D.C. (Hanlon and Pickett, 1979).

Governmental Involvement in Mental Health

The federal government first became involved in the financing of mental health services with the 1935 passage of the Social Security Act. This shift in responsibility from the state to the federal government grew out of the notion during the depression that if local communities could not care for their ill people, then the government should undertake this responsibility. The impact of World War II on community mental health was unprecedented; 875,000 draftees out of 15 million, or almost 6%, were rejected from military service because of existing mental illness (Snow and Newton, 1976). The end of the war witnessed a significant increase in the government's role for the mentally ill; in 1946 Congress enacted the National Mental Health Act, making grants available to states to develop programs outside of state hospitals. This legislation sought to apply a community health approach to the treatment of mentally ill people; in reality, individual psychotherapy based on a medical model was the primary mode of treatment used (Ramshorn, 1971). The act did establish the National Institute of Mental Health (NIMH) in 1949 and designated it as the agency responsible for mental health in the United States. Also during the 1940s, two important types of treatment facilities came into existence: outpatient clinics and psychiatric units in general hospitals.

The next major piece of legislation to affect mental health was the creation in 1955 of the Joint Commission on Mental Illness and Health (Snow and Newton, 1976). This commission consisted of representatives of 36 organizations and agencies chosen by NIMH. Five years after its inception, the Joint Commission submitted its report to Congress. This historical document, *Action for Mental Health,* was published in 1961 as a 338-page report emphasizing the need for better training of personnel, providing early and intensive treatment for the acutely ill, and carrying out research activities. The report also recommended the development of additional facilities, including units in general hospitals and clinics and programs for aftercare, rehabilitation,

---

Essential and Supplementary Services of Community Mental Health Centers as Specified in Federal Legislation

Essential services

- Inpatient care for patients requiring short term hospitalization
- Partial hospitalization including day and night care
- Outpatient treatment
- Emergency services on a 24-hour basis
- Consultation and education for members of the community

Supplementary services

- Diagnostic services including the making of treatment recommendations
- Rehabilitation services and vocational counseling
- Precare and aftercare
- Training for all kinds of personnel and
- Research and evaluation

From Landsberg, G., and Hammer, R.: Community Ment. Health J. 13:63-70, 1977.

and mental health education (Joint Commission, 1961).

Following the publication of this report, President John F. Kennedy appointed a cabinet-level committee to review the report and make recommendations regarding the need for federal action. Based on this report, in 1963, Kennedy made the first Presidential address on behalf of the mentally ill and called for a "bold new approach" to maintain and return patients to their local community. These actions culminated in the community mental health centers concept (Rubin, 1971).

Legislation for Community Mental Health

Community mental health centers became a reality in October 31, 1963, when Congress enacted Public Law 88-164, the Mental Retardation Facilities and Community Mental Health Centers Construction Act of 1963, authorizing federal matching funds of $150 million over a 3-year period to be used by states in construction of centers. This act sought to provide comprehensive mental health services to all residents in a specific area known as a *catchment area*. Each catchment area was to comprise of 75,000 to 200,000 people. Besides providing five essential services to qualify for funding, centers were encouraged to implement five additional services. Both the essential and supplementary services are listed in the box above.

The original legislation envisioned that funding would be provided to centers to enable them to get started, at which time federal funds would decrease as state and local funds increased. This plan did not work in many areas, since state and local funds rarely increased sufficiently to take over much of the federal portion. To keep the centers operational, Congress extended Public Law 89-105 (the 1964 legislation to establish the "seed money" concept of financing centers based on a declining formula of federal support over a 51-month period) nine times. In 1965 Congress overrode a Presidential veto to pass the Community Mental Health Centers Amendments of 1975 (PL 94-63). These amendments provided a more stable source of funding for centers, made available distress grants, and extended the funding cycle to a maximum of 12 years. The amendments also provided grants for specialty areas, including child care, aging, court screening, care for discharged mentally ill people, transitional services, and substance abuse. Actually the 1975 amendments legally defined the components of a community mental health center's services and documented those which must be provided. These amendments have been severely criticized because of their lack of flexibility and limited responsiveness to the unique needs of individual communities (Citizens Guide, 1977). For example, each center was required to offer the same essential and supplemental services regardless of the unique needs of the population within the catchment area. The needs of an aging population would be different from those families with young or adolescent children.

The 1977 report of the President's Commission on Mental Health recommended strengthening the community mental health system and again extended funding. The 117 recommendations of the report were divided into eight sections: community support systems, service delivery, financing, personnel, patient's rights, research, prevention, and public understanding. The main thrust of the recommendations was to establish a new federal grant program for community mental health services where they were inadequate and increase the flexibility of communities in planning a comprehensive network of services. In general the report called for many of the same priority areas as mentioned in the original legislation of the 1960s (President's Commission, 1978).

Following publication of the President's Commission on Mental Health report, legislation passed in 1980 emphasized the need for communities to be flexible in planning services to meet their unique needs. This legislation gave states greater authority over mental health funds, allowed flexible and innovative program planning and development, and emphasized prevention as well as the development of new approaches to meet the mental health needs of priority populations.

Communities became eligible to plan according to their needs and not be restricted to federally mandated services. Linkages were also supported among agencies to promote coordination and reduce duplication (Nation's Health, 1981).

State and Local Roles in Mental Health

Currently all states provide some kind of mental health services, although the responsible agency varies among the states. Some states have separate departments of mental health, whereas in other states mental health programs are administered through a division of mental health, which is a branch of the state health or welfare department (Wilner et al., 1978). Placement of the agency may affect the amount of power it has as well as its ability to solicit state funds.

In recent years many states have established and authorized local mental health authorities to develop mental health programs. In these states the state agency plans and coordinates programs, whereas the local agency carries out the activities of finding cases, diagnosis, treatment, education, consultation, and rehabilitation (Wilner et al., 1978).

The passage of the Community Mental Health Centers Act of 1963 provided states with new responsibility for planning and administering mental health services. Community health nurses must know what agencies exist within a state as well as within the local area. Information to secure regarding mental health services includes the type and location of available agencies, eligibility requirements, fee schedule and accepted method of payment, ease of access to agency, whether clients are seen immediately on request or if the demand for services necessitates that clients sign a waiting list, what type of providers see clients, and how clients make initial contact with the agency.

Criticism of Community Mental Health Centers

Despite two decades of federal and local funding, few centers have met the dreams of their architects to provide comprehensive, accessible mental health services at the local level. The community mental health movement has been plagued with requirements and stipulations for funding that have largely ignored the unique needs of the communities being served. Centers often fail to define program boundaries and priorities. Frequently they are accused of trying to be all things to all people regardless of program priorities, personnel, and other resources. The legislation mandated services with no consideration to community characteristics or needs. Despite an initial wish of applying public health principles to mental health, few centers assessed the needs of their community and planned accordingly.

The concept of catchment areas is often rigid and fails to take into account unique needs of the service area. In many centers catchment areas are rigidly adhered to in defining the eligible population even when these boundaries seem unworkable. A person could live across the street from a boundary line and perhaps have to drive 5 miles to a center rather than cross the boundary and use the nearby center. The catchment concept has caused additional problems when rural versus urban populations are examined. Seventy-five to 200,000 people in Wyoming are found in a far larger geographical area than in New York City. Further, catchment areas have ignored duplication of services and accessibility. Each center provides its own range of services, with minimal coordination among centers. The catchment concept is problematic for a mobile population in which many may not have a legal residence.

Community mental health centers have also failed to achieve financial independency by excessively relying on federal funds and not developing adequate mechanisms to obtain third party reimbursement. Although many insurance policies do cover treatment for mental illness, centers have not made use of all opportunities to recover fees for their services. Inpatient care is most easily recovered; often outpatient and community-focused services are not covered by third party payers and clients or participants are not required consistently to participate in the payment scheme. In addition, the consultative and educational efforts of prevention tend to receive limited attention, and even less is done with evaluation of program effectiveness. Centers are also criticized for using poorly trained staff unqualified to provide care to clients seeking services.

Further, many centers are managed by health care providers untrained in the administrative skills of marketing, finance, economics, accounting, labor relations, organizational behavior, and other basic managerial skills. Lacking a managerial orientation, centers have been unable to reduce dependence on governmental funding. Time and energy are frequently directed toward program offerings designed to receive grant funding rather than toward developing programs that can best serve the community and possibly increase third party reimbursement.

In many geographical areas centers have severe image problems by being viewed as a treatment facility for the mentally ill who are poor or chronically ill. Centers do not consistently call to mind the image of a place where people of all walks of life would choose to seek services. For these reasons, in many areas centers have failed to achieve their initial goals. Community health nurses need to be aware of these criticisms to understand client reluctance to seek mental health services. In addition to the stigma of mental illness, centers are not always conveniently located. Clients often have to change buses several times to reach a center only to find that all clients are scheduled at the same time, and there will be a 2-hour wait.

Benefits of Community Mental Health Centers

Despite the criticisms leveled against centers, supporters acknowledge their good points. The greatest accomplishment may be demystification of mental illness. In previous decades mentally ill people were sent to long-term care hospitals and had limited contact with friends, family, and other community residents. Fear of the unknown influenced many people to develop stereotypes about the mentally ill; hence, providing treatment in the community tended to reduce the mystery. Increasingly, children and adolescents receive psychiatric treatment in centers. There is a renewed hope that trends in legislative flexibility may enable centers to implement the original vision of a community-based and community-oriented approach to the treatment of mentally ill people.

■ ■ ■

The history of the development of community mental health, even with its unfulfilled dreams, sets the stage for examining the most prevalent problems dealt with by community health nurses. The next section focuses on contemporary challenges in the United States that increase the risk of developing emotional problems.

CHALLENGES TO THE MAINTENANCE OF MENTAL HEALTH

Rapid social and technological changes in contemporary society have strained resources for human adaptation. Maintaining health, especially mental health, is particularly difficult in times of rapid change, under intense social, economic, and environmental pressures, and amid an escalating climate of personal responsibility for health. During the 1970s many American dreams vanished as energy became scarce and as crisis after crisis called attention to the flaws and false promises of technology. Every gain in life-style pleasure and comfort seemed to exhort a high price in terms of the long-range implications for health. Despite rapidly accelerating health care costs, the overall health indexes of morbidity and mortality failed to drop noticeably. Further, clear-cut data supported the notion that health really does result from "what you eat, how you think and feel and what you do."

Although each of these social conditions has implications for mental health, the effects of inflation of the mental health of the American family deserves special attention because of the far-reaching effects. According to Johnson (1979), the psychological effects of inflation are insidious as it slowly erodes the family's standard of living. The American Dream, although tarnished, continues to purport that hard work leads to economic achievement and greater personal success and satisfaction. For the first time in recorded history, it seems unlikely that parents can hope their children will have a better life. Currently only 20% of the American population will change their social status: 5% will move downward socially, and 15% will increase their status. Expectations for success have a limited chance of realization despite talent, intelligence, education, and hard work.

A wide discrepancy between expectations and the actual potential for social mobility leads to feelings of anomie, (alienation and loneliness) depression, and decreased self-esteem. A variety of social conditions challenge the maintenance of mental health; these include inflation, more women in the labor force, changing roles for both men and women, a heightened self-awareness, and a desire to "feel good" despite the method or cost. Levi (1979) summarizes four high risk psychosocial conditions as being (1) uprooting of families caused by mobility and family disruption; (2) dehumanization of societal institutions to the extent that services are provided in an impersonal, noncaring way that devalues the worth of people; (3) psychosocial side effects of innovations so that improved technologies or products change the behavior of people in either an unexpected or a hazardous way; and (4) psychosocial factors as constraints on health programs and activities, for example, the interference to service delivery caused by the stigma attached to mental illness. A framework for prevention is described in preparation for a detailed description of major mental health stressors, high risk groups, and nursing implications.

FRAMEWORK FOR MENTAL ILLNESS PREVENTION

Leavell and Clark (1965) described levels of prevention in 1953 when they identified the approaches to preventive medicine as primary, secondary, and tertiary. In the 1960s psychiatrist Gerald Caplan described levels of prevention specific to psychiatry. Caplan (1974) defined primary prevention as efforts directed toward reducing the incidence of mental disorders in a community; secondary prevention referred to decreasing the duration of disorders; and tertiary prevention referred to reducing the level of impairment.

More recently Bloom (1979) described intervention to prevent mental disorders according to prevalence and incidence figures. The first type of intervention is

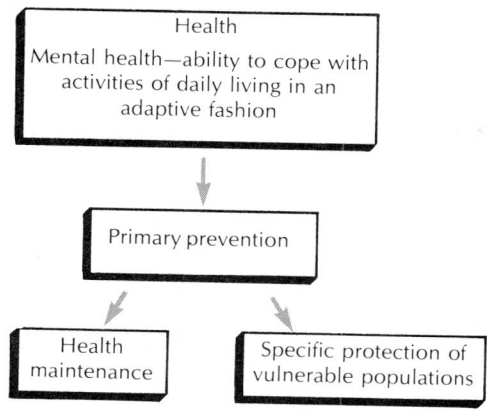

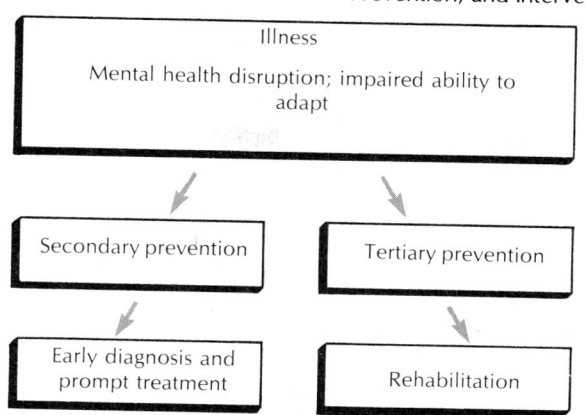

Fig. 18-1. Mental health–mental illness continuum.

designed to reduce the number of persons with the disorder in a given population (prevalence). Primary prevention attempts to reduce the onset of new cases by reducing incidence through programs aimed at either an entire population group or only at persons at risk. Techniques for mental illness control focusing on early case finding and prompt treatment are secondary prevention. Tertiary prevention is unrelated to incidence and may actually increase the prevalence as it increases life expectancy for people with chronic illness. Fig. 18-1 depicts the mental health–mental illness continuum and includes levels of prevention.

Bloom (1979) distinguished between disease prevention and health promotion. For example, some disorders are prevented by highly specific measures that do not affect anything other than the targeted disease. In contrast, many nonspecific activities seem to have a positive effect on mental health in general, but their exact prevention of a specific disease cannot be documented. Stress management techniques seem to improve the overall quality of life, but proof is generally not available that one specific stress-related illness was prevented.

Critics say mental illness prevention lacks scientific specificity and is like a "shot in the dark." Since the actual cause of most mental illness is seldom known, prevention is often viewed as an activity distracting from the real business of mental health care: treating sick people. From a community mental health perspective it seems obvious that treating sick people is only one aspect of the total range of mental health efforts.

The *public health paradigm* for disease prevention is based on Leavell and Clark's model (1965), which describes the interaction between host, agent, and environment as the period of prepathogenesis. Pathogenesis extends from the person's first contact with the disease-producing stimuli to the actual change in functioning.

The combination of prepathogenesis and pathogenesis makes up the natural history of the disease. Based on this tracing of disease development, specific interventions can be established. This approach holds that each disorder has a necessary and identifiable precondition.

Although this classic public health paradigm explains many forms of mental illness, an approach developed by Bloom (1979) offers more promise for community health nursing. The basis for the *new mental health paradigm* is that stressful life events affect mental health, especially the mental health of vulnerable people. This new approach does not begin by searching for the cause of each disorder but rather ". . . preventive intervention programs can be organized around facilitating the mastery or reducing the incidence of particular stressful life events without undue regard for the prior specification of which forms of disability might be prevented" (Bloom, 1979, p. 183). The steps of this paradigm can be summarized as follows:

1. Identify a stressful life event that seems to have undesirable consequences for health and develop methods to identify people at risk.
2. Study the consequences of the event and develop intervention approaches.
3. Implement and evaluate the success of intervention.

Seemingly, the most effective primary prevention approach requires a union of public health and mental health concepts. Such a model blends the classic public health triad of host, agent, and environment as described in Chapter 7 but adds the paradigm developed by Bloom. Fig. 18-2 demonstrates this combined model. The nursing goal in relation to this triad is to help people (hosts) strike a balance between factors that might disrupt mental health (agents) and the available supports (environment). Both Chapters 7 and 12 provide additional ways of looking at this triad.

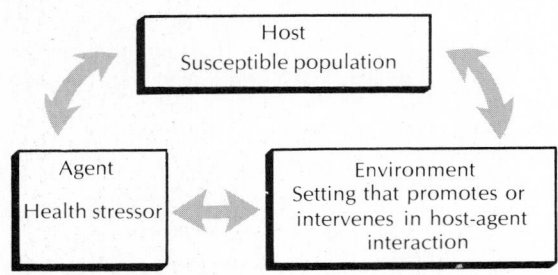

Fig. 18-2. Epidemiological triad.

Factors such as crowding, poverty, inflation, racism, mobility, family disintegration, type of occupation, and level or threat of crime and violence potentially decrease host resistance to mental health disruption. In contrast, timely and effective physical and psychological care and support, police protection, social and family support networks, and educational opportunities increase resistance on a community level. On a personal or small group basis, mental health education, anticipatory guidance, crisis intervention, counseling, and support groups decrease host susceptibility. Community health nurses are in key positions to identify individual family and group needs, conflicts, and stressors.

Additional factors deserve consideration in establishing a framework for examining mental health. First, it is unlikely that all mental illness will ever be prevented. Unlike the relationship between vitamin C and scurvy, predisposing factors for mental illness are difficult to pinpoint. Second, how people respond to life events depends on the interaction of inherited characteristics, previous experience, perception, and environment. It is also important to recognize that prevention deals with both high risk groups and high risk situations.

GOALS OF COMMUNITY MENTAL HEALTH NURSING

Goals of community mental health nursing are multifaceted and are only summarized here. The first goal deals with primary prevention and seeks to prevent the occurrence of mental disorders by strengthening individual, family, and group coping abilities. Several examples of primary prevention are discussed later in this chapter in relation to specific high risk populations such as divorced people or members of two-career families.

The second goal, consistent with secondary prevention, aims to detect early signs of mental health disruption so that prompt counseling, treatment, and referral can be provided. In clinics, schools, home health care, and the work place, community health nurses detect early signs of increased levels of anxiety, decreased ability to cope with stress, and failure to perceive self, the environment, and/or reality accurately. Finding cases in mental health, as in all other areas of community health nursing, is a major goal.

In terms of tertiary prevention, community health nurses play vital roles in monitoring the progress of discharged persons, especially their medication regimen, coordination of care, use of advocacy, and response to referral.

An additional goal that cuts across all levels of prevention is coordination among agencies serving mental health clients. Frequently, support, encouragement, and interpretation of agency resources help clients become more comfortable with the facilities they must visit and the often multiple types of care they must seek.

MAJOR RISK FACTORS WORKING AGAINST MENTAL HEALTH

Changes in social situations carry an increased risk for some people because of their coping ability, the nature and quantity of stressors, and the amount and availability of support networks. Further, because of the complex, interactive nature of factors leading to mental illness, it is impossible to precisely assign events to a particular risk category. This section describes several physiological and psychosocial factors influential in mental health status. The adage "all people are created equal" is not true. Some are born with physical and psychological handicaps, and the odds in life seem stacked against them. The choices discussed in this section are not meant to be inclusive; rather, they set forth examples of risk factors often seen in community health.

Severe Mental Deficiency

Severe mental deficiency, different from mental illness, is often defined as an IQ less than 50. This disorder occurs in all socioeconomic groups and frequently results from structural or biochemical abnormalities of the developing brain. Many causes of severe mental deficiency are the result of prenatal insults, which are often genetic or chromosomal in origin. The financial and emotional costs associated with these deficiencies are high, and in many cases documented forms of prevention are known. Some of the examples cited in this chapter do have known preventive measures. Chapter 29 presents detailed information about developmental disabilities. This chapter highlights selected forms of mental deficiency not covered in detail in Chapter 29.

Metabolic Abnormalities

Screening often prevents severe mental deficiency caused by metabolic abnormalities. Early detection and prompt treatment minimize brain disruption. These disorders include phenylketonuria (PKU), galactosemia, and congenital hypothyroidism. Screening of newborns indicates that PKU occurs in approximately 1 in 11,500 live births, galactosemia in 1 in 40,000 to 60,000, and congenital hypothyroidism in 1 in 3500. Untreated, each disorder can produce a severely defective child, yet effective dietary or medication treatment enables these children to develop at a normal or nearly normal rate (Eisenberg and Parron, 1979).

Noxious Substances

In addition to population screening and intervention in metabolic disorders, other high risk situations for severe mental deficiency occur when pregnant women are exposed to noxious substances either in the environment or through direct consumption. For example, exposure to radiation, environmental pollutants, and certain medications produces detrimental effects on a developing fetus. Pregnant women should be advised to take as few medications as possible during the first trimester and to avoid drinking alcoholic beverages and smoking cigarettes.

Consumption of more than 3 ounces of absolute *alcohol* (about six drinks/day) has been shown to result in a defined abnormality known as the fetal alcohol syndrome (Healthy People, 1979). It is estimated that 4000 to 5000 such infants are born annually, and they tend to have low birth weight, be mentally retarded, and often suffer behavioral, craniofacial, skeletal, neurological, cardiac, or genital abnormalities. The risk of this syndrome increases with the level of alcohol consumption. In one study 32% of infants born to heavy drinkers had congenital defects, compared to 14% for moderate drinkers and 9% among nondrinkers (Oulette et al., 1977). Chapter 22 presents more detailed information about the hazardous effects of substance abuse.

Lead poisoning also contributes to severe mental retardation and death. Even low doses of lead can cause impaired cognitive, verbal, perceptual, and motor skills. Screening for the presence of lead, especially in paint, is a major community health nursing role. In a 3-month period, the Childhood Lead Poisoning Program tested 90,000 children and found 7000 with high blood lead levels. Although chelation therapy is a useful treatment, efforts must be directed toward environmental sources to prevent the occurrence of lead poisoning (Richmond and Filner, 1979).

Developmental Attrition

Developmental attrition, or children's cumulative loss of intellectual and emotional potential, results from many sources, including unwanted pregnancies, complications of pregnancy and parturition, malnutrition, infection, insufficient cognitive stimulation, inadequate emotional support, poor schooling, and racial or class discrimination. The last trimester of pregnancy and the first 2 years of life are susceptible times for the effects of malnutrition and infection (Richmond and Filner, 1979).

Learning disorders may result from the fetal and neonatal deficiencies described earlier. Although the etiology of learning disorders is complex and often involves a variety of factors, several patterns are noted. For example, pregnancy-related factors include "maternal malnutrition, or toxemia during pregnancy, difficult labor or delivery producing anoxia and prematurity" (Richmond and Filner, 1979, p. 322). Similarly, childhood-related factors, such as head injury, fever, meningitis, encephalitis, lead poisoning, drug intoxication, and severe nutritional deficits, can cause learning disorders. Just as with lead poisoning and malnutrition, prevention is essential.

Nursing Implications for Mental Deficiencies

The implications for nursing are numerous, since many types of mental deficiency are preventable. Special target areas include health education to inform the public of risk factors, careful assessment to detect potential high risk individuals and groups, early identification, treatment, and follow-up. Specific interventions would be directed toward the following:

1. Preparation for parenthood through education in the schools and community
2. Availability of family planning services and screening of high risk pregnancies
3. Prenatal care throughout the pregnancy beginning in the first trimester
4. Optimal nutrition during pregnancy as well as the developmental stages of childhood and adolescence
5. Prevention and treatment of congenital abnormalities and inborn errors of metabolism, and early detection and treatment of developmental disabilities

Schizophrenia

Although the etiology of schizophrenia, a psychotic disorder characterized by disturbances of thought, mood, and behavior, remains unclear, there is an increasing correlation with a genetic predisposition. The likelihood of having a schizophrenic child is 10% when one parent is so diagnosed and rises to 40% with two schizophrenic parents (Anthony, 1974). It is also thought that schizophrenia may be the result of ineffective parenting and faulty family communication instead of, or as well as, heredity. In spite of the relatively low incidence of schizophrenia, the impact of this disease is significant because of its often chronic nature and early age of onset, usually in the teenage or young adult years. About 100,000 new cases are diagnosed annually, with an overall prevalence between 0.7% and 1.0% (President's Commission, 1978).

Studies of children born to schizophrenic parents have indicated some differences between those who do and those who do not develop the disorder. Those who later become schizophrenic are more likely to have experienced vulnerability in infancy, such as early separation from the mother or being born when the mother was in an acute stage of the disease. Poor school performance, low peer acceptance, and disruptive behavior tend to characterize the children of depressed or schizophrenic mothers (Tableman, 1981). Watt's study (1974) of schizophrenic families demonstrated that girls tend to be introverted, immature, and quietly maladjusted while boys were negativistic, unpleasant, antisocial, and actively maladjusted.

Genetic counseling is not effective as a prevention measure in schizophrenia, since the adult-onset disorder usually follows the age at which the first child is born, and childhood schizophrenia is less common than adult-onset schizophrenia. Measures currently being used for schizophrenic families include day-care services, after-school enrichment programs, homemaker services, and supportive social service efforts during episodes of acute illness. Although these efforts do not prevent schizophrenia, they can relieve stress and potentially prevent additional mental health problems.

Tableman (1981) reported on enrichment projects for children of schizophrenic parents which supplement regular day-care programs. The aim of the supplemental services is to assist children with motor development, self-care, receptive language development, cognitive development, graphic and prereading skills, social behavior, and speech.

Schizophrenics are often hospitalized during acute episodes. However, many schizophrenic individuals are poorly managed once they leave the hospital because the concept of deinstitutionalization discussed in the following section, has not been adequately implemented across the nation.

Abuse of Deinstitutionalization

Providing nursing care to families with a chronically ill member is a complex process. Of the chronic psychi-

atric illnesses, schizophrenia is most frequently seen in the community. In recent years deinstitutionalization affected the services provided by community health nurses. Deinstitutionalization sought to move long-term psychiatric patients out of the warehouse atmosphere of large, public hospitals and back to their communities. However, many communities failed to plan in advance of this trend and were unable to provide coordinated and comprehensive services; instead patients were "dumped" onto the community with no systematic plan for aftercare.

One of the basic premises of community health is continuity of care, yet this critical component is often overlooked in planning for the chronically mentally ill population. If community-based programs are to be successful for this population, someone must serve as advocate and coordinator. Often after many years of hospitalization, people are discharged with little self-confidence and substantial deficits in problem-solving ability or basic skills required for daily living. Also, the society to which they return has changed so drastically, it is hard for them to cope.

In addition, several myths and stereotypes hinder the delivery of care to chronically ill psychiatric patients. Examples include the following: (1) Once psychotic, always psychotic. Such a belief connotes a hopeless and incurable nature to the illness and tends to be reflected in attitudes and treatment approaches. (2) Chronic means that no active treatment is indicated. This stereotype perpetuates the notion of warehousing patients primarily to separate them from society; namely, since local treatment centers are for acute illness, chronically ill patients should be sent to hospitals for long-term custodial care. (3) Chronically ill patients do bizarre things and are often dangerous to themselves and others. Few of these individuals are dangerous, and with supervision and guidance, their dress and behavior can be directed into appropriate channels (Tarail, 1980).

In contrast to these beliefs, mounting evidence indicates that psychotic persons can be maintained effectively outside the hospital if acute episodes are carefully monitored and treated and if medications and both directive and supportive treatment are provided.

Continuity of Care Program

Davies (1981) describes a continuity of care program that incorporates a full range of services designed to help chronically ill psychiatric patients return and remain in the community following hospitalization. The components of this program have implications for community health nurses, who are often in key positions for implementation. The program begins during hospitalization, with the selection of a primary clinician who coordinates care and community services following discharge. The specific services include a continuum of care designed to meet individual needs, allowing easy access to and reentry into the community, and crisis intervention. Three major service categories are provided: direct, community network, and case management.

Direct services include individual, group, and/or family counseling as well as assessment of basic skills. If essential community survival skills are absent, a teaching plan is developed to overcome this deficit. Outreach services in the form of home visits and telephone calls comprise the direct service component. The *community network* component works with community residents and other health care providers to increase awareness of mental health needs and discuss better ways to integrate former psychiatric patients back into the community. *Case management* includes coordination of services for maintaining the person in the community and flexibility so the plan of treatment is modified as the person's needs and abilities change. Community health nurses can become active participants in such a program by first serving as client advocates, then as coordinators of care.

A continuity of care program for chronic psychiatric patients would include at least five major components: (1) community acceptance, (2) client advocacy, (3) individual supervision, (4) client education, and (5) group supervision. For a continuity of care program to be successful, community residents must accept the presence of discharged psychiatric patients in their midst. Residents often fear these patients and believe their presence will decrease property values or bring harm to community members.

Community acceptance can be fostered by open dialogue, public education programs, and support from local radio, television, or newspapers. Mental health volunteers such as representatives from the local mental health association can speak to community groups to convey the message that the majority of chronically ill psychiatric patients are withdrawn rather than violent, and they need acceptance, support, and encouragement.

Client advocacy, as discussed in Chapter 32, is especially useful for discharged persons. In an organized continuity of care program, one person, typically a community health nurse, makes regular visits to clients to determine their needs relative to obtaining community services. These clients often have difficulty being sufficiently assertive to get through the "red tape" of some agencies and secure information or services.

Home visits provide *individual supervision* and typically emphasize medication maintenance, discussed in detail later in this chapter. In addition to monitoring medication usage, nurses observe the client's appearance, nutritional status, level of cleanliness (both of person and environment), and clarity of thought processes.

Client education is essential for many discharged psychiatric patients who must relearn basic living skills. These skills are appropriately taught prior to discharge, but if community health nurses note clients who are unable to perform services for themselves, such as cooking, cleaning, shopping, or paying bills, then a referral to the mental health center or a community program is indicated. Client education is essential to aid clients relearn previously known skills that may have been forgotten during a lengthy hospitalization.

Many clients benefit from *group supervision* where they can share feelings and experiences with understanding peers and staff. Some groups are nondirective, and members discuss any topic of interest; others focus on a specific topic and are lead by a member or outside resource person.

Affective Disorders

Affective disorders comprise one of the most common psychiatric syndromes and are essentially of three types: depressive disorder; manic disorder; and bipolar affective disorder, in which episodes of manic and depressive behavior alternate. As with the schizophrenias, the etiology of affective disorders is not clearly understood but does seem to result from multiple factors, including genetic predisposition, stressful life events, high risk for stress based on personality characteristics, and either inherited or acquired biological abnormalities (President's Commission, 1978). There is growing evidence of genetic transmission, with the risk being 20 times greater for developing an affective disorder if there is a family history of such among first-degree relatives (Perris, 1973).

According to Eisenberg and Parron (1979) the overall prevalence rate for depression is between 16% and 20%, with greater risk being among women, nonwhites, separated, divorced, poor, and less educated people. Two classes of antidepressants (the tricyclics and monoamine oxidase inhibitors) currently are used to successfully treat 70% to 80% of depressive episodes. Similarly, phenothiazines and lithium are effective for treating manic episodes. Regular maintenance doses of lithium tend to decrease the recurrence of bipolar affective disorders. (See the section on drugs on p. 427 for further information.)

Depression

For purposes of this discussion, only the affective disorder of depression is elaborated on. It is estimated that one in five Americans (20%) has at least a moderate amount of depressive symptoms, and all people will experience some depression from time to time. It is magnitude and constancy that make depression a community health problem.

The clinical manifestation of depression results from the interaction of at least three sets of variables: stress factors, concomitant precipitating factors, and predisposing genetic and personality characteristics. Life stressors tending to precipitate depressive episodes generally relate to a loss of something valuable, for example, a divorce, death, or a threat to self-image. In general the greater the number of stressors, the greater the likelihood of depression. Marital stressors seem most difficult for women and job-related ones for men (Jacobsen, 1980). Unmarried women are at high risk for depression because of economic pressures, social isolation, and responsibilities for children. Poverty seems to be the most difficult stressor. Lower-class women are five times as likely to become depressed as are middle-class women. Females are twice as likely as males to become depressed, and both young adults (16- to 24-year-olds) and the elderly (60- to 79-year-olds) constitute high risk groups.

While genetic factors seem to partially explain depressive predisposition, especially when manic episodes are also present, there does appear to be considerable environmental influence. It is well established that early parenting behaviors contribute to level of self-esteem, personal belief system, and feelings of security and trust of others. Currently, a number of social influences contribute to depression. As mentioned previously, economic conditions can precipitate depression and feelings of inadequacy. The media present the American life-style as happy, carefree, and always smiling and purchasing things, yet many people are confronted with a variety of unpleasant and often painful life stressors that dispute this image.

The role of women in society also has implications for the development of depression. Despite numerous social forces to the contrary, women continue to be characterized as loving, faithful wives and mothers. Many women are electing not to adhere to this stereotype but instead are pursuing careers and life goals of their own choosing. The stress and ambivalence associated with trying to blend careers with raising a family often support depressive symptoms.

The primary prevention of depression is directed toward building adaptive strengths and coping resources in people, especially those at high risk. Thus addressing broad social issues and initiating programs are indicated as primary preventive measures for depression. People need to learn more effective ways to cope with life events before a crisis to self-esteem and personal worth develops. In addition, attention should be devoted to high stress periods, such as the early child-rearing years when parents' worth and competency may be threatened when children do not conform to social expectations. For example, not all children are healthy, normal, attractive, intelligent, and well-mannered regardless of parental behaviors. Parents can become involved in educational programs for parenting or support groups to help them cope with family responsibilities more effectively.

Community health nurses see clients at risk for depression in a variety of settings, including clinics, the home, the work place, and schools. Group education as well as individual counseling can be carried out by community health nurses for people at risk for depression. For example, classes in stress management, parenting, assertiveness, and coping with crises can decrease the tendency to become depressed by enriching self-esteem and teaching skills needed for successful coping.

PSYCHOSOCIAL FACTORS INCREASING THE RISK OF MENTAL ILLNESS

Psychosocial factors increasing the risk of mental health disruption refer to the accumulation of psychological, social, economic, and cultural forces affecting adaptation. People do not respond to one stimulus at a time but react to the cumulative impact of variables in their lives. Of particular interest is the effect of life events on the maintenance of psychosocial stability. As Hamburg and Killilea (1979, p. 257) point out, "life change events of predictable and unpredictable nature are an inevitable aspect of human experience. These events may produce life stress that exceeds an individual's coping ability." Changes in life events are inevitable; it is the rapidity at which they occur, the significance they hold for those involved, and each person's coping ability that determine their influence. In general, factors that influence whether life events are viewed as disruptive to psychological equilibrium include the following (Hamburg and Killilea, 1979):

1. A person's biological and psychological characteristics
2. The social and environmental context of the life event
3. Individual coping ability
4. The rate and number of changes occurring at a given time

As mentioned in Chapter 38, Holmes and Rahe (1976) devised a social adjustment rating scale in which numbers are assigned to the effect of predictable life events.] Examples of life events having either a negative or positive effect included marriage, moving to a new home, assuming a mortgage, death of a spouse, divorce, or a minor traffic violation. Each change event had a different numerical outcome, depending on the way the researchers determined its effect on their study sample. In addition, the outcome of each event depended on both the perception of the people involved and their ability to cope with the change. For people with limited competence in handling change, even minor life events such as receiving a traffic ticket can be disruptive, while more adaptive people may seem barely affected by what appear to observers to be major life disruptions. Four broad approaches for dealing with stressful circumstances include the following (Hamburg and Killilea, 1979):

1. Containing distress within limits that are personally tolerable
2. Maintaining self-esteem
3. Preserving interpersonal relationships and a sense of belonging to a valued group
4. Meeting the conditions and demands of the new situation and simultaneously preparing for the future

Various interventions and coping strategies are available for dealing with change. The strategy chosen depends on the developmental and family history of the person, the specific circumstances surrounding the event, including the number of stressors at any one time, and the nature of the available support system.

Before discussing specific community mental health nursing interventions, two mental health stressors—divorce and two-career families—that are increasing both in number and impact on family stability are discussed. By no means are these stressors meant to represent an inclusive list but rather they are two common life events in typical communities that are not ordinarily addressed in community health nursing literature.

Divorce as a Life Change Stressor

In recent years the divorce rate has increased dramatically, confronting individuals and families with new and often multiple problems. In 1979, women initiated divorce proceedings at twice the rate of 1955. According to the National Center for Health Statistics, the number of divorces per year in the United States tripled between 1959 and 1979, to reach 1.181 million in 1979. Interestingly, nearly one third of these divorces, 439,000 or 6.1 per 1000, occurred in the 17 states counted as the South—traditionally considered a section of the nation with a slower pace of living and a greater commitment to family ties. These figures were compared to 6.1 divorces per 1000 population in the West, 5 per 1000 in the North Central states, and 3.6 per 1000 in the Northeast.

In a divorce each person must examine and often alter an established way of coping. In a 5-year study of 60 families, Kelly and Wallerstein (1977) found that the first year after a divorce was the most critical. More than 1 million children annually in the United States experience the disruption and stress accompanying the dissolution of a family. While not all people experience continuing difficulties from the divorce, everyone involved can benefit from support during this transition period.

The community health nursing role is that of supporting all members of families going through a divorce as each attempts to reestablish psychological stability. Before looking at each member's possible reactions, it is useful to note several key components and reactions to the experience. For all involved, divorce is both a disorganizing and reorganizing process that may take several years to resolve. Divorce is both a maturational and a situational life crisis, and like other life crises, the potential for growth and personal development exists, although considerable support and understanding may be needed. At this time, all involved need acceptance and nonjudgmental understanding. People going through or adapting to a divorce often behave in ways that seem contrary to societal expectations; it is essential to accept the person while recognizing that the observed behavior is an effort to cope with a threat to stability.

For example, divorced women often feel worthless, helpless, or physically unattractive. Many have only known a role as someone's wife; when a divorce occurs, they may temporarily lose their sense of identity. The challenge facing these women is to find meaning and purpose in their own life experiences, such as through work or school. Children both help and hinder the process of divorce adjustment. They help in that the pattern of life goes on much the same as before, since children's needs remain constant or become intensified by the experience. Meals must be prepared, carpools driven, and schedules met. On the other hand, children deplete energy reserves when one parent has major responsibility for meeting their needs. Frequently mothers retain custody of children. Wilk (1979), reporting on a study of single divorced mothers who attended a Planned Parenthood Center, found through interviews that these women, when asked to describe themselves, used terms such as "lost," "flighty," "lonely," "floating," and "trying to make it through one day at a time." Compounding these feelings of loneliness, the women felt considerable pressure from the greater parenting responsibilities than that experienced in two-parent families. In many instances a major concern stemmed from not having someone to talk with about their problems. Those interviewed requested that a group be formed to help them deal with problems related to parenting, community resources, housing, transportation, and child care.

Men, too, experience pain and disruption to their lives when a divorce occurs. Regardless of the events and feelings surrounding a divorce, there is a threat to stability and a necessity for learning new ways to adapt. Both men and women seek validation of their worth from members of the opposite sex. Also, in most divorces men leave their familiar home and often miss the furniture and treasured items they were accustomed to seeing and using. Barhopping, staying out all night at singles parties, buying fancy clothes and cars, and spending hours on the telephone reflect efforts to cope with feelings of alienation, loneliness, and rootlessness. No matter how stressful and strained a marriage is, it does represent a familiar way of life; being single requires an entirely different set of behaviors.

Individual and/or group counseling helps people cope with the feelings, fears, and need to develop new personal resources. Such sessions, for both children and adults, assist the involved parties to disengage from their past relationships with a minimum of pain and destructive feelings. Many of the feelings surrounding a divorce are similar to the grief over the death of a loved one. People need to express and deal with feelings of denial, anger, depression, acceptance, and resolution in an unbiased environment. While family and friends are immensely needed, they are rarely unbiased in their views, which limits their ability to assist in the resolution of feelings.

The children of divorcing parents comprise a special concern for community health nurses, both because of the numbers involved and because of the disruption and stress attendant on family disruption (Tableman, 1981). The research of Kelly and Wallerstein (1977) indicates that all children initially react to family disruption with aberrant behavior, and all profit from support during this stress period. Some children experience continuing problems, and community health nurses need to assess whether children's reactions are within normal ranges or if more extensive counseling is indicated. In general, children's reactions vary according to the child's age, sex, developmental stage, and amount of conflict surrounding the event. Table 18-1 provides information about age-specific reactions to divorce.

Children often are delayed in their progress in working through their feelings of loss because they become immobilized in denial by maintaining the fantasy that their divorced parents will someday reconcile and they will live "happily ever after." Moreover, Kelly and Wallerstein (1977) found that stresses and/or resources in the environment, including parental interactions and the availability of the noncustodial parent, influenced coping ability. Based on their research, they developed a "divorce-specific" assessment guide, which is modified and shown in Table 18-1. This guide provides

critical information for nurses working with families who are involved in a divorce by identifying typical behaviors that occur at each stage of growth and development.

Over time the characteristics of a child's response to divorce depend on the parents' reaction to the experience and their ability to recognize and provide support for the child's needs. Frequently parents are so caught up in dealing with their own feelings related to the divorce that they have limited resources available to share with their children. Lack of parental nurturance is particularly detrimental to preschool children who under normal circumstances have substantial dependency needs. According to Tableman (1981), preschool girls are particularly vulnerable to the decreased parental attention, especially from the mother, that may occur during a divorce. Typically during the later preschool years children form identities with the same sex parent. Lack of time and attention at this developmental stage disrupts this process.

Children are also at risk for mental health disruption when they are caught in the middle of parental conflict. Frequently there are legal contests over custody, visitation rights, amount of child support, and decisions about who gets which of the joint possessions. For children caught in the middle of parental hostilities and battles, resolution of the divorce trauma is difficult; rather than coping with a single crisis, their emotions are kept in a turmoil through an ongoing experience. Children from divorced families tend to be overrepresented in the caseloads of psychiatric facilities. Common presenting symptoms are depression, aggressive outbursts, and behavioral problems in school (Kalter, 1977; Shanok and Lewis, 1977).

Divorce is considered by many to be the most potentially serious mental health disrupter of the next decade. When a divorce occurs, each family member is confronted with the task of resisting mental health disruption and yet responding to multiple changes and demands for new roles. Divorce frequently tends to be both a disorganizing and a reorganizing process for all people involved. Counseling, support, and guidance can be provided to each person to reinforce host resistance by strengthening coping ability.

Two-Career Families
Adaptations and Adjustments

Historically, few models exist for the two-career family. While women have in the past helped with farming or with the family business, only since World War II have women comprised a significant portion of the work force. Also, women, as they become better educated, are pursuing careers demanding of time, attention, and energy. Both men and women are taking jobs

Table 18-1. Age-specific reactions to divorce

Observed behavior	Nursing intervention
Early preschool (2½-3½ years)	
Acute regression, heightened aggression and irritability, fearfulness, separation anxiety, bewilderment, acute sadness, tearfulness	Provide guidance to the custodial parent, who serves as the child's best support person Teach communication skills to parents so they can assist the child to interpret the meaning of divorce Help parent look at alternatives for intervening in the child's regressive behavior
Later preschool (3½-6 years)	
Fear, excessive worrying, heightened anxiety, whininess, restlessness, moodiness, general irritability, and symptomatic behaviors, including phobias, sleep disturbances, compulsive eating, aggressiveness, and temper tantrums Difficulty understanding what is happening Frequently asking where the absent parent is Increasing use of fantasy to substitute for absent parent Some experience considerable feelings of guilt and self-blame	Help parent become increasingly consistent and predictable about visitation, discipline, and support Provide support and encouragement to parents and babysitter (when appropriate) concerning child's need for reassurance that he is loved and will be cared for
Early latency (6-9 years)	
Behavioral changes in school Obvious pain, suffering, and fear Often immobilized by the divorce Less able to use denial than are younger children, yet open confrontation with reality is painful Nearly insatiable need to maintain contact with both parents Frequent outbursts of anger Feelings of deprivation; focused on fantasies of getting new toys, clothes, or pets Feelings of responsibility	Open discussions may be too threatening but these children can talk about how "other kids react to . . ." Help parents support the child's need for contact with them; for assurance that he is loved and that anger is all right Respect the child's need for the defenses of denial or repression; let children verbalize on *their* timetable Use "divorce monologue" to discuss common reactions of many children; this lets the child know that his reactions are all right and does not force him to talk before he is ready
Later latency (9-12 years)	
Behavioral changes in school Torn in loyalty between parents Considerable worrying Have the ability to express their feelings and can also channel them into organized activities Child's superego controls may be threatened as external controls are decreased or become inconsistent because of parental stress Have an increased need to discuss the divorce experience with someone outside the family, but they feel very loyal to at least one parent and often have trouble talking about that parent At first may appear poised and calm about family situation as they actively try to make order of their lives Anger well organized and object directed (expressed outwardly and also as demandingness; a dictatorial attitude)	Encourage the child to talk with both parents about fears and worries, hurts and anger Support children as they express pain and anger; help them channel these feelings into socially accepted outlets Help parents become increasingly consistent and firm in their approach to the children Listen, listen, listen
Adolescence (12-18 years)	
Intense feelings of pain (anger, sadness, sense of loss and betrayal) Strong feelings of shame and embarrassment Concern about their future as a marital partner Concern about adequacy as a sexual partner in their current dating or future married life Often unrealistic concern about finances Shortened disengagement from and shift in perceptions of parents Accelerated individuation of parents Heightened awareness of parents as sexual objects Loyalty conflicts Strategic withdrawal as a defense against pain	Provide an opportunity for open discussion of feelings, including helping adolescents plan ways to express their feelings directly and constructively Discuss feelings of shame, embarrassment, and fear of the future Use communication strategies such as role-playing or psychodrama to help adolescents learn new ways to deal with feelings Practice improved, honest, and open communication patterns

Based on data from Wallerstein, J.S., and Kelly, J.B.: Am. J. Orthopsychiatry **47**:4-22, Jan. 1977.

that do not end at five o'clock; problems and challenges of the work place are felt at home as people carry projects and problems home with them.

Also, job-related travel has increased in the last few years for both men and women, leading to additional responsibilities for the parent who remains at home. If one spouse travels considerably more than the other, there may be feelings of resentment or the common ground for discussion of work events may be altered. The one who stays at home may feel put-upon when the spouse is perceived as having so much fun. In contrast, travel is tiring, often hectic, and usually not as exciting as it seems to observers. Hence, the traveling spouse may come home tired and irritable and desire peace and quiet, which may conflict with the expectations of other family members.

Men may feel threatened by highly successful and visible women. The traditional family prototype has been for husbands to gain recognition for their achievements outside the home and for wives to be supportive of the husband's career and provide a family environment that enriches the entire family. As women gain recognition and acclaim for their career accomplishments, even the most enlightened men may feel twinges of envy and discomfort. There have been few role models for men to turn to in regard to learning how to be a participant in a successful two-career family. Thus men may need as much, if not more, support than women do in adapting to contemporary family lifestyles. Opportunities to discuss what it is like to be a man in today's society can be helpful, such as in support groups led by a knowledgeable nurse. Many communities have begun such groups by using volunteer professionals who provide services to various agencies and community programs.

Working Women

According to Schecter (1979), as more women have entered the labor market in response to economic necessity, a new version of the "battered woman" has emerged. For many women taking a job outside the home necessitates the juggling of multiple roles with minimal family or other help. Schecter postulates that the stress inherent in the juggling of several roles has led to the psychological battering of women in the form of symptoms of exhaustion, migraine, hypertension, peptic ulcer, and ulcerative colitis. Most of the women entering the labor force are in the 25 to 44 age group, and nearly two thirds are in clerical, service, or sales jobs where pay rates are low. Currently women who work full-time earn 57 cents for every dollar earned by men. This gap has widened from 64 cents for women per male dollar since 1955 (Schecter, 1979). In addition, two thirds of all women who work do so either because

they are separated, widowed, or divorced or because their husbands' earnings are below the poverty line.

Working Mothers

The nature of parental work is critical for family adaptation. Evidence suggests that working affects both the marriage and the parent-child relationship. The decisive variable seems to be whether women work because they want to or because they have no other alternative. Also, the degree of satisfaction derived from outside employment influences family relationships. Generally, when people gain satisfaction from their work, they feel less frustration and irritability.

In regard to child bearing, there is little evidence that working per se has harmful effects. Children often profit from the increased opportunities for being responsible members of the family (Johnson, 1979). There is evidence, however, that working mothers do experience considerable guilt over being away from their children. Society continues to blame mothers for any misconduct or aberrations in the behavior of their children. Also, most working women, even in two-parent families, continue to retain responsibility for the majority of the family's upkeep. Despite publicity about new family roles, not all husbands share equally in family maintenance functions. Husbands may be threatened and unclear about female employment, especially if the wife has an obviously superior job or if meals are not on time or social events are discouraged. A wife's employment often affects the relative power in the marital relationship. The power relationship centers on the resources brought in by each partner. With more women employed, the degree of total economic dependence on men has lessened notably. This means that two-career couples must continually renegotiate the power base of their marriage, even to mundane activities such as who does the dishes or drives the carpool. Since the average American woman who holds down a full-time job also puts in an additional 26 hours a week in work at home, there is fertile ground for family conflict. Being tired, feeling put-upon, and experiencing guilt for leaving small children with sitters compound the coping needs of the working woman.

Working mothers often employ one or a combination of three defense mechanisms to assist them in coping with guilt. *Rationalization* is noted when women say "I may as well work, I would just spend my time playing cards or tennis." The second defense mechanism, *projection*, is seen when the woman blames others for her need to work such as "If my husband had a better job, I would not have to work." On the other hand, the most potentially dangerous defense mechanism, *overcompensation*, is seen when women try to atone for the "sin of working" by buying the child's forgiveness for her absence through toys, other treats, and lack of limits and discipline. This defense mechanism is often heard in a phrase such as "I am gone so much, that I just hate to make little Susie. . . ."

The role of the community health nurse is to assess parental reactions to working and help parents adapt more positively to these experiences. To do this some key steps need to be identified as stages in managing coping with work and a family. First, mothers need to acknowledge their feelings about working. It is all right to just enjoy getting out of the house and pursuing personal life and career goals. Mothers are not negligent of their families if they admit their own needs and goals. It is the denial of this human aspect that potentially causes family stress.

A second area in which parents often need help includes child care arrangements. A critical issue includes finding someone to care for the children who is similar or who will be consistent with parental goals and expectations. Children find different sets of rules confusing, so maximal amounts of consistency should be attempted. Various child-care arrangements are possible, including household help, babysitters, and day-care centers. The choice should be both economically and emotionally satisfactory to parents. Nurses can be of considerable help in aiding parents explore alternatives, weigh the pros and cons of each, and select a child-care arrangement that fits their unique needs. At one time or another all working mothers feel guilt, but these episodes can be minimized by self-assessment, careful planning, and the support and encouragement of others, including both family and health care providers.

MANAGEMENT OF PSYCHOTROPIC DRUG REGIMENS

Over the past 20 years the number of individuals in the community using psychotropic drugs, or medications to treat psychiatric symptoms, has increased. There are several reasons for this increase, including advancements in psychopharmacology, development of community-based mental health centers, and an attempt to keep in or return to the community those people with psychiatric problems who would have been institutionalized only 15 to 20 years ago. Another reason for this increase is the excessive prescribing of psychotropic drugs for minor or nonpsychiatric problems. An example of this would be the excessive prescribing of diazepam (Valium). For many years diazepam has been the most prescribed drug in the United States.

The management of individuals using psychotropic drugs presents several problems for health care providers. Individuals being treated for psychiatric problems may be reluctant to tell others about their treatment for fear of being labeled "crazy" and not having their other problems or concerns taken seriously. This reluctance to tell others about their treatment could extend to physicians and other health care providers. As a result, medications that adversely interact with psychotropic drugs are prescribed. When antipsychotic drugs that have anticholinergic properties are used in combination with other anticholinergic drugs, they can produce severe anticholinergic side effects.

The frequency of psychological problems in the elderly population is increasing, and the changing metabolic characteristics of this age group make them more susceptible to medication overdosages. Elderly people take an average of six or seven medications at at given time (Linton, 1980). This adds to health care providers' problem of managing medications.

Community health nurses can assess clients in a variety of settings less threatening than physicians' offices or hospital rooms. People are less likely to feel threatened in their own homes or in a community-based clinic and more likely to communicate information openly and freely.

This sense of security and control makes establishing rapport more easily accomplished. Building a trusting relationship and gathering a complete medication history are two important steps in the management of psychotropic drug regimens.

Community mental health clients need to take all medications as prescribed and to keep follow-up appointments. Also, if the community health nurse observes a deteriorating mental status, appropriate referrals should be made for further evaluation and any necessary changes or modifications in treatment.

This portion of the chapter will describe psychotropic drugs commonly used in the management of psychiatric problems in the community setting. The discussion will include the use of these drugs, how they may work, their side effects, and objectives of maintenance of individuals taking these medications. There are also several appendixes that will provide information about the usual dosages of these various drugs.

As mentioned earlier, one of the first items necessary for the maintenance of people taking psychotropic drugs is a thorough medication history. The initial data base should include information about past medical problems, medication history, vital signs, and a mental status examination. This information is presented in the box on the next page. In addition, certain psychotropic medications need further routine evaluations.

This section will not totally prepare community health nurses to manage psychiatric illnesses but is intended to provide information about the management of individuals in the community receiving psychotropic medications.

Data Base for Medication Management
- Psychiatric/medical diagnosis
- Vital signs
  - Blood pressure
  - Pulse
- Medication history
  - Present medications
    - Routine and PRN medications
    - Name of the medication
    - Prescribed dosage
    - Frequency of administration
    - How long the individual has been taking the medication
  - Past medications (especially those that caused the individual problems)
    - Name of the medication
    - How long the individual was taking the medication
    - Any side effects from the medication
  - Over-the-counter medications frequently taken
    - Sleep aids
    - Laxatives
  - Leftover medications that the individual may take occasionally
- Past medical history
  - Liver disease
  - Glaucoma
  - Kidney disease
  - Visual problems
  - Alcohol or drug abuse
- Mental status examination

Antipsychotics

Antipsychotics (neuroleptics or major tranquilizers) help control acute and chronic psychotic conditions such as schizophrenia, mania, paranoid symptoms, agitated psychotic depression, involutional or senile psychosis, organic dementia, and psychotic reactions to amphetamines. Nonpsychiatric conditions include intractable hiccups, alcohol withdrawal, and pain control; antipsychotics also depress emesis. These medications are used as adjunctive therapy in various disorders having psychogenic components, such as arthritis, peptic ulcer disease, and severe asthma. Symptoms controlled by antipsychotic drugs include hyperactivity, hostility, delusions, hallucinations, negativism, and poor sleep (Krupp and Chatton, 1982).

Classification and Action

About two thirds of the classes of antipsychotics are in the phenothiazine derivative class. Thioxanthenes, similar in structure to phenothiazines, are the second class of antipsychotics. The remaining classes are butyrophenones, dihydroindoles, dibenzoxazepines, and diphenylbutyl piperdines. The major antipsychotic drugs commonly used are listed in Appendix E.

The discovery of phenothiazine derivatives arose from antihistamine research in 1951 (Bergersen, 1976). Chlorpromazine hydrochloride (Thorazine) was the first phenothiazine and is the reference compound for all other compounds in this class.

It is thought that psychotic symptoms may be related to an excess of dopamine in the central nervous system (Smythies, 1980). The antipsychotics increase the rate of dopamine turnover (synthesis and destruction) and may block dopamine-mediated transmission (Bergersen, 1976) or receptor sites in the limbic system as well as the hypothalamus and extrapyramidal system tract (Newton and Godbey, 1978). These actions possibly account for the extrapyramidal side effects of the antipsychotics. Antipsychotic drugs are eliminated slowly from the body because of the hepatic formation of active metabolites and accumulation in body tissues, particularly fatty tissues. Therefore when the medication is stopped, clients may continue to experience therapeutic as well as side effects for weeks afterward. Antipsychotics do not produce euphoria, there is no tolerance to their antipsychotic effects, and they are not addicting (Harris, 1981b).

Side Effects and Complications

Phenothiazine derivatives produce a wide variety of untoward effects. Table 18-2 lists these effects. Phenothiazines can cause unpleasant behavioral effects, including feelings of lassitude, fatigability, and depression. This depression may account for the greater incidence of suicide in psychotics undergoing drug therapy than in those receiving only institutional care (Bergersen, 1976).

Some clients taking antipsychotics, commonly the elderly or those taking several anticholinergics, can develop a syndrome often called *atropine psychosis* (Harris, 1981b). The symptoms associated with this syndrome (listed in the box on the next page) can be corrected by discontinuation of the medication.

Although some of the side effects of antipsychotics are common, they are usually not severe or dangerous (Harris, 1981b). Postural hypotension and sedation are the most troublesome, and tolerance is developed after a few weeks. Extrapyramidal symptoms (EPS), discussed in greater detail later in this chapter, are frequent side effects of antipsychotics. EPSs include akathisia, acute dystonias, drug-induced parkinsonism, and tardive dyskinesia.

Pigmentation of the skin and eyes has also been re-

Table 18-2. Antipsychotic drug side effects

System or organs	Effects
Cardiovascular system	Orthostatic hypotension
	Hypertension
	Tachycardia
	Bradycardia
	Fainting
	Dizziness
	Pallor
	T wave changes, prolonged PR intervals, and QRS complex reflecting slowed conduction
Central nervous system	Drowsiness
	Sedation
	Headache
	Convulsions
	Extrapyramidal symptoms
	Electroencephalographic changes
	Cerebral edema
Ear, eye, nose, and throat	Blurred vision
	Pigmentation of eyes after sun exposure
	Nasal congestion
Gastrointestinal system	Anorexia
	Constipation
	Cholestatic jaundice
	Excessive salivation
	Weight changes
	Dyspepsia
	Diarrhea
	Paralytic ileus
	Increased appetite
	Dry mouth
Genitourinary system	Dark urine
	Incontinence
	Menstrual irregularities
	Changed libido
	Inhibited ejaculation
	Gynecomastia
	Difficult urination
	Delayed ovulation
	Impotence
	Glycosuria
	Lactation
Metabolic system	Hyperglycemia and hypoglycemia
	Hyperthemia and hypothermia
Blood	Blood dyscrasias (agranulocytosis usually)
Skin	Photosensitivity
	Excessive sweating
	Dermatoses (erythematous and eczematous)
	Pigmentation after sun exposure

Symptoms of Atropine Psychosis

Purposeless overactivity
Agitation
Confusion
Disorientation
Dry, flushed skin
Tachycardia
Sluggish dilated pupils
Bowel hypotmotility
Dysarthria
Memory impairment

ported as a rare occurrence in long-term treatment (3 to 10 years) with phenothiazines or thioxanthenes. This dark purplish brown or blue-gray pigmentation of the skin occurs after exposure to the sun. Pigmentation of the conjunctiva, sclera, lens, and cornea can also occur and usually does not impair vision. The pigment is reabsorbed after the drug is discontinued (Harris, 1981b). However, pigmentation of the retina can produce pigmentary retinopathy and cause blindness. Rarely, some blood dyscrasias, usually agranulocytosis, can occur. Immediate discontinuation of the medication and reverse isolation should be initiated. Blood dyscrasias can prove fatal if not corrected.

Maintenance Objectives

Community health nurses must know their clients' medication treatment regimen. Only after the nurse knows what medications the client is taking and in what amounts can an accurate assessment be made.

Psychiatric clients receiving antipsychotic drugs will in most cases have received initial treatment during a psychotic episode requiring hospitalization. Most of the side effects from these medications occur early in the course of treatment and may not be seen by the community health nurse. It is possible, though, that the individual began taking antipsychotics as an outpatient before becoming severely psychotic, or was taking them for a nonpsychiatric medical problem, or has not adhered to the prescribed drug regimen. Also, some side effects associated with anitpsychotic drugs can appear months after initial treatment. The community health nurse therefore needs to be familiar with the side effects of specific medication(s) the client is taking. Side effects should be suspected and evaluated if symptoms are present. In addition to routine monitoring, testing should be done periodically to avoid serious side effects associated with long-term use. Monitoring and testing should include complete blood count to detect dyscrasias, hepatic function studies to detect liver function abnormalities, blood sugar tests for hyperglycemia, opth-

Symptoms Present in Most Depressions

Appetite disturbances (either weight gain or weight loss)
Lowered mood (varying from mild sadness to intense feelings of guilt and hoplessness)
Difficulty thinking
Inability to concentrate or make decisions
Loss of interest in work, recreation, or activity
Somatic complaints (headache, sleep disturbances, insomnia or hyposomnia, decreased sexual drive)
Psychomotor retardation or agitation
Suicidal ideation

almic testing to rule out increased intraocular pressure or pigmentary retinopahy as causes for impaired vision, and observation for extrapyramidal symptoms. In addition, periodic renal function tests for individuals receiving fluphenazine dihydrochloride (Prolixin) should also be considered.

Antidepressants

As mentioned earlier in this chapter, depression is one of the most common psychiatric disorders, with potential effects on many body systems. In general there are three major groups of depression: reactive, affective, and depression secondary to illness and drug use. All three groups may exhibit similar symptoms. Symptoms associated with depression are listed in the box above.

Reactive depression occurs in response to some outside (exogenous) stress factors such as loss of a significant person by death or divorce, loss of status, or loss of financial stability. Depression associated with reactive disorders generally does not require medication and can be treated with psychotherapy and the passage of time.

The three subclassifications of affective disorders include major depressive episode, manic episode (to be discussed later in this chapter), and cyclic combination of the two, called bipolar disorder (Krupp and Chatton, 1982). Affective depressions (endogenous) are periods of mood depression that occur relatively independently of the person's life situation or events. There are also depressive neuroses or dysthymic disorders that vary in severity and duration and are differentiated from major affective disorders in their severity of symptoms and lack of psychotic features.

In depression secondary to chronic illness and drug use, any chronic illness such as rheumatoid arthritis or chronic heart disease can cause depression. Also, the use of reserpine, corticosteroids, oral contraceptives, antihypertensive drugs, appetite-suppressing drugs alcohol, opiates, sedatives, and psychodelic drugs can cause depression (Krupp and Chatton, 1982).

Classification and Action

Depression is associated with low brain levels of norepinephrine and abnormalities in serotonin function (Smythies, 1980). Antidepressant drugs fall into three categories: tricyclic antidepressants, the tetracyclics, and monoamine oxidase inhibitors (MAOIs). The commonly used drugs in these categories are listed in Appendix E.

The tricyclic compounds are the most widely used antidepressant drugs. Recent studies have demonstrated that 70% of people with depressive disorders respond favorably to tricyclic antidepressants (DeGennaro et al., 1981). These compounds bear close structural resemblance to the phenothiazine compounds, but the actual mechanism of their action is not known. It is hypothesized that these drugs may affect brain amine levels by interfering with their reuptake into nerves, thereby potentiating the action of catecholamines (Bergersen, 1976). These drugs also have atropine-like actions.

The second category of antidepressant drugs are the tetracyclics, which are chemically different from the tricyclics but present a similar picture in clinical practice. These drugs are relatively new and although not yet rigorously tested do seem to relieve depression quickly. Examples of tetracyclics are trazodone, amoxapine, and maprotiline; these drugs have a lower incidence of anticholinergic and cardiovascular side effects than other antidepressants.

The third category of antidepressant drugs are the MAOIs. MAO enzymes normally destroy neurohormones such as epinephrine, norepinephrine, and serotonin. The MAOIs prevent this destruction, thus increasing motor activity.

Side Effects and Complications

Antidepressants can produce a wide variety of side effects, some of which are fatal. The side effects of tricyclic compounds are similar to those of antipsychotics but with fewer EPSs and no pigment deposition. Side effects seen with antidepressent drugs are listed in Ta-

Table 18-3. Frequent side effects of selected antidepressants

System or organs	Effects	
	Tricyclics	MAOIs
Cardiovascular system	Hypotension, tachycardia, palpitations, arrhythmias, first-degree heart block, myocardial infarction	Orthostatic hypotension, arrhythmias, paradoxical hypertension, flushing
Central nervous system	Sedation, dizziness, fatigue, weakness, headache, disorientation, disturbed concentration, insomnia, restlessness, nightmares, ataxia, tremors, numbness, electroencephalographic changes, EPSs, mania	Restlessness, dizziness, vertigo, headache, insomnia, confusion, fatigue, paresthexias, mania
Ear, eye, nose, throat	Blurred vision, tinnitus, increased intraocular pressure, mydriasis	Blurred vision, tinnitus
Gastrointestinal system	Dry mouth, nausea, vomiting, upset stomach, constipation, diarrhea	Dry mouth, nausea, constipation, diarrhea, anorexia
Genitourinary system	Urinary retention, gynecomastia, galactorrhea, altered sexual drive	Urinary retention, altered sexual drive
Blood	Bone marrow depression (agranulocytopenia and others)	
Skin	Rash, urticaria, pruritus	Rash, flushing
Other	Cholestatic jaundice, photosensitivity, edema, weight changes, facial sweating	Hepatitis, weight changes, peripheral edema, sweating

ble 18-3. Some of the effects of MAOIs can be dangerous or even fatal. Paradoxical hypertension can occur when certain foods rich in amines (such as tryramine) or in amino acids (such as tryosine) are ingested. The pressor amines are normally inactivated by MAO but because MAO is inhibited, they can produce hypertension and intracranial bleeding. Foods that contain these amines include liver, aged cheeses, yogurt, alcholic beverages, excess caffeine and chocolate, and foods that have been aged, pickled, or smoked. These foods should be avoided for at least 2 to 3 weeks after discontinuation of drug therapy because of continued MAO inhibition. Jaundice and leukopenia are also known side effects of MAOIs. Because of these possible complications, use of MAOIs is usually reserved for hospitalized patients. Suicidal tendencies also occur more often near the end of the depressive cycle; thus clients warrant close attention at this time (Bergersen, 1976).

Maintenance Objectives

As with phenothiazines, community health nurses should observe for side effects and make referrals when the person's status indicates the need for such action. Client education is essential, especially when MAOIs are used. Monitoring includes routine evaluation using those guidelines mentioned earlier. Additionally, close attention should be paid to changes in mental status indicating suicidal tendencies. Periodic blood cell counts

and hepatic function tests are recommended when MAOIs are used.

Antianxiety Agents

Antianxiety drugs (minor tranquilizers or sedative-hypnotics) are used for treatment of symptoms associated with psychoneurotic and psychosomatic conditions. These drugs are widely used and often abused. Use of these drugs without careful assessment of causes behind the presenting symptoms often masks more serious physical and psychological problems. For example, anxiety can be secondary to hyperthyroidism and sleep disturbances caused by depression. Antianxiety drugs are also used for treatment of insomnia, sedation, anxiety, nausea and vomiting, hyperbilirubinemia or chronic cholestasis, acute seizure disorders, and muscle spasms.

Classification and Action

Antianxiety drugs as a group vary in chemical structure but have similar pharmacological and behavioral effects. All depress the central nervous system, but they differ in their secondary central and peripheral effects. These drugs can be divided into three groups: barbiturates, benzodiazepines, and nonbarbiturate-nonbenzodiazepines. Commonly used antianxiety drugs are listed in Appendix E.

Barbiturates depress the neurons and synapses of the

Table 18-4. Side effects of antianxiety agents

System or organ	Effects
Cardiovascular system	Hypotension, palpitations, tachycardia, swelling of the feet, arrhythmias, flushing
Central nervous system	Fatigue, drowsiness, ataxia, headache, vertigo, dizziness, slurred speech, electroencephalographic changes, sleep disturbances, hallucinations, lethargy, muscle weakness, insomnia, paradoxical rage reaction, fainting
Ear, eye, nose, throat	Blurred vision, diplopia, tinnitus
Gastrointestinal system	Nausea, vomiting, anorexia, dry mouth, constipation, diarrhea, epigastric distress, weight changes
Genitourinary system	Libido changes, urinary frequency/retention/decreased flow, minor menstrual irregularities, acute hepatic necrosis or disfunction
Blood	Decreased hematocrit, blood dyscrasias
Skin	Rash, petechiae, pruritus, urticaria, jaundice, bullous dermatitis, Stevens-Johnson syndrome

ascending reticular formation of the brainstem. This effect may be responsible for the reduction in electrical activity of the cortex (Bergersen, 1976). As a result of this reduction in stimuli the need for wakefulness and alertness is decreased. Small doses produce a calming effect, whereas larger doses induce sleep. Barbiturates do not have analgesic properties; they will not induce sleep when people are in pain.

The disadvantages of barbiturates far outweigh their advantages. While less expensive than other antianxiety drugs, tolerance often develops and can lead to physical and emotional addiction, in which clients take increasingly larger doses to achieve the desired effect. Barbiturates suppress the rapid eye movement (REM) stages of sleep, which can produce an adverse rebound effect when the drug is discontinued. This leads to restless sleep, nightmares, and intense dreaming (Harris, 1981a). These drugs are often used in suicides; they have a narrow margin of safety, and overdose can be accidental. People taking barbiturates may awaken in a confused state, forget they previously took the medication, and repeat their dosage (Holvey, 1972). Because of the disadvantages, barbiturates are seldom indicated as antianxiety agents.

Benzodiazepines, for the treatment of anxiety, are among the most widely used drugs (Bergersen, 1976). Chlordiazepoxide (Librium) was the first to be developed, followed by diazepam (Valium). The benzodiazepines reduce anxiety, induce sedation and sleep, have anticonvulsant effects, and produce skeletal muscle relaxation (Anderson, 1980). All benzodiazepines have similar chemical structures and clinical properties. They depress certain reflexes of the spinal cord, which in turn reduce skeletal muscle tension. Their antianxiety action may be caused by inhibiting the stimulation of portions of the limbic system (amygdala and hippocampus) that influence behavior (Bergersen, 1976). Insomnia, tension, and anxiety, prominent in many psychoneurotic and psychosomatic conditions, are relieved by these effects.

Side Effects and Complications

Side effects of barbiturates and other antianxiety drugs are listed in Table 18-4. Acute poisoning from barbiturates can occur when 15 to 20 times the usual therapeutic dose is absorbed. In the early stage of acute poisoning, excitement and confusion precede deep sleep or stupor. Death usually results from respiratory failure but can result from hypostatic pneumonia or pulmonary edema. Chronic barbiturate poisoning can be caused by increasing tolerance and the development of drug dependency. Symptoms of chronic barbiturate poisoning include slowness of thought, mental depression, incoherent speech, failing memory, skin rash, weight loss, gastrointestinal upset, and anemia. Often there is ataxic gait; coarse tremors of the lips, fingers, and tongue; increased emotional instability; and mental confusion. Injury and death can result from falls, from burns caused by fires set by falling asleep while smoking, or from falling asleep while working with or driving heavy machinery. Accidental overdose occurs when drugs used in combination with barbiturates interact in a negative way.

Benzodiazepines have fewer disabling side effects than phenothiazine derivatives. Although initially considered safe, effective, and not likely to cause dependency, these drugs are often abused and can become addictive. Krupp and Chatton (1982) indicate that while the "safer" benzodiazepines are replacing barbiturates for use in inducing sedation, there have been no significant reductions in suicides caused by drugs. These drugs must be carefully dispensed and closely monitored.

The third category, nonbarbiturate-nonbenzodiazepine compounds, defines a group of older drugs that offer no advantages over barbiturates or benzodiazepines and may lead to serious toxicity. They have a narrow margin of safety, suppress REM sleep, and have a high risk of abuse and physical dependency.

Maintenance Objectives

Maintenance of clients taking antianxiety drugs centers on monitoring for side effects and giving clients information about the drug's use and contraindications. Treatment for most side effects is dosage related; as the dosage exceeds levels necessary for sedation, side effects develop. Serious side effects result from large doses or chronic use of the drug. The elderly and debilitated are especially susceptible to overdoses because of their metabolic changes. Client assessment should elicit information about possible contraindications for use of these drugs. For example, diazepam is contraindicated for people suffering from acute narrow-angle glaucoma and chloral hydrate for people with hepatic or renal impairments.

Client teaching should include proper use of drugs as well as safety during their use. The operation of machinery before the client's condition has stabilized is contraindicated. Alcohol use can potentiate the effects of antianxiety drugs and may lead to injury or accidental overdose. Clients should be informed of the addiction potential of chronic excessive use and be cautioned about symptoms associated with sudden withdrawal of the drug. It is important for chronic users of these drugs to be periodically reevaluated by their physician(s) concerning the need for their continued use.

Antimanic Agents

Lithium is the drug of choice for the short-term management of the manic phase of bipolar disorder, also referred to as manic-depressive illness, and for long-term prophylaxis of bipolar disorder (Harris, 1981a). Lithium, the lightest known solid element, exists in its natural form as a salt and is also manufactured in client use as a salt. This drug was introduced in 1970 for use in terminating manic and hypomanic episodes of bipolar disorder.

Classification and Action

Lithium's exact mechanism of action has not yet been defined, but it may slow the flow of neurotransmitters by speeding the inactivation of norepinephrine within certain central nervous system fibers. Lithium is

Table 18-5. Side effects of lithium carbonate

Metallic taste in the mouth
Fine tremor of the hand
Nausea
Polyuria
Polydipsia
Diarrhea or loose stools
Muscular weakness or fatigue
Faulty coordination
Dizziness
Slurred speech
Blurred vision
Edema of the face, hands, feet, or abdominal wall

given orally and reaches peak serum levels in 1 to 3 hours. It is more effective in terminating or treating manic episodes than depressive episodes; therefore tricyclic or MAOI antidepressants often are added to the treatment regimen.

Lithium has a narrow therapeutic index; therefore, blood levels of lithium need to be monitored regularly. Additionally, no two people respond in the same way to lithium. What may be a therapeutic dose for one person can be lethal for another. Because of the narrow therapeutic index, lithium is given in at least two divided doses daily, usually starting with 900 to 1200 mg per day. As the dosage is raised slowly in increments of 300 mg, serum blood levels are tested two to three times a week until the blood level of lithium is stable. Once stability is reached, serum blood levels are checked less frequently and often can be monitored once every 3 months.

Lithium is used in combination with both antidepressants and antipsychotic drugs. Lithium is the drug of choice for manic episodes, however, because of the lag between the onset of symptoms and symptom reduction; phenothiazine drugs are often used to quickly reduce symptoms and prevent people from harming themselves through their hyperactivity.

Side Effects and Complications

The severity of side effects parallels the serum lithium levels. At therapeutic levels (0.6 to 1.4 mEq/L), mild gastrointestinal symptoms, fine tremor, slight muscle weakness, thirst, and polyuria may be experienced. At toxic levels (greater than 2.0 mEq/L), side effects are more severe and are often the result of sodium loss. Side effects associated with lithium are listed in Table 18-5. Sodium and lithium are reabsorbed at the same location in the proximal tubules of the kidneys. Any sodium loss, such as occurs with diarrhea, use of diuretics, or excessive perspiration, results in increased lithium levels (Krupp and Chatton, 1982).

Side effects usually disappear when the drug is discontinued for 24 hours, and the drug can then be restarted at a lower dose (Newton & Godbey, 1978). If lithium levels are allowed to stay high or rise, the severity of the symptoms will increase and stupor, coma, or convulsions may result.

Maintenance Objectives

Because the effectiveness of lithium is directly related to serum levels and thus dosage, it is important that the person take the drug as prescribed. The long-term use of lithium has adverse effects on renal function (Tryer et al., 1980). It occasionally induces a nephrogenic diabetes insipidus and infrequently thyrotoxicosis. For these reasons thyroid (T_4) and renal function (urinalysis, BUN, serum creatine) tests should be checked at 3- to 6-month intervals (Krupp and Chatton, 1982).

Lithium in combination with some antipsychotic drugs can produce severe neurotoxicity. Haloperidal (Haldol) has been reported to produce an encephalopathic syndrome in combination with lithium. Spring (1979) reported that lithium and thioridazine (Mellaril) can produce a neurotoxic episode. Clients given such combinations should be watched closely for early signs of neurotoxicity—drowsiness, confusion, ataxia, disorientation, and slurred speech.

Antiextrapyramidal Symptom Agents

Extrapyramidal symptoms (EPSs) are side effects that occur in about a third of the individuals receiving antipsychotic drugs (Newton and Godbey, 1978). The frequency of EPSs varies with the drug used. A list of psychotropics and their incidence of EPSs is given in Table 18-6. These side effects probably result from the blockage of dopamine receptor sites in the extrapyramidal system tracts. There are four classes of EPSs: akathisia, acute dystonias, drug-induced parkinsonism, and tardive dyskinesia.

Akathisia, the most common EPS, is the symptom often leading to noncompliance with drug treatment (Van Putten, 1974). It typically occurs early in treatment (2 to 4 weeks), peaks in 6 to 10 weeks, and declines in 12 to 16 weeks. It is characterized by a subjective desire to be in constant motion, followed by an inability to sit or stand still; thus pacing often results.

Acute dystonias also appear early in the course of treatment (2 to 3 days), peak in 1 week, and decline in 2

Table 18-6. Frequency (highest to lowest incidence) of antipsychotic agents causing extrapyramidal symptoms

Generic name	Trade name
Fluphenazine	Permitil, Prolixin
Trifluoperazine	Stelazine
Perphenazine	Trilafon
Prochlorperazine	Compazine
Thiopropazate	Dartalan
Acetophenazine	Tindal
Triflupromazine	Vesprin
Chlorpromazine	Thorazine
Carphenazine	Proketazine
Butaperazine	Repoise
Piperacetazine	Quide
Thiothixene	Navane
Thioridazine	Mellaril
Mesoridazine	Serentil

weeks. In acute dystonias, clients often experience bizarre muscle spasms of the head, neck, back, and tongue. Torticollis (sideways twisting of the neck), oculogyric crisis (backward rolling of the eyes in the socket), tics, and grimaces frequently occur. These symptoms are sometimes painful and extremely frightening to the person.

Drug-induced parkinsonism is indistinguishable from idiopathic parkinsonism. Its symptoms are first seen at 24 days, peak in 2 to 6 weeks, and decline in 8 to 16 weeks (Harris, 1981c). Clients with drug-induced parkinsonism tend to have a reduction of facial and arm movement, festinating gait, and pill-rolling tremor of the hands.

Tardive dyskinesia is a serious side effect because it is irreversible in many cases. Tardive dyskinesia is characterized by involuntary movements of the face, mouth, jaw, and tongue. This syndrome is not relieved when the psychotropic drug is discontinued and may even get worse. Krupp and Chatton (1982) report indications that the incidence is increasing and that reported prevalence varies from 3% to 50% of clients undergoing long-term antipsychotic therapy. Symptoms that may appear after months or (usually) years of treatment include involuntary sucking, chewing, licking, and pursing movements of the tongue and mouth. Also, puffing of the cheeks, eye blinking, and abnormal movement of the extremities are symptoms of tardive dyskinesia.

Table 18-7. Side effects of antiextrapyramidal symptom agents

System or organ	Effects
Cardiovascular system	Tachycardia, paradoxical bradycardia, transient hypotension
Central nervous system	Disorientation, nervousness, weakness, irritability, headache, hallucination, euphoria, delusions
Ear, eye, nose, throat	Blurred vision, mydriasis, increased intraocular pressure, dilated pupils, photophobia, difficulty swallowing
Gastrointestinal system	Dry mouth, nausea, vomiting, constipation, sore mouth and tongue
Genitourinary system	Urinary hesitancy/retention
Skin	Rash

Classification and Action

Drugs used to treat EPSs are antiparkinsonian agents that inhibit or block the effect of acetylcholine at the junction between the nerve endings and the effector organs. Commonly used anticholinergic antiparkinsonian agents are listed in Appendix E.

Side Effects and Complications

Side effects of these drugs are anticholinergic in nature and are listed in Table 18-7. Caution should be exercised when administering anticholinergics to individuals with prostatic hypertrophy or glaucoma. The gastrointestinal symptoms associated with these drugs can be minimized by giving the drugs with meals. Large doses may cause disorientation, agitation, hallucinations, psychotic episodes, and acute delirium, which can be mistaken for failure to respond to antipsychotic therapy (Holvey, 1972).

Maintenance Objectives

The use of antiparkinsonian agents for the treatment of EPSs is usually of short duration. After 4 to 6 weeks the drugs can be discontinued, usually with no recurrent symptoms.

As stated earlier, tardive dyskinesia associated with long-term antipsychotic agents is not alleviated by antiparkinsonism agents and may be worsened by them (Krupp and Chatton, 1982). Prevention and early detection are, at present, the best interventions available.

Community health nurses are in a position to educate and observe the patient for early symptoms of tardive dyskinesia Early manifestations include fine, wormlike movements of the tongue at rest and facial tics or jaw movements of recent onset. The incidence of tardive dyskinesia increases with age, and the syndrome is three times more common in patients over 40 years. It is also more common in women. Patients who had early EPSs at the onset of therapy seem most prone to tardive dyskinesia later (Newton and Godbey, 1978). Clients with suspected tardive dyskinesia or EPSs should be referred to the physician or treatment center for further evaluation.

SUMMARY

The pressures and stresses of the twentieth century are taking their toll on the mental health of the population. People are increasingly succumbing to stress-related ills, thereby impairing their ability to cope and adopt to changing life events. In the early 1960s tremendous financial resources were channeled into the development of community mental health centers, yet critics contend that these centers have not fulfilled their original promises. Instead of being truly community oriented, the mental health system is accused of being a "revolving door" where clients are treated briefly in the hospital then released to the community, often without adequate advance preparation. As pointed out by Davies (1981), some communities have been able to develop comprehensive programs to adequately meet the needs of the returning psychiatric client; however, this has by no means been a universal realization. In too many instances, clients are returned to the community only to be housed in inadequate boarding or nursing homes. Critics contend that all that has changed over the years in regard to community-based treatment for psychiatric clients has been "who pays the bill." The implications for community health nursing are evident: Who, more than community health nurses, have access and visibility in the community? Who can better serve as a client advocate to help the chronically ill navigate a complex social and health care system? For many, the tasks of locating health care facilities and arranging transportation are overwhelming responsibilities. Advocacy, caring, and coordination are imperative challenges for the community health nurse.

Like the chronically ill psychiatric client, those who are coping with numerous and often taxing life struggles need the attention of the community health nurse. Families are changing, and the ability to adapt to new roles is not as easy as it might seem at first glance. Mutual support groups are a special kind of assistance that can be provided in communities to help people obtain primary mental health services before any disruption in the ability to cope effectively. Just talking about life pressures with a group of similar and concerned people is often a major source of relief. Considerable problem solving can also be provided in support groups as people share with one another what has helped them. Nurses can be instrumental in serving as catalysts or leaders of such groups.

BIBLIOGRAPHY

Anderson, G. D.: Benzodiazepines, Nurse Pract. 5(1):47-51, Jan.-Feb. 1980.

Anthony, E.: A risk-vulnerability intervention model for children of psychotic parents. In Anthony, E., and Koupernick, C., editors: The child and his family, New York, 1974, John Wiley & Sons, Inc., pp. 99-121.

Bergersen, B.: Pharmacology in nursing, ed. 13, St. Louis, 1976, The C.V. Mosby Co.

Bloom, B. L.: Prevention of mental disorders: recent advances in theory and practice, Community Ment. Health J. 15(3):179-191, 1979.

Caplan, G.: Supprt systems and community mental health, New York, 1974, Behavioral Publications.

Citizens guide to the Community Mental Health Centers Amendment of 1975, Washington, D.C., 1977, U.S. Government Printing Office.

Davies, M. A.: Continuing care unit; a model of services for chronic psychiatric patients. J. Psychiatr. Nurs. 19:42-45, Feb. 1981.

DeGennaro, M., et al.: Antidepressant drug therapy, Am. J. Nurs. 81(7):1304-1310, July 1981.

Eisenberg, L., and Parron, D.: Strategies for the prevention of mental disorders. In Healthy people: the Surgeon General's report on health promotion and disease prevention; background papers, Washington, D.C., 1979, U.S. Government Printing Office, pp. 135-155.

Harris, E.: Psychtropic drugs: lithium, Am. J. Nurs. 81(7):1310-1315, July 1981a.

Harris, E.: Antipsychotic medications, Am. J. Nurs. 81(7):1316-1323, July 1981b.

Harris, E.: Extrapyramidal side effects of antipsychotic medications, Am. J. Nurs. 81(7):1324-1328, July 1981c.

Harris, E.: Sedative-hypnotic drugs, Am. J. Nurs. 81(7):1329-1334, July, 1981d.

Hamburg, B., and Killilea, M.: Relation of social support, stress, illness, and use of health services. In Healthy people: the Surgeon General's report on health promotion and disease prevention; background papers, Washington, D.C., 1979, U.S. Government Printing Office, pp. 254-276.

Hanlon, J., and Pickett, G.: Public health: administration and practice, ed. 7, St. Louis, 1979, The C.V. Mosby Co.

Healthy people: the Surgeon General's report on health promotion and disease prevention DHEW Pub. No. (PHS)79-55071 Washington, D.C., 1979, U.S. Government Preinting Office.

Holmes, T., and Rahe, R.: The social readjustment rating scale, J. Psychosom. Res. 11(2):213-218, 1976.

Holvey, D.: The Merck Manual of diagnosis and therapy, ed. 12, Rahway, N.J., 1972, Merck, Sharp, and Dohme Research Laboratories.

Jacobson, A.: Melancholy in the 20th century: causes and prevention, J. of Psychiatr. Nurs. 7(18):11-21, 1980.

Joint Commission on Mental Illness and Health: Action for mental health, New York, 1961, Basic Books, Inc., Publishers.

Johnson, C.: The American family during inflationary times, Psychiatr. Opinion 16(9):13-16, 1979.

Kalter, N.: Children of divorce in an outpatient psychiatric population, Am. J. Orthopsychiatry. 47:40-51, Jan. 1977.

Kelly, J. B., and Wallerstein, J. S.: Brief interventions with children in divorcing families, Am. J. Orthopsychiatry 47:23-39, Jan. 1977.

Kelly, J. B., and Wallerstein, J. S.: Divorce counseling: a community service for families in the midst of divorce, Am. J. Orthopsychiatry 47:4-22, Jan. 1977.

Krupp, M., and Chatton, M.: Current medical diagnosis and treatment, Los Altos, Calif.: 1982, Lange Medical Publications.

Lancaster, J.: Coping mechanisms for the working mother, Am. J. Nur 75:1322-1323, Aug. 1975.

Lancaster, J.: Community mental health nursing: an ecological perspective, St. Louis, 1980, The C.V. Mosby Co.

Landsberg, G., and Hammer, R.: Possible programmatic consequences of community mental health center funding arrangements: illustrations based on inpatient utilization data, Community Ment. Health J. 13:63-70, 1977.

Leavell, J., and Clark, E.: Preventive medicine for the doctor in his community: an epidemiological approach, New York, 1965, McGraw-Hill Book Co.

Levi, L.: Psychosocial factors in preventive medicine. In Healthy people: the Surgeon General's report on health promotion and disease prevention, Washington, D.C., 1979, U.S. Government Printing Office, pp. 207-252.

Linton, P.: Psychopharmacology of the aging, Ala. J. Med. Sci. 17(2):155-159, 1980.

Marmor, J., and Pumpian-Mindlin, E.: Toward an integrated conception of mental disorders, J. Nerv. Ment. Dis. 3:19-29, Jan. 1950.

National Institute of Alcohol Abuse and Alcoholism: Critical review of the fetal alcohol abuse syndrome, Rockville, Md., 1977, Department of Health, Education and Welfare.

Nation's Health, Washington, D.C., 1981, U.S. Government Printing Office.

Newton, M., and Godbey, K.: How you can improve the effectiveness of psychotropic drug therapy, Nurs. '78 8(7):46-55, 1978.

Oulette, E., et al.: Adverse effects on offspring of maternal alcohol abuse during pregnancy, N. Engl. J. Med. 297:538-540, 1977.

Perris, C.: The genetics of affecting disorders. In Mendels, J., editor: Biological psychiatry, New York, 1973, John Wiley & Sons, Inc., pp. 385-415.

President's Commission on Mental Health; Report of the task panel on the nature and scope of the problem, vol. 2, Appendix, Washington, D.C., 1978, U.S. Government Printing Office.

Rachlin, S.: When schizophrenia comes marching home, Psychiatr. Q. 50(3):202-210, 1978.

Ramshorn, M.: The major thrust in American psychiatry: past, present, and future, Perspect. Psychiatr. Care 9(4):144-154, 1971.

Richmond, J., and Filner, B.: Infant and child health needs and strategies: In Healthy people: the Surgeon General's report on health promotion and disease prevention: background papers, Washington, D.C., 1979, U.S. Government Printing Office, pp. 305-323.

Rubin, J.: The community mental health movement in the United States circa 1979, Am. J. Psychoanal. 31(1):68-79, 1971.

Schecter, D.: Women in the labor force: some mental health implications, Psychiatr. Opinion 16(9):17-19, 1979.

Shanok, S., and Lewis, D.: Juvenile court versus child guidance referral: psychological and parental factors, Am. J. Psychiatry 134(10):1130-1133, 1977.

Smythies, J.: The neurochemical basis of psychiatry, Ala. J. Med. Sci. 17(2):156-161, 1980.

Snow, D., and Newton, P.: Task, social structure and social process in the community mental health center movement, Am. Psychol. **31**(8):582-594, 1976.

Spring, G.: Neurotoxicity with combined use of lithium and thioridazine, J. Clin. Psychiatry **40**(3):135-138, 1979.

Tableman, M.: Overview of programs to prevent mental health problems of children, Public Health Rep. **96**(1):38-44, 1981.

Tarail, D.: Current and future issues in community mental health, Psychiatr. Q. **52**:27-38, 1980.

Taylor, C.: Mereness' essentials of psychiatric nursing, ed. 11, St. Louis, 1982, The C.V. Mosby Co.

Tryer, S., et al.: Lithium and the kidney, Lancet **1**(8159):94-95, Jan. 12, 1980.

Van Putten, T.: Why do schizophrenic patients refuse to take their drugs? Arch. Gen. Psychiatry **31**(7):67-73, 1974.

Watt, N.F.: Childhood and adolescent routes to schizophrenia. In Ricks, D.F., Thomas, A., and Ruff, M., editors: Life history research in psychopathology, vol. 3, Minneapolis, 1974, University of Minnesota Press, pp. 194-208.

Wilk, J.: Assessing single parent needs, J. Psychiatr. Nurs. **116**(6):21-22, 1979.

Wilner, D. M., Walkley, R. P., and O'Neill, E. J.: Introduction to public health, ed. 7, New York, 1978, Macmillan Publishing Co., Inc.

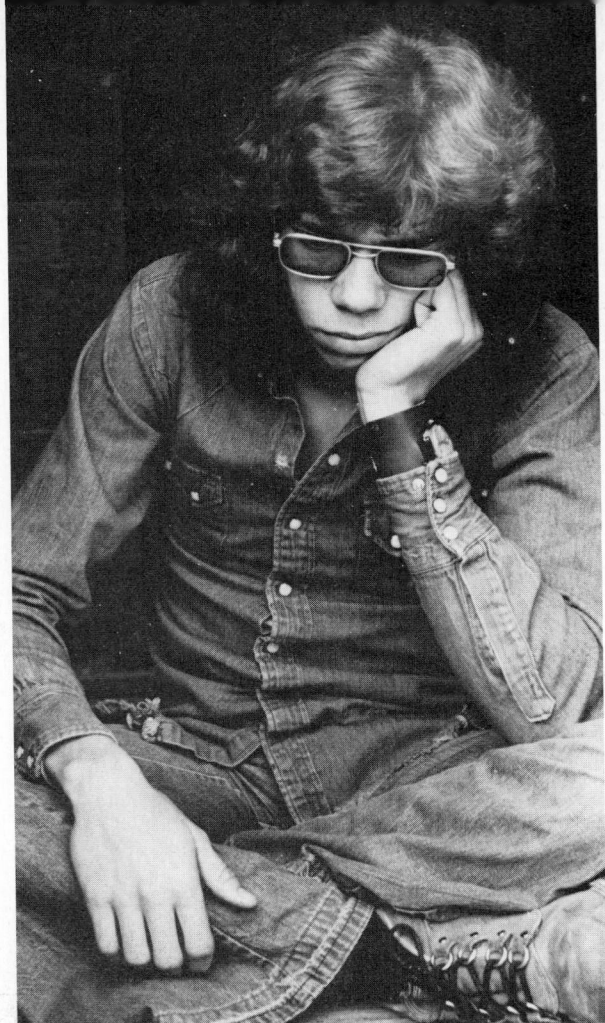

Chapter 19

PHYLLIS GRAVES

INTERVENING IN CRISES

Crisis is a term commonly used in our society for instances in which circumstances are suddenly altered. Headlines may reveal that a city has no more funds and is in crisis or that there is an unexpected interruption of an energy source and thus a crisis. Events are not crises, but they may lead to crisis. The nature and characteristics of crises are distinctive and set apart from other changes in circumstances. In addition, crises progress through a series of identified phases, each with its own possibilities for intervention.

Anticipated and unanticipated events predispose individuals, families, and communities to crises. Crisis intervention techniques can be used by health professionals, nonhealth professionals, and volunteers trained to assist individuals, families, and communities in crisis. Crisis intervention assists clients in resolving situations so that the state after the crisis reflects an improvement over the state before the crisis. Responsible community health nurses know about facilities available for crisis prevention and intervention, and they know how clients may gain entry to those resources.

This chapter considers the nature, characteristics, and phases of crisis as well as the types of crises that can occur in individuals, families, and communities. An overview of crisis intervention is presented, and the concepts of primary, secondary, and tertiary prevention as they relate to the crisis are discussed. A case is used to illustrate how community health nurses can use the nursing process in crisis intervention. Community resources for crisis are considered in the last section of the chapter.

NATURE OF CRISIS

Caplan (1964), a leader in the development of crisis theory, described crisis as an "upset" or disequilibrium in a steady state occurring when usual problem-solving strategies are ineffective. Typically a problem situation causes a change in equilibrium, whereby the person initiates a previously successful problem-solving or coping strategy to reinstitute a state of balance. Because of the magnitude of the crisis, usual problem-solving strategies are often ineffective, leading to an intense level of disequilibrium.

New strategies for problem solving must be initiated to alleviate the disruption. The effectiveness of the new strategies leads to one of three potential outcomes. First, effective strategies often lead to a better state of functioning than before the crisis. Crises provide opportunities for people to learn new coping mechanisms that can later be applied to other situations. In this instance, the crisis proves to be a growth situation. In the second potential outcome, the person returns to the level of functioning before the crisis with no appreciable gain or loss in functioning. In the third outcome, there is a loss in that the person reaches a less favorable state than previously existed. When the new strategies are ineffective or the problem continues or intensifies over time, the risk of major psychological disorganization increases.

Crises may result in psychological growth, return to a previous level of equilibrium, or reach a new level of psychological functioning that is maladaptive. These possibilities are reflected in the Chinese characters used for the word *crisis* (Aguilera and Messick, 1982). The characters mean danger and opportunity. In a crisis, previous coping strategies are not effective in solving the problem, and there is opportunity for growth through the development of new ways of coping. However, there is also the danger that ineffective problem solving results in psychological maladaptation.

An essential property of the concept of crisis is the potential for promoting growth. Crises present challenges and call for new responses (Rapoport, 1965). Assisting those in crisis to achieve growth is an inherent role for community health nurses.

Not only individuals but families and communities face crises. As with individuals, when families and communities incur problems that are not solved by usual coping strategies, a crisis occurs. The upset of the steady state of a family or community also offers the possibility for growth and improved function and the danger of developing major disorganization. Whether the crisis occurs to the individual, family, or community, the situation is one in which a problem not solved by usual coping strategies is present, disequilibrium exists, and there is opportunity for growth through the development of new coping strategies.

CHARACTERISTICS OF CRISIS

In a crisis an event occurs and brings about problems for which usual coping strategies are inadequate, and a state of disequilibrium ensues. During this state of disequilibrium people confront hazardous situations that at the time cannot be avoided or solved with usual problem-solving skills. People in crisis feel helpless and often desire assistance in relieving their misery. Duration of the state of disequilbrium, the individual's perception of the event and problems, and the functioning pattern of the individual (each of which is discussed in the following paragraphs) are characteristic of crises. In addition, cognitive processes may be altered, subjective feelings tend to be present, and in many people physiological symptoms occur.

The concept of disequilibrium is related to duration; most crises last between 4 and 6 weeks. Crises tend to be temporary and self-limiting. Individuals in crisis are in disequilibrium that cannot be tolerated indefinitely, and successful or unsuccessful resolution is reached within a relatively short period of time. For the community health nurse this means that intervention must be prompt and must be concentrated in a brief time span.

To the individual in crisis the event and accompanying problems are perceived as having serious consequences. Whether or not an event and its problems lead to crisis depends on the perception of the individual and the coping abilities of that person. For example, if a person loses his job after being with a company for 20 years and having no experience with unemployment, crisis is a possible result. However, for a high school student who works only for additional spending money, job loss is much less likely to be followed by crisis.

The pattern of functioning is also a feature of those in a state of crisis (Caplan, 1964). In crisis there is a decrease in the level of function and associated disorganization. In the disequilibrium state of crisis even routine tasks may not be effectively completed. The recognition of this impairment of functioning level is exemplified by the custom in many communities to take food to the homes of families who have experienced events such as death, accident, or serious illness. Families in crisis are not expected to perform at the same level of function as others.

Lindemann's (1979) research with survivors of the Coconut Grove fire is a classic study of individuals in crisis. Fire engulfed a Boston nightclub on November 28, 1942, while the Harvard-Yale football game was being celebrated. The magnitude of the fire was tremendous, and the death toll reached 491; only 39 people in the nightclub survived the fire. Responding to a request for psychiatric assistance, Lindemann worked with the burn victims, their relatives, and the relatives of those who died.

Physical and psychological reactions were noted. Frequent physical responses included sighing respiration, exhaustion, lack of strength, and altered gastrointestinal patterns. For example, usual activities such as walking resulted in a feeling of exhaustion. However, even with the exhaustion, there were feelings of restlessness and the need for activity. Routine tasks were sought and carried out with much effort. Psychological responses in the crisis of acute grief included guilt, hostility, and preoccupation with the image of the deceased. Several people reported intense visual images of their dead relatives.

Although Lindemann found that reactions to the crisis usually closely followed the precipitating event, there were instances of delayed responses. An individual's need to deal with an important problem was a factor in the later grief response. One example involved an adolescent girl who was burned and whose parents were killed in the Coconut Grove fire. Two younger siblings were her chief concern during her hospitalization and resettlement time. Only after more than 2 months did she show depression, frequent crying, and other symptoms of grief.

Lindemann's work with the victims of the Coconut Grove fire and with others in crisis provides an understanding of psychological and physiological responses. Further, he was a pioneer in developing interventions that promote growth through successful resolution.

The problems resulting in crisis stem from events of loss, threat of loss, or overwhelming challenge (Spradley, 1981). Not only undesirable events such as the death or serious illness of a significant other but also desirable events like an important new job may produce problems for a person who lacks effective coping strategies. The problems that could arise following a much desired promotion include establishing relations with new peers, relations with former co-workers, changes in family life-style, and changes in social obligations. Once a significant event has occurred, the associated problems are inevitable, and without adequate coping strategies, crisis can result.

Another feature of crisis is "cognitive uncertainty" (Spradley, 1981). The individual in crisis cannot predict the outcome of the situation. This uncertainty has the effect of increasing the tension experienced by the person in crisis who subjectively experiences many feelings; those of helplessness and ineffectuality are characteristic (Caplan, 1964). The helplessness that is present when there is an uncertain outcome to a problem for which usual coping mechanisms have been ineffective can readily be understood. In addition, depending on the situation, feelings of anxiety, guilt, fear, or shame can be involved. For instance, if a child is severely injured while playing, the parents may feel guilty and think that if they had been more attentive, the accident could have been prevented.

Physiological symptoms may become manifest in individuals in crisis. Physiological responses to crisis vary from person to person and depend on the individual's response to stressors. Sleep disturbances, gastrointestinal symptoms, muscle tension, shortness of breath, irritability, need for routine activity, and exhaustion are among the possible manifestations of crisis. For example, a widow whose husband had died 2 days before said that the night he died she had been able to sleep only intermittently, and at 4 AM she had begun cleaning the kitchen.

Summary of Characteristics

Crisis in an individual, family, or community is characterized by the presence of an inevitable problem, uncertain outcome, perception of disequilibrium, and decrease in the level of functioning. The person in crisis experiences feelings of helplessness and somatic symptoms. The time a crisis lasts is limited to an average of 4 to 6 weeks.

PHASES OF CRISIS

Progression of an individual through a crisis is described by Caplan (1964) as occurring in four phases. In phase 1 a problem is encountered, and there is an initial rise in tension, which causes the person to recall coping strategies that have been successful in the past. When past strategies do not solve the problem and it remains, phase 2 occurs with a further rise in tension. In phase 2 upset of the steady state or disequilibrium is evident with the appearance of the characteristic psychological and physiological crisis responses; ability to function is impaired. Phase 3 with another rise in tension stimulates the individual to mobilize resources. Activities in phase 3 can include bringing into awareness previously overlooked aspects of the problem, redefining the problem, setting aside irrelevant aspects, and developing new problem-solving mechanisms. If the strategies used in phase 3 are successful, the problem will be resolved and the individual will either return to the previous state of equilibrium or move to an improved level of functioning. If the strategies of phase 3 are not successful, phase 4 follows. With continuation of the problem, lack of success in resolution, and increased tension, a breaking point is reached, and major disorganization results.

Fig. 19-1, developed by Schwenk and Bittle (1979)

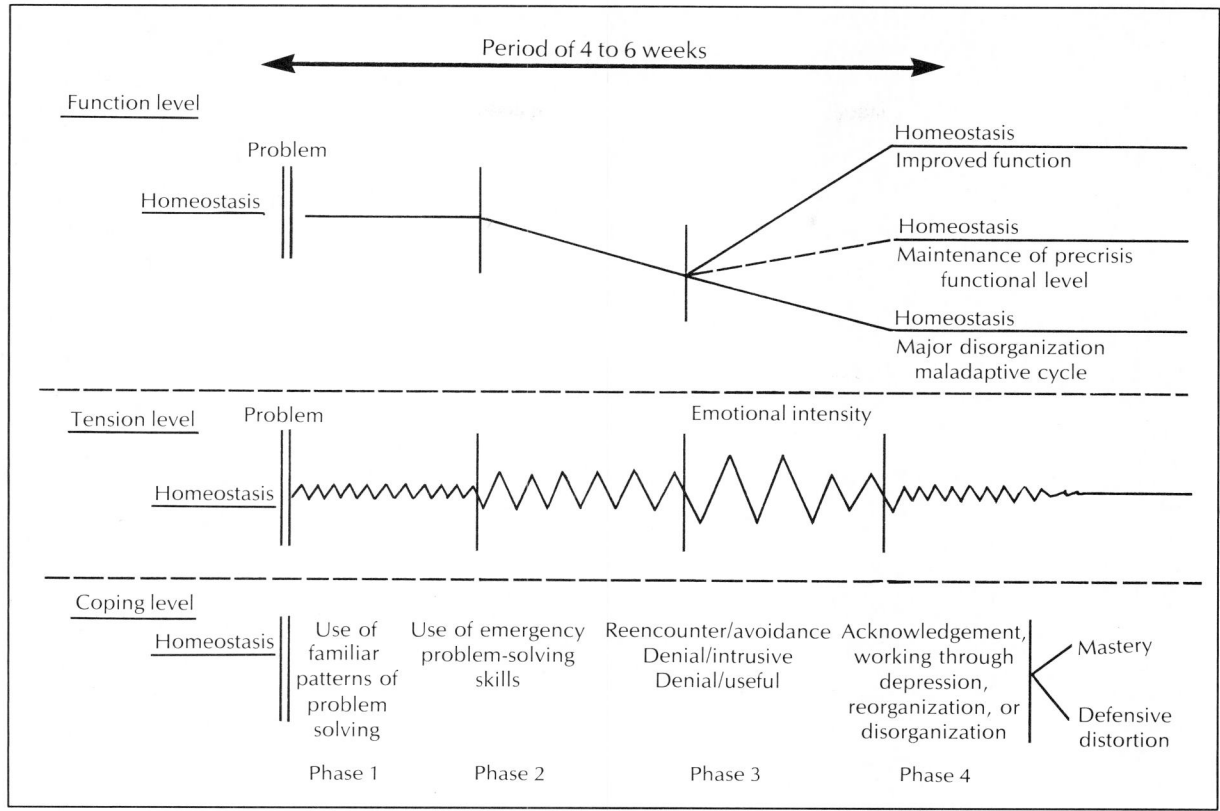

Fig. 19-1. Characteristics of function and tension in crisis. (Modified from Schwenk, T. L., and Bittle, S. P.: J. Fam. Pract. **8**:115, 1979.)

illustrates the four phases of crisis with their levels of function and tension. Tension begins in phase 1 and increases with each phase until either the problem is solved or a threshold is crossed and major disorganization results. Level of function begins to decrease in phase 2 (disequilibrium) and continues to decrease until either major disorganization occurs or the problem is resolved. With the use of successful coping strategies, function may be regained at the level before the crisis, or an improved level of function may be achieved.

Fig. 19-1 illustrates the coping level across the four phases of crisis. Homeostasis is disturbed, and familiar coping patterns are attempted. When previous problem-solving methods fail, either new effective skills are used, resulting in mastery, or ineffective skills are used, resulting in maladaptation.

TYPES OF CRISIS

Crisis may be categorized into two types, maturational and situational. Maturational crises or developmental crises occur at the time of natural transitions in the developmental process. Successful coping with a maturational crisis leads to the next developmental level. The popularity of publications like the book *Passages: Predictable Crises of Adult Life* (Sheehy, 1976) demonstrates a public awareness of and concern about transition periods. Entering school for the first time, marriage, and retirement are examples of events that can lead to maturational crises. Situational crises, also called accidental crises, follow unanticipated sudden events over which no control can be expected. Divorce, death, illness, and flood are examples of events that can lead to situational crises. Both maturational and situational crises may affect individuals, families, and communities.

Individuals and Crisis

Across the life span individuals continue to develop and are faced with transition when moving from one stage of development to the next. Because the transitions can be anticipated, measures can be taken to lessen their impact. Developmental psychologists like Erikson (1950) have identified normal major states of transition in humans (see above).

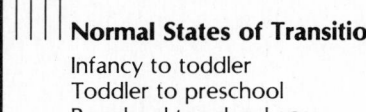

Normal States of Transition

Infancy to toddler
Toddler to preschool
Preschool to school age
School age to adolescence
Adolescence to adult
Adult to middle age
Middle age to old age

From Erikson, E.: Childhood and society, New York, 1950, W. W. Norton & Co., Inc.

Seven Stages of Family Life

Stage

1   Early marriage: intimacy or games?
2   Coping with parenthood
3   When children go to school
4   Families with adolescents
5   Shrinking family
6   Empty nest
7   Three generations together

From Rhodes, S., and Wilson, J.: Surviving family life, New York, 1981, G.P. Putnam's Sons.

Maturational Crises

In moving from one developmental stage to the next, individuals are at risk of experiencing maturational crisis. As with all crises, maturational crises hold the possibility for growth and the danger of stagnation or regression. For example, in adolescence, issues concerning dating, sexual activity, and career choice are confronted. Young adults face establishing their own households, securing jobs, and possibly parenting. (In Part Four of this text, problems across the life span are considered.)

Because transition periods are predictable, there is opportunity to assist individuals to anticipate and cope. For example, discussion groups for those in their early teens can ease the transition into adolescence. Programs before retirement can assist older individuals cope with the problems of old age.

Situational Crises

Unlike maturational crises, situational crises affecting individuals are frequently sudden and unexpected. The death of a significant other, disabling injury, rape, job loss, and divorce are examples of events that can result in situational crisis. Because these events are unexpected, anticipatory guidance is not possible. With situational crises prompt contact and early intervention can assist the individual to cope with the event. Centers for battered women, laryngectomy self-help groups, and rape crisis centers are examples of organizations developed to assist individuals in coping with specific events that can lead to situational crisis.

Both transition from one developmental stage to the next and occurrence of a significant unanticipated event can stimulate an individual crisis. For maturational and situational crises, the individual must acquire new coping strategies to effect successful resolution.

Families and Crisis
Maturational Crises

Family life is a dynamic cycle requiring readjustments as one phase is passed and another entered (Duvall, 1977). Typically there are periods of relative calm followed by more intense activity at transition times in the life of the family. As with individuals, families may face either maturational or situational crises. Like individuals, families progress through developmental stages with each one presenting a unique set of circumstances and requiring new coping strategies. For successful progression through the developmental stages, all family members must cope with the new situations. Each developmental stage (seven, described in the box above) of family life requires members to relinquish some roles previously held and to assume new roles.

Stages may be altered depending on the age and past experience of the couple getting married. The following paragraphs provide general guidelines; however, variations are found in different couples depending on their unique characteristics and life situations during each stage. In stage 1, early marriage, new couples often establish a household separate from their families of origin, develop effective ways of settling differences, and decide on patterns of living together on a daily basis. If there are children from a previous marriage of either or both partners, additional negotiations take place to form a blended family.

With the birth of children, stage 2, each family member assumes new roles and relationships. Parents must learn to effectively meet the needs of an initially totally dependent person. The way the parents previously spent their time, money, and energy may change dramatically. Not only the roles of parents but also those of each child change as subsequent children enter the family. As additional children are born, the child who was the baby in the family becomes an older brother or sister. New responsibilities may be added to the older child's daily activities with the birth of additional children.

As children enter school, the family enters stage 3. During the school years, as children gain independence and establish relationships outside the home, the roles of parents and siblings change again. Parents must often work through situations in which they are no longer the whole world to their children. Teachers, church workers, club leaders, coaches, and others become increasingly important to the children.

Stage 4 involves children in adolescence experiencing rapid physiological and psychological changes and brings a distinct set of challenges to the family. As adolescents cope with problems of sexuality and selection of an occupation, parents must set limits that protect the adolescent while simultaneously allowing freedom for the individual to successfully complete the developmental tasks.

In late adolescence as children leave home, parents in stage 5 face new life situations. They are once again a couple and must reestablish a previous relationship. If parents essentially led parallel lives with little attention devoted to their relationship as a couple during the years of raising children, they may be relative strangers to one another when the children begin to leave home. An additional stressor during both stages 5 and 6 is that of aging parents. Whereas in earlier years the older generation provided for and nurtured the younger generation, problems of aging (as described in Chapter 28) may reverse these roles, thereby necessitating new coping strategies by both generations.

The extent to which the developmental tasks of stage 5 were met largely determines the nature and quality of stage 6. If parents adjusted to the departure of the children and either continued or learned meaningful ways to occupy themselves, the empty nest can be a time of freedom of choice and exercise of creativity. Adults often travel and engage in hobbies and career pursuits that were previously omitted during the busy years of raising children.

As family development continues, children marry and have families of their own, bringing three generations into the family structure. Parents in stage 7 have the new roles of in-laws and grandparents. Relationships in this situation include not only the children's spouses and the grandchildren but also the spouses' families of origin.

Stages of family development are predictable, and nursing intervention in the form of anticipatory guidance can be provided to assist families in coping with the inherent problems of each stage. Programs designed to promote growth through the family developmental process include premarital conferences that are often sponsored by churches, preparation for parenthood classes, and parenting groups. If a family successfully progresses through the developmental stages, the individual family members and the family as a whole benefit from growth.

Situational Crises

Situational crises affecting families can occur in any of the developmental stages. Stressful unanticipated events precipitating a family crisis may include the birth of a premature infant, the death of a family member, a diagnosis of serious illness, and relocation. A crisis ensues when family resources are insufficient for effective coping. Although anticipatory guidance is not always possible for family situational crises, resources are available to assist families confronted with stressful situations. People who have experienced a particular event often band together to form an organization of support for others facing the same situation. Organizations for families of retarded children, hyperactive children, cancer victims, children lost as a result of sudden infant death syndrome, and so forth have been useful as crisis intervention strategies.

Not all families who encounter a stressor event experience crisis. Some families are more prone to crisis than others. Whether or not crisis occurs depends on interaction of the event, the family's perception of the event, and the family's coping resources (Hill, 1965). If a family defines an event as threatening and impossible to overcome, crisis is more likely than if an event is seen as a challenge to be met. Families in which there is effective communication, coalition formation, and the ability to work together toward a goal have internal resources that aid them in averting crises (Hall and Weaver, 1974). Nurses can assist families to cope by using interventions such as objective clarification of events, promotion of the development of internal family resources, and referral to community resources.

An organized effort to aid families at risk of situational crises occurred in Israel during the Yom Kippur War (Caplan, 1976). During military conflicts soldiers are killed, and families must deal with the deaths. Caplan, an expert in crisis intervention, worked in Israel at the time and implemented principles of intervention for families of casualties.

The first principle Caplan used was to ensure that families were linked to significant others who could provide emotional support and create assistance. This began by bringing family members together in one location to inform them of the death. External support was simultaneously provided by friends, neighbors, and members of religious congregations. Nurses in the community and other health care providers monitored the status of bereaved families to identify those who needed additional attention. For most families, no additional crisis intervention was required.

Five other principles served as guides for families needing further assistance. The second principle called for limiting further aid to only those families truly needing help. This meant that careful assessment was required to determine families at greatest risk for disequilibrium from the effects of the war.

The third principle dealt with avoiding psychiatric labels for families struggling to cope with their loss. Families were treated and referred to as normal people under stress rather than dysfunctional families or people to whom a label connoting an illness was assigned.

The fourth crisis intervention principle called attention to the need to use professional and nonprofessional volunteers who were members of the community to act as interveners. By being community members they could understand the nature of the crisis and convey sincere empathy; they were easily accessible and were usually knowledgeable about resources and services available. Community health nurses were among the health professionals who provided crisis intervention.

The fifth principle suggested that mutual self-help groups and support networks be established. By joining other families who had experienced the same loss, energy could be mobilized to cope and group support gained.

The last principle dealt with providing assistance to the supporters. People helping others to cope with crises often feel drained of their energy. Unless the supporters receive some nurturance, they are prime candidates for burnout or high stress reactions themselves. Expert consultation was made available to community health nurses and others working with bereaved families in crisis. The crisis intervention program for families of soldiers killed in battle was organized to provide efficient and effective assistance from members of local communities.

Situational and maturational crises can occur in families, and they may happen simultaneously. For example, job loss at the time a family's first child is born would require adaptation to a developmental and situational event. Both types of crises require involvement of all family members and additional strategies to cope successfully.

Communities and Crisis
Maturational Crises

Communities are also at risk for both maturational and situational crises. Growth, expansion, and retrenchment are developmental stages that can lead to maturational crisis in communities. Growth early in the life of a community often takes place by people in the region moving to a concentrated area. As growth in a community occurs, there is a need for formal governmental structure and services to meet such basic needs of citizens as health care, education, safe water supply, sewage disposal, utilities, public safety, fire protection, and transportation. Unless problems resulting from growth are successfully solved, stagnation or loss of population will result. The West is dotted with ghost towns that did not cope with developmental events.

During expansion there is a diversification and continued growth. A community originally established on one or two economic bases such as manufacturing or agriculture expands and becomes a center for a variety of activities such as education, medical care, trade, and industry. The diversification brings people of different cultural backgrounds, talents, and experiences into the community. While expanding, there is a further need for basic services and a need for the blending of the newcomers into the life of the community. During successful expansion, basic needs are met and the community is richer for the contribuitons of the newcomers. Crisis can arise when any basic need is not met or when there is conflict among the various segments of the population.

With retrenchment, loss of population and therefore loss of economic support for basic needs occur. Loss of population can result from movement to suburbs and/or loss of economic bases, such as industries closing. Individuals who are elderly, poor, or have few job skills are less likely to leave a community. If the needs of those remaining in a community are not met, crisis can result.

Young people predominate in growing communities; thus maternal and child services are especially needed. These services include facilities for prenatal care, well-child care, handicapped children, appropriate day-care, and school health. As communities and their populations mature, there is greater need for chronic illness services and programs for the elderly.

Anticipatory preparation to avoid crisis in the growth and expansion stages of a community can include forecasting the population growth and planning and providing facilities to accommodate that growth. In retrenchment, financial support must be found to provide basic services. One example of a revenue source for such communities is a local tax on all income earned within the community. In this way people who are employed in the community but choose to live outside the area contribute to meeting the needs of the community. Communities in retrenchment as a result of the loss of an economic base often begin aggressive programs to attract new businesses and industry to the area.

By being active members of boards and committees charged with the responsibility for planning and providing basic services, community health nurses make health needs known and play a part in developing coping strategies to prevent a maturational crisis in the community. Political activity by nurses can also influence the development of a community. By election to public office or support of candidates for public office, nurses can play an active part in the developmental life of a community.

Situational Crises

Situational crises in a community can result from events such as floods, tornadoes, hurricanes, fires, or the sudden influx of a large number of refugees. When these unexpected events lead to crisis, resources beyond the community are needed to successfully resolve the situation.

Intervention in situational crises in communities includes mobilization of local disaster plans and assistance from governmental and voluntary agencies. Community health nurses are involved in maintaining the health of citizens affected by disaster. In shelters they work to assist parents to care for their children under adverse conditions, to meet the needs of the chronically ill so that complications do not occur, and generally to either provide support or identify support systems to prevents individual and family crisis. As part of the health department, the Red Cross, or voluntary organizations, community health nurses work at all levels, from making policy to rendering direct service in a community crisis.

Summary of Types of Crisis

Communities, families, and individuals are at risk of maturational and situational crisis. All crises have in common an event, often sudden and unexpected, which results in significant problems for which usual coping resources are inadequate. For maturational crises, anticipatory guidance is possible, but for situational crises (because they are unpredictable), intervention can occur only after the event. Community health nurses are in a position to provide care for individuals, families, and communities in maturational and situational crisis.

CRISIS INTERVENTION

Because crisis is a temporary state of upset, the aim of intervention is to promptly assist the individual, family, or community to resolve the situation so that growth with an improved level of function is achieved when equilibrium is regained. In crisis intervention clients are not viewed as harboring pathological conditions but as needing to acquire support and coping mechanisms to resolve a specific situation. The summary of crisis intervention that follows is based on the work of several authors (Aguilera and Messick, 1982; Caplan, 1964; Hoff, 1978; Schwenk and Bittle, 1979).

Crisis intervention is a short-term method focused on solving immediate problems. The usual length of a crisis with or without intervention is 4 to 6 weeks. To be effective in preventing an outcome of disorganization, intervention must take place while disequilibrium is present. Unlike psychotherapeutic techniques, such as psychoanalysis, which are long term and focus on the past, crisis intevention is short term with one to six contacts and focuses on the present.

Crisis intervention is a method that can be used by health professionals, nonhealth professionals, and volunteers after special training. Nurses, physicians, psychologists, and social workers are among the health professionals who use crisis intervention. Many nonhealth professionals in the course of their work are confronted with crisis situations and are able to use intervention. Police, clergy, and teachers are among the nonhealth professionals for whom crisis intervention is useful training. Frequently, trained volunteers using crisis intervention can provide the necessary care. Some examples of places using volunteers include rape crisis centers, drug abuse facilities, and self-help groups in which people who have experienced a traumatic event like a mastectomy or the birth of a handicapped child help other in similar predicaments.

To provide specific crisis intervention services, crisis teams may be formed. The composition of the team is dependent on the purpose of the service and the resources available. A crisis team at a drug abuse facility could consist of a psychiatrist, nurse, social worker, and former drug abuser. Members of a team bring their own unique backgrounds plus crisis intervention expertise. For any one client, leadership of the team is assumed by the member who can best assist the client in resolving the crisis. As discussed earlier in the chapter, present crisis intervention techniques are based on the work of Caplan (1964), Hill (1949), Lindemann (1979), and other pioneers in the field. For example, after working with the Coconut Grove fire victims, Cobb and Lindemann (1979) described a three-phase model for crisis intervention. Objective presentation and clarification of the event occur in phase 1. In phase 2 the care giver assists the person in crisis to work through the problems resulting from the stressor event. Phase 3 deals with readjustment, with the care giver assisting the individual to plan for the future.

Community health nurses and other health professionals with training function as crisis intervention therapists. In crisis intervention, assessment of the client and the problem is the first step during the initial contact. Information is gathered on the following: (1) precipitating event, (2) resulting problem(s), (3) onset of the crisis, (4) impact of the crisis on the life of the client, (5) impact of the crisis on the life of significant others, (6) coping strategies used in the past, (7) strengths of the client, (8) individuals in the client's life who can provide support, and (9) risk of homicide or suicide.

The stressor event and its meaning to the client and the family are explored. The resultant problems, attempts to deal with them, and coping mechanisms used in the past are reviewed. In addition, strengths of the client and external supports are identified.

To assess potential for suicide or homicide, direct and specific questions are asked (Aguilera and Messick, 1982). Are you considering suicide? Are you planning to kill someone else? If so, how and when? The more specific the plan and the more lethal the method, the greater the risk of suicide (Dixon, 1979). Clients at risk of harming themselves or others are not candidates for crisis intervention and should be referred for psychiatric evaluation and possible hospitalization.

With candidates for crisis intervention, information obtained during assessment is organized and presented to the client so that the relation between the event, problems, and crisis is evident. This organized summary of information allows for client validation and serves as a therapeutic technique for a person who does not recognize the relation among the components of the crisis. To plan the intervention the problem must be broken into manageable parts.

The intervention techniques used in crisis are varied. Techniques used include listening actively with concern, helping the client express feelings, exploring new ways of coping, helping the person find and use supports, and assisting him to gradually accept reality. With the client immediate goals are set, workable plans of action are explored, and specific actions are chosen. The client leaves the session with certain tasks to perform. In crisis intervention the therapist is an active and direct participant. For example, the therapist may contact community agencies that require referral from a health professional. However, the resolution of the crisis rests with the client.

In the first contact it is important to maintain focus on the crisis. The therapist and client should be aware that crisis intervention lasts only a few weeks at most. For some clients one contact provides the assistance necessary for resolution of the problem. In future contacts progress in using new coping methods and meeting goals is reviewed, and the therapist provides rein-

Assess
- Clarify precipiting event
- Explore meaning of event to the client
- Identify problems
- Identify present and past coping strategies
- Identify resources

Diagnose
- Clearly define the problems
- Label the problem

Plan
- Separate problems into manageable pieces
- Explore alternative coping methods
- Set goals
- Define specific tasks to meet goals

Intervene
- Formulate an objective statement of the situation
- Carry out tasks to meet goals
- Mobilize resources

Evaluate
- Appraise progress toward goals
- Evaluate the success of coping methods used
- Reinforce the progress made

forcement for client successes. Other aspects of the crisis problem, in manageable pieces, are explored, and ways of coping are considered. Throughout crisis intervention individuals and/or groups who can provide support are identified and mobilized. The length and frequency of client contacts with the therapist depend on the nature of the crisis but usually range from one to six.

In the terminal interview a summary of new strategies attempted—successful and unsuccessful—and progress made reinforces the gains of the client. To help the individual maintain the achieved level of function, realistic plans for the future are discussed. The client who achieves resolution of a crisis at an improved level of function has experienced growth and gained coping mechanisms that can prevent a crisis in the future.

The familiarity of the crisis process to the community health nurse lies in its parallelism to the nursing process of assessment, nursing diagnosis planning, intervention, and evaluation. Steps in crisis intervention as they occur in the initial nursing process are shown in the box above.

In crisis intervention the assessment has a present orientation and remains focused on the crisis situation. As with care in other community health nursing inter-

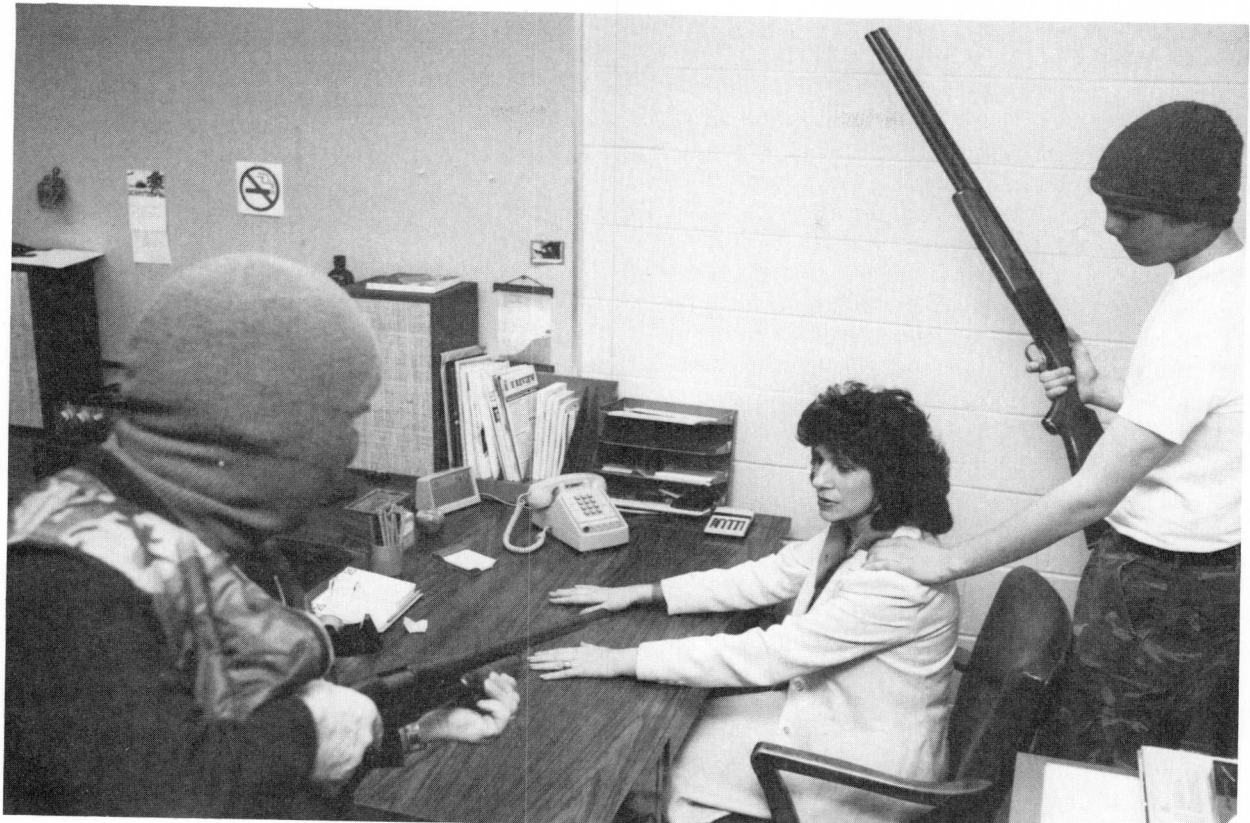

Fig. 19-2. Hostage.

actions, the client is an active participant in planning, intervention, and evaluation.

Crisis intervention may be provided in individual, family, or group settings, with the choice depending on the need of the client and the availability of services. An example of group intervention following a community disaster with crisis potential was the efforts of a Washington, D.C., area Health Maintenance Organization (HMO) after a Hanafi Muslim sect seized and held hostages for more than 1½ days (Sank, 1979). Mental health professionals from the HMO offered the released hostages eight group sessions that began 4 days after the ordeal. During the group sessions former hostages discussed their perceptions of the event, their feelings while being held hostage, problems they were having since their release as a result of the experience, and methods of coping with those problems. The aims of the intervention were to provide support for the ex-hostages and assist them in developing the coping skills necessary to deal with problems resulting from the traumatic event.

Three aspects of crisis add to the possibility of favorable resolution through crisis intervention (Caplan, 1964). First, the crisis outcome is determined most often not by the client's past experiences or the nature of the event leading to crisis but by internal and external factors during the course of the crisis. Crisis intervention through the use of techniques such as developing new ways of coping and mobilizing support can provide internal and external factors that tilt the resolution in favor of a successful outcome. Second, the client in crisis has an increased desire for help. Therefore the client in crisis is more likely to seek and accept crisis intervention. Third, clients in crisis are more likely to be influenced by others than they are in periods of equilibrium. Because of these aspects of crisis, therapists skilled in crisis intervention have a unique opportunity to influence crisis outcome.

Because of their educational backgrounds, acceptance by clients, and frequent encounters with individuals and families in crisis, community health nurses can be an integral part of a community's crisis intervention efforts. They may provide crisis intervention to individuals, families, and groups; participate on crisis intervention teams; and serve on committees that manage crisis programs.

PRIMARY, SECONDARY, AND TERTIARY PREVENTION

The aim of *primary prevention* is to avert the occurrence of an illness or situation. For example, immunizations for communicable diseases are a measure of primary prevention used to avert diseases such as rubella, mumps, and poliomyelitis. Primary prevention aims to avert crises in stressful maturational and situational circumstances. Primary prevention for maturational crisis is based on the knowledge of the problems accompanying transitions across the life span. Community health nurses working with individuals and families can provide anticipatory guidance for individual and family developmental transitions. In settings such as prenatal classes, parenting groups, and adolescent discussion groups there is also opportunity to discuss transition problems and helpful coping mechanisms. By sitting on community boards, participating in civic and voluntary organizations, and speaking at public functions, community health nurses contribute to the primary prevention of developmental crises in communities.

To prevent crisis following a stressful situational event, prompt action is needed. The group sessions for ex-hostages are one example of an effort to provide primary prevention for a group who experienced a traumatic event. A situational event for which some communities provide primary intervention is rape. Comprehensive rape crisis intervention considers care of the victim from the time of the assault through courtroom appearances testifying against the assailant (McCombie, 1980). Community health nurses encounter many individuals and families at risk of situational crisis and have the opportunity to use primary prevention. Individuals who have experienced the loss of meaningful relationship through death or disease, birth of a high risk infant, or loss of income are among those who may benefit from primary prevention of crisis. Either by providing direct assistance or by referral, the community health nurse can use primary prevention.

Secondary prevention entails finding cases early to prevent sequelae. Early identification of those in crisis and prompt institution of crisis intervention can promote a favorable outcome. Recalling that a crisis has a limited duration emphasizes the need for intervention without delay. The client in crisis needs an appointment today, not next week. If referral to an agency is needed, the nurse should be certain the agency is aware that the client is in crisis and is not to be deferred.

Tertiary prevention consists of rehabilitation when sequelae of a situation have occurred. In crisis this means that resolution has resulted in a level of function that is lower than the level before crisis, and there is

major disorganization. To assist clients whose resolution of crisis is not successful, referral to mental health specialists is needed. Whereas the goal of primary prevention is to avert crisis and the goal of secondary prevention is to successfully resolve the crisis, the goal of tertiary prevention is to return to the former level of function or a higher one following an unsuccessfully resolved crisis.

The Nursing Process

The following example illustrates crisis intervention by a community health nurse with a client in crisis. A summary of the nursing process used in this situation is described after the example.

Susan Jones, a community health nurse employed by a county health department, had been given several new clients. Among them was Betty Steward, who was a 23-year-old unmarried mother of a 4-year-old girl and expecting her second child. A review of Betty's record revealed that she was in her 39th week of pregnancy and had missed her clinic visit the previous week; a home visit was planned. On arriving at the home, Susan was greeted by a young woman with uncombed hair and a rumpled housecoat; she was obviously not pregnant. Betty said she had delivered twin boys 3 days ago, and she and her sons had arrived home earlier in the day. Betty's daughter, Karen, was at home and eager to show her brothers to the nurse. Susan's examinations of Betty and the infants revealed no physical problems.

As Susan talked with Betty, she noted Betty's slow movements and sad expression. Susan told Betty she appeared to be sad and asked if there was a problem. Betty began to cry and said that throughout the pregnancy she had planned to give the infant up for adoption, but when the twins were born, she thought they were "special" and changed her mind. Now she was uncertain of her decision and felt overwhelmed.

Although Betty's only income had been child support from Karen's father, Betty felt that Karen needed her at home during the preschool years and was unemployed at the time of the pregnancy. However, Betty looked forward to the time when Karen would enter school, Betty would get a job, and their situation could improve. Keeping the infants meant loss of a goal to Betty. In addition, she expressed concern about her ability to provide for the infants. Not expecting to keep the infant, no care items were available; the only formula was the take-home package from the hospital, and there was little food in the house. Repeatedly Betty said she needed to decide whether or not to keep the twins.

Susan inquired about individuals in Betty's life who had helped when she had decisions to make in the past. Betty said she had neither family nor friends with whom she could discuss the situation about the twins. However, Betty's minister was a person she trusted and who had been of help previously.

The plan developed by Susan and Betty was for Betty to contact her minister and meet with him and for Susan to contact a community agency to arrange for emergency formula, supplies for the infants, and food for Betty and Karen. If Betty's decision was to keep the infants, further plans would be made on the next visit. They agreed that Susan would return in 2 days, and if Betty needed her before then, she would call.

On Susan's next visit Betty was smiling and said that after talking with her minister she had made a final decision and would keep the twins. Her biggest problem was how she would provide for them because she did not want to leave them to work. Susan informed Betty about Aid to Families with Dependent Children and told her how to go about contacting the social worker. Susan was to call the social worker so that he would expect Betty's call, and Betty would arrange for an appointment. The next visit was scheduled for 1 week later.

By the next visit Betty had seen the social worker; interim assistance was arranged, and she would soon receive regular benefits. Betty's concern now was providing a suitable environment for the children. When asked what kind of place she would like, she referred to a clean place that did not have roaches and mice, which were her main objections to the present house. They discussed options for the problem, and the action planned was for Betty to contact the landlord and request that he have the pests exterminated. Because Betty had little experience taking assertive action with someone she considered an authority figure, they role played the contact with the landlord. The next visit was scheduled for 3 weeks.

At the next visit Betty, neatly dressed, met Susan at the door and began to tell her about the telephone call to the landlord. She related that she had been firm in her request for extermination services, and as a result, the landlord agreed. She proudly showed Susan the twins and her cleaner house. Susan commended Betty for the progress she had made and spoke of her recent achievements. Although life with her daughter and the infants was not without problems, Betty was successfully coping with the situation. As a result of her contact with her minister, members of the congregation had come to visit, and Betty talked of her plans to participate in church activities. With the present situation resolved, routine health care plans for the family were agreed on, and Betty was to contact Susan if assistance was needed in the future.

The steps in the nursing process—assessment, nursing diagnosis, planning, intervention, and evaluation—are reviewed here as carried out in the previous example. The first step in the nursing process is assessment, and Susan began assessment of the Steward family by checking the biophysical status of the mother and infants. Assessment of the emotional status revealed problems subsequent to the birth of twins. Further assessment revealed lack of coping strategies and loss of a life goal leading to a diagnosis of crisis.

There was no evidence that Betty was suicidal or would have harmed another. Using crisis intervention, the remainder of the first visit focused on the problems associated with the crisis. Assessment included identification of individuals who could be a support, and this revealed Betty's minister.

Plans were developed jointly by Susan and Betty with priorities established so that problems of greatest importance were dealt with first. Consistent with crisis intervention, problems were considered in manageable parts. Implementation of the plans involved active participation by the nurse and client and allowed Betty to develop new coping skills. The role playing to prepare Betty for the contact with the landlord was an example. In the last contact Betty's successful efforts and achievement were reviewed and reinforced, and plans for the future were discussed.

Throughout the crisis period, reassessment, client participation in planning, intervention, and evaluation occurred. The last visit reviewed progress and future plans. In this case study the client successfully resolved the problems resulting from the birth of twins and developed new coping strategies.

Community Resources

Crisis resources available in a community depend on the size of the community, crisis needs, and the interest and expertise present. The community health nurse in a rural community may be the only health care professional available but need not be the only resource. Other professionals, such as ministers and cooperative extension agents or home economists employed by the agricultural component of a state university, may provide primary and secondary prevention. For example, the cooperative extension agent works on a daily basis with homemakers and has an educational background that includes knowledge of individual and family development. Parenting classes and groups to discuss transitions in family life are examples of activities aimed at primary prevention of crisis and may be conducted by cooperative extension agencies. In organizing crisis resources in a rural community, the community health nurse should consider the roles that could be played by both professionals and volunteers.

In larger communities, resources for crisis include both official and voluntary agencies. Among official agencies, the health department and mental health center may offer programs of primary and secondary prevention for individuals and families. In health departments, community health nurses participate in assessing needs for crisis services, diagnosing specific areas for intervention, planning, intervening, and evaluating actions. Tertiary prevention is offered by mental health centers and private psychiatric facilities for clients in whom crisis resolution resulted in a decreased level of function with disorganization.

Voluntary agencies in a community are concerned with a wide variety of conditions including infertility, drug abuse, birth defects, mental retardation, hyperactivity, cancer, kidney disease, child abuse, battered women, and rape. Services provided by these agencies range from distributing information to sponsoring support groups to offering crisis intervention. In some communities traditional agencies are expanding their scope of services to include crisis assistance. For example, some Young Women's Christian Associations (YWCA) offer help to battered women. Religious institutions may also offer programs of primary prevention and less often secondary prevention of crisis. Community health nurses have opportunities to support voluntary crisis efforts through joining the membership, serving as consultants, accepting board membership, and providing direct services through the agency.

Minimally, community health nurses provide primary prevention services and have knowledge of the resources for secondary and tertiary crisis prevention. For effective referral to a community resource, the community health nurse must know the specific services of the agency, eligibility requirements for clients, and the procedures for obtaining services. If the community health nurse does not provide crisis intervention, a prompt and appropriate referral of clients in crisis is needed.

SUMMARY

Crisis is an upset in a steady state, a disequilibrium, resulting from problems that follow an event of significance to the client and for which coping skills are inadequate. With crisis there is both the opportunity for growth and the achievement of a higher level of psychological functioning if successful resolution occurs and the danger of a decreased level of psychological function and disorganization if resolution is not successful. The disequilibrium of crisis cannot be long endured; with or without intervention a new state of equilibrium is reached in 4 to 6 weeks.

The individual in crisis perceives the event, which may be desirable or undesirable, as having serious consequences. The person also perceives a state of upset, an uncertainty of outcome, and feelings of helplessness and ineffectuality. Physiological manifestations of crisis are varied and depend on the individual's response to stressful situations.

As defined by Schwenk and Bittle (1979) the four phases of crisis are characterized by changes in tension and function levels. As the crisis progresses, the individual experiences increased tension and decreased function levels.

Maturational and situational crises may affect individuals, families, and communities and are not mutually exclusive; situational crisis may be imposed maturational crisis. Because transitions in individual, family, and community life are predictable, anticipatory guidance to provide effective coping skills is possible for situations having the potential for maturational cri-

sis. With situational crisis, often sudden and unexpected, intervention quickly following the traumatic event can provide coping mechanisms sufficient for prevention.

Crisis intervention is a short-term treatment modality by which clients in crisis are assisted in developing coping mechanisms and are provided support to resolve the situation so that the client reaches equilibrium at an improved level of psychological function after the crisis. With training the techniques of crisis intervention are suitable for use by health professionals, nonhealth professionals, and volunteers. In crisis intervention the focus remains on the present situation, and there is a present orientation. The steps of the crisis process are essentially those of the nursing process—assessment, diagnosis, planning, intervention, and evaluation. Throughout crisis intervention the client and therapist play active roles. The client deals with the crisis problems in manageable parts, and progress made is reinforced.

The concepts of primary, secondary, and tertiary prevention are useful in organizing crisis services in a community. With primary prevention, efforts are directed at averting the occurrence of crisis. Secondary prevention entails finding cases early and instituting crisis intervention promptly. If crisis resolution is unsuccessful, tertiary prevention with rehabilitation by mental health specialists is necessary.

By working with official and voluntary agencies, community health nurses can participate in assessment, diagnosis, planning, intervention, and evaluation of crisis services for individuals, families, and communities. Community health nurses may provide direct intervention for clients in crisis or may refer them to resources best able to meet their needs.

BIBLIOGRAPHY

Aguilera, D., and Messick, J.: Crisis intervention theory and methodology, ed. 4, St. Louis, 1982, The C.V. Mosby Co.

Caplan, G: Principles of preventive psychiatry, New York, 1964, Basic Books, Inc., Publishers.

Caplan, G: Organization of support systems for civilian populations. In Caplan, G., and Killilea, M., editors: Support systems and mutual help: multidisciplinary explorations, New York, 1976, Grune & Stratton, Inc.

Cobb, S., and Lindemann, E.: Neuropsychiatric observations after the Coconut Grove fire. In Lindemann E.: Beyond grief, New York, 1979, Jason Aronson.

Dixon, S: Working with people in crisis, St. Louis, 1979, The C.V. Mosby Co.

Duvall, E: Marriage and family development, ed. 5, New York, 1977, J.B. Lippincott Co.

Erikson, E: Childhood and society, New York, 1950, W.W. Norton & Co.

Hall, J., and Weaver, B., editors: Nursing of families in crisis, Philadelphia, 1974, J.B. Lippincott Co.

Hill, R: Families under stress, Westport, Conn., 1949, Greenwood Press, Publishers.

Hill, R.: Generic features of families under stress. In Parad, H.: Crisis intervention: selected readings, New York, 1965, Family Service Association of America.

Hoff, L.A.: People in crisis understanding and helping, Menlo Park, Calif., 1978, Addison-Wesley Publishing Co.

Lindemann, E.: Symptomatology and management of acute grief. In Lindemann, E.: Beyond grief, New York, 1979, Jason Aronson.

McCombie, S., editor: The rape crisis intervention handbook, New York, 1980, Plenum Press.

Rapoport, L. The state of crisis: some theoretical considerations. In Parad, H.: Crisis intervention: selected readings, New York, 1965, Family Service Association of America.

Rhodes, S., and Wilson, J.: Surviving family life, New York, 1981, G.P. Putnam's Sons.

Sank, L.I.: Psychology in action: community disasters, Am. Psychol. **34:**334, 1979.

Schwenk, T.L., and Bittle, S. P.: Applicability of crisis intervention in family practice, J. Fam. Pract. **8:**1151, 1979.

Sheehy, G: Passages: predictable crises of adult life, New York, 1976, Dutton.

Spradley, B.W.: Community health nursing: concepts and practice, Boston, 1981, Little, Brown, & Co.

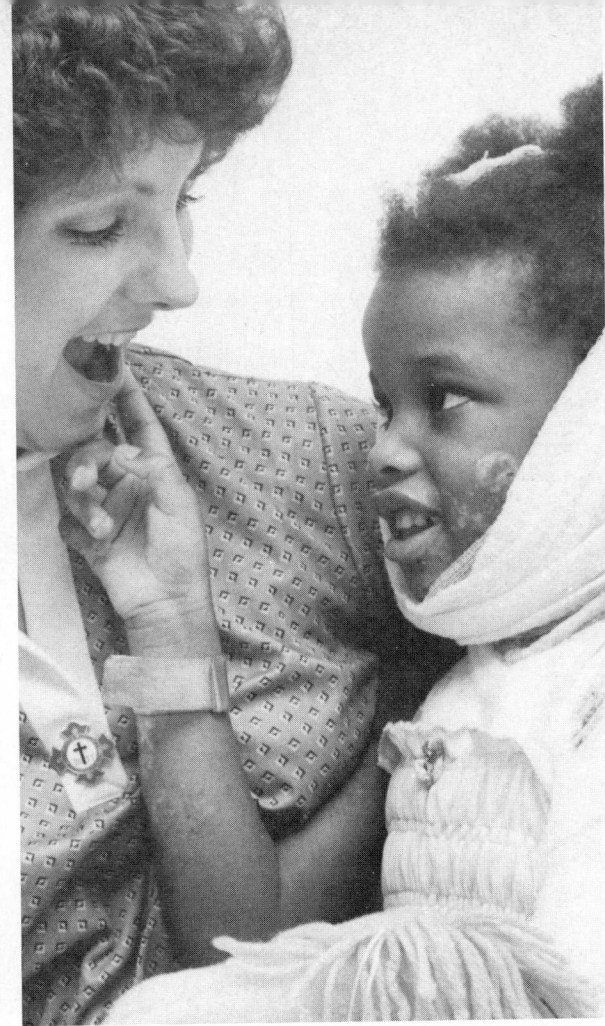

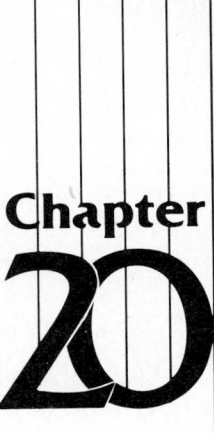

Chapter
20

JEANETTE LANCASTER
DAVID KERSCHNER

VIOLENCE AND HUMAN ABUSE AS COMMUNITY HEALTH PROBLEMS

The most powerful obstacle to culture, according to Freud (1955) is the human innate, independent, and instinctual tendency toward aggression. Other scholars have argued that aggression and violence are not innate, but rather are learned behaviors. Violence seems to be ever present. Headlines in newspapers report political kidnappings, terrorist attacks, and senseless killings. Television news displays in vivid color the capture of a rape suspect, victims of a family shooting, and battles among Third World countries. Statistically the major causes of death for young males in the United States are all violent. White males are more likely to die from vascular accidents, suicide, and homicide, whereas black males are at greater risk for homicide, vehicular accidents, and drowning accidents (Hanlon and Pickett, 1979). People are increasingly harming and killing others as well as themselves.

In the fast-paced era of the 1980s people may have either harbored more hostility or used fewer constructive channels for venting pent-up feelings. Underlying most violence toward oneself or others is a deep-seated sense of hostility, which the affected individual may or may not recognize. Hostility tends to be a motivating force and is exhibited in impulses, urges, and tendencies to behave in ways that lead to injury or destruction for either animate or inanimate objects. Hostility includes active aggression, anger, and hatred as well as passive gestures such as gossip, neglect, and the withholding of affection and fair treatment.

All people, to some degree, are pulled by two opposing forces: to be acceptable to self and society, and to exhibit strong asocial and antisocial tendencies. To understand community violence, one must recognize the presence of these opposing forces in all people. Each

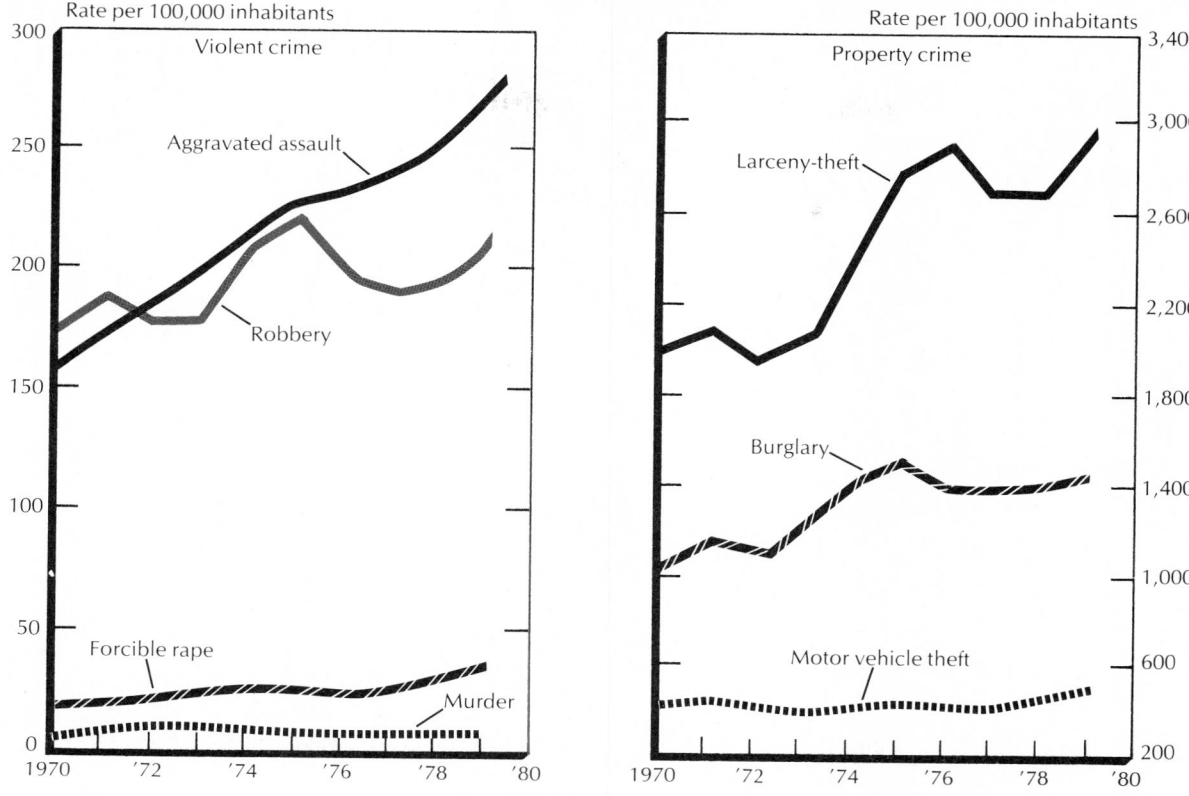

Fig. 20-1. Selected crime rates from 1970 to 1979. (From Statistical abstracts of the United States, Bureau of the Census, Washington, D.C., 1981, U.S. Government Printing Office.)

person has an innate ability to lash out and harm or destroy self or others. The crucial factor lies in what causes some people to unleash these forces while others keep their hostility and aggression in check.

This chapter examines violence and human abuse as a community health problem. A systems theory framework is used to aid in organizing content as well as to order information needed by community health nurses into a systematic format. As described in Chapter 6, a variety of frameworks could be used to organize content to systematically assess, plan, implement, and evaluate nursing actions.

Systems theory, as described in Chapter 6, looks at the whole by way of careful examination of the parts. To look at violence and human abuse from a holistic perspective one should discuss the subsystems that lead to violence. Specifically, social, community, family, and individual factors influencing violence are described, followed by an overview of commonly seen types of violence and suggested actions community health nurses can take.

SCOPE OF THE PROBLEM

Violence and human abuse are not new phenomena but are increasingly becoming public health concerns. Communities around the country are voicing anger and fear about rising crime and violence rates. According to the 1980 *Uniform Crime Reports,* overall crime in the United States increased 50% from the previous decade. In 1980, 1 of every 15 urban dwellers and 1 of 45 people in rural areas were the victims of crime (Uniform Crime Reports, 1980).

Also in 1980, violent crimes (homicide, forcible rape, robbery, and aggravated assault) and property crimes (burglary, larceny, theft, motor vehicle theft, and arson) increased 11% and 9%, respectively, over 1979 crime rates (Uniform Crime Reports, 1980). Between 1971 and 1979 violent crimes surged 60% and property crimes escalated 54%. Fig. 20-1 depicts this increase. This rising trend was also seen in the first 6 months of 1981, with an increase of 5% in violent crimes and 2% in property crimes over the same period in 1980 (Uniform Crime Reports, 1981). An average increase in

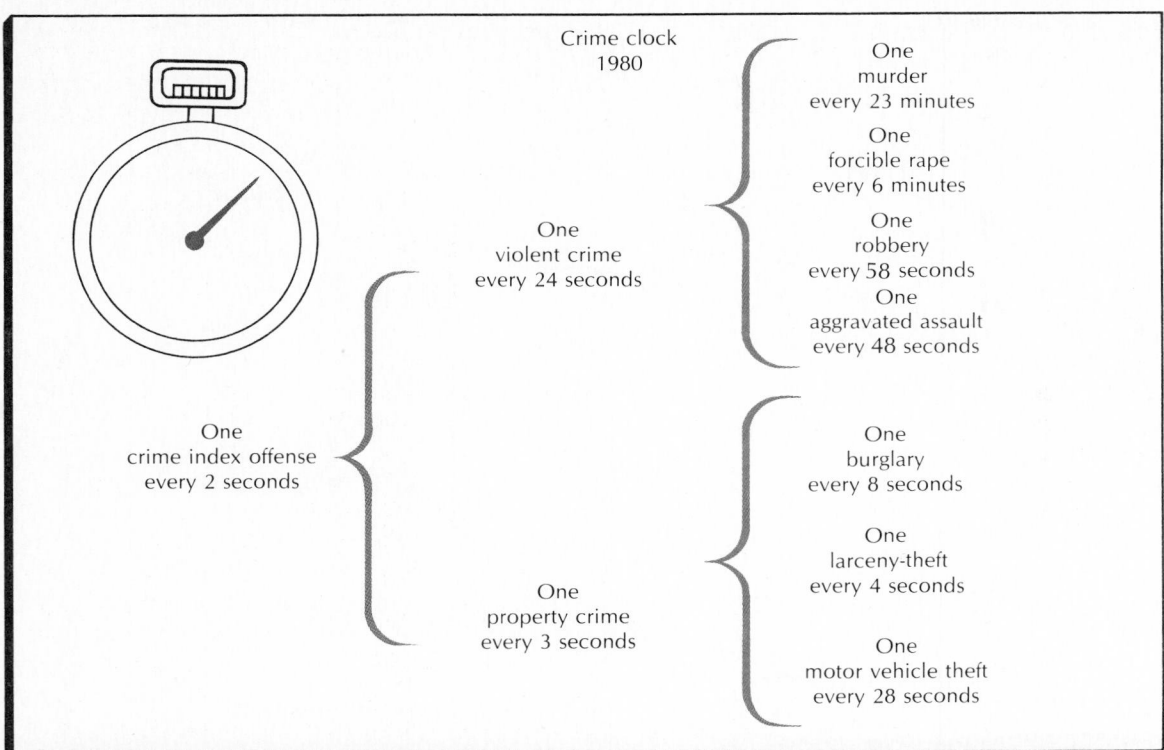

Fig. 20-2. Crime clock. (From Uniform crime reports, for the United States, Federal Bureau of Investigation, Washington, D.C., 1980, U.S. Department of Justice.)

crime for all size cities and suburban counties for the first half of 1981 occurred. Fig. 20-2 demonstrates the daily rate at which forms of crime occur.

Violence against family members is more difficult to measure, since many crimes of this nature go unreported. However, the extent of this community health problem should not be underestimated. For example, in one national survey it was found that of the persons interviewed, 20% said they had hit a child with some object, 4.2% admitted to having beaten a child, and an additional 2.9% said they had used a knife or gun on a child (Hendrix, 1981). Helfer and Kempe (1976) estimate that about 600 children are killed annually by their parents and approximately 25% of all fractures seen in a child's first 2 years and 10% to 15% of other trauma in children under 3 are the result of parental abuse.

Most killings, about 50% or more, occur between people who know one another (Allen, 1981) and about 30% occur within the family (Newman, 1979). Domestic disputes account for over half of all police night calls and often result in violent encounters with the police as they answer these calls (Allen, 1981).

Detection of family violence and abuse can be partic-

ularly difficult because of the nature of the problem, guilt, and the possibility of punishment. Community health nurses, like social workers, are in key positions to detect and intervene in community and family violence, since they have access to clients in a wide variety of settings, including the home.

The roots of human abuse and violence lie both in the people directly involved and in the social system in which they live. Violent behavior is a reflection of a society that endorses violence as a means of achieving goals, dealing with frustrations, and controlling the actions of its members. The next section presents several ways the community as a social system supports, reenforces, and at times encourages violence.

FACTORS INFLUENCING SOCIAL AND COMMUNITY VIOLENCE

Numerous variables within a community can support or minimize violence. Changing social conditions, multiple demands on people, worsening economic conditions, and the institutions that make up a given society or community influence the level of violence and human abuse. To understand key factors that affect people so that they inflict abuse on themselves and/or others, selected contemporary social conditions are reviewed.

Work

The American way of life reinforces competition for goods and services as an essential and valued aspect of free enterprise. People are expected to be productive, contributing, and self-sufficient. The American work ethic dates to the Industrial Revolution when arduous child and adult labor was expected. People are expected to work hard to enjoy the "good life." However, in inflationary times when unemployment is high, willing people are not always able to find sufficient work to maintain a satisfactory standard of living.

Work as an institution cannot be relied on to meet basic human needs. Jobs can be repetitive, boring, and nearly lacking in stimulation. Also, even in jobs with the potential for stimulation, supervisors and other forms of organizational control may discourage creativity and reward conformity and "following the rules." In many work settings people try to get ahead regardless of the cost to others. Adults often go home feeling physically and psychologically drained. They may have worked at a back-breaking pace all day only to be yelled at by the boss for what seemed like a trivial oversight. It is hard to separate feelings generated at work from the home environment. The father arrives home tired, angry, and generally feeling inadequate because of a series of reprimands. Soon after he sits down, his 4-year-old son runs through the house pretending to fly a wooden airplane. After about three loud trips past his father, who keeps shouting for the child to be quiet and go outside, the airplane hits the father in the head. This provides a fertile setting for striking out in frustration and anger.

In addition, in times of economic constraints people are often afraid to give up even those jobs that are frustrating, are boring, or create great stress; at such times any job seems better than none. People feel trapped; their family needs necessitate that they keep the hated job, which often engenders resentment toward those who are dependent on them, such as children, unemployed spouses, older relatives, and handicapped or sick family members.

People also abuse the social system in relation to work. For example, welfare recipients, such as mothers receiving Aid to Families of Dependent Children, may earn more money through welfare than by working. This becomes a vicious cycle: the mother is often unskilled, uneducated, and therefore unable to secure profitable employment; dependency occurs as the mother remains on welfare rather than take a menial job; and the abuse continues. Other people abuse society by feigning disability to receive funds, by misrepresenting the number of people in their home or the presence of a father in the home, or even by continuing to receive Social Security payments after the eligible person dies.

Unemployment often precipitates abusive outbursts. The inability to secure or maintain a job may lead to feelings of inadequacy, guilt, boredom, dissatisfaction, and frustration.

Education

In recent years schools have assumed many responsibilities traditionally assigned to the family. Schools teach sexual development, discipline children, and often serve as holding stations for children who have no other place to go. Large classes often mean that teachers spend more time and energy monitoring and disciplining children than challenging and stimulating them to learn. In large classes isolation is often the primary method of dealing with children who do not conform to norms of expected behavior. The nonconforming child is simply removed from the classroom because time does not permit concerted efforts directed toward helping the child learn alternative ways of behavior.

Ironically, children are often punished for hitting or biting other children by being spanked. Such punishment only reinforces the child's tendency to strike out at others because adults are seen as directing the forbidden action toward the child.

Prince (1981) contends that five basic human needs—stimulation, power, intimacy, interdependence, and "anger outlets"—could be provided by major social institutions but in most cases are not. She believes that the educational system, especially in urban areas, fails to meet these needs largely because of a lack of financial resources. Schools, according to Prince, are often lonely, boring places where the expression of anger is discouraged by the threat of punishment and where children gain feelings of self-esteem from achievement on tests.

Media

Television, movies, newspapers, and magazines portray happy, fun-loving people. Television parades in front of 6 million eyes, in brilliant living color, all the wonders money can provide. Yet for many Americans the hope of buying many of the nonessentials seems unrealistic. Such polarization between what is available and what is possible provides fertile ground for the development of abusive patterns. Frustration, unfilled dreams, and unmet wishes are often handled through hurting someone who is limited in the ability to fight back.

The media cater to children by presenting products intended to stimulate their curiosity and desire to purchase. Parents subsequently may get angry when their children frequently request the foods, toys, and clothes they see on television, in magazines, or in newspapers or hear advertised on the radio.

Not only do the media tantalize children and adults with the vast array of possible items to buy and things to do, but they often portray the world as a violent place. Hitting, kicking, stabbing, and shooting are seen daily as ways to handle anger, frustration, and so forth. The media sanctions violence when the good guys conquer the bad ones. Thus violence is often seen as being justified when the perpetrator views the cause to be worthy.

Organized Religion

Three of the human needs cited by Prince (1981) are often provided by the church—stimulation, a sense of worth or power, and some degree of closeness and intimacy. Interestingly, throughout history a seemingly contradictory relationship has existed between abuse and religion. For example, many religious groups uphold the philosophy of "spare the rod, spoil the child." Also, some faiths uphold victimization of people with their disapproval of divorce. Families may stay together, although at emotional or physical war with one another, because of religious commitments (Prince, 1981).

Although controversial in nature, the role of guilt as a form of victimization needs to be considered. Although every society has its own rules and sanctions for what is acceptable, rigid guidelines complete with predictions of dire spiritual consequences can produce guilt and lower self-esteem. The dividing line seems to be between those religious bodies that offer guidelines and encouragement for behavior and those that exercise their beliefs to keep members "in line" (Bruhn and Fuentes, 1981).

Population: Density and Characteristics

A community's population, size, location, and surroundings can influence the potential for violence. A major metropolitan area like Los Angeles may have a density of 6000 people per square mile compared to 23,000 per square mile in New York City, but density alone does not determine violence. It is the type of high density area that determines the nature and amount of crime (Newman, 1979).

High population density communities with a *sense of cohesiveness* may have a lower crime rate than areas of similar size, which lack social and cultural groups to support unity among members. Bonds formed among church groups, clubs, and professional organizations may promote harmony rather than violence among members. Such groups allow members an opportunity to talk about stressors rather than to respond through violence. For example, residents of public housing projects often form neighborhood associations to deal with situations common to many or all residents. Tension can often be released in a productive way through projects carried out by the association.

Some high population density areas experience a community *feeling of powerlessness and helplessness* rather than one of cohesiveness. Fear and apathy may cause community residents to withdraw from social contact. Withdrawal can foster crime, since everyone assumes someone else will report suspicious behavior and all fear reprisals for such reports.

Youth often attempt to deal with feelings of powerlessness and helplessness by forming gangs. In many cities these gangs have been highly destructive, as adolescents and young adults have attempted to deal with their feelings by turning to crime against people and property to release frustration.

Other high population density areas may be characterized by a *sense of confusion* resulting in disintegration and disorganization. These areas often have a transient population who have limited physical or emotional investment in the community. Lack of community concern allows crime and violence to go unchecked and may become a norm for the area. Also, as crime increases, residents who are able to move and who desire a safer way of life will leave the area. This often reduces the capability for increasing community integration, since the residents who leave a disintegrating neighborhood are often the most capable members of the population.

The potential for violence tends to increase among highly heterogeneous populations. Differences in age, socioeconomic status, ethnicity, religion, or other cultural characteristics may lead to system stress and disrupt community stability. Highly divergent groups may neither accept nor understand one another. They may not communicate effectively, and many such groups become hostile and antagonistic toward one another. Isolation or hostile attacks can occur, thereby increasing tension and decreasing the potential for community cohesiveness and integration. Each group may see the other as different and not belonging. The alienated group may become the focal point for the other's frustrations, anger, and fears.

Community Facilities

As discussed in Chapter 17, communities differ in the resources and facilities they provide to residents. Some are far more desirable as places to live, work, and raise families. With regard to the potential for crime and violence in a community, recreational facilities, such as playgrounds, parks, swimming pools, movie theaters, tennis courts, and other areas for exercise and play, provide socially acceptable outlets for a variety of feelings, including aggression.

Spectator sports, organized by the community, such as football or hockey, also allow members of the community to vicariously express feelings of anger and frustration. However, viewing sports can often encourage a sense of violence as participants hit or shove one another or take balls or other items from participants against whom they are competing. Educational institutions such as schools and libraries also provide places and resources for constructive use of time.

Religious institutions can provide spiritual and social support as well as aid in forming a sense of community unity. While the absence of such facilities can increase the likelihood of violence, their presence alone does not prevent violence or crime. These facilities are adjuncts and resources to be used by residents for pleasure, personal enrichment, and group development. Chapter 17 provides information about community health assessment.

■   ■   ■

Familiarity with factors contributing to a community's violence or potential for violence enables community health nurses to recognize them and intervene accordingly. When factors are discovered that need correction or improvement, it is the nurse's role to work with the citizens and agencies of the community to correct or improve these deficits. The next section moves from violence in the community to violence in the family. It examines the family as a social system both influencing and influenced by the larger social system and the subsystems or individual family members.

FAMILY VIOLENCE

Society has traditionally considered the family one of the most powerful examples of social unity. The family unit in society shapes and is shaped by all the forces surrounding it. In the past, many of the behaviors and actions sanctioned within the family were severely punished by society if they occurred elsewhere. Roman law gave fathers the power of life and death over their sons. For centuries female offspring were considered parental property to be sold or forced into marriage. Once married, women became the property of their husbands.

Family violence takes many forms: it can be directed against one's child, one's spouse, elderly family members, or developmentally disabled family members.

Violence within the Family

No member of the family is guaranteed immunity from abuse and neglect. Spouse abuse, child abuse, abuse of the elderly family member, serious violence among siblings, and mutual abuse by members all occur. While these examples are not inclusive, they demonstrate the scope of family violence.

Recognizing the battered child or spouse in the emergency room is painfully simple after the fact. Unfortunately, by the time medical care is sought, serious physical and emotional damage may have been done. Community health nurses are in a key position to predict and deal with abusive tendencies. By understanding factors contributing to the development of abusive behaviors the nurse can identify abuse-prone families.

Families differ in their degree of effectiveness as a system. Effective families are able to promote the growth and development of members while maintaining cohesion as an identifiable system (Taylor, 1982). An effective family is not necessarily free from problems but rather has developed a structure and method of functioning that allows it to deal with problems as they arise. Learning to be a responsible family member does not come naturally to all people. Most people receive minimal, if any, preparation for parenthood. They therefore repeat the patterns learned in their own family. In many instances, patterns of family interaction are passed from one generation to another, leading to ineffective family members who are unable to handle stress, frustration, and anger constructively. Family stress may be manifested by the entire system, with overt tension and hostility among members, or may be directed primarily toward one member.

Development of Abusive Patterns

Several factors characterize people who become involved in family violence, including the way in which individual members were raised, the unique characteristics of members, and/or a crisis.

Previous Exposure to Violence

Of all the factors that characterize the background of abusers, the most predictably present is previous exposure to some form of violence. Past episodes of family violence are almost universal in the history of abusers. As children, abusers were often beaten themselves or witnessed the beating of siblings or a parent. Children raised in this fashion may abhor the use of violence, but they have had no experience with other models of family relationships.

Abused children learn early which behaviors lead to abuse and which do not. Typically they relate to their parents in either of the following two ways or in a combination of the two. Compliance is one pattern whereby the child learns what the parent expects and behaves accordingly. This type of child begins at an early age to take care of the parents, such as by bringing them coffee, cigarettes, and so on (Scharer, 1979). Other children learn that they only get attention when they are being noncompliant, so they provoke abuse to avoid being totally ignored. They seem to feel that any attention is better than no attention.

People who become abusers learn parenting skills from dysfunctional role models. Their parents may have set unrealistic goals, and when the children failed to perform accordingly, they were criticized, demeaned, and punished and affection was often withheld. The children were told how to act, what to do, and how to feel, thereby discouraging the development of autonomy, problem-solving skills, and creativity (Scharer, 1979). Children raised in this fashion grow up feeling unloved and worthless and may want a child of their own so they will feel assured of someone's love.

To protect themselves from feelings of worthlessness and fear of rejection, these children form a protective shell and increasingly grow hostile and distrustful of others. The behavior of potential abusers reflects a low tolerance for frustration, emotional instability, and the onset of aggressive feelings with minimal provocation. Because of their emotional insecurity, they often depend on a child or spouse for meeting their needs so that they may be valued and feel secure. When their needs are not met by others, they become overly critical. Critical, resentful behavior and unrealistic expectations of others lead to a vicious cycle. The more critical these people become, the more they are rejected by and alienated from others.

Abuse-prone people are emotionally labile, often adopting behaviors that reflect a belief that nothing in life is stable or permanent. Aggression is their primary mode of responding to others, since they only know one way of dealing with internalized resentment, fear, and anger. Lacking personal acceptance, abuse-prone people are suspicious of others and question overtures of kindness as well as authority. Almost predictably, abuse-prone people marry one another, and neither partner knows how to relate in a mature fashion to the spouse.

Characteristics of Abusers

Certain traits characterize abusers and the families in which they were raised. Many abusers were previously regarded as "problem children" in their families. Often they were labeled as special or unwanted because of a birth defect, feeding problem, or developmental handicap or delay.

Many abusers were socially isolated because of family mobility. Abusive parents often feel guilty for being unable to cope smoothly with the needs of an exceptional child, and they deal with their feelings of guilt, frustration, embarrassment, or helplessness with violence.

Perceived or Actual Crisis

A perceived or actual crisis typically precedes the onset of an abusive episode. Abuse-prone people generally are not adept at problem solving; even a small crisis can seem overwhelming. Since crisis reinforces feelings of inadequacy and low self-esteem, it is often the number of events occurring in a short time span that precipitates abusive patterns. Factors such as unemployment, strains in the marriage, or an unplanned pregnancy may set off violence.

Mobility also constitutes a precipitating stimulus, since frequent moves disrupt social support systems and tend to isolate people, at least briefly. For the abuse-prone family the difficulty of mobility is keen in that they do not readily seek out new relationships, which means that they only have the family to turn to for support. Resources may be unfamiliar to them because of the location, name, or inaccessibility of the resources. They are alone in a new place and cannot find resources, yet they hesitate to ask for help.

Crowded living conditions may precipitate abuse. The presence of numerous people in a small space tends to heighten tensions and to reduce the possibility of any privacy. Tempers flare because of the constant stimulation from others.

VIOLENCE AGAINST INDIVIDUALS OR ONESELF

The potential for violence against individuals (e.g., murder, robbery, rape and assault) or oneself (e.g., suicide) is directly related to the level of violence in the community. Persons living in areas of high crime and violence are more likely to become victims than those in more peaceful areas. Identification and correction of factors affecting the rates of community violence (violence against individuals) is one way of reducing violence against the family.

First, persons can take measures to reduce their vulnerability to violence by improving the physical security of their home and learning personal defense measures. Community health nurses can encourage people to keep windows and doors locked, trim shrubs around their home, and keep lights on during high crime periods. Many neighborhoods organize crime watch programs and post signs to the effect, as well as signs indicating that certain homes will assist children who need help; these homes are identified by the sign of a hand, usually posted in a window. Other neighbors informally agree to monitor one another's property and safety. Also, many law enforcement agencies evaluate homes for security and teach individual or neighborhood safety programs. Individuals install home security systems, participate in personal defense programs such as judo or karate, and purchase firearms for their protection. The method of protection chosen should be carefully evaluated and meet the family's needs and abilities. Personal defense methods and owing firearms can be dangerous if proper instruction is not included.

Homicide

Homicide is a term that includes any violent death that is neither a suicide nor an accident. Homicide includes deaths cause by murder, nonnegligent manslaughter, justifiable homicide (self-defense), and legal executions. In 1980 there were over 22,500 homicides in the United States (Statistical Abstracts, 1982). Of all homicides, murder is by far the most common. During 1980 there were nearly 22,000 murders committed (Statistical Abstracts, 1981). Hanlon and Pickett (1979) point out that murder represents only a small fraction of all homicides; 80% of all homicides are committed to resolve a conflict and are not premeditated. Often individual's inability to deal with a minor conflict develops into an intense emotional response, leading to the homicidal act. Abuse-prone individuals are at risk for homicidal acts because of their inability to deal with stressful situations in nonviolent ways. .

Rape

Currently rape is one of the most underreported yet fastest growing forms of human abuse in the United States. The rate of occurrence of this crime is rising annually. In 1970 there were over 37,000 cases of reported rape (Uniform Crime Reports, 1970) compared to 75,989 reported cases in 1979 and 82,088 in 1980 (Uniform Crime Reports, 1980).

Since many rapes are not reported because of fear of retaliation, public ridicule, and guilt about having somehow provoked the attack, the actual incidence is many times higher than reported.

For reported rapes, cities constitute higher risk areas than rural settings, and the hours between 8 PM and 2 AM, on weekends, and during the summer are the most critical times. In about one half of the rapes the victim and offender meet on the street, while in the remaining attacks the rapist either gains entry to the victim's home or somehow entices or forces the victim to accompany him.

Primary, secondary, and tertiary preventions are needed. Specifically, primary prevention refers to averting the occurrence of rape; secondary involves early treatment to prevent complications; and tertiary prevention is aimed at stopping the progression of the results of the initial health problem.

Primary prevention of rape includes providing information about the dangers involved in going places with strangers, avoiding high risk locations, and safeguarding one's home against possible entry. Primary prevention of rape, as in other forms of human abuse, requires a broad-based community focus for educating both the community as a whole and key groups such as police, health care providers, educators, and social workers. Public awareness is directed toward increasing knowledge about rape, raising questions about beliefs and attitudes about victims, and discussing and developing intervention alternatives.

Secondary prevention for rape victims begins with an understanding of the commonly accepted dynamics. Rape is generally more an aggressive than a sexual activity. The underlying issues are more often hostility, power, or control than sexual desire, with the defining issue being lack of consent of the victim. The danger that accompanies rape is keen; often, resisting victims are hit, kicked, or stabbed. Although the act of rape is sexual, it is the violence that traumatizes the victim because of the fear to her life, helplessness, lack of control, vulnerability, and experience of being the living target for someone's wrath.

People react to rape differently, depending on their personality, past experiences and background, and support received after the trauma. Some victims cry, shout, or discuss the experience, while others withdraw and fear discussing the attack. During the immediate as well as the follow-up stages, victims need to talk about what happened and to express their feelings and fears in a nonjudgmental atmosphere. No matter what people think or feel, they are entitled to these views. Therefore nonjudgmental listening is an essential nursing measure.

In any psychological trauma the right to privacy and confidentiality is of the utmost importance. Victims should not be expected to answer questions in an area where others can hear them. Nurses are responsible for providing continuous care once the victim enters the health care system, including monitoring the actions of other workers who may be less sensitive to the psychological needs of the victim (Dietz, 1978).

Since rape is a situational crisis for which advance preparation is rarely possible, nursing efforts are directed toward helping victims maximize their ability to cope with the stress and disruption of their lives caused by the attack. Counseling is oriented to the present, focusing on the crisis and the concomitant fears, feelings, and issues involved. The goal is to help the victim use problem-solving skills to develop ways to regroup personal forces. Counseling includes assessing the appropriateness of the reaction to the event. Is the person distorting reality? Is the anxiety level so high that it interferes with coping and problem solving? How much has this crisis affected the person's daily life?

The next major area to assess is the nature, availability, and quality of the victim's support system. It is important to determine if family and friends are part of the support network or whether they hold the victim somehow responsible for the crisis. Whom has the victim told about the experience? The victim of rape may need assistance in talking with and asking for support from family and friends because of fear of rejection, anxiety, or guilt.

Five key areas that are crucial nursing interventions include the following:

1. Avoid viewing the woman as a victim and begin to think of her as a client. In a crime such as rape people often have difficulty moving out of a victim role and seeing themselves as coping, capable people. The crime has been committed; the person must reorganize personal resources and learn new ways of adapting.

2. Help the individual confront the reality of the crisis and deal with the attendant feelings. The emotional wound, just like a cut or burn, cannot heal until it has been cleaned. The emotions must be opened up, cleaned out, and treated.

3. Assist the person to confront the crisis one step at a time. Problem solving, reorganizing emotional resources, and planning new coping strategies take time and should be attacked one at a time.

4. Help the person gain an understanding of the crisis. Often people who experience a situational crisis will ask "why me?" Such questions may indicate a cause-and-effect kind of reasoning where the person keeps saying "If only I had (not) done_____, this would not have happened." If the woman used poor judgment before the rape, such as leaving a bar with a stranger or walking down a dark street, help her examine alternative behavior for the future, while reinforcing that her behavior did not justify the violence brought against her.

5. Examine alternative actions for coping with current situations. One residual effect of situational crises is to reduce the victim's ability for dealing with daily occurrences and problems. When this happens, these people need to turn to their sources of support and evaluate alternatives while mobilizing their resources and relearning previous coping abilities.

The activities of the secondary prevention phase often continue into the phase of *tertiary prevention*, when rape victims are helped to deal with the crisis of rape so their lives are not emotionally scarred for the future. Just as during secondary prevention, victims must be reminded that they may have delayed reactions to the rape. They need to recognize that they are not emotionally decompensating but rather their phobias, nightmares, or increased motor activity (reflected in moving, taking trips, or frequently changing telephone numbers) are reactions to a crisis. Many rape victims need follow-up mental health services to help them cope with the long-term effects of the crisis. They may be hesitant to ask for help or follow through on these services, so community health nurses must not only make appropriate referrals but also take the initiative in calling the victim to check on her and remind her of appointments. Rape victims need support, encouragement, and acceptance from those with whom they come in contact.

Suicide

Suicide can be viewed in much the same way as homicide with relation to the abuse-prone individual. Not only can suicide be a means of escape for the abused family member but also for the abuser as well. Suicide ranks as the second leading cause of death among persons 15 to 45 years of age in the eight most industrialized countries of the world (Hanlon and Pickett, 1979). For the victim of abusive behavior the pain, humiliation, and despair created by an inability to get away from the abusive environment may be too much to bear. For these individuals homicide may be unthinkable, but they may be capable of turning their anger and frustration inward, leading to self-destructive acts. At the same time the abuse-prone individual may find his uncontrollable violence too great a burden to tolerate, and being unable to seek help, he chooses to commit suicide rather than repeat the abusive patterns.

The leading factors associated with suicidal attempts are listed by Hanlon and Pickett (1979) as broken homes or frequent moves during childhood, marital disharmony, emotional immaturity, cruelty to children, and jealousy bordering on the pathological. One can clearly see how the abuse-prone family could have one or more of these factors present in their lives.

Behavioral Indicators of Potential Abusive Parents

The following characteristics, while not inclusive or definitive indicators of abuse, do comprise warning signs in couples expecting a child that abuse may be present or may occur at some future time.

1. Denial of the reality of the pregnancy as evidenced by a refusal to talk about the impending birth or to think of a name for the child.
2. An obvious concern or fear that the baby will not meet some predetermined standard: sex, hair color, temperament, or resemblance to family members.
3. Failure to follow through on the desire for or seeking of an abortion.
4. An initial decision to place the child for adoption and a change of mind.
5. Rejection of the mother by the father of the baby.
6. Family beset by stress and numerous crises, so that the birth of a child may be the "straw that broke the camel's back."
7. Initial and unresolved negative feelings about having a child.
8. Lack of support for the new parents.
9. Isolation from friends, neighbors, or family.
10. Parental evidence of poor impulse control or fear of losing control.
11. Contradictory history.
12. Appearance of detachment.
13. Appearance of misusing drugs or alcohol.
14. Shopping for hospitals or health care providers.
15. Unrealistic expectations of the child.

FAMILY ABUSE

There are many factors that may precipitate an abusive episode. Community health nurses may be able to predict a potential abusive episode and refer the person to a social or health care agency. The box on the next page summarizes behavioral indicators of potentially abusive parents. Many of these characteristics pertain to all aspects of family abuse, specific types of which are discussed later.

Child Abuse

The presence of child abuse signifies ineffective family functioning. Abusive parents who recognize their problem are often reluctant to seek assistance because of the stigma attached to being considered a child abuser. Child abuse ranges from violent, physical attacks, resulting in severe injury, to passive neglect, resulting in insidious malnutrition or other problems. It is not limited to physical maltreatment but includes emotional abuse such as yelling at or continually demeaning and criticizing the child.

Children are frequent victims of abuse because they are small and relatively powerless in the family hierarchy. In many families only one child is subjected to abuse. Parents may identify with this particular child or the child may have certain qualities, such as looking like a relative, being handicapped, or being particularly

bright and capable, that provoke the parent.

Reliable statistics are not available to clearly depict the extent of child abuse. However, it is known that the highest fatality rate occurs in children under 3 years—children who are too young to explain their cuts, bruises, and fractures (Hanlon and Pickett, 1979). The box above depicts behavioral indicators of potentially abusive parents. These indicators do not show the pain and often poor emotional stability of the parents. As described in the previous section on family patterns supportive of violence, abusive parents are typically emotionally impoverished people with many unmet needs and poor impulse control (Taylor, 1982).

It is essential that community health nursing recognize the physical and behavioral indicators of abuse and neglect. The box on the next page summarizes indicators of physical abuse, physical neglect, sexual abuse, and emotional maltreatment. The sections that follow describe additional characteristics of child abuse.

Child neglect in general can be divided into two categories: physical and emotional. Physical neglect is defined as failure to provide adequate food, proper clothing, shelter, hygiene, or necessary medical care (Leaman, 1979). The child is not valued to the extent that even basic requirements for successful adaptation are met. In contrast, emotional neglect is the omission of

---

Factors That May Indicate Presence or Potential for Abuse

The following characteristics, while not inclusive of all possible behaviors leading to abusive patterns, serve as cues that abuse may be present or could occur at some future time.

Abuse should be investigated when the child:

1. Has an unexplained injury
   a. Skin: burns, old or recent scars, ecchymosis, soft tissue swelling, human bites
   b. Fractures: recent or ones that have healed
   c. Subdural hematomas
   d. Trauma to genitals
   e. Whiplash (caused by shaking small children)
2. Seems dehydrated or malnourished without obvious cause
3. Is given inappropriate food or drugs (alcohol, tobacco, medication prescribed for someone else, foods not appropriate for the child's age)
4. Shows evidence of general poor care: poor hygiene, dirty clothes, unkempt hair, dirty nails
5. Is unusually fearful of nurse and others
6. Is considered to be a "bad" child
7. Is not dressed appropriately to the season or weather conditions
8. Reports or shows evidence of sexual abuse
9. Has injuries not mentioned in history
10. Seems to need to take care of the parent and speak for the parent

---

basic nurturing, acceptance, and caring essential for healthy personal development. These children are largely ignored or in many cases treated as nonpersons. Such neglect usually affects the development of self-esteem in that it is difficult for a neglected child to feel a great deal of self-worth because no one ever seems to care. Neglect is much more difficult to assess and evaluate than abuse because it is more subtle and may go unnoticed. Astute observations of children, their homes, and the way in which they relate to their care givers can provide clues of neglect.

Physical abuse refers to one or more episodes of extreme disciplining or displaced aggression or frustration often resulting in serious physical damage to the internal organs, bones, central nervous system, or sense organs. This form of abuse is most often seen in episodes of beating, burning, kicking, branding, or shaking the child.

Emotional abuse includes extreme debasement of a child's feelings so that the child feels inadequate, inept, uncared for, and worthless. Examples are constant criticism and ridiculing directed toward some children who ultimately may believe themselves to be "bad" people. Victims of emotional abuse learn to hold in their feelings to avoid incurring additional scorn. Repressing feelings can lead to symptoms of hyperactivity, withdrawal, overeating, psychosomatic dermatological problems, vague and often difficult-to-pinpoint complaints, stuttering, truancy, or general hostility and aggression toward others or themselves.

Sexual abuse ranges from fondling to rape. A particularly destructive form of sexual abuse, incest, deserves attention because of the nature and magnitude of the problem. Incest is not limited to "backwoods" people but occurs in all races, religious groups, and socioeconomic classes. Incest is receiving greater attention because of mandatory reporting laws, yet all too often its incidence remains a family secret. Victims of incest are unprotected, unsupported, and often made to feel responsible. Even when the experience is not at the time especially frightening to the child, conflicts often develop later. Sexual abuse robs children of control over their own bodies and emphasizes their vulnerability.

While the long-range effects of incest are unknown, it is believed that this behavior is as devastating for males as for females. Additionally, there is a disproportionate representation among clients in psychiatric hospitals of people who were sexually abused as children. Incest seems to cause later difficulty in the maintenance of healthy adult relationships. According to Rubinelli (1980) as many as three fourths of prostitutes may have been victims of incest. Frequently incest victims are hindered in dealing with this situation because health professionals are uncomfortable with the topic and do not encourage its discussion. To detect incest and provide victims an opportunity to deal with their feelings, community health nurses can ask questions that convey that the speaker will both be heard and helped.

Spouse Abuse

Spouse abuse is an increasing social problem requiring the attention of nurses and other health care professionals. Only recently has this phenomenon been openly talked about; in the past, spouse abuse was often considered a family secret. Spouse abuse is defined as any physical attack by one marital partner against another, ranging from a slap to homicide. Although spouse abuse usually refers to instances in which husbands behave in a violent way toward wives, it must be remembered that wives do abuse husbands. Wives emotionally and physically strike out at their husbands and leave scars on the mind and body which are difficult to heal. Although this discussion focuses on battered women, a more common occurrence than battered husbands, many of the dynamics apply to either situation.

Spouse abuse is not only a physical act but also is seen in the emotional abuse of another adult. Emotional abuse takes many forms, but it is often seen is the overly critical attitude of a spouse in which the marital partner, seemingly, does nothing right. Criticism is demeaning and tends to lower the self-esteem of the one who is criticized. Emotional abuse occurs also when a person is hampered in accomplishments in accordance with innate potential by the limits and restrictions of another. For example, spouses often demand that the marital partner not do something, like go to school or secure a job; a husband may fear that his wife will intellectually or socially surpass him if she gets a college education or finds a satisfactory job. Likewise, a wife may limit her husband's potential by complaining when the husband is away from home on business trips or to pursue a degree.

Battered women often have bruises, lacerations, and broken bones. Similar to families with a history of child abuse a large portion of spouse abuse victims and victimizers have a violent family history. Interviews with battered women indicate the batterer comes from all socioeconomic levels and professions. Batterers are typically described as moody, angry, impulsive, tense, suspicious, and resentful (Weingourt, 1979).

Many battered women have low self-esteem and a general sense of worthlessness. They often remain in a fear-filled marriage for reasons such as an innate cultural or religious belief that it is the woman's role to make the marriage a success. To admit that they are battered is to admit failure as a wife. Other women use the rationalization of "'oh-but-he-needs-me', how can I desert him?" (Weingourt, 1979). The woman thus sees herself as worthy only when she is taking care of a dependent, needy man. The sicker he gets, the more he needs her; hence her basic human worth is validated by remaining in this pathological marriage.

In a study of 150 battered women, Roy (1977) documented the [seven] highest priority factors that kept the women in their marriages. In order of importance these reasons were (1) hope that the husband would reform, (2) feelings of no place to go, (3) fear of reprisals from the husband, (4) children making it difficult to find an alternative place to live, (5) financial problems because of unemployment and lack of money, (6) fear of living alone, and (7) belief that divorce is a shameful state.

Women often experience animosity from parents, friends, neighbors, the police, and health care providers when they openly acknowledge that they cannot keep their own house in order. To avoid society's reaction to being battered, women may hide injuries by staying at home until bruises and scratches heal or by wearing concealing clothing. Because of unpredictable reactions, battered women may hesitate to discuss how their injuries occurred.

Battering is often evidenced in physical signs such as bruises, lacerations, or broken bones. A swollen face, reddened hands, and bruises and cuts on the legs are key signs. Frequently the injuries are carefully inflicted on those parts of the body which can easily be disguised by concealing clothing, such as the abdomen, upper thigh, and back.

It is important to recognize that spouse abuse often accompanies child abuse (Hendrix, 1981). Van Stolk (1976) contends that many women are beaten along with their children or are beaten when they try to shield their children from injuries. Beating a pregnant woman may reflect the man's desire to terminate the pregnancy and thereby relieve him of the impending burden of another dependent. Some batterers are emotionally disturbed and unable to recognize the consequences of their actions. This lack of awareness may result from mental illness or the influence of drugs or alcohol.

Prince (1981) described a three-phase cycle often present in spouse abuse. During the first phase, *tension building*, the victim tries to calm the abuser by being compliant, nurturing, and generally nonoffensive. Despite the presence of complaint behavior, *battering* may ensue, motivated by rage as the abuser punishes the woman for "misbehavior." Severe injury or death can occur during this second phase. During the third phase, however, the batterer is *apologetic* and contrite, even attempting to convince the victim that the out-of-control episode will not be repeated. Often victims are misled by this behavior, especially since they are trying to convince themselves that "things will work out and we'll live happily ever after." The hopes and dreams of the past for a happy, loving relationship tend to overshadow the reality of recent behavior and reinforce the continuation of the relationship.

It is important to understand this cyclical pattern so as to curb the impatience felt toward women who are reluctant or unwilling to remove themselves from such a harmful situation. If abuse is suspected, the person should be asked directly about such a possibility. Because of shame and fear, women are hesitant to volunteer such information, but they often feel relieved to discuss their fears and life realities. Women are often defensive and apologetic about their spouse's behavior. A listening, nonjudgmental approach is useful in encouraging a description of past events and planning for the future.

Victims of abuse are often reluctant to leave the familiar, abusive situations because they do not envision themselves as having options. Although they may keenly fear for their safety, at least their present life-style is familiar. In providing care for these women, community health nurses should help them identify and set priorities for their alternatives. Individual or marriage counseling may help some, while others must leave the abusive situation and begin a new life. It is not uncommon for women to simply refuse to do anything, besides worry about the future. When this occurs, the most useful preventive effort is to assist the woman to plan ahead by considering what the quickest escape route is if violence erupts. Where could she go? Who could she call? The most critical step is for the woman to regain some mastery over her life. She must plan ways to take care of herself in the event that the battering recurs. These plans must include income, shelter, legal aid, and child care.

Abuse of the Elderly

Abuse of the elderly seems to be more prevalent than reported cases would indicate. Abuse of the elderly includes neglect as well as physical or psychological assault. The elderly are neglected and abused when others fail to provide adequate food, clothing, shelter, and physical care and to meet physiological and safety needs.

Roughness in handling elderly people can lead to bruises and bleeding into tissue because of the fragility of their skin and vascular systems. It is often difficult to determine if the injuries of the elderly result from abuse, falls, or other natural causes. Careful assessment both through observation and discussion assists in determining the cause of injuries. Other ways in which the elderly are physically abused occur when caretakers impose unrealistic toileting demands, as well as when the special needs and previous patterns of the elderly person are ignored.

The elderly are also abused with regard to nutrition. They may be given food that they cannot chew or swallow or that is contraindicated because of dietary restric-

tions. Care givers may overlook food preferences or social or cultural beliefs and patterns about food. Elderly people may become undernourished if they can neither prepare their own food nor eat that prepared for them.

Care givers occasionally give elderly people medication to induce confusion or drowsiness so they will be less troublesome, need less care, or allow others to gain control of their financial and personal resources. Once medicated, the elderly have few means to act in their own behalf.

The most common form of psychological abuse is rejection or simply ignoring elderly people, conveying that they are worthless and useless to others. On incorporating these feelings into their self-view the elderly regress and become increasingly dependent on others, who tend to resent the imposition and demands on their time and life-style. The pattern becomes cyclical: the more regressed the person becomes, the greater the dependency, and so on. Further, the elderly people's past accomplishments and present abilities are not consistently acknowledged, causing them to feel less capable than they may actually be.

Care givers abuse elderly people for a variety of reasons. The elderly family member may impose a physical, emotional, or financial burden on the care giver, leading to frustration and resentment. The abuser may be reversing earlier family patterns, whereby the abuser was previously abused by the elderly person (Elder Abuse, 1980).

Elderly people need to retain as much autonomy and decision-making ability as possible. Community health nurses have multiple avenues for detecting abuse among the elderly and have skills and responsibility for finding cases, giving treatment, or making referral. Many families caring for elderly members exhaust their resources and coping ability. Community health nurses can assist in finding new sources of support and aid. Block and Sinnott (1979) identified the following resources for easing stressors of both care takers and elderly people: (1) home-related services such as home aides, medical and/or nursing care, meal delivery service, home repair, and home visits; (2) monetary assistance; (3) day-care and respite day-care centers; (4) transportation services; (5) counseling and other mental health services; and (6) educational programs focusing on the care of the aged.

Abuse of Developmentally Disabled People

Many of the same aspects of child abuse apply to abuse of developmentally disabled people. The term *developmental disabilities* refers to a variety of mental and physical impairments that interfere with an individual's ability to function in an acceptable manner in society because of limitations in the ability to care for oneself, learn, speak, or accomplish other self-care. Several unique characteristics cause this group to be at a high risk for abusive treatment. For example, developmentally disabled people tend to require more attention and supervision than their normal counterparts, which may increase care-giver frustration because of the seemingly never-ending needs and demands. Parents may perceive themselves as trapped with responsibility and feel resentment, anger, and guilt toward their developmentally disabled children.

In addition, these children often fail to live up to the hopes and expectations of their parents. With normal children, parental self-esteem tends to increase because of the accomplishments of their children. Children with developmental delays may not enhance parental status and esteem because their achievements are limited and not comparable to those of normal children.

Infants who begin life by being premature or having mental or physical deficits are especially vulnerable to abuse by both parents and care givers (Sandgrund et al., 1974). These children are viewed as sickly, demanding, and in general "problem children." Their care is expensive in both energy and time; because of the differences from other children, parents tend to worry about their ability to provide adequate care. Also, these children are often less responsive or respond negatively to attention provided, causing care givers to feel insecure in their abilities. As parents become insecure and frustrated and feel inept in eliciting the normal responses of smiling, cooing, and so on, they may be tempted either to ignore the child or strike out physically.

Interventions by community health nurses working with families with a developmentally disabled member are similar to those mentioned for child abuse (p. 460). Community services to assist families in dealing with the stress and crisis associated with the child's handicap and referral to agencies able to assist with education and child care are key ingredients of nursing action. Families may need to learn how to seek outside diversions to provide them strength to cope with their life situation. Homemaker services, day-care, or sitters may be realistic aids for many of these families. Chapter 30 presents additional information about this group.

NURSING ACTIONS IN ABUSE CASES

Community health nurses are in a key position to identify abuse victims in homes, schools, clinics, work settings, and many other places. In the preceding sections, specific types of abuse were discussed. The actions taken by nurses are determined by many factors, including the nature and extent of the abuse, the interest and willingness of the victim and abuser to learn new ways of behaving, the resources available for referral, and the nurses' own ability to predict, recognize, and intervene in abusive situations.

As mentioned, several types of abuse, especially those involving neglect and emotional abuse in contrast to physical abuse, are often difficult to detect. Victims may not realize they are being abused but rather think that the demeaning or neglectful treatment is all that can be expected from others. Many hesitate to acknowledge the abuse directed toward them, fearing the abuser will seek some form of retaliation.

For the purposes of this discussion, nursing interventions directed toward all forms of abuse are combined. More commonalities than differences exist in planning interventions. Community health nurses should know about available community resources for abuse victims. Most larger cities have community resource directories available for a nominal fee. If no such directory is available, then a group of nurses can work together to compile information on what services are available for various clients' needs, who the contact person is, who will be served, and if a fee is charged.

Questions to be raised regarding services for abused people include the following: Are temporary shelters available, and if so, what population do they serve? What emergency funds, transportation, and legal aid are available? How do police and courts respond to abuse and violence? Do they show concern, empathy, and a sincere wish to help, or is the attitude accusatory, punitive, and judgmental?

If attitudes and resources are inadequate, what are the nursing implications? For example, it is often helpful to work with local radio and television stations and newspapers to provide information about the nature and extent of human abuse as a community health problem and also to acquaint people with available services and resources. Frequently people fail to seek services early in an abusive situation because they simply do not know what is available to them. Ideally a program or planned emphasis for abused people begins with a needs assessment to identify potential clients and determine how to effectively serve this group. Not only can community health nurses serve as catalysts for getting programs started and a major source of public education, but they often treat both the abused and abusers.

Preventive Measures

Consistent with public health philosophy, the direct role of the community health nurse begins with prevention. Prevention has two components. Ideally prevention militates against the onset of human abuse. However, when prevention of the occurrence of abuse has not been possible, community health nurses can initiate preventive measures to reduce or terminate further abuse.

Prevention of psychosocial problems cannot easily be documented; however, many clinicians believe that providing support and psychological enrichment to at-risk individuals and families prevents the onset of health disruption. For example, community health nurses have varied opportunities to strengthen and even teach parenting abilities. Parenting skills do not come naturally to all people. Basic skills such as diapering, feeding, quieting, and even holding and rocking a baby can comprise a class or home or clinic visit. Parents also need to learn acceptable and workable ways to discipline children so that limits are maintained without breaking the child's spirit or causing physical harm.

Mutual support groups are valuable for new parents, families with special children, or abused people themselves. Such groups have variable formats and can provide information, support, and encouragement. Nurses can help begin such groups or can actually serve as group leaders. Chapter 17 describes the role of the community health nurse in working with community groups.

Abusers generally do not like their behavior. The abuser has failed to live up to society's expectations of a good parent, good spouse, or good child. When abuse becomes apparent or even suspected, there are at least two needy people involved: one is the abused person and the other is the abuser. Scorn and disdain for abusers will further alienate them from any potential help. Nursing action needs to take into account the needs of *all* who are involved in the abusive situation. This often necessitates a careful and honest examination of personal values and beliefs. It is essential to recognize that the abuser is a needy person who behaves in a dysfunctional manner out of a multitude of needs and life frustrations. Abusers have difficulty trusting; they are frustrated, frightened people with little faith that anyone actually cares about them. The nursing role is multifaceted, including assessment, direct care to the abused person, enlistment of the abuser in a program to receive help, and implementation of broad-based community education and direct services to meet the many and varied needs of this group.

In addition, community health nurses bring to client encounters their own past experiences, attitudes, and values. As a child or young adult the nurse may have been a victim of abuse or may have had classmates, friends, or family members who were abused. The emotional investment and sheer drain of energy required for effectively working with abusers and victims of abuse cannot be disregarded. Abusers present difficult clinical challenges because of their reluctance to

seek help or to remain actively involved in the helping process.

Preventive measures are most useful when potential abusers recognize their tendency to be abusive and seek help. For children, in addition to the general measures described, there is often a need for 24-hour child protection services or care givers, where parents can take the child until the acute family or individual crisis has been resolved. Telephone crisis lines can be used to provide immediate emergency assistance to families.

Protective Measures

Nursing interventions for victims of abuse assist clients to either change the circumstances that have previously led to abuse or remove themselves from the abusive environment. Protection of victims of abuse is a primary goal of any intervention. As mentioned, not only the abused person but the abuser needs to be protected. Paying attention to only the abused person reinforces the abusive person's feelings of hopelessness, lack of trust, and belief that no one really cares.

Protective measures are called forth especially when child abuse occurs. All states have some type of child abuse reporting law. In most states the nurse suspecting a child has been abused must report the case to the authorities. Deliberate failure to report abuse cases may result in further injury or death for the child and criminal punishment for the nurse. The community health nurse needs to check local and state laws governing the definition and reporting of child abuse. Despite the fact that child abuse must be reported, some health care providers are reluctant to accept the responsibility for making the decision to report it.

Physicians and nurses often hesitate to report a suspected battered child even though they know not to do so is illegal. All state statutes provide protection from civil suit for anyone making or participating in the reporting of child abuse (Cazalas, 1978). The child's protection must be the first concern of health care providers once any emergency medical concerns have been treated. Only through proper notification of authorities can the child's protection be assured. Once the child's health and safety are provided for, measures can be started to help the family members deal with their abusive behavior.

Therapeutic Intervention

Therapeutic intervention requires a longer period of time than other types of intervention. It involves dealing with the psychological damage caused by being abusive and having been abused. Dealing with the guilt of abusing a child and developing new resources for coping with crisis are not easy tasks. Referral to community mental health or social work services is necessary and may even be required by the authorities.

The community health nurse can meet the families' therapeutic needs in a variety of ways. Besides referral to appropriate community agencies, nurses can act as role models for the family. During clinic and home visits nurses can demonstate constructive adult-child interactions. Nurses often teach mothers child care skills such as proper feeding, calming a fretful child, effective discipline, and constructive communication. Nurses not only give parents information about how to feed a child, but should go a step farther and demonstrate this skill. Parents are often frustrated when they try to feed an infant or young child who spits back most of the food. The nurse can calmly show how to offer small amounts of food, use finger foods where appropriate, and remain calm when all efforts at feeding are met with rebellion.

When nurses see families in any setting, they can demonstrate good communication skills and discipline by teaching both parents and children in a calm, respectful, and informative manner. Also, if children behave in undesirable ways, such as handling equipment destructively, the nurse can model appropriate discipline by removing the equipment from the child and redirecting the child's attention to areas or items more suitable for play. Parents watch and listen to what nurses say and do. Talking about children in their presence should be avoided; parents and children should be shown positive types of communication.

Role modeling can be used with abuse victims of all ages. When provided nursing care to abused spouses or to the elderly, nurses can demonstrate communication skills, conflict resolution, and skill training. For example, adult children often become abusive toward their parents when they become frustrated and taxed in their abilities to care for the elderly person. Nurses, during home visits, can demonstrate ways to physically and psychologically care for family members. For example, some elderly people resist having baths, having their clothes changed, taking medications, eating, or exercising. The nurse can work with care givers to assist them develop approaches that will be acceptable to the individual elderly person. No standard set of approaches applies to all people. Assessment, creativity, and critical thinking help the nurse, family, and client together devise ways of meeting client and family needs without causing undue stress and frustration. The following case study shows these factors.

Mrs. Smith, a 75-year-old bedridden woman, consistently became rude and combative when her daughter attempted to bathe and change her clothes each morning. During a home visit, the daughter told the nurse, Mrs. Jones, that she had gotten so frustrated with her mother on the previous morning that she had hit her. The daughter felt terrible about her behavior but also knew that her mother's incontinence made it essential that Mrs. Smith be kept clean.

Mrs. Jones, in taking Mrs. Smith's vital signs and examining her skin turgor, engaged Mrs. Smith in a conversation where she learned that Mrs. Smith felt stiff and seemed to have more joint pain resulting from arthritis in the mornings. By late afternoon, her joints were more flexible and less painful. Nurse, daughter, and client discussed their options and decided that the daughter would only wash her mother's anal area in the morning and put clean pads under her if indicated. Total hygienic care was scheduled for the late afternoon. By careful assessment, listening, and problem solving, early intervention served to reduce the possibility of further abuse for Mrs. Smith.

Likewise, between marital partners, abuse often occurs when people are unable to communicate with one another, when one or both partners have either poor impulse control or high levels of frustration, or when they simply know no other avenues for getting the partner's attention. Just as nurses can model communication and conflict resolution strategies for children and the elderly, they can do the same for spouses. Adults do not always speak clearly, honestly, and directly to one another. People give mixed or confused messages, then wonder why the listener misunderstood them. Often nurses can refer potential or actual abusers and victims to community mental health centers, family service centers, or private practice counselors.

Tools for Working with Abusive Persons

Scharer (1979) applies the six subroles of nursing originally described by Peplau (1952) as tools for working with abusive persons. These subroles apply to abusive situations regardless of the age of the victim. Abusers often fear they will be condemned for their actions, so it is often difficult to make and maintain contact with abusive families. Although community health nurses convey an attitude of caring and concern for them, families may doubt the sincerity of this concern. They may avoid being home at the scheduled visit time out of fear of the consequences of the visit or an inability to believe that anyone really wants to help them. If the victim is a child, parents may fear that the nurse will try to remove the child.

The subroles mentioned earlier to help nurses deal with abuse situations are as follows: mother-surrogate, managerial, technical, teacher, counselor, and socializing. These subroles do not necessarily occur in a sequential or hierarchical order. More than one subrole may occur simultaneously, or they may occur in random order. For example, the sixth subrole, socializing, may be the first one incorporated in the nurse-client interaction.

Mother-surrogate, the first subrole, is used in developing the nurse-client relationship and continues to some degree throughout the duration of the relationship. To convince the family that the nurse really wants to help them, the initial focus should be on the needs of the abusers. By responding first to their difficulties and conflicts, nurses convey an understanding, nonjudgmental attitude. Generally abusers do not want to hurt their victims, and when abuse is discovered, they often feel ashamed of their actions. When nurses convey willingness to listen to the fears, conflicts, and pain of the abuser, a trusting relationship often develops. This interaction may represent the first time someone has devoted time, concern, and energy to listening to the abuser's fears and concerns. Frequently abusers strike out in times of intense frustration. They lose control of their own actions and are later appalled by what they have done.

As a mother-surrogate the nurse teaches basic parenting or adult-to-adult interaction and care-giving skills. Often both abusers and victims need assistance in locating community resources where they can learn skills such as shopping, budgeting, meal preparation, and ways to manage stress, be assertive, or seek a job.

Care givers, especially those caring for children, handicapped people, or the elderly, may need to learn age-appropriate expectations. It is unreasonable to expect a 14-month-old to have moral judgment and be able to differentiate between what is right and wrong. Children at this age do not deliberately annoy care givers by breaking delicate pieces of china. Nor do they set out to spill things; toddlers and young children simply do not always have fine motor coordination. Likewise, a person with poor sphincter control does not willingly soil clothes or bedding. Care givers must learn to deal with their frustrations when soiling occurs and take appropriate preventive measures, such as using thick underwear or bed padding.

Additionally, families do not always know how to have fun. Nurses can assess how much recreation and opportunities for tension release are integrated into the family's life-style. Through community assessment the nurse will know what resources and facilities are available and how much they cost. Families may need counseling about the value of recreation and play in reducing tension and appropriately channelling aggressive impulses.

In the *managerial subrole* the nurse organizes and coordinates activities with the family. Examples include helping the family to schedule and arrange clinic appointments, transportation, and babysitters; to find job training programs; to explore career choices and op-

portunities and pursue them; or to establish linkages with neighbors or social agencies. Nurses should avoid doing for families what they can do for themselves because this can call forth old memories of dependency and lack of autonomy. Doing for other people what they are capable of doing for themselves is not growth producing. Families and community health nurses should jointly plan ways to increase the family's responsibility for their own well-being.

The use of the *technical subrole* depends on family needs and abilities. For example, if abuse has caused injuries, the nurse may need to teach basic skills such as dressing changes, cast care, or vital sign monitoring. Although this role is usually minimal, the nurse does assess the family's care-giving and person care skills. If a handicapped or elderly person was abused when the care giver tried to provide physical care, the care giver may not have the technical competence to perform necessary skills. In such an instance the nurse should teach the skill and provide an opportunity for the care giver to practice it with supervision and feedback as to the accuracy of the performance.

The *teacher subrole,* like the technical, also includes many traditional nursing actions, such as role modeling, anticipatory guidance, and health education. It is important not to overwork this role, since abusers are often told what they should do. Giving advice should be avoided, since this may undermine the person's ability to be responsible and make informed choices while living with the consequences of the decisions. The teacher subrole includes careful listening to problems and concerns, helping people clarify their needs, and helping to examine possible solutions and alternatives for action (Scharer, 1979).

For example, if a mother were unable to discipline her son without resorting to abuse, the nurse could listen carefully to the mother's recounting of an example where discipline failed. Together they could examine the past situation and determine what other actions the mother could have tried. If the 2-year-old broke a favorite vase and the mother spanked the child, finding that her rage increased as the spanking continued, the nurse and mother might consider other forms of discipline. Restricting the environment so the child does not come into contact with valuable items would be an alternative to spanking. The mother might send the child to a quiet place for 10 minutes instead of spanking him, or breakable items might be eliminated from the environment until the child has better impulse control.

The *counselor subrole* comes into play once a trusting relationship has been established. In this subrole the nurse helps abusers explore feelings and look at alternative ways of coping. For example, if adults are involved in marital conflicts, the nurse helps them explore feelings, decide what is expected from one another, identify how the spouse's behavior differs from the expected, describe previous responses to one another, and determine less destructive ways to respond.

Socializing is the sixth and final subrole. It is evidenced by focusing on abusers as people, such as by providing them with opportunities to talk about their interests or what they have been doing that has been enjoyable. Abusers may be inept at social skills; they may profit from opportunities to practice socializing in a safe environment. This does not mean that nurses merely chat with clients, but after determination that a client or family lacks social skills, the nurse systematically engages the client in such interaction. This stage of the nurse-client relationship may occur quite early and increase comfort and trust among participants.

Child Abuse

Therapeutic intervention in child abuse also includes the children. The nurse must assess the child's physical and mental status during visits. Studies by Jones (1977) have found that abused children are at a higher risk for damage to the central nervous system and maldevelopment of ego function. Reports of mental retardation, learning disorders, perceptual-motor dysfunction, cerebral palsy, impaired speech and language, growth failure, and emotional disturbances have been documented in abused children. Any of these would require referral and further evaluation or treatment. It is important to remember that early treatment of emotional problems in abused children may have significant impact on breaking the intergenerational cycle of abuse (Kinard, 1980).

■   ■   ■

Intervention in human abuse requires a multidisciplined and coordinated team approach, since many facets of human existence are involved. Often the nurse serves as the coordinator of the team and ensures that appropriate disciplines are included in the plan of care.

SUMMARY

The potential for human abuse and neglect is acquired over many years and stems from a multitude of factors, including societal influences, family history, behavioral characteristics of both the abuser and the abused, and a number of specific precipitating events. Community violence is also influenced by many factors such as unemployment, dysfunctional community interactions, and lack of cultural activities. Increasing attention is being focused on these age-old problems as varying groups seek to establish a safe environment to live and work in. Women, children, and the elderly are

no longer content to be considered the property of others. All people have rights, including being able to live without abuse directed toward them. Because of the stigma attached to the occurrence of human violence, there has historically been poor reporting mechanisms, yet the occurrence seems significant and also increasing in the face of rapidly changing events and social conditions.

Community health nurses must play a key role in prevention, early detection, and prompt intervention. Helping people learn parenting skills as well as ways to care for their elderly relatives are only two examples of prevention. It is erroneous to assume that everyone knows about the normal childhood milestones or the changes that typically occur with aging. Prevention of abuse and violence is the most critical task for community health nurses.

BIBLIOGRAPHY

Allen, J.: Violence in the family, Fam. Community Health **4**(2):19-33, 1981.

Block, M., and Sinnott, J., editors: The battered elderly syndrome: an exploratory study, College Park, Md., 1979, University of Maryland Press.

Bruhn, J., and Fuentes, R.: Child Abuse: a societal paradox, 1981, Unpublished data.

Cazalas, M.: Nursing and the law, Germantown, Md., 1978, Aspen Systems Corp.

Dietz, P.: Social factors in rapist behavior. In Roda, R., editor: Clinical aspects of the rapist, New York, 1978, Grune & Stratton, Inc.

Elder abuse, Washington, D.C., 1980, National ClearingHouse on Aging.

Freud, S.: Civilization and its discontents. In Strachey, J., editor: The complete psychological works of Sigmund Freud, London, 1955, Hogarth Press, Ltd.

Hanlon, J., and Pickett, G. : Public health administration and practice, ed. 8, St. Louis, 1983, The C.V. Mosby Co.

Helfer, R., and Kempe, C.: Child abuse and neglect: the family and community, Cambridge, Mass., 1976, Harvard University Press.

Hendrix, M.: Home is where the hell is, Fam. Community Health **4**:(2)53-59, 1981.

Jones, C.: The fate of abused children. In Franklin, A., editor: The challenge of child abuse, New York, 1977, Academic Press, Inc.

Kinard, E.: Mental health needs of abused children, Child Welfare **59**(8):451-462, 1980.

Leaman, J.: Recognizing the abused child, Nurs. '79 **9**(2):65-67, 1979.

Newman, G.: Understanding violence, New York, 1979, J.B. Lippincott Co.

Peplau, H.: Interpersonal relations in nursing, New York, 1952, G.P. Putnam's Sons.

Prince, J.: A systems approach to spouse abuse. In Lancaster, J.: Community mental health nursing: an ecological perspective, St. Louis, 1981, The C.V. Mosby Co.

Roy, M.: A current survey of 150 cases. In Roy, M., editor: Battered women, New York, 1977, Van Nostrand Reinhold Co.

Rubinelli, J.: Incest: it's time we face reality, J. Psychiatr. Nurs. **18**(4):17-18, 1980.

Sandgrund, A., Gaines, R., and Green, A.: Child abuse and mental retardation: a problem of cause and effect, Am. J. Ment. Defic. **79**(3):327-330, 1974.

Scharer, K.: Nursing therapy with abusive and neglectful families, J. Psychiatr. Nurs. **17**(9):12-21, 1979.

Silver, L., Barton, W., and Dublin, C.: Child abuse laws: are they enough? JAMA **1**:65-68, 1967.

Statistical abstracts of the United States: 1981, Bureau of the Census, Washington, D.C., 1981, U.S. Government Printing Office.

Statistical abstracts of the United Sttes: 1981, Bureau of the Census, Washington, D.C., 1982, U.S. Government Printing Office.

Taylor, C.: Mereness' essentials of psychiatric nursing, ed. 11, St. Louis, 1982, The C.V. Mosby Co.

Uniform crime reports for the United States, Federal Bureau of Investigation, Washington, D.C., 1970, U.S. Department of Justice.

Uniform crime reports for the United States, Federal Bureau of Investigation, Washington, D.C., 1980, U.S. Department of Justice.

Uniform crime reports for the United States, Federal Bureau of Investigation, Washington, D.C., Jan.-June, 1981, U.S. Department of Justice.

Van Stolk, M.: Beaten women, beaten children, Children Today **5**(2):9-12, 1976.

Weingourt, R.: Battered women: the grieving process, J. Psychiatr. Nurs. **17**(4):40-47, 1979.

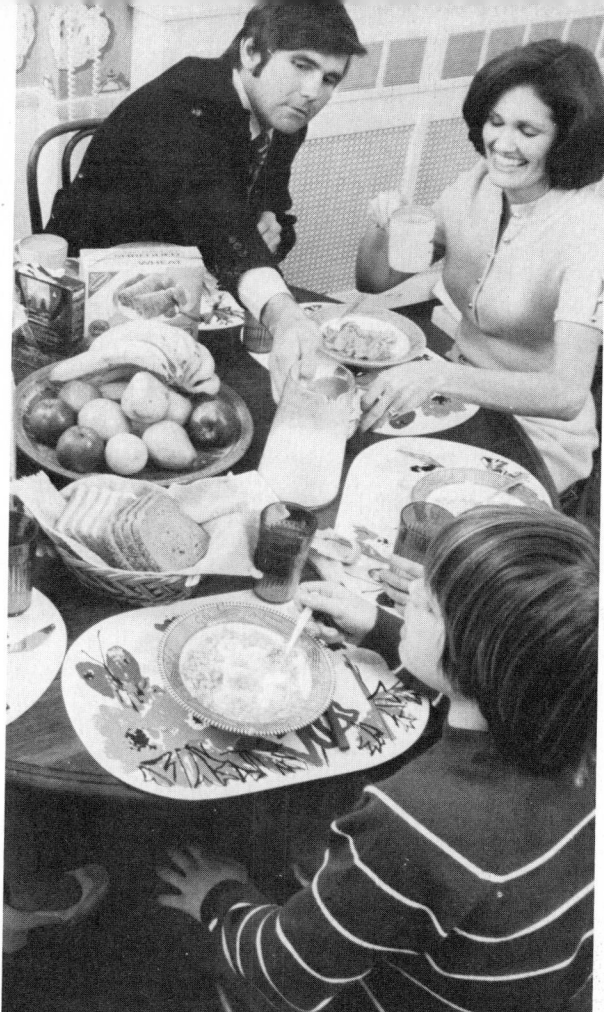

Chapter 21

NANNETTE WOREL

PROMOTING HEALTH THROUGH NUTRITION AND EXERCISE

Fitness has recently become a major community health priority. Joggers and bicyclers seem to be everywhere, and the waiting lines at the tennis and racquet ball courts are growing longer every day. The media instruct the public to eat right and get plenty of exercise, yet rarely provide practical information about doing so. This chapter describes current trends in nutrition and exercise, and nursing's role in promoting health through these means is explored.

PROMOTING HEALTH THROUGH NUTRITION

Historical Perspectives on Nutrition

National concerns regarding nutrition have shifted drastically during the twentieth century. For example,

nutritional deficiencies (especially those related to vitamins) were the focus of national attention during the 1920s and 1930s. As World War II approached, Americans became interested in discovering improved and more efficient ways to use food supplies at home and in needy allied countries (Caliendo, 1981).

At the end of the war the focus remained on providing food to the needy in other countries until the late 1960s when Americans realized that much hunger and malnutrition existed in their own land. This concern continued through the 1970s when it became apparent that another aspect of malnutrition existed and that was "overnutrition" or people eating more food than necessary to satisfy normal body requirements. The late 1970s and early 1980s brought increasing evidence that simple changes in the dietary habits and life-styles of many Americans could have important impact on the severity and incidence of many of the leading causes of death in the United States. As has been discussed in other chapters, coronary heart disease, high blood pressure, diabetes mellitus, dental caries, liver disease, and obesity have been identified as diseases believed to be linked to diet. Coronary heart disease is the nation's number one killer and has been linked with an excessive intake of saturated fats and cholesterol; high blood pressure has been associated with excessive calories and dietary salt; diabetes mellitus has been associated with excessive caloric intake and obesity; dental caries has been linked to excessive sugar intake; liver disease has been associated with heavy alcohol intake; and obesity has been linked with excessive caloric intake (Caliendo, 1981).

This growing relation between disease occurrence and excess consumption of alcohol, sugar, salt, saturated fats, and cholesterol has prompted many nutrition experts to suggest that simple changes in the dietary habits and life-styles of Americans may result in significant

reductions in the incidence of the leading causes of morbidity and mortality (Caliendo, 1981).

Is There a Perfect Diet?

It would be wonderful if a nurse had a simple, straightforward answer to the question of what to eat to remain healthy. Unfortunately, for all so-called experts who offer the American public the benefit of their wisdom, other equally vocal individuals contradict the first. For example, for every expert who suggests that Americans need to eliminate fiber from their diets, another purports that fiber is the answer to America's ills. Research in the area of nutrition is rapidly producing new information to contradict the old. In addition, political, social, and economic influences on the growing, marketing, distributing, and consuming of food products greatly affect the messages received by the American consumer. Many times the consumer is able to exert little control over such significant aspects of food consumption as availability and pricing. As can be seen in Fig. 21-1, income, educational level, and life-

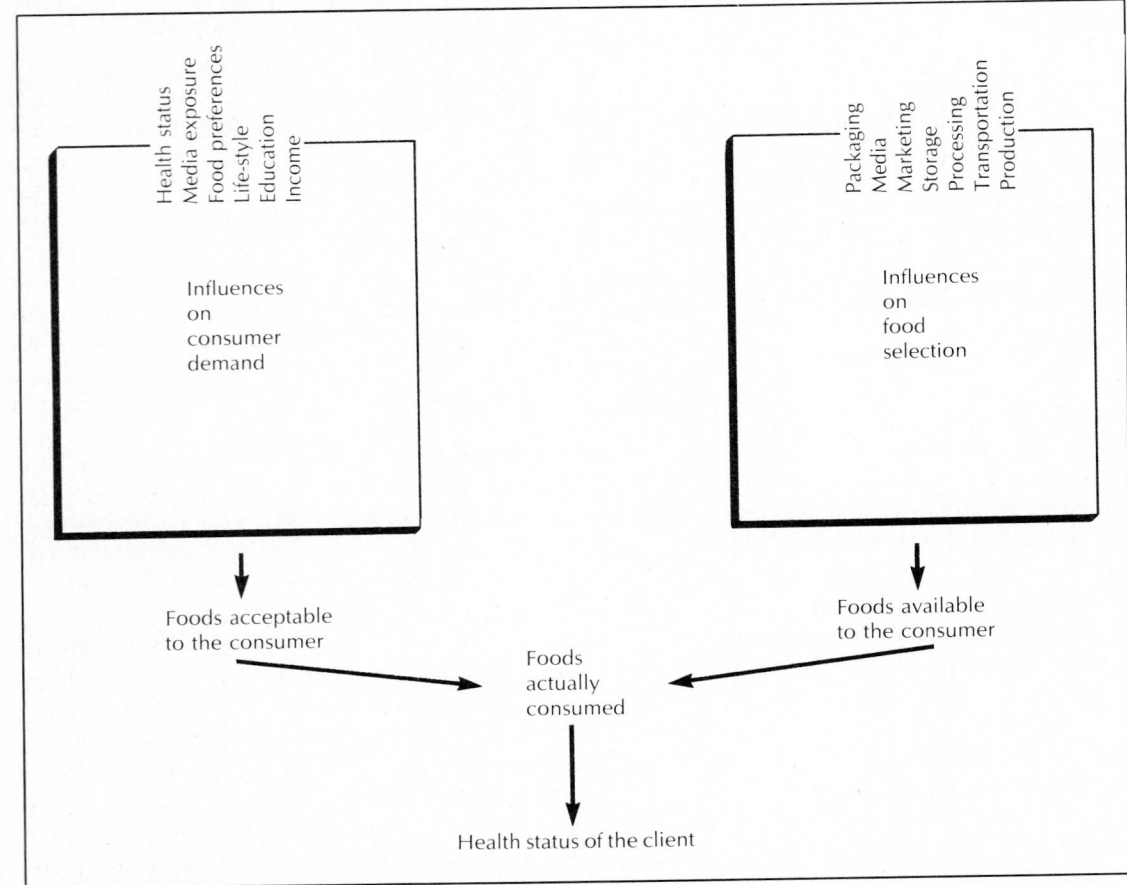

Fig. 21-1. Influences on food selection and ultimate health status.

style are but a few of the factors influencing food selection.

Frequent and extended contact with clients in the community affords the nurse an excellent opportunity to provide information and counseling regarding the role of nutrition in the promotion of health and the prevention of illness. However, before providing such counseling, it is essential that the nurse develop an understanding of the biological, psychological, sociocultural, and environmental factors influencing food selection and eating behaviors.

Biological Factors

The body's requirements for nutrients are one biological determinant of eating behavior. These nutrients provide the necessary energy for the metabolic processes provide the structural components of bones and tissues; and regulate physiological processes (Pender, 1982). Nutrients important for human growth and development include the following:

- Protein to support growth
- Fats for energy and the absorption of fat-soluble vitamins
- Carbohydrates as an energy source for activity and metabolic processes
- Vitamins and minerals to serve a variety of functions, including bone and tissue development

Outward indicators such as fatigue, apathy, or listlessness are the most often noted biological determinants of eating behaviors. These symptoms can indicate that caloric intake is insufficient to meet the energy demands placed on the body. One final important biological determinant of food selection is thought to be the hypothalamus and its potential malfunction in the physiological regulation of food intake (Pender, 1982).

Psychological Factors

Positive emotions such as enjoyment and tranquility as well as negative feelings like anger and insecurity often affect the eating behaviors of individuals. Food may represent rewards, comfort, and security to clients experiencing a variety of emotions, and the important role these emotions play in food selection cannot be stressed enough. For example, when a life situation such as an argument with a spouse results in increased anxiety, the person is likely to choose to eat foods that are empty in calories, junk foods, in search of some personal security.

Habits such as regular midmorning coffee breaks with pastries are another important factor in determining eating behavior. They require little or no conscious thought and often result in poor dietary practices. Habits depend on foods that are ready to eat with minimal preparation and often result in the selection of fast foods with little nutritional value.

Two other important psychological factors are self-esteem and knowledge about nutrition. One study (Schafer, 1979) showed a positive correlation between the quality of the diet consumed and the self-esteem of the individual. In addition, a study conducted by Stein in 1976 demonstrated that knowledge about the benefits of good nutrition influences food selection.

Sociocultural Factors

The cultural and ethnic backgrounds of clients play a major role in food selection and eating behaviors. Respect for and recognition of these food preferences are important for nurses in dealing with clients in the community. Boykin (1975) offered the following suggestions for dealing with various ethnic and cultural groups:

1. Recognize food preferences and habits
2. Determine frequency of consumption of ethnic foods
3. Recognize and reinforce positive aspects of the ethnic foods
4. Provide information to the client(s) regarding the nutritional value of ethnic foods
5. Include the client in dietary planning endeavors
6. Tailor recommended changes as much as possible to ethnic and cultural practices
7. Encourage major changes in dietary practices only when foods are clearly hazardous to the health of clients

Working with clients of a particular ethnic group for whom a specific diet has been recommended can be quite a challenge for the community health nurse. For example, the diet recommended for a client with hypertension who is of Mexican descent would most likely be quite different from that recommended for a client with hypertension who is of Japanese descent. Attempting to incorporate foods that are low in sodium while staying within cultural limitations necessities close teamwork between nurse and client.

Environmental Factors

Cost, accessibility, and convenience are the major factors influencing food selection and subsequent eating behavior. With food prices on the rise, consumers are constantly attempting to get the most for their money. Unfortunately, foods high in nutritional value, such as fruits and grains, appear to be more expensive than highly refined sugar products. The consumer ends up with foods that are high in calories but have only minimum nutritional value. By being familiar with cultural limitations and the available resources, the nurse can assist clients in selecting menus that are sound nutritionally. For example, the nurse may recommend that less expensive cuts of meat be purchased or navy beans be used as a source of protein in the diet of a low-income family. The nurse may recommend seasonal fruits and vegetables to not only minimize cost but to maximize nutritional value as well.

Accessibility is a major factor in food selection. Many low-income families may have limited mobility and must rely on local merchants for their food choices. In addition, seasonal variations affect the availability of fruits and vegetables. Clients often need guidance in selecting foods high in nutritional value that are available all year.

Finally, convenience plays a large part in food selection. It has been estimated that "30 percent of meals are eaten outside the home and convenience foods constitute 60 percent of the American diet" (Pender, 1982, p. 275). As a result, nurses are faced with the challenge of assisting clients select nutritious foods that require minimum preparation and look appealing.

Dietary Recommendations

In light of the many variables influencing food selection and the conflicting opinions regarding the benefits of almost all nutrients, it seems that attempting to outline a diet plan that is universally agreed on and applicable to all consumers at all times is an impossible task. However, in 1977 the U.S. government became involved and the Assistant Secretary for Health and Surgeon General, Julius Richmond, suggested that "individuals have the right to make the informed choices and the government has the responsibility to provide the best data for making a good dietary decisions" (p. 2621). That same year the U.S. Senate Select Committee on Nutrition and Human Needs published a report that made the following dietary recommendations to the American consumer:

1. Eat a variety of foods
2. Maintain ideal weight
3. Avoid too much saturated fat and cholesterol
4. Eat foods with adequate starch and fiber
5. Avoid too much sugar
6. Avoid too much sodium
7. If you drink alcohol, do so in moderation

Though the recommendations of the committee seemed at first glance to be vague and innocuous, they nonetheless evoked quite an uproar from powerful lobbies such as cattle farmers and those who process food. Suddenly cholesterol, salt, sugar, and fiber became hotly debated topics from health food stores to cocktail parties. Opposing groups were consoled by the fact that the recommendations advocated moderation rather than elimination of certain aspects of the American diet, and

the recommendations have become widely accepted as a *starting point* for dietary planning.

Although each of the committee's recommendations is valuable, clients are often unable or unwilling to adhere to them without more specific how-to advice. The nurse may incorporate the following tips when assisting clients with dietary planning (USDHEW, 1980):

1. *Eat a variety of foods.* Clients often are unsure of exactly what constitutes a balanced diet, and a review of the basic food groups—fruits and vegetables; bread and cereal; milk and cheese; and meat, fish, and poultry—might be helpful. Clients should be encouraged to select items from each of the major food groups on a daily basis to ensure variety. By varying foods selected on a daily basis, clients are less likely to develop a deficiency in or excess of single nutrients while ensuring an adequate diet. The recommended daily dietary allowances (RDAs) seen in Table 21-1 are invaluable when assisting clients in evaluating the adequacy of present dietary practices. For example, if an analysis of a client's diet demonstrates a consistent lack of protein, the nurse could use the table to assist the client in determining the recommended daily protein allowance according to age, sex, weight, and height and then comparing the recommended intake with the actual intake. Appropriate nursing interventions could then be mapped out and implemented.

2. *Maintain ideal weight.* [The 1973 DHEW Conference on Obesity offered suggested body weights for adult women and men.] Though the figures seen in Table 21-2 are not absolutes, they do provide a starting point for assisting clients in setting realistic goals for weight gain, loss, or maintenance. Suggestions on ways to improve eating habits (such as eating slowly, preparing smaller portions, and avoiding "seconds") may be useful to clients.

3. *Avoid too much saturated fat and cholesterol.* To assist the client in complying with this recommendation the nurse may suggest the following USDHEW, 1980, p.12):

■ Choose lean meat, fish, poultry, dry beans and peas as protein sources.
■ moderate use of eggs and organ meats (such as liver)
■ limit intake of butter, cream, hydrogenated margarines, shortenings and coconut oil, and foods made from such products
■ trim excess fat off meats
■ broil, bake or boil rather than fry
■ read labels carefully to determine both amount and types of fat contained in foods

4. *Eat foods with adequate starch and fiber.* To assist clients in selecting carbohydrates, it is important for the

Table 21-1. Recommended daily dietary allowances (RDAs)* (Designed for the maintenance of good nutrition of practically all healthy persons in the United States.)

Sex-age category	Age (yr) From	To	Weight Kg	lb	Height cm	in	Food energy (calories)	Protein (g)	Calcium (mg)	Phosphorus (mg)	Iron (mg)	Vitamin A (IU)	Thiamin (mg)	Riboflavin (mg)	Niacin (mg)	Ascorbic acid (mg)
Infants	0	0.5	6	14	60	24	kg × 117.0 / lb × 53.2	kg × 2.2 / lb × 1.0	360	240	10	1,400	0.3	0.4	5	35
	0.5	1	9	20	71	28	kg × 108.0 / lb × 49.1	kg × 2.0 / lb × 0.9	540	400	15	2,000	0.5	0.6	8	35
Children	1	3	13	28	86	34	1,300	23	800	800	15	2,000	0.7	0.8	9	40
	4	6	20	44	110	44	1,800	30	800	800	10	2,500	0.9	1.1	12	40
	7	10	30	66	135	54	2,400	36	800	800	10	3,300	1.2	1.2	16	40
Males	11	14	44	97	158	63	2,800	44	1,200	1,200	18	5,000	1.4	1.5	18	45
	15	18	61	134	172	69	3,000	54	1,200	1,200	18	5,000	1.5	1.8	20	45
	19	22	67	147	172	69	3,000	54	800	800	10	5,000	1.5	1.8	20	45
	23	50	70	154	172	69	2,700	56	800	800	10	5,000	1.4	1.6	18	45
	51+		70	154	172	69	2,400	56	800	800	10	5,000	1.2	1.5	16	45
Females	11	14	44	97	155	62	2,400	44	1,200	1,200	18	4,000	1.2	1.3	16	45
	15	18	54	119	162	65	2,100	48	1,200	1,200	18	4,000	1.1	1.4	14	45
	19	22	58	128	162	65	2,100	46	800	800	18	4,000	1.1	1.4	14	45
	23	50	58	128	162	65	2,000	46	800	800	18	4,000	1.0	1.2	13	45
	51+		58	128	162	65	1,800	46	800	800	10	4,000	1.0	1.2	12	45
Pregnant							+300	+30	1,200	1,200	+18†	5,000	+0.3	+0.3	+2	60
Lactating							+500	+20	1,200	1,200	18	6,000	+0.3	+0.5	+4	80

Adapted from Recommended Dietary Allowances, ed. 8, 1974, Food and Nutrition Board, National Academy of Sciences–National Research Council, Washington, D.C.

* Also available in libraries. This publication tabulates the RDAs for eight more nutrients, discusses the basis for all the RDAs, and reviews current knowledge of the dietary needs for other nutrients.

† This increased requirement cannot be met by ordinary diets; therefore the use of supplemental iron is recommended.

NOTE: The Recommended Daily Dietary Allowances (RDAs) should not be confused with the U.S. Recommended Daily Allowances (U.S. RDAs). The RDAs are amounts of nutrients recommended by the Food and Nutrition Board of the National Research Council and are considered adequate for maintenance of good nutrition in healthy persons in the United States. The allowances are revised from time to time in accordance with newer knowledge of nutritional needs.

The U.S. RDAs are the amounts of protein, vitamins, and minerals established by the Food and Drug Administration as standards for nutrition labeling. These allowances were derived from the RDAs set by the Food and Nutrition Board. The U.S. RDA for most nutrients approximates the highest RDA of the sex-age categories in this table, excluding the allowances for pregnant and lactating females. Therefore a diet that furnishes the U.S. RDA for a nutrient will furnish the RDA for most people and more than the RDA for many. U.S. RDAs are protein, 45 g (eggs, fish, meat, milk, poultry), 65 g (other foods); vitamin A, 5,000 IU; thiamin, 1.5 mg; riboflavin, 1.7 mg; niacin, 20 mg; ascorbic acid, 60 mg; calcium, 1 g; phosphorus, 1 g; iron, 18 mg. For additional information on U.S. RDAs, see the Federal Register, vol. 38, no. 49 (Mar. 14, 1973), pp. 6959-6960, and Agriculture Information Bulletin 382, Nutrition Labeling — tools for its use, p. 8.

Table 21-2. Suggested body weights

| Height | | Men (lb) | Women (lb) |
ft	in		
4	10		92 to 119
4	11		94 to 122
5	0		96 to 125
5	1		99 to 128
5	2	112 to 141	102 to 131
5	3	115 to 144	105 to 134
5	4	118 to 148	108 to 138
5	5	121 to 152	111 to 142
5	6	124 to 156	114 to 146
5	7	128 to 161	118 to 150
5	8	132 to 166	122 to 154
5	9	136 to 170	126 to 158
5	10	140 to 174	130 to 163
5	11	144 to 179	134 to 168
6	0	148 to 184	138 to 173
6	1	152 to 189	
6	2	156 to 194	
6	3	160 to 199	
6	4	164 to 204	

From DHEW Conference on Obesity, Washington, D.C., 1973.

nurse to differentiate between simple and complex carbohydrates. Simple carbohydrates (sugars) provide little in the way of nutrients but do add calories. Complex carbohydrates are foods such as beans, peas, whole grain cereals, fruits, and vegetables that provide essential nutrients in addition to calories. The nurse can provide invaluable assistance to clients by offering suggestions of foods that stretch food dollars and are high in nutritional value.

5. *Avoid too much sugar.* To avoid excessive sugars it is recommended that clients do the following (USD-HEW, 1980, p. 16):

- use less of all sugars, including white sugar, brown sugar, raw sugar, honey and syrups
- eat less of foods containing these sugars, such as candy, soft drinks, ice creams, cakes, cookies
- select fresh fruits or fruits canned without sugar or with light syrup rather than heavy syrup
- read food labels for clues in sugar content—if the names sucrose, glucose, maltose, dextrose, lactose, fructose, or syrups appear first, then there is a large amount of sugar
- remember, how often you eat sugar is as important as how much sugar you eat

6. *Avoid too much sodium.* Clients can effectively lower their sodium intake by:

- cooking with small amounts of salt
- adding little or no salt to food at the table
- limiting intake of salty foods, such as chips, nuts, and condiments
- reading labels to determine the amount of sodium in processed foods

7. *If you drink alcohol, do so in moderation.* This recommendation is self-explanatory, yet clients may benefit from understanding that alcoholic beverages tend to have little nutritional value but are high in calories. In addition, heavy drinking has been linked to cirrhosis of the liver and neurological disorders.

Analyzing Dietary Information

The community health nurse is frequently asked to comment on information clients receive about food products in lay magazines and the media. As has been previously discussed, controversy continues to mount regarding the benefits of nearly every nutrient. Fortunately, in 1979 the American Society for Clinical Nutrition presented a step-by-step approach to analyzing nutritional data. Such an approach requires that the individual consider three questions when evaluating information regarding nutrition:

1. What kind of evidence has been presented relating a specific nutrient to a certain disease process?
2. What is the quality (strength) of this evidence?
3. What are the possible risks and benefits of increasing, reducing, and/or eliminating the specific nutrient from the diet?

The answers to these questions assist the nurse in determining the validity of claims made about dietary practices. By combining a sound background in nutrition principles with the analysis of information just outlined, the community health nurse is in a strategic position to assist clients in understanding the difference between factually based and nonsubstantiated nutrition information.

Using the Nursing Process in Promoting Sound Nutrition

Because most meal planning and preparation occur in the home, the community health nurse has an ideal opportunity to provide nutrition education. In addition, although physicians, dietitians, nutritionists, and home economists often assist in resolving nutritional problems and related diseases, the responsibility for identification frequently rests with the community health nurse. It is through the nursing process that community health nurses are able to detect and intervene in nutritional difficulties encountered by individuals, families, and groups within the community.

Assessment

Any assessment tool that focuses only on the foods eaten and ignores the cultural, environmental, and economic influences on dietary habits does not provide an adequate basis for planning nursing interventions. Information regarding food preferences, preparation time, cost, availability, daily meal patterns, physical limitations, and environmental constraints (such as lack of running water) must be obtained. In addition, the client's relation to the family and community as a whole must be considered in the assessment phase to gain an understanding of all influences in food selection and eating behaviors. For example, before helping a client with hypertension to select a low sodium diet, the nurse would gather information regarding such variables as the client's eating patterns (is most of the food prepared at home or eaten out); family support of the dietary changes of one member (are other family members willing to alter their diets somewhat); and cultural influences (does the client's ethnic background dictate a diet high in sodium).

Finally, the nurse may use a food diary during the assessment phase. For this activity the client is asked to keep a record for a specified period of time (usually 1 week) of all foods and beverages consumed, the time of day the foods are eaten, and any emotions (such as anger, happiness, frustration) that are present when the eating behavior takes place. The diary can be jointly reviewed by the nurse and client, eating and food selection patterns identified, and interventions planned.

Planning

The information gathered in the assessment process guides the planning aspect of nutrition education. Whether working with individual clients, families, or large groups, the community health nurse must consider the concerns, interests, and priorities of the potential audience when planning nursing interventions. Individuals, families, and groups may have limited food choices because of the cost and availability of foods and the confusion over advertising claims of many products.

It is essential in the planning phase of the nursing process to include all individuals who the proposed nutritional changes may affect. For example, in assisting an adolescent in planning a weight reduction diet, the nurse would benefit by including the family member responsible for selecting food as well as the individual responsible for financing the diet. Inclusion in the planning process generally encourages participation in the implementation of the diet.

It is in the planning phase that additional resource persons such as nutritionists, physicians, and dietitians are consulted to assist in meeting the identified needs of the individual, family, or community group. For example, the community health nurse may involve the physician of a client with diabetes or a nutritionist when assisting the individual in planning a reducing diet.

Special needs of clients may be met by community nutrition resources or governmental aid programs. For example, mothers with low birth weight infants may the eligible for the Special Supplemental Food Program for Women, Infants and Children (WIC). Such a program provides vouchers to be used only for specified foods that are high in nutritional value. Elderly clients confined to their homes may benefit from a local Meals on Wheels program in which one hot meal a day is brought to their home. Through the use of community resources, the nurse is able in the planning phase to assist the client in meeting needs identified in the assessment phase.

Implementation

The nursing process culminates in the implementation and evaluation of the plan jointly developed by the nurse and client(s). It is during implementation that client motivation and teaching abilities of the nurse become essential. Involving the client in the planning phase, setting reasonable and achievable goals, and suggesting the individual incorporate self-rewards (e.g., a new outfit when weight loss reaches a certain point) into the plan often assist in keeping the client interested and motivated during implementation of the nursing plan. Teaching strategies such as those described in Chapter Ten are useful during implementation of a nutrition education program with individuals, families, or groups.

Evaluation

Regardless of the strategy selected for implementation, constant awareness of how the client is perceiving the benefits of the proposed change is essential to success. Thus evaluation in the form of continuous feedback cannot be forgotten. Progress can be monitored throughout and corrections made to ensure maximum benefit from the nursing interventions. An evaluation completed at the conclusion of the nursing intervention provides the nurse with valuable information as to the degree that objectives and client needs have been met.

To evaluate the clients' progress the community health nurse may ask them to keep a daily diary of food intake to be checked at each client-nurse encounter. The community health nurse can use the data in the diary to continually educate the clients about nutritious foods for a balanced diet.

Requests for assistance in controlling weight are frequently received from individuals, families, and groups. Thus it is essential for the nurse to have a basic understanding of weight control.

Weight Control

"Obesity is generally defined as being 20 percent or more overweight by standard height and weight tables" (Pender, 1982, p. 294). With two out of every five Americans estimated to be obese, the potential for nursing intervention in obesity is endless. Heredity, interpersonal factors such as family problems, anxiety, unrealistic expectations of self and others, sociocultural factors (e.g., food selection practices), and environmental factors have been identified as probable causes of obesity. Thus according to Pender (1982, p. 295),

> Results of numerous studies suggest it is more important to deal with personal, social, and environmental influences, rather than biochemical causes of obesity. Research has yielded definitive information on biochemical etiology except in relation to a limited number of metabolic disorders.

Assessment of the individual(s) desiring weight loss is essential to developing an individualized, effective program. In addition to gathering data regarding current dietary practices and sociocultural influences, the nurse may also consider the client's past weight loss program. The nurse should recall that:

> Studies have shown that individuals who derive the greatest benefits from a weight reduction program exhibit adult-onset rather than adolescent-onset obesity, report few previous attempts to achieve weight loss and are more adept at self-reinforcement (Pender, 1982, p. 296).

In planning a weight loss program, the nurse may incorporate the following suggestions (Pender, 1982):

1. The diet must be individualized and realistic.
2. A slow, gradual weight loss is preferable to a rapid loss. A reduction of no more than 2 to 3 pounds per week should be instituted.
3. Food should be served in small portions.
4. The diet should contain all the minerals and vitamins essential for body functioning.
5. Eating habits can be changed. Accepting control over eating habits is essential for continued client success.

Because weight loss involves expending more calories than are consumed, obese individuals should be encouraged to participate in an exercise program to facilitate weight loss. The exercise serves to provide continuous motivation throughout the weight loss period and assists in preventing protein loss from muscle that may occur when inactivity accompanies dieting (Pender, 1982). In counseling the obese individual regarding exercise, the nurse should stress the following:

1. Weight loss is the primary goal of exercise.
2. Correct breathing to maximize ventilatory efficiency is essential.
3. A slow, gradual program is best. Obese individuals should progress more slowly in exercise programs than their normal-weight counterparts.
4. Swimming is excellent for obese individuals. It not only permits maximum oxygen uptake by the tissues but the water provides support and buoyancy to the individual.

■   ■   ■

Though controversy exists regarding the value of many nutrients, little doubt seems to remain that nutrition plays a vital role in maintaining health. Attempts have been made to link diseases with dietary practices, and the government has made recommendations regarding the elimination of excesses from the American diet. The responsibility of the consumer in selecting nutritious foods at the lowest possible price is being advocated in professional and lay publications alike. It seems that nutrition is indeed essential to health promotion.

The concept of physical fitness and its relation to health promotion and maintenance is also receiving much attention. The remainder of this chapter focuses on the promotion of health through exercise.

PROMOTING HEALTH THROUGH EXERCISE

The Industrial Revolution helped to create a world in which sedentary life-style is not only possible but encouraged. Most Americans either drive or ride to work and once there are involved in occupations that require little if any vigorous physical activity. Even recreational activities have become sedentary as people elect to be spectators rather than participants.

Fortunately, the past decade has shown an encouraging resurgence of interest in physical fitness and exercise. Research has attempted to determine the positive (and negative) effects of fitness on health. Problems such as obesity, coronary artery disease, hypertension, and anxiety have been linked with a sedentary life-style; the term *diseases of hypokinesis* was coined to describe diseases that have been associated with inactivity. In 1977 a Gallup poll discovered that almost half of the American adults claimed to exercise regularly to keep fit (Healthy People, 1979). A recent Harris Poll found that 50 million American or approximately 23% were involved in some sort of systematic exercise, and another 25 million Americans (11%) claimed to run regularly (Mann, 1981).

Exercise and Physical Fitness Defined

Exercise has been defined as the "regular or repeated appropriate use of physical activity for the purpose of training or developing the body and mind for the sake of health" (Halfman and Hojnacki, 1981, p. 1). Such a definition indicates that exercise provides healthful benefits physiologically and psychologically as long as it is performed on a regular basis.

The term *physical fitness* merely expands on the concept of exercise. Fitness takes into account the efficiency of the cardiac, pulmonary, and circulatory systems and examines the ability of these systems and others to respond to physical demands. Getchell (1979) identified the following basic components of fitness:

- Cardiorespiratory endurance—capability of heart, blood vessels, and lungs to function at optimum efficiency in delivering nutrients and oxygen to tissues and removing wastes
- Muscular strength—capacity of muscles to exert maximum force against a resistance
- Muscular endurance—capacity of muscles to exert force repeatedly over a period of time
- Flexibility—ability to use muscles and joints through maximum range of motion
- Motor skill performace—ability of nerves to receive messages that result in smooth coordinated muscle movement

Thus exercise conditions the various body systems to respond in a physically fit manner to demands placed on them.

Effects of Exercise
Physiological Effects

Nurses have long been aware of the detrimental effects of prolonged bed rest and the resultant lack of exercise. Venous thrombosis, orthostatic hypotension, a progressive increase in heart rate, and a reduction in the strength of skeletal muscles are a few of the problems associated with prolonged bed rest. In recent years much research has been conducted in an attempt to demonstrate a cause and effect relationship between physical inactivity in ambulatory populations and specific disease processes. Though no unequivocal relationships have been demonstrated, physiological responses and benefits to exercise have been determined, as can be seen in Table 21-3.

In addition, risk factors for specific diseases have been identified, and studies have shown exercise to be effective in reducing many of them. For example, 15 factors have been identified as increasing the likelihood of suffering a heart attack (Fixx, 1980). These factors include blood pressure, activity, weight, mood and coping style, fasting blood sugar level, serum triglycerides, fibrinolysins, cigarette smoking, diet, abnormal electro-

cardiogram readings, uric acid, pulmonary function, glucose tolerance, heredity, and cholesterol. Of the 15 factors, exercise has been shown to influence all but one, heredity. Serum triglycerides, blood pressure, and psychic stress have been shown to decrease with regular exercise, whereas the levels of high-density lipoproteins (thought to protect individuals from coronary heart disease) have been shown to increase. In addition, individuals involved in regular exercise have been shown to adopt a more health-conscious life-style, with resultant decreases in smoking, obesity, and alcohol consumption (Fixx, 1980).

Psychological Effects

In 1979 Harris (p. 130) pointed out that "although the physiologic mechanisms by which physical exercise relieves tension and improves the psychological state and mental health require further investigation, there is evidence of a relationship between the individual's mood and muscle condition and posture." It has been proposed that exercise can improve the psychological state of humans by providing a means through which a person can express the evolutionary need to engage in physically aggressive, large muscle activities (Walker, 1975). In a study conducted by De Vries (1972) of the University of Southern California's School of Medicine, it was discovered that neuromuscular tension in a group of volunteers was more effectively decreased with moderate exercise than with the use of tranquilizers. Although the psychological benefits of exercise and physical fitness have been extensively researched in a variety of settings, no exact mechanism of action has been discovered. Individual differences in expectations, beliefs, and coping patterns have been identified as having potential effects on the psychological benefits received from exercise (Folkins and Sime, 1981).

In short, exercise has been cited as a means through which an individual can attain physiological and psychological benefits. The community health nurse is in a prime position to observe the activity patterns and resultant problems of individuals and groups. By recognizing the potential benefits of exercise and promoting physical fitness, innovative and vitally important nursing interventions can be planned. The elderly constitute a group with whom nursing interventions can be especially beneficial in preventing the diseases of hypokinesis.

Exercise Benefits to the Elderly Population. Our society has unfortunately tended to create a stereotype for the majority of healthy older individuals. This stereotype encourages older people to sit back, take it easy, and enjoy life. A problem arises when it becomes apparent that the ability to enjoy life depends in part on

Table 21-3. Physiological responses and benefits to body systems from exercise

System	Physiological responses to exercise	Physiological benefits
Cardiovascular	Increased cardiac output as a result of increased heart rate and stroke volume (caused by increased contractility of the heart muscle, increased preload, and decreased afterload Maximum muscle blood flow during exercise increases to approximately 90% of the total cardiac output Blood flow to muscle groups is enhanced because of alterations in resistance and capitance of the vessels composing the peripheral vascular bed Widened arteriovenous oxygen difference resulting from an increased number of cellular mitochondria Cerebral blood flow remains constant Skin blood flow fluctuates with the intensity of the exercise Blood pressure fluctuates according to the type of exercise and the muscle groups involved	Increased exercise tolerance resulting from increased efficiency in the delivery of oxygen to exercising muscles Strengthened cardiac muscle that produces lowered exercising and resting heart rates Increased development of collateral circulation Increased efficiency in the peripheral vascular system resulting in sustained improvement in oxygen extraction
Coronary	Increased heart rate Increased contractility Increased myocardial oxygen consumption	Strengthened cardiac muscle
Pulmonary	Increased pulmonary perfusion Increased ventilation rate and depth Increased rate of oxygen and carbon dioxide diffusion Increased perfusion of alveoli, which results in enhanced exchange of oxygen and carbon dioxide	Improved pulmonary function measurements of peak flow and residual volume May help individuals reduce their smoking habits through increased ventilatory stress
Musculoskeletal	Increased bone strength Postulated increase in collagen content of the connective tissue surrounding muscle fibers Increased density of muscles Increased number of mitochondria	Improved resistance to fractures as a result of increased bone strength Improved healing if fractures occur Increased force of muscle contraction before tearing Reduced body fat Increased lean body mass Faster muscle contraction Prolonged work of muscles because of delay in tiring
Metabolic	Body produces adenosine triphosphate (ATP) through anaerobic or aerobic metabolism Body begins through training to burn fats rather than carbohydrates for glycogen Hypothalamus regulates temperature and dissipates heat	Increased number of calories expended Reduced body fat Increased proportion of lean body mass

the level of health of the individual, which in turn is influenced by the level of physical fitness.

Recent studies have indicated that an older individual can minimize the losses that accompany aging and thereby improve the quality of life through physical activity (Price and Luther, 1980). Some normal effects of aging, such as a decreasing maximum oxygen uptake level and capacity for physical work, can be reversed to some extent through exercise. In addition, the loss of lean tissue, strength, and flexibility can be minimized if an individual remains active throughout the aging process. As has been indicated for the general population,

exercise may also provide the elderly with some degree of immunization against the diseases of hypokinesis. Finally, studies have indicated that physical activity can positively influence the general self-image of an older individual (Price and Luther, 1980).

By combining knowledge regarding the normal aging process with that of exercise principles, the community health nurse is in a prime position to assist elderly clients in promoting health through exercise. As with the general population, realistic goals must be set; programs must be designed to avoid overstressing clients during the first session; and individual limitations must be considered. For example, through normal aging the maximum oxygen uptake ability declines linearly. The nurse can capitalize on this knowledge by understanding that a lower heart rate is necessary for an older individual to achieve the maximum benefit from exercise. Thus walking is an activity the nurse may "prescribe" to elderly clients. Considering individual differences, the nurse may assist them in setting realistic goals in terms of distance and pace.

Fitness Evaluation

For decades governmental agencies and various community health organizations have encouraged Americans to check with their physicians before embarking on an exercise program. In recent years the National Heart, Lung and Blood Institute and various consumer groups have begun to question this advice. More and more consumers are dissatisfied with the level of knowledge that their personal physicians possess regarding exercise; the specialty of exercise physiology has gained popularity. In addition, some researchers feel that for adults under 60, failing to begin an exercise program because of an unwillingness or inability to consult a physician first is far more detrimental than embarking on a sensible exercise program without obtaining medical approval (Ryan, 1981).

Pender (1982, p. 237) seems to have reached a reasonable compromise between the two schools of thought by suggesting that "all individuals who have a family or personal history of cardiovascular disease or are over 35 years of age should obtain a complete physical examination before beginning an exercise program." Such an examination not only facilitates early detection of problems, but encourages a 'team approach' (physician-nurse-client) to developing an exercise program. Whereas the nurse may be actively involved in developing exercise programs for adults in the community and for children in schools, a close collaborative effort from the nurse, physician, and client in the development of the physical activity program facilitates early screening and detection of problems the person may experience in the exercise program.

In using the nursing process to assist clients in incorporating physical activity into their life-styles, an assessment of the present level of fitness must be completed. In addition to obtaining information about beliefs related to exercise, interest areas, and present life-style, the nurse may assist the client in attaining one or more physical measures of personal fitness. These measures include but are not limited to resting heart rate, maximum heart rate, blood pressure, joint and muscle flexibility, forced vital capacity, and residual volumes.

Assessing the level of fitness of an individual assists the nurse in answering these common questions: How much should I exercise? What kind of exercise should I do?

How Much Exercise is Enough?

Individuals who participate in physical activity on a regular basis often report that they feel better physically, have more energy, and even require less sleep. However, an individual wishing to initiate an exercise program is often confused about how and where to begin.

In 1979, the U.S. Department of Health, Education and Welfare published a report entitled *Healthy People: the Surgeon General's Report on Health Promotion and Disease Prevention*. In that report (p. 133) it was concluded that:

> The kind of physical activity probably most beneficial to the cardiovascular system is sometimes called aerobic—exercise requiring large amounts of oxygen for energy production. Examples include brisk walking, climbing stairs, running, cross-country skiing and swimming.

The report went on to suggest that beneficial effects from aerobic exercise could be achieved in 15 to 30 minutes of exercise at least three times per week.

Aerobic exercise demands oxygen and forces the body to process and deliver it. It is when the body is maximizing the uptake of oxygen that the "aerobic effect" occurs. To assist the client in determining the level at which the aerobic effect will occur, a simple formula is provided. By using the formula, a community health nurse and a 45-year-old male client would discover that to achieve the minimum aerobic effect, the man would need to increase his heart rate to [114 beats per minute.] As the client became conditioned, he could aim for 85% of the maximum heart rate or 149 beats per minute.

The formula for determining minimum and maximum aerobic effect is:

$$220 - \text{Client's age} = \text{Maximum heart rate}$$
$$\text{Maximum heart rate} \times 0.65 = \text{Minimum aerobic effect}$$
$$\text{Maximum heart rate} \times 0.85 = \text{Maximum aerobic effect}$$

Components of a Fitness Program

Any exercise program should include these four aspects (Pender, 1982): (1) a warm-up period, (2) stretching exercises, (3) aerobic exercise, and (4) a cool-down period. The exercise session should gradually progress from a low to a vigorous level of activity and then slowly return to a low activity level. All four aspects are of equal importance in a fitness program and are considered individually.

Warm-Up Period

"Warming up" before attempting more strenuous exercise provides an opportunity for the body to increase the blood flow to the heart, enhance tissue oxygenation, and decrease muscular tension. A warm-up period of 10 to 15 minutes is more than adequate, and exercises such as arm circles, head rotations, lateral waist bends, and side leg raises can be used.

Stretching Exercises

Once major muscle groups are warmed up, the client is ready for stretching exercises. These exercises put more strain on muscles than do the warm-up exercises and therefore should be done slowly with the positions held for only a few seconds. Stretching exercises that concentrate on the hamstring or back increase the body's readiness to proceed to the aerobic phase of the exercise program. For a description of specific stretching exercises, see the bibliography at the end of the chapter.

Aerobic Exercise

Any exercise that is rhythmical, is continuous, and increases the uptake of oxygen can be termed *aerobic*. Brisk walking, running, or swimming are examples of aerobic activities, whereas golf and softball are not considered as such. The heart rate of an individual walking, running, or swimming could be maintained at a consistently high level for a period of time, but the heart rate of an individual playing golf or softball would fluctuate as the sport demanded. The aerobic exercise should be done for 15 to 30 minutes at least three times each week.

Clients should be instructed by the nurse in the following self-care activities before engaging in aerobic activity (Pender, 1982):

1. Exercise should never be engaged in during the hottest or most humid parts of the day.
2. The client should wait 1½ to 2½ hours after exercising to eat a large meal.
3. Adequate salt and potassium intakes should be maintained to prevent muscle cramps.
4. Clear liquids should be taken before, during, and after a workout to prevent dehydration.

In addition to counseling the client in the preceding self-care activities, the nurse should instruct the person in how and when to check his pulse and should emphasize the importance of seeking medical attention if the following symptoms develop (Pender, 1982, p. 263):

- chest or arm pain
- marked increase in shortness of breath
- irregular heartbeat
- light-headedness, fainting
- nausea and vomiting
- unexplained weight changes
- muscle or joint problems
- prolonged fatigue
- muscle weakness
- unexplained changes in exercise tolerance

Cool-Down Period

A cool-down period of 5 to 10 minutes, following aerobic activity, is necessary to allow body temperature and heart rate to slowly decrease while promoting the removal of the waste product, lactic acid, from the muscles. Exercises such as walking and deep breathing and the stretching exercises previously discussed in this section are excellent for the cool-down period. The key is to select exercises that do not allow a rapid change in heart rate but rather a gradual decrease.

Designing an Exercise Program

The nurse and the client should determine the major intent of any exercise program before its design. For example, is program being designed to help the client lose weight, improve cardiovascular fitness, or gain psychological benefits? Such information, when combined with data regarding the client's present physical condition and past medical history, facilitates the design of an exercise program. Hojnacki (1981) identified the following criteria for designing an individualized exercise plan:

1. Type of exercise desired (i.e., walking, running, etc.)
2. Heart rate desired to achieve aerobic effect
3. Intensity of activity
4. Duration (length) of activity
5. Frequency (number of sessions each week)

The importance of individualizing exercise programs cannot be stressed enough and neither can the importance of setting realistic goals. Embarking on an exercise program without firm, realistic goals may cause the individual to become frustrated, lose interest, or potentiate the hazards of exercise.

Potential Hazards of Exercise

Although exercise has demonstrated benefits, it also has associated risks of which the client needs to be aware. Common problems associated with exercise and related nursing interventions can be seen in Table 21-4.

Incorporating Fitness into Work Place and Life-Style

Approximately one third of an American adult's time is spent in the work place, yet recent technological advances have produced a largely sedentary American work force. Few jobs demand physical activity sufficient to promote a high level of physical fitness (Blomquist, 1981). It has been estimated that over 132 mil-

Table 21-4. Common exercise-related problems and suggested nursing interventions

Problem	Probable causes	Nursing interventions
Nausea and/or vomiting	Delayed gastric emptying secondary to exercise	Encourage client to exercise on an empty stomach
Dehydration	Inadequate fluid intake	Encourage individual to consume fluid (preferably water) during exercise; it is a myth that a person can become "waterlogged"; enough fluid should be consumed to produce 200 ml of urine per hour (Mann, 1981)
Injury related to heat	Inadequate training Inadequate precautions	Educate clients in signs and symptoms and first aid for heat stroke and heat exhaustion; encourage clients to exercise during cool parts of the day
Injuries (i.e., sprains, tears, sore muscles)	Overuse Misuse	Instruct individuals in appropriate first aid and follow-up measures

lion workdays (or $25 billion) are lost each year as a result of the illness and premature deaths of employees (Kondrasuk, 1980). Many of these workdays need not be lost if more employees become physically fit.

In view of the length of time an individual spends in the work place and the importance of attempting to incorporate fitness into the daily activities of Americans, a challenge has been presented to employers to protect the health of employees whose replacement would be costly (in terms of time and money). The community health nurse can effectively work with business and industry to promote health in the work place. Assessment of employee fitness levels, needs, and desires as well as the planning, implementation, and evaluation of employee fitness programs are activities that fall well within the scope of community health nursing practice.

Unfortunately, many places of employment do not have employee fitness programs. The programs that presently are in existence vary widely. For example, one company's idea of a fitness program for employees may consist of sponsoring employee athletic teams, whereas another in the same community may offer a gymnasium complete with exercise rooms, swimming pool, and an in-house exercise physiologist.

When attempting to design an employee fitness program, the nurse must consider the available facilities, the financial support obtainable, the characteristics of potential participants, and the attitude and commitment of the management toward physical fitness. The extent to which the management of a firm or industry supports employee fitness programs greatly affects the success of any endeavor by the nurse to improve the health of employees.

Unfortunately, however, simply making exercise programs available in the work place has not proven to be an exceptional motivation to individuals. Firms with extensive employee exercise programs report between 15% and 60% participation (Blomquist, 1981). As a result, companies are now trying such things as monetary rewards, public recognition, planned competition, and information on self-management techniques as potential incentives.

If a client is unwilling or unable to incorporate more physical exercise in the work place, the nurse can assist the individual in determining other areas in which additional activity can be made part of a daily routine. For example, the client may be encouraged to park in the far corner of a shopping mall rather than fighting for a space directly in front of the entrance. Such an action forces the individual to walk farther than normal, thereby accomplishing the goal of adding more exercise without requiring extra equipment or significantly long periods of time. Additional suggestions for incorporating more activity into the daily routine include walking up and down stairs instead of taking the elevator, taking a walk around the block after lunch or on a coffee break instead of lingering in the cafeteria, performing yard work personally instead of delegating it to someone else, and arising 15 minutes earlier to perform stretching and breathing exercises before the rigors of the day begin.

Promoting Exercise in the Community

With the growing public interest in exercise and physical fitness and the strong epidemiological and clinical evidence that supports exercise as a means of disease prevention, the community health nurse has become increasingly involved in promoting community health through exercise. Although such a task cannot be undertaken alone, nursing activities in a community campaign to promote fitness center around getting community members interested in exercise, keeping their interest, assisting them in locating facilities for exercise, and directing their efforts.

Getting People Interested

Mass media campaigns have demonstrated their effectiveness in reducing specific risk factors in target populations (Thomas, 1979). By enlisting the support of community groups and governmental agencies, the nurse could at very little cost spearhead a campaign to educate community residents about the need for, benefits of, and simple how-to's of starting an exercise program.

In addition, the community health nurse assigned to a school district can be instrumental in promoting exercise in the schools. Because exercise habits that span the life cycle are best formed in childhood, the place to initiate such habits is in the schools. Stressing the importance of lifetime fitness and teaching basic fitness skills to schoolchildren could produce dramatic results in future years. Recent cuts in the funding of school physical fitness programs call for lobbying and educational efforts on the part of the nurse.

Finally, the nurse must focus on obtaining the interest and support of other health professionals in the community. The importance of exercise cannot be stressed enough. A concerted, coordinated effort by all the health professionals in a community has far greater impact than any one individual working alone.

Keeping People Interested

Even the best exercise program will fail if the individual or group is not motivated to adhere to it. Finding "just the thing" that prompts an individual or group to continue an exercise program in spite of aching muscles and time limitations is difficult at best. Though there are no motivators that work in all situations, the following suggestions may assist the nurse in fighting what Fixx called "the war on sloth" (1980):

1. *Involve* the clients in the planning process. The clients are able to provide the nurse with clues as to the types of activities they may enjoy as well as any stumbling blocks that may inhibit their participation.
2. *Select* activities the individuals have already mastered. The clients may become discouraged and quit if they are unable to master a new skill (such as swimming) in the exercise program.
3. *Plan* the exercise activities at the same time every day to help in establishing a routine.

4. *Include* others in the exercise program. Individuals may find it more difficult to stop the program if others are depending on them. The old adage "misery loves company" was never truer than in the initial stage of an exercise program.
5. *Develop* realistic, achievable goals. The clients may be more apt to continue participation when a particular goal is in sight. Some clients enjoy plotting their progress on a graph so that achievement is easy to see. Plotting on a chart the number of minutes of exercise or the miles walked is one way of determining how close goals are to being met.
6. *Encourage,* encourage, encourage! Let the clients know that the positive aspects of exercising are readily apparent in their physical appearance, modification of habits (such as smoking), or other outward measures.
7. *Acknowledge* the disadvantages of exercise. Preparing clients for the daily aggravations of exercise and at the same time expounding on the positive aspects not only protect the nurse's credibility with clients, but also help to prevent discouragement during the initial phases of the program.
8. *Financial rewards* are extremely effective with some clients. At the beginning of the week the individuals may set goals and fine themselves a predetermined amount (e.g., 25¢) if the goals are not met. The fine could be placed in a fund to be used only when the goals have been met for four consecutive weeks.
9. *Integrate* music into the exercise program if at all possible. Music often facilitates movement, relieves boredom, and may distract the individual from the repetitive nature of some exercises. For example, when jumping rope or doing sit-ups in time to a jazzy tune, clients are often amazed at the number of repetitions they are able to complete during a given musical selection. The music helps to distract them from the otherwise boring, repetitive task.
10. *Devise* the exercise program to fit into the individual's present life-style. Programs that require minimum alterations in an individual's life-style may meet with less resistance than those demanding greater changes.
11. *Enlist* the support of companies and community organizations to provide additional motivations. Discounts on insurance rates, free group exercise programs, and free clinics in which exercise-related problems can be discussed are a few examples of additional incentives to exercise.

Locating Places to Exercise

Through the assessment process, the community health nurse is well aware of existing gaps in exercise programs. The interests of the target groups and the existing facilities give the nurse direction in expanding and creating exercise programs. The nurse could coordinate efforts to create bicycle and fitness trails, open school gymnasiums to adults in the evening, and encourage the use of neighborhood parks and recreational facilities.

Directing Efforts

In spite of the increasing number of Americans participating in exercise programs, the 1979 report by the Surgeon General pointed out that "most participants do not exercise often or vigorously enough to achieve maximum health benefits" (Healthy People, p. 134). The report also found that:

Participation rates are higher among whites than minorities; among males than females; among younger than older persons; among the more educated than the less educated; among professionals than blue collar workers; among the affluent than the poor; and among suburbanites than city dwellers.

These facts, combined with data gathered in a community assessment, give the nurse direction in planning interventions. Target groups are identified through the assessment process, and programs specific to their needs can then be designed and implemented.

APPLICATION OF THE NURSING PROCESS

The use of the nursing process in the areas of nutrition and exercise can be seen in the following example:

A 23-year-old female college student contacted the local public health agency for assistance in weight loss. Because of budgetary limitations, no nutritionist was available, and the woman was referred to the community health nurse.

Assessment revealed that the client lived alone, socialized rarely, and ate only convenience foods. In addition, she had a limited income, did not participate in a regular exercise program, and had a limited knowledge of basic nutritional facts. The food diary indicated that feelings of anxiety related to schoolwork and frustration over the lack of social life often accompanied binge eating of high calorie, low nutrition snack foods.

In planning nursing interventions, the community health nurse involved the client. Behavior patterns were identified and alternatives were suggested by the nurse and client, who was assisted in setting short- and long-term goals. The nurse planned interventions accordingly. For example, one goal the client set was to lose 25 pounds and another was to exercise three times each week. The nurse

was challenged to plan interventions that assisted the client in attaining and maintaining her ideal weight.

In implementing the planned interventions, the nurse had to stay attuned to difficulties that the client was experiencing in carrying out the desired plan of action. For example, when the client was unable to cease snacking while studying, as she had originally planned, the nurse assisted her in selecting low calorie, nutritious snacks such as raw vegetables.

The effectiveness of the nursing interventions were evaluated in terms of the number of pounds lost, alterations made in eating patterns, and improved muscle tone attained. The client and nurse alike were able to monitor the results of the diet and exercise regimen and make modifications as indicated.

SUMMARY

This chapter has described current trends in nutrition and exercise. Although there is yet to be discovered a single product or activity that is a panacea for all Americans, useful benefits from improved nutrition and increased exercise have been shown.

Perhaps in no other area does nursing have a brighter future than in that of health promotion. The roles nursing can and will play in health promotion are endless. Identification of risk factors, education and motivation of individuals and groups, and interpretation of research findings and claims made in lay publications are only a few of the contributions community health nurses can make. Though other disciplines such as medicine and nutrition are essential to health promotion, it is often the community health nurse who first comes into contact with individuals and groups in need of nutritional and exercise guidance. That nurse must be acutely aware of the impact that the role modeling of nutritional habits and exercise programs can have on clients. Obese nurses have little effectiveness encouraging clients to diet and exercise if the nonverbal message conveys that these activities are unimportant to the care giver.

There is no diet plan or exercise prescription that works for all people at all times, but through the use of the nursing process, clients can be assisted in developing individualized plans for health promotion.

BIBLIOGRAPHY

Blomquist, K.: Physical fitness programs in industry: applications of social learning theory, Occup. Health Nurs. **29**:30-33, July 1981.

Boots, S., and Hogan, C.: Creative movement and health, Top. Clin. Nurs. **3**:23-31, July 1981.

Boykin, L.S.: Soul foods for some older Americans, J. Am. Geriat. Soc. **23**:380-382, 1975.

Bray, G.: Dietary guidelines: the shape of things to come, J. Nutr. Educ. **12**(suppl. 2):92, 1980.

Caliendo, M: Nutrition and preventive health care, New York, 1981, Macmillan Publishing Co., Inc.

De Vries, H.,: and Adams, G.M. Electromyographic comparison of single doses of exercise and meprobamate as to effects on muscular relaxation, Am. J. Phys. Med. **51:**130-141, 1972.

Edwards, S., and Gettman, L.: The effect of employee physical fitness on job performance, Per. Adm. **13:**41-44, Nov. 1980.

Fadiman, J.: food and nutrition. In Hastings, A., Fadiman, J., and Gordon, J., editors: Health for the whole person, Boulder, Colo., 1980, Westview Press, Inc.

Fixx, J.: The complete book of running, New York, 1977, Random House, Inc.

Fixx, J.: Jim Fixx's second book of running, New York, 1980, Random House, Inc.

Fleming, P., and Brown, J.: Using market research approaches in nutrition education, J. Nutr. Educ. **13:**4, 1981.

Folkins, C.H., and Sime, W.E.: Physical fitness training and mental health, Am. Psychol. **36:**373-389, April 1981.

Getchell, B.: Physical fitness: a way of life, New York, 1979, John Wiley and Sons, Inc.

Halfman, M.A., and Hojnacki, L.H.: Exercise and the maintenance of health, Top. Clin. Nurs. **3:**1-10, July 1981.

Harris, D.: Fat: no deposit no return, Women Sports **50:**54, Oct. 1977.

Harris, L.: The Perrier study: fitness in America, New York, 1979, Great Waters of France.

Harvey, M., and Harvey, W.: Running: immunization against the diseases of hypokinesis, Top. clin. Nurs. **3:**41-51, July 1981.

Healthy People: the Surgeon General's report on health promotion and disease prevention, DHEW Pub. No. 79-55071, Washington, D.C., 1979, U.S. Department of Health, Education and Welfare.

Heyn, D.: The nutrition free-for-all, Fam. Health **13:**24, 1981.

Hickey, N., et al.: Study of coronary risk factors related to physical activity in 15,171 men, Br. Med. J. **3:**507-509, 1975.

Hojnacki, L.H.: Fitness evaluation, Top. Clin. Nurs. **3:**11-22, July 1981.

Kannel, W., and Sorlie, P.: Some health benefits of physical activity, Arch. Intern. Med. **139:**857-861, 1979.

Kelly, K.L.: Evaluation of a group nutrition education approach to effective internal control, Am. J. Public Health **69:**813-816, 1979.

Kondrasuk, J.: Company physical fitness programs: salvation or fad? Per. Adm. **25:**47-50, Nov. 1980.

Mann, G.: Medical care for the fitness revolution, South. Med. J. **74:**261-263, March 1981.

Metress, J., and Kart, C.: A system for observing the potential nutritional risks of elderly people living at home, J. Geriatr. Psychiatry **11:**67, 1978.

Pender N.J.: Health promotion in nursing practice, New York, 1982, Appleton-Century-Croft.

Peterson, E.: Making nutrition education really work, J. Nutr. Educ. **12**(suppl. 2):92, 1980.

Pollock, M., and Blair, S.: Exercise prescription, J. Phys. Educ. Res. **52:**30-35, Jan. 1981.

Price, J.H., and Luther, S.L.: Physical fitness: its role in health for the elderly, J. Gerontol. Nurs. **6:**517-523, Sept. 1980.

Richmond, J.: Forward, Am. J. Clin. Nutr. **32:**2621, 1979.

Ryan, B.: The government's surprising new position, Parade Nov. 15, 1981.

Robinson, C., and Lawler, M.: Normal and therapeutic nutrition, ed. 16, New York, 1982, Macmillan Publishing Co., Inc.

Schafer, R.B.: The self-concept factor in diet selection and quality, J. Nutr. Educ. **11:**37-39, 1979.

Senate Select Committee on Nutrition and Human Needs: Dietary goals for the United States, Washington, D.C., 1977, U.S. Government Printing Office.

Stein, M.P., et al.: Results of a two year health education campaign on dietary behavior: the Stanford three-community study, Circulation, **54:**826-832, 1976.

Thomas, G.: Physical activity and health: epidemiologic and clinical evidence and policy implications, Prev. Med. **8:**89-103, 1979.

U.S. Department of Health, Education and Welfare: Nutrition and your health, Washington, D.C., 1980.

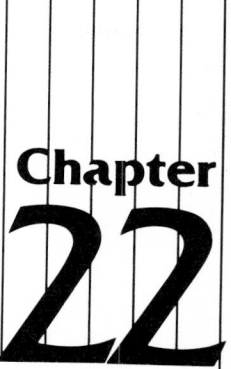

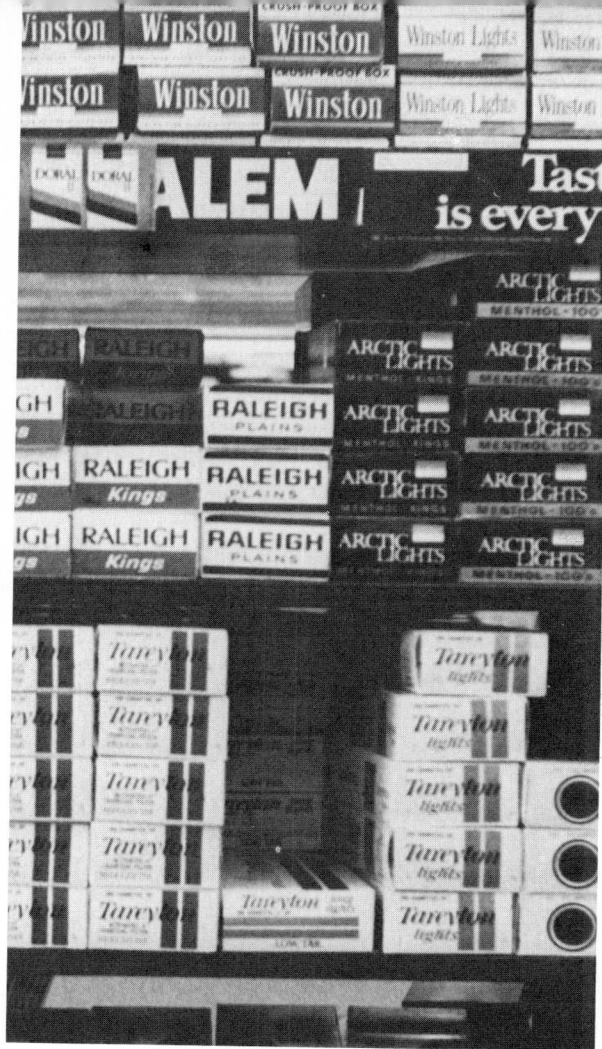

Chapter 22

JEANETTE LANCASTER

SUBSTANCE ABUSE AND COMMUNITY HEALTH NURSING

Heavy tobacco, alcohol, and drug use has been linked to numerous forms of morbidity and mortality. In 1978, 1 of the 12 health status goals established by a task force of the Department of Health, Education and Welfare called for reducing the incidence of alcohol and drug abuse. Likewise, in *The Surgeon General's Report on Health Promotion and Disease Prevention* (Healthy People, 1979), the first two challenges for prevention addressed cigarette smoking and alcohol and drug use. This report cited cigarette smoking as the single most preventable cause of death, and alcohol as a factor in over 10% of all deaths in the United States.

Substance abuse, or the use of chemicals having undesirable effects on people, is a major target area for community health nurses to address. Given the role of community health nurses as promoting the health of individuals, families, and communities, substance abuse is an essential component of the scope of practice. Staying healthy is neither an easy nor a static task. The diseases affecting particular age groups tend to differ from one another, as do the major risk factors. In one way or another substance abuse affects all ages, all races, both sexes, and all segments of society. Directly or indirectly few people are immune to the hazards of substance abuse either through direct consumption or through indirect avenues such as secondhand smoke, increased accident potential for abusers, and family disruption when one or both parents or a child abuses drugs or alcohol.

This chapter examines ways to minimize health disruptions either directly or indirectly attributed to substance abuse. The first section briefly depicts the scope of the problem and its attendant effect on nursing, health care, and society. Following sections discuss in detail alcohol abuse, drug abuse, and smoking. Each describes groups at greatest risk for becoming involved in abuse, behavioral and physiological implications of abuse, and avenues of intervention.

OVERVIEW OF SUBSTANCE ABUSE IN MODERN SOCIETY

The necessity for community health nurses to become actively involved in the prevention and cessation of substance abuse is underscored when one considers the numerous and far-reaching consequences attributed to these habits. Heavy tobacco, alcohol, and drug use has been associated with low birth weight and congenital abnormalities in the children of users; accidents, homicides, and suicides; chronic diseases, such as cardiovascular diseases, cancer, and lung disease; violence and family disruption.

Attitudes and Social Conditions Influencing Substance Abuse

Historically confusion has existed as to whether substance abuse is a problem for the health care or the criminal justice system. Abusers have often been viewed as weak, misguided people who could do better if they would only "pull themselves up by their bootstraps." Substance abuse has typically been associated with a perceived lack of self-control, and victims of these maladies are viewed negatively by health care professionals and members of the lay community. Many people hold negative attitudes toward substance abusers, attitudes that influence their actions.

Attitudes are reflected in a tendency to behave either positively or negatively toward a person, group, object, situation, or value (Community Health Nurse, 1978a). Attitudes significantly influence small and large matters of life. Attitudes develop over a period of years and are greatly influenced by the family. Membership in groups throughout life also influences attitudes, and in some groups strong forces urge conformity to group norms of thinking about selected objects, events, people, or ideas. Education and the media also influence attitude development.

Attitudes toward alcohol and drug abuse tend to be more severe than those toward smoking. In general, smoking is viewed as an unnecessary habit harmful both to the smoker and those forced to inhale smoke by-products. In contrast, attitudes toward alcohol and drugs tend to be harsher, with users of these substances often viewed as weak-willed, immoral, and irresponsible people.

Research studies of nurses' attitudes toward alcoholic clients reflect an overwhelming predominance of ambivalent, moralistic, and pessimistic attitudes (Community health nurse, 1978a). Although most nurses intellectually recognize alcohol abuse as a disease as well as a community health problem, they often retain a core of deeply entrenched negative attitudes derived from previous learning, experiences, and peer group associations. These same attitudes are reflected in beliefs about people addicted to substances other than alcohol. While on one hand nurses acknowledge that most substances that are abused are addictive, they also think that people could give up this dependency if they would only try harder.

Ambivalence or negative attitudes toward substance abusers reinforce a tendency to deny the magnitude of the problem or avoid abusers. Abusers tend to seek help; when they are unable to give up their dependency yet continually reappear for help, nurses are inclined to feel frustrated and helpless. Nothing seems to help, so providers turn away. This perceived rejection then reinforces the person's already damaged self-image and often motivates increase reliance on chemicals.

Attitudes are usually reflected in words and actions. If community health nurses are to help chemically dependent people, it is essential to recognize them as individuals with health problems who cannot always clearly ask for help. Substance abuse, because of its addictive nature and effect on both physiological and psychological functioning, is a complex phenomenon. Treatment and rehabilitation are possible, and substance abusers are and can be worthwhile, productive members of society. Goals should be realistic, mutually established, and implemented in a gradual fashion, with continuous support and reinforcement for positive steps taken.

Also, in thinking about attitudes toward substance abuse, consider how society categorizes "good" and "bad" drugs. Good drugs are those prescribed by a health care provider, yet this makes them no less addictive and problematic. Americans have come to rely heavily on legal drugs to relieve (or mask) fear, tension, and physical and/or emotional pain. We have sanctioned the "path of least resistance." Rather than learning to cope with stress, hurt, and so forth, people take pills to blot out feelings. Hence a new culture of substance abusers has arisen and been sanctioned by society.

Children grow up witnessing parental models of substance abuse. Note the parent who can only get one foot out of bed before groping for a cigarette on the bedside table. After lighting a cigarette, albeit with shaking hands, this same bleary-eyed parent lumbers to the kitchen to plug in the coffee pot for the second jolt of stimulant. Children see addiction in their own homes and learn that certain substances help people get through the day.

Additionally, many social conditions have hastened dependence on a variety of chemicals. The mass media often create and magnify social problems. Recall when the threat of war or international uprising was absent? Society marches at a fast pace. We hurry just to wait in line on crowded freeways, airports, and shopping areas. Americans have become a foot-tapping society—rushed, anxious, and harried. Little wonder people seek to escape from pressure.

Cultural values of achievement, competition, profit, and mobility have shifted emotional gratification. Who really believes the adage "It is not who wins or loses but how you play the game that matters"? Tell that to a group of parents of 9-year-old Little Leaguers and watch their incredulous expressions. The pressure to be best is often overwhelming and typically stressful. People have a drink at noon and 5 o'clock PM to calm their frayed nerves. Coffee and cigarettes serve as crutches for making it through the day. The problem is complex; the cost is great. Community health nurses must play a role in promoting health by minimizing substance abuse. To do so, it is necessary to understand selected abusive patterns. Alienation from family and friends often occurs. The dependent person may go to great lengths to assure a supply of the drug, including securing it from a variety of sources to avoid embarrassment and detection; substitute chemicals may be used; meals tend to be neglected, as does grooming.

During the advanced stages severe .physical problems or psychological symptoms occur. Drug usage becomes continuous, and afflicted individuals become increasingly dependent on others to organize and manage their lives.

Chemical Dependency Syndrome

Various components make up chemical dependency, including psychological, social, medical, economic, and legal aspects. Generally more males than females are involved; the greatest incidence is among young and middle-aged adults. Exposure, availability, and price are key determinants in the rates and distribution of chemical dependency. The various drugs used can lead to similar problems, including unemployment, bankruptcy, family disruption, neglect of children, and traumatic injury or death. Some chemicals because they are highly addictive, expensive, or run the risk of being contaminated, have significant potential consequences.

Westermeyer (1976) divided the clinical course of chemical dependency into three stages: early (problematic heavy use); middle (chronic dependence and addic-

tion); and advanced. During the early stage, greater doses are taken and the drug assumes an increasingly important role in the person's life. The person thinks more and more about the drug and structures activities to maximize drug benefit. Problems often encountered during this phase include traumatic injury (from falls, fights, accidents) or legal problems (from assaults, child abuse, and automobile accidents).

During the middle phase, as the dosage is increased, the cost of acquiring the drug rises, and longer periods of intoxication ensue. The drug is required to prevent the onset of withdrawal. People close to the chemically dependent person notice personality changes when he is under the influence of the drug or compared to behavior when he is sober. Family- and job-related problems are frequent at this time because of the lack of predictability of behavior when using the drug.

Community health nurses hold health promotion as a major goal. Effective health promotion and intervention begin with an understanding of the psychological dynamics of both the chemically dependent person and the family. Typically, chemically dependent people have many negative feelings toward themselves. While on the exterior they may appear either hostile, aggressive, and blaming of others, or charming and gracious, inside they are likely to feel fear, hurt, pain, guilt, or shame (Tarrant Council on Alcoholism and Drug Abuse, 1981). To withstand these negative self-feelings, spontaneous defenses often arise and develop with no conscious recognition on the person's part. The major defenses seen in chemical dependency include the following (Tarrant Council on Alcoholism and Drug Abuse, 1981, p. 1):

1. Regression, or the spontaneous forgetting of shameful and painful memories
2. Rationalization, or the intellectual process of making irrational behavior seem rational
3. Projection, or the unconscious unloading of personally unacceptable thoughts, feelings, and attitudes about self onto others

These defenses cause chemically dependent people to be out of touch with the severity of their symptoms in that they forget, explain away, and blame others for their problems. As can be seen in the following box the chemically dependent person goes through a complex series of feelings and behavior during each stage of the dependency process.

Families play a crucial role in chemical dependency. Frequently they deny the problem and minimize in their own minds the degree to which the family member abuses drugs or alcohol. The family often assumes a protective function, trying to hide the problem from others. They make excuses for absences or tardiness to

Guidelines for Self-Management of the Process of Recovery in the Family Illness of Chemical Dependency

■ The end (it appears)
■ The chemically dependent person
Come to a feeling of powerlessness
↓
Desire for help
↓
Ask for help
↓
Gain knowledge and understanding skills and awareness of personal power resources
↓
Gain knowledge of the personal role in the family illness
↓

Very few families have the resources to deal with this illness alone.

Friends and unskilled concerned others do not possess these resources.

You are not alone unless you choose to be. Professional and skilled support is available. The chemically dependent person has an illness and needs understanding and support, *as does the family.*

Concerned others and the chemically dependent person must learn how to deal with the illness effectively for their sakes. *Education classes at councils or treatment facilities, treatment at treatment facilities, private counseling, literature, and peer support groups provide for meeting these needs.*

Family and concerned others are part of the process. They develop the same symptoms and problems as the chemically dependent person, though they are not using a chemical. Family and friends must give equal attention to their own symptoms. As the chemically dependent person is dysfunctional because of drug-induced behavior, the family becomes dysfunctional because of emotionally induced behavior. The recovery for the chemically dependent person will not begin until his system changes. Being part of that system, the family has power to cause a change in the system.

■ The family and concerned others
Come to a feeling of powerlessness
↓
Desire for help
↓
Ask for help
↓
Gain knowledge and understanding skills and awareness of personal power resources
↓
Gain knowledge of the personal role in the family illness
↓

Used with permission of S. Brooke, Tarrant Council on Alcoholism and Drug Abuse, Fort Worth, Tex.

work, school, or social activities and support rationalization about the use of chemicals. Every time they say that the chemically dependent person has "the flu," they reinforce their wall of self-deception.

The process of chemical dependency becomes a self-perpetuating cycle. As the dependent person uses more chemicals, spontaneous projections such as "Maybe if you cooked once in a while, I wouldn't need to get high" occur, instilling guilt and feelings of inadequacy in the family. To prove their own worth, then, the family continues to protect the dependent member by apologizing for him, excusing him, and doing for him what he is capable of doing himself.

As the process progresses, and if intervention has not occurred, the family may move to the middle stage as defined by Westermeyer (1976), where they monitor the dependent person's intake of chemicals, hide or throw away the supply, and plead with him to quit.

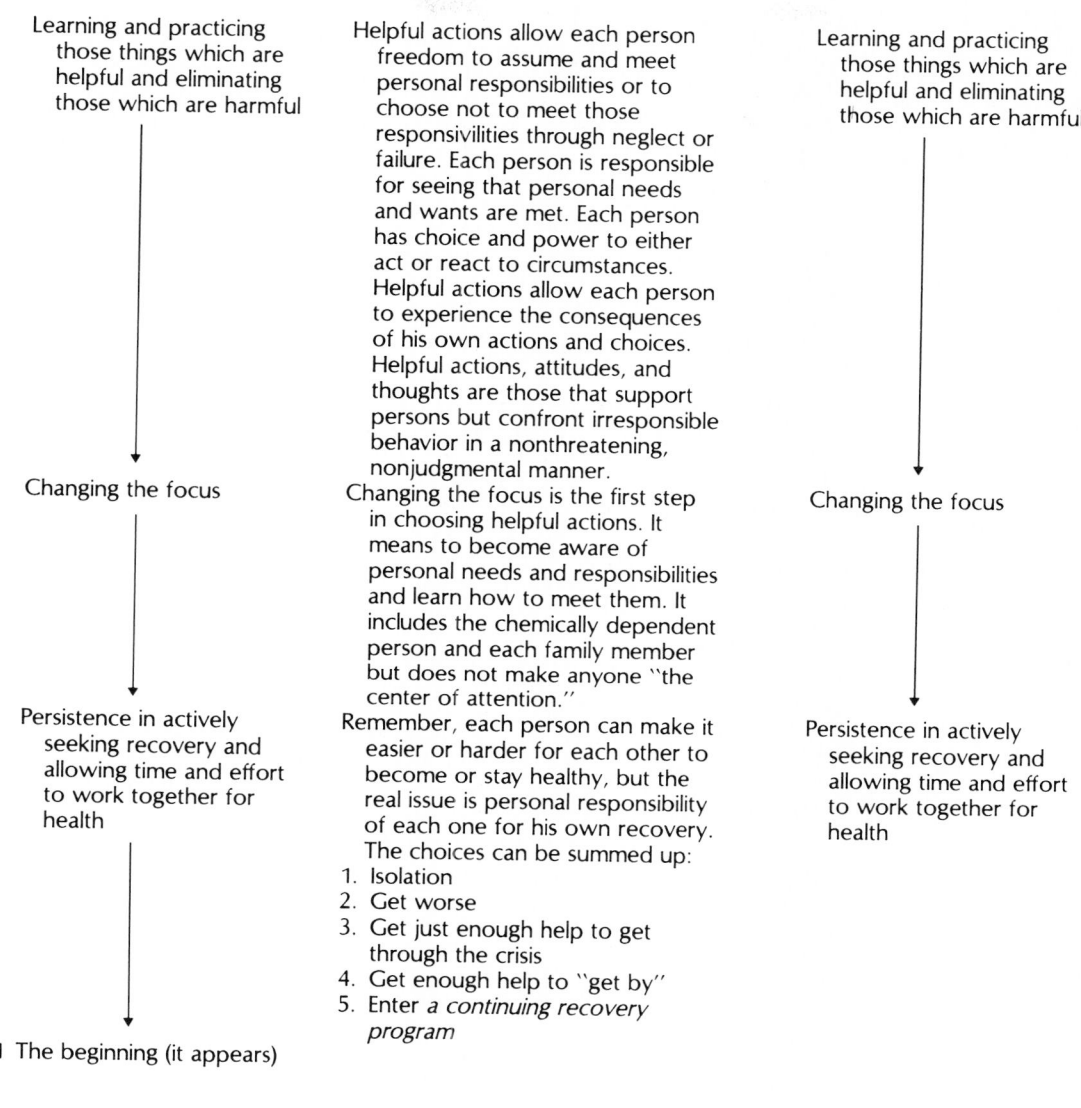

Learning and practicing those things which are helpful and eliminating those which are harmful

↓

Changing the focus

↓

Persistence in actively seeking recovery and allowing time and effort to work together for health

↓

■ The beginning (it appears)

Helpful actions allow each person freedom to assume and meet personal responsibilities or to choose not to meet those responsivilities through neglect or failure. Each person is responsible for seeing that personal needs and wants are met. Each person has choice and power to either act or react to circumstances. Helpful actions allow each person to experience the consequences of his own actions and choices. Helpful actions, attitudes, and thoughts are those that support persons but confront irresponsible behavior in a nonthreatening, nonjudgmental manner.

Changing the focus is the first step in choosing helpful actions. It means to become aware of personal needs and responsibilities and learn how to meet them. It includes the chemically dependent person and each family member but does not make anyone "the center of attention."

Remember, each person can make it easier or harder for each other to become or stay healthy, but the real issue is personal responsibility of each one for his own recovery. The choices can be summed up:

1. Isolation
2. Get worse
3. Get just enough help to get through the crisis
4. Get enough help to "get by"
5. Enter *a continuing recovery program*

Learning and practicing those things which are helpful and eliminating those which are harmful

↓

Changing the focus

↓

Persistence in actively seeking recovery and allowing time and effort to work together for health

However, typically the more the family attempts to control substance use, the more the dependent person uses chemicals, and the more inadequate the family feels.

During the advanced stage, families often compensate for their low self-worth by blaming the dependent member for all their troubles. The family's attempts to control and manipulate the chemical dependency actually support the abuse and perpetuate the cycle. To re- verse this process the family must gain some insight into how the disease affects them and the dependent person as well as what they are doing to perpetuate the cycle. The box above depicts the progression of chemical dependency within the family.

Community health nurses are often in a key position to detect the early onset of chemical dependency and to guide clients and families to appropriate referral sources such as a mental health center, private practitioner, or hospital clinic. Through home visits, clinic appointments, and various screening activities nurses can detect the presence of chemical dependency. With regard to chemical dependency the first goal is prevention followed by early intervention. The next section examines the type of preventive efforts that hold the greatest potential.

Prevention

The most effective way to handle chemical dependency is to prevent its onset. The role of prevention, however, is by no means held only by community health nurses but is a responsibility of multiple types of health care, social service, and education providers. Chemical dependency is thought to result from a variety of social, psychological, cultural, and physiological factors. Prevention efforts are directed toward reducing stress, teaching people ways to constructively spend leisure time, reinforcing abstinence from drugs as a positively valued characteristic, and informing people of the untoward effects of substance abuse.

Prevention starts early, and community health nurses in many parts of the country play active roles in schools. Nurses can either work directly in prevention by meeting with classes and others groups of children or can provide teachers with information and resources for substance abuse prevention. Since peers play a vital role in influencing the onset of substance abuse, a useful prevention strategy involves getting youth to work with other young people and help them learn and feel comfortable refusing to become involved with substances. The National Institute on Drug Abuse developed a series of booklets on drug abuse for use in the classroom and in other youth groups. Since this chapter cannot provide in-depth discussion of the myriad of prevention possibilities, readers are referred to the following booklets: "Saying No: Drug Abuse Prevention in the Classroom" (1981); "Beyond the Three R's: Training Teachers for Affective Education" (1980); and "Doing Drug Education: The Role of the School Teacher" (1980). Each has many valuable prevention suggestions.

With children, prevention centers primarily on providing education about the potential hazards of alcohol abuse and providing affective education, which helps children learn to deal effectively with feelings and needs. Adults, however, typically know about the effects of alcohol. They have already been provided with information about the consequences of excessive drinking. Prevention of alcohol abuse in adults is complex and requires a multifaceted, societal approach.

To date, no one theory of causation for alcoholism has been identified. Primary factors leading to or supporting the development of alcoholism are thought to be largely psychological, sociological, and/or physiological in nature. The most effective prevention efforts rely on major shifts in social functioning, whereby the positive aspects of alcohol consumption are minimized and the deleterious aspects emphasized. The media portray alcohol as a substance to aid in relaxation and socialization. As people become increasingly hurried, tired, and stressed, alcohol use seems more acceptable and inviting as a method for coping with life's demands.

Prevention lies more with social institutions such as the work place, churches, and community groups and organizations than with health care professionals. However, health care professionals often serve as catalysts to encourage industry to begin stress-reduction programs, remain alert to the needs of high risk employees (those with multiple needs, health problems, and limited or no support networks), and detect early signs of alcohol abuse. Similarly, community health nurses can encourage churches and community groups to recognize the needs of their members and the greater community for encouragement, support, and assistance in times of increased stress. Additionally, each of these organizations and many others can provide programs to teach participants ways to cope more effectively with life's demands and thereby decrease the need to turn to alcohol as a crutch for coping.

Early Detection

If prevention has not been accomplished, the next phase is early detection and treatment. To do this it is important to recognize the major risks associated with drug dependence. Diet is often associated with drug dependence for several reasons. Opiates such as morphine or codeine serve as appetite suppressants, as do psychostimulants or amphetamines, including Benzedrine, pesoxyephedrine and methamphetamine (Desoxyn). Alcohol-dependent people consume many nonnutritious calories in their beverages. Additionally, drug dependence is expensive, and chemicals rather than food may receive priority for limited funds. Chemically dependent people also tend to transfer their behavior from one item to another. For example, on giving up cigarettes, ex-smokers may overeat or drink to excess to compensate for unmet needs. Thus people who abuse substances should be carefully monitored as they attempt to cease one habit, lest they transfer the needs onto another one.

Many severely drug-dependent people neglect their appearance and hygiene as they increasingly focus their attention on the chemicals they tend to use. Particular health risks from these tendencies include skin disorders, dental caries, and gum disease. Living conditions often suffer, thereby predisposing people to additional diseases associated with filth and pest infestation. The

---

General Behavior Characteristics of Substance Abuse

- Abrupt changes in school or work attendance, quality of work, grades, discipline, work output
- Unusual flare-ups or outbreaks of temper
- Withdrawal from responsibility
- General changes in overall attitude
- Deterioration of physical appearance and grooming
- Furtive behavior regarding actions and possessions
- Wearing of sunglasses at inappropriate times (to hide dilated or constricted pupils)
- Continual wearing of long-sleeved garments (to hide injection marks)
- Association with known users of drugging substances
- Unusual borrowing of money from parents or friends
- Stealing small items from home, school, or employer
- Attempts to appear inconspicuous in manner and appearance (to avoid attention and suspicion)
- May frequent odd places without cause, such as storage rooms, closets, basements (to take drugs)

From Signs of use of substances for drugging effects, Washington, D.C., 1978, Pharmaceutical Manufacturers Association.

---

box above lists general behavior characteristics of substance abusers.

Sleep deprivation and disturbances are associated with barbiturates and other hypnotic agents. Although one of the clinical uses of these substances is to induce sleep, chronic use leads to sleep impairments. To achieve the desired effect, the drug-dependent person may increase the dosage, thereby leading to a vicious cycle. Sleep deprivation then leads to an entirely new set of symptoms, including feelings of depersonalization, memory, and concentration disturbances, with severe deprivation leading to a psychotic state.

Pain suppression is associated with narcotic addiction, and central nervous system depressants with analgesic properties. Many diseases go unnoticed because pain is not experienced; some reach an irreversible state, when earlier detection and treatment could have effected relief.

Biorhythms tend to be interrupted by chemical dependency and affect many complex functions, including secretion of hormones, production of enzymes, metabolism of food and drugs, and usual levels of activity

(Westermeyer, 1981). In addition, the life-style associated with drug dependence and acquisition (crime) often increases stress.

The drug-dependent person often experiences various types of physical pathology, including skin, musculoskeletal, respiratory, cardiovascular, blood and lymphatic, gastrointestinal, genitourinary, and central nervous system disorders as described by Milby. Many body systems are at risk from substance abuse, with specific systems at greater risk depending on the substance being used.

■　　■　　■

It is not possible to describe in detail each substance that may be abused; however, attention is focused on the abuse of alcohol, tobacco, and selected other drugs, including marijuana, cocaine, and heroin. The restriction of drugs to these categories by no means negates the importance of abuse of other substances, such as barbiturates, hallucinogens, and amphetamines. These merely serve as prototype substances.

ALCOHOL ABUSE

Alcoholism is a chronic disease characterized by repetitive and often compulsive drinking that produces injury to the drinker's health and other aspects of life, including martial status, career, interpersonal relationships, or other required societal adaptations. Over the years alcoholism has been considered a social problem, a medical problem, and an illegal condition. The effects of alcoholism are widespread and cost individuals, families, communities, and employers considerably in terms of direct costs, lost revenues, pain, and human suffering.

Scope of Alcohol Abuse

There are approximately 10 million problem drinkers in the United States, and of these at least 6 million may be alcoholics (Disease Prevention and Health Promotion, 1979). The problem is compounded when one considers that between 3% and 4% of all alcoholics are homeless and rely on institutional support. Such dependence results in a substantial drain on public and private resources. Additionally, alcohol annually indirectly causes many deaths as a result of accidents, homicides, suicides, or other related events or disorders.

Alcohol abuse costs individuals, families, and communities billions of dollars annually because of lost productivity, health care costs, accidents, crime, and demands on the social welfare and judicial systems. Table 22-1 depicts the estimated annual costs associated with alcohol.

In addition to these economic costs, there are many

Table 22-1. Costs resulting from and associated with alcohol use

Item	Estimated cost (billions of dollars)
Sources of cost related to alcohol use	
Lost production	
Among males aged 21-59	$15.46
Among the military	0.41
Premature mortality	3.77
Health care costs	12.74
Motor vehicle crashes	5.14
Fire losses	0.43
Social responses	
Social welfare system	1.27
Alcohol programs	0.08
Highway safety	0.03
Fire protection	0.39
Criminal justice system (nonviolent crime)	0.17
Sources of associated costs	
Violent crime	2.10
Criminal justice system (violent crime)	0.76
TOTAL	$42.75

Modified from The community health nurse and alcohol-related problems, Pub. No. 017-024-00753-6, Rockville, Md., 1978a, National Institute on Alcohol Abuse and Alcoholism, Public Health Service, Department of Health, Education, and Welfare.

social costs of alcohol-related problems that are nearly impossible to estimate. The families of the estimated 10 million people who misuse alcohol suffer economic hardships, broken homes, and at times physical harm.

Many of the long-range effects of alcohol are discussed in depth later. However, several are highlighted here to emphasize the magnitude of this problem. For example, community health nurses should realize that cirrhosis of the liver is the fifth leading cause of death in the United States, and alcohol is related to this disease in approximately 95 out of 100 instances. Alcoholism reduces life expectancy 12 years and is related to several types of cancer, heart disease, and other illnesses. Alcohol use is associated annually with 25,000 traffic fatalities, 15,000 homicides and suicides, and almost half of all police arrests (Disease Prevention and Health Promotion, 1979).

Increased Risk Factors

Statistically, people with alcohol-related problems have a mortality and suicide rate 2.5 times greater than the average and are 7 times more prone to become involved in accidents (Community Health Nurse, 1978b). Health problems associated with alcohol abuse include higher rates of cancer of the larynx, oral cavity, liver, and esophagus. It is unclear whether the lack of adequate nutrition often associated with alcohol abuse increases susceptibility to the effects of alcohol or whether the alcohol itself causes the damage. However, it is known that alcoholic individuals with cancer have lower survival rates and a greater susceptibility for developing another primary tumor compared to nonalcoholics with the same type of cancer.

People at greatest risk for lung and esophageal cancer are those who combine heavy alcohol intake with heavy smoking. The risk of esophageal cancer is 44 times greater for those who consume more than six drinks and one or more packs of cigarettes daily (Community Health Nurse, 1978b).

Physiological Effects of Alcohol

Although there are several kinds of alcohol, ethyl alcohol, or ethanol, is the substance contained in alcoholic beverages. The ethanol concentration in a beverage indicates the relationship between the amount of alcohol in the drink and the total volume of liquid. *Proof* when applied to distilled spirits describes the concentration of ethanol and is usually based on a 2:1 ratio. That is, an 80-proof liquor contains 40% alcohol.

Alcohol, like sugar, is a simple, incomplete food with limited nutritional value. Although it lacks vitamins, amino acids, and minerals, alcohol does provide calories for heat and energy. Alcohol goes directly to the stomach, and its absorption is slowed if food, especially fatty food, is present. However, if a drink is diluted with a carbonated beverage, it will be absorbed more rapidly (Community Health Nurse, 1978a).

Soon after consumption, alcohol moves into the bloodstream and small intestine, where it is absorbed at variable rates by the organ's tissues. The *brain* is highly sensitive to alcohol, where it initially serves as a stimulant and later becomes a depressant. Extensive use of alcohol can result in premature aging of the brain. A well-known central nervous system effect of excessive alcohol is "blacking out." This episode is different from "passing out" in that it is a period of total amnesia during which the person may or may not appear to others to be under the influence of alcohol (Gitlow, and Peyes, 1980). After coming out of a blackout, the person is usually aware of a void during which memory does not fill in the details of what occurred. People may spend vast amounts of money during these episodes with no recall of doing so.

Alcohol consumption affects *emotions* by decreasing cognitive functions, thereby giving the emotions free reign. With inhibitions released, people may display emotions previously held back and become hostile, tearful, or "the life of the party." Some people drink to dull emotions. Drinking provides temporary relief, and the underlying emotions reappear when the effects of the alcohol wear off.

Small amounts of alcohol induce *sleep*, whereas larger amounts interfere with sleep by shortening the period of rapid eye movement (REM) sleep. Alcohol consumption does not affect tactile responses but does decrease *sensitivity to pain*, resulting in an increased incidence of burns, cuts, scrapes, and bruises among problem drinkers.

Nutritional deficiencies, especially deficits of the B vitamins lead to a variety of *alcohol-related neurological disorders*. These deficiencies are the result of decreased taste for food, decreased appetite (since alcohol is high in calories), and faulty absorption of nutrients because of irritation to the lining of the stomach and small intestine. Peripheral polyneuropathy subsequent to nutritional deficiency is characterized by weakness, numbness, partial paralysis of extremities, pain in the legs, and impaired sensory reactions and motor reflexes (Community Health Nurse, 1978a). This condition is reversible with adequate diet and supplemental B vitamins. However, if untreated, polyneuropathy can progress to Wernicke's encephalopathy, which is more serious although reversible. Wernicke's encephalopathy is characterized by ophthalmoplegia, nystagmus, ataxia, apathy, drowsiness, and confusion, as well as the inability to concentrate. Without treatment this disease can be fatal.

Another disease often manifested after improvement from Wernicke's encephalopathy is Korsakoff's psychosis. This condition is characterized by disorientation and memory defect whereby clients usually fill in the gaps in their memory (confabulation). Many people with Korsakoff's psychosis show limited improvement with treatment.

Alcohol is an irritant to the *gastrointestinal system*; it can damage the mucosa and result in esophagitis and gastritis. Increased capillary fragility can result in gastric bleeding, and ulcers often result. Excessive alcohol intake can cause weight gain because of the concentrated sugar and calorie content.

Alcohol also significantly affects the *cardiovascular system*. By causing vasodilation of peripheral vessels, alcohol produces flushing, heat loss, and a sense of warmth, while simultaneously causing vasoconstriction of the great vessels, producing resistance and increasing the work of the heart.

Prolonged alcohol use has been associated with enlargement of the *liver*, probably because of an accumulation of triglycerides in the hepatic cells (Community Health Nurse, 1978a). This fatty liver condition tends to be reversible with abstinence from alcohol and the assumption of a nutritious diet. Two serious alcohol-related hepatic diseases are hepatitis and cirrhosis. *Hepatitis* is an inflammation of the liver resulting either from a virus or from a toxic reaction. Similarly, *cirrhosis* is a chronic liver disease that leads to severe liver degeneration. Both of these ailments are thought to result largely from the direct effects of alcohol on liver tissue, and they may occur even in the presence of adequate diet. Lack of an adequate diet in the presence of heavy alcohol consumption increases the likelihood that cirrhosis will occur.

Pancreatitis is another condition resulting from prolonged alcohol consumption, with symptoms ranging from gastritis-like sensations to severe pain with nausea, vomiting, and rigidity of the abdomen. Usually abstinence from alcohol and consumption of adequate food and fluids relieve the symptoms.

Alcohol-dependent people frequently have decreased immunity and are thus highly susceptible to infections. Because of the depression of white blood cells, they have decreased ability to fight diseases and are highly susceptible to upper respiratory infections.

Development and Effects of Alcohol Addiction

Large doses of alcohol consumed over an extended time lead to decreased sensitivity to alcohol's effects. This phenomenon, *tolerance*, or the need to continually increase the dosage to achieve the desired effect, is common to all potentially addictive drugs. The withdrawal reaction, or acute abstinence syndrome, occurs when the addicted person suddenly stops or markedly decreases the intake of the addicting drug. Withdrawal symptoms are usually not seen unless a person has consumed the equivalent of a pint of distilled spirits for at least 10 consecutive days (Butz, 1981).

Withdrawal signs include hyperexcitability, anxiety, anorexia, insomnia, and tremor. Vital signs are usually elevated, and the person may feel irritated and shaky inside. This stage develops a few hours after alcohol intake is stopped, peaks in 24 to 36 hours, and may end abruptly with no further problems.

More severe withdrawal problems include hallucinosis and delirium tremens. In hallucinosis, the alcohol-dependent person maintains clarity of consciousness but typically experiences vivid auditory hallucinations usually within 48 hours after the cessation or reduction of heavy alcohol intake. The most severe reaction to alcohol withdrawal, delirium tremens, is characterized by disorientation, paranoia, and outbursts of irrational behavior, leading to threat of self-harm. Tachycardia is common and may be accompanied by fever, rapid breathing, sweating, vomiting, and diarrhea (Community health nurse, 1978a). Unless vigorous treatment is initiated, death can ensue because of shock, malignant hyperthermia, or secondary to complicating illness, infection, or injury. The delirium condition peaks usually the third day after cessation of drinking and persists 2 to 3 days, often ending abruptly and dramatically (Butz, 1981). During withdrawal some people experience grand mal seizures, usually during the first 48 hours. Because of the potentially severe physiological component of delirium tremens, treatment should be carried out in an inpatient facility.

Signs that indicate a person has been drinking considerably include tremulousness, nervous sweating, and tachycardia. Also, small bruises are often found, especially on the alcoholic housewife; these are the result of running into things and falling. There may be cigarette burns on fingers, chest, and legs. Alcoholics are especially susceptible to severe periodontal disease. As a group they do not neglect their physical or oral hygiene; however, they are for some unexplained reason particularly susceptible to acute necrotizing ulcerative gingivitis (Vincent's disease) and pyorrhea (Gitlow and Peyes, 1980).

Groups at Risk

People with a family history of alcoholism, those experiencing grave personal problems or stressful life events, or people with a history of other addiction are most likely to develop an alcohol-related problem. It is unclear whether the drinking patterns that seem to "run in families" result from hereditary predisposition or attitudes and patterns learned during the early formative years. Drinking problems occur less frequently in families where drinking occurred in association with meals or special occasions than where drinking was strictly prohibited. In the latter instances, a strong aura seems to surround drinking, and often during adolesence this behavior is thoroughly explored.

People with emotional problems or those beset with numerous life changes are particularly susceptible to alcohol abuse. Conditions such as desertion, divorce, separation, parental rejection, aging, role change, or role conflict comprise prime events for the onset of problem drinking. Alcohol becomes an "easy" answer for the complexities of coping with life's problems.

Women are at risk for alcohol-related problems because of conflicts in role definition as well as lack of consistency between personal and others' expectations. Also, women who are alone, such as widows, "isolated-feeling housewives," and divorcees, are often at risk for excessive drinking to cope with loneliness. Other at risk groups of women include those belonging to minority groups.

Adolescents are at risk. As discussed in Chapter 25,

developmentally this is a stage of searching, testing, and defining oneself. As adolescents try to be like others, they often incorporate alcohol abuse into their repertoire of skills. Substance abuse in general has been steadily increasing among young people. Approximately 20% of 12- to 17-year-olds report having had a drink; about half of these claim to drink at least once a month, and nearly 3% report drinking daily (Healthy People, 1979). Although young people tend to drink less frequently than adults, they seem to consume larger quantities and are more likely to become intoxicated. It is not difficult to see why the leading cause of death in the 15- to 24-age group is attributed to alcohol-related accidents and 60% of all alcohol-related traffic fatalities are among young people.

The elderly are at risk because of mandatory retirement and the necessity for living on a fixed income, which may restrict choices. Older people are often lonely and unhealthy and lack feelings of worth and purpose. Drinking fills in the voids in their lives. However, it should be noted that most elderly alcoholics drank before they reached old age.

Women and Alcohol

The drinking patterns of women are changing. Forty years ago it was virtually unheard of for women to drink, while today over 60% of all American women and almost 90% of all college-age women drink. Estimates of the ratio of women alcoholics to men alcoholics vary from 1:4 to 1:2 (Hennecke and Fox, 1980).

There do seem to be several differences between men and women in regard to alcohol and related problems. For example, with alcohol, as with many other behaviors, a double standard prevails. Men who drink heavily tend to be more readily accepted than are women. Hence, women are more likely to try to hide their drinking; less likely to seek help, they tend to become seriously ill before the disease is detected.

A commonly seen pattern among women who become alcohol abusers is that they begin as social drinkers. Finding that a couple of drinks helps them deal with feelings of anxiety and shyness and allows them to more comfortably "be themselves" in unfamiliar situations, they accelerate their drinking to avoid painful feelings and difficult situations (Sandmaier, 1977). Before they realize it, these women are daily relying on alcohol. Why don't they seek help? Partly because they do not recognize the warning signals of problem drinking and also because they are ashamed to admit they may be drinking to excess. Rather than bear the stigma of being a "fallen woman," they hide their drinking habits from people who might offer help.

Although no single cause of alcoholism for women has been found, several variables have been identified.

Table 22-2. Drug use during pregnancy

Drug	Effect on fetus	Safe use of drug
Nicotine	Heavy smoking can lead to low birth weight babies, which means that the baby may have more health problems. Especially harmful during second half of pregnancy.	Should be avoided.
Alcohol	Daily drinking of more than two glasses of wine, or a mixed drink, can cause fetal alcohol syndrome. Babies tend to low birth weight, mental retardation, physical deformity, and behavioral problems, including hyperactivity, restlessness, and poor attention span.	Should be avoided.
Aspirin	During last 3 months of pregnancy frequent use may cause excessive bleeding at delivery and may prolong pregnancy and labor.	Under physician's supervision.
Tranquilizers	Taken during the first 3 months of pregnancy may cause cleft lip or palate or other congenital malformations.	Avod if possibility of pregnancy and during early pregnancy. Use only under physician's supervision.
Barbiturates	Mothers who have taken large doses may have babies who are addicted. Babies may have tremors, restlessness, and irritability.	Only under physician's supervision.
Amphetamines	May cause birth defects.	Only under physician's supervision.

From Deciding about drugs: a woman's choice. DHEW Pub. No (ADM) 80-820, Rockville, Md., 1979, National Institute on Drug Abuse, Department of Health, Education, and Welfare.

The traditional social role of women has enhanced the reliance on alcohol and other drugs. Historically, women have derived their sense of self-worth primarily through relationships with men. Women typically earn less money for the same work as men, and are often known as "_____'s wife" and perhaps "_____'s mother." Although many women derive great pleasure from the role of wife and homemaker, others find this a boring, lonely existence offering few rewards and little or no enrichment or self-worth. Many feel trapped at home; they married prior to preparing themselves for a rewarding career and therefore have limited opportunities to find challenging employment.

The working woman, likewise, has her unique set of stresses. While loneliness and boredom may not be among the feelings experienced, pressure, conflicting demands, and sensory overload often exist. This is not to imply that working women are not lonely but rather that they have additional stressors related to the work setting as well as the demands of juggling multiple roles.

Alcoholic women can usually identify a particular life crisis that set off their drinking pattern. Examples include family or marital stresses such as separation, divorce, financial pressures, children, loss of a significant person, blow to self-esteem, health crisis, feeling of lack of meaning and fulfillment in life, and sexual problems. All women experience some of these problems; however, some cope more effectively than others.

Effects on the Fetus. An added problem in alcohol abuse among women is the potential for alcohol-induced birth defects. It is estimated that such birth defects occur in 1 of every 100 women consuming more than 1 ounce of alcohol daily during early pregnancy. Heavy use of alcohol by pregnant women, described as 3 ounces of absolute alcohol or about six drinks per day, may result in fetal alcohol syndrome (FAS). Fetal alcohol syndrome thus accounts for approximately 1 birth defect in every 5000 births. Infants suffering from this defect tend to be of low birth weight, to be mentally retarded, and to have behavioral, facial, limb, genital, cardiac, or neurological abnormalities (Healthy People, 1979).

FAS seems to be caused by the ethanol intake rather than by caloric insufficiency. A high blood alcohol level during critical periods of embryonic development leads to FAS. The average alcohol intake may not be as important as the amount consumed during heavy episodes of drinking. Malformations are most likely to occur as a result of heavy drinking during the first trimester, and growth retardation caused by heavy drinking occurs during the third trimester of pregnancy.

Table 22-2 presents the effects of drug use, including alcohol, during pregnancy.

Effects of Alcohol on the Family

The effects of alcohol are by no means limited to the drinker. In many instances families suffer multiple and long-lasting problems because of the alcohol abuse of one member. In dealing with their alcoholic relative, families often rely on denial to cope with the overwhelming implications of their problem. Feeling embarrassed, humiliated, and helpless, family members may simply ignore the existence of the problem. Family members struggle to avoid conflicts and try to control the environment so alcohol is not present; when these efforts fail, they often plead with, threaten, or attempt to punish the alcoholic.

As family members become more ashamed of the behavior of their alcoholic relative, many avoid contact with friends and relatives. With increasing social isolation, the family has fewer resources on which to draw for their own support.

As described in the section on chemical dependency, families frequently blame themselves for the drinking habits of their relatives and feel acute guilt for the role they may have played in the development or continuation of this problem. The family typically lives in a state of continuous anxiety about what will happen next—an accident, loss of income, or loss of esteem and status in the community. Alcoholics typically create ongoing crises for themselves and their families through unpaid bills, loss of job, and embarrassing social situations (Community Health Nurse, 1978a).

Although most alcoholics behave as though they were quite independent, many are heavily dependent on those around them. When their drinking propels them into a crisis, their usual response is to do nothing about this, but rather wait until someone comes along to bail them out. Each time the alcoholic is bailed out the cycle of drinking → crisis → dependency is rewarded. Additionally, once the crisis is over it is easy to deny the existence of a problem, and the rescuers are often regarded with hostility for interfering.

Families of alcoholics are usually angry. Their rage may be repressed; if so, however, it is ultimately expressed in a more covert fashion, such as via ulcers or inappropriate outbursts toward strangers. The anger also may be suppressed and perceived as boredom, depression, chronic fatigue, and disinterest.

Nonalcoholic family members often make great efforts to maintain some semblance of family stability. The nonalcoholic parent may become an overachiever, trying to be sure the children are well fed and involved in age-related activities and that the home is clean and comfortable. To maintain family order, the alcoholic member is often unconsciously excluded. Order, however, is rarely maintained for lengthy periods because of the disruptive behavior brought on by the drinking. When drinking, alcoholics are often hostile, belligerent, irresponsible, self-centered, and violent; sober, these same people can be remorseful, kind, generous, affectionate, and solicitous. The startling contrast between drinking and nondrinking behavior and the lack of predictability keep families confused as to what to expect.

Children have difficulty understanding how a parent can seem like a cruel, overbearing monster one day and come home all smiles and bearing gifts the next time. Also, the longer families go without seeking help, the greater the likelihood that the family will disintegrate. The divorce rate among alcoholics is four times the national average (Community Health Nurse, 1978a).

Children are particularly susceptible to the effects of alcoholism in the family. These youngsters are frequently the victims of child abuse because of poor parental control of emotions. They fear the unpredictability of their parent's behavior and may avoid bringing friends to their home. Children often assume many of the adult responsibilities of their alcoholic parent and must work at home or care for siblings when they would prefer to play with peers.

Children cope with alcoholism by fleeing, fighting, or being either "super good" or a "super coper" (Community Health Nurse, 1978a). They flee by literally escaping physically—hiding under the bed, hiding in closets, or staying away from home as much as possible—or by fleeing mentally—emotionally insulating themselves from the family.

Other children react to adult alcoholism by physical and/or verbal agression. They strike out at other children or act out in school or at home. In contrast, some children try either to be perfect or to rescue and help the family cope, thereby increasing their level of stress by this added responsibility.

Role of the Community Health Nurse

Since community health nurses come in contact with families of alcoholics in a variety of settings, they play a vital role in prevention, assessment, intervention, and referral. As described in Chapter 32, community health nurses are responsible for coordinating client care both via appropriate referrals and through careful monitoring, coordination of services and resources, and follow-up. Because of their lowered level of tolerance, many alcoholics (and other substance abusers) become lost in the health care system. For example, if care is not provided satisfactorily in agency A, the abuser may give up rather than seek alternative sources of care. Community health nurses can guide clients from one agency to another and offset feelings of "no one will (or can) help me."

Not only do community health nurses serve as a source of referrals and coordinators of care, but they also assess the potential for and/or presence of alcohol-related problems and provide direct intervention, including counseling and health education. In assessment, the guide by Heinemann and Estes (1976) provides a thorough tool. Alcoholics are generally poor historians, especially about their drinking habits, since

Table 22-3. Indications of alcohol-related problems

Family	Social	Physical	Occupational	Drinking behavior	Legal
Quarrels over drinking	Loss of interest in activities not directly associated with drinking	Hangover (malaise, red eyes, hand tremor)	Work pace more spasmodic	Gulping drinks	Driving while under the influence of alcohol
Physical abuse	Not seeing customary friends	Alcohol or mouthwash on breath	Avoiding boss/associates	Shifting from one alcoholic beverage to another	Frequent automobile accidents
Decreased socialization with friends	Seeking out new "friends" with similar drinking preferences	"Accident prone"—fractures, cuts, burns, etc.	Neglecting details formerly attended to	Admits drinking more than peer group	Other offenses—assault, disorderly conduct, property crimes, public drunkenness, reckless driving
History of divorce	Marked behavior change after drinking	Vague, minor complaints, especially in women	Job changes (frequent)	Drinks to relieve anger, depression, etc.	Referral to an alcohol safety action program
Withdrawal of children	Irritability	Blackouts (no memory of events though not passing out)	Frequent absences from work	Repeated conscious efforts at abstinence	Underage purchasing of alcoholic beverages
Reluctance of children to bring friends home	Sensitive to comments from others about drinking	Injuries, especially when treatment is delayed 24 hours	Disappears in afternoon	Blatant, indiscriminate use of alcohol	
School or other behavioral problems in children; "super straight"	Inappropriate telephone calls	Hospitalization for peptic ulcer, gastritis, pancreatitis	Neglects household tasks	Drinking alone	
Family history of alcoholism, abstinence, broken home	Personality change, poor judgment, inability to concentrate, memory impairment	Laboratory findings (early): BSP retention 10%-15%	Falling grades	Hiding bottles	
Woman recently separated, divorced, children leaving home		Serum enzymes	Frequent absence from school	Not measuring drinks	
Signs of fetal alcohol syndrome in newborns and young children		Uric acid 10%-15%		Drinking before going to a social function	
Financial worries				Not knowing how many drinks one has had	
				Intoxication	

From The community health nurse and alcohol-related problems, Pub. No. 017-024-00753-6, Rockville, Md., 1978a, National Institute on Alcohol Abuse and Alcoholism, Public Health Service, Department of Health, Education, and Welfare.

they often deny the extent of the problem. Specific questions are suggested, including what, when, where, and who. Questions asking how and why tend to increase defensiveness and are less desirable (Heinemann and Estes, 1976). During the assessment, the client should stay focused on the topic, and digressions into lengthy descriptions of past drinking episodes are discouraged.

Information derived from the assessment may lead to nursing interventions directed toward maintaining adequate nutrition and hydration, providing a safe environment in the home, promoting rest and sleep, and teaching new ways to handle stress and to cope with conflict and other possible problems (Schultz and Dark, 1982).

As seen in Table 22-3 there are multiple implications and areas for intervention in alcohol-related problems. Community health nurses often counsel family members and provide support as well as teach them new ways to deal with their alcoholic relative.

In addition, children of alcoholics are often recognized in school because of their many absences, signs of physical or emotional abuse, or behavior problems in the classroom. Often the nonalcoholic parent can be contacted via the school-age child and referrals made for all or several family members. For teens, Alateen, a nation-wide program addressing the needs of adolescent children of alcoholics, has been helpful. This type of support is sponsored by Al-Anon, a self-help group for adult relatives and close friends of alcoholics, and is based on the principles of Alcoholics Anonymous. The purpose of Al-Anon is to facilitate discussion and resolution of common problems related to being closely associated with an alcoholic.

In both industries and the community, nurses are in key positions to design prevention programs, detect alcohol-related problems, and make appropriate referrals. The first step is to know the available community resources for the treatment of alcohol-related problems. Community resource directories and telephone books are places to start in identifying if there are facilities for acute care of alcohol-related problems. Questions to ask include the following: Which hospitals or clinics run detoxification units? Does the community mental health center have a special program or unit for alcohol addiction? What resources are available in both the public and the private sector? Who is eligible for the various resources?

Not only should the health-related resources be assessed but the availability of lay support and self-help groups is vitally important. It is generally recognized that Alcoholics Anonymous (AA) has done more for the treatment of this disease than have health care providers. Basically, AA treatment consists of 12 steps leading toward recovery. In the first three the alcoholic acknowledges the crux of the problem and makes a commitment to work toward resolution. During the next four steps the person takes an honest look at self, shares this information with a special person, and begins to modify behavioral deficiencies. In the succeeding four steps the alcoholic continues self-scrutiny. Finally in the last step he reaches out to help others. The fellowship, support, and encouragement among AA members, all of whom are abstaining alcoholics, is tremendous. Members are available to one another day and night to aid in crisis intervention and to respond to other calls for support and aid.

Al-Anon and Alateen are similar self-help programs for spouses, parents, children, or others involved in a painful relationship with an alcoholic. *Al-Anon* family groups are available to anyone who has been affected by their involvement with an alcoholic. Local groups meet regularly to help members learn the facts about alcoholism as an illness, the types of treatment available, ways that can help the alcoholic, and how to reduce their own tension. In addition, many cities have *Alateen* groups for youth between 12 and 20 years who live in an alcoholic family situation. These groups are of vital importance, since children who live in alcoholic families are at risk for emotional problems. The purposes of Alateen include providing a forum for discussing family stressors, learning coping skills from one another, and gaining support and encouragement from knowledgeable peers.

Alcohol-Drug Interactions

Not only must nurses be aware of the effects of alcohol on individuals and families but special attention needs to address possible alcohol-drug interactions, since many mixtures can be accidentally fatal. The physical and behavioral effects of drug and alcohol combinations must be recognized by community health nurses. Many frequently prescribed drugs contain at least one ingredient known to interact adversely with alcohol. Most adverse effects resulting from such combinations are accidental, yet the death and morbidity tolls are high.

It is important to carefully assess clients as to their present and previous drinking patterns and determine if they are impulsive drinkers or have a chronic dependence on alcohol. In addition, even when not drinking, chronic alcoholics may have altered drug effects because of liver damage. For example, among chronic heavy drinkers there is an increased metabolism rate for phenytoin (Dilantin), which necessitates larger than normal doses to achieve the desired effect.

Specific drugs to be aware of include analgesics, anesthetics, antialcohol preparations, antianginal and antihypertensive agents, anticoagulants, anticonvulsants, antidepressants, stimulants, antihistamines, antidiabetic agents, antiinfectives, barbiturates, tranquilizers, and narcotics. Clients taking any of these medications should be queried as to their alcohol consumption patterns. While great detail cannot be provided here, several examples of drug-alcohol interaction are cited to focus attention on the magnitude of this problem. Table 22-4 presents selected interaction effects of alcohol with several commonly used drugs.

Even when used alone, *salicylate*-type analgesics can cause mild gastrointestinal bleeding. Combined with alcohol, bleeding can be greatly aggravated. Also, community health nurses need to understand the use and possible consequences of *disulfiram* (Antabuse) as an agent to encourage abstinence. This drug is given as a useful chemical barrier to alcohol consumption. If a client is taking disulfiram and subsequently takes a drink, the results are extremely unpleasant and can be dangerous. Such combinations will cause a rise in blood pres-

Table 22-4. Interaction effects of alcohol with other drugs

Type of drug	Generic name	Trade name	Interaction effect with alcohol
Analgesics Nonnarcotic	Salicylates	Products containing aspirin Bayer Aspirin Bufferin Alka-Seltzer	Heavy concurrent use of alcohol with analgesics can increase the potential for gastrointestinal bleeding. Special caution should be exercised by individuals with ulcers. Buffering of salicylates reduces possibility of this interaction.
Narcotic	Codeine Morphine Opium Oxycodone Propoxyphene Pentazocine Meperidine	 Pantopon Paregoric Percodan Darvon Darvon-N Talwin Demerol	Narcotic analgesics and alcohol interact to reduce functioning of the central nervous system (CNS) and can lead to loss of effective breathing function or respiratory arrest: death may result.
Antianginal	Nitroglycerin Isosorbide dinitrite	Nitrostat Isordil, Sorbitrate	Alcohol in combination with antianginal drugs will cause the blood pressure to lower—creating a potentially dangerous situation.
Antibiotics Antiinfective agents	Furazolidone Metronidazole Nitrofurantoin	Furoxone Flagyl Cyantin Macrodantin	Certain antibiotics, especially those taken for urinary tract infections, have been known to produce disulfiramlike reactions (nausea, vomiting, headaches, hypotension) when combined with alcohol.
Anticoagulants	Sodium warfarin Acenocoumarol Coumarin derivatives	Coumadin, Panwarfin Sintrom Dicumarol	With chronic alcohol use, the anticoagulant effect of these drugs is inhibited. With acute intoxication the anticoagulant effect is enhanced; hemorrhaging could result.
Anticonvulsants	Phenytoin	Dilantin	Chronic heavy drinking can reduce the effectiveness of anticonvulsant drugs to the extent that seizures previously controlled by these drugs can reoccur if the dosage is not adjusted appropriately. Enhanced CNS depression may occur with concurrent use of alcohol.

From Blum, S., and Kreblein, K.: Interaction effect of alcohol with other drugs, Lincoln, Neb., 1977, Nebraska Division on Alcoholism; compiled from Lipman, A.G.: Drug interactions with alcohol, Mod. Med. **44**(4):67-69, Feb. 15, 1976; Fact sheet — Drug interactions with alcohol, National Clearinghouse for Alcohol Information (Feb. 1976); It's dangerous to mix alcohol and drugs, National Clearinghouse for Alcohol Information; and The whole college catalog about drinking, U.S. Department of Health, Education, and Welfare, NIAAA.

Continued.

Table 22-4. Interaction effects of alcohol with other drugs—cont'd

Type of drug	Generic name	Trade name	Interaction effect with alcohol
Antidiabetic agents, hypoglycenics	Chlorpropamide Acetohexamide Tolbutamide Tolazamide Insulin	Diabinese Dymelor Orinase Tolinase Iletin	The interaction of alcohol and either insulin or oral antidiabetic agents may be severe and unpredictable. The interaction may induce hypoglycemia or hyperglycemia; also disulfiram-like reactions may occur.
Antidepressants	Nortriptyline Amitriptyline Desipramine Doxepin Imipramine	Aventyl Elavil, Endep Pertofrane Sinequan Tofranil	Enhanced CNS depression may occur with concurrent use of alcohol and antidepressant drugs.
Antihistamines	For example, chlor-pheniramine	Many cold & allergy remedies Coricidin Allerest	The interaction of alcohol and these drugs enhances CNS depression.
Antihypertensive agents	Rauwolfia preparations Resperine Guanethidine Hydralazine Pargyline Methyldopa	Rauwiloid Serpasil Ismelin Apresoline Eutonyl Aldomet	Alcohol, in moderate dosage, will increase the blood pressure–lowering effects of these drugs and can produce postural hypotension. Additionally, an increased CNS depressant effect may be seen with the rauwolfia alkaloids and methyldopa.
Antimalarials	Quinacrine	Atabrine	A disulfram-like reaction and severe CNS toxicity will result if antimalarial drugs are combined with alcohol.
CNS depressants Barbiturate hypnotics	Phenobarbital Pentobarbital Secobarbital Butabarbital Amobarbital	Luminal Nembutal Seconal Butisol Amytal	Since alcohol is a depressant, the combination of alcohol and other depressants interact to further reduce CNS functioning. It is extremely dangerous to mix barbiturates with alcohol. What would be a nondangerous dosage of either drug by itself can interact in the body to the point of coma or fatal respiratory arrest. Many accidental deaths of this nature have been reported. A similar danger exists in mixing the nonbarbiturate hypnotics with alcohol
Nonbarbiturate hypnotics	Methaqualone Glutethimide Bromides Flurazepam Chloral Hydrate	Quaalude Doriden Neurosine Dalmane Noctec	Disulfiram-like reactions have been reported with alcohol use in the presence of chloral hydrates.
Tranquilizers (major)	Thioridazine Chlorpromazine Trifluoperazine Haloperidol	Mellaril Thorazine Stelazine Haldol	The major tranquilizers interact with alcohol to enhance CNS depression, resulting in impairment of voluntary movement, such as walking or hand coordination; larger doses can be fatal.
Tranquilizers (minor)	Diazepam Meprobamate Chlordiazepoxide-HCL Oxazepam	Valium Equanil Miltown Librium Serax	The minor tranquilizers depress CNS functioning. Serious interactions can occur when using these drugs and alcohol.

Table 22-4. Interaction effects of alcohol with other drugs — cont'd			
Type of drug	**Generic name**	**Trade name**	**Interaction effect with alcohol**
CNS stimulants	Caffeine Amphetamines Dextroamphetamine Methamphetamine	In coffee and cola Vanquish Benzedrine Dexedrine Desoxyn	The stimulant effect of these drugs can reverse the depressant effect of alcohol on the CNS, resulting in a false sense of security. They do not help the intoxicated person gain control over coordination or psychomotor activity.
Disulfiram (antialcohol preparation)	Disulfiram	Antabuse	Severe CNS toxicity follows ingestion of even small amounts of alcohol. Effects can include headache, nausea, vomiting, convulsions, rapid fall in blood pressure, unconsciousness, and — with sufficiently high doses — death.
Diuretics (also antihypertensive)	Hydrochlorthiazide Chlorothiazide Furosemide Quinethazone	Hydrodiuril Esidrix Diuril Lasix Hydromox	Interaction of diuretics and alcohol enhances the blood pressure — lowering the effects of the diuretic; could possibly precipitate postural hypotension.
Monoamine oxidase inhibitors (MAOI)	Pargyline Isocarboxazid Phenelzine Tranylcypromine	Eutonyl Marplan Nardil Parnate	Alcoholic beverages (such as beer and wines) contain tyramine, which will interact with MAOI to produce a hypertensive, hyperpyrexic crisis. Frequent use of alcohol with MAOIs may result in enhanced CNS depression.

sure, flushing of face, tachycardia, pounding headache, sense of apprehension, dizziness, rapid breathing, nausea, vomiting, weakness, and fainting (Interaction Effect of Alcohol with Other Drugs, 1977). Similarly, diabetics taking oral hypoglycemic drugs such as *tolbutamide* (Orinase) can develop an adverse reaction to alcohol similar to that of disulfiram (Heinemann and Estes, 1976).

Tolbutamide has different effects for chronic versus occasional alcohol users. Whereas short-term consumption of large amounts of alcohol increases the half-life of tolbutamides, chronic alcoholism causes a significant decrease in tolbutamide half-life.

The last example cited here, but certainly not the least dangerous combination, occurs when alcohol is mixed with antihistamines. Drowsiness, a common side effect of antihistamines, is increased to the extent that performance skills such as driving or operating machinery are impaired.

DRUG ABUSE

Americans continue to use drugs, both legal and illicit ones, to cope with life stressors. Several commonly used drugs are discussed in some detail to highlight the problem. Marijuana, cocaine, and heroin uses are discussed because these substances are commonly abused in most American communities. See Table 22-5 for signs of drug use.

Abuse of Illicit Drugs
Marijuana

Typical marijuana smokers are practically indistinguishable from their nonsmoking peers. The use of this substance cuts across all demographic lines, with a higher incidence among college students and college graduates than the general population. Professional and higher income adults rank among the highest occupational groups involved in the experimental use of marijuana (Carr and Meyers, 1980). Use is more frequent among males, in cities, and in the western part of the United States, followed by states in the Northeast, North Central, and South. The first marijuana experience for users tends to occur between the ages of 14 and 21 years.

Increased use in recent years can be attributed to a variety of factors. During the social and political upheavals of the 1960s, marijuana was a symbol of protest against the Vietnam War and the "establishment." It became a common form of recreation on campuses and

Table 22-5. Possible signs of use of specific substances for drugging effects

Substances	Signs
Glue, vapor-producing solvents, propellants	Odor of substance on breath and clothes Excess nasal secretions, watering of eyes Poor muscular control Drowsiness or unconsciousness Increased preference for being with a group, rather than being alone Plastic or paper bags or rags containing dry plastic cement or other solvent found at home or in lockers at school or at work
Depressants (barbiturates, tranquilizers, "downs")	Symptoms of alcohol intoxication with one important exception: no odor of alcohol on breath Staggering or stumbling Falling alseep unexplainably Drowsiness; may appear disoriented Lack of interest in school and family activities
Stimulants (amphetamines, cocaine, "speed," "bennies," "ups")	Pupils may be dilated (when large amounts have been taken) Mouth and nose dry; bad breath; user licks his lips frequently Goes long periods without eating or sleeping Excess activity; user is irritable, argumentative, nervous; has difficulty sitting still Chain smoking If injecting drug, user may have hidden eyedroppers and needles among possessions
Narcotics (heroin, morphine)	Lethargic, drowsy Pupils are constricted and fail to respond to light Inhaling heroin in powder form leaves traces of white powder around nostrils, causing redness and rawness Injecting heroin leaves scars, usually on the inner surface of the arms and elbows, although user may inject drugs in body where needle marks will not be seen as readily Users often leave syringes, bent spoons, bottle caps, eyedroppers, cotton, and needles in lockers at school or at work, or hidden at home
Marijuana	In the early stages of intoxication, may appear animated with rapid, loud talking and bursts of laughter In the later stages, may be sleepy or stuporous Whites of eyes may appear inflamed; pupils may be dilated Odor (similar to burnt rope) on clothing or breath Remnants of marijuana, either loose or in partially smoked "joints," in clothing or possessions NOTE: Unless under the influence of the drug at a time of observation, marijuana users are difficult to recognize; infrequent users may not show any of the general symptoms. Marijuana is greener than tobacco. Cigarettes made of it (called "joints," "sticks," or "reefers") are rolled in a double thickness of brown or off-white cigarette paper. Smaller than a regular cigarette, with the paper twisted or tucked in at both ends. the butts (called "roaches") are not discarded but saved for later smoking if not consumed at initial usage. Marijuana also may be smoked in a pipe (very small bowl, long stem) or cooked in brownies and cookies.
Hallucinogens (LSD, PCP, mescaline)	Senses of sight, hearing, touch, body image, and time are distorted Mood and behavior are affected, the manner depending on emotional and environmental condition of the user Users may become fearful and experience a degree of terror Users of LSD may have unpredictable flashback episodes without use of the drug NOTE: It is unlikely that persons using hallucinogens will do so in school, at work, or at home at a time when they might be observed. At least in the early stages of usage, these drugs generally are taken in a group situation under special conditions designed to enhance their effect. LSD is odorless, tasteless and colorless. It usually is taken orally in tablets, capsules, or a wide variety of substances (impregnated with liquid LSD). PCP is most frequently found in tablets, powder, or mixed with leaf mixtures for smoking. Even though declared to be different chemicals, many illicit drugs may contain PCP.

From Signs of use of substances for drugging effects, Washington, D.C., 1978, Pharmaceutical Manufacturers Association.

among servicemen and spread across all age groups and social classes. While 1 in 5 youth and adults report use of marijuana, only 1 in 20 say they have used it more than 100 times (Carr and Meyers, 1980).

As marijuana use legally moved from a felony to a misdemeanor, emphasis on the medical risks associated with its use increased. Despite numerous efforts to prove otherwise, the majority of research on this substance points to its being less of a health hazard than the indiscriminate use of either alcohol or tobacco (Carr and Meyers, 1980).

Despite the fact that marijuana has not been documented as a major community health hazard, it does have a number of effects that influence individuals and the community. For example, users experience a short-term increase in heart rate, "reddening of the eyes, drying of the mouth, and dose-related distortions of sensory information—touch, smell, taste, and vision may become intensified and perceived by many as pleasurable" (Carr and Meyers, 1980, p. 166). Because of distortions in perception and vision, driving becomes difficult and the risk of accidents increases. Inhibitions may be reduced, allowing people to behave in ways normally avoided.

Tolerance, the need for increasingly large doses to achieve the same effect, and dependence are not usually associated with marijuana use. However, this substance does temporarily affect psychomotor skills, although to a lesser extent than alcohol.

Marijuana has been used for centuries as a therapeutic substance. References to cannabis use date back to the fifteenth century, and cannabis was included in the *U.S. Pharmacopoeia* until 1941. It has recently been used to help reduce intraocular pressure in the eyes of glaucoma patients; to relieve the pain of cancer patients; to reduce or eliminate loss of appetite, nausea, and vomiting following chemotherapy; to relieve asthmatic distress by temporarily dilating the bronchial passages; and to facilitate sleep as a sedative-hypnotic (Carr and Meyers, 1980).

Cocaine

In recent years interest in cocaine use in the United States has increased; approximately 4 million people between the ages of 18 and 25 were thought to have used this substance in 1976. Cocaine is one of several alkaloids found in the leaves of the coca plant native to the "eastern watershed of the Andes Mountains in Peru, Columbia, and Bolivia" (Carr and Meyers, 1980, p. 183). The street-level purity of cocaine in the United States is about 13% by the time it has been cut with substances such as lactose, glucose, and mannitol. Also, one never knows what else has been mixed with the cocaine; hence the risk in using such a drug is great.

Cocaine can be fatal when ingested in large doses or taken by people with a particular sensitivity to this drug. However, there is little scientific evidence to prove there is physiological dependence and tolerance to cocaine. The potential does exist for psychological dependence (Carr and Meyers, 1980). Cocaine is a central nervous system stimulant, and the desired effect is excitation; irritability and hyperactivity have been associated with its long-term use. Cocaine may be injected, sniffed, or swallowed. When sniffed, the user frequently complains of a runny nose.

Besides the direct hazards associated with cocaine use, indirect effects relate to poor eating and sleeping habits. Likewise, because of the expense involved, substance abuse is often related to theft and other types of crime. Withdrawal symptoms include depression, lassitude, headache, excessive sleeping, convulsions, and seizures. It is estimated that cocaine use alone or in combination with other drugs leads to 350 deaths annually, with the greatest hazard coming from drug interactions.

Heroin

Heroin addiction, while less prevalent than in the past, is still a major health problem. There are an estimated 240,000 drug treatment "slots" in the United States, with 60% devoted to heroin users. Nearly 85% of those receiving drug treatment do so on an outpatient basis, 8% are in residential programs, and the remaining 7% are in hospitals, prisons, or day-care settings (Lewis and Sessler, 1980).

Over the decades a variety of techniques have been developed to treat heroin addiction. The therapeutic communities of the late 1950s took a variety of forms. A forerunner of this treatment approach, Synanon, was "the first organized efforts by addicts themselves to solve their problems through self-help techniques" (Lewis and Sessler, 1980, p. 99). This program, while controversial because of its approach and some of its leaders, required total immersion into a thoroughly prescribed and disciplined life-style, including indefinite residence in a Synanon facility.

The greatest effort in treating heroin addiction has been the development of methadone, a synthetic opiate for use in the maintenance of heroin addicts. Although used since the 1940s as a drug to aid withdrawal at the Lexington, Kentucky, Public Health Service Hospital, it was not used as a maintenance drug until the 1960s. In 1964 researchers Vincent Dole, an internist and biochemist, and Marie Nyswander, a psychiatrist, noticed a difference in the behavior of chronic heroin addicts maintained on methadone compared to those on heroin. Those maintained on methadone seemed more alert, energetic, and interested in constructive social activities compared to the ones on heroin, who became lethargic after an infection and underwent withdrawal as it wore off (Lewis and Sessler, 1980). A treatment program was devised to offer methadone maintenance, counseling, job training, and other forms of support.

From a social perspective, many inner-city heroin users have been raised in broken homes, live in inadequate housing, are poorly educated, and often are unemployed. It is frequently difficult to determine which comes first: the poor social conditions or the addiction. The key factor is that treatment programs must include social rehabilitation components. Community health nurses are in key positions to coordinate the needs of clients with available and accessible services. Many of these people are unskilled, unemployed, and undereducated.

Treatment of Illicit Substance Abuse

Historically "drug epidemics" have occurred during periods of job shortages and high labor surpluses (Lewis and Sessler, 1980). Many of the federal programs that previously have aided these people have recently been reduced, thereby decreasing the rehabilitation options. In the future, industry may be called on to take a more active role in social rehabilitation as the federal government's involvement diminishes in this arena.

Widely varying types of treatments have been attempted for substance abuse. Selected types are summarized here to give an overview of community health nursing implications. The most severe event associated with substance abuse is overdose. Often this is a life-threatening situation requiring immediate emergency care. Community health nurses do not tend to be involved in the acute stages of drug overdose, but they are often involved in coordinating care when the person returns to the community.

Likewise, detoxification usually takes place in a controlled hospital setting where withdrawal from the drug can be accomplished on a regular schedule and where staff members are trained to recognize and deal with the physical and emotional problems faced during withdrawal. However, detoxification from opiates often takes place in outpatient programs (Milby, 1981). The dose schedule may be reduced over a 6-week period, providing less disruption of life routines than caused by hospitalization. Detoxification, or gradual withdrawal, allows for a less painful method of abstinence than going "cold turkey."

Currently there are four major heroin treatment methods: maintenance programs using methadone and L-alpha acetyl methadol (LAAM, a long-acting form of methadone), detoxification programs, outpatient drug-free programs, and drug-free therapeutic communities. The first three are generally outpatient programs and the fourth is residential. There are also inpatient hospital programs and those in prisons.

Maintenance Programs. As mentioned, methadone is a synthetic opiate used as a maintenance drug for heroin addicts. Its effect lasts approximately 24 hours, compared to 3 to 4 for heroin. Additionally, the effect of LAAM lasts 2 to 3 days, but LAAM does not produce the same subjective effects as methadone, thereby being less desired by clients. The Federal Drug Administration has set criteria for admission to methadone maintenance programs that carefully define eligible patients. The criteria require objective evidence of 2 consecutive years of opiate addiction, evidence of current addiction, and a minimum age of 18 years (Milby, 1981).

Detoxification Programs. Detoxification programs are used to relieve withdrawal symptoms and to enable addicts temporary freedom from their addiction. The ordinary course of treatment is 21 days, although some programs have reported success in 7 to 14 days (Lewis and Sessler, 1980). The primary goals of these programs are to withdraw addicts from drugs and engage them in follow-up treatment. These programs seem to have a good short-term effect but the rate of relapse is high. Programs are increasingly structuring their efforts to provide maximal amounts of supportive care and follow-up. For example, some addicts become depressed after detoxification and can be effectively treated with antidepressants. Other drugs currently being tested (naltrexone) are narcotic antagonists that block the effects of heroin.

Outpatient Drug-Free Programs. Outpatient abstinence programs seek to help people via counseling, group therapy, employment assistance, job training, and other supportive services (Lewis and Sessler, 1980). These clinics seem more effective in treating persons using illicit drugs other than heroin. Many of these programs are offered in association with community mental health centers and other forms of comprehensive care. The nursing role in these programs is multifaceted and often includes counseling, observation, and referral.

Therapeutic Communities. "Therapeutic community (TC) is a generic term for an institution that treats and rehabilitates individuals with relatively severe behavioral problems like drug addiction and alcoholism" (Milby, 1981, p. 205). Most therapeutic communities assume that addiction results from long-term psychological problems, and the community becomes the main source for meeting the physical and emotional needs of residents.

Federal Government's Response to Illicit Drug Use

During the twentieth century the federal government has made many attempts to decrease the use of illicit drugs. In spite of billions of dollars spent and millions of hours devoted to curbing drug abuse, there are as many abusers of illicit drugs as ever before and a rapidly increasing population who are misusing legally available drugs.

The first piece of drug legislation was the District of Columbia Pharmacy Act of 1906, which set a precedent for other acts. This act "permitted a physician to prescribe narcotics to addicts but only when 'necessary for the cure' of addiction; the prescription of narcotic drugs to non-addicted persons was limited to the treatment of injury or disease" (Goldberg, 1980, p. 21).

Subsequently, the Harrison Narcotics Act of 1914 marked the official entry of the government into narcotic control. This act simplified record keeping on narcotics and required standard forms to be kept for 2 years on the sale of narcotic drugs. In 1929 the Porter Act called for the development of two federal drug treatment centers—one at Lexington, Kentucky (1935), and the other in Forth Worth, Texas (1938).

In 1930 the first federal agency devoted to the control of illicit drugs, the Federal Bureau of Narcotics (FBN), was established to control the most dangerous drugs (Goldberg, 1980). Later the Boggs Act of 1951 and the Narcotic Control Act of 1956 increased penalties for all drug law violators.

As a result of the Advisory Commission on Narcotics and Drug Abuse (the Pettyman Commission) appointed by President Kennedy in 1963, drug abuse came to be viewed as a health concern rather than an entirely legal issue. The Narcotic Addict Rehabilitation Act of 1966 (NARA) officially considered addiction a medical problem

The Nixon Administration afforded drug abuse high priority because of increases in urban crime ascribed to drug use. The public's increasing concern about heroin addiction and the development of new approaches to treat heroin addiction occurred. The Comprehensive Drug Abuse Prevention and Control Act of 1970 provided support for drug treatment, rehabilitation, education, and enforcement. In 1970 the federal government allocated $101.9 million to drug abuse, compared to $5,712.9 million in 1978. Numerous drug abuse milestones were reached during the Nixon administration, culminating in the establishment of the National Institute on Drug Abuse (NIDA) within the Department of Health, Education, and Welfare (Goldberg, 1980).

The emphasis on drug abuse diminished during the Ford Administration. President Carter supported treatment, rehabilitation, and job-training programs for former heroin addicts, better coordination of research efforts, and concern for the prescribing of addictive drugs such as barbiturates and other sedative-hypnotic drugs. Drug abuse efforts are presently receiving limited national attention, yet the problem remains.

Abuse of Legal Drugs

Substance abuse includes the use of both illicit and legally sanctioned drugs. It is becoming increasingly common in responding to the rush and stresses of life for people to rely on tranquilizers, pain relievers, antidepressants, and sedatives. Community health nurses have multifaceted goals in dealing with this problem. First, careful assessment is essential to accurately determine a person's pattern and mix of substances. People do not always tell health care providers about all of the medications they are taking, thereby allowing for possible inadvertent prescribing of adversely related combinations.

Assessment includes determining exactly what prescribed and nonprescribed drugs are being taken as well as the symptoms that prompt their use. Rather than relying on drugs to relieve tension, clients may need to be referred to an agency or source providing psychological counseling, stress reduction, exercise, and so forth. The community health nurse must know what resources are available, as well as who is eligible and the specific type of assistance offered by each.

The focus of this text is on health promotion, and many chapters have addressed the multiple changes in society requiring continuous adaptation. As mentioned in Chapter 38, stress is a frequent companion to changing roles, responsibilities, and life-styles. Men, women, and children are engaged in constant life changes as they create and/or adapt to an ever-changing society. The use of either prescribed or nonprescription drugs is a poor choice for dealing with change, stress, and general life pressures.

Prevention of Substance Abuse

Prevention of substance abuse begins with learning factual information about drugs and their effects and then identifying alternative ways to fill one's life. For those who already have problems with drugs, "early intervention with personal counseling and support is essential" (Deciding about Drugs, 1979, p. 9). Many people have not consciously acknowledged their dependence on drugs. The questions in the following box can be included in an interview to determine whether addiction is present or imminent. If the person answers yes to a number of these questions, he may be misusing drugs or alcohol.

> ### ⫿⫿⫿ Danger Signals of Addiction
>
> - Do those close to you often ask about your drug use? Have they noticed any changes in your moods or behavior?
> - Are you defensive if a friend or relative mentions your drug or alcohol use?
> - Are you sometimes embarrassed or frightened by your behavior under the influence of drugs or alcohol?
> - Have you ever gone to see a new doctor because your regular physician would not prescribe the drug you wanted?
> - When you are under pressure or feeling anxious, do you automatically take a tranquilizer or drink or both?
> - Do you take drugs more often or for purposes other than those recommended by your doctor?
> - Do you mix drugs and alcohol?
> - Do you drink or take drugs regularly to help you sleep?
> - Do you have to take a pill to get going in the morning?
> - Do you think you have a drug problem?

From Deciding about drugs: a woman's choice, DHEW Pub. No. (ADM) 80-820, Rockville, Md., National Institute on Drug Abuse, Department of Health, Education, and Welfare.

On learning that a client abuses alcohol or prescribed or nonprescription drugs, the next step is to assist the person to identify alternatives for dealing with the circumstances or problems leading to substance abuse. The community resource directory can provide sources of assistance, as can many of the specific suggestions found in other chapters of the text.

SMOKING AND HEALTH

Cigarette smoking is the single most preventable factor contributing to illness, disability, and death in the United States. Despite widespread public knowledge about the hazardous affects of smoking and general acceptance that smoking is indeed harmful, there are still many adult and young smokers in the United States (Healthy People, 1979). In 1979 there were more than 50 million smokers in the United States. The prevalance of smoking declined substantially between 1965 and 1970. In addition, in 1978 the prevalance of cigarette smoking among adults reached its lowest point in over 30 years. Although the percentage of adults who are regular smokers fell from an estimated 41.7% in 1965 to an estimated 33.2% in 1978, the total number of smokers over age 17 increased because of population increases. In 1978 an estimated 54 million men and women smoked 615 billion cigarettes (Smoking and Health, 1979).

Cigarette smoking is a costly and preventable hazard to health. Smoking is a primary factor in lung cancer as well as cancer of the larynx, pharynx, oral cavity, esophagus, pancreas, and bladder. In addition, cigarette smoke interacts with certain substances involved in occupational exposure, such as asbestos and uranium, to aggravate the risk that might accrue from occupational exposure or smoking alone (Disease Prevention and Health Promotion, 1979). Smoking also doubles the risk of heart attack for men.

Health care costs in 1979 were documented as being $205 billion per year, with the federal government paying $59 billion. Smoking is estimated as accounting for $5 to $8 million in health care expenses aside from indirect costs resulting from lost productivity, absenteeism, and wages. These indirect costs are estimated to be between $12 and $18 million annually (Smoking and Health, 1979). A substantial portion of these costs is borne by nonsmokers through effects on health insurance premiums, disability payments, and other private and tax payer–supported programs. The adverse health effects of smoking vary considerably in their nature and severity, depending on duration and frequency of smoking, presence or absence of concurrent illness, environmental exposures to other toxic substances, age, and sex (Smoking and Health, 1979).

Short-Term Effects

The lungs retain more than 85% of the compounds actually inhaled through the nose, mouth, and trachea. Cigarette smoke and the 2000 known chemicals in it escape the body's first lines of defense, the mouth and nose, because of the way inhaled. As the smoke travels through the mouth, it affects the taste buds on the tongue so that foods can taste different.

As the smoke continues down the throat through the trachea, the mucosa becomes inflamed. The outer layer of cells along the trachea are damaged and transformed over time into types of cells not effective in protecting the body.

Smoke changes the elasticity of the bronchioles and causes them to constrict. Smoke also impairs the cilia, considerably reducing efficient washing of the tracheobronchial tree. The cilia are paralyzed, and mucus cannot be cleared from the lungs. Excessive amounts of mucus are also produced and begin to clog airways. People who smoke are much more likely to be able to cough up some of this mucus when asked to than are people who do not smoke. This is because of the excessive amount of mucus produced and its collection in the airways.

Changing Cigarettes

Considerable changes have occurred in cigarettes in recent years. In 1954 the average tar yield of most cigarettes was 37 mg and the average nicotine yield was 2 mg. In contrast, in 1980 the comparable figures were 14 mg tar and less than 1 mg nicotine (Health Consequences of Smoking, 1981). Smokers have turned to these reduced tar and nicotine cigarettes out of concern for health, yet new hazards have arisen. For example, cigarette yields measured by machine are different from those the consumer actually obtains by smoking the cigarette because of differences in patterns of smoking between people and testing machines. Additionally, to make cigarettes palatable when tar and nicotine are reduced, manufacturers have introduced a variety of flavorings and other chemical additives. Since manufacturers do not have to reveal what additives they use, it is impossible to assess the current risks of cigarettes (Health Consequences of Smoking, 1980).

Maintenance of the Smoking Habit

The component of cigarette smoke responsible for the biological dependence on and tolerance to tobacco has not been clearly identified, although nicotine seems to be the most likely culprit. Tolerance is seen in the need for an increasing dose of a substance to receive the desired effect. Tolerance toward carbon monoxide and tar has also been identified (Smoking and Health, 1979).

Many smokers maintain this undesirable habit because they had seen or previously experienced the tobacco withdrawal syndrome. The onset of this syndrome is rapid, and several characteristic behaviors are usually seen. Changes in mood and performance are obvious in the outbursts of temper; lack of tolerance for people, events, and things; impaired performance because of lack of concentration; and episodes of daydreaming. Other effects of cessation include craving for tobacco, irritability, restlessness, anxiety, dullness, sleep disturbance, and impaired judgment and psychomotor performance (Smoking and Health, 1979).

There is, however, a hopeful social trend in America in that the number of adult cigarette smokers is steadily declining. More people than ever before are knowledgeable about the risks associated with smoking. In fact, "today's cigarette smokers are a troubled minority"; 9 out of 10 would like to quit (Smoking Digest, 1977, p.1). Smokers are worried about their health, are seeking help, and need the understanding, support, and encouragement of knowledgeable community health nurses.

To understand smoking as a community health problem and to plan effective health promotion strategies, it is necessary to explore the scope of smoking as a health hazard by describing who and how many people smoke, the known health hazards associated with smoking, and successful efforts at smoking prevention and cessation.

Involuntary Smoking

Involuntary smoking is the "inhalation of tobacco combustion products in smoke-filled atmospheres by a nonsmoker" (Smoking Digest, 1977, p. 23). In these instances the nonsmoker can involuntarily breathe toxic components of tobacco smoke. The chemical components of tobacco smoke are derived from two sources: *mainstream* and *sidestream* smoke. "Mainstream smoke is the smoke inhaled and then exhaled by the smoker, and sidestream smoke is the smoke which is generated by the cigarette while it smolders" (Smoking Digest, 1977, p. 24). Even when a smoker inhales, two thirds of the smoke goes into the environment (Fig. 22-1).

Although a debated topic (Diamond and Forrester, 1983), involuntary smoking may be dangerous, since the sidestream smoke contains higher levels of toxins than the mainstream smoke. Sidestream smoke has 5 times as much carbon monoxide, 50 times as much ammonia, and twice as much tar and nicotine as the mainstream smoke (Smoking Digest, 1977).

Over 90% of mainstream smoke is in the form of a gas. Seventy percent of this gas is oxygen and nitrogen, which are normally inhaled, while the remaining 20% is a combination of chemicals toxic to people. Examples of chemicals in this collection of gas include formaldehyde, hydrogen cyanide, ammonia, and carbon monoxide.

Carbon monoxide is particularly dangerous to health, since it bumps oxygen molecules out of the red blood cells and forms a new compound—carboxyhemoglobin. As the level of this new compound increases in the blood, body cells become starved for oxygen. Nonsmokers, on inhaling carbon monoxide, evidence impairments in preforming visual, auditory, and manual tasks.

Cigarette smoke causes eye irritation, headaches, nose and throat discomfort, and a variety of other allergic-like reactions. After only 30 minutes in a smoke-filled room, the carbon monoxide inhaled by a nonsmoker will increase the person's heartbeat and blood pressure. Many people suffer from chronic cardiovascular and respiratory symptoms and are highly susceptible to the effects of smoke.

Pipe and Cigar Smoke

Pipe and cigar smokers do not tend to inhale as vigorously as cigarette smokers; thus they are at less risk of developing lung cancer. However, the risk equals that

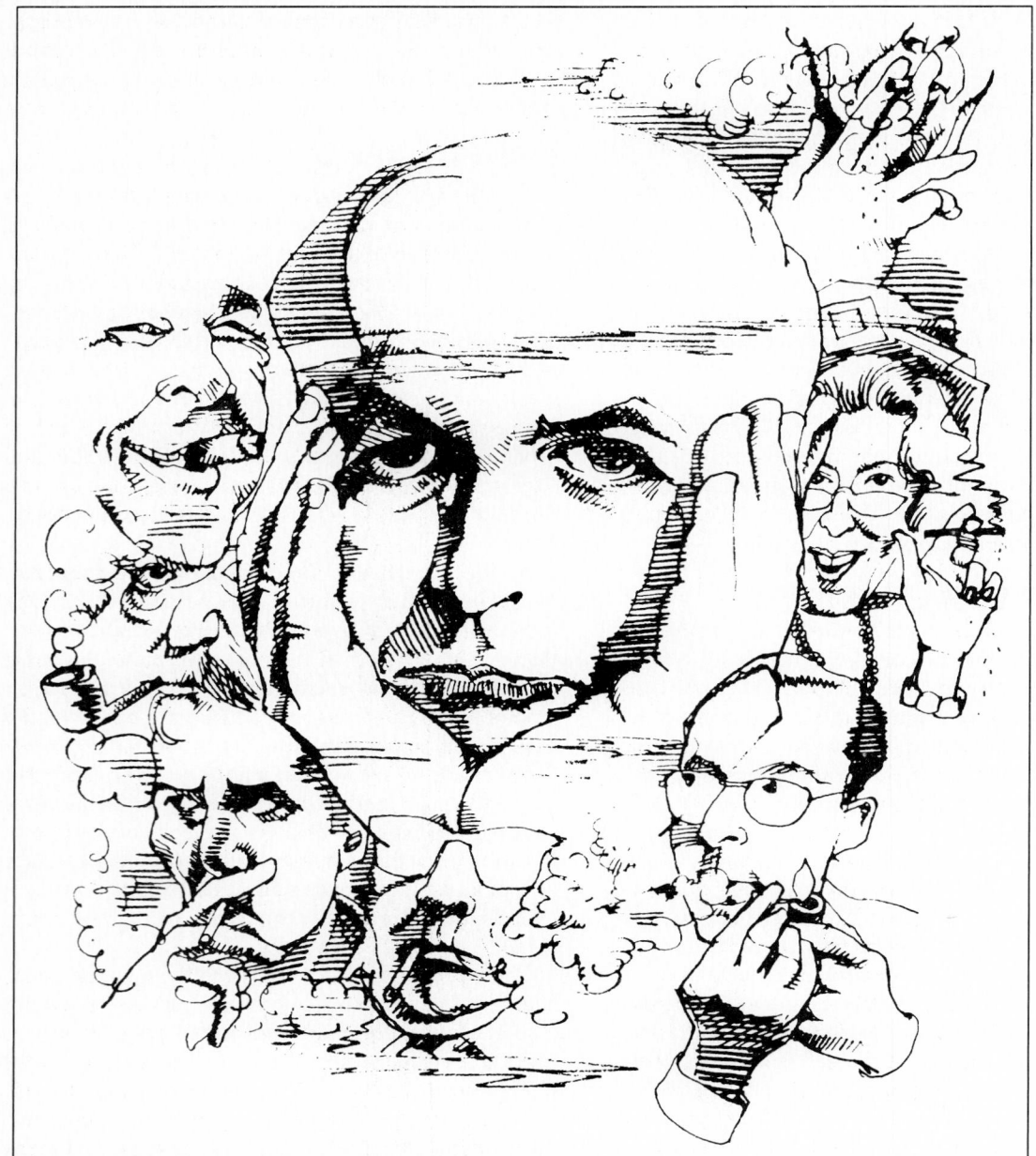

Fig. 22-1. Involuntary smoking is the inhalation of tobacco combustion products—by a nonsmoker. (Smoking digest: progress report on a nation kicking the habit, Bethesda, Md., 1977, Public Health Service, Department of Health, Education, and Welfare.)

of cigarette smoking when inhaling occurs. Smoke exposure in the upper respiratory tract is approximately equal for all smokers and comprises a major health risk. This means that all smokers have about the same chance of developing cancer of the esophagus, pharynx, larynx, and oral cavity. Additionally, pipe and cigar smokers are at higher risk for developing chronic obstructive pulmonary disease (COPD) than are nonsmokers.

Smokeless Tobacco

Smokeless tobacco is not a new creation. This habit was especially popular in the 1800s and early 1900s as a form of tobacco consumption. Over the years the habit of spitting came to be viewed as unsanitary. However, in recent years the tobacco industry has recognized that chewing could become equated with a macho image and yield lucrative returns for them. Numerous television and movie personalities have publicly endorsed this habit, and it is being promoted as the ideal habit for active people who use their hands in their work or in pursuing hobbies or leisure activities (Christen, 1981).

Approximately 22 million Americans now use smokeless tobacco, and a portrait of the typical "chewer" ranges from the young to the old and includes students, athletes, and professional and blue collar workers in urban and rural settings. It is not uncommon for young males to start dipping or chewing by the age of 10 years. In youth circles a worn imprint of a circular can on the hip pocket is considered a symbol of virility, maturity, and toughness.

Like other forms of tobacco use, chewing and dipping have addictive properties. About 5 minutes after putting chewing tobacco or snuff in their mouth, users begin to feel a "buzz" as the nicotine gets into their system. Most regular users chew or dip every 20 to 30 minutes during their working hours to maintain the desired nicotine level. People who dip or chew become nicotine dependent; as with cigarettes, pipes, and cigars, nicotine and other chemicals are absorbed through the lungs as well as the mucus areas of the mouth and nose.

The mechanical effects of smokeless tobacco on the mouth and teeth make this habit especially harmful. Tobacco is generally grown in sandy soil, and after several years of its use, people who chew and dip often wear down the tips of their teeth because of the continuous association with grit. Frequent use of tobacco increases the risk of cancer of the mouth and oral leukoplakia, or lesions of the soft tissues of the mouth characterized by a white patch or plaque. These lesions are not easily differentiated from other mouth diseases, since their texture varies from a "smooth, somewhat translucent white area to a thickened, cracked, and hardened lesion" (Christen, 1981, p. 10). Currently, leukoplakia is considered precancerous and does lead to cancer in about 5% of cases. Even though the incidence is low, this is a serious condition.

In addition, like other forms of tobacco, smokeless tobacco contains a substance called N-nitroso-nornicotine (NNN), which is a proven cancer-causing agent in animals. The amount of NNN is higher in snuff and chewing tobacco than in cigarette smoke.

Interaction between Smoking and Substances Involved in Occupational Exposures

While many studies have examined the effects of either smoking or occupational hazards on health, few have looked at the cumulative effects of these agents. However, six ways in which smoking may act with physical and chemical agents to produce or increase adverse health effects are as follows:

1. Tobacco products may serve as vectors by be-

coming contaminated with toxic agents found in the work place, thus facilitating entry of the agent by inhalation, ingestion, and/or skin absorption.
2. Work place chemicals may be transformed into more harmful agents by smoking.
3. Certain toxic agents in tobacco products and/or smoke may also occur in the work place, thus increasing exposure to the agent. Examples include carbon monoxide, methylene chloride, acetone, acrolein, aldehydes, arsenic, cadmium, formaldehyde, hydrogen sulfide, ketones, lead, methyl nitrite, nicotine, nitrogen dioxide, phenol, and polycyclic compounds (Smoking and Health, 1979).
4. Smoking may contribute to an effect comparable to that resulting from exposure to toxic agents found in the work place, thus causing an additive biological effect. Coal dust and cigarette smoke appear to have an additive effect in the production of obstructive airway disease. Similarly, smoking cotton workers show an increased prevalence of byssinosis when compared to nonsmoking cotton workers. Cotton dust inhalation produces an acute clinical picture of chest tightness, cough, and shortness of breath. Previously this syndrome was know as "Monday morning fever," since it occurred on the first day after a 2-day absence from the cotton dust. Also, chlorine and cigarette smoke seem to have a cumulative effect. The rate of chronic nonspecific respiratory disease among smoking firefighters is higher than among their nonsmoking counterparts.
5. Smoking may act synergistically with toxic agents found in the work place to cause a much more profound effect than that anticipated simply from the separate influences of the agent and smoking added together. Asbestos provides one of the most dramatic illustrations of synergism with smoke. Asbestos insulation workers who smoke are at a far greater risk of developing bronchogenic carcinoma than their nonsmoking counterparts. It has been determined that asbestos workers who smoke have 8 times the lung cancer risk of all other smokers and 92 times the risk of nonsmokers not exposed to asbestos (Smoking and Health, 1979). Synergistic effects also occur in rubber industry workers because of the fumes, dust, and smoke interaction, and uranium and gold miners show synergistic effects.
6. Smoking may contribute to accidents in the work place. Injuries attributed to smoking are caused by lack of attention, preoccupation of the hand used for smoking, irritation of the eyes, and soughing. Smoking also contributes to fire and explosions in the work place.

Health Consequences of Smoking for Women

According to the 1980 Report of the Surgeon General (Health Consequences of Smoking for Women, 1980), the first signs of an epidemic of smoking-related diseases among women is now appearing. Since women did not begin smoking in great numbers until World War II, most women smokers are between 30 and 60 years of age. It is predicted that as these women grow older and continue to smoke, their burden of smoking-related diseases will increase. Major prospective studies of smoking and mortality have reached consistent conclusion: "Death rates from coronary heart disease, chronic lung disease, lung cancer, and overall mortality rate are significantly increased among both women and men smokers" (Health Consequences of Smoking for Women, 1980, p. v). The risks are increased with the amount smoked, duration of smoking, depth of inhalation, and tar and nicotine content. Specifically, women cigarette smokers have more than three times the risk of dying of stroke resulting from subarachnoid hemorrhage and twice the risk of having a heart attack as nonsmoking women. Of critical importance is recognition among women of the synergistic effect of smoking and the use of oral contraceptives. Their combination causes a 22-fold increase in the risk of subarachnoid hemorrhage stroke and a 20-fold increase in heart attacks in heavy smokers (Health Consequences of Smoking for Women, 1980). Female smokers also report more acute and chronic conditions, including chronic bronchitis and/or emphysema, chronic sinusitis, peptic ulcers, and arteriosclerotic heart disease, than women who have never smoked (Health Consequences of Smoking for Women, 1980).

Further, the age-adjusted incidence of acute conditions such as influenza for female smokers is 20% higher than for nonsmokers. As might be expected, smokers lose more days of work and report more limitations of activity than their nonsmoking counterparts.

Cigarette smoking is causally associated with cancer of the lung, larynx, oral cavity, esophagus, and kidney in women. It is estimated that cigarette smoking accounts for 18% of all newly diagnosed cancers and 25% of all female cancer deaths. These women have 2.5 to 5 times as great a likelihood of developing lung cancer as nonsmoking women. Lung cancer death rates of all histological types are highest in industrialized countries where there has been a higher prevalence of smoking for a longer time.

It should also be noted that women are increasing their risk for laryngeal cancer. This type of cancer is most prevalent in the fifth through seventh decades of life and is highly correlated with heavy alcohol consumption. When women quit smoking, their risk of developing larngeal cancer decreases until 10 years after cessation; then the rate approaches that of nonsmokers. Similarly, women who both smoke and drink have an increased susceptibility to cancer of the oral cavity (lip, tongue, gums, buccal mucosa, hard and soft palate, salivary glands, floor of the mouth, and laryngopharynx (Health Consequences of Smoking for Women, 1980).

Spontaneous abortions are increased, and there is a greater incidence of bleeding during pregnancy and premature rupture of membranes for women who smoke. This association is independent of socioeconomic and racial factors as well as parity. There is also a greater incidence of premature and prolonged rupture of amniotic membranes, abruptio placentae, and placenta previa. In addition, women who smoke during pregnancy have more fetal and neonatal deaths than nonsmoking pregnant women, and a relationship has been established between sudden infant death syndrome and smoking (Health Consequences of Smoking for Women, 1980).

Of key importance are health hazards of maternal smoking to the unborn fetus and neonates. The effects of smoking on infant health are increased by heavier smoking and reduced if a woman stops smoking during pregnancy. A variety of toxic substances in cigarette smoking, including nicotine and hydrogen cyanide, cross the placenta and directly affect the fetus. Similarly, carbon monoxide generated from cigarette smoking is transported into fetal blood and interferes with oxygen supply to the fetus. Additionally, fetal growth is directly retarded by smoking. Babies born to women smokers are, on the average, 200 g lighter than those born to comparable nonsmokers (Health Consequences of Smoking for Women, 1980). This relationship is independent of the other factors known to influence birth weight, such as race, parity, maternal size, socioeconomic status, sex of the child, and gestational age. However, if a woman gives up smoking early in the pregnancy, her risk of delivering a low birth weight baby approaches the nonsmoker's rate. Fetal growth retardation caused by maternal smoking is reflected in a decrease in all dimensions, including body length and chest and head circumference.

The direct effects of maternal smoking on children extend beyond the fetal and neonatal stage. Children of mothers who smoked during pregnancy lag measurably in physical growth, and some evidence points to behavioral and cognitive effects. Nicotine, which is a known poison, has been found in the breastmilk of smoking mothers. Also, children whose parents smoke have

Table 22-6. Estimates of the percentage of current, regular, adolescent, (aged 12 to 18 years) cigarette smokers, United States, 1968-1979

Year	Ages 12 to 14		Ages 15 to 16		Ages 17 to 18		Ages 12 to 18	
	Male	Female	Male	Female	Male	Female	Male	Female
1968	2.9	0.6	17.0	9.6	30.2	18.6	14.7	8.4
1970	5.7	3.0	19.5	14.4	37.3	22.8	18.5	11.9
1972	4.6	2.8	17.8	16.3	30.2	25.3	15.7	13.3
1974	4.2	4.9	18.1	20.2	31.0	25.9	15.8	15.3
1979	3.2	4.3	13.5	11.8	19.3	26.2	10.7	12.7

From The health consequences of smoking for women. A report of the Surgeon General, Pub. No. 326-003, Washington, D.C., 1980, Office on Smoking and Health, Department of Health and Human Services.

NOTE: Current regular smoker includes respondent who smokes cigarettes at least weekly.

more respiratory infections and hospitalizations during the first year of life. It is difficult to document a relationship between maternal smoking and long-term growth and development of children because of the interaction of numerous external factors as the child grows.

Morbidity and Mortality

Specific categories of health disruption, discussed in this section, are aggravated by smoking.

Cardiovascular disease is the major cause of death in the United States for both men and women. Smokers are at greater risk for these diseases, with the risk being compounded when oral contraceptives are also used. Smoking seems to increase the level of high-density lipoprotein (HDL), a protein complex that transports cholesterol in the blood. Women smokers also experience an increased risk for subarachnoid hemorrhage, and the risk is even greater when oral contraceptives are used (Health Consequences of Smoking for Women, 1980). Additionally, rates are higher in urban versus rural areas because of the potentiating effect of pollution and smoking (Health Consequences of Smoking for Women, 1980). Low tar and nicotine cigarettes reduce the risk of lung cancer, and ex-smokers experience a decrease in their relative risk of developing lung cancer. About 15 years after smoking ceases, the ex-smoker's risk of developing lung cancer approximates that of the nonsmoker.

While the relationship between smoking and cancer of the esophagus is not as straightforward as it is for cancer of the lung or larynx, there is an association. This disease is serious, since the median survival after diagnosis is 6 months, and the 5-year survival rate is only 3%. Alcohol use is also correlated with the onset of

cancer of the esophagus, and smoking and alcohol seem to have a synergistic effect.

Chronic *nonneoplastic bronchopulmonary disorders* are a major cause of morbidity and mortality in the United States. The majority of these illnesses are chronic obstructive lung diseases (COPDs), including chronic bronchitis and emphysema. Cigarette smoking has been found to be a major cause of COPD. Women seem to be at less risk for COPD than men, possibly because of differences in prior smoking habits.

Adolescent Smoking

The chief characteristics of adolescence are growth, transition, and change. The rate of physical growth is more rapid than at any other stage of development except the neonatal stage. During this period adolescents are trying to find themselves and become an integral part of their peer group. The specific developmental changes of adolescence have already been discussed (Chapter 26); hence only those differences directly related to smoking are emphasized.

There are some developmental differences between boys and girls that may account for the increased rate of female adolescent smokers. Girls seem to have "greater susceptibility to expressed anxiety, greater need for help and reassurance, greater closeness to friends, and more concern for what is socially desirable" (Health Consequences of Smoking for Women, 1980, p. 273).

As can be seen in Table 22-6 there has been a significant increase in the percentage of female smokers since 1968. There has also been a slight decline in the age of onset of smoking in the younger two groups.

Adolescents tend to smoke lower tar cigarettes than their adult counterparts, with girls being slightly ahead of boys in this characteristic. In addition, an association between cigarette smoking (in the 12- to 17-year age range) and the reported use of alcohol, marijuana, and/or hashish, or stronger substances, such as hallucinogens, cocaine, heroin, and other opiates, has been found (Abelson et al., 1977).

Several demographic and psychosocial factors place adolescents at greater risk for beginning to smoke. A number of studies have found smoking to be correlated with lower parental income and education (Borland and Rudolph, 1975; Reeder, 1979). Adolescent smoking is twice as high in single-parent homes as in households with both parents present. This may be influenced by the higher incidence of smoking among divorced or separated adults and the tendency of adolescents to model the behavior of their parents. Additionally, adolescents are more likely to smoke if one or both of their parents smoke, as well as if older siblings smoke.

Adolescent smoking behavior is highly correlated with having friends who smoke. When correlating parental smoking, socioeconomic status, and scholastic performance, Borland and Rudolph (1975) found the greatest influencer to be scholastic performance. High scholastically rated students were less likely to smoke than students earning lower grades. Also, studies of achievement, aspirations, and expectations have demonstrated reduced motivation and lower aspiration to be associated with a higher prevalence of smoking (Allegrante et al., 1977-1978; Johnston et al, 1977). High school students in college preparatory classes were far less likely to smoke than students in other types of curricula.

Smoking Cessation

Information from public opinion and attitude polls indicates that 90% of smokers have either tried to quit smoking or would like to do so if they could find an effective method. These people need help! Smoking cessation is a difficult and painful process because of the often agonizing effects of physical and psychological withdrawal. People who continue to smoke do so in the "face of rising concern from their families and friends, hostility from nonsmokers, and a proliferation of restrictions on smoking in public places" (Smoking Digest, 1977).

People seem to continue smoking for one or more of the following reasons (Smoking Digest, 1977):
- A sense of increased energy or stimulation
- The satisfaction of handling or manipulating things
- The accentuation of pleasure and relaxation
- The reduction of negative feelings (anger, anxiety, fear, etc.)

- "Craving" or psychological addiction
- Habit

Helping people quit smoking requires an understanding of their motivation for smoking as well as knowledge of a variety of potential programs that may be successful. In addition, various characteristics have been identified to describe people who successfully quit smoking.

Specifically, higher levels of education are associated with greater success in quitting. "Among those with a college education or higher, 52.1 percent of the men and 48.1 percent of the women who have ever smoked have quit" (Health Consequences of Smoking for Women, 1980, p. 304). For all other educational levels, 40.5% of men and 31.3% of women have quit. As might be expected from the advanced education statistics, smoking cessation is also associated with higher levels of income and professional rather than technical work.

Men are more likely than women to remain successful abstainers. Light smokers have the greatest success in stopping, as do those with a great commitment to change, those who use behavioral techniques, and those who have access to a social support system. Examples of behavioral techniques include the substitution of candy and gum for cigarettes. One man used peppermint disks to curb the urge to smoke. These low-calorie pieces of hard candy were easy to keep on hand, and their sharp flavor aided in smoking cessation. While the candy did not curb the physiological withdrawal, it did ease the psychological loss of a cigarette in his hand and mouth. Successful quitters also have friends, family, and co-workers who provide support and encouragement during this high stress time.

Regardless of treatment type or smoking cessation approach used, women have more difficulty giving up cigarettes than men. Women frequently report symptoms of anxiety and depression when they alter their smoking habits; they also tend to fear overeating and subsequent weight gain if they cease their smoking.

Public Health Educational Campaigns

No doubt the public health campaign against cigarettes has produced substantial changes in public attitudes. As noted, most people realize smoking is dangerous, and the majority of smokers would like to terminate this habit. These campaigns have clearly emphasized specific health hazards associated with smoking. However, while effective in informing the public of the dangers of smoking, public health education has not been as effective in inducing people to change this habit.

Self-Help and Smoking Cessation Clinics

Of the 29 million Americans who quit smoking between 1964 and 1975, approximately 95% of them quit on their own. A variety of smoking cessation programs have been developed by voluntary health agencies, profit-making corporations, and health professionals. The approaches used include group therapy, individual counseling, physical messages, and self-help guides. Methods in these approaches range from the use of drugs, electric shock, or hypnosis to acupuncture.

National voluntary health organizations such as the American Cancer Society, the American Heart Association, and the American Lung Association for several years have sponsored group smoking cessation clinics through their local community chapters. Several profit-making corporations have entered this area in recent years, including SmokEnders, the National Association on Smoking and Health, and the Schick Centers. These three programs tend to be far more expensive than the programs offered by voluntary health organizations. Additionally, the Seventh Day Adventist Church offers a 5-day program for a modest fee. This program includes lectures by a clergy-health team, films on the harmful effects of smoking, explanations of smoking cessation procedures, and group interaction.

A variety of physicians have developed their own methods to help clients stop smoking. For example, physicians at the Mayo Clinic offer eight sessions of lectures, films, group discussions, and a "buddy system" (Smoking Digest, 1977). However, most physicians do not inform clients that they need to quit smoking or offer ways to attempt cessation. Both the American Cancer Society and the Federal Government have developed packets of informative materials to aid in smoking cessation.

Since a majority of ex-smokers quit without any involvement in a formal smoking cessation program, a number of organizations have developed written materials to provide smokers with information about the physical, emotional, social, and economic effects of smoking. Materials have included, in addition to information, self-tests and self-help modules.

Evaluative data on clinics have been sporadic and therefore have not provided a clear picture of the potential usefulness of these mechanisms. In most clinics there is a reasonable abstinence rate (often between 30% and 60%) following each session; however, this rate tends to drop appreciably on long-term follow-up.

Attitude Changes

The most successful programs to date in reducing adolescent smoking have been those emphasizing a positive, constructive approach to health (Fisher, 1980). In contrast to programs designed to impress on adolescents the risks of smoking, positively oriented programs emphasize skills for fending off the temptation and for handling peer pressure to smoke. In the positive programs for smoking prevention, there is no attempt to induce guilt, shame, or dread about current or future smoking habits.

Techniques for instilling nonsmoking values in teens include the use of values clarification, assertiveness skills, and other educational strategies designed to increase resistance to peer pressure to smoke Greenberg and Deputat, 1978; Purcell et al., 1979). These techniques are also used with abuse of alcohol and other drugs. Scare techniques where youth are presented with cancerous laboratory animals to demonstrate the effects of smoking and also lectures and films on the effects of smoking seem less effective as a long-range prevention tool than do the enrichment and attitude change approaches. Success has also been reported from having peers help one another learn to understand the effects of smoking and avoid succumbing to peer pressure for conformity. Peer assistance also works for adults and can easily be incorporated into self-help programs.

The nursing role is one of helping clients choose the program that best suits their unique needs, is readily available, and is affordable. Nurses also serve as group leaders or resource persons in groups offered by health care agencies and voluntary associations.

SUMMARY

The abuse of a variety of substances poses health problems for Americans. Alcohol, drugs, and cigarettes comprise major abusive chemicals and constitute health hazards both for those directly involved and for people indirectly involved. Prevention of substance abuse is the prevailing goal. To provide information about prevention, community health nurses must know the signs, patterns, and effects of substance abuse.

Attitudes are of critical importance in health promotion relative to substance abuse, since the way people think and feel is conveyed in verbal as well as nonverbal messages. When nurses think that people who abuse drugs are weak and could help themselves if they would only try harder, this attitude is conveyed to the client. Attitudes toward substance abuse are most helpful to clients when based on the premise that people use chemicals to deal with life. People need acceptance, understanding, and commitment to help them deal constructively with their health hazards. The health consequences of substance abuse are in many instances life threatening; most people who abuse alcohol, drugs, and cigarettes know about the consequences. What they need is consistent help in dealing with the life events leading to and encouraging this habit and support as they try to quit if that is their choice.

Numerous programs are available for dealing with the problems of substance abuse. The community health nurse needs to know what programs and resources are available in the local area, what they charge, who is eligible, and what degree of success has been reported with each one. Major roles include support, encouragement, teaching, and referral.

BIBLIOGRAPHY

Abelson, H.I., Fishburne, P.M., and Cisin, I.: National survey on drug abuse: 1977. A nationwide study—youth, young adults and older people, DHEW Pub. No. (ADM) 78-618, Washington, D.C., 1977, Public Health Service, Department of Health, Education, and Welfare.

Allegrante, J.P., O'Rourke, T.W., and Tuncalp, S.: A multivariate analysis of selected variables on the development of subsequent youth smoking behavior, J. Drug. Educ. 7(3):237-248, 1977-1978.

Beyond the three R's: training teachers for affective education, DHHS Pub. No. (ADM) 80-233, Rockville, Md., 1980, Prevention Branch, Division of Resource Development, National Institute on Drug Abuse, Department of Health and Human Services.

Borland, B.R., and Rulolph, J.R.: Relative effects of low socioeconomic status, parent smoking and poor scholastic performance among high school students, Soc. Sci. Med. 9:27-30, 1975.

Botwin, G.J., and Eng, A.: A comprehensive school-based smoking prevention program, J. School Health 50(3):209-213, 1980.

Butz, R.H.: Intoxication and withdrawal. In Estes, N.J., and Heinemann, M.E., editors: Alcoholism: development, consequences, and interventions, ed. 2, St. Louis, 1981, The C.V. Mosby Co., pp. 102-108.

Carr, R.R., and Meyers, E.J.: Marijuana and cocaine: the process of change in drug policy. In Drug Abuse Council: The facts about drug abuse, New York, 1980, The Free Press, pp. 153-189.

Christen, A.G.: The facts about smokeless tobacco, Listen 34:7-11, June 1981.

The community health nurse and alcohol-related problems, Pub. No. 017-024-00753-6, Rockville, Md., 1978a, National Institute on Alcohol Abuse and Alcoholism, Public Health Service, Department of Health, Education, and Welfare.

The community health nurse and alcohol-related problems, instructor's curriculum planning guide, Pub. No. 017-024-00754-4, Rockville, Md., 1978b, National Institute on Alcohol Abuse and Alcoholism, Public Health Service, Department of Health, Education, and Welfare.

Critical review of the FAS, Rockville, Md., 1977, National Institute on Alcohol Abuse and Alcoholism, Department of Health, Education and Welfare.

Deciding about drugs: a woman's choice, DHEW Pub. No. (ADM) 80-820, Rockville, Md., 1979, National Institute on Drug Abuse, Department of Health, Education, and Welfare.

Diamond, G.A., and Forrester, J.S.: Clinical trials and statistical verdicts: probable grounds for appeal, Ann. Intern. Med. 98(3):385-394, 1983.

Disease prevention and health promotion. Federal programs and prospects, Washington, D.C., 1979, DHEW Pub. No. (PHS) 79-55071B, Department of Health, Education, and Welfare.

Doing drug education, the role of the school teacher, DHHS Pub. No. (ADM) 80-232, Rockville, Md., 1980, Prevention Branch, Division of Resource Development, National Institute on Drug Abuse, Department of Health and Human Services.

Estes, N.J.: Counseling the wife of an alcoholic spouse, Am. J. Nurs. 74:1251-1255, 1974.

Fisher, E.B.: Progress in reducing adolescent smoking, Am. J. Public Health. 70:7, pp. 678-679, 1980.

Gitlow, S.E., and Peyes, J.S.: Alcoholism: a practical treatment guide, New York, 1980, Grune & Stratton, Inc.

Goldberg, P.: The federal government's response to illicit drugs, 1969-1978. In Drug Abuse Council: The facts about drug abuse, New York, 1980, The Free Press, pp. 20-62.

Gordon, L.V., and Haynes, D.K.: Smoking-related attitudes of parents of fourth graders, J. School Health 11:403-412, Aug., 1981.

Greenberg, J.S., and Deputat, Z.: Smoking intervention: comparing three methods in a high school setting, J. School Health 48(8):498-502, 1978.

The health consequences of smoking. The changing cigarette. A report of the Surgeon General, DHHS (PHS) Pub. No. 81-50156, Washington, D.C., 1981, Department of Health and Human Services.

The health consequences of smoking for women. A report of the Surgeon General, Pub. No. 326-003, Washington, D.C., 1980, Office on Smoking and Health, Department of Health and Human Services.

Healthy people: the Surgeon General's report on health promotion and disease prevention, PHS Pub. No. 79-55071, Washington, D.C., Dec. 1979, Department of Health, Education and Welfare.

Heinemann, E., and Estes, H.J.: Assessing alcoholic patients, Am. J. Nurs. 76:786-794, 1976.

Hennecke, L., and Fox, V.: The woman with alcoholism. In Gitlow, S.E., and Peyser, H.S.: Alcoholism: a practical treatment guide, New York, 1980, Grune & Stratton, Inc.

Interaction effect of alcohol with other drugs, Lincoln, Neb., 1977, Nebraska Division on Alcoholism.

Johnston, L.D., Bachman, J.C., and O'Malley, P.M.: Drug use among American high school students, 1975-77, DHEW Pub. No. (ADM) 78-619, Washington, D.C., 1977, Alcohol, Drug Abuse and Mental Health Administration, Public Health Service, Department of Health, Education, and Welfare.

Lewis, D.C., and Sessler, J.: Heroin treatment: development, status, outlook. In Drug Abuse Council: The facts about drug abuse, New York, 1980, The Free Press, pp. 95-125.

McAlister, A.L., et al.: Adolescent smoking: onset and prevention, Pediatrics 63(4):650-657, 1979.

Milby, J.: Addictive behavior and its treatment, New York, 1981, Springer Publishing Co., Inc.

Mishara, B.L., and Kastenbaum, R.: Alcohol and old age, New York, 1980, Grune & Stratton, Inc.

Purcell, I., et al.: Children and smoking, Aust. Fam. Physician 8(12):1284-1286, 1979.

Reeder, L.G.: Sociocultural factors in the etiology of smoking behavior: an assessment. In Jarvik, M.E., et al.: Research on smoking behavior. NIDA Research Monograph 17, DHEW Pub. No. (ADM) 80-820, Washington, D.C., 1979, Public Health Service, Department of Health, Education and Welfare.

Sandmaier, M.: Alcohol abuse and women: a guide to getting help, Rockville, Md., 1977, National Clearinghouse for Alcohol Information.

Saying no: drug abuse prevention ideas for the classroom, DHHS Pub. No. (ADM) 81-916, Washington, D.C., 1981, National Institute on Drug Abuse, Department of Health and Human Services.

Schultz, J.M., and Dark, S.L.: Manual of psychiatric nursing care plans, Boston, 1982, Little, Brown & Co.

Signs of use of substances for drugging effects, Washington, D.C., 1978, Pharmaceutical Manufacturers Association.

Smoking and health, DHEW Pub. No. 79-50066, Washington, D.C., 1979, Department of Health, Education and Welfare.

Smoking digest: progress report on a nation kicking the habit, Bethesda, Md., 1977, Public Health Service, Department of Health, Education, and Welfare.

Tarrant Council on Alcoholism and Drug Abuse: The family illness, Fort Worth, Tex., 1981, The Council.

Teenage smoking: national patterns of cigarette smoking, ages 12 through 18, in 1972 and 1974, DHEW Pub. No. (NIH) 76-931, Washington, D.C., 1976, Public Health Service, National Institutes of Health, Department of Health, Education and Welfare.

Westermeyer, J.: Primer on chemical dependency, Baltimore, 1976, The Williams & Wilkins Co.

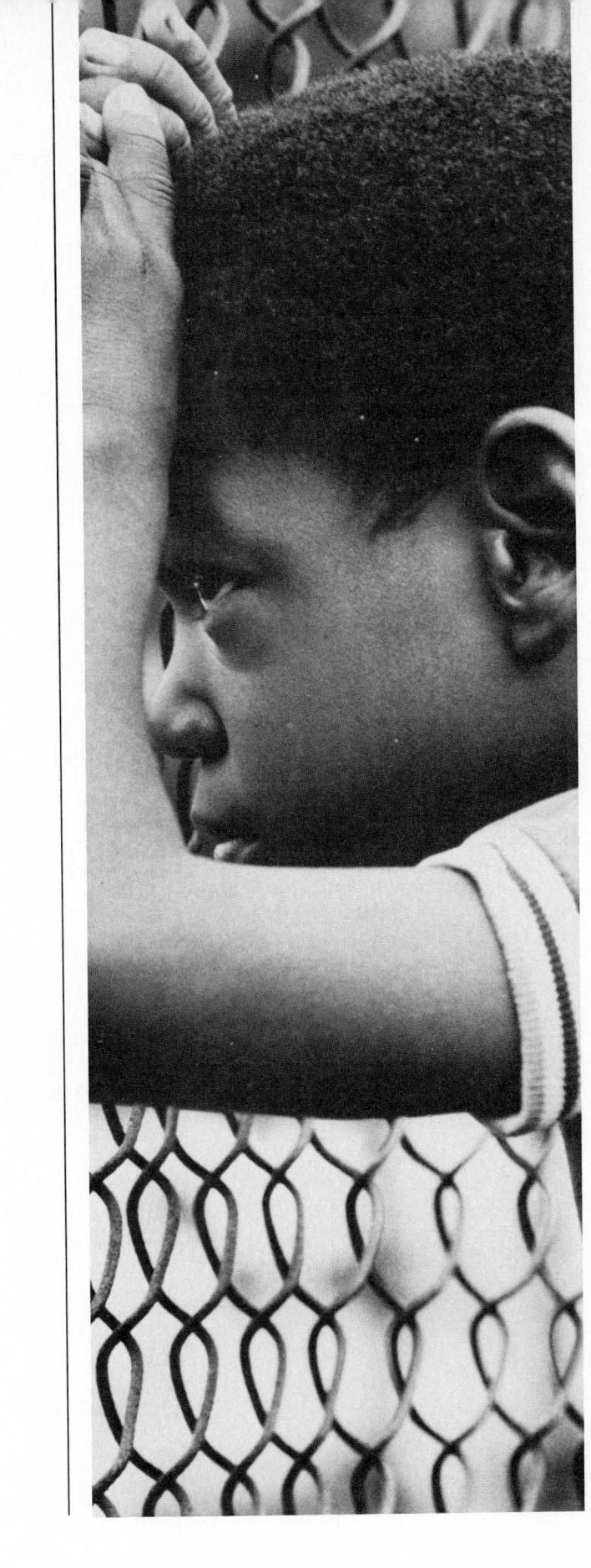

Part Four

COMMUNITY HEALTH PROBLEMS: A DEVELOPMENTAL APPROACH

The family is a major influence on the individual's concept of health and illness. It influences the action taken by or for the person with a health problem. The environmental, social, and economic factors as well as the resources of the community to meet health needs influence the individual's health risks and reactions to health.

The community health nurse has the opportunity to influence the actions and reactions to health of all individuals of the community from birth through senescence. The community health nurse may influence the health of the neonate and infant by introducing healthy parenting behaviors, risk factor appraisal, and interventions at this stage of life. Likewise the community health and/or school health nurse is in a position to introduce illness prevention and health promotion activities to the school age and adolescent populations. Appropriate influences during these developmental stages have the potential for changing the future outlook for the nation's health.

The young and middle-aged adults are faced with many life changes and challenges that they may find rewarding or demanding. Previous life-styles and increases in stress from social, environmental, and economic constraints often result in risk for major health problems during this life stage.

Continued.

Part Four

The community health nurse's primary function with persons of all ages should be to promote quality as well as quantity of life. As the elderly population continues to increase (grow), the health care delivery system and nursing must address and plan strategies to cope with increasing longevity, chronic health problems, and technological advances as well as twentieth century economic, social, and health issues.

Major health problems of individuals can be identified and related to their developmental phase. This factor becomes evident when age-specific morbidity and mortality data are reviewed. Chapters 23 to 27 explore the major developmental tasks, health needs, and risk factors for individuals from birth through senescence.

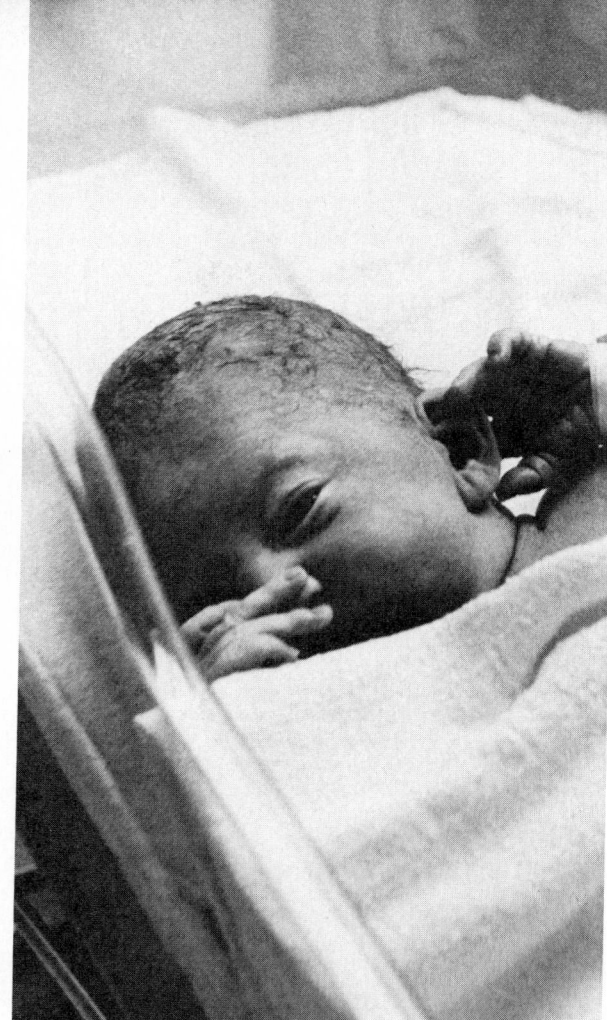

Chapter 23

NANCY DICKENSON-HAZARD
DENISE GEOLOT

THE FIRST YEAR OF LIFE

Children are one third of our population and all of our future . . . their health is our foundation.

The promotion of child health provides society with an opportunity to be well. Since children must learn health practices, the opportunity to teach health promotion and maintenance is greater for children than any other population.

The period of life known as childhood is fraught with many dimensions of human behavior on the part of the child and parent. The community health nurse has the unique opportunity to become an integral part of this period of life and to assist these human beings in expressing positive health behaviors.

This chapter provides information on the assessment of child health within the community for the child from birth through age 1 year. The content includes age-specific growth, development, definition of major health problems, and the tools and techniques of health promotion activities.

PRENATAL ENVIRONMENT

Assessing the quality of the atmosphere in which a fetus grows is the first step in ensuring a healthy childhood. The community health nurse has the opportunity to make this assessment in a variety of settings. Being aware of the prenatal factors that promote wellness facilitates the scope of the nurse's assessment.

Before Conception

At the moment of conception some aspects of wellness are determined. Influential in their effect on fetal health before and at the time of conception are genetic and chromosomal abnormalities, blood group incom-

Table 23-1. Nursing implications: facilitating parental knowledge regarding genetic disorders

Before conception	After conception
Identify parents at risk	Identify parents at risk prenatally
Provide educational programs on common genetic disorders	Implement data collection including medical history, family pedigree, and laboratory data
Provide individual explanation sessions for parents at risk	Implement individual counseling session regarding the disorder with parents
Implement data collection, including medical history, family pedigree, and laboratory data	Refer parents for genetic counseling
Implement an education session on the specific disorder	Refer parents to local groups
Refer parents for detailed genetic counseling	

Factors Influencing Fetal Growth

Factors at conception
Maternal physical health during pregnancy
Maternal nutrition
Maternal drug/substance ingestion
Maternal weight gain during pregnancy
Previous pregnancy history
Use of prenatal services
Circumstances of conception and pregnancy
Adjustment to pregnancy including past experiences, attitudes, and expectations

patibilities, and maternal age and state of health. The education and counseling of prospective parents about these factors are important aspects of the nurse's role.

Of primary concern is that up to 5% of all births in the United States involve birth defects, the majority of which are inherited (Healthy People, 1979). Although prevention of genetic defects is the primary objective when advising the parents at risk, facilitating parental knowledge regarding the disorder becomes a priority once conception has occurred. Nursing's assessment and referral are essential elements of the complex process of genetic counseling. Table 23-1 describes appropriate nursing interventions before and after conception.

After Conception

Once conception has occurred, fetal growth becomes dependent on the intrauterine environment as provided by the expectant mother. The physical and psychosocial well-being of the mother is influenced by many elements (see following box). The role of nursing at this point of life is to facilitate the quality of maternal health, thereby ensuring fetal health.

Nursing activities that promote maternal health and the environment after conception include implementation of a:

Complete data collection mechanism

Physical assessment and appropriate laboratory studies

Plan of care in collaboration with parents-to-be, focusing on their physical and psychosocial needs

Fetal Assessment and Parent Education

Despite efforts to ensure fetal health through maternal health promotion, fetal difficulties can and do arise. Modern technology has improved the health professional's ability to detect these difficulties. Sonography, amniocentesis, and mechanical fetal monitoring are a few of the mechanisms that may be used antenatally. Knowledge of their implications can facilitate the nurse's assessment of fetal health.

As the pregnancy progresses, education about the neonate and parenting must begin in addition to continued monitoring of maternal and fetal physical health. The pediatric prenatal visit is an effective health promotion activity in which expectant parents, with the nurse's help, can lay the groundwork for positive influences on the child's health.

The prenatal period of life requires nursing assessment and intervention. The nurse needs to be aware of the scope of factors that affect fetal growth and development to incorporate them into a data collection system and to use them in the development of a plan of care. Thorough fetal assessment facilitates child health.

PHYSICAL GROWTH AND DEVELOPMENT

The terms *growth* and *development* incorporate two distinct concepts: (1) quantitative or measurable aspects of the increase in the size of individuals (growth) and (2) qualitative or observable aspects of the progressive changes in the individuals as they adapt to their environment (development) (Waechter, 1976).

Human growth and development are orderly, predictable processes that begin with the embryo and continue until death. Individuals progress through definite

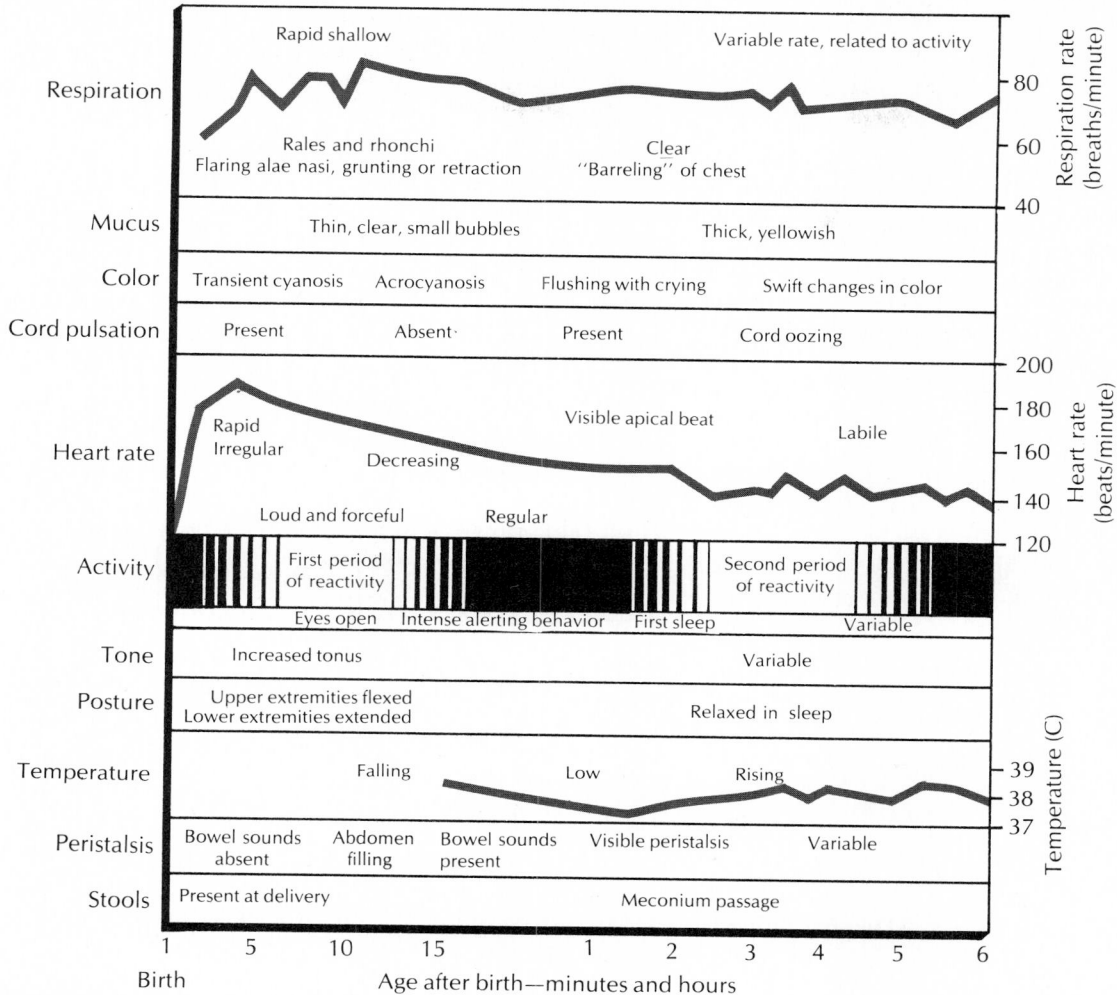

Fig. 23-1. Vital signs and activity fluctuations during the neonatal transition. (From Clark, A.L., and Affonso, D.D.: Childbearing: a nursing perspective, ed. 2, Philadelphia, 1979, F.A. Davis Co.)

phases of growth and development in their lifetime. These phases are influenced by a multitude of hereditary and environmental factors.

When assessing the measurable and observable aspects of growth and development, the nurse must be cognizant of the overall process as well as the factors that influence it. In addition, each person progresses through the different phases of growth and development in his own manner and at his own pace, demonstrating behaviors that are clearly individual to him. These individual variations within orderly growth and development processes must also be considered when assessment is implemented.

The Neonate

The period of life from birth to 1 month is commonly referred to as the *neonatal period*. During this phase of

life the newborn's functioning and behavior are mostly reflexive. Stabilization of major body functions is the primary task of the neonate.

The behavior of a newborn is at best described as erratic. However, there is a definite sequence of events through which a neonate progresses as stability is achieved in the first hours of life (Fig. 23-1). Nursing needs to be aware of the normalcy of this sequence and to be alert to the subtle physical changes it produces when making an assessment.

Physical Assessment

Physical examination of the newborn is one of the most important tools for assessing neonatal health. Using the data obtained from a physical examination provides the nurse with an opportunity to implement preventive health activities.

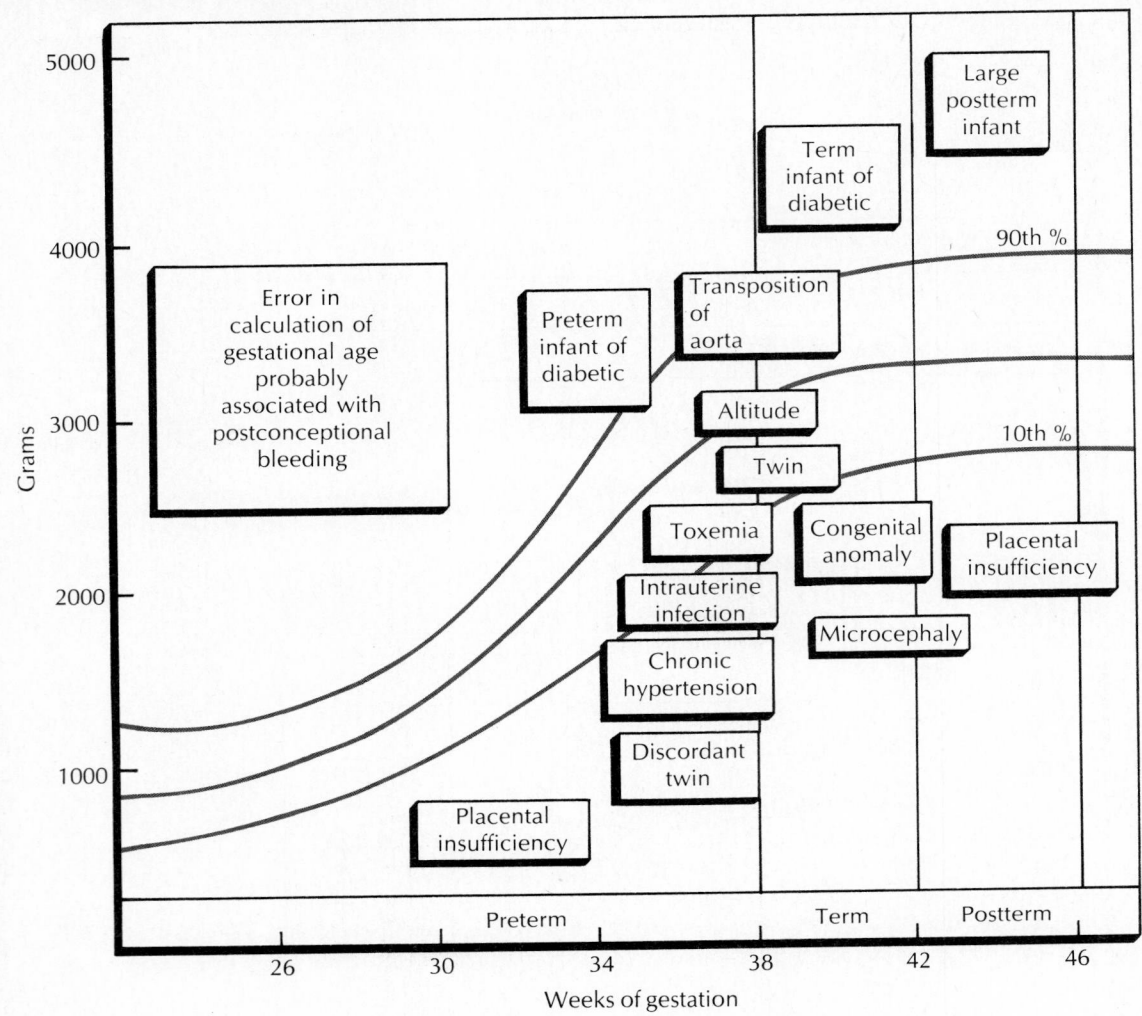

Fig. 23-2. Conditions associated with deviations of intrauterine growth and weight. (From Brown, M.S., and Murphy, M.A.: Ambulatory pediatrics for nurses, used with permission of McGraw-Hill Book Co., New York, 1975.)

With the trend toward early discharge after delivery (within 24 to 48 hours), the community health nurse frequently conducts a neonatal assessment. Though the physical examination of a newborn does not differ greatly from the general pediatric physical assessment, the nurse needs to be aware of normal variations and minor abnormalities that may be apparent, especially in the home setting. Appendix J provides a compilation of these normal variations and guidance for appropriate anticipatory nursing procedures. (Brown and Murphy 1975; Chow et al., 1979; DeAngelis, 1979; Scipien et al., 1979; Tackett and Hunsberger 1981; Vaughan et al., 1979.)

Though these variants place the newborn in no immediate danger, they are usually a cause of worry and concern for parents. Understanding their origin, presence, and course enables the nurse to facilitate parental coping. Provision of education regarding these abnormalities and variations is nursing's responsibility. This parental education coupled with support and reassurance is nursing's most important function in assisting parents to adjust to these normal occurrences.

Apgar Scoring

Neonatal physiological function at birth is assessed through observation scoring of the newborn characteristics of appearance, pulse, grimace, activity, and respirations (Apgar, 1966). (See a basic pediatric text for a complete discussion of Apgar scoring.) Although the community health nurse does not perform this assess-

Table 23-2. Formulas for approximate average height and weight of normal infants and children (after Weech)

| Age | Weight | | Age | Height | |
	kg	lb		cm	in
At birth	3.25	7	At birth	50	20
3-12 months	$\dfrac{\text{Age(mo)} + 9}{2}$	Age(mo) + 11	At 1 year	75	30
1-6 years	Age(yr) $\times$ 2 + 8	Age(yr) $\times$ 5 + 17	2-12 years	Age(yr) $\times$ 6 + 77	Age(yr) $\times$ 2½ + 30
6-12 years	$\dfrac{\text{Age(yr)} \times 7 - 5}{2}$	Age(yr) $\times$ 7 + 5			

From Vaughan, V.C., McKay, R.J., and Behrman, R.E., editors: Nelson textbook of pediatrics, ed. 11, Philadelphia, 1979, W.B. Saunders Co., p. 23.

ment, knowledge of the data obtained provides information pertinent to the management of well-infant care.

Gestational Age

Gestational age (GA) is defined as the number of weeks spent in utero to the time of birth (Dubowitz, 1970). Estimates of GA serve as indicators to physical maturity and are an important aspect of evaluating neonatal physical growth and development. Indications for making GA estimates include (1) determining problems that may occur for the premature or small infant; (2) assessing actual GA before labeling as large, small, or average; (3) distinguishing malnourished from dehydrated infants; and (4) using GA as an educational tool for parents (Chow, 1979).

Assessing the GA of a neonate assists the nurse in facilitating the neonate's health. It provides a method for identifying potential problems and taking preventive action. Conditions associated with variations in the intrauterine growth and age are shown in Fig. 23-2.

Physiological Changes

The average newborn weighs 7 lb 1 oz (3200 g), is 19⅓ inches (49 cm) in length, and has a head circumference of 13½ inches (34 cm). As the neonate develops physically, an individual and identifiable pattern of growth begins to appear. The normal newborn can lose up to 10% of his birth weight in the first few weeks of life. This weight reduction occurs primarily as a result of fluid losses through respiration, urination, defecation, and decreased intake. Generally between the second and third week of life, birth weight is regained. By 1 month the neonate should be beginning a pattern of weight gain of 5 to 7 ounces per week, a gain in length of ½ to 1 inch per month, and an increase of 2 cm per

Table 23-3. Head circumference in term infants*

Period	Head circumference increments	
First 3 months	2.0 cm/month =	6 cm
4-6 months	1.0 cm/month =	3 cm
6-12 months	0.5 cm/month =	3 cm
First year		12 cm

From McMillan, J.A., The whole pediatrician catalog, Philadelphia, 1977, W.B. Saunders Co., p. 6.
*Expected head circumference during infancy can be estimated by remembering that the average full-term infant shows the following increments in head growth.

month in head circumference. Table 23-2 approximates height and weight of infants and children. Table 23-3 outlines the expected increases in head circumference in full-term infants.

As the neonate begins to establish vital organ functioning, many physiological changes occur. The transition from fetal to independent neonatal physiology is quite complex, and survival outside the protected uterine environment is the result of embryonic and fetal growth. At birth major organ systems are functional though not advanced.

Central Nervous System

The peripheral and autonomic nervous systems are adequately developed at birth, permitting the neonate to survive outside the uterine environment. Except for the optic and olfactory nerves, all cranial nerves are present and myelinated.

Cardiovascular System

The heart lies transverse with a shift to the right side at birth. The neonate's heart has three additional openings at birth. Under normal circumstances, the ductus venosus closes at birth, the foramen ovale within 3 to 4 weeks of birth, and the ductus arteriosus between 1 and 8 days of life. The newborn heart rate gradually decreases to 130 to 140 from the fetal rate of 130 to 160. Systole and diastole are of shorter duration, greater intensity, and higher pitch. The newborn's respiratory movements are primarily abdominal and vary in rate and rhythm.

Gastrointestinal System

Some of the salivary glands are functional at birth with the majority maturing around 3 months of age. The newborn's stomach lies horizontally and is filled with fluid. The liver is palpable, and the large intestine is filled with sterile meconium. Meconium is generally passed within the first 24 hours of life.

Genitourinary System

At birth bladder capacity is 60 ml, and voiding is involuntary. The first voiding usually occurs within 48 hours. The kidneys may be palpable at birth, and genitalia may be slightly to moderately enlarged.

Skeletal System

The cartilage of the newborn's hands and feet are present at birth with ossification of phalangeal shafts,
metacarpals, and metatarsals beginning. Although eruption does not occur for several months, a newborn's lower central incisors and first molars show evidence of calcification.

Physiological stabilization is a long-term process affected not only by birth but by the rapid continued growth of the neonate. The changes in physiology are evidenced through the monitoring of vital signs. Community health nurses should be aware of these subtle changes in respiration, heart rate, and blood pressure to make an accurate assessment of the newborn's physiological functioning. (See a basic text in pediatric nursing for a review of these values.)

Danger Signs

Although most newborns adjust to functioning outside the uterine environment without incident, the possibility of neonatal difficulty exists. The nurse should therefore be alert to the danger signs indicating a need for referral and management when assessing the newborn (Chow, et al. 1979). These danger signs are presented in the box below.

Reflex Activity

Reflex activity of the neonatal period and early infancy stage is dominated by a large number of primitive reflex patterns. These reflexes are generally present at or shortly after birth. Absence or asymmetry of reflexive response or abnormal persistence of response beyond the time of voluntary motor function is an indication of

---

Danger Signs in the Newborn

A positive family history for major disease or illness
Gestational or delivery complications
Abnormal positioning of baby
Congenital malformations
Rapid or difficult respirations
Rapid, slow, or irregular pulse
Abnormal cry
Unusual cough
Cyanosis
Sweating
Vomiting of bile
Delayed or inadequate voiding
Bleeding, specifically noting cord and circumcision
Single umbilical artery

Full, bulging fontanel
Small head size
Convulsions, twitching, excessive irritability
Lethargy
Fever or hypothermia
Paralysis
Jaundice
Pallor
Petechiae
Behavior or appearance change
Excess salivation
Diarrhea
No meconium passage in first 48 hours
Cord odor or exudate

Adapted from Chow, M.P., et al.: Handbook of pediatric primary care, New York, 1979, J. Wiley & Sons, Inc., pp. 122-123; and Vaughan, V.C., McKay, R.J., and Behrman, R.E., editors: Nelson textbook of pediatrics, ed. 11, Philadelphia, 1979, W.B. Saunders Co., pp. 415-418.

Table 23-4. Infant reflexes

Reflex	How to elicit	Response of infant	Clinical implications
Acoustic blink	Produce a sharp loud noise (a clap of the hands) about 30 cm from the head.	By second or third day of life infant blinks both eyes. Disappearance of reflex is variable.	Absence may indicate decreased hearing.
Ankle clonus	Flex the leg at the hip and knee, sharply dorsiflex the foot, and maintain pressure.	Rhythmic flexions and extensions of the foot at the ankle.	Abnormal if more than 10 beats during the first 3 months or more than 3 beats after 3 months. Sustained clonus indicates upper motor neuron disease.
Babinski	Stroke lateral aspect of the plantar surface of foot from heel to toes. Use a blunt object.	Hyperextension or fanning of toes occurs. As myelinization is completed, the normal response becomes flexion (downward curling) of all toes; the positive (pathological) sign is hyperextension (dorsiflexion) of the great toe with or without fanning of the remaining toes.	After 2 years of age, a positive sign is the most significant clinical symptom of the presence of an upper motor neuron (pyramidal tract) lesion.
Blinking	Shine a light suddenly at the infant's open eyes.	Eyelids close in response to light. Disappears after first year.	Absence may indicate poor light perception or blindness.
Landau	Suspend infant carefully in prone position by supporting infant's abdomen with examiner's hand.	By 3 months of age the expected response consists of extension of head, trunk, and hips. Head is slightly above horizontal plane. Disappears by 2 years of age.	If newborn collapses into a limp concave position, it is abnormal.
Moro	With infant in supine position gently support head and lift it a few centimeters off the surface. As soon as neck relaxes, suddenly release the head and let it drop back to the surface. *or* Produce sudden loud noise, or jar the table or crib suddenly.	Normal response is present at birth and is one in which the arms extend outward, the hands open, and then are brought together in midline. The legs flex slightly. Usually disappears by 3 to 4 months. Infant may cry.	Asymmetry indicates possible paralysis. Absence suggests severe neurological problem. Persistence beyond 4 months may indicate neurological disease. If it lasts longer than 6 months, it is definitely abnormal.
Neck righting	With infant in supine position turn head to one side.	Infant's trunk rotates in direction in which head is turned. Appears at 4 to 6 months. Disappears at 24 months.	Absent or decreased reflex may indicate spasticity.
Palmar grasp	With infant's head positioned in midline place examiner's index fingers from ulnar side into infant's palm and press against palm.	Normal response is flexion of all fingers around examiner's fingers. Present at birth and disappears by 4 months when infant is ready to reach.	Note symmetry and strength. Persistence of grasp beyond 4 months suggests cerebral dysfunction.
Parachute	Infant is held in a prone position and is quickly lowered toward the surface of the examining table or floor.	Normal response is extension of arms, hands, and fingers, as if to break a fall. Appears by 9 months and persists.	Asymmetry or absence of response is abnormal.

From Chow, M.P., et al.: Handbook of pediatric primary care, New York, 1979, John Wiley & Sons, Inc., pp. 735-737; as adapted from Erickson, M.L.: Assessment and management of developmental changes in children, St. Louis, 1976, The C.V. Mosby Co., pp. 62-66; and Conway, B.L.: Pediatric neurological nursing, Philadelphia, 1977, The C.V. Mosby Co.

Continued.

Table 23-4. Infant reflexes — cont'd

Reflex	How to elicit	Response of infant	Clinical implications
Perez	Infant is held in a suspended prone position in one of the examiner's hands. The thumb of the other hand is moved firmly from sacrum along entire spine.	Normal response is extension of head and spine, flexion of knees on the chest, a cry, and emptying of the bladder. Present at birth and disappears by 3 months.	Absence indicates severe neurological disease.
Placing	Infant is held erect and the dorsum of one foot touches the undersurface of the examining table top.	Infant flexes hip and knee and places stimulated foot on top of the table. Present at birth and disappears by 6 weeks or variable.	Absent in paralysis or in infants born by breech delivery.
Plantar grasp	Examiner's finger is placed firmly across base of infant's toes.	Toes curl downward. Present at birth and disappears by 10 to 12 months.	Absent in defects of lower spinal column. Infant cannot walk until this reflex disappears.
Rooting	Infant is held in supine position with head in midline and hands against chest. Examiner strokes perioral skin at corner of mouth or cheek.	Infant opens mouth and turns head toward stimulated side. Present at birth and disappears by 3 to 4 months (awake); by 7 months (asleep).	Absence indicates severe central nervous system disease or depressed infant.
Rotation test	Infant is held upright facing examiner and rotated in one direction and then the other.	Infant's head turns in the direction in which the body is being turned. If head is restrained the eyes will turn in the direction in which the infant is turned.	If head and eyes do not move, it indicates a vestibular problem.
Spontaneous crawling (Bauer's response)	Infant is lying prone and examiner presses soles of feet.	Infant makes crawling movements. Present at birth.	Crawling is absent in weak or depressed infants.
Stepping	Infant is held upright and soles of feet are put in touch with solid surface.	Infant "walks" along surface. Present at birth and disappears at 6 weeks.	Absence indicates depressed infant, breech delivery, or paralysis.
Sucking	With infant in supine position place nipple or finger 3 to 4 cm into mouth.	Vigorous sucking of finger or nipple. Present at birth and disappears by 3 to 4 months (awake) and 7 months (asleep). Tongue action should push finger up and back. Note rate of suck, amount of suction, and patterns or groupings of sucks.	Absence in term infants indicates central nervous system depression. Weak reflex may lead to feeding problems.
Tonic neck	With infant in supine position passively rotate head to one side.	Arm and leg on side to which head is turned extend, and opposite arm and leg flex (fencer's position). Present sometimes at birth but usually by 2 to 3 months. Disappears by 6 months.	Obligatory response is always abnormal. Persistence beyond 6 months is abnormal and indicates central motor lesions (e.g., cerebral palsy).
Trunk incurvation (Galant's)	Infant is held prone in examiner's hand. With the other hand the examiner moves a finger down the paravertebral portion of the spine, first on one side, then on the other.	Infant's trunk should curve to the side being stimulated. Present at birth and disappears by 2 months.	Presence of spinal cord lesions interrupts this reflex.
Vertical suspension positioning	Infant is held upright, head is maintained in midline.	Legs are flexed at the hips and knees. Present at birth and disappears after 4 months.	Scissoring or fixed extension indicates spasticity.

a serious health problem. Since the newborn, later the infant, is largely dependent on his reflexive ability, assessment of these response characteristics and their timing of appearance and disappearance becomes vital to the infant's health. (See Table 23-4 for a summary of reflexes and techniques of assessment.)

Sensory Function

Sensory function of the newborn is primitive. The neonate perceives and responds to tactile stimulation that is soothing and painful. Although visual acuity is poor, the newborn can fixate both eyes for a short period of time as well as follow large moving objects and blink in response to bright light (Table 23-5). Auditory stimulation evokes changes in motor activity as evidenced by the startled reaction to loud, sudden noises. Taste is also primitively developed in the newborn, demonstrated by a response to sweet and sour stimulation. Additional techniques for screening infant sensory function can be found in Appendix K.

Table 23-5. Landmarks of visual development

Age	Characteristic development	Age	Characteristic development
Birth	Pupils react to light. Blink reflex in response to light stimulus. Corneal reflex in response to touch. Rudimentary fixation on objects with ability to follow to the midline.	44 weeks to 12 months	Exhibits smooth visual pursuit of objects and sound in the vertical and horizontal planes. Visual acuity exceeds 20/200. Transverse diameter of the cornea is 12 mm, the adult size. Amblyopia may develop with lack of binocularity. Fixates intently on facial expressions.
2 to 4 weeks	Fixation ability advances; stares at light source. Follows to midline more reliably. Tear glands begin to function.	12 to 18 months	Discriminates simple geometric forms. Visual acuity 20/100. Full binocular vision developed. Able to identify forms. Associates with visual experiences. Displays an intent interest in pictures. Able to scribble on a paper. Convergence becomes well established.
4 to 12 weeks	Convergence appears. Binocular fixation is established. Follows moving object with head and eye movements through 180 degrees. Fascinated by bright colors and lights. Tear glands display response to emotion.	18 months to 2 years	Depth perception remains crude. Accommodation well developed. Visual acuity 20/40.
12 to 20 weeks	Begins to inspect his own hands. Accommodation begins to develop. Able to fixate on objects more than 3 feet distant. Foveal pit becomes distinguishable as macula development proceeds. Pigmentation of fundus not developed; appearance of fundus is pale. Visual acuity 20/200.	2 to 3 years	Convergence smooth. Fixation on small objects or pictures should approach 50 seconds. Able to recall visual images. Visual acuity 20/30.
20 to 28 weeks	Able to rescue a dropped block. Hand-eye coordination is developing. Binocular fixation becomes fully developed. Ultimate color of iris is established. Discrimination between simple geometric forms is beginning to develop. Color preference for reds and yellows develops.	3 years to 4 years	Able to copy geometric figures. Reading readiness is present. Lacrimal glands are fully developed.
		5 years	Minimum potential for amblyopia to develop. Color recognition is well established.
28 to 44 weeks	Depth perception begins to develop. Displays interest in tiny objects. Tilts head backward to see upward.	6 years	Visual acuity approaches 20/20. Color shading may be differentiated. Astigmatism may develop at any point throughout life. Depth perception fully developed.

From Chinn, P.: Child health maintenance: concepts in family-centered care, St. Louis, 1979, The C.V. Mosby Co., p. 67; as adapted from Whipple, D.V.: Dynamics of development: euthenic pediatrics, New York, 1966, McGraw-Hill Book Co.; Liebman, S.D., and Gellis, S.S.: The pediatrician's ophthalmology, St. Louis, 1966, The C.V. Mosby Co.; and Keeney, A.H.: Development of vision. In Falkner, F., editor: Human development, Philadelphia, 1966, W.B. Saunders Co.

Table 23-6. Normal sleep patterns

Age	Number of hr/24 hr	Comments about sleeping habits
Newborn	Low: 10 Average: 16½ High: 23 (7-8 short naps)	No child fits into a routinely prescribed sleep pattern.
8-12 weeks	(2-4 naps)	Release into sleep varies with infants. Some are more tense than others.
2-4 months	Low: 8-10/night High: 11-12/night 2-3 naps/day	Although there is no correlation with solid food intake and sleeping through the night, the parent's attitude may make the difference.
6-12 months	11-12/night 2-3 naps/day	There should be an established routine for bedtime. Baby may wake because of illness, teething, or separation anxiety.
12-18 months	8-12/night 1-2 naps/day	There may be waking problems after the mother returns to work, even after several months.
2-3 years	8-12/night 1 nap/day	There is a need for rituals and consistency at bedtime. Active children may not nap after 2½ years.
3-4 years	8-12/night May take 1 nap/day	Some children wake with dreams. (One fifth of the night is spent dreaming.) Many children wake and wander at night. Some children accept a net over the crib or a locked half-door on the bedroom. The habit of sleeping with parents should be discouraged. This is a good time to shift from crib to bed.
4 years	8-12/night	Some dreaming and waking may result.
4½-5 years	8-12/night	There may be an increase in bad dreams and night terrors. The child may need considerable attention to get back to sleep. The child may enjoy reading at bedtime before lights out. Dreams may be at a low peak.

From Chow, M.P., et al.: Handbook of pediatric primary care, New York, 1979, John Wiley & Sons, Inc., p. 319.

The Infant

Infancy extends from 1 month to 1 year, and during this period of time major physical growth is occurring. Generally infants double their birth weight by 6 months and triple it by 12 months of age. By the end of the first year, an infant grows between 10 and 12 inches in length.

Physiological Stability

Physiological functioning becomes more sophisticated at this time. Brain growth is quite rapid with myelination occurring in a cephalocaudal direction. Visual ability becomes more refined, and by 1 year an infant can focus, follow, distinguish detail, and demonstrate color preference (Table 23-5). Heart rhythm and rate are stabilized.

Although fetal hemoglobin persists until 20 weeks, adult hemoglobin begins to appear around 13 weeks. Neonatal red blood cells are replaced by adult red blood cells, increasing the red blood cell life expectancy from 100 to 120 days. Salivary glands mature around the third month, and the stomach capacity increases to 360 ml by 1 year.

Sleep

The infant's physiological abilities are evidenced by the patterns of body functions that develop over the first year. The average newborn sleeps approximately 16 hours a day. During his wakeful periods, his attention span is quite short (7 to 10 minutes) and focuses primarily on gratification of needs. The timing and pattern of newborn sleep is generally quite unpredictable and without routine (Table 23-6).

Sleeping patterns become more predictable over the next few months, and by 3 months of age the infant is generally sleeping through the night and taking several naps during the day. By 12 months nighttime sleep is extended to 11 to 12 hours, naps are decreased to 1 to 2 per day, and a quite predictable routine of sleep and activity has developed. The attention span of a 12-month-old also has increased, demonstrated by an ability to remain engaged in an activity up to 30 to 45 minutes versus 15 to 20 minutes at 6 months.

Elimination

The elimination patterns of the infant also change throughout the first year. The first stools are called meconium. They are dark green to black, sticky, odorless, and generally passed within the first 48 hours. Transitional stools that are yellowish green appear about the third or fourth day. Subsequent stool frequency and consistency are dependent on the type and amount of oral intake an infant receives. Breast-fed babies tend to have bright mustard yellow stools that are soft and unformed with curdlike matter and very little odor. Bottle-fed babies tend to have yellow to yellowish green stools that are more formed and odoriferous. Frequency of stool elimination is largely dependent on gastrointestinal absorption and mobility and is thus individualized from infant to infant. In general, breast-fed babies have fewer stools per day (one to three) than bottle-fed babies (four to six) in the first weeks. This pattern reverses after 2 to 3 weeks, and the frequency of stool elimination increases in breast-fed babies and decreases in bottle-fed babies.

Bladder capacity increases from 600 ml at birth to 840 ml by 1 year. Most newborns urinate involuntarily within the first 24 hours and have between six to eight wet diapers per 24 hours in the first weeks. As bladder capacity increases, frequency tends to decrease, and volume of voiding increases.

Feeding

During the first year of life feeding behavior and patterns become a function of physiological development. The stomach capacity for fluids at birth is 30 to 60 ml (1 to 2 oz). Caloric and fluid requirements of the newborn are 130 to 100 calories/kg and 130 to 200 ml/kg. Hence the neonate feeds often in small amounts. As stomach capacity for fluids increases from 90 to 150 ml (3 to 5 oz) at 1 month to 240 ml (8 oz) at 1 year and caloric and fluid requirements stabilize, the feeding frequency of an infant decreases, and the amount per feeding increases.

In general, newborns are unpredictable in regard to how often they want to feed. Some require feeding every 2 hours, whereas others extend to every 4 hours. However, a pattern of feeding every 3 to 4 hours should begin to appear by 12 weeks of age. By 6 months an infant wants to eat 3 to 5 meals per day, and by 12 months most have developed a pattern of 3 meals a day and a snack.

Growth Spurts

Physical growth in the first year is evidenced by periods of time called growth spurts. During these spurts patterns of infant behavior change in a chain-reaction type of response to the process of physical maturation. During these periods of growth, physiological functioning and subsequent metabolic requirements increase. The growing body's demand for additional energy through calories prompts the infant to alter his feeding patterns by increasing the amount as well as the frequency of feeding. If his new energy and hunger demands are met, a few changes in behavior may be noted. However, the most frequent occurrence is that these needs are initially not met, and the parental complaint of a fussy, always hungry baby results.

Changes Created by Growth Spurts. Sleeping patterns may be altered during growth spurts. For some infants this may mean sleeping more; for others sleep may be interrupted and fretful because of hunger. Elimination patterns may also be affected during periods of growth. Generally there is a decrease in the frequency and amount of body waste, since intake is used to its maximum for growth. However, if the infant's feeding needs are overmet, his elimination patterns may increase or remain the same.

Growth spurts are most frequent and noticeable by parents in the first 6 to 8 months of life but continue to occur periodically until adolescence.For parents who have not been prepared to expect this normal growth occurrence the changes in the infant's behavior can be stressful. Nursing can prevent this potential stress for parents and infants by providing (1) early anticipatory guidance and education regarding the origin and course of growth spurts, (2) counseling on how to manage them, and (3) support and reassurance when they do occur.

The first evident spurt occurs approximately at 6 weeks of age, and the behavior patterns that accompany the growth appear every 6 to 8 weeks thereafter until approximately 6 months of age. The behavioral changes stimulated by the growth spurt usually last 4 to 7 days, after which the infant demonstrates a new pattern of behaviors.

Neuromotor Assessment

Neuromotor development in the first year occurs in a cephalocaudal direction of head to foot progression. The average infant can be assessed for performance of specific progressive behaviors when evaluating physical development (Table 23-7).

As the infant progresses through this pattern of physical development, he gains more voluntary control over the use of his body. His activity and behavior by 1 year have become more purposeful and less reflexive.

PSYCHOSOCIAL DEVELOPMENT

A child's growth process includes not only physical development but emotional and social development as well. Many variables influence the child's psychosocial growth. Psychological variables generally relate to interpersonal and cognitive characteristics, as well as per-

Text continued on p. 530.

Table 23-7. Waechter developmental guide: summary of average development during the first year

Age	Physical and motor development	Intellectual development	Socialization and vocalization	Emotional development
1 month	Physiologically more stable than in newborn period Waves hands as clenched fists Objects placed in hands are dropped immediately Momentary visual fixation on objects and human face Tonic neck reflex position frequent and Moro reflex brisk Able to turn head when prone, but unable to support head Responds to sounds of bell, rattle, etc. Makes crawling motions when prone Sucking and rooting reflex present Coordinates sucking, swallowing, and breathing	Reflexive No attempt to interact with environment External stimuli do not have meaning	Cries, mews, and makes throaty noises Responds in terms of internal need states Interested in the human face	Response limited generally to tension states Panic reactions, with arching of back and extension and flexion of extremities Derives satisfaction from the feeding situation when held and pleasure from rocking, cuddling, and tactile stimulation Maximum need for sucking pleasures Quiets when picked up
2 months	Moro reflex still brisk Posture still toward tonic neck reflex position Has visual response to patterns Eye coordination to light and objects Follows objects vertically and horizontally Responds to objects placed on face Listens actively to sounds Able to lift head momentarily from prone position Turns from side to back Able to swallow pureed foods	Recognition of familiar face Indicates inspection of the environment Begins to show anticipation before feeding	Begins to vocalize; coos Beginning of social smile Actively follows movement of familiar person or object with eyes Crying becomes differentiated Vocalizes to mother's voice Visually searches to locate sounds of mother's voice	Maximum need for sucking pleasures Indicates more active satisfaction when fed, held, rocked
3 months	Frequency of tonic neck reflex position and vigor of Moro response rapidly diminishing	Shows active interest in environment Can recognize familiar faces and objects such as bottle; how-	More ready and responsive smile Facial and generalized body response to faces	Maximum need for sucking pleasure Wishes to avoid unpleasant situations Not yet able to act in-

From Waechter, E.H., and Blake, F.G.: Nursing care of children, ed. 9, Philadelphia, 1976, J.B. Lippincott Co.

Table 23-7. Waechter developmental guide: summary of average development during the first year — cont'd

Age	Physical and motor development	Intellectual development	Socialization and vocalization	Emotional development
3 months — cont'd	Uses arms and legs simultaneously but not separately Able to raise head from prone position; may get chest off bed Holds head in fairly good control Begins differentiation of motor responses Hands are beginning to open, and objects placed in hands are retained for brief inspection; able to carry objects to mouth Indicates preference for prone or supine position "Stepping" reflex disappears Landau reflex appears Eyes converge as objects approach face Has necessary muscular control to accept cereal and fruit	ever, objects do not have permanence Recognition is indicative of recording of memory traces Begins playing with parts of body Follows objects visually Begins to be able to coordinate stimuli from various sense organs Shows awareness of a strange situation	Preferential response to adult voices Has longer periods of wakefulness without crying Begins to use prelanguage vocalizations, babbling and cooing Laughs aloud and shows pleasure in vocalization Shows anticipatory preparation to being lifted Turns head to follow familiar person Ceases crying when mother enters the room	dependently to evoke response in others
4 months	Ability to carry objects to mouth Inspects and plays with hands Grasps objects with both hands Turns head to sound of bell or bottle Reaches for offered objects Eyes focus on small objects Begins to demonstrate eye-hand coordination Ability to pick up objects Rooting reflex disappears; tonic neck reflex disappearing Sits with minimum support with stable head and back Turns from back to side Breathing and mouth	Recognizes bottle on sight Becomes bored when left alone for long periods of time Actively interested in environment Indicates beginnings of intentionality and interest in affecting the environment Indicates beginning anticipation of consequences of action	Vocalizes frequently and vocalizations change according to mood Begins to respond to "no, no" Enjoys being propped in a sitting position Turns head to familiar noise Chuckles socially Demands attention by fussing; enjoys attention	Interest in mother heightens Is affable and lovable Shows signs of increasing trust and security

Continued.

Table 23-7. Waechter developmental guide: summary of average development during the first year — cont'd

Age	Physical and motor development	Intellectual development	Socialization and vocalization	Emotional development
4 months — cont'd	activity coordinated in relation to vocal cords Holds head up when pulled to sitting position Begins to drool			
5 months	Ability to recover near objects Reaches persistently Grasps with whole hand Ability to lift objects Begins to use thumb and finger in "pincer" movement Able to sustain visual inspection Able to sit for longer periods of time when well supported Begins to show signs of tooth eruption Ability to sleep through night without feeding Moro reflex and tonic neck reflex finally disappear	Able to discriminate strangers from family Turns head after fallen object Shows active interest in novelty Attempts to regain interesting action in environment Ability to coordinate visual impressions of an object Begins differentiation of self from environment	Enjoys play with people and objects Smiles at mirror image More exuberantly playful but also more touchy and discriminating	Other members of the family become important as the baby's emotional world expands Begins to be able to postpone gratification Awaits anticipated routines with happy expectation Begins to explore mother's body
6 months	Ability to pick up small objects directly and deftly Ability to lift cup by handle Grasps, holds, and manipulates objects Ability to pull self to sitting position Begins to "hitch" in locomotion Momentary sitting and hand support When lying in prone position, supports weight with hands Weight gain begins to decline Ability to turn completely over	Increasing awareness of self Responds with attentiveness to novel stimuli Begins to be able to recognize mother when she is dressed differently Objects begin to acquire permanence; searches for lost object for brief period	Very interested in sound production Playful response to mirror Laughs aloud when stimulated Great interest in babbling, which is self-reinforcing Begins to recognize strangers	Begins to have sense of "self" Increased growth of ego
7 months	Ability to transfer objects from one hand to another Holds object in one hand Gums or mouths solid foods; exploratory behavior with food	Ability to secure objects by pulling on string Repeats activities that are enjoyed Discovers and plays with own feet Drops and picks up objects in exploration	Vocalizes four different syllables Produces vowel sounds and chained syllables Makes "talking sounds" in response to the talking of others Crows and squeals	Begins to show signs of fretfulness when mother leaves or in presence of strangers Shows beginning fear of strangers Orally aggressive in biting and mouthing

Table 23-7. Waechter developmental guide: summary of average development during the first year — cont'd

Age	Physical and motor development	Intellectual development	Socialization and vocalization	Emotional development
7 months —cont'd	Ability to bang objects together Palmar grasp disappears Bears weight when held in standing position Sits alone for brief periods Rolls over adeptly	Searches for lost objects outside perceptual field Has consciousness of desires Growing differentiation of self from environment Rudimentary sense of depth and space		
8 months	Ability to ring bell purposively Ability to feed self with finger foods Begins to experience tooth eruption Sits well alone Ability to release objects at will	Uncovers hidden toy Increased interest in feeding self Differentiation of means from end in intentionality Has lively curiosity about the world	Listens selectively to familiar words Says "da da" or equivalent Babbles to produce consonant sounds Vocalizes to toys Stretches out arms to be picked up	Plays for sheer pleasure of the activity Anxiety when confronted by strangers indicates recognition and need of mother; attachment behavior begins to be obvious and strong
9 months	Rises to sitting position Creeps and/or crawls; maybe backward at first Tries out newly developing motor capacities Ability to hold own bottle Drings from cup or glass with assistance Begins to show regular patterns in bladder and bowel elimination Good ability to use thumb and finger in pincer grasp Pulls self to feet with help	Ability to put objects in container Examines object held in hand; explores objects by sucking, chewing, and biting	Responds to simple verbal requests Plays interactive games, such as peek-a-boo and patty cake	Mother is increasingly important for her own sake; reacts violently to threat of her loss Begins to show fears of going to bed and being left alone Increasing interest in pleasing mother Active search in play for solutions to separation anxiety
10 months	Ability to unwrap objects Pulls to standing position Uses index finger to poke and finger and thumb to hold objects Finger feeds self; controls lips around cup Plantar reflex disappears Neci-righting reflex disappears Sits without support; recovers balance easily Pulls self upright with use of furniture	Begins to imitate Looks at and follows pictures in book	Extends toy to another person without releasing Responds to own name Inhibits behavior to "no, no" or own name Begins to test reactions to parental responses during feeding and at bedtime Imitates facial expressions and sounds	Has powerful urge toward independence in locomotion, feeding; beginning to help in dressing Experiences joy when achieving a goal and mastering fear

Continued.

Table 23-7. Waechter developmental guide: summary of average development during the first year — cont'd

Age	Physical and motor development	Intellectual development	Socialization and vocalization	Emotional development
11 months	Ability to hold crayon adaptively Ability to push toys Ability to put several objects in container; releases objects at will Stands with assistance; may be beginning attempts to walk with assistance Begins to be able to hold spoon "Cruises" around furniture	Works to get toy out of reach Growing interest in novelty Heightened curiosity and drive to explore environment	Repeats performance laughed at by others Imitates definite speech sounds Uses jargon Communicates by pointing to objects wanted	Reacts to restrictions with frustration, but has ability to master new situations with mother's help (weaning)
12 months	Turns pages in book; can make marks on paper Babinski sign disappears Begins standing alone and toddling "Cruises" around furniture Lumbar curve develops Hand dominance becomes evident Ability to use spoon in feeding	Dogged determination to remove barriers to action Further separation of means from ends Experiments to reach goals not attained previously Concepts of space, time, and causality begin to have more objectivity	Jabbers expressively Has words that are specific to parents Few, simple words Experimentation with "pseudo-words" of great interest and pleasure	Ability to show emotions of fear, anger, affection, jealousy, anxiety Is in love with the world

sonality and temperament differences. Social and cultural variables include such factors as family structure, familial attitudes, beliefs, and economic status.

Critical Periods

As with physical development, individual differences must be considered when assessing the child's psychosocial development. The individuality of a child's progression through the developmental phases is also influenced by the concept known as "critical periods of development." A critical period is a specific span of time during which the environment has its greatest impact on a child's development. The nature of the stimuli provided by the environment varies among children. The child's developmental progression depends on the timing and degree of environmental stimuli and his readiness to be stimulated by the environment (Sutterly and Donnelly, 1978). For example, an infant cannot learn to ride a bike regardless of the intensity of the stimuli, whereas a 6-year-old has the readiness and ability to learn.

Temperament

Children differ in personality temperament. *Temperament*, defined as an individual's behavior style, is usually one of the following three types: easy, slow to warm, and difficult (Thomas and Chess, 1977). Characteristics are shown in Table 23-8. Children have been found to demonstrate temperamental characteristics in the first weeks of life. Though the environment can influence a child's behavior, the basic temperament is unique to him.

Developmental Theories

Many theories of growth and development have evolved to explain this human process. Most familiar are the theories of Erikson and Piaget. The framework of these developmental hypotheses is used throughout this section.

Erikson

Erikson's theory of psychosocial development is based on the process of socialization. He theorizes life

Table 23-8. Temperament and personality characteristics

Temperament	Characteristic
Easy	Positive mood
	Regular body functions
	Low to moderate intensity of reaction
	Adaptability to new situations
Slow-to-warm up	Low activity level
	Tendency to withdraw on first exposure to new stimuli
	Slow adaptability
	Somewhat negative mood
	Low intensity of reaction to situations
Difficult	Irregular body functions
	Intensity in reactions
	Withdrawal from new stimuli
	Slow adaptation
	Negative mood

Adapted from Thomas, A., and Chess, S.: Pediatr. Ann. **6**:26-45, Sept. 1977.

development as a continuous struggle for an emotional-social equilibrium. Though Erikson's theory acknowledges the presence of an id, ego, and superego as defined by Freudian theory, it adds the further dimension of environmental influences on personality development. According to Erikson, each stage of life has its own tasks to be mastered, each has negative counterparts. Equilibrium occurs when the primary task of the stage is mastered. However, Erikson stresses that the negative counterparts are never completely mastered and must be reevaluated at subsequent times throughout life (Erikson, 1963).

Piaget

Piaget's theory of development focuses on cognition, which undergoes a gradual qualitative growth over the childhood years. According to Piaget, a variety of new experiences (or stimuli) must exist for learning to occur. The individual response to these stimuli occurs through assimilation and accommodation. *Assimilation* is the process of incorporating new experiences into current activities or thinking (i.e., experiences are adapted to the individual). *Accommodation* is the process of responding to the environment through a new means of activity and thinking (i.e., the individual is adapted to experiences). The combination of these processes allows the child to organize his world by ordering and classifying his experiences. The end result is

adaptation or the balance between the individual and his environment through new and expanded thoughts, behaviors, and problem-solving methods (Piaget, 1951).

Psychosocial Competency

Much of the foundation for psychosocial competency is built during the first year of life. According to Erikson, this first stage of life from birth to 1 year is charged with the task of developing trust versus a sense of mistrust. The newborn enters the world dependent on others for meeting his needs. If his basic needs are met through a close, warm, comforting relationship, a sense of trust develops. If his needs are not met or are only met sporadically, a sense of mistrust develops, since a child is never certain that his needs will be met. The caretaker-infant relationship therefore becomes an important factor in the infant's development of a sense of trust. The quality of this relationship has a direct impact on the infant's sense of well-being as influenced by the behavioral consistency and motivation of the caretaker.

Traditionally, the caretaker in our society is the infant's mother. However, becoming a mother does not necessarily mean being motherly. A *mother* is defined as a biological parent, whereas *mothering* is the means necessary to care for the infant. *Motherliness* is the capacity of the mother to be gratified by the exchange between herself and her infant and to use this gratification for her own growth. Mothering and motherliness are the qualitative characteristics that are necessary for the infant's development of a sense of trust (Klaus and Kennell, 1976). However, these qualities do not spontaneously occur at the moment of conception or birth but are developed as the mother and infant learn to respond to each other. The synchornization of maternal and infant responses, which results in a unique emotional relationship is termed *bonding* or *attachment*.

Maternal-Infant Bond. Attachment occurs when mother and infant elicit behaviors from each other that are reciprocal and complimentary. Maternal attachment behaviors are largely centered on a mother's attentiveness to her infant and her maintenance of physical contact (Leifer, 1972). Infant attachment behaviors center on maintaining focus or contact with the mother (Bowlby, 1969). The box on p. 532 outlines attachment behaviors identified in mothers and infants.

The infant's process of attachment occurs in developmental phases for the infant (Bowlby, 1969). Phase 1 is a period of orientation and signaling without discrimination of the person. Characteristic behaviors include tracking, smiling, reaching, and ceasing to cry when hearing the voice or seeing the face. Phase 2 is a continued period of orientation and signaling but is di-

Maternal and Infant Attachment Behaviors

Maternal behaviors

1. Prenatal period
   a. Expression of attitude about changing body image
   b. Verbalization about fetus
   c. Response to quickening
   d. Preparations for baby
   e. Degree of anxiety and fear about labor and delivery
   f. Desire for knowledge about labor and delivery
   g. Degree of emotional lability
2. Intrapartum period
   a. Spontaneity of verbal response at delivery
   b. Attempts to see and touch baby
   c. Questions about condition, appearance, and behavior of infant
   d. Reaction to sex of baby
3. Postpartum period: claiming and identification through
   a. Touch—proximal, ventral (close to body), affectionate
   b. Distal contact—talking to and about infant
   c. Eye contact
   d. Recognization of individualization of infant
   e. Performance of caretaking responsibilities in a positive manner

Infant behaviors

1. Sucking
2. Rooting
3. Grasping
4. Clinging
5. Regular changes between sleep, wakefulness, activity, and crying
6. Smiling and babbling
7. Normal activity level
8. Response to ministrations by calming
9. Visual alertness
10. Response to sensory stimuli
11. Quiets when presented with mother's face, voice, touch
12. Response to feeding

Adapted from Bowlby, J.: Attachment and loss, vol. 1, Attachment, New York, 1969, Basic Books, Inc., Publishers; Clark, A.L., and Affonso, D.D.: Childbearing: a nursing perspective, ed. 2, Philadelphia, 1979, F.A. Davis Co.; and Klaus, M.H., and Kennell, J.H.: Maternal-infant bonding, St. Louis, 1976, The C.V. Mosby Co.

rected toward a discriminated person. This phase begins at about 3 months of age and extends to 9 to 10 months. Behaviors are similar to those of phase 1, but the infant now displays a differential reaction to the mother, such as responding only to her voice or touch when he is crying.

In phase 3, the infant attempts to maintain closeness to the discriminated person by means of locomotion as well as by behavior signals. This phase lasts from approximately 10 months to 3 years of age. Characteristic behaviors include following, climbing on, exploring and then hurrying back to mother's side and clinging.

Phase 4 is the formation of a reciprocal relationship and occurs at about 4 years of age. Characteristic behaviors include the child's ability to predict the mother's movements, separating with ease from the mother, and attempting to change the mother's behavior to meet his own needs or goals (Ainsworth, 1969, Bowlby, 1969).

As with any process of human development, the interaction between mother and infant and subsequent attachment are influenced by a wide variety of factors. These variables include not only maternal and infant characteristics but environmental factors as well. These factors are outlined in Table 23-9 and should be considered when assessing the maternal-infant bond.

Father-Infant Bond. Although the maternal-infant bond is the primary influence on the infant's sense of well-being, the importance of the father-infant bond cannot be negated. This attachment occurs in much the same manner as the maternal-infant bond. Infant and father progress through an acquaintance process. Initially in this process, father and infant acquire information about each other through behaviors and signals. Once signals are received and responded to, each assesses the other's responsiveness to the signals. Finally, as infant and father begin to relate in a reciprocal man-

Table 23-9. Factors affecting maternal-infant attachment

Maternal factors	Infant factors	External factors
Past experiences	**Physical**	**Environment**
Relationship with own mother	Size: weight, height	Economic state
Genetic and cultural background	Sex	Housing
Significance of cultural values and expectations	Gestational age	Hospital policy and routines
Interpersonal interaction skills	General health	Behavior and attitude of staff
Relationships and experience with family and spouse	Appearance	
Parity	Presence or absence of visual blemishes	**Support systems**
Experience with previous pregnancy and infants	**Psychosocial responsiveness**	Father's response to mother and infant
Self-concept, self-image, and level of motherliness	Activity level	Presence of support from father, family, and peers
Current pregnancy experience	Perceptual and sensory abilities to receive, attend, discriminate, and respond to stimuli	Cultural support and values
Planned or unplanned	Threshold of sensory sensitivity	Family goals
Acceptance of pregnancy	State of alertness, sleep patterns, and crying behaviors	Response of siblings
Perception of fetus as individual	Ease of pacification	**Other**
Fantasies and expectations of newborn	Ability to initiate and elicit mothering interaction	Pending responsibilities
Age of parents-to-be	Response and reaction to mother's caretaking	Course of labor, delivery and postpartum period
Health of mother		Time of initial contact with infant
Degree of fear and worry about fetus, labor, and delivery		Multiple births
Actual labor and delivery experience		
Neonatal period		
Perception of labor and delivery		
Degree of physical comfort		
Hormonal levels		
Comparison of real to fantasized infant		
Ability to identify and accept infant as separate individual		
Ability to perceive infant cues		
Feelings about competence to care for infant		

Adapted from Chow, M.P., et al.: Handbook of pediatric primary care, New York, 1979, John Wiley & Sons, Inc.; Clark, A.L., and Affonso, D.D.: Childbearing: A nursing perspective, ed. 2, Philadelphia, 1979, F.A. Davis Co. and Klaus, M.H., and Kennell, J.H.: Maternal-infant bonding, St. Louis, 1976, The C.V. Mosby Co.

ner, further aspects of personality become known to each other and serve to validate or negate previous responsiveness.

The development of a paternal-infant bond is especially important in our society today. Extended families are less available to new parents, thereby increasing the father's support role within the nuclear family. Bonding of father and infant facilities the development of this paternal role, allowing the father to provide for the emotional and physical needs of the infant (Rapoport, 1977).

The father's participation in meeting the demands of child rearing and nurturing is further facilitated when the opportunity for bonding occurs early in the infant's life. A father's image of a baby is one of separateness, contrary to the mother who views the baby as an integral part of herself. Therefore the father's attachment to the infant is not as strong initially. Early exposure, especially at birth, provides the father with the needed opportunity to begin developing a bond with his new child.

Parent-Child Bond. In addition to the individual bonds mother and father develop with their infant, they also need to nurture a bond as a parental unit (Duvall, 1977). Working in unison to promote healthy growth and development of their infant needs to be a focus of new parents, but often feelings of insecurity intervene. The nurse can assist parents in developing as a unit by being an empathetic listener, by teaching parenting skills that gratify the infant's and parents' needs, and in understanding normal growth and development.

Cognitive Competency

Cognitive competency is another area of development that is rapidly expanding in the first year of life. Piaget views the first 2 years of life as the sensorimotor period. During this period the infant moves from reflexive to symbolic behavior, when expression and communication originate from the infant's body. During the first 24 months a child progresses through six stages toward cognitive competence. Stage 1 from birth to 1 month is characterized by the use of reflexes and random body movements. A neonate has no awareness of himself or of a world outside of himself. Stage 2 from 1 to 4½ months is characterized by habits of behavior that are learned by chance and repeated for their pleasurable benefit. These new behaviors or habits are the result of physical maturation as well as repetitive use of reflexes and random movements. In stage 3 an infant of 4½ to 9 months achieves eye-hand coordination. New behaviors that were accidentally discovered initially are repeated as a means of making the environment more interesting. Stage 4 brings the coordination of more complex behaviors as perception begins to develop in

the 9- to 12-month-old. The infant learns to get around obstacles or to use a new means to get what he wants.

By 12 to 18 months the toddler is demonstrating experimentation behaviors. Through trial and error the toddler discovers different ways to achieve the desired result. The evidence of beginning reasoning, memory, and retention appears in these activities. Between 18 and 24 months the child develops the ability to form mental images, and his thought is characteristically symbolic. Imitation becomes apparent in this stage, and permanency of objects is a well-developed thought.

Nursing Role

Stimulation of an infant's psychosocial and cognitive environment is an important parenting skill that nurses can teach. The need for visual, sensory, and tactile stimulation in promoting healthy development is as essential for the infant as food. Appendix J provides age-appropriate stimulation suggestions that can be used in the first year.

Knowledge and assessment of developmental milestones are also important aspects of infant development. Fine and gross motor skills were previously reviewed in this chapter. An appropriate focus when assessing psychosocial and cognitive development centers on an infant's social and language behaviors. Characteristic behaviors are reviewed in Table 23-7.

FACTORS AFFECTING GROWTH AND DEVELOPMENT

Mastery

Human growth and development are continuous processes that are complex yet predictable. Although the exact age for accomplishing the specific tasks of each stage varies from child to child, a chronology of events does exit, which involves a wide range of norms, allowing for individual differences. The individual pace of a child through the developmental stages is set by a variety of factors. Of primary importance in this progression from one stage to another is the successful mastery of the tasks and milestones of the preceding stage (Erikson, 1963). Because development is a sequential process, a child must successfully complete, in his own individual style, the particular task of the specific developmental stage. For example, a 15-month-old cannot run unless he can walk. Similarly a 2-year-old cannot separate easily from his mother unless he has come to trust her. Although a child never completely finishes all the developmental tasks in a given stage, some degree of mastery and comfort must be achieved before proceeding successfully to the next stage (i.e., a child continues to learn to trust other people throughout his life but must have developed a basic trust of his mother to separate and expand his world).

Adequacy of Attachment Process

A number of factors affect the child's ability to progress through and master the developmental stages. Of importance early in the child's life are the nature and adequacy of the maternal-infant bond. The quality of this bond and the parental-child relationship and its management have been found to have the most profound effect on the child's developmental progress. Significant psychosocial variables that influence bonding and attachment are summarized in Table 23.9. Other important nurturing influences that have been described as having a significant impact on development include the prenatal environment, ordinal position, and societal attitudes, expectations, and culture as interpreted within the child's home (Sutterly, 1978). Parental income, socioeconomic class, and family structure are further identified as influences on growth and development.

Health Environment

Additional influences stem from the physical status of the individuals as well as the environment. The health of a child affects not only his responsiveness in the developmental process but the responsiveness of others to him as well. Similarly, the adequacy of nutrition as it influences health affects a child's development. Factors within the physical environment also play an important part in this process, including adequacy of housing, season and climate of the home, geographical location, and availability and exposure to physical exercise.

Heredity

Hereditary variables must be considered as factors that influence growth and development. In assessing such variables the nurse must be cognizant of the physical and psychosocial results of an individual's genetic makeup. Physical characteristics and diseases are inherited as are some aspects of the individual's behavioral temperament (Thomas, 1977). Therefore the nurse should assess these genetic forces through an evaluation and history of the genetic makeup of several generations (Table 23-1).

COMMON CAUSES OF MORBIDITY AND MORTALITY

Major strides have been made over the past 20 years to improve the safety of life for infants. The infant mortality in 1977 was a record low 14 infant deaths per 1000 live births. This reduction in infant mortality is attributable to improved nutrition, housing, and prenatal, obstetrical, and pediatric care. Provided current trends continue, the mortality for infants in the United States will be reduced to 12 deaths per 1000 live births in 1982 and will drop further to 9 per 1000 by 1990 (Healthy People, 1979).

Despite a 32% drop in the infant mortality over the past 8 years, significant problems still exist. The first year of life is the most hazardous period until age 65. Black infants remain at risk. Nearly twice as many black infants die before their first birthdays than do white infants (24 per 1000 in 1977) (Healthy People, 1979). Similarly, infants from low-income situations and certain regional areas demonstrate higher morbidity and mortality.

The primary threats to infant health and survival are low birth weight (immaturity), congenital anomalies with associated problems, and sudden infant death syndrome (SIDS). In 1977 the leading cause of death in children under 1 year of age was congenital anomalies and the secondary effects of such birth defects (8420 deaths). The second leading cause of death in 1977 was SIDS (4751 deaths), followed by immaturity (3714 deaths) (Healthy People 1979).

Congenital Anomalies

A congenital anomaly is any deviant organ or part existing before or at birth in an abnormal form, structure, or location but not necessarily detected at birth (Vaughan, et al., 1979). Congenital anomalies involving the heart and circulatory system occur in approximately 1 of every 100 infants. The chance of a congenital heart defect in the newborn sibling of an affected child is 1 per 50 live births (Healthy People, 1979). The need for genetic counseling of the parents of an affected child is apparent, with referral to genetic resources as appropriate.

Cardiovascular Anomalies

Since congenital anomalies, particularly those of the cardiovascular system, pose the greatest mortality threat to infants, the nurse should be familiar with the major signs and symptoms of congenital heart disease. Early recognition and referral facilitate early management and potentially reduce the threat of death. The physical findings in newborns and infants with congenital heart disease include anorexia, cyanosis, delayed development, enlarged heart or liver, dyspnea during feeding, failure to gain weight, heart murmurs, tachycardia (up to 150 to 200 beats per minute at rest), tachypnea (up to 50 to 60 respirations per minute at rest), and recurrent repiratory infections and distress.

Major Organ Systems

Congenital anomalies of other major organ systems may also pose a threat to infant health. (See a basic pediatric nursing text for a review of the major organ system anomalies and their accompanying signs and symptoms.) Although the incidence of these birth defects is less frequent and in some cases not as life threatening as those of the cardiovascular system, the nurse has a responsibility to be knowledgeable of the symptoms when making an assessment. Those most likely to be lethal to the infant in addition to the congenital heart defects are malformations of the brain and spinal conditions involving the combination of several malformations, such as spina bifida and hydrocephalus.

Genetic Disorders

Also included under the diagnosis of birth defects are the genetic diseases. About one fourth of these defects are thought to be genetic in origin. The five types of genetic or inherited disease factors that cause the most illness and death include Down's syndrome, brain and neural tube defects, defects related to ethnic groups (e.g., Tay-Sachs disease, sickle-cell anemia, cystic fibrosis), sex-linked defects (e.g., hemophilia, muscular dystrophy), and metabolic disorders (Healthy People, 1979).

External Factors

Birth defects may also result from exposure of the fetus to toxic agents during pregnancy. External factors that increase infant mortality and morbidity include infections, particularly rubella; exposure to radiation and chemicals; and maternal alcohol or drug abuse.

Sudden Infant Death Syndrome

Sudden infant death syndrome (SIDS) is responsible for approximately one third of all deaths (8000 to 10,000) occurring in infants from ages 1 week to 1 year (Healthy People, 1979). It occurs most often between 2 and 4 months of age and is found to be uncommon before 1 month and after 8 months. SIDS occurs more frequently in males, low birth weight infants, twins, and low socioeconomic groups. It often occurs during normal sleep periods and happens during times of the year when the incidence of upper respiratory illnesses is increased.

Definition

SIDS is the sudden death of any infant or young child, which is unexpected by history and in which a thorough postmortem examination fails to demonstrate an adequate cause of death (Bergman, 1972). Its etiology has eluded identification; multiple theories of causation have evolved over the years. Table 23-10 reviews disproven and current theories regarding SIDS etiology.

Table 23-10. Theories regarding SIDS

Insufficiently proven causes of SIDS	Currently demonstrated causes of SIDS
Myocardial conduction abnormalities	Depressed CO_2 sensitivity, resulting in failure to stimulate respirations
Accidental suffocation	
Allergic reactions or immunopathology	Interruption in respiratory and/or cardiac central control function
Nutritional deficiency	
Infection	
Traumatic, endocrine, or toxic causes	Nasal obstruction
	Neurological problem in which laryngeal sensory receptors reflexively inhibit breathing
	Oropharyngeal occlusion

Adapted from Chow, M.P., et al.: Handbook of pediatric primary care, New York, 1979, John Wiley & Sons, Inc., p. 994.

Since the nurse is frequently in a position to provide counsel and answer questions of concerned clients, familiarity regarding these theories is essential.

Clinical Presentation

The clinical picture presented by the family of a SIDS victim is relatively unremarkable, as most infants die at home, during the night while sleeping, without difficulty, and unobserved. Parents often discover their infant lying lifeless in the crib, often in a state of disarray, with a blood-stained fluid in the nose and mouth (Shaw, 1970).

Nursing Role

Nursing's role in this perplexing and agonizing experience is to assist the family in coping. The grief reaction is acute, and severe stress is felt by the entire family. The initial reactions are the predictable symptoms and behavior of the grief process: shock, denial, anger, guilt. A sense of emotional numbness may develop in the parents immediately after the initial response, and frequently insomnia, anorexia, fatigue, depression, and preoccupation with the SIDS event occur (Patterson and Pomeroy, 1974). During this time of responding to an unexplained, unexpected loss, the parents and family require tremendous support. The nurse is in a position to provide this through the therapeutic relationship. Interventions need to be made at the time of

---

Nursing Interventions in SIDS Management

Recommended management* at the time of SIDS death

- Performance of autopsies on all infants dying suddenly and unexpectedly
- Prompt notification of the results of that autopsy to the parents
- Use of the term *sudden infant death syndrome* on the death certificate
- Follow-up information and counseling for all families provided by a knowledgeable health professional

Appropriate management within 1 week of infant's death includes a home visit with the following objectives for care:

- Provide emotional support during the grieving period
- Listen empathetically
- Provide information on SIDS to the family members as they are generally ready for it
- Anticipate normal grief reactions, and reassure parents that their reactions are normal
- Answer all questions asked by parents, and give printed material on SIDS
- Assist parents in dealing with siblings and relatives
- Put parents in touch with parent groups and the National Foundation of Sudden Infant Death
- Support the whole family during the pregnancy and infancy period of a subsequent child
- Refer parents for psychiatric help if abnormal reactions exist and persist

Indications for referral

- Parent(s) shows no emotion
- Parent(s) overintellecutalizes (e.g., is obsessed with scientific details)
- Parent(s) persistently denies the infant's death
- Continuing inability of parent(s) to resume previous responsibilities and level of functioning

*Recommended by National Foundation of Sudden Infant Death (NFSID) from Mile, M., editor: Mental health aspects of SID, Report of a conference sponsored by NFSID and National Institute for Mental Health, Kansas City, July 30, 1075, U.S. Department of Health, Education, and Welfare. Adapted from Chow, M. P., et al.: Handbook of pediatric primary care, New York, 1979, John Wiley & Sons, Inc., p. 998; and Tackett, J. J., and Hunsberger, M.: Family centered care of children and adolescents, Philadelphia, 1981, W. B. Saunders Co., p. 686.

death as well as after the cause of death has been confirmed (see the box above). The family should be contacted at home within 5 to 7 days after the death. During this and subsequent visits the nurse should focus on providing empathetic support and assisting the family in coping and progressing through the grief process.

Significant studies in managing potential SIDS victims have been made through research of SIDS, and preventive measures are being instituted in major neonatology centers across the United States. Of primary importance is early recognition and referral of infants at risk to such tertiary care centers. Management generally involves home apnea monitoring, parental education regarding SIDS and cardiopulmonary resuscitation, and close frequent follow-up (Bergman, 1976). Although this approach has not solved the mystery of SIDS, it has prevented deaths. Community health nurses should be knowledgeable about the availability of such resources and may be involved in the implementation of the management plan.

Health Problems Associated with Immaturity

Two thirds of all infant deaths occur in those newborns weighing less than 5½ lb (2500 g) at birth (Healthy People, 1979). Consequently, the potential of death to the low birth weight and frequently premature infant poses one of the greatest health hazards.

Definition of Immaturity

There are several definitions for infants based on gestation and weight with which the nurse should be familiar. The *premature* or *preterm* infant is one born before the end of the thirty-seventh week of gestation, regardless of birth weight. Low birth weight infants (less than 2500 g) are classified as follows (Dubowitz et al., 1970):

- Appropriately grown for gestational age (AGA); that is, infants whose rates of intrauterine growth are normal at birth, but who are small because they are born before the end of the thirty-seventh week.
- Small for gestational age (SGA); that is, infants whose rates of intrauterine growth are slow but who are born at or later than term (38 to 41 weeks).
- Small for gestational age *and* premature; that is, infants whose rate of intrauterine growth is retarded, and who are delivered before 37 weeks.

In general, infants who are born prematurely are SGA, weighing less than 2500 g, although they may be AGA or LGA (large for gestational age).

Factors Disposing to Prematurity

Chronic hypertensive disease
Toxemia
Placenta previa
Abruptio placentae
Cervical incompetence
Low socioeconomic status, including poor
  nutrition, chronic infection, fatigue, and
  generally poor personal and
  environmental hygiene
Absence of prenatal care
Multiple pregnancies
History of previous premature delivery
Age (highest incidence under age 20)
Order of birth (highest incidence in first
  pregnancies)

From Chow, M.P., et al.: Handbook of pediatric primary care, New York, 1979, John Wiley & Sons, Inc., p. 143.

Predisposing Factors

Factors disposing infants to premature delivery are identified in the box above. The circumstance of prematurity creates additional health problems for these infants. Premature infants (80% to 90%) are at risk in the first year because of an increased incidence of anorexia, birth injuries, hyaline membrane disease, septicemia, and respiratory and other infections. The primary causes of morbidity in the premature infant are hemorrhage, kernicterus, anemia, and infection.

Nursing Follow-up Care

Follow-up care of premature infants is the primary management. A plan of care is directed toward preventing the health problems associated with immaturity and facilitating the family's coping by providing support and anticipatory guidance to the parents concerning the physical and psychosocial development of the infant. Community health nurses are in a position to implement such a plan of care through home and clinic contacts, while providing the necessary element of continuity of care.

Though a premature infant requires more frequent follow-up visits, the preventive pediatric care does not differ significantly from that of a full-term infant. However, during the follow-up care of a preterm infant or the infant who has experienced complications or prolonged illness of the family of the infant, extra attention in certain areas of physical and developmental assessment is required. Table 23-11 provides an appropriate plan of care for such infants.

Table 23-11. Nursing implications in follow-up care for premature infants

Nursing goal	Nursing implication
Prevent neurological function impairment	Scheduling frequent follow-up visits (initially 1 to 2 times a week, advancing to once a month when a normal pattern of growth is identified)
	Complete physical and neurological assessment at each visit
	Referral as appropriate
Promote physical growth and prevent function impairment	Monitoring of height, weight, and head circumference at each visit
	Nutritional monitoring and education; use of supplemental nutrients and calories to ensure adequate nutrition; suggested techniques for feeding
	Education regarding skin care because of maceration proneness
	Education regarding maintenance of thermal environment
	Education regarding proneness to and avoidance of infections
	Education regarding infant need for rest and gentle handling
	Referral as appropriate, especially early dental assessment and hearing and ophthalmological examinations
Promote maximum development	Routine developmental screening
	Education regarding sensory stimulation
	Promotion of maternal-infant bond and paternal-infant bond
	Promotion of normal newborn experiences and avoidance of overprotection
	Referral as appropriate, especially to community resource support groups

Adapted from Korones, S.B., and Lancaster, J.: High risk newborn infants, ed. 3, St. Louis, 1981, The C.V. Mosby Co.; and Tackett, J.J., and Hunsberger, M.: Family centered care of children and adolescents, Philadelphia, 1981, W.B. Saunders Co.

Cause of Neonate Morbidity

Although infectious diseases no longer pose the major life threat they once did 20 years ago, they do remain the leading cause of illness and restricted activity for children under 6 years of age. Neonates are particularly susceptible to sepsis, a bacterial infection involving the bloodstream and frequently the meninges. Gram-negative bacilli and group B- beta hemolytic streptococci are the most common agents of sepsis in neonates. Sites vulnerable to entry of the infectious agents are the umbilicus, skin, and nasopharynx, and infections may spread rapidly with few signs or symptoms. The neonate is particularly susceptible to these agents and subsequent sepsis for a number of reasons, such as exposure to contaminated equipment and environment, unrecognized infections in other persons, an immature immune system, and the body's inability to carry out effective phagocytosis.

The signs and symptoms of sepsis are subtle and difficult to detect. However, neurological involvement may occur rapidly. Since community health nurses may have the first contact with an infant developing sepsis, they should be alert to its symptoms, which include the following (Chow et al., 1979; Korones, 1981):

Full anterior fontanel that lacks normal pulsations
Hypothermia
Continued lethargy, anorexia
Persistent apneic spells or seizures
Feeding poorly with a weak suck
Persistent diarrhea, vomiting, spitting up
Jaundice and liver enlargement between the fourth and eighth day of life
Petechia, shrill cry, or abdominal distension

The mortality for neonatal sepsis is high, and meningitis is responsible for 60% to 70% of the fatalities. In addition, up to 80% of those who survive sepsis suffer serious neurological complications resulting in brain damage, retardation, and developmental and growth delays.

Nursing Role

The nurse's role is early recognition and assessment. Preventive measures can be implemented by the nurse in an attempt to reduce the incidence and spread of the agents of speticemia. Community health nurses can initiate prevention through parental and family education in hygiene techniques. Potential environmental sources of the bacteria can be identified by the community health nurse who can then refer the client for treatment.

Finally, the nurse has a responsibilty to provide support to the parents of an infant who develops sepsis. Particular attention to the disruption in the bonding process is needed if hospitalization occurs. The nurse should identify measures that facilitate bonding and

Table 23-12. General measures for symptoms of infectious disease

Symptom	Measure
Fever	1. Antipyretic medication 2. Tepid sponge baths 3. Liberal fluid intake 4. Rest and limited activity
Upper respiratory symptoms	1. Liberal fluid intake 2. Cool mist vaporizers 3. Decongestants 4. Warm gargles, saline solution mouth and throat irrigations, cool liquids, and soft foods for sore throat as appropriate to age 5. Petrolatum jelly to protect the skin around the nares 6. Cough preparations generally ineffective and contraindicated in infants and young children
Generalized aching and malaise	1. Rest and limited physical activity 2. Warm baths 3. Body massage 4. Cold compresses for headache 5. Analgesic medication
Anorexia	1. Small, frequent feedings of favorite foods and liquids 2. Relaxed attitude about oral intake; forcing foods and fluids is usually counterproductive
Rash	1. Proper hygiene and bathing to reduce incidence of secondary infection 2. Cool baths, local applications of calamine lotion, and mild anesthetic ointments or systemic antihistamines to relieve pruritus 3. Fingernail care, including frequent cutting and cleaning, to reduce effects of scratching; gloves or mittens may be used at night on younger children 4. Saline mouthwashes if mucous membranes are involved

Adapted from Chow, M.P., et al.: Handbook of pediatric primary care, New York, 1979, John Wiley & Sons, Inc.; and Krugman, S., Ward, R., and Katz, S.L.: Infectious diseases of children, ed. 6, St. Louis, 1977, The C.V. Mosby Co.

parental involvement in the care of the infant. (See Table 23-12 for additional follow-up suggestions.) The community health nurse can be most instrumental in a successful resolution by acting as a client advocate and supporter.

Causes of Infant Morbidity

For the infant 1 month to 1 year of age, infection remains the greatest cause of illness. (This is also true of children up to 6 years of age, although the causative agent for each age group may differ as a result of host susceptibility and development of immunity.) Of greatest significance is the incidence of influenza and pneumonia in infants.

The origin of an infectious disease such as influenza or pneumonia may be viral or bacterial. The symptoms generally fall into specific categories such as fever, upper respiratory symptoms, generalized ache and malaise, anorexia, and exanthem. Early recognition and management of these symptoms serve to abate their severity and complications (Table 23-12).

Nursing Role

The community health nurse frequently encounters infants and children with infectious diseases. Assisting parents through education in recognition and responsible symptomatic management can prevent further complications. In addition, facilitating client knowledge in the prevention of infectious disease spread is well within the community health nurse's role. Health promotional activities that need to be stressed include adequate nutrition, avoidance of sources of infection or ill persons, use of responsible hygiene measures, and early intervention if symptoms occur.

MAJOR HEALTH PROBLEMS

During the process of physical and emotional maturation, a child passes through many stages. Each presents risks to health and well-being. Nurses should provide anticipatory guidance, and when indicated, assist parents with the management of these problems.

Major health problems during the neonatal period include the phenomenon of jaundice and regulation of body temperature. With infants the health problems of major concern include upper respiratory tract infections, otitis media, allergies, and gastorintestinal illnesses.

Jaundice

Jaundice refers to the yellowish color of the skin and results from the breakdown of red blood cells plus the immaturity of liver enzymes to conjugate and excrete bilirubin. Bilirubin must be conjugated to bind with al-bumin for excretion. Unbound (indirect) bilirubin cannot be excreted from the body and is subsequently absorbed into the fatty tissue and the brain.

Physiological jaundice (icterus neonatorum) is a normal occurrence between the second and fourth day of life and appears in approximately 50% of all full-term newborns. Bilirubin levels may reach 6 to 10 mg/dl, and resolution generally occurs by the seventh to eight day. A bilirubin level exceeding 10 mg/dl for the full-term infant is suggestive of more than normal physiology and would be considered hyperbilirubinemia (Vaughan, 1979).

Hyperbilirubinemia

Hyperbilirubinemia of the newborn appears in the first week of life but persists rather than resolving. Among the causes may be a more severe form of physiological jaundice, blood group incompatibility (hemolytic disease), or breast-feeding jaundice. The primary cause of the problem is elevated levels of unconjugated bilirubin resulting from deficiency or inactivity of bilirubin glucuronyl transferase, a liver enzyme that conjugates bilirubin. The immediate danger is kernicterus when bilirubin levels exceed 15 to 20 mg/dl.

Hyperbilirubinemia resulting from breast-feeding occurs in one of every 200 infants and is believed to be caused by the secretion of a substance in breast milk that inhibits the activity of bilirubin glucuronyl transferase (Chow et al., 1979). Increased bilirubin levels begin by the seventh day and may peak and persist at 2 to 3 weeks of age.

Hyperbilirubinemia caused by hemolytic disease is the result of excessive red blood cell destruction because of Rh incompatibility or ABO incompatibility. In both instances jaundice appears in the first 24 to 72 hours. The hemolytic process that occurs because of Rh incompatibility creates a more severe jaundice and an increased danger of kernicterus.

Kernicterus

Kernicterus refers to neurological damage that occurs when unconjugated bilirubin is deposited in brain tissue. The mortality is high, and survivors generally demonstrate signs of central nervous system damage. When serum bilirubin levels reach 18 mg/dl and above, the risk of kernicterus exists (Vaughan, 1979). Low birth weight and premature infants are particularly at risk and at lower levels.

Nursing Role

With the advent of early discharge after delivery, the community health nurse may encounter newborns with signs of jaundice. Early recognition and intervention thus become responsibilities that the community health nurse must assume. Observation is the primary tool nurses can use when assessing a neonate for jaundice. Progressive hyperbilirubinemia is accompanied by the appearance of jaundice in a cephalocaudal advancement. The yellow appearance shows first in the head and neck, advances to the trunk and umbilicus, and progresses to the groin, upper thighs, knees, ankles, elbows, and finally to the palms of the hands and soles of the feet. As the yellow appearance progresses downward and outward, the level of bilirubin progresses upward. Management common to all causes of jaundice and hyperbilirubinemia involves adequate hydration and support, education, and counseling of the parents.

Temperature Control

Temperature control is the result of heat production and heat loss function. In newborns the heat production function is unreliable as are the controls for the rate and amount of heat loss. Since the environment influences the amount of heat loss, regulation and maintenance of the thermal environment are critical to the newborn.

The instability of thermal regulatory functioning in the neonate is caused by a number of factors including the immaturity of perspiring and shivering mechanisms, small amounts of subcutaneous fat, and a relatively great body surface area (Korones, 1981). By controlling the immediate environment of the newborn, some degree of this thermal imbalance can be offset. The normal infant temperature should be 97.5° to 98.6° rectally. This body temperature can be maintained by keeping a warm room temperature of 74° to 76° and by providing external warmth such as blankets.

The premature or low birth weight infant requires special attention to thermoregulation. As the weight (body mass) of the baby decreases, the body surface area becomes proportionately greater. In addition, the lesser the amount of subcutaneous fat, the greater the degree of heat loss. For the preterm infant this means a constant effort needs to be made to control his body temperature through environmental measures.

Upper Respiratory Tract Infections

Over half of all acute illnesses treated in ambulatory settings include infections of the upper respiratory tract (URIs). Infants and children are particularly susceptible to URIs because of their immunological immaturity; small, easily obstructed airways; underdeveloped accessory muscles; and ineffectual coughing ability (Vaughan, 1979).

Nursing role

Nursing's primary responsibility in URIs is prevention, which includes providing anticipatory guidance in nutrition, rest, and hygiene. In addition, community health nurses should identify infants and children at risk because of numerous URIs, institute preventive measures, and implement close follow-up. Careful assessment is essential. Data retrieved from the assessment determine nursing's management.

Assessment begins with a chronological picture of the present complaint, including data regarding the presence, character, and severity of cough, fever, respiratory difficulty, rhinorrhea, other discharge, pain, and sore throat. The physical assessment should focus on determining the severity and location of the illness (Table 23-13). In addition, measurement of vital signs, particularly the respiratory rate, character, and rhythm, facilitates determination of severity.

Though the management of upper respiratory infections varies according to the severity and location, several general measures can be appropriately instituted. These measures include hydration through generous amounts of fluids, humidification through cool mist or steam vaporizers, and symptomatic relief measures such as bulb syringing for nasal discharge, use of antipyretics for fever reduction, and warm saline gargles for sore throat in older children.

Otitis Media

Suppurative otitis media, a bacterial infection of the middle ear, is a significant complication of URIs in infants and children. Frequently, serous otitis media, an accumulation of fluid in the middle ear, is the sequela of suppurative otitis media.

Serous otitis media, generally caused by allergy or nasopharyngeal inflammation, is characterized by marked conductive hearing loss persisting for weeks. The fluid produces a "popping" sensation with swallowing and a feeling of fullness. On examination the tympanic membrane is retracted, translucent, and dull. Fluid may be evident behind the drum as may air bubbles. A decrease in drum mobility is a definitive finding (Bruch, 1979). Management is directed toward identification of cause and alleviation of discomfort. The fullness may be alleviated by the Valsalva maneuver (holding nose and blowing) or the use of decongestants, although their efficacy has yet to be proven.

Causes and Management. The common causes of suppurative otitis media vary with age. In infants 6 to 8 weeks of age and younger, gram-negative bacilli and staphylococci are most prevalent. In older infants and children Pneumococci, *Haemophilus influenzae,* and *mycoplasma pneumoniae* are common causative organisms. Nasal congestion, irritability, and cough are characteristic. Other associated symptoms may include fever, vomiting, diarrhea, and hearing difficulties. Physical examination reveals outward bulging of the

Table 23-13. Signs helpful in localizing respiratory tract abnormality

Site of abnormality	Signs evident from simple observation	Signs evident on further examination
Upper Respiratory Obstructions		
Nose	Noisy respirations (nasal congestion)	Nasal mucosa edematous and either red (suggesting infection) or pale (suggesting allergic rhinitis)
	Rhinorrhea	
	Occasional cough (secondary to postnasal drip or associated pharyngitis)	Nasal discharge (usually thin, clear)
	No signs of respiratory distress except in young infants who may have obligatory nasal breathing	Chest clear to auscultation except for transmitted sounds
Paranasal sinuses (ethmoid and maxillary sinuses clinically most significant in children < 6 years of age)	Mucopurulent nasal discharge	Nasal mucosa usually red, edematous
	Choking cough (↑ at night, occasionally productive of mucopurulent material)	Mucopurulent nasal discharge
	Older children may report postnasal drip and/or pain—frontal, temporal, retroorbital, or in upper incisors	May see mucopurulent discharge in midline of pharynx (postnasal drip)
Pharynx, tonsils	Dysphagia (in severe tonsillopharyngitis)	Pharynx red
	Older children may complain of sore throat; however, sore throat may also result from pain referred from the middle ear, parotid gland	Tonsils enlarged, red, with or without whitish or yellow exudates
		Petechiae on soft palate (suggesting streptococcal infection)
		Discrete ulcers on anterior tonsillar pillars or pharynx (suggesting enteroviral infection, herpangina)
		Anterior cervical lymph node enlargement (with or without tenderness)
Larynx (edema, spasm)	Normal chest configuration	Respiratory rate rarely over 60/min
	Hoarseness	Decreased breath sounds
	Barking ("croupy") cough	Supraclavicular and suprasternal retractions relatively more pronounced (compared to intercostal and subcostal retractions)
	Inspiratory stridor	
	Dysphagia, drooling (in epiglottitis)	
	May have signs of respiratory distress	
	Prolonged inspiratory phase	
Lower Airway Obstructions		
Trachea and bronchi (edema, mucus)	Deep ("hacking") cough	Rhonchi
	No signs of respiratory distress unless other areas of respiratory tract are also involved	Respiratory rate more rapid (over 60/min)
	Normal voice	
Bronchioles (edema, mucus, spasm)	Wheezing (expiratory whistling sound); may be absent in severe airway obstruction	Hyperresonance to percussion
		Decreased breath sounds
		Prolonged expiratory phase
	Hyperexpansion of chest, with increased anterior-posterior diameter and shallow respirations	Musical rales: sonorous sibilant
	May have signs of respiratory distress	Pronounced intercostal and subcostal retractions
Alveoli (exudate, edema, collapse)	May have signs of respiratory distress	Overinvolved lung, *may* have: dullness to percussion decreased breath sounds coarse and fine rales
Pleura	"Splinting" of chest	Overinvolved pleura, *may* have: dullness to percussion decreased breath sounds friction rub
	May have signs of respiratory distress	

Adapted from Chow, M.P., et al.: Handbook of pediatric primary care, New York, 1979, John Wiley & Sons, Inc., pp. 548-549; as reprinted with permission from Rowe, D.S.: Unpublished material, 1973.

drum with redness and obscured visualization of bony landmarks and light reflex (Bruch, 1979).

Management involves the use of antibiotics appropriate to the age and causative organism. Decongestants are frequently used in conjunction with antibiotic therapy. Follow-up for both serous and suppurative otitis media is essential. The status of the middle ear's response to treatment, as well as the hearing response, should be evaluated.

Allergies

Allergies pose a health problem for approximately 20% of the pediatric population. Though allergies can appear at any age, infants and children at ages 5, 10, and 15 appear to be more susceptible. Over 80% of these allergic children achieve symptom relief if intervention is instituted (Rapaport and Linde, 1970). For this reason nurses must be aware of the origin and symptoms of allergies as well as the appropriate treatment and preventive activities.

Causes

Allergy can be defined as a hypersensitivity to a substance or the environment, which ordinarily causes no response in other persons. When the offending substance (antigen) produces symptoms in an individual, it is designated an allergen. Allergens gain entry into the body through inhalation, ingestion, injection, or direct contact. A list of common allergy-producing substances is outlined in the following box. The degree of the body's response to the allergen is primarily dependent on the frequency and duration of exposure. Other factors such as state of health, age, and genetic predisposition also affect the allergic response. In addition, variables such as the season, weather, emotional state, and time of day appear to affect the intensity of the response.

Symptoms

The most common allergic manifestations in infancy are atopic dermatitis, gastrointestinal disturbances, and mild rhinorrhea. Foods are the most common allergies with milk the most frequent offending substance followed by eggs, orange juice, wheat, corn, and beef (Feingold, 1973).

In later childhood environmental substances are the leading cause of allergic conditions with symptoms developing more frequently in those with an infantile allergic history. Symptoms suggestive of allergies in older children include those previously described for infancy with the potential for development of the following (Feingold, 1973; Rapaport and Linde, 1970):

Tension-fatigue syndrome including listlessness, irritability, fatigue, facial pallor without anemia, cir-

Common Allergy-Producing Substances

Inhalants
Pollen
Mold
House dust
Animal dander
Fabric fiber
Feathers
Dyes
Chemicals

Injectants
Vaccines
Injected drugs
Animal serum
Animal saliva
Animal venom
Insect stings

Bacterial infectants

Ingestants
Food
  Cow's milk
  Eggs
  Wheat
  Chocolate
  Cola products
  Fish, pork, chicken, legumes
  Corn
  Citrus fruits, strawberries
Drugs
  Aspirin
  Antibiotics
  Barbiturates
Food additives

Contactants
Plants
Topical drugs
Resins
Metals
Cosmetics
Dyes
Chemicals

Other environmental factors
Sunshine
Temperature changes
Air pollution

From Tackett, J.J., and Hunsberger, M.: Family centered care of children and adolescents, Philadelphia, 1981, W.B. Saunders Co., p. 494.

Procedure for an Elimination Diet

The procedure is as follows:

1. A diary of each food, beverage, or medication that is ingested at meals or between meals without alteration in customary patterns is to be recorded for 7 to 10 days.
2. Constituents of all home-prepared foods must be listed as well as ingredients of all packaged foods. Concealed foods may be included in prepared products.
3. Symptoms are also recorded for 7 to 10 days. By correlating symptoms with the information in the diary, the nurse frequently can determine the elimination diet suitable for the particular case; for example, milk-free, salicylate-free, or others.
4. The elimination diet is initiated.
5. Two weeks following the start of an elimination diet, the client is interviewed, and the diet is reviewed. Improvement can be expected within 2 to 3 weeks if the correct food has been eliminated.
6. Two weeks later another interview and review are conducted.
7. If symptoms have not subsided, the program is abandoned, and another diet regimen is implemented.
8. If the diet is successful in eliminating symptoms it should be continued for at least 2 months before attempting additions of new foods to the diet.
9. New foods can then be added individually every 5 to 7 days.
10. If symptoms return, the food should be discontinued.
11. If the second attempt at introducing the food is not successful, the food should be permanently excluded from the diet.
12. This procedure is repeated with other foods, each one taken individually, until a well-balanced and varied diet is provided for the client.
13. The diet diary should be continued for a few months, if possible, in the event of a recurrence of symptoms.
14. All labels, especially of prepared foods, must be read carefully.
15. Home-prepared foods are preferable because the ingredients can be controlled.
16. Absolute adherence to the diet is imperative. If undesirable weight loss occurs, more of the prescribed carbohydrates, sugar, fats, and oils must be taken. This may require eating four to five meals a day.
17. Caution should be taken not to place a child on a nutritionally deficient diet for long periods of time when no specific results have been obtained.

From Chow, M.P., et al.: Handbook of pediatric primary care, New York; 1979, John Wiley & Sons, Inc., pp. 831-832.

---

cles of discoloration under the eyes ("allergic shiners")

Recurrent otitis or serous otitis media

Upper respiratory symptoms including:

Allergic salute—itching and rubbing of nose upward, which leads to a crease across the nose just above the tip

Excoriated nares and sometimes epistaxis

Rhinorrhea with seromucoid discharge

Postnasal mucoid discharge leading to a tickling, productive cough

Nasal congestion that causes mouth breathing and pursing of lips

Recurrent laryngitis

Lower respiratory tract problems including allergic bronchitis and bronchial asthma

Skin problems including urticaria and types of dermatitis

Assessment and Management

Assessment of the allergic condition requires a detailed history and complete physical examination. Of primary importance to the assessment is securing a detailed nutrition or diet history as well as information regarding family history. The probability of inheriting allergic problems based on familial incidence is 75% if both parents are allergic, 50% if one parent is allergic, and less than 10% if neither parent is allergic.

Management of allergies is dependent on the identified allergen source (see box on p. 543). Most frequently, for infants this management requires diet control. Such control in the form of an elimination diet is instituted when sufficient evidence from a history and physical examination warrants removing the suspected substance from the child's diet. The above box illustrates the procedure for instituting an elimination diet (Feingold, 1973).

Under circumstances in which environmental allergens are suspected, particularly with the home, desensitization or allergy-proofing measures can be implemented (Table 23-14), (Rapaport, 1970). Though it is virtually impossible to eliminate all allergens from a child's environment, avoidance of known offending substances and partial relief from exposure can benefit the allergic child.

Table 23-14. Home allergy-proofing techniques	
Potential antigen	**Proofing actions**
House dust (leading cause of respiratory allergy)	1. Restrict use of bedroom to sleeping. 2. Use shades instead of blinds or curtains. 3. Place washable plastic over mattresses. 4. Use no carpeting or wool scatter rugs. 5. Damp dust daily with child out of room. 6. Allow no stuffed animals or knickknacks. 7. Have minimum furniture; if stuffed, it should be foam rubber. 8. Either close off heat ducts or cover with cheesecloth. (Wash often.) 9. Keep doors and windows closed. 10. Avoid storing wool in closets or use of wool blankets.
Mold, mildew	1. Eliminate plants and aquariums from child's bedroom and play area; keep to minimum throughout home. 2. Avoid use of cellars as play or living area. 3. Clean bathroom and tile areas with antimold agent (Lysol) regularly. 4. Cleanse vaporizers or humidifiers frequently. 5. Use dehumidifier in humid or damp areas.
Danders, feathers	1. Use Dacron or foam rubber pillows and mattresses. 2. Get rid of pets or limit to outdoors. 3. Allow no stuffed animals or furniture and no clothing stuffed or insulated with feathers (down).
Contactants	1. Buy no wool clothing. 2. Wash all new clothing and linens before using. 3. Double-rinse infant's clothing and diapers. 4. Wash baby articles in mild soap. 5. Use mild soap to bathe baby and rinse well. 6. Avoid use of perfumed lotions, powders, oils.

From Tackett, J.J., and Hunsberger, M.: Family centered care of children and adolescents, Philadelphia, 1981, W.B. Saunders Co., p. 497.

Vomiting and Diarrhea

Another health problem of concern during infancy is the vomiting and diarrhea syndrome. The etiology of this illness, whether symptoms occur together or singularly, is varied (Table 23-15).

When assessing an infant for vomiting and diarrhea it is often necessary to verify the meaning of these terms with parents. Frequently vomiting, which is forceful, projectile, or nonprojectile retching of gastric contents, is confused with regurgitation, a common benign occurrence in the first year of life involving nonforceful, nonprojectile, effortless expulsion of gastric contents generally after feeding. Similarly, diarrhea is defined as watery, copious bowel movements that are usually green in color and have a foul odor, but the term is frequently misinterpreted by parents.

Management of vomiting and diarrhea is directed toward control of symptoms and prevention of dehydration. *Dehydration* is defined as the percentage of body weight lost as water. For example, a child who is 5% dehydrated has lost 50 ml of water for every kilogram of body weight. Though the majority of children with vomiting and/or diarrhea are less than 5% dehydrated, it is imperative that nurses be knowledgeable of the clinical signs of dehydration, which may include dry mucous membranes, reduction in tear formation, decreased urination, decreased skin turgor, and sunken eyes and fontanel.

Nursing Role

Nursing measures directed toward resolution of vomiting and diarrhea are primarily diet modifications. Clear liquids such as apple juice; flat, diluted ginger ale; Lytren; or Pedialyte are recommended for the first 24 hours. Liquids should be given in small amounts and frequently (1 to 2 oz every 30 to 60 minutes). If fluids are retained or diarrhea does not worsen and/or improves, solids such as rice cereal, applesauce, and bananas can be added to the diet. Generally medications such as sedatives, antiemetics, and antidiarrheals are not recommended for younger children, since they can mask the progression of vomiting and diar-

Table 23-15. Etiology of vomiting and diarrhea

Causes of diarrhea	Causes of vomiting
Nonbacterial, nonspecific, or viral	Chalasia
Dietary mismanagement	Intestinal obstruction
Symptom of other illnesses such as otitis media, urinary tract infection, meningitis (in infants)	Overfeeding
	Pyloric stenosis
Complication of antibiotic therapy (ampicillin, neomycin, tetracycline)	Gastroenteritis
	Meningitis
Bacterial such as *Salmonella, Shigella,* enteropathic *Escherichia coli*	Parasites
Malabsorption such as monosaccharide and disaccharide deficiencies, cystic fibrosis, celiac disease	Respiratory
	Septicemia
Milk allergy	Urinary tract
Food poisoning	Congenital adrenal hyperplasia
Chronic ulcerative colitis	Diabetic acidosis
Chronic giardiasis	Drugs such as digitalis, aspirin, some antibiotics, sulfonamides
Intestinal obstruction	Increased intracranial pressure

Adapted from American Academy of Pediatrics, Report of the Committee on Infectious Disease, 1982, ed. 19, Evanston, Ill., 1982, Red Book; Chow, M.P., et al.: Handbook of pediatric primary care, New York, 1979, John Wiley & Sons, Inc.; and Krugman, S., Ward, R., and Katz, S.L.; Infectious diseases of children, ed. 6, St. Louis, 1977, The C.V. Mosby Co.

rhea. In addition, these medications tend to make children drowsy and in this way decrease fluid intake because of induced sleep.

Nurses must also counsel and educate parents in monitoring of symptoms and their progression as well as assess parental knowledge and compliance with dietary management. Further education in techniques that reduce spread or severity is important, particularly in the home environment. Following the course of illness is essential as referral may be required if symptoms are not successfully abated by the management plan.

COMMON CONCERNS OR PROBLEMS

A common problem might be defined as a child's behavior, which elicits concern on the part of parents. Frequently parents have behavioral expectations of their children, which may be in regard to some physical or psychosocial aspects of their growth or development. When the infant or child does not demonstrate the expected behaviors, parents often respond in an emotional, anxious, or insecure manner. The child then reacts to the parents' response, creating additional stress in the family situation. For example, the mother of a 1-month-old infant expects the baby to feed every 4 hours and sleep through the night. When the infant wants to eat every 2 hours and is up three times a night, the mother becomes concerned, anxious, and maybe insecure about her mothering abilities. This response subsequently affects her ability to be relaxed and motherly toward her infant, and the infant responds by being more demanding. Table 23-16 outlines common childhood behaviors that normally occur yet may create parental concern.

Many factors contribute to the occurrence of common problems. Significant variables include the following:

Parental expectations of a child's behavior and of their own behavior as parents, which are frequently unrealistic

Lack of parenting experience and knowledge

Emotional impact of becoming a parent

Age, sex, and temperament of the child as it affects the parents and family

Too much concern and emphasis on the part of parents toward common problems.

The most frequently identified common concerns or problems of infancy include colic, feeding, sleeping and elimination patterns and behaviors, crying, gas, hiccups, teething, spoiling, weaning, and stranger or separation anxiety. Appendix J describes these problems and appropriate anticipatory guidance and management.

SAFETY AND ACCIDENT PREVENTION

Accidents are the most preventable cause of mortality and morbidity in infants and children. During the first year of life accidents are the sixth leading cause of death and become the leading cause after the first year.

Practice of age-appropriate safety measures can significantly reduce and prevent most accidents. Nursing

Table 23-16. Common childhood behaviors

Age (years)	Behaviors
1	Sucks thumb, smears stools, shakes bed, bangs and rocks, and masturbates
2	As above; has temper tantrums, tears books or wallpaper, tears bed apart, removes clothes, runs around, and has many demands before sleep
2½	Above behavior to a lesser degree; stutters and has disruptive aggressive attacks such as hitting and biting
3	Less of the above behaviors
3½	Again an increase in some of the above behaviors; spits, picks nose, bites fingernails, and whines
4	Runs away, kicks, spits, bites nails, grimaces, calls names, boasts, brags, uses silly language, has nightmares and fears, needs to urinate in moments of emotional distress, has ''belly'' pains and may vomit
5	A decrease in some behaviors, blinks eyes, shakes head, clears throat, and sniffles
5½ to 6	All the above behaviors and increased clumsiness
7	Tries to control behaviors and may have headaches
8	Picks at fingers, cries with fatigue, and makes faces
9	Stamps feet, fiddles, drops and breaks things, picks at self, growls and mutters

From Chow, M.P., et al.: Handbook of pediatric primary care, New York, 1979, John Wiley & Sons, Inc., p. 322.

in its emphasis on health promotion and supervision can have a significant impact on accident prevention. The counseling and education of parents on the developmental abilities and related safety measures needed to provide an accident-free environment are responsibilities that nursing must meet when delivering well-child care. Appendix J provides information regarding developmental abilities according to age, implications in terms of incidence of accidents, and appropriate nursing interventions.

TOOLS FOR ASSESSMENT

The nursing process involves the assessment, diagnosis, planning, implementation, and evaluation of the health needs of a patient. An accurate assessment through data collection is the basis for any further plan of intervention. The tools and techniques used for assessment vary depending on the child's age. However, basic methods provide nursing with a uniform and reliable approach to assessment of an individual child's health needs.

History

The history and subsequent assessment of the child and his family begin at the moment of contact through observation. This technique of data collection provides information regarding the physical as well as psychosocial, developmental, and interactional growth and development of the child and his family. A more formal interview should be directed toward gathering data relative to the child's immediate health status. Traditional information gathered in an initial pediatric health history is reviewed in Appendix A.

Physical Examination

Data collected from the physical assessment of a child serve as verification for information collected from observation and the history interview. For example, observation may reveal that a 6-year-old is limping; the history may reveal the child is complaining of pain in the right ankle after falling off his bicycle 1 day earlier. The physical examination verifies these data through findings of edema, bruising, and limited range of motion. Similarly, data collected during a health maintenance visit can verify the observation and history that a child is in good health.

Approaches in conducting a physical examination for a pediatric client are most important and must be adapted to the child's age and developmental level. Suggested approaches and sequence of conducting the physical examination according to age are summarized in Table 23-17.

Health Assessment

Combining the components of history taking and physical assessment with the elements of physical and psychosocial growth and development pertinent to a specific age results in a total health assessment. In pediatrics, health assessments are generally implemented at specific time intervals. In the first 6 years of life, health assessment visits for the normally developing child are generally recommended at the following ages: 2 to 4 weeks, 2, 4, 6, 9, 12, 15, 18, and 24 months, and annually until 6 years. Outlines for the content of these health visits are included in Appendix A. Health promotion activities for the specific age groups are discussed later in this chapter.

Recording of the data collected during health assess-

Table 23-17. Approach to the routine physical examination

Physical examination*	Approach
0 to 4 months	
1. Observe general appearance, body proportions, and development	Approach while asleep or quiet
2. Observe color and respirations	
3. Count respirations, auscultate heart, count apical pulse, auscultate chest	
4. Palpate anterior and posterior fontanels	Place infant in parent's arms
5. Measure head circumference	
6. Palpate the abdomen and femoral pulses	Give infant bottle; have infant supine on table or in mother's lap
7. Examine genitalia and rectum	
8. Examine eyes, ears, nose, mouth, and throat	Place infant in mother's arms or supine on table
9. Examine extremities	Observe and examine infant on table
10. Test central nervous system development — test primary reflexes	
4 to 12 months	
1. Observe general appearance, body proportions, and development	Place infant in parent's lap
	Distract infant with bottle, rattle, or toy
2. Observe color and respirations	
3. Auscultate heart and chest	Place infant in upright position first in parent's lap and lying down after this
4. Palpate anterior and posterior fontanels and measure head circumference	
5. Examine abdomen, genitalia, and rectum	In parent's lap
6. Examine eyes, ears, nose, mouth, and throat	
7. Test central nervous system development	
1 to 3 years	
1. Observe for general appearance, body proportions, and development	Allow child to play with familiar tools (e.g., tongue blade, flashlight, stethoscope, or toy)
2. Examine extremities and nervous system	Have child in parent's lap or walking in examining room
3. Examine neck	
4. Examine chest and heart	Allow child to have a security object and be in parent's lap or on examining table
5. Examine abdomen	
6. Examine genitalia and rectum	
7. Examine head, eyes, ears, nose, throat, and mouth	Use parent's and examiner's lap before using the examining table for examination of the abdomen and genitalia and, in some cases, eyes, ears, nose, throat, and mouth
3 to 6 years	
1. Evaluate nervous system development	Talk to the child
2. Examine head, neck, chest, heart, abdomen, extremities	Use flattery
3. Genitourinary and rectal last	Allow child to sit in parent's lap if so desired
	Use familiar instruments (e.g., stethoscope)
	Allow child to play with instruments
6 to 9 years	
1. Perform physical examination in orderly fashion with genitourinary and rectum last	Give patient choice whether parents should remain in room for examination
	Use flattery
	Ask child questions
	Familiarize patient with instruments
	Encourage cooperation
9 years to adolescence	
1. Perform physical examination in orderly fashion with genitourinary and rectum last	Give patient choice whether parents should remain in room for examination
	Ask patient questions
	Educate patient regarding body, instruments, and findings
	Encourage patient to ask questions or talk about himself and his activities

From Barnard, M.M., et al.: Handbook on comprehensive pediatric nursing, New York, 1981, McGraw-Hill Book Co., pp. 20-22; as adapted from Scipien, G.M., et al.: Comprehensive pediatric nursing, ed. 2, New York, 1979, McGraw-Hill Book Co., p. 25. Used with permission.
*Developmental assessment is done throughout entire history and physical examination and should be used first on physical examination for building rapport. Educate patient and/or parents regarding body, instruments, examination, and findings throughout physical.

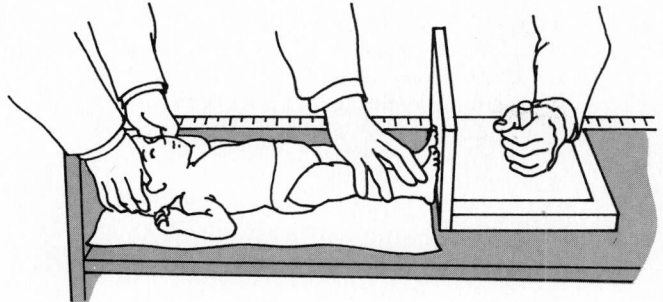

Fig. 23-3. Measurement of infant height. (From Maternal and Child Health Program: evaluation of body size and physical growth of children, Washington, D.C., 1976, Department of Health, Education and Welfare.)

ment visits is as vital as the assessment itself. The documentation of care through recording provides a means for review and evaluation. Consequently, using a tool that facilitates documentation and communication about a child's health status becomes essential to the provision of quality, comprehensive care.

In addition to the history and physical examination, other tools are useful in the monitoring, screening, and evaluation of the growth and development of children and are discussed in the following pages.

Monitoring Physical Growth and Development

Measurement of the child's height, weight, and head circumference is most important in the health assessment process because growth is a major characteristic of childhood. Since atypical patterns of growth are common indicators of pathology, these measurements should be made between five and six times in the first year and annually thereafter. Additionally, these measurements need to be recorded on a growth chart and compared to the norms for the child's age and his own previous growth pattern. Appendix K illustrates commonly used growth charts.

Accuracy and correct measuring techniques are basic to measurement usefulness as evaluators of growth. Height, as a measure of skeletal and muscular growth, is most accurately measured in the supine position for children until they are 2 to 3 years old, (Fig. 23-3). The appropriate technique requires two people. The top of the head must touch the headboard perpendicular to the table while the sliding footboard rests against the soles of the feet. Weight, as an indicator of general growth and nutritional status, is measured on an infant scale without clothing (except diaper) for children until they are approximately 2 years of age.

The head circumference is a particularly important measurement, especially in the first year of life when brain growth is most rapid. A nonstretchable measuring tape should be used for the calibration of head size and placed around the largest circumference of the head (around occiput and just above eyebrows).

Vital Signs

Vital sign measurement is another indicator of health status. Temperature readings, though not routinely done on health assessment visits, should be measured for every ill child. The choice of thermometer type depends on the child's age, but generally rectal or axillary measurements are done on children under 5 to 6 years with oral temperatures taken after this age. Regardless of the thermometer type, sufficient time for registering of the nonelectronic temperature must be allowed. In general, rectal temperatures require approximately 4 minutes to register, axillary 5 minutes, and oral 4 to 5 minutes. In addition, it is important to recognize the differences in temperature measurement according to method, and the method must be recorded. The normal oral temperature is 96° to 99° F (36° to 37° C), whereas rectal temperatures are generally 1° higher than oral, and axillary temperatures are 1° lower.

Pulse. The pulse rate directly reflects the heartbeat and is a means of evaluating the circulatory system. Pulse readings should be made at every visit whether the child is sick or well. Because an infant's pulse is so rapid, it is best felt in the femoral areas and auscultated for in the apical area.

Respiration. Observation and measurement of the respiratory rate should be done at every encounter. Resting or sleeping respiratory rate measurements are the most reliable. Palpating or auscultating the infant's chest makes counting easier; the count should be done for a full minute because of the infant's normally irregular breathing pattern.

Blood Pressure. Blood pressure is an indirect measure of pressure exerted against arterial walls during ventricular contraction and relaxation. Accurate measures of an infant's blood pressure are difficult to obtain. Current recommendations are to include measurement and recording of blood pressure at the health assess-

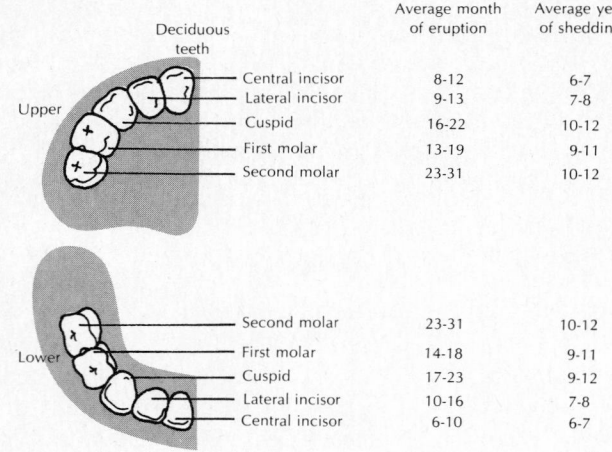

Deciduous teeth	Average month of eruption	Average year of shedding
Upper		
Central incisor	8-12	6-7
Lateral incisor	9-13	7-8
Cuspid	16-22	10-12
First molar	13-19	9-11
Second molar	23-31	10-12
Lower		
Second molar	23-31	10-12
First molar	14-18	9-11
Cuspid	17-23	9-12
Lateral incisor	10-16	7-8
Central incisor	6-10	6-7

Average ages at which children acquire and lose deciduous (primary) teeth.

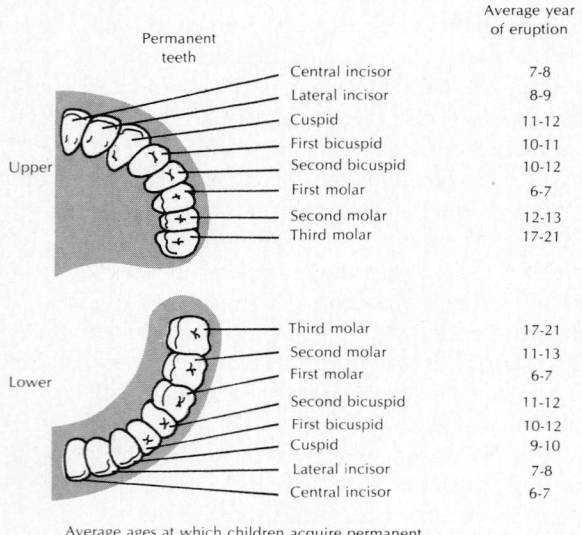

Permanent teeth	Average year of eruption
Upper	
Central incisor	7-8
Lateral incisor	8-9
Cuspid	11-12
First bicuspid	10-11
Second bicuspid	10-12
First molar	6-7
Second molar	12-13
Third molar	17-21
Lower	
Third molar	17-21
Second molar	11-13
First molar	6-7
Second bicuspid	11-12
First bicuspid	10-12
Cuspid	9-10
Lateral incisor	7-8
Central incisor	6-7

Average ages at which children acquire permanent (secondary) teeth.

Fig. 23-4. Ages of tooth eruption. (From Barnard, M.M., et al.: Handbook on comprehensive pediatric nursing, New York, 1981, McGraw-Hill Book Co., p. 57. Taken from materials distributed by the American Dental Association.)

such as diagnosis of a health problem and subsequent monitoring.

Dental Age

Dental age is assessed through knowledge of normal patterns of tooth eruption (Fig. 23-4). Most humans develop two sets of teeth in a lifetime. By knowing the approximate age of eruption and shedding of teeth, assessment of normal growth for age can be made. In general, an infant's primary (deciduous) teeth begin to erupt around 6 months, and this set is complete by 3 years of age. The primary teeth begin shedding around age 6 and are replaced by permanent teeth. This replacement process is usually completed by 18 to 25 years of age

Screening Tools

See Appendixes A and K for information on additional tools for screening physical growth and development.

Monitoring Psychosocial Development
Developmental Scales

Of the most useful tools available to nursing are those designed to assess psychosocial and/or developmental skills. Children generally follow similar patterns of development. Subsequently, developmental standards have been established based on studies of the age levels at which the average child masters various motor, language, adaptive, and social behaviors. The Waechter Developmental Guides provide comprehensive summaries of growth and development during infancy and should be a component of the essential knowledge base for nurses involved in pediatric care (Table 23-7).

Purpose of Screening Tests

Developmental and psychosocial screening tests are designed to assess how an individual child is developing compared to the average standard. These tests are a means for determining the need for intervention and perhaps more comprehensive evaluation. Screening tests used most frequently in pediatrics are selected primarily for their ease of administration, economic feasibility, and accuracy and reliability of results. Interpretation of their results requires recognition of the range of

ment visit after 3 years of age, unless otherwise indicated. The flush method of obtaining a blood pressure reading is generally used for children under 1 year.

Laboratory Studies

Further means for monitoring physical growth and development include the use of laboratory studies on blood and urine. These studies can be used for (1) monitoring of health status (i.e., hemoglobin, and hematocrit determinations in monitoring anemia); (2) screening for health problems (i.e., Sickledex to identify the presence of sickle-cell trait); or (3) diagnosis of health problems (i.e., Coombs to identify presence of abnormal antigen-antibody levels). In addition, data from laboratory studies may be used for multiple purposes normalcy, individual variations, and the variables present in the test situations. Some of the more popular and frequently used screening tests are discussed next.

Overview of Screening Tests

Denver Developmental Screening Test. The Denver Developmental Screening test (DDST) was developed to screen children from birth to 6 years for early detection of developmental lags (Appendix J). It can be used at one time or for periodic screening and assesses personal, social, fine motor, adaptive, language, and gross motor developmental skills and behavior (Frankenburg, et al., 1971).

Neonatal Perception Inventory. The Neonatal Perception Inventory (NPI) (Appendix K) was developed to determine a new mother's concept of what an average baby's behavior is like and what her assessment is of her own infant's behavior. It is primarily used to identify infants and mothers at risk for developing an unhealthy bond. The NPI is administered in two parts. Part I questionnaire is completed on the first or second day postpartum. Part II questionnaire is administered when the infant is 1 month of age (Broussard and Hartner, 1971).

Degree of Bother Inventory. The Degree of Bother Inventory is generally used in conjunction with Part II of the NPI (Appendix K). This inventory questionnaire is administered at 1 month of age and requires the mother to indicate to what degree the listed infant behaviors in her own baby are bothersome or create concern. The purpose of the tool is to identify and rank those behaviors that the mother finds particularly bothersome so that interventions may be initiated. The Degree of Bother Inventory is most useful for first-time mothers as is the NPI (Broussard and Hartner, 1971).

Carey Infant Temperament Scale. The Carey Infant Temperament Scale (CITS) is designed to obtain a profile of an infant's temperament. It is appropriate for use in infants 4 and 8 months of age and provides information useful in planning the child's well care and in initiating parental anticipatory guidance. The scale is a questionnaire completed by parents in areas such as feeding, sleep, elimination and play patterns as well as infant response to different stimuli (Carey, 1972).

Home Observation for Measurement of Environment. Home Observation for Measurement of Environment (HOME) is a unique tool using both clinical and home visit observations. It is designed to identify characteristics of the environment of children from birth to 3 years and from 3 to 6 years (Appendix B). HOME consists of an inventory for each age group. Each inventory scale identifies certain aspects of the quality and quantity of the social, emotional, and cognitive environments available to the child in his home.

This tool is particularly valuable to the community health nurse as a means of assessing environmental adequacy for development and for initiating interventions.

The inventory for newborns to 3-year-olds measures the following six subscales: emotional and verbal responsiveness to the mother, avoidance of restriction and punishment, organization of physical and temporal environment, provision of appropriate play materials, involvement of the mother with child, and opportunities for variety in daily stimulation. Inventory items for 3- to 6-year-olds measure the provision of stimulation through equipment, toys, and experience; stimulation of mature behavior; provision of physical and language stimulation; avoidance of restriction and punishment; provision of pride, affection, and thoughtfulness, masculine stimulation; and independence from parental control (Caldwell, 1976).

IMMUNIZATIONS

Immunity is defined as the body's resistance to the effects of harmful agents. The protection of immunity can be received through active or passive means. (See Chapter 12 for a discussion of active or passive immunity.)

Active artificial immunization is initiated for infants and children to protect them against the once common and dangerous infectious diseases such as measles, mumps, rubella, tetanus, diphtheria, and pertussis. The neonate enjoys a relatively short period (first few weeks to 2 months) of natural passive immunity as a result of placental transfer of maternal antibodies. However, this protection is only against those diseases for which the mother has developed sufficient antibodies, and it is temporary. The young infant then becomes rapidly at risk for infection because of the short-term passive immunity of his own poorly developed and immature immune system. In normal infants the immune system is capable of responding with adequate antibody production by 2 months of age. This is generally the recommended age to begin artificial immunizations.

Active immunization is conferred through two basic types of agents. Antibody production for tetanus and diphtheria is stimulated through the use of a toxoid, which is a bacterial toxin that has been heated or chemically treated to decrease the virulence but not the antibody-producing ability. The use of vaccines, a suspension of attenuated or killed microorganisms, provides an active immunity response for pertussis (a killed bacteria), measles, mumps, rubella, and polio (i.e., Sabin and Salk vaccines, attenuated and killed viruses, respectively). Appendix E provides information regard-

Table 23-18. Recommended immunization schedules for infants and children not initially immunized at usual recommended times in early infancy

Timing	Recommended schedules				Comments
	Preferred schedule	Alternatives*			
		1	2	3	
First visit	DTP[†] 1, OPV[‡] 1, Tuberculin test (PPD)[§]	MMR,[‖] PPD	DTP 1, OPV 1, PPD	DTP 1, OPV 1, MMR, PPD	MMR should be given no younger than 15 months old
1 month after first visit	MMR	DTP 1, OPV 1	MMR, DTP 2	DTP 3,	
2 months after first visit	DTP 2, OPV 2	—	DTP 3, OPV 2	DTP 3, OPV 2	—
3 months after first visit	(DTP 3)	DTP 2, OPV 2	—	—	In preferred schedule, DTP 3 can be given if OPV 3 is not to be given until 10 to 16 months
4 months after first visit	DTP 3 (OPV 3)	—	(OPV 3)	(OPV 3)	OPV 3 optional for areas for likely importation of polio (e.g., some southwestern states)
5 months after first visit	—	DTP 3 (OPV 3)	—	—	
10 to 16 months after last dose	DTP 4, OPV 3 or OPV 4	DTP 4, OPV 3 or OPV 4	DTP 4, OPV 3 or OPV 4	DTP 4, OPV 3 or OPV 4	—
Preschool	DTP 5, OPV 4 or OPV 5	DTP 5, OPV 4 or OPV 5	DTP 5, OPV 4 or OPV 5	DTP 5, OPV 4 or OPV 5	Preschool dose not necessary if DTP 4 or 5 given after fourth birthday
14 to 16 years old	Td[¶]	Td	Td	Td	Repeat every 10 years

From American Academy of Pediatrics: Report of the Committee on Infectious Diseases, ed. 19, Evanston, Ill., 1982, The AAP, pp. 18-19. Copyright American Academy of Pediatrics, 1982.

* Alternative 1 can be used in those more than 15 months old if measles is occurring in the community.
Alternative 2 allows for more rapid DTP immunization.
Alternative 3 should be reserved for those whose access to medical care is compromised by poor compliance.
[†] DTP, Diphtheria and tetanus toxoids with pertussis vaccine.
[‡] OPV, Oral, attenuated poliovirus vaccine contains types 1, 2, and 3.
[§] Tuberculin test, Mantoux (intradermal PPD) preferred. Frequency of tests depends on local epidemiology. The Committee recommends annual or biennial testing unless local circumstances dictate less frequent or no testing.
[‖] MMR, Live measles, mumps, and rubella viruses in a combined vaccine.
[¶] Td, Adult tetanus toxoid (full dose) and diphtheria toxoid (reduced dose) in combination.
NOTE: For all products used, consult manufacturer's brochure for instructions for storage, handling, and administration. Biologics prepared by different manufacturers may vary, and those of the same manufacturer may change from time to time. The package insert should be followed for a specific product.

ing the basic immunization agents and their administration schedule in pediatrics.

The interval between immunizations is important to the immunity response. After the first injection, antibodies are produced slowly and in small concentrations (primary response). However, the antibody-producing mechanism has been altered in response to this first injection so that subsequent injections with the same antigen are recognized by the body. Once this recognition occurs, antibodies are produced much faster and in higher concentration (secondary response). Because of this secondary response, once an initial immunization series has been started, *it does not need to be restarted if interrupted, regardless of the length of time elapsed.*

Once the initial series is completed, boosters are required at the appropriate time intervals to maintain an adequate concentration level of antibodies.

Occasionally, children are encountered who have received no immunizations. The immunization schedule for these children is listed in Table 23-18. However, if compliance with this schedule and follow-up care are doubtful, it is valid to simultaneously administer diphtheria, tetanus, pertussis (DPT) or tetanus, diphtheria, (Td) if the child is over 6 years of age, trivalent oral polio virus vaccine (TOPV), measles, mumps and rubella (MMR), and tuberculin test (PPD [Mantoux]).

Contraindications

Contraindications for the administration of immunizations are relatively few. Vaccines should not be administered to children with acute febrile illness or to those who have had severe reactions to the previous dose. Minor illnesses or infections are not contraindications for administration. Specific circumstances for nonadministration of a particular agent are listed in Appendix E. In addition, those with the following conditions are not routinely immunized and require medical consultation before the agent is administered, especially the live virus vaccines: pregnant women, persons with a generalized malignancy, those on immunosuppressive therapy or with immunodeficiency disease, persons with marked sensitivity to eggs or chicken, or persons who have had recent immune serum globulin or plasma or blood administration, (a wait of 3 months is advised).

Parent Education

An important component of implementing an immunization program is parental preparation and education regarding the program, what responses or reactions to expect, and how to manage these common reactions. Although much discussion has occurred over these issues, parents should be informed of the risks and benefits of each immunizing agent in addition to the common side effects. Appendix E discusses potential reactions to specific immunizations and appropriate treatment measures that parents can institute to minimize discomfort.

NUTRITION

One of the most important components of maintaining a child's health is the promotion of good nutrition and dietary habits. The quality and quantity of nutrition influence the growth and development of a child. Nursing's role involves the use of a sound knowledge base to promote and assist parents in implementing nutritional adequacy for the child.

Basics

Proteins, fats, carbohydrates, vitamins, and minerals are the essential ingredients of a basic diet. These elements must be combined in sufficient quantities to meet the energy or caloric needs of a child, and quantities vary according to age and individual differences. In addition, water requirements must be balanced with the energy produced or the calories metabolized.

Nurses find it useful to be familiar with the terminology of nutrition. A nutrient's *requirement* is the least amount of the specific nutrient that promotes optimum health (Fomon, 1974). Requirements are expressed in minimum terms, and their values are estimated. Therefore they are not used as recommended intakes because variables such as race, age, and socioeconomic status make their estimates uncertain for all circumstances.

The recommended daily allowances (RDAs) are values of levels of intake of essential nutrients considered by the Food and Nutrition Board of the National Academy of Sciences, National Research Council, to be adequate to meet the nutritional needs of almost every person (Table 23-19). The estimates are intended for general use as based on the needs of average individuals expending average amounts of energy. These advisable intakes are generally higher than the actual requirement and represent a safe amount of nutrients.

Factors Influencing Nutrition

As with every aspect of human behavior, nutritional habits that affect nutritional states of health are influenced by a wide variety of variables, which are derived from parents as well as the child. Though some habits may be changed, others have to be accepted and accounted for when nursing implements a sound nutrition program. Among the parental factors most influential to food preferences and eating patterns are the ethnic, racial, cultural, and socioeconomic variables. How and what parents eat and their attitude toward nutrition are invariably passed on to their child. The child also brings individual variables to the nutritional situation (i.e., a slow eater, a picky eater, periods of disinterest, development of preferences, presence of food allergy, and alterations in eating patterns during periods of growth).

No one diet is effective for all children or even for one age group. Nurses must accept and be knowledgeable about individual styles, methods, and approaches to child nutrition to assist parents in providing the appropriate nutrients for their child.

Types of Infant Feeding

Supplying essential nutrients to an infant is done primarily through breast- and/or bottle-feeding. The method of feeding is a choice that must be made by

	Age	**Weight**		**Height**		**Energy needs**	
Category	years	kg	lb	cm	in	kcal	with range
Infants	½	6	13	60	24	kg × 115	(95-145)
	½-1	9	20	71	28	kg × 105	(80-135)
Children	1-3	13	29	90	35	1300	(900-1800)
	4-6	20	44	112	44	1700	(1300-2300)
	7-10	28	62	132	52	2400	(1650-3300)
Males	11-14	45	99	157	62	2700	(2000-3700)
	15-18	66	145	176	69	2800	(2100-3900)
	10-22	70	154	177	70	2900	(2500-3300)
Females	11-14	46	101	157	62	2200	(1500-3000)
	15-18	55	120	163	64	2100	(1200-3000)
	19-22	55	120	163	64	2100	(1700-2500)
Pregnancy						+300	
Lactation						+500	

Table 23-19. Mean heights and weights and recommended energy intake

From Tackett, J.J., and Hunsberger, M.: Family centered care of children and adolescents, Philadelphia, 1981, W.B. Saunders Co.; as adapted from Food and Nutrition Board, National Research Council: Recommended dietary allowances, ed. 9, Washington, D.C., 1980, National Academy of Sciences.

parents with guidance and without pressure. The advantages and disadvantages of both methods should be discussed with parents prenatally, and the differences between the basic forms of milk should be reviewed. In addition, parents should also be aware of the need for vitamin and mineral supplementation as well as current recommendations on infant nutrition methods.

With the first choice of whether to breast-feed or bottle-feed, nurses can offer counsel to parents. In addition to providing nutritional facts, nursing must be prepared to instruct, encourage, reassure, and support parents in the method of their choice. For breast-feeding, this means helping the mother establish a successful routine by discussing comfortable positioning, appropriate techniques, feeding frequency, the let-down reflex, care of breasts, and length of feedings. In addition, assessing the mother's feelings about nursing her infant and providing support and encouragement are important in allaying anxieties regarding the adequacy and effectiveness of her chosen method.

For bottle-feeding, parents require instruction regarding preparation and care of the equipment and formula, positioning of the person feeding as well as the infant and bottle, in addition to the factors of frequency, length, and feelings about the method of feeding. When solids are introduced, nurses need to provide guidance regarding the types, amount, frequency, and progression of foods offered. In addition, nurses must be aware that parents can become overly concerned about their child's eating habits when the child does not meet parental expectations. Overfeeding or underfeeding can

ensue, and the nurse can prevent such feeding difficulties by being aware of these attitudes and expectations and of parental nutritional knowledge in general. Appendix J provides suggestions for anticipatory guidance for common feeding problems.

Currently there is a trend for the new mother to breast-feed her infant. Breast milk is recommended by many health professionals as the preferred method of feeding an infant in the first 6 months of life. Recent studies document the nutritional efficacy and soundness of breast-feeding. However, some supplementation is necessary. For the infant who is solely breast-fed, the following need to be supplemented (Fomon, 1974):

1. Vitamin D. Although breast milk contains adequate amounts of vitamins A and B complex, there is an inadequate amount of vitamin D to meet the 400 IU/day RDA. Additionally, vitamin C in human milk is adequate, provided that the maternal diet contains sufficient vitamin C.

2. Iron supplementation. The normal birth weight infant has sufficient iron stores until 4 to 6 months of age, at which time body stores must be supplied. Breast milk contains adequate amounts of absorbable iron to meet requirements. An infant who is exclusively breast-fed does not require exogenous sources of iron unless breast-feeding is discontinued before 6 months. Use of iron-fortified cereals and formula is recommended in this circumstance. (See Table 23-20 for a listing of the iron content of selected foods.)

3. Fluoride. Breast milk contains inadequate

Table 23-20. Iron content of selected foods fed to infants in the United States

Food	Elemental iron	
	mg/100 g of food	mg/100 kcal
Milk or formula		
Human milk	0.05	0.07
Cow milk	0.05	0.07
Iron-fortified formula	0.9-1.3	1.2-1.8
Formula unfortified with iron	<0.05	<0.05
Infant cereals		
Iron-fortified (dry) mixed with milk*	7-14	7-14
Wet-packed cereal-fruit	1-6	1.3-7.5
Strained and junior foods		
Meats		
Liver and a few others	4-6	4-6
Most meats	1-2	1-2
Egg yolks	2-3	1.0-1.5
"Dinners"		
High meat	<1	<1.
Vegetable-meat	<0.5	<0.5
Vegetables[†]	<0.5	<0.5
Fruits[†]	<0.5	<0.5

From Fomon, S.J.: Infant nutrition, ed. 2, Philadelphia, 1974, W.B. Saunders Co., p. 314.

* Assuming that one part by weight of dry cereal is mixed with six parts of milk.

[†] A few varieties of vegetables and fruits provide 1 to 2 mg of iron/100 g (1 to 3 mg/100 kcal).

amounts of fluoride, and supplementation is recommended.

Milks other than human milk have been used successfully for infant feeding. Commercially prepared formulas are most popular because they are convenient, contain standard ingredients, and are fortified with vitamins and minerals, negating the need for supplements. However, a formula prepared at home with evaporated or condensed milk or use of forms of cow's milk requires supplementation, generally of vitamins A, D, and C, fluoride, and iron (Fomon, 1974). Additionally, skim, lowfat, or 2% milk is not recommended for infants under 1 year of age because of insufficient fat and caloric contents.

Advanced Feeding

Infants receiving breast milk or formula with the appropriate supplementation do not require additional foods before 6 months of age. There are no nutritional, developmental, or psychological advantages to starting infants on solids before this time. However, the trend toward early introduction of solids does exist, and changing this trend does not occur easily. Nurses can make a significant contribution to the nutritional adequacy of infants and children primarily through parental education and support. This requires being up to date on current nutritional findings and also being accepting of parents who for a variety of reasons wish to implement early introduction of solids. Providing parents with sound factual information regarding the best nutrition for their child is the basis for nursing education and ideally for parental decisions.

Development of Feeding Behavior

Feeding behaviors are the outcome of motor development. For example, an infant's ability to swallow solid food is dependent on his fine oral motor skills; an older infant cannot feed himself until he has achieved fine and gross motor skills of the upper body. Consequently, from a developmental perspective, infants are not physically able to handle solid food consumption until 5 to 6 months of age. Correlating developmental abilities as they relate to feeding behaviors and subsequent readiness for solid foods may help parents decide when to introduce solids. Table 23-21 provides information regarding the developmental sequence of feeding behaviors.

Nutritional Considerations

Other factors should be considered by parents when making decisions regarding solid food introduction. One such factor is the way calories are distributed in solids versus human milk or formula. Generally solid baby foods are high in carbohydrates, moderate in protein, and low in fat, whereas human milk or formula is high in fat and carbohydrates and lower in protein. When infants are fed solids and also switched to whole, 2%, or low-fat cow's milk, the diet becomes excessively high in protein, sodium, and other solutes. Since the infant cannot excrete these large solutes efficiently unless large amounts of body fluid are used, this type of diet is hazardous for the infant. Hence, breast-feeding is physiologically and nutritionally sounder than other feeding methods.

Parents should know the diversity of composition and nutritional quality of commercially prepared infant foods. Reading labels carefully and evaluating brands as to their nutritional content are important ar-

Table 23-21. Development of feeding skills

Age	Oral and neuromuscular development	Feeding behavior
Birth	Rooting reflex	Turns mouth toward nipple or any object brushing cheek
	Sucking reflex	
	Swallowing reflex	Initial swallowing involves the posterior of the tongue; by 9-12 weeks anterior portion is increasingly involved, which facilitates ingestion of semisolid food
	Extrusion reflex	Pushes food out when placed on tongue; strong the first 9 weeks.
		By 6-10 weeks recognizies the feeding position and begins mouthing and sucking when placed in this position
3-6 months	Beginning coordination between eyes and body movements	Explores world with eyes, fingers, hands, and mouth; starts reaching for objects at 4 months but overshoots; hands get in the way during feeding
	Learning to reach mouth with hands at 4 months	Finger sucking—by 6 months all objects go into the mouth
	Extrusion reflex present until 4 months	May continue to push out food placed on tongue
	Able to grasp objects voluntarily at 5 months	Grasps objects in mittenlike fashion
	Sucking reflex becomes voluntary, and lateral motions of the jaw begin	Can approximate lips to rim of cup by 5 months; chewing action begins; by 6 months begins drinking from cup
6-12 months	Eyes and hands working together	Brings hand to mouth; at 7 months able to feed himself biscuit
	Sits erect with support at 6 months	Bangs cup and objects on table at 7 months
	Sits erect without support at 9 months	
	Development of grasp (finger to thumb oppostion)	Holds own bottle at 9-12 months
		Pincer approach to food
		Pokes at food with index finger at 10 months
	Relates to objects at 10 months	Reaches for food and utensils including those beyond reach; pushes plate around with spoon
		Insists on holding spoon not to put in mouth but to return to plate or cup
1-3 years	Development of manual dexterity	Increased desire to feed himself
		15 months—begins to use spoon but turns it before reaching mouth; may hold cup, likely to tilt cup rather than head, causing spilling
		18 months—eats with spoon, spills frequently, turns spoon in mouth; holds glass with both hands
		2 years—inserts spoon correctly, occasionally with one hand; holds glass; plays with food; distinguishes between food and inedible materials
		2-3 years—self-feeding complete with occasional spilling; uses fork; pours from pitcher; obtains drink of water from faucet

From Scipien, G.M., et al.: Comprehensive pediatric nursing, ed. 2, New York, 1979, McGraw-Hill Book Co., p. 163. Used with permission.

eas of parent learning. Parents also need to know that the cost per unit of calories is considerably higher for commercially prepared foods than formula. In addition, the incidence of constipation in infants is greater when solid food intake is high, and the introduction of solids too early may possibly lead to overfeeding and later overeating. Finally, a greater possibility of food allergy exists for infants when solids are introduced too early as the foreign proteins in foods become antigens because of insufficient IgA production until after the age of 6 months.

Once parents have made the decision to start solid foods, nurses can assist them in developing a program for introducing appropriate foods in sensible amounts and in the best sequence. For example, it is not nutritionally sound to give an infant eggs as the first solid food, primarily because of difficulties in digesting and a high incidence of allergy to the egg protein. Dry cereal fortified with iron is a more appropriate starter food because of the ease of digestion and iron fortification (at a time when newborn iron reserves are low). Table 23–22 provides guidelines for feeding infants birth to 1 year.

Nutrition for the Preterm or Low Birth Weight Infant

The low birth weight or preterm infant requires a special plan for nutrition. Basically these infants require increased calories, protein, vitamins, and minerals for growth. Though able to absorb protein and carbohydrates efficiently, preterm infants absorb fat poorly and readily lose fat-soluble vitamins and calcium through fecal fat loss. In addition, iron stores are depleted much earlier than they are in full-term infants, and stores of vitamin E and folic acid are deficient in the first 3 months of life (Committee on Nutrition, 1977).

Because of these nutritional deficiencies and added requirements, the feeding of a low birth weight infant must be managed very closely. This infant requires approximately 110 to 150 calories/kg/day with vitamins A, C, D, and B group supplementation. Calcium needs to be supplemented as well as iron. Additional vitamin E and folic acid are required in the first 3 months of life.

Promoting Good Eating Habits

The first 5 years of life are most important in developing sound eating habits in children. Many nursing activities to assist parents in choosing the most nutritionally sound methods of feeding their children have been discussed. However, an additional activity is initiating the diet history.

Soliciting a diet or nutritional history from parents is one of the most useful tools nurses have. A diet assessment provides information regarding the adequacy of the diet and facilitates identification of areas of parental concern. Such an assessment should take place at every well-child visit, and the data obtained should be used in conjunction with current nutritional information to educate and guide parents in providing a well-balanced diet for their infant or child (Appendix A).

HEALTH PROMOTION ACTIVITIES

Health is a state each of us wishes to experience, and some take for granted. However, it is not a guaranteed commodity but rather one that must be achieved and maintained. A person must be able to demonstrate behaviors that assist him in adapting in a healthy manner to his individual life circumstance. Promotion of health is evident in a person when he is able to identify and accept realities, adjust to changes in his environ-

ment, maintain a wholesome attitude toward himself and life, and assume responsibility for managing his own health as appropriate for his age and development.

Nursing Role

The role of nursing is to facilitate and support individuals in endeavors for health. Nurses can provide the means and specific activities that promote and maintain an individual's health. This interaction with nursing is especially important for children, who are dependent on others for health. Through objectives that promote health motivation and assist family members in using their own resources in identifying health needs and assuming responsibility for their own care, nurses can assist parents in learning and adapting health promotion behaviors that positively affect the health of their children.

Health Assessment Visits

Many of health promotion activities have been discussed throughout this chapter. Of singular importance, however, are the well-child or health maintenance visits. Through these encounters nurses can assess, guide, counsel, and teach parents the basics of child health care.

The specific components of the health assessment visits include (1) gathering of health history information pertinent to the age and needs of the child; (2) collecting physical assessment data pertinent to the history; (3) developing a plan to meet health needs and to promote health in collaboration with parents; (4) implementing the plan of action; and (5) evaluating the plan through follow-up. Of utmost importance to the success of a health assessment and promotion visit is collaboration with the parents and/or child. Their involvement throughout the process is essential for compliance and can be achieved by active listening; soliciting parental thoughts, feelings, and opinions; verifying parental knowledge; and promoting parental participation. Appropriate health assessment tools are included in the Appendix.

Group Education and Home Intervention

To provide and promote health for their children, parents require guidance and counseling. The health assessment encounter is only one setting in which this educational counseling can occur. Parent groups and home encounters are additional ways in which community health nurses can facilitate health.

Group health education is a popular, effective, and time-efficient means of health promotion. Parenting groups often focus on a specific age, developmental stage, or health problem. However, before program de-

Table 23-22. Feeding guidelines for infants

	0-2 wk	2 wk-2 mo	2 mo	3 mo	4-5 mo	5-6 mo
During the first 6 months*						
Formula						
Per feeding	2-3 oz	3-5 oz	5 oz	6-6½ oz	7-8 oz	7-8 oz
Average total	22 oz	28 oz	30 oz	32-34 oz	32 oz	28 oz
Number of feedings	6-8	5-6	5-6	5	4-5	4-5
Food texture	Liquids	Liquids	Liquids	Liquids	Baby soft	Baby soft
Food additions						
Apple juice†						3-4 oz
Baby cereal, enriched					2-2½ tb. B and S	3 tb. B and S
Strained fruits					1½-3 tb. B, L, and S	2-3 tb. B, L, and S
Strained vegetables					1-2 tb. L	2-3 tb. L
Strained meats						1-2 tb. L
Egg yolk or baby egg yolk						½ med or 1 tb.
Teething biscuit						½-1
Total calories	440	560	600	660-680	729-788	791-870
Recommended calories 117 cal/kg	410	410-608	608	667	725-784	784-878
Oral and neuromuscular development related to food intake	Rooting, sucking, swallowing	Rooting, sucking, swallowing	Rooting, sucking, swallowing	Extrusion reflex diminishes; sucking becomes voluntary	Learning to put hands to mouth; develops grasp	Chewing begins; can approximate lips to rim of cup

From Scipien, G.M., et al.: Comprehensive Pediatric Nursing, ed. 2, New York, 1979, McGraw-Hill Book Co., p. 162. Used with permission.
*Calculations based on male growing at the 50th percentile for height and weight.
†Offer small amounts (2-4 oz) when milk is presented from the cup.
NOTE: B, breakfast; L, lunch; S, supper.

	6-7 mo	7-8 mo	8-9 mo	9-10 mo	10-11 mo	11-12 mo
For infants 6 to 12 months of age						
Formula						
Per feeding	8 oz†	8 oz	8 oz	8 oz	8 oz	8 oz
Average total	28 oz	28 oz	24 oz	24 oz	24 oz	24 oz
Number of feedings	3-4	3-4	3	3	3	3
Food texture	Gradual increase ———————		Mashed at table ———————			Cut fine
Food items						
Orange juice	4 oz	4 oz	4 oz	4 oz	4 oz	4 oz
Fortified cereal	⅓ cup, B	⅓ cup, B	½ cup, B	½ cup, B	½ cup, B	½ cup, B
Fruit, canned or fresh	4 tsp. B, L, and S	4 tsp. B, L, and S	2 tb. L and S	2 tb. L and S	3 tb. L and S	3 tb. L and S
Vegetables	1½ tb. L and S	2 tb. L and S	2 tb. L and S	2 tb. L and S	3 tb. L and S	3 tb. L and S
Meat, fish, poultry	1 tb. L and S	2 tb. L and S	2 tb. L and S	2 tb. L and S	2½ tb. L and S	2½ tb. L and S
Egg yolk or baby egg yolk	1 med yolk, or 2 tb.	1 med yolk, or 2 tb.	1 med yolk, or 2 tb.	1 whole egg	1 whole egg	1 whole egg
Teething biscuit or bread	1 biscuit	1 biscuit	½ slice bread	½ slice bread	½ slice bread	½ slice bread
Starch — potato, rice macaroni			2 tb, S	2 tb, S	2 tb, S
Dessert — custard, pudding						2 tb, S
Butter			1 tsp	1 tsp	1 tsp	1 tsp
Total calories	859	876	937	974	1037	1069
Recommended calories (108 kcal/kg)	810-864	864-918	918-972	972-1015	1015-1048	1048-1083
Oral and neuromuscular development related to food intake	Begins using cup ———————————————————					
		Sits erect with support ———————		Without support———————		
		Feeds himself biscuit ———————				
				Holds bottle	Picks up small food items and releases	Holds and licks spoon after dipped into food; self-feeding

velopment, as discussed in Chapter 9, nurses must assess the learning needs of clients and avoid duplication of current classes or health education resources already available in the community. (See Chapters 8 and 9 for a detailed discussion of program planning for health education.)

Intervention in the home should be based on the health needs of the client and directed toward health promotion. The reasons for initiating a home visit vary. It may be prompted by the birth of a premature infant or may be the result of follow-up needed for a major health problem such as congenital heart disease. Regardless of the originating cause, being in the client's home provides an opportunity for the nurse to assess and teach, using the resources of the client's environment. In addition, observational data gathered while in the client's home provide insights that can greatly influence the overall assessment of the client's health status.

Other Activities

Parental knowledge and understanding of child growth and development are means to ensure child health. To promote this healthy view of children, the development of reading bibliographies for parents is a useful resource. Such readings can focus on a specific age (eg., toddlers) or a specific problem (e.g., the allergic child) These resources can include materials related to parenting approaches or coping with the responsibilities of being a parent. When developing such bibliographies, they should be kept short, be specific to an age or problem, and consist of accurate, pleasant, and easy-to-read material.

Community Resources

Promoting the health of children is largely dependent on the use of available community resources. To identify resources for a specific area or region, nurses should consider the following potential services or interest groups:

Children's services centers or clinics
Well-child clinics
Woman-infant-child programs
Immunization clinics
Communicable disease clinics
Crippled children's services
Child abuse centers or councils
School heatlh programs
Project Grow
Head Start
Parents Anonymous
Youth services bureaus
Crisis or hotlines for parents and/or children
Parent discussion groups

Adult education groups on aspects of parenting (e.g., infant care, coping)
Child development classes
Infant/child stimulation classes
Prepared childbirth and classes or groups on raising children
Local community advocate groups (e.g., single parents,
Working mothers, nursing mothers)
Day care nurseries

BIBLIOGRAPHY

Ainsworth, M.D.S.: Object relations, dependency, and attachment: a theoretical review of the infant-mother relationship, Child Dev. **40**:969-1026, Dec. 1969.

Alexander, M.M., and Brown, M.S.: Pediatric history taking and physical diagnosis for nurses, ed. 2, New York, 1979, McGraw-Hill Book Co.

American Academy of Pediatrics: Report of the Committee on Infectious Diseases, ed. 19, Evanston, Ill., 1982, The AAP.

American Dental Association: Your child's teeth, Chicago, 1971, The Association.

Apgar, V.: The newborn (Apgar) scoring system, Pediatr. Clin. North Am. **13**:645-650, 1966.

Barnard, M.M., et al.: Handbook on comprehensive pediatric nursing, New York, 1981, McGraw-Hill Book Co.

Bergman, A.B.: Sudden infant death, Nurs. Outlook **20**:775-777, Dec. 1972.

Berman, A.B.: Sudden infant death syndrome: an approach to management, Primary Care **3**:1-18, March 1976.

Bowlby, J.: Attachment and loss, vol. 1, Attachment, New York, 1969, Basic Books, Inc., Publishers.

Broussard, E.R., and Hartner, M.S.: Further considerations regarding maternal perception of the firstborn. In Hellmuth, J., Jr., editor: Exceptional infant: studies in abnormalities, vol. 2, New York, 1971, Brunner/Mazel, Inc.

Brown, M.S., and Murphy, M.A.: Ambulatory pediatrics for nurses, New York, 1975, McGraw-Hill Book Co.

Bruch, W.M.: Otitis media, Pediatr. Nurs. **5**:9-14, Jan.-Feb. 1979.

Bureau of Maternal and Child Health and Nutrition: Diet history questionnaire, Washington, D.C., 1978, U.S. Department of Health, Education and Welfare.

Caldwell, B.: Home observations for measurement of the environment, Little Rock, 1976, University of Arkansas Center for Child Development and Education.

Carey, W.B.: Clinical application of infant temperament measurements, J. Pediatr. **81**:823-828, Oct. 1972.

Chinn, P.: Child health maintenance: concepts in family centered care, St. Louis, 1979, The C.V. Mosby Co.

Chow, M.P., et al.: Handbook of pediatric primary care, New York, 1979, John Wiley & Sons Inc.

Clark, A.L. and Affonso, D.D.: Childbearing: a nursing perspective, ed. 2, Philadelphia, 1979, F.A. Davis Co.

Committee on Nutrition, American Academy of Pediatrics: Nutritional needs of low birth weight infants, Pediatrics **60**:519-527, Oct. 1977.

Conway, B.L.: Pediatric neurological nursing, Philadelphia, 1977, The C.V. Mosby Co.

Curtis, J.: Working mothers, New York, 1976, Simon & Schuster, Inc.

DeAngelis, C.: Pediatric primary care, ed. 2, Boston, 1979, Little, Brown & Co.

Dietrich, H.F.: Accident prevention in childhood is your problem too, Pediatr. Clin. North Am. **1**:759-769, 1954.

Dubowitz, L., Dubowitz, V., and Goldberg, C.: Clinical assessment of gestational age in the newborn infant, J. Pediatr. **77**:1-10, July 1970.

Duvall, E.: Marriage and family development, Philadelphia, 1977, J.B. Lippincott Co.

Erickson, M.L.: Assessment and management of developmental changes in children, St. Louis, 1976, The C. V. Mosby Co.

Erikson, E. Childhood and society, New York, 1963, Jeffrey Norton Publishers, Inc.

Feingold, B.F.: Introduction to clinical allergy, Springfield, Ill., 1973, Charles C Thomas, Publisher.

Fomon, S.J.: Infant nutrition, ed. 2, Philadelphia, 1974, W.B. Saunders, Co.

Food and Nutrition Board, National Research Council: Recommended dietary allowances, ed. 9, Washington, D.C., 1980, National Academy of Sciences.

Frankenburg, W.K., and Dodds, J.B.: Denver Developmental Screening Test, Denver, 1969, University of Colorado Medical Center.

Frankenburg, W.K., Goldstein, A.D., and Camp, B.W.: The revised Denver Developmental Screening Test: its accuracy as a screening instrument, J. Pediatr. **79**:988-995, Dec. 1971.

Healthy People: Public Health Service, DHEW Pub. No. (PHS) 79-55071, Washington, D.C., 1979, Department of Health, Education and Welfare.

Keeney, A.H.: Development of vision. In Falkner F., editor: Human development, Philadelphia, 1966, W.B. Saunders Co.

Klaus, M.H., and Kennell, J.H.: Maternal-infant bonding, St. Louis, 1976, The C.V. Mosby Co.

Korones, S.B.: High risk newborn infants, ed. 3, St. Louis, 1981, The C.V. Mosby Co.

Krugman, S., Ward, R., and Katz, S.L.: Infectious diseases of children, ed. 6, St. Louis, 1977, The C.V. Mosby Co.

Lancaster, J.: Coping mechanisms for the working mother, Am. J. Nurs. **8**:1322-1324, Aug. 1975.

Leifer, A.J.: Effects of mother-infant separation on maternal attachment behavior, Child Dev. **43**:1203-1218, Dec. 1972.

Liebman, S.D., and Gellis, S.S.: The pediatrician's ophthalmology, St. Louis, 1966, The C.V. Mosby Co.

Lowell, J.D.: Congenital hip dysplasia, Clin. Pediatr. **3**:279-287, May 1964.

Lynn, D.B.: The father: his role in child development, Monterey, Calif., 1974, Brooks/Cole Publishing Co.

Maternal and Child Health Program: Evaluation of body size and physical growth of children, The Maternal and Child Health Program, Washington, D.C., 1976, U.S. Department of Health, Education and Welfare.

McMillan, J.A.: The whole pediatrician catalog, Philadelphia, 1977, W.B. Saunders Co.

Miles, M., editor: Mental health aspects of SIDS. Report of conference sponsored by the National Foundation for Sudden Infant Death and the National Institute of Mental Health, Kansas City, July 30, 1975, U.S. Department of Health, Education and Welfare.

Patterson, K., and Pomeroy, M.K.: Nursing care begins after death when the disease is Sudden Infant Death Syndrome, Nursing '74 **4**:85-88, May, 1974.

Piaget, J., and Inhelder, B.: La Genese do l'idee de hasard chez l'enfant, Paris, 1951, Presses Universite de France.

Pipes, P.L.: Nutrition in infancy and childhood, St. Louis, 1981, The C.V. Mosby, Co.

Rapaport, H.G., and Linde, S.M.: The complete allergy guide, New York, 1970, Simon & Schuster, Inc.

Rapoport, R.: Father, mother and society, New York, 1977, Basic Books, Inc., Publishers.

Ross Laboratories: NCHS growth charts, Columbus, Ohio, 1976; as adapted from National Center for Health Statistics: NCHS growth charts, 1976, Monthly vital statistics report, Vol. 25, no. 3, Suppl. (HRA) 76-1120, Health Resources Administration, Rockville, Md. June 1976. Data from the Fels Research Institute, Yellow Springs, Ohio.

Rowe, D.S.: Signs helpful in localizing respiratory tract abnormality, San Francisco, June 1973, University of California, (Unpublished material.)

Scipien, G. M., et al.: Comprehensive pediatric nursing, ed. 2, New York, 1979, McGraw-Hill Book Co.

Shaw, E.B.: Sudden unexpected death in infancy syndrome, Am. J. Dis. Child. **119**:416-418, May 1970.

Sutterly, D., and Donnelly, G.: Perspectives in human development: nursing throughout the life cycle, Philadelphia, 1978, J.B. Lippincott Co.

Tackett, J.J., and Hunsberger, M.: Family centered care of children and adolescents, Philadelphia, 1981, W.B. Saunders Co.

Thomas, A., and Chess, S.: Temperament and the parent-child interaction, Pediatr. Ann. **6**:26-45, Sept. 1977.

Vaughan, V.C., McKay, R.J., and Behrman, R.E., editors: Nelson textbook of pediatrics, ed. 11, Philadelphia, 1979, W.B. Saunders Co.

Waechter, E. H., and Blake, F.G.: Nursing care of children, ed. 9, Philadelphia, 1976, J.B. Lippincott Co.

Whipple, D.V.: Dynamics of development: euthenic pediatrics, New York, 1966, McGraw-Hill Book Co.

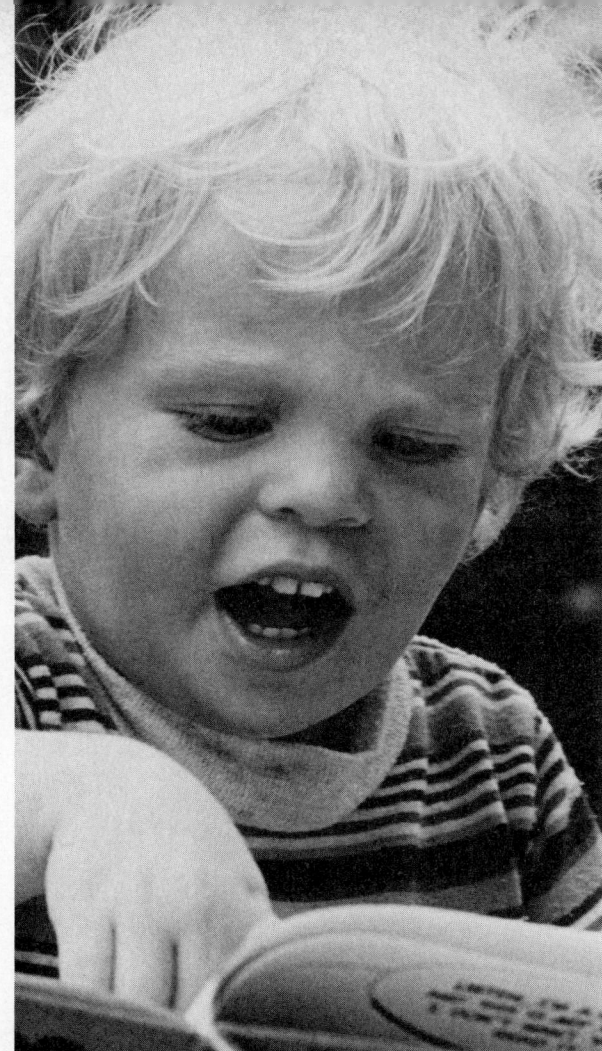

Chapter 24

NANCY DICKENSON-HAZARD

THE SECOND THROUGH SIXTH YEARS OF LIFE

Toddlers and preschool children are mobile, curious, and adventuresome. As their developmental abilities expand, so do their environments and life experiences. Through the use of newly acquired physical language and social skills, these children become more adept in mastering and manipulating the world in which they live. The experimentation and learning of these age groups, however, can present obstacles to the child's well-being. The health goal for these children thus becomes the provision of opportunities for maximal growth and development while maintaining a healthy, safe environment. Parents and health care professionals will find a challenge in accomplishing this goal.

This chapter will focus on the health assessment, maintenance, and promotion of children in their toddler and preschool years. Significant physical and psychosocial aspects of health will be reviewed as well as the factors that can influence the health goal.

PHYSICAL GROWTH AND DEVELOPMENT

The Toddler

The toddler years span 1 to 3 years of life. During this time, physical growth and development rates decelerate from the rapid growth rate of infancy, and by 2 years of age the growth rate has stabilized. A toddler gains approximately 5 lb (2.6 kg) annually. Birth weight is usually quadrupled by 2½ years. The average toddler gains 5 in (12.7 cm) in the second year and 3 to 4 in (7.6 to 10.2 cm) in the third year. A toddler's height at 2 years of age generally represents 50% of eventual adult height.

Physiological Functioning

Physiological functioning becomes more competent during the toddler years. The physiological changes of these years are not as dramatic as those of infancy and occur at a slower rate. However, development is continuing throughout all major organ systems. Major changes are discussed in the following paragraphs.

Cardiovascular System. The cardiovascular system has stabilized. Heart rate is generally 70 to 130 beats per minute and total hemoglobin volume is close to adult values. In addition, the respiratory rate of a toddler has slowed to 20 to 30 respirations per minute, although respiratory movements continue primarily in the abdominal area.

Gastrointestinal System. Growth in the gastrointestinal system includes an increased stomach capacity to 500 cc, mature salivary glands, and liver maturity and efficiency, which facilitates vitamin storage, glucogenesis, amino acid changes, and ketone body formation. In addition, as diet progresses to adult foods and proportions, and as the lower intestines mature, stools produced by the toddler become similar to those of an adult.

Urinary Function. The increased physiological competency of toddlerhood will create changes in the ability to control urinary function. For example, the bladder capacity of a 2-year-old is 500 to 600 cc, thereby decreasing the number of voidings per day while promoting bladder tone in preparation for voluntarily controlled voidings.

Lymphoid Tissue. During the toddler years, lymphoid tissue increases in size as evidenced by the presence of peripheral nodes and enlarged tonsils and adenoids. The increased incidence of infections in the toddler years creates hyperplasia of the lymphoid tissue, a normal physiological occurrence, which persists long after the primary infection has been resolved.

Skeletal Growth. Skeletal growth is evidenced by the closure of the anterior fontanel by 18 months and the addition of epiphyses to the long bones. A phenomenon of normal physiological genu varum (bowlegs) and genu valgum (knock-knees) occurs in the toddler years (Fig. 24-1) as a result of skeletal growth (Bunch, 1979). The broad-based gait of a toddler is created by a long trunk, short arms and legs, and large head. To compensate for weight distribution, the spine curves anterioposteriorly (lordosis) and legs bow. This bow-legged appearance generally persists until approximately 18 months of age and is followed by a physiological genu valgum (knock-knee) with protective toeing-in of the foot. See Appendix K and accompanying figures, which provide information regarding screening for orthopedic problems. The use of such procedures in a screening clinic situation will be most helpful to com-

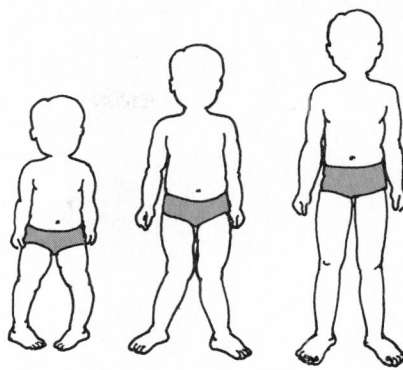

Fig. 24-1. Progression from bowlegs to profound knock-knees to correction. This sequence is perfectly normal and represents the normal patterns of development. (From Bunch, W.H. Reprinted with permission of the publisher of Pediatric Nursing, Vol. 5, No. 4, July/August 1979.)

munity health nurses when assessing young children for potential health problems.

Dental Growth. Dental growth continues with the calcification of first and second bicuspids and second molars. The number of primary teeth by the end of the second year has increased to a complete set of 20 (see Fig. 23-4). Preventive dental care should begin as soon as primary teeth erupt. Early care requires parents to wipe the teeth clean daily. By 18 months to 2 years brushing with a fluoride toothpaste should be done daily. Teaching children to do this activity themselves should also be begun at this age. An initial visit to the dentist needs to be scheduled at 3 to 4 years of age.

Sleeping Patterns. The sleeping patterns of a toddler become more routine and there is often a need for bedtime rituals. The average toddler will sleep 8 to 12 hours a day and by 3 years has usually relinquished the afternoon nap for nighttime sleep only.

Feeding Behaviors. Feeding behaviors of toddlers also change. They are able to express distinct food preferences, and the 2- to 3-year-old is frequently an on-the-run, picky eater. The toddler becomes disinterested in food, his appetite falls, and food jags are common. The development of fine and gross motor skills also influence the ability to eat (see Table 23-21). Nonetheless, the toddler's nutritional requirements need to be met.

The toddler requires between 1000 and 1500 kcal/day because of increased body size. The protein requirement is 1.8 g/kg/day and can be met if a balanced diet is consumed. Additionally, the water requirement for the 1- to 3-year-old is 115 to 125 ml/kg/day as a result of the high metabolic rate.

Motor Skills. The toddler years are a time for achieving physical competency in both fine and gross motor skills. Refinement of previous motor skills and mastery

Table 24-1. Developmental behaviors

Age	Fine motor skills	Gross motor skills	Social behavior	Language ability
15-18 months	Uses spoon and cup with little spilling; builds 2-cube tower; can undress; has refined pincer grasp	Stoops and recovers; walks well; pushes furniture to climb; walks up stairs one at a time with assistance	Rolls ball back and forth with 1 other person; imitates household chores; indicates desires without crying; drinks from a cup	Vocabulary of 10 to 20 words; understands simple questions; forms 2-word phrases; beginning to name pictures
2 years	Builds a 6-cube tower; turns pages of a book one at a time; begins to dress self; washes and dries hands	Runs; walks up and down stairs alone; walks backwards; jumps in place; throws ball overhand	Removes clothes; awareness of ownership; helps out; eats with family but cannot sit through entire meal	Points to body parts; has 300-400 word vocabulary; uses ''my'' pronouns and prepositions; forms 3- to 4-word phrases
3 years	Opens and closes doors using knob by self; uses fingers to hold pencil; builds 8- to 10-block tower; zips zippers; does simple buttoning	Walks up and down stairs alternating feet; rides tricycle; broad jumps; dresses with assistance	May have imaginary playmates; can put on simple garment; washes and dries hands; likes to have a choice	Uses plurals; forms 3- to 4-word sentences, using correct grammatical structures
4 years	Draws a 3-part man; buttons easily; can cut out pictures	Catches ball with hands; broad jumps; climbs up and down stairs, alternating feet; balances on one foot momentarily	Separates easily from mother; can button clothing; plays interactive and associative games, demonstrating some control; able to share	Comprehends and uses opposites; has increased vocabulary and about 90% comprehensibility; speaks in full sentences, using prepositions, pronouns, adverbs, and adjectives
5 years	Copies a square accurately; draws a 5-part man; begins to tie shoelaces	Runs with speed and agility; dresses without supervision; skips crudely	Developing attachment outside of family; engages in cooperative play; strives for independence	Vocabulary expanding to 3-syllable words; composition increasing to spoken paragraphs

of new ones make the toddler a very mobile, busy person. The average toddler should be assessed for motor performance when evaluating physical development. Table 24-1 describes landmark behaviors and abilities for the toddler and preschooler.

The Preschooler
Physiological Growth

The world of the 3- to 6-year-old rapidly expands because of increased physical abilities. Preschool children become active members of a world both in and out of the family unit. Growth patterns for each individual preschooler are fairly well established by the age of three. During these years, most children increase their weight annually by approximately 5 lb (2.6 kg). The average height gain is 3 to 4 in (7.6 to 10.2 cm) in the third year and 2 to 3 in (5.1 to 7.6 cm) per year until prepubescence.

Physical and physiological growth continues but at a slower pace than previously. Some preschoolers appear to grow gradually over the years, whereas others demonstrate growth spurts.

Musculoskeletal Growth. Skeletal growth primarily is further bone ossification and epiphysis development. Visible dental growth is minimal until the sixth through eighth year when primary teeth are lost and replaced by deciduous adult teeth. The lower central incisors are generally lost and replaced first. Musculoskeletal development is aided by central nervous system progression, as evidenced by a more coordinated and adept preschooler.

Visual acuity matures as well. The normally hyperoptic (farsighted) toddler develops into a preschooler with 20/30 vision by 5 or 6 years (Table 23-5).

Cardiovascular Refinement. Cardiovascular refinement occurs during preschool years as evidenced by a heart rate drop to 70 to 110 beats per minute. The hemoglobin stabilizes at 12 to 13 g and respiratory rates continue at 20 to 30 respirations per minute. Respiratory movement remains primarily abdominal until the end of the fifth or sixth year when it becomes diaphragmatic.

Gastrointestinal System. The gastrointestinal system is sufficiently developed so that the child can chew and swallow in an adult manner. Stomach capacity continues to increase and urinary bladder capacity is 600 to 750 cc in 24 hours, creating voiding patterns similar to an adult.

Feeding Habits. Eating and sleeping habits stabilize over the preschool years. The 3- to 5-year-old usually regains appetite and interest in food. Caloric intake requirement ranges from 90 to 100 kcal/kg/day and the average daily water requirement is 1½ to 2 oz lb (100 to 125 ml/kg). The protein requirement for the preschooler increases to 3 g per kg. These requirements can be met with a planned, balanced diet focusing on the preschooler's food preferences.

Sleeping Patterns. The sleeping patterns of a preschooler are generally predictable. Most sleeping time is at night, although occasional daytime naps are not unusual. By 3 years most children have graduated from crib to bed, have developed definite bedtime routines, and display few sleep problems (Table 23-6).

Motor Skills. The fine and gross motor skills of a preschooler also continue development. The clumsiness and oftentimes ineptness of the toddler vanishes, and the preschooler becomes a master of physical abilities. The average 3- to 5-year-old needs to be assessed for performance of these skills when physical development is evaluated (see Table 24-1).

PSYCHOSOCIAL GROWTH AND DEVELOPMENT

The Toddler

During the second to fourth years of life, a child's personality comes into its own. The individuality of the child becomes more apparent and his psychosocial development is enhanced by his improved physical prowess as well as his expanding communicative ability.

Erikson's Concepts

This toddler age period is stage 2 of Erikson's theory of life development. During this time a toddler is charged with the task of developing a sense of autonomy versus one of shame or doubt. This task is partially accomplished through the discovery of the difference between dependence and independence. A toddler is able to make this discrimination if a sense of trust has developed in a significant caretaker. Trusting allows the child to see the separateness of oneself and caretaker (usually the mother).

In viewing themselves as separate, the toddlers will begin to explore their world. This exploration is facilitated by their physical abilities of walking, climbing, and running. They quickly learn that their own behaviors have an impact on their environment and the people within that world. They are no longer a passive contributor to the family, and their newfound ability to affect change in their world facilitates a sense of autonomy and independence.

At the same time a toddler still needs and desires closeness and dependency, especially to significant persons. The exploration and independence is fun and challenging but it is also full of unknowns, at times intimidating, at times frightening. Consequently, toddlers must begin to balance those behaviors and actions, which meet both dependent and independent needs.

Learning to Balance Needs

Achieving this balance is accomplished in a variety of ways. First the toddler learns to tolerate separation from the mother. As children learn more about themselves and their capabilities, they are able to separate from others for longer periods of time. Initially the separation may be merely across the room, but gradually the distance and time length of separation increases as the toddler becomes more secure with this independence.

Communication Skills

The ability to communicate further facilitates achievement of the balance between autonomy and doubt. Language is an important aspect of psychosocial as well as intellectual development, and its development involves comprehension (receptive) as well as speaking (expressive) skills (Lenneberg, 1967). The stages of language development are found in Table 24-2.

Receptive Skills

Receptive language skills are known to be achieved earlier than expressive skills, as evidenced by toddlers' early ability to follow simple instructions (Lenneberg, 1966). During this time toddlers are absorbing the language of their environment. They are passive partici-

Table 24-2. Age ranges of language developmental stages

Stages	Age
Cooing stage	0-2 months
Babbling stage	2-6 months
First word, usually imitated	12-18 months
Rapid vocabulary acquisition	18 months-3 years
Open and pivot words	
Telegraphic sentences	
Steady word acquisition	3-5 years
Multiword sentences	
Basic mastery of language by end	
Progressively complex sentences	6-11+ years
Use of pronouns, proper nouns, prepositions	
Basic grammatical mastery by end	

From Tackett, J.J., and Hunsberger, M.: Family centered care of children and adolescents, Philadelphia, 1981, W.B. Saunders Co., p. 151.

pants in the communication process and their behavioral responses to the language of their world reinforces their sociability, sense of autonomy, and subsequent participation. For example, a toddler responds to mother's request to put the toy in the toybox by doing so. Mother responds with praise, and the toddler feels a sense of pleasure and accomplishment. The act has been an independent one, which increases social acceptability with mother and contributes to wanting to participate in future interactions.

Expressive Skills

Expressive language skills make the toddler an active participant in the communication process (Lenneberg, 1966). Through speech, the toddlers expand the scope of their interactive ability. They can now respond to their environment through verbal and behavioral expression, thereby having a greater impact. For example, imagine the affect the toddler will have if the mother is told "I did it" by the child after being asked to put the toys away. Both mother and child feel a sense of accomplishment, but the child is now able to verbalize this feeling as well as act it out.

Play

Finally, the dimension of play becomes an integral part of the toddler's life and serves as a tool to achieve developmental tasks. Play reflects a child's physical, cognitive, and psychosocial development and serves as a medium for the child's orientation to self and the world. Learning is accomplished through play, and play provides the child with a safe, self-controlled means to explore feelings and the environment. In addition, play contributes to a child's development in all spheres: the physical activity of play contributes to coordination; the explorative activity of play contributes to reality orientation; and the experimental activity of play contributes to self-awareness and emotional expressions (Caplan, 1973).

Play undergoes development as well, based on the child's abilities and environmental changes and opportunities. The progression of play reflects varying degrees of sociability from playing alone to playing alongside to playing cooperatively. The younger child spends the most time playing alone or parallel with another child, whereas the 5-year-old is able to play cooperatively. Types of play have been categorized by Parten (1932) as follows:

Unoccupied behavior: Child occupies self with watching whatever happens to be of momentary interest. When nothing exciting is occurring, play is initiated with own body (e.g., sitting, standing, rolling).

Onlooker: Child watches other play. May make inquiries or give suggestions but does not interact in play with others.

Solitary independent: Child plays alone and independently with toys different from those used by other children who are within speaking distance. Child does not get close but pursues own activity without concern for what others are doing.

Parallel: Child plays beside other children, not with them, using similar toys and choosing activities that bring others close.

Associative: Child plays with other children in a common activity. Borrowing and lending occur but there is no organization, division of labor, or control by any one child which shapes direction of play.

Cooperative: Child plays in a group that is organized for a purpose. Roles and tasks are assigned, activity is organized, and leadership and control are evidenced.

Nurse's Role

These characteristics of play are most useful in assessing the productivity and purpose of play as related to the child's developmental stage. Since play is a child's work, it is important for nurses to be knowledgeable in ways to stimulate play. Concrete, practical suggestions from nurses to parents can promote healthy productive play. Principles useful in assisting parents to promote play are as follows:

Parents should be taught characteristics and content of play.

Opportunities for play should be provided which are appropriate to the child's age.

Expense of toy is not necessarily an indicator that it will promote development. Common household items such as plastic cartons provide as much stimulation as an expensive set of stackables.

Parents need to play with their child.

Parents need to be aware of the child's response to play, that is, when to stimulate and when to rest

Play should be pleasurable.

Toys should be safe, durable, and suitable to child's developmental abilities.

Toys should promote child's own creativity and resourcefulness and not be excessive, confusing, or overwhelming.

In addition to adhering to these principles, nurses can assist parents in directing play and selecting toys through suggested readings and provision of information appropriate to child's age and safety needs.

Piaget's Concepts

Children of toddler or preschool age see things only from their point of view. Lifelike qualities are given to inanimate objects and everything is considered real. They believe they can make things happen just by thinking of them and that the world exists for them alone.

Piaget views this characteristic egocentric thought pattern as the preoperational period of cognitive development. This period, which lasts from 2 to 7 years of age, makes the child appear quite illogical. The child's task is to utilize language and memory and to understand past, present, and future happenings. Specifically, the 2- to 4-year-olds are in stage 1 of this period, or the preconceptual phase. During this time they are able to form mental images that stand for things they cannot see (symbolic thought). Play becomes the primary tool for the development of these images and, coupled with language and imitation, assists children to establish their place in relationship to their environment. Since they are egocentric, much of their play is parallel because they cannot readily focus on what someone else may want. As they become more aware of other influences in their world, children of this age will display more socialized behavior at the end of this period.

Nurse's Role. Assessment of developmental milestones continues to be an important responsibility of nurses at this age. While much of a child's development has occurred, personality formation is ongoing. Fine and gross motor skills have previously been reviewed in this chapter. Knowledge and assessment of social

and language skills are also appropriate (see Table 24-1).

The Preschooler
Erikson's Concepts

Ages 4 to 8 mark the entry into the third stage of development according to Erikson. During this phase children must learn to develop a sense of initiative versus a sense of guilt as they broaden the scope of their environment. They will come in contact with more peers, more authoritarian figures, and more new life experiences and societal rules than ever before. In their eagerness to explore, the preschoolers rush in to accomplish new skills, tasks, and capabilities in the expanded world of home, school, and neighborhood. They begin to initiate themselves and their personalities in a world away from home. They may also have some feelings of guilt for wanting to be dependent and to be close to familiar surroundings and persons. Resolving this conflict and achieving a psychosocial balance requires parental sensitivity in knowing when to comfort and allow dependency and when to encourage independency.

The preschoolers' own developmental progression assists them in resolving this conflict. The comfortable expansion of their social sphere and skills occurs when the 4 to 6-year-old has mastered some degree of self-control. It is at this age that all aspects of psychosocial development begin to have the greatest interaction, because social, emotional, physical, and cognitive development must all come forth in order to be acceptable in social spheres outside the home.

Piaget's Concepts

Cognitive development impacts greatly on this total developmental interaction. According to Piaget, the 4- to 6-year-olds begin to move away from egocentricity. At the same time they achieve control over bodily functions and to some degree behavior. In stage 2 of the preoperational period, the preschooler becomes more perceptual and intuitive. Prelogical reasoning appears and experiences and objects are judged by outside appearances and results. As an example, that father will be angry if father's newly planted flowers are pulled up is deduced by 4-year-old *before* the act is carried out, thereby demonstrating prelogical reasoning. As for objects being judged by outward appearances, a preschooler will insist there are more oranges than tangerines when shown an equal number because the oranges are bigger.

Cognition is further enhanced by the child's increasing use of language to express self rather than acting out feelings or desires. This development influences the child's play, which subsequently becomes more social. In sum, as the preschoolers move into spheres outside of the home, they are equipped to deal with forthcoming experiences because cognition, language, and control have increased while egocentrism and dependency have decreased.

Sociability

With exposure to new life experiences, the preschooler will begin to test out social behaviors for safety and effectiveness. Some of these behaviors will be retained and reused, and others will be adapted for better efficacy. Always the preschooler will continue to develop psychosocially and cognitively, beginning with the foundation acquired in early years and building upward.

A developmental assessment of this age must take into account the basic skills with which the preschooler should be equipped. Fine and gross motor milestones have been previously reviewed. Appropriate social behaviors and language skills are outlined in Table 24-1.

FACTORS AFFECTING GROWTH AND DEVELOPMENT

An overview of pertinent factors that influence the growth and development of children has been discussed in the preceding chapter. These factors continue to be influential in the toddler and preschool years.

Expansion and Expertise

Of singular importance to the toddler and preschool children is the expansion of experiences created by their own increasing developmental abilities. A type of feedback mechanism ensues whereby the child is able to do more physically and psychosocially, which expands the manipulative and learning opportunities in the environment. Once new elements in the environment are mastered, the child uses this expertise to practice and expand further to include interactions with people and experiences outside the home. As an example, the toddler, having learned to climb, will push a chair to the countertop to reach a cookie. Once the climbing is mastered in the home, the toddler will then use this skill at the playground where climbing up the slide will be attempted.

Integration

As the child advances through the preschool years, all the developmental skills will be integrated into the whole personality. Rather than focusing on a specific skill, such as the 2-year-old learning to climb or the 3-year-old mastering language, the child at the end of preschool years will have incorporated all skill spheres into a repertoire of effective behaviors. Although a distinct individual person exists in the child as an infant, this individual becomes more apparent by the end of the fifth year as a result of this integration process.

Additional Factors

The trends toward two-career families and increased use of child care alternatives are added influences to the toddler and preschooler's developmental experiences.

Working mothers constitute a large portion of the U.S. work force today (Curtis, 1976). The primary motive for working is monetary need. With this trend many changes occur within the family (e.g., chores and day-to-day parenting must be shared) and many feelings and emotions ensue (mother may feel guilty; father may feel relieved to have added income) (Curtis, 1976; Lancaster, 1975). In all changes that may occur, the child's need for care must be arranged. For some families this may mean home care; for others day care will be the solution. Frequently the family will consult with the nurse for advice.

Nurse's Role

The nurse can implement intervention at several points in the family's decision-making process regarding mother's return to work. First, parents may need assistance in identifying the need for mother to return to work and possible alternatives. For example, part-time work by one spouse may be sufficient to meet financial need, or work in the home by one parent may be an alternative.

Second, once the decision has been made, assisting parents to identify child care alternatives is a responsibility nurses can assume. Care options appropriate to the child's age should be explored with parents (e.g., care in the home, day care centers or homes, nursery school, play schools or groups, kindergarten). To facilitate the choice of child care options, the nurse should advise parents to consider (1) the philosophy, attitude, and emotional tone to and around children expressed by the person acting as primary caretaker; (2) the physical environment, its safety, its appeal and diversity, materials and equipment, and access or proximity to parents; (3) other participants in the setting, their health, their response to caretaker and environment, and their age and developmental level. In addition, it is wise for nurses to counsel parents of the need to visit and observe the care setting before final selection and to periodically evaluate the setting and its effects and influence on the child.

A third activity nurses can implement is facilitating parental coping and adjustment to the two-career family situation. Appropriate nursing intervention would focus on reallocating of chores and responsibilities to include all family members; assisting parents to identify feelings (e.g., inadequacy, guilt, anger, resentment, relief, freedom) regarding return to work and the influence they have on the child's attitude toward this change; and assisting the family to identify stresses created by the change which may produce tension and to improve inadequate coping management.

COMMON CAUSES OF MORBIDITY AND MORTALITY

Since causes and factors are generally studied for the 1- to 5-year-old range, mortality and morbidity will be discussed in terms of both the toddler and preschooler age groups. Problems relevant to one specific age group will be defined as such.

Mortality

Children over 1 year of age are enjoying better health today than ever before. The death rate for children has fallen to 43 per 100,000 population in 1977 versus 330 per 100,000 in 1925. By 1990 this mortality rate is expected to be reduced further to 34 per 100,000 (*Healthy People,* 1979).

The primary cause of death formerly was infectious and communicable disease. Now cases of these once-dreaded diseases (polio, diphtheria, measles, and rubella) are seldom seen. Instead, accidents and injuries have become responsible for 45% of childhood deaths. In descending order of incidence, the most common causes of fatal injuries are motor vehicle accidents, burns, drowning, choking, falls, and poisoning. Among children ages 1 to 5, over 3400 died from injuries in 1976, 40% being attributable to motor vehicle injuries and 20% to burns. No other preventable cause poses such a threat to life as accidents. In addition, the segments of the childhood population most at risk have been identified as boys, who demonstrated an annual death rate higher than females, and blacks, who demonstrated an overall higher mortality rate (*Healthy People,* 1979).

Nurse's Role

Clearly the goal of nursing should be provision of preventive measures for these major health threats. Using safety measures can prevent most accidents. Appendix J provides age-appropriate accident prevention interventions that should be a primary component of every nurse's management plan.

Community health nurses have the opportunity to implement education in the home, clinic, and school settings. A reduced number of accident-related deaths and injuries can be realized by the provision of organized education programs from community health nurses.

Morbidity

For children in the toddler and preschool age group, infections continue to be the most common cause of restricted activity. Although resistance to many causative agents of infectious diseases is developing in children from 1 to 6 years, their exposure and subsequent immunity are by no means complete. The toddler and preschooler are frequently plagued with upper respiratory infections and secondary complications such as pharyngitis, otitis media, bronchitis, and bronchiolitis. The incidence of influenza and pneumonia as well as allergies can also be high for this age group. See Chapter 23 for a detailed discussion of these health problems.

Nurse's Role

The role of the nurse clearly is to implement preventive measures. These nursing activities may be directed toward primary prevention (i.e., reducing the incidence of the problem for the child) or they may be directed toward secondary prevention (i.e, reducing the incidence of secondary complications). Specific nursing interventions for the health problems mentioned earlier which affect toddlers and preschoolers have been discussed in Chapter 23. The reader is referred to that chapter for a review (Tables 23-12 through 23-14 and boxed material on pp. 543 and 544).

MAJOR HEALTH PROBLEMS

The Toddler and Preschooler

Although the major health problems of infants discussed in Chapter 23 have significant incidence rates in the 2- to 6-year-old, the toddler and preschool groups are also at risk of developing additional illnesses. Of significance are the viral illnesses and exanthems.

Viral Illnesses

Viruses are the most common causative organism of infectious disease in children. Of particular significance is the incidence of viral hepatitis, influenza, roseola, and varicella. Appendix J reviews their presentation and management as well as these features for other common infectious diseases.

Hepatitis. Up to 70,000 cases of viral hepatitis are reported each year in the United States. There are two types of viral hepatitis, type A and type B. Clinical features are compared in Table 24-3. Since children are less likely to demonstrate jaundice and generally have milder symptoms, their symptomatic and supportive care can be managed easily at home with the proper counseling.

Influenza. Influenza is an acute disease of the respiratory tract caused primarily by A, B, and C influenza viruses. Since these viruses have the ability to change (become mutants), epidemics can be anticipated as well as difficulties in implementing an influenza immunization program.

Roseola and Varicella. Roseola is the most common exanthem in infants and young children ages 6 months to 2 years of age; 95% of the cases of this benign viral illness occur in these ages. Roseola demonstrates a seasonal pattern with peak incidence in the spring and autumn. Varicella, commonly known as chickenpox, is a highly contagious disease caused by the varicella-zoster virus. Children between 2 and 8 years demonstrate the highest incidence, whereas infants are generally protected in the first few months through maternal passive immunity. Varicella occurs more frequently in the winter and spring months. Appendix J reviews the common exanthematous diseases.

Measles, Mumps, Rubella. With the introduction of the measles, mumps, and rubella vaccines, the incidence of these once-common childhood illnesses has been reduced significantly. However, the unimmunized populations are at risk, with the highest incidence of disease occurring in school age children. Prevention of these infectious diseases is the primary goal, and education and promotion of immunization is well within the nurse's role. See Appendix E for a discussion of immunizations.

Child Abuse and Neglect

The phenomenon of child abuse is a recent and unfortunate one. The battered and neglected children in the United States account for many injuries, burns, and accidents, as well emotional problems, brain damage, and even death. Although the actual number of cases of

Table 24-3. Hepatitis A and hepatitis B: comparison of major features

Features	Hepatitis A	Hepatitis B
Synonym	Infectious hepatitis	Serum hepatitis
Incubation period	15-40 days	50-180 days
HB Ag (Australia antigen in blood)	Absent	Present in incubation period
Age group	Usually children and young adults	All age groups
Mode of transmission	Primarily fecal-to-oral route; some parenteral spread (blood products); contaminated water, food, infected shellfish	Primarily parenteral (transfusion of blood or blood products, drug inoculation); some nonparenteral (body fluids of infected persons)
Seasonal	Fall and winter predominantly but also throughout the year	Any season
Onset	Usually acute	Usually insidious
Fever	Common; precedes jaundice	Less common
Jaundice	Rare in children; more common in adults	Rare in children; more common in adults
Severity	Usually mild	Often severe
Abnormal SGOT	Transient; 1-3 weeks	More prolonged; 1-8 months
Thymol turbidity	Usually elevated	Usually normal
IgM levels	Usually increased	Usually normal
Virus excretion		
Blood	Present during late incubation period and early acute phase	Present during late incubation period and acute phase; may persist for months and years
Feces	Present during late incubation period and acute phase	Probably present but no direct proof
Value of gamma globulin prophylaxis	Good	Uncertain
Immunity		
Homologous	Present	Present
Heterologous	None	None

From Chow, M.P., et al.: Handbook of pediatric primary care, New York, 1979, John Wiley & Sons, Inc., p. 915; as adapted from Krugman, S., et al.: Infectious diseases of children, ed. 6, St. Louis, 1977, The C.V. Mosby Co., p. 101.

child abuse and neglect is elusive because of difficulties in identification, estimates range from 200,000 to 4 million a year. Minimally, 2500 children die annually from circumstances associated with abuse or neglect (*Healthy People*, 1979).

Incidence and Predisposing Factors

Children under three are the most frequent victims and women the most frequent abusers, although men abuse more severely and are involved in sexual assault. All races and socioeconomic groups are involved, but statistics indicate a higher incidence in lower socioeconomic classes (Kempe and Helfer, 1972).

The psychodynamics involved in an abusive situation are characterized by the following factors:

A crisis precipitating the occurence, preceded by multiple frustrations, problems, and inability to cope

A premeditated injury

Parents who were abused as children, who lack support systems, and who display a lack of trust

A child who has been "labeled" as different by the parent, possibly as a result of unplanned pregnancy, illness, or prematurity

Common clinical findings associated with child abuse as given by Chow (1979) are listed in the box in the preceding column.

Nurse's Role

Prevention is the primary goal when considering child abuse (Kempe and Helfer, 1972). Nurses have the responsibility to use their knowledge and skill to identify potential abusive situations. Risk screening should be implemented prenatally and postnatally and periodically throughout well child care (see boxed material below and on next page). If a family at risk is identified, additional supportive measures need to be implemented in the interest of prevention (see box on next page)

Managing a situation of child abuse is difficult and will require a multidisciplinary approach (Fontana and

---

Common Clinical Findings of Child Abuse

Skin: burns, old scars, ecchymosis, soft tissue swelling, human bites
Fractures: skull, rib, limb, presence of old fractures on x-ray films, epiphyseal separations
Subdural hematomas
Intestinal injuries
Trauma to genitals
Growth retardation
Poor hygiene
Whiplash: shaken infant syndrome caused by manual shaking of trunk or extremities resulting in intraocular and intracranial hemorrhage (Caffey, 1974, p. 396)

From Chow, M.P., et al.: Handbook of pediatric primary care, New York, 1979, John Wiley & Sons, Inc., p. 1030.

Observations of Parents-to-Be in Physician's Office or Prenatal Clinic

1. Are the parents overconcerned with the baby's sex?
2. Are they overconcerned with the baby's performance? Do they worry that he will not meet the standard?
3. Is there an attempt to deny that there is a pregnancy (mother not willing to gain weight, no plans whatsoever, refusal to talk about the situation)?
4. Is this child going to be one child too many? Could he be the "last straw"?
5. Is there great depression over this pregnancy?
6. Is the mother alone and frightened, especially by the physical changes caused by the pregnancy? Do careful explanations fail to dissipate these fears?
7. Is support lacking from husband and/or family?
8. Where is the family living? Do they have a listed telephone number? Are there relatives and friends nearby?
9. Did the mother and/or father formerly want an abortion but not go through with it or waited until it was too late?
10. Have the parents considered relinquishment of their child? Why did they change their minds?

From Kempe, C.H.: Approaches to preventing child abuse, Am. J. Dis. Child. **130:**941–947, 1976; copyright 1976, American Medical Association.

Observations to Be Made at Postpartum Checkups and Pediatric Checkups

1. Does the mother have fun with the baby?
2. Does the mother establish eye contact (direct en face position) with the baby?
3. How does the mother talk to her baby? Is everything she expresses a demand?
4. Are most of her verbalizations about the child negative?
5. Does she remain disappointed over the child's sex?
6. What is the child's name? Where did it come from? When did they name the child?
7. Are the mother's expectations for the child's development far beyond the child's capabilities?
8. Is the mother very bothered by the baby's crying? How does she feel about the crying?
9. Does the mother see the baby as too demanding during feedings? Is she repulsed by the messiness? Does she ignore the baby's demands to be fed?
10. What is the mother's reaction to the task of changing diapers?
11. When the baby cries, does she or can she comfort him?
12. What was/is the husband's and/or family's reaction to the baby?
13. What kind of support is the mother receiving?
14. Are there sibling rivalry problems?
15. Is the husband jealous of the baby's drain on the mother's time and affection?
16. When the mother brings the child to the physician's office, does she get involved and take control over the baby's needs and what's going to happen (during the examination and while in the waiting room) or does she relinquish control to the physician or nurse (undressing the child, holding him, allowing him to express his fears, etc.)?
17. Can attention be focused on the child in the mother's presence? Can the mother see something positive for her in that?
18. Does the mother make nonexistent complaints about the baby? Does she describe to you a child that you don't see there at all? Does she call with strange stories that the child has, for example, stopped breathing, turned color, or is doing something "on purpose" to aggravate the parent?
19. Does the mother make emergency calls for very small things, not major things?

From Kempe, C.H.: Approaches to preventing child abuse, Am. J. Dis. Child. **130:**941-947, 1976; copyright 1976, American Medical Association.

Special Well-Child Care for High-Risk Families

1. Promote maternal attachment to the newborn.
2. Phone the mother during the first 2 days at home.
3. Provide more frequent office visits.
4. Give more attention to the mother.
5. Emphasize nutrition.
6. Counsel discipline only for accident prevention.
7. Emphasize accident prevention.
8. Use compliments rather than criticism.
9. Accept phone calls at home.
10. Arrange for regular home visits by a public health nurse or a lay health visitor.

From Kempe, C.H.: Approaches to preventing child abuse, Am. J. Dis. Child. **130:**941-947, 1976; copyright 1976, American Medical Association.

Robinson, 1976). Nurses will be an integral part of this team by offering support to the parents and child, teaching parents how to nurture and parent, and investigating community services available to the family. Both child and parents will require health care interventions. The goal of management is directed toward the protection of the child, support and rehabilitation of parents, and the return of the child to the home when deemed safe. In addition, it is mandatory that all cases of suspected abuse and neglect in the United States be reported to appropriate authorities. Although this responsibility is generally the physician's, reporting by other health professionals is permitted in some states. Although failure to report suspected cases can result in prosecution, reporters of such cases are immune from court action for civil liability. Generally, child abuse or neglect is reported to local or state government child protection agencies. Abused children usually are temporarily removed from the home until the family situation restabilizes and the parents have demonstrated a willingness to continue care as well as a positive caring attitude toward their child.

A plan of follow-up is essential to any circumstance of child abuse. Nurses can contribute in this follow-up by assisting parents to deal with the frustrations of parenthood, teaching parenting approaches, providing support and encouragement, and facilitating the identification and use of community resources. Appropriate community services may include the following (Chow et al., 1979):

Crisis hotlines
Parents Anonymous
Single parents' groups
Lay community organizations
Crisis nurseries or child care centers
Day care centers
Parent education groups
Health visitor groups

COMMON CONCERNS AND PROBLEMS

Parents continue to experience concern over common problems as their children grow. This occurrence was discussed in Chapter 23, and Table 23-21 gives an overview of common childhood behaviors.

Specific to the toddler and preschool years, behavioral habits that evoke parental concern may include biting, hitting, masturbation, sleep and eating disturbances, negativisim, temper tantrums, toilet training, discipline, and limit setting.

Nurse's Role

Nurses have the responsibilities of educating parents in understanding the normalcy of these behaviors, as-

sisting parents to identify effective coping behaviors when dealing with the behavior of concern, identifying with parents appropriate approaches to handling the child and the behavior, and providing support and reassurance to parents. Appendix J provides information pertinent to the nursing assessment and management of the these common problems.

TOOLS FOR ASSESSMENT

The basic tools and techniques of a pediatric assessment, including monitoring physical and psychosocial aspects of health, were discussed in Chapter 23. Since these principles apply throughout childhood, the reader is referred to that chapter for a review. Additionally, Appendix A presents the components of a health assessment, including health promotion activities that are specific to the toddler and preschool age group. Variations of these tools and techniques relevant to the toddler or preschool child are discussed in the following section.

Monitoring Physical Growth and Development

Measurements of a child's height and weight continue to be valuable tools for assessing growth. For children old enough to stand (generally over 3 years), a traditional scale or yardstick may be used (Fig. 24-2). The

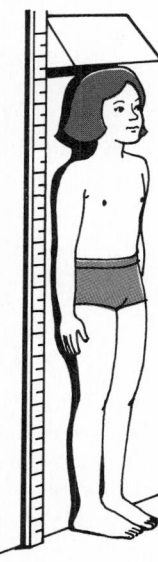

Fig. 24-2. Measurement of height. Child's heels, shoulder blades, and occiput touch wall. (From Evaluation of body size and physical growth of children, The Maternal and Child Health Program, Washington, D.C., 1976, Department of Health, Education, and Welfare.)

child's heels, shoulder blades, and occiput should touch the wall. Older children can be weighed accurately on an adult-type scale, wearing only underwear. Monitoring growth by plotting measurements on growth charts should also continue (Appendix K).

Vital Signs

Continued measurement of vital signs provides data pertinent to the assessment of the state of health and should be implemented at each encounter with the child. For older children, reliable pulse measures may be taken in the radial area, and respiratory rate can be counted as they sit, either through auscultation or observation. For blood pressure measurements, the standard sphygmomanometer can be used for children over 3 years. The important point of technique which must be remembered is that a blood pressure cuff should cover two thirds of the upper arm to gain an accurate reading.

Other Indicators of Physical Growth and Development

Additional methods of monitoring physical growth in the young child include assessment of skeletal or bone age and dental age. In addition, laboratory studies may be useful in monitoring healthy growth. While these assessment methods are not widely used on a routine basis, familiarity with their purpose and interpretation may be useful (see Chapter 23 for a discussion of dental age and laboratory studies).

Skeletal Age. The skeletal system demonstrates that definite developmental stages in the growth of connective tissue, cartilage, and bone can be used in assessing growth. Skeletal age is obtained by radiological examination of the wrist and hand bones. Interpretation is made by noting the ossification centers present, their size, and the morphological stage of each center. Based on this interpretation of skeletal development, a child's growth can be classified as average, early maturation, short, or tall (Todd, 1937).

Screening Tools

Assessment of a child's vision, hearing, and speech is an essential component of any health assessment. Although it is impossible to test all ages for all the specific aspects of vision, hearing, and speech development, age-appropriate methods for determining general abilities are available and should be used. As the child's ability develops and participation in screening procedures becomes more cooperative, the more complete and accurate the assessment of vision, hearing, and speech will become. For example, an infant can be assessed for an overall ability to see, focus, hear, and utter sound, whereas a preschool or school age child, because

Table 24-4. Development of speech sounds

Age	Sounds
3 to 4 years	Lip sounds — *m, p, b, w, h*
4 to 5 years	Tongue contact sounds — *n, t, d, ng, k, g, y*
5 to 6 years	*f*
6 to 6½ years	*v, th* (voiced, as in *then*), *ch, sh, l*
6½ to 7 years	*z, s, r, th* (voiceless, as in *this*)

From Brown, M.S., and Murphy, M.A.: Ambulatory pediatrics for nurses, ed. 1, New York, 1975, McGraw-Hill Book Co., p. 226.

of a higher level of development, can be assessed for visual activity, visual fields, near and far vision, color vision, hearing acuity, vocabulary, articulation and syntax. Incorporating the appropriate age-specific screening method of vision, hearing, and speech development is well within the nurse's role. Appendix K discusses appropriate vision and hearing screening methods. Table 24-4 reviews age-appropriate development of normal speech sounds.

A useful speech assessment tool is the Denver Articulation Screening Examination (DASE) (Appendix J). The DASE is a screening tool that requires no special training to administer. It is used to detect speech disorders in children from 2½ to 6 years of age. This word imitation test consists of 22 items complete with pictures. Administration of the test requires the examiner to say the words and have the child repeat them.

Monitoring Psychosocial Development

The need to implement developmental screening and the purpose of such screening has been discussed in Chapter 23. The continued monitoring of psychosocial development remains important during the toddler and preschool years. Several of the developmental scales previously discussed can be used in the assessment of children in this age group (i.e., DDST and HOME). In addition to these, tools specific to the toddler and preschooler are discussed below.

Preschool Readiness Experimental Screening Scale (PRESS)

The PRESS was designed to assess the maturational level of children between 4 and 5 years of age. It does not assess intellectual capacity but focuses on knowledge of color, numbers, ability to draw, comprehension, coordination, and personal-social maturity. This

Table 24-5. Psychosocial screening tests commonly used in childhood

Test name	Quality measured	Child's age	Comments
Bayley Scales of Infant Development (California First Year Mental Scale)*	Mental age	1 mo-3½ yr	Developed and used in the famous longitudinal Berkeley Growth Studies, which began in the 1930s. Heavily based on the Gesell Developmental Schedules.
The Blacky Pictures	Psychosexual adjustment; personality traits	3 or 4 yr-adult	A projective test consisting of 10 cards with cartoonish pictures of a dog (Blacky) in interactions with parents and siblings and in other everyday situations (eating, etc.) Child is asked to tell a story about each picture. Story content ostensibly reveals child's attitudes, fears, jealousies, aggressive tendencies, etc.
Cattell Infant Intelligence Scale*	Mental age, IQ	2-30 mo	Often considered the best of the infant IQ tests. Developed as a downward extension of the Stanford-Binet.
Children's Appreception Test (CAT)	Psychosexual adjustment; personality traits	3-10 yr	A projective test of 10 cards with drawings of young animals usually interacting with, watching, or being watched by adult animals (young dog being spanked by female adult dog in bathroom, young rabbit alone in crib in darkened room, baby bear and adult bear engaged in tug-of-war with another adult bear, etc.). Child is asked to tell a story about each picture. Story content ostensibly reveals child's attitudes, fears, jealousies, aggressive tendencies, etc. A supplemental form (CAT-S) includes some pictures related to health situations (young rabbit being examined by rabbit doctor, young kangaroo with bandaged leg and tail.
Gesell Developmental Schedules*	Developmental quotient (DQ)	1 mo-3 yr	One of the earliest developmental tests (devised in the 1920s), widely adapted in several subsequent tests. Includes motor, adaptive, language, and personal-social behavior. Test items much like those of Denver Developmental Screening Test. No longer in widespread use.
Goodenough-Harris Drawing Test	IQ	3-12 yr	Originally the Goodenough Draw-A-Man Test (1926), this revised and restandardized version asks a child to make 3 drawings—a man, a woman, and a representation of self. Tests interpretation is based on the fact that children use more detail in their human figure drawings as they grow older. This revision is reportedly more accurate than the Draw-A-Man but lacks the older test's ease and simplicity of scoring. Should be used as a screening test only, not as means to diagnose retardation or acceleration.
House-Tree-Person Test (H-T-P)	Psychosexual adjustment; personality traits	4 yr-adult	Child is asked to make 3 separate drawings—a house, a tree, and a person. The tester notes the style and order of parts drawn, omissions, comments made while drawing, size, etc. The house is said to represent the home and family relationships; the tree, perceptions about oneself and relationship to the environment; and the person, either one's ideal (wished-for) self or a significant other.
Merrill-Palmer Scale	Mental age, per centile, standard score	2-6 yr	Predominantly a performance test (peg board, form board, building blocks, jigsaw puzzle, buttons and buttonhole, etc.) with some verbal tasks ("What does a doggie say?" "What flies?" . . . swims? . . . bites?" etc.) Many test items are timed. An interesting and attractive test to most children—examination goes at a fast pace and test items come packaged in individual, colored boxes.

From Barnard, M.U., et al.: Handbook of comprehensive pediatric nursing, New York, 1981, McGraw-Hill Book Co., p. 113.
*Mental age and IQ measurements of children under 4 years are poor predictors of mental age and IQ at later ages. To some extent this is because tests for young children must rely heavily upon motor skills, whereas "intelligence" as measured in older children and adults is a different highly verbal and cognitive phenomenon.

Continued.

Table 24-5. Psychosocial screening tests commonly used in childhood—cont'd

Test name	Quality measured	Child's age	Comments
Minnesota Pre-school Scale	IQ	1½-6 yr	Includes a verbal IQ test and a nonverbal test. Verbal items include naming objects, telling what is happening in a picture, pointing to pictured objects and body parts, vocabulary questions, digit span questions, problem-solving about everyday situations (''What should you do when you are hungry?'', etc.). Nonverbal items include copying geometric shapes, block building, picture puzzles, spatial arrangements, etc.
Peabody Picture Vocabulary Test*	Mental age, IQ, percentile	2½ yr-adult	Vocabulary is tested against age norms as a measure of mental age and IQ. Test consists of a booklet of pictures given to the child (there are 4 drawings on each page) and a list of vocabulary words read to the child (one word to go with each page). As the word is read for each page, the child is instructed to print to (or otherwise signify) the one of the 4 drawings that best matches the word. As an IQ test for young children, should be considered a screening instrument only.
The Quick Test (QT)	Mental age, IQ after 20 years of age	1½ yr-adult	Designed to provide a rough estimate (screening) of IQ in childhood, although IQs vary from those provided by general intelligence tests. Child is asked to indicate which of 4 pictures on a page best matches a spoken vocabulary word
Rorschach Test	Psychosexual adjustment; personality traits	3 or 4 yr-adult	The famous and controversial projective test utilizing inkblots to study personality and diagnose psychiatric disorders. Child is shown a series of 10 cards, each with a bilaterally symmetrical inkblot, and is asked to describe what the picture could represent (what he or she ''sees'' in it). Content of reports is analyzed, along with child's emotional responses, incidental remarks, etc.
Slosson Intelligence Test*	IQ	1 mo-adult	Largely similar to the Gesell Developmental Schedules for young children and to the Standford-Binet for older children and adults. A convenient, brief, screening test for children from 4 years on.
Stanford-Binet Intelligence Scale*	IQ	2 yr-adult	The original (although much revised) IQ test, generally considered the most accurate and the standard by which other tests are evaluated. Test items include eye-hand coordination and manipulation tasks (blocks, form board, beads for stringing, etc.), object identification, identification of missing parts of pictures, problem solving in everyday situations (''What should you do if . . . ?''), recognition of absurdities in stories or pictures, memory tests, etc., and extend upward through the range of verbal, computational, and logical problems for older children and adults.
Vineland Social Maturity Scale	Independence (self-reliance)	Birth to adult	Information about self-help skills and responsibility for self-care is gathered either from an adult who knows the child well or from the child. Scale items include, for example, reach, grasp, large motor mobility, following instructions, chewing food, using eating utensils, dressing and undressing, toileting, using writing utensils, bathing, routine household chores, reading and letter writing, and money management. Social age and social quotient are calculated by comparing child to age norms.
Wechsler Intelligence Scale for Children (WISC)	IQ	5-15 yr	WISC has verbal and performance subtests and produces verbal, performance, and full-scale IQs. Items include digit span, vocabulary, arithmetic, general information and comprehension, mazes, picture completion, picture puzzles, etc. Scores for average and above-average children are generally a few points higher than Stanford Binet scores.
Wechsler Pre-school and Primary Scale of Intelligence (WPPSI)	IQ	4-6½ yr	WPPSI is a downward extension of WISC and is of similar format. Also generally produces higher scores than the Stanford-Binet.

tool is easy to administer and score and provides information indicative of a child's overall readiness to attend kindergarten (Rogers and Rogers, 1972).

Additional Psychological and Intellectual Tests

Many screening tests have been developed with the intent of measuring various psychological and intellectual traits of childhood. Table 24-5 provides a summary of such screening tools that may be useful for the nurse dealing with pediatric patients within the community.

Immunizations

Continuation of the basic immunization schedule implemented in infancy is indicated for the toddler and preschooler. The reader is referred to the immunization section of Chapter 23 and Appendix E for a full discussion of immunizations.

Nutrition

The promotion of nutritionally sound dietary habits remains important during the toddler and preschool years. (See the section on nutrition in Chapter 23 for a review of the basic nutrition principles indicated for children.) Throughout the first year infants will develop significantly in the types and amounts of food they can eat. They will progress from having to be fed to insisting on feeding themselves. As a child progresses through the toddler and preschool years, nutritional status and eating is affected by a decreasing physical growth rate, motor maturity, and cognitive and personality factors. They can now feed themselves and demonstrate food preferences and individual eating habits, thereby exerting an influence over their nutritional status. In assisting parents to maintain nutritional adequacy for their toddler or preschooler, the following suggestions can be made:

Offer a balanced diet that meets recommended daily allowances for age (Table 23-24), incorporating food preferences and variety.

Offer food several times a day (i.e., five to six times versus three regular meals).

Limit milk intake to 16 ounces a day to avoid a filling up on milk instead of eating solids as well as milk.

Offer suggested amounts of food as listed in Table 24-6.

Emphasize favorites that are nutritional and can be self-fed.

Continue to avoid nuts, bony fish, popcorn because of risk of aspiration.

Generally vitamin and iron supplements are not required. However, during periods when appetite and intake decrease, temporary use is appropriate. During this period, nutritionally sound foods (es-

pecially those high in iron and low in sugar) should be offered more frequently.

Diet Assessment

Since toddlers and preschoolers can be unpredictable in regard to the quantity as well as the quality of what they eat, periodic assessment is indicated in determining nutritional adequacy. Appendix A illustrates age-appropriate diet histories. Factors specific to this age group which require consideration in the nurse's assessment and management include the need for (1) increased caloric intake; (2) 10% to 15% protein, 50% carbohydrate, and 35% fat caloric distribution; and (3) increased water intake.

HEALTH PROMOTION ACTIVITIES

The community health nurse can assist families to promote toddler and preschooler well-being in a variety of ways and settings. Many of these activities have been discussed throughout this chapter, but several warrant reemphasis.

Health Assessment

The continuation of an orderly assessment of health is essential during the toddler and preschool years. (Appropriate health assessment tools are included in the appendix section of this text.) The health assessment visit needs to be implemented on a regular basis and should focus on promoting health-oriented behaviors in the parent and child. Parent education and anticipatory guidance from nurses are two means for promoting such behaviors, as is emphasis on preventive health measures, particularly safety and accident prevention (see Appendix J). In addition, the nursing management plan for health maintenance activity needs to include the child's participation. For example, even at the age of 2 to 3 years, a child can be taught and encouraged to brush his teeth, thereby promoting dental health. Finally, the use of screening tools during the health assessment visit, which are designed to assess physical and psychosocial development, are particularly important in the rapidly changing toddler and preschooler. Age-appropriate tools were discussed earlier in the text and in Appendixes A and J.

Parenting Groups

Parenting groups are an additional way the community health nurse can promote health. Being the parent of a toddler or preschooler can be stressful for both parent and child. Assisting parents to understand and be knowledgeable about their child's developmental phase should be a nursing focus. Courses on parenting techniques are a possible mechanism nurses can use. Table

Table 24-6. Recommended food intake for good nutrition*

Food group	Servings per day	Average size of servings					
		1 year	2-3 years	4-5 years	6-9 years	10-12 years	13-15 years
Milk and cheese 1.5 oz cheese = 1 cup milk (1 cup = 8 oz or 240 gm)	4	½ cup	½-¾ cup	¾ cup	¾-1 cup	1 cup	1 cup
Meat group (protein foods)	3 or more						
Egg		1	1	1	1	1	1 or more
Lean meat, fish, poultry (liver once a week)		2 tb	2 tb	4 tb	2-3 oz (4-6 tb)	3-4 oz	4 oz or more
Peanut butter			1 tb	2 tb	2-3 tb	3 tb	3 tb
Fruits and vegetables	At least 4, including:						
Vitamin C source (citrus fronts, berries, tomato, cabbage, cantaloupe)	1 or more (twice as much tomato as citrus)	⅓ cup citrus	½ cup	½ cup	1 medium orange	1 medium or- ange	1 medium or- ange
Vitamin A source (green or yellow fruits and vegetables)	1 or more	2 tb	3 tb	4 tb (¼ cup)	¼ cup	⅓ cup	½ cup
Other vegetables (potato and legumes, etc.) or	2	2 tb	3 tb	4 tb (¼ cup)	⅓ cup	½ cup	¾ cup
Other fruits (apple, banana, etc.)		¼ cup	⅓ cup	½ cup	1 medium	1 medium	1 medium
Cereals (whole-grain or enriched)	At least 4						
Bread		½ slice	1 slice	1½ slices	1-2 slices	2 slices	2 slices
Ready-to-eat cereals		½ oz	¾ oz	1 oz	1 oz	1 oz	1 oz
Cooked cereal (including macaroni, spaghetti, rice, etc.)		¼ cup	⅓ cup	½ cup	½ cup	¾ cup	1 cup or more
Fats and carbohydrates	To meet caloric needs						
Butter, margarine, mayonnaise, oils: 1 tb = 100 calories (kcal)		1 tb	1 tb	1 tb	2 tb	2 tb	2-4 tb
Desserts and sweets: 100-calorie portions as follows: ⅓ cup pudding or ice cream, 2 3-inch cookies, 1 oz cake, 1⅓ oz pie, 2 tb jelly, jam, honey, sugar		1 portion	1½ portions	1½ portions	3 portions	3 portions	3-6 portions

From Vaughan, V.C., and McKay, R.J.: Nelson textbook of pediatrics, ed. 11, 1979, W.B. Saunders Co. p. 189. 1979, ed. 11
*Based on food groups and the average size of servings at different age levels.

Table 24-7. Content outline for group of parents of toddlers

Session	Topic and content
First	Introduction and getting to know each other Discussion of development theories and tasks of age group Review of mastery, investigation, testing, and manipulating
Second	An age of activity: in or out of control Discussion about toddler behaviors: temper tantrums, negativism, jealousy, sibling rivalry, ritualism, separation behaviors, regression
Third	Approaches to toddler behaviors Discussion about limit setting and discipline
Fourth	Changing physically and learning to control body functions Discussion about toilet training, sleeping, eating, and self-comforting behaviors and patterns Considerations about how to handle safety considerations
Fifth	The necessity of play and learning sex role Discussion of learning through play Review of ideas about toys, television, playmates, play groups, and nursery school Discussion of sex role identification and factors influencing this
Sixth	Speech and learning to express self Discussion of timetable, reinforcement, nonverbal activities

24-7 illustrates an overview of course content for a group of parents of toddlers.

Additional health promotion mechanisms appropriate for the toddler or preschool child are discussed in Chapter 23 under this heading.

COMMUNITY RESOURCES

Identification of available community resources is the nurse's responsibility. Groups or services that may be beneficial for parents of a child in this age group are listed in Chapter 23.

BIBLIOGRAPHY

American Academy of Pediatrics: Report of the Committee on Infectious Diseases, ed. 19, Evanston, Ill., 1982, The Academy.

Barnard, M.U., et al.: Handbook of comprehensive pediatric nursing, New York, 1981, McGraw-Hill Book Co.

Brown, M.S., and Murphy, M.A.: Ambulatory pediatrics for nurses, ed. 1, New York, 1975, McGraw-Hill Book Co.

Bunch, W.H.: Common deformities of the lower limb, Pediatr. Nurs. **5:**18-25, July-Aug. 1979.

Caffey, J.: The whiplash shaken infant. Manual shaking by the extremities with whiplash-induced intracranial and intraocular bleedings, linked with residual permanent brain damage and mental retardation, Pediatrics **54:**396-403, Oct. 1974.

Caplan, F., and Caplan, T.: The power of play, New York, 1973, Anchor Press.

Carver, D.H., and Seto, D.S.Y.: Hepatitis A and B, Pediatr. Clin. North Am. **21:**674, Aug. 1974.

Chow, M.P., et al.: Handbook of pediatric primary care, New York, 1979, John Wiley & Sons, Inc.

Curtis, J.: Working mothers, New York, 1976, Simon & Schuster, Inc.

DeAngelis, C.: Pediatric primary care, ed. 2, Boston, 1979, Little, Brown & Co.

Drumwright, A.F.: Denver Articulation Screening Examination: scoring and interpretation instructions, Denver, 1971, University of Colorado Medical Center.

Ducroquet, R., Ducroquet, J., and Ducroquet, P.: La marche et les boiteries, Paris, 1965, Masson. English translation: Walking and limping, Philadelphia, 1968, J.B. Lippincott Co.

Duvall, E.: Marriage and family development, Philadelphia, 1977, J.B. Lippincott Co.

Erikson, E.: Childhood and society, New York, 1963, W.W. Norton & Co., Inc.

Fontana, V.J., and Robinson, E.: A multidisciplinary approach to the treatment of child abuse, Pediatrics **57:**760-764, May 1976.

Fraiberg, S.: The magic years, New York, 1959, Charles Scribner's Sons.

Furlong, G.P., and Lawn, G.W.: Evaluation of foot deformities in the newborn, Gen. Practitioner **31:**89-87, Nov. 1965.

Healthy people: Public Health Service, DHEW (PHS) Pub. No. 79-55071, Washington, D.C., 1979, Department of Health, Education and Welfare.

Kempe, C.H.: Approaches to preventing child abuse, Am. J. Dis. Child. **130:**941-947, Sept. 1976.

Kempe, C.H., and Helfer, R.: Helping the battered child and his family, Philadelphia, 1972, J.B. Lippincott Co.

Kempe, C.H., and Hopkins, J.: The public health nurse's role in the prevention of child abuse and neglect, Public Health Curr. **15:**1-4, May 1975.

Krugman, S., Ward, R., and Katz, S.L.: Infectious diseases of children, ed. 6, St. Louis, 1977, The C.V. Mosby Co.

Lancaster, J.: Coping mechanisms for the working mother, Am. J. Nurs. **8:**1322-1324, Aug. 1975.

Lenneberg, E.H.: The natural history of language. In Smith, F., and Miller, G.A., editors: The genesis of language, Cambridge, Mass., 1966, The M.I.T. Press.

Lenneberg, E.H.: Biological foundations of language, New York, 1967, John Wiley & Sons, Inc.

Lowell, J.D.: Congenital hip dysplasia, Clin. Pediatr. **3:**279-287, May 1964.

Maier, H.: Three theories of child development, New York, 1969, Harper & Row Publishers, Inc.

Maternal and Child Health Program: Evaluation of body size and physical growth of children, The Maternal and Child Health Program, 1976, Washington, D.C., Department of Health, Education and Welfare.

Parten, M.: Social participation among preschool children, J. Abnor. Soc. Psychol. **4:**242-245, March 1932.

Pipes, P.L.: Nutrition in infancy and childhood, St. Louis, 1981, The C.V. Mosby Co.

Rogers, W.B., Jr., and Rogers, R.A.: A new simplified preschool readiness experimental scale (PRESS), Clin. Pediatr. **11:**558-562, Oct. 1972.

Scipien, G., et al.: Comprehensive pediatric nursing, ed. 2, New York, 1979, McGraw-Hill Book Co.

Spector, R.E.: Cultural diversity in health and illness, East Norwalk, Conn., 1979, Appleton-Century-Crofts.

Stanisavljeuic, S.: Diagnosis of congenital hip pathology in the newborn, Baltimore, Md., 1964, Williams & Wilkins.

Tachdjian, M.O.: Pediatric orthopedics, vol. 1, Philadelphia, 1972, W.B. Saunders Co.

Tackett, J.J., and Hunsberger, M., editors: Family centered care of children and adolescents, Philadelphia, 1972, W.B. Saunders Co.

Todd, T.W.: Atlas of skeletal maturation, St. Louis, 1937, The C.V. Mosby Co.

Vaughan, V.C., McKay, R.J., and Behrman, R.E., editors: Nelson textbook of pediatrics, ed. 11, Philadelphia, 1979, W.B. Saunders Co.

Waechter, E., and Blake, F.: Nursing care of children, ed. 9, Philadelphia, 1976, J.B. Lippincott Co.

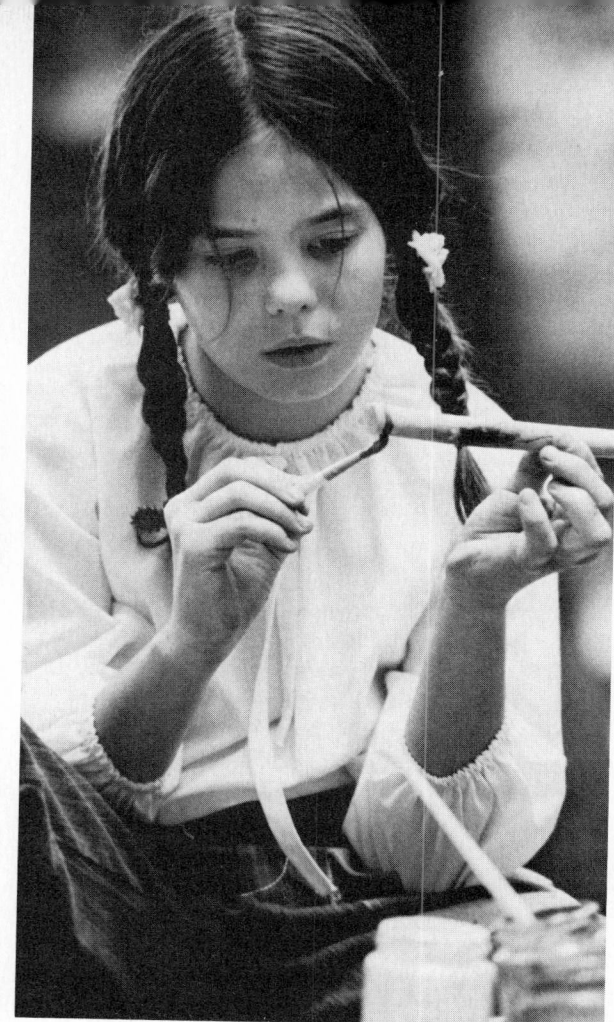

Chapter 25

NANCY DICKENSON-HAZARD

SCHOOL AGE CHILDREN AND ADOLESCENTS

Both the school age child and the adolescent live in rapidly expanding worlds. The life experiences confronting them are diverse and complex. Although the health of this nation's children and adolescents is better than ever, school age and adolescent persons are confronted with health problems more complex than those of preceding generations. School and societal influences create multiple dilemmas for these age groups. Nurses in community health settings are in a position to educate school age children and adolescents regarding these dilemmas and the subsequent influence on health. These educational encounters may occur in the school, the clinic, or in the home. It is hoped that the promotion of positive health behaviors by community health nurses during this period of life will contribute to establishing a healthy nation.

This chapter will focus on the health assessment, maintenance of health, and health promotion activities germane to the school age child and adolescent. The physical and psychosocial aspects of health will be reviewed as well as significant factors that can positively or negatively influence health behavior.

PHYSICAL GROWTH AND DEVELOPMENT OF SCHOOL AGE CHILDREN

The period of life from 6 to 12 years is characterized by steady physical growth, neuromuscular refinement, and rapid expansion of cognitive and social skills. During this phase of life, physical, and psychosocial mastery of the expanding environment is the primary task.

Physical Competency

Physical competency of the school age child is assessed through measures of physical growth and indicators of normal development, that is, neuromuscular ability, sensory organ development, and tooth shedding and eruption. However, the developmental pace within each of these areas is highly individualized from child to child. The nurse's awareness of the factor of individuality as well as knowledge of "usual" development provides the basis of an accurate assessment.

Changes in Height and Weight

Physical growth in the younger school age child is reflected by an average annual gain of 2 in (5.5 cm) in height and 5.5 lb (2.5 kg) in weight. In general, boys are an average of 1 inch taller and 2 pounds heavier than girls until approximately ages 9 to 10. At this time girls begin to grow more rapidly in height and weight, and by age 12, girls are generally 2 pounds heavier and 1 inch taller than boys. The preadolescent growth spurt usually occurs between 9 and 14 years for girls and between 12 and 16 years for boys (Tanner, 1962).

Skeletal Growth

Physiological changes continue through school age years, which reflect continued maturation and refinement. Skeletal growth in the trunk and extremities is steady, with most of the hand and feet bones present but not complete. Evidence of small and long bone ossification is present. Remodeling of the facial bones is evidenced by visualization of frontal sinuses on x-ray film and a change in eustachian tube positioning to a more downward, anterior direction. As skeletal growth progresses over the school age years, changes in overall body appearance and posture occur. The stoop shoulder, slightly lordotic posture with a prominent abdomen develops into a more erect posture by the end of this period.

Dental Growth

Dental growth is most prominent during the school age years. By the tenth year, all primary teeth have been shed and permanent teeth have erupted, with the exception of the second and third molars (see Fig. 23-4). The sequence of shedding and eruption is important to proper occlusion, or the alignment of the chewing surface of the maxillary teeth to the mandibular teeth when the jaws are closed.

Cardiovascular Functioning

Cardiovascular functioning continues to be refined. The heart rate drops to an average of 65 to 90 beats per minute, the hemoglobin stabilizes around 12 to 13 g, and arterial blood pressure normalizes. The heart size has increased six times the original newborn size and growth is fairly complete. Respiratory function and rates have stabilized and lung growth is minimal.

Gastrointestinal System

Physical changes to the gastrointestinal system are few although the stomach capacity continues to expand. The liver is high within the abdominal cavity and normally cannot be palpated. The urinary system has expanded, increasing bladder capacity to 1000 ml/24 hours. Bowel and bladder control is usually well established.

Patterns of Sleep and Eating

The sleeping and eating patterns of the school age child are relatively stable. The sleep requirement varies from 8 to 10 hours a night, and the number of meals is usually three plus one or two light snacks. Nutritional needs will increase slightly for quantity rather than quality (see Tables 23-19 and 24-6). These patterns are disrupted, however, during the preadolescent and adolescent growth spurt when caloric and water requirements increase along with appetites.

Sexual Growth

The ages of 10 to 12 are generally considered the prepubertal years. Before this age sexual growth is minimal. However, during the prepubertal period sexual characteristics become visible and maturation begins. A detailed discussion follows in the section on adolescent physical growth and development.

Neuromuscular Development

The central nervous system continues to mature slowly. Neuromuscular skills are refined and expanded. Sensory organ development is fine tuned and cognitive skills increase. The school age child should be able to perform a wide range of physical skills. Table 25-1 presents an overview of all aspects of school age growth and development on which a nursing assessment should be based.

PHYSICAL GROWTH AND DEVELOPMENT OF THE ADOLESCENT

The period of life from 13 to 18 years is characterized by a steady progression of physiological changes. The resultant changes in physical appearance and body function require adolescents to adapt their body image and to adjust to the maturing body. These physical changes, coupled with the emotional, psychological, and social adaptations of adolescence, push the young person to learn to develop coping mechanisms that will be carried throughout life.

Age (years)	Physical competency	Intellectual competency	Emotional-social competency	Nutrition	Play	Safety	Immunizations
6-12 (General)	Gains an average of 2.5-3.2 kg/year (5½-7 lb/yr). Overall height gains of 5.5 cm (2 in) per year; growth occurs in spurts and is mainly in trunk and extremities. Loses deciduous teeth; most of permanent teeth erupt. Progressively more coordinated in both gross and fine motor skills. Caloric needs increase with growth spurts.	Masters concrete operations. Moves from egocentrism; learns he is not always right. Learns grammar and expression of emotions and thoughts. Vocabulary increases to 3000 words or more; handles complex sentences.	Central crisis: industry vs. inferiority; wants to do and make things. Progressive sex education needed. Wants to be like friends; competition important. Fears body mutilation, alterations in body image; earlier phobias may recur, nightmares; fears death. Nervous habits common.	Fluctuations in appetite result from uneven growth pattern and tendency to get involved in activities. Tendency to neglect breakfast caused by rush of getting to school. Though school lunch is provided in most schools, child does not always eat it.	Plays in groups, mostly of same sex; "gang" activities predominate. Books for all ages. Bicycles a must. Sports equipment. Cards, board, and table games. Most of play is active games requiring little or no equipment.	Enforce continued use of safety belts during car travel. Bicycle safety must be taught and enforced. Teach safety related to hobbies, handicrafts, mechanical equipment.	
6-7	Depth perception developed. Vision reaches adult level of 20/20. Gross motor skill exceeds fine motor coordination. Balance and rhythm are good—runs, skips, jumps, climbs, gallops. Throws and catches ball. Dresses self with little or no help.	Vocabulary of 2500 words. Learning to read and print; beginning concrete concepts of numbers, general classification of items. Knows concepts of right and left; morning, afternoon, and evening; coinage. Intuitive thought process. Verbally aggressive, bossy, opinionated, argumentative. Likes simple games with basic rules.	Boisterous, outgoing, and know-it-all, whiney; parents should sidestep power struggles, offer choices. Becomes quiet and reflective during 7th year; very sensitive. Can use telephone. Likes to make things: starts many, finishes few. Give some responsibility for household duties.	Preschool food dislikes persist. Tendency for deficiencies in iron, vitamin A and riboflavin; 100 ml/kg of water per day; 3 gm/kg protein daily.	Still enjoys dolls, cars, and trucks. Plays well alone but enjoys small groups of both sexes; begins to prefer same sex peer during seventh year. Ready to learn how to ride a bicycle. Prefers imaginary, dramatic play with real costumes. Begins collecting for quantity, not quality. Enjoys active games such as hide-and-seek, tag, jump rope, roller skating, kickball. Ready for lessons in dancing, gymnastics, music. Restrict TV time to 1-2 hours/day.	Teach and reinforce traffic safety. Still needs adult supervision of play. Teach to avoid strangers, never take anything from strangers. Teach cold prevention and reinforce continued practice of other health habits. Restrict bicycle use to home ground; no traffic areas; teach bicycle safety. Teach and set examples regarding harmful use of drugs, alcohol, smoking.	TOPV and DPT boosters if not received by age 6.

Adapted from Smith, E.C.: Growth and development of school age child: maintaining wellness. In Tackett, J.J., and Hunsberger, M., editors: Family centered care of children and adolescents, Philadelphia, 1981, W.B. Saunders Co., pp. 1086-1087.

Continued.

Table 25-1. Competency development of the school age child – cont'd

Age (years)	Physical competency	Intellectual competency	Emotional-social competency	Nutrition	Play	Safety	Immunizations
8-10	Myopia may appear. Secondary sex characteristics begin in girls. Hand-eye coordination and fine motor skills well established. Movements are graceful, coordinated. Cares for own physical needs completely. Constantly on move; plays and works hard; enforce balance in rest and activity. Vision and hearing fully developed.	Learning correct grammar and to express feelings in words. Likes books he can read by himself; will read funny papers, scan newspaper. Enjoys making detailed drawings. Mastering classification, seriation, spatial and temporal, numerical concepts. Uses language as a tool; likes riddles, jokes, chants, word games. Rules guiding force in life now. Very interested in how things work, what and how weather, seasons, etc., are made.	Strong preference for same-sex peers; antagonizes opposite-sex peers. Self-assured and pragmatic at home; questions parental values and ideas. Has a strong sense of humor. Enjoys clubs, group projects, outings, large groups, camp. Modesty about own body increases over time; sex conscious. Works diligently to perfect skills he does best. Happy, cooperative, relaxed and casual in relationships. Increasingly courteous and well-mannered with adults. Gang stage at a peak; secret codes and rituals prevail. Responds better to suggestion than dictatorial approach.	Needs about 2100 calories/day; nutritious snacks. Tends to be too busy to eat. Tendency for deficiencies in calcium, iron, and thiamine. Problem of obesity may begin now. Good table manners. Able to help with food preparation.	Likes hiking, sports. Enjoys cooking, woodworking, crafts. Enjoys cards and table games. Likes radio and records. Begins qualitative collecting now. Continue restriction on TV time.	Stress safety with firearms. Keep them out of reach and allow use only with adult supervision. Know who the child's friends are; parents should still have some control over friend selection. Teach water safety; swimming should be supervised by an adult.	TD vaccine if series not previously received.

| 11-12 | Vital signs approximate adult norms. Growth spurt for girls; inequalities between sexes increasingly noticeable; boys attain greater physical strength. Eruption of permanent teeth complete except for third molars. Secondary sex characteristics begin in boys. Menstruation may begin. | Able to think about social problems and prejudices; sees others' points of view. Enjoys reading mysteries, love stories. Begins playing with abstract ideas. Interested in whys of health measures and understands human reproduction. Very moralistic; religious commitment often made during this time. | Intense team loyalty; boys begin teasing girls and girls flirt with boys for attention; best friend period. Wants unreasonable independence. Rebellious about routines; wide mood swings; needs some times daily for privacy. Very critical of own work. Hero worship prevails. "Facts of life" chats with friends prevail; masturbation increases. Appears under constant tension. | Male needs 2500 calories/day; female needs 2250 (70 calories/kg/day); 75 ml/ kg of water per day; 2 g/kg protein daily. | Enjoys projects and working with hands. Likes to do errands and jobs to earn money. Very involved in sports, dancing, talking on phone. Enjoys all aspects of acting and drama. | Continue monitoring friends; Stress bicycle safety on streets and in traffic. |

Puberty

Puberty refers to the biological stage of development during which physical changes occur that make reproduction possible. Adolescence refers to the psychological maturation of this stage (Tackett and Hunsberger, 1981). Young persons mature at different rates and will complete puberty and adolescence at varying times.

Height and Weight

Physical growth during adolescence is accelerated, with both males and females achieving their final mature height by the end of puberty. The majority of this growth occurs over a 2- to 3-year span and begins 2 years earlier for females than males. For females, this growth spurt normally begins at approximately 9½ years, peaks at 12 years, and stops by 14 years. The height spurt for boys begins at approximately 10½ years, peaks at 14 years, and ends at 16 years. Boys will average an 8-inch height gain while girls average a 3-inch gain during this time (Tanner, 1962). In addition, growth follows a pattern for both sexes. Initially legs lengthen first, followed by widening of thighs, broadening of shoulders, and trunk growth.

Skeletal Growth

As skeletal mass doubles during adolescence, significant gains in weight are noted. In addition, muscle (lean body mass) and primarily fat (nonlean body mass) double. Muscles increase in number of cells and in size for males whereas only an increase in size is noted in females. Conversely, females average twice as much body fat as males when physical maturation is completed (Vaughan et al., 1979).

Cardiovascular Function

During this growth period the body is changing physiologically as well. The heart demonstrates a rapid increase in size, resulting in the same size, shape, and location as the adult heart. The heart rate stabilizes at 60 to 90 beats per minute with males having a slightly faster rate than females. Although hemoglobin and hematocrit levels in boys may elevate slightly, they are generally stabilized for girls. The lungs and respiratory system demonstrate growth as evidenced by the adult-shaped chest, the addition of tissue, and thicker chest walls. Respiratory rates slow to 16 to 20 for both sexes.

Gastrointestinal Tract

The gastrointestinal tract matures rapidly during puberty, and the stomach capacity may increase to 900 cc. The liver attains adult size and position as do other internal organs (spleen, pancreas, uterus). Bladder capacity also increases to up to 1500 ml/24 hours.

Sexual Maturation

Of great significance in the adolescent is the process of sexual maturation that occurs during puberty. Sexual maturation involves the development of primary and secondary sexual characteristics. Primary sex characteristics are those physical and hormonal changes necessary for reproduction. Secondary sex characteristics externally differentiate male from female (Tanner, 1962).

Females

Sexual growth is rapid during puberty and follows a specific sequence of events. In females, puberty occurs in the following sequence (Committee on Adolescence, 1968):

Initial enlargement of breasts
Appearance of straight pigmented pubic hair
Maximum physical growth
Appearance of kinky pubic hair
Menstruation
Growth of axillary hair

The timing of this sequential phenomena is highly individualized. However, menarche, in general, is occurring earlier with each generation (Daniel, 1977; Kreutner and Hollingsworth, 1978). Presently adolescent females are beginning to menstruate at an average age of 12 years with menarche occuring about the time the growth spurt ends. This timing of menstruation generally occurs within 5 years of beginning breast development (Tanner, 1962).

Males

In males, puberty occurs in the following sequence (Committee on Adolescence, 1968):

Beginning growth of the testes
Straight pigmented pubic hair
Beginning enlargement of the penis
Early voice changes
First nocturnal ejaculation
Kinky pubic hair
Age of maximum growth
Growth of axillary hair
Marked voice changes
Development of facial beard

The sequence of pubertal events in males follows a timetable as well. Generally the male growth spurt occurs at about the same time as penile growth and about a year after the increase in testicular size. These events usually occur at approximately 14 years of age (Tanner, 1962).

Hormonal Mechanism

All of the pubertal events are created by hormonal changes within the body when the hypothalamus begins to produce releasing factors. The gonadotrophic-releasing hormones then signal the pituitary to secrete gonadotrophin hormones. Once secreted, the gonadotrophic hormones stimulate cells in the ovary to produce estrogen and cells in the testes to produce testosterone. These hormones (estrogen and testosterone) are responsible for the development of secondary sex characteristics. See a basic text in physiology for a more detailed discussion.

Nurse's Role

Evaluation of normal sexual development is essential to the assessment of adolescent growth. The nurse must be able to determine the stage of sexual development, evaluate normal progression, identify any abnormalities of development, and educate adolescents in regard to the changes created by their sexual development. Tanner staging in the most widely used assessment tool. It defines sexual development in stages according to sex and developing secondary and primary sex characteristics. See Tanner (1962) for a detailed discussion.

PSYCHOSOCIAL DEVELOPMENT OF SCHOOL AGE CHILDREN

Erikson's Concepts

From the ages of 6 to 12 children expand their social and cognitive spheres. Erikson regards this stage as a period of striving to develop a sense of industry versus a sense of inferiority. To achieve this balance, school age children direct their energies (industry) toward becoming competent in these skill areas. Physical and cognitive abilities, however, are often lacking, and a sense of inadequacy and inferiority can result (Erikson, 1963). This sense of inferiority is inevitable for most school age children at some point in this phase of development. However, achieving the positive component of competency generally outweighs the negative aspect of inadequacy, because assets and liabilities are recognized and coping behaviors are developed which do not compromise self-esteem.

During this phase of development a child learns to become a productive member of a peer group. Peers of the same sex become important for judging one's success. Learning to contribute, collaborate, and work cooperatively in relationships toward a common goal becomes a measure of a child's success. In addition, the child works diligently to achieve and improve skills, because success at whatever task is being attempted is desired.

The achievement of these individual and group member competencies occurs gradually over the school age years. Table 25-2 outlines this progression.

Table 25-2. Competencies of the school age child

Age (years)	Typical behaviors
6	Constant activity; enjoys group activities
	Spontaneously dramatic
	Indecisive, explosive behavior; rudeness
	Strict literal conscience
	Cheating common; behaves differently at school than at home
	Eager to learn and help out
7	Cautious in play
	Self-critical; anxious to do things right
	Talkative; expressive language
	Beginning to understand time and money
	Assumes responsibility; concerned about what is right and wrong
	Sensitive to feelings of others; concerned about fairness
	Aware of sexuality; modest
8	Seeks out and initiates group activity
	Accepts responsibility with greater ease
	Friendships are tenuous and friendly; segregated by sex
	Begins to collect items
	Can recognize individual differences; evaluates own self
	Relates to past and present (time concepts)
	Begins to resent authority of parents but needs their support
9	Generally responsible and dependable
	More reasonable and independent
	Peer group and conformity as well as hero worship quite important
	Begins to see parents more realistically (they can be wrong, etc.)
	Expanding interests; increased ability to plan and to see a project through to completion
	Self-sufficient and self-critical; strong sense of right and wrong
	Increased awareness of sexuality and reproduction
10	Cooperative projects and activities dominate; follows and submits to rules
	Friends of same sex; companions and activities most important
	Beginning sexual maturation for girls
	Girls more socially mature than boys
	Develops distinct hobbies and interests
	Continues to appraise parents
11-12	Development of ``best friends''
	Feelings of opposition and dislike for opposite sex
	Characteristic sexual maturation more apparent, especially for girls
	Increase in physical and intellectual curiosity
	Group or clubs popular
	Secretive; demands privacy yet can be unruly, slovenly, and disrespectful
	Ambivalent feelings regarding parents and independence versus dependence
	May develop annoying overt behaviors, e.g., hair twirling and nail biting

Piaget's Concepts

The thought processes of school age children undergo significant change over this period of development. Piaget characterizes the cognitive competencies of 6- to 7-year-olds as intuitive. Thinking is based on the immediate unanalyzed relationships between events in the environment and the child's point of view. The child cannot consider wholes or parts simultaneously but focuses only on the whole or the part. A 6- or 7-year-old continues to consider and interpret things and events in relation to self. Consequently, organization and reasoning are not apparent in thought processes or conversation (Maier, 1969).

Between the ages of 8 and 10, cognitive abilities increase in reasoning and realism. According to Piaget, this state of concrete operations allows children to realize their way of thinking is not the only way. They are able to consider more parts of the whole while maintaining a concept of the whole. In addition, 8- to 10-year-olds are able to logically consider a problem or event, arriving at a conclusion or solution. This increased cognitive development allows children to expand their social and intellectual capacity by using the newly acquired abilities to differentiate, categorize, problem solve, conceptualize time and space, and understand causality (Maier, 1969).

The period of development from 6 to 12 years results in major changes for children physically, emotionally, and intellectually. Since these changes are gradual, the overall affect on abilities does not appear as dramatic as viewed for other developmental periods. However, the degree of growth in the child as a person is phenomenal. Table 28-1 provides an overview of the developmental accomplishments of this age group.

PSYCHOSOCIAL DEVELOPMENT OF THE ADOLESCENT

Erikson's View of Adolescence

Between the ages of 13 and 20, a person has the task of leaving childhood and becoming an adult. According to Erikson, adolescents must establish their own identity or be caught in confusion regarding their role (Erikson, 1963). As they approach adulthood, teenagers will contend with establishing intimate relationships or remaining socially isolated. Decisions regarding life-style and vocation are eminent. Peer and social spheres are expanding, and adult social and cognitive skills need to be developed. In addition, adolescents need to establish an emotional independence and equilibrium with their families as well as to adjust to and master their sexuality.

Developmental Tasks

Nine developmental tasks have been defined for adolescence (Havinghurst, 1972). These tasks include (1) accepting one's body and consolidating sex role; (2) expanding peer relationships to include both sexes; (3) gaining emotional independence from family members; (4) achieving economic independence; (5) selecting and preparing for a vocation; (6) developing adult intellectual skills and concepts; (7) becoming socially responsible; (8) preparing for marriage and family responsibilities; and (9) developing realistic values in harmony with the world.

Accomplishing these tasks demands concentrated energy and thought on the part of the teenager. When considering the profound nature of what must be achieved during this period, it is little wonder that the following behaviors and attitudes are characteristic: emphasis on importance of peers, submission and conformity to peer group, preoccupation, ambivalence, idealism, egocentricity, feelings of inferiority, rebelliousness, moodiness, noncommunication, and feelings of insecurity.

Piaget's View of Cognition

In the area of cognition adolescents expand their ability to reason logically at a concrete level and move into the stage of formal operation. According to Piaget, formal thinking involves thinking about thoughts and separating the real from the possible. At this stage, adolescents develop the ability to use abstract logic, examine relationships, construct hypotheses, and through deductive reasoning, logically test them (Maier, 1969).

These new cognitive abilities allow the adolescent to examine issues and values from differing points of view and to construct individual ideas and values. Thus teenagers can realistically plan their life events, fully understanding time sequence and consequence of their actions.

Morality

Moral development also changes during this period of formal thinking. Behaviors now reflect individual conscience and internalized principles rather than acceptance of rules of those in authority. Adolescents now make decisions based on what they perceive as best for them and as the conclusion of introspective thinking. The moral behaviors adolescents display are the result of their own thinking, conscience, and decision to act.

Adolescents struggle during this phase to establish their own identity. The final integration of physical, emotional, and cognitive skills will be evident in the adolescent development and demonstration of social behaviors. Table 25-3 provides an overview of the psychosocial development of the adolescent and school age child.

FACTORS INFLUENCING GROWTH AND DEVELOPMENT

As the child continues to grow and develop throughout the school and adolescent years, exposure to a multitude of new factors will influence progression through these stages. As for the earlier years, growth and development are affected by the degree of success or failure a child has had in mastering the tasks of preceding stages. (See Chapter 23 for an overview of factors affecting growth and development for preceding stages. These factors continue to be influential throughout the life span). However, unlike earlier years, a child is now equipped with more complex cognitive, physical, and social skills, and more complex tasks are faced. In addition, the degree of difficulty a child or adolescent experiences in accomplishing these more complex tasks during these current stages influences overall developmental expression.

Table 25-3. Social behavior development

	School age child	Adolescent
Love	Learns parents can be wrong. Sometimes can be disillusioned with own parents and would like to trade them in or is certain he or she is adopted. Learns to share some of own thoughts only with peers. Parents and home a place to return to for some companionship, comfort, and security.	Vascillating and expanding Within home: parents wonderful, wise, understanding, and deceitful, dishonest, and stupid. With peers: relationships intense and unstable. With world: idealistic and shallow.
Fears	Is superstitious.	Worries about loss of identity (bodily, emotionally). Worries about failure (in school, career, friendship). Is uncertain.
Play	Games show superstitions, teasing, insults Cooperative play—baseball, jacks, hopscotch. Peers of same sex important. Collections—a type of hoarding.	Develops skills in individual and group (games, sports, activities). Joins clubs, groups, sports. Cliques important—involve peers of same sex but with activities associated with opposite sex.
Dependency	Rejects some ideas of parents and tries own ideas, but usually returns to home base Reduces need for dependency by using rituals—bedtime, mealtime, bathtime.	High ambivalence between wanting limits and freedom. Discovers responsibility that comes with freedom.
Morality	Thinks of own needs first and is out to satisfy them. Can think of relationship between the act and following consequences. Begins to develop an idea of what it means to live by a label (good boy, good girl, bad boy, bad girl). Peer group begins to influence morality with fixed rules and rituals.	Begins to see that own actions effect a large group of individuals rather than just self. Beginning logical thought about own principles, rights, justice as compared with rest of community.
Self-image	Begins to see self within a label given by world (boy, girl, mean, nice, bully, cute, etc.)	Learned through group contact. Desire to be just like everyone else but more so. Try on many different roles. Hypochondriasis (excessive worry over body and bodily functions).
Habits	*Eating:* Eats meals with family and can sit through entire meal. Has definite likes and dislikes, but may change suddenly. Has rituals around mealtime—same location at table, same silverware, same food. *Bowels:* Needs no help from adults. *Sleeping:* May spend night away from home. *Dressing:* Can decide on own clothing and dress self, but may ask for help and then ignore it. Can comb own hair.	*Eating:* Many food fads. Constant eating. Worry over bodily functions leads to fad diets to correct specific problems. Would rather eat with peers than family. *Sleeping:* May get wound up in activities and sleep very little. May have trouble going to bed and getting up in morning. *Dressing:* Conforms with peers—clothing, hair, makeup, jewelry.

From Brown, M.S., and Murphy, M.A.: Ambulatory pediatrics for nurses, ed. 1, p. 311-312. Copyright 1975, McGraw Hill Book Co., New York. Used with permission of the publisher.

Role of Peers

Of singular importance to influences on growth and development is the role of peers. With the exception of one's family, a child's or adolescent's peer group exerts the greatest influence on development (Damon, 1977). It is with and through the peer group that a variety of developmental tasks are accomplished. Peers permit the individual to try out and even fail in new skills, to validate thoughts, feelings, and concepts, and to receive acceptance and support as a unique person. Conversely, a peer group can place demands and pressure on the individual to conform which create feelings of being uncomfortable or even inferior. The balanced affect of this peer influence can be positive at times, negative at others, and almost always lasting.

Role of Family

As the child's world expands outside of the home, the role of family influence changes. Since the child has and is developing individual thoughts and perceptions, parents no longer are viewed as the ultimate, all-knowing authority. A child and particularly the adolescent learn that parents are human; they make mistakes and do not have all the answers. Frequently parental values and ideas are questioned and differences and conflicts arise. Despite these confrontations, however, the child still needs parental love and support. Parental guidance, knowledge, and experiences continue to be used by their children as resources for verification of their own fast-developing repertoire of behaviors. Parental values, ideas, and expectations become a springboard for adolescents to develop their own. Although adolescents may diverge or digress from parental points of view, the influence remains and eventually affects decisions and behaviors (Sutterley and Donnelly, 1973)

Physical Well-being

The state of health and nutrition will affect a child's ability to grow and develop. Optimal mastery of skills and tasks occurs when physical well-being is optimal. Deficiencies in nutrition and problems with health alter an individual's sense of wellness and perceptions of self. Functioning at a diminished capacity creates difficulties in accomplishing complex tasks. Therefore promotion and maintenance of health and nutrition become important components in the normal developmental progression.

COMMON CAUSES OF MORBIDITY AND MORTALITY

Early Childhood

While the health of children in the United States is better now than 10 years ago, the slow decline in mor-tality remains of concern. A major contributor to this slow decline is the fact that 45% of all deaths occur as a result of accidents (Healthy People, 1979). This preventable cause of death requires the attention of health care professionals if the health of children is to continue to improve.

In addition to accidents, children ages 1 to 14 are victims of cancer, birth defects, influenza, and pneumonia (Healthy People, 1979). Although the mortality for these is relatively low as compared to accidents, their threat remains. Early recognition of symptoms and preventable measures are largely responsible for minimizing these problems. See Chapters 23 and 24 for a detailed discussion of birth defects and respiratory illness.

Screening for cancer through history and physical assessment is an important aspect of the nurse's role. Table 25-4 presents historical data indicative of childhood malignancies, which require immediate referral.

School Age Health Problems

School age children face significant health problems including learning and school difficulties; behavioral disturbances; speech, hearing, and vision problems; and infectious diseases of protozoan and bacterial origin. In addition, children today are rapidly developing risk factors that may eventually lead to adult disease and disability. For example, as many as 40% of the children ages 11 to 14 already demonstrate potential characteristics of heart disease, such as overweight, high blood pressure, and high cholesterol (Healthy People, 1979). To enhance healthy growth and development, the health care professional must be aware of these potential preventable risks and direct efforts toward their significant reduction.

Health in Adolescence and Early Adulthood

As measured by the usual mortality and morbidity indicators, the health of adolescents is relatively good. The death rate for adolescents and young adults is substantially below other age groups. However, this improvement in the death rate over other groups and over the years has not been sustained. In fact, individuals aged 15 to 24 years now have a higher death rate than 20 years ago. In 1960 the adolescent mortality was 106 deaths per 100,000. In 1977 this rate had increased to 117 deaths per 100,000, representing approximately 48,000 deaths in that year alone (Healthy People, 1979).

Violent death and accidents, particularly motor vehicle accidents, account for the majority of deaths in this age group. Three fourths of all deaths are specifically attributable to homicide, suicide, and accidents (Healthy People, 1979). The greater risk-taking that occurs in this age group leads to behaviors that are charac-

Table 25-4. Historical data for screening for childhood malignancies

	Family history	Review of systems
Leukemia	Related syndromes or diseases (i.e., Down's syndrome, immune deficient disease) Carcinogen exposure (e.g., radiation, immunosuppressive drugs)	Signs of anemia: pallor, excessive tiredness, decreased exercise tolerance Bleeding tendencies; excessive bleeding, nosebleeds, petechiae Recurrent infections—local or systemic
Central nervous system disorders	Congenital spine or skull defects Presence of CNS-related disorders (e.g., neurofibromas, tuberous sclerosis)	Signs of CNS dysfunction: headaches; visual problems, i.e., diplopia, nystagmus, decreased acuity; ataxia; vomiting without nausea and on waking; palsies and paresis
Wilms' tumor	Associated congenital anomalies (e.g., hemihypertrophy, hypospadias, cryptorchism, renal masses)	Signs of gastrointestinal dysfunction: abdominal pain, distention or enlargement, diarrhea, anorexia Signs of urinary dysfunction: hematuria General signs: fever, lethargy

Adapted from Wolf, W.J., and Bancroft, B.: Early detection of childhood malignancies, Pediatr. Nurs. 5;43-48, Jan.-Feb., 1980.

terized by aggressiveness, errors in judgment, and ambivalence, which more frequently result in death or injury.

Men of this age group are at particular risk. Their death rate is almost three times that of young women (Healthy People, 1979). Although chronic disease is not a leading cause of death, the behaviors and life-styles displayed by this young population may create a later susceptibility.

Adolescents also face other potential threats to health. Substance abuse, pregnancy, and sexually transmissible diseases are among the most common health-related problems for this age group. In 1977 between 60% and 75% of all adolescents reported experiences with alcohol and/or drug consumption. One fourth of American teenage girls have had at least one pregnancy by age 19 and between 8 to 12 million cases of sexually transmitted diseases are reported annually (Healthy People, 1979). To some extent the presence of these problems represents failure to assist adolescents to secure the help and information they require to solve problems and make decisions. Hence, when dealing with this age group, nurses in the community health setting should center priorities around preventive health and self-care education.

MAJOR HEALTH PROBLEMS OF SCHOOL AGE AND ADOLESCENT PERSONS

Among the major health problems affecting both school age children and adolescents are accidents and injuries. Since in few other areas of concern can prevention and health education play a major role, nursing's responsibility becomes one of promoting health through prevention.

Accidents

Motor vehicle accidents are responsible for more than 20% of all childhood deaths and 37% of adolescent mortality. Alcohol consumption has been implicated in many of the adolescent fatalities (Healthy People, 1979). Prevention of these accidents will require changes in behavior on the part of parents as well as children. The incorporation of safety education and accident prevention is a necessary component of each health maintenance visit. In addition, educational efforts need to be directed toward and involve the child or adolescent as well as parents. Appropriate anticipatory guidance is discussed in Appendix J.

Recreational Accidents

Most accidents among older children are related to recreational activity and equipment. Bicycles, swings, and skateboard injuries account for the most accidental morbidity. (See publications from the U.S. Consumer Product Safety Commission for information on toy and play equipment safety and maintenance.) For the preadolescent and adolescent, injuries from contact sports such as football and basketball are the primary causes of injury. Teaching and reinforcing the need to use and maintain proper recreational and sports equipment as well as safe participation are important factors in implementing safety education. In addition to educating the sports participant, nurses should also include sports personnel and teachers in this safety education. Although emphasis should remain on safety and accident prevention, such programs may also include advice on immediate management (first aid) of the sports injury and appropriate transport of the injured athlete (Smith, 1979).

Motorcycle Accidents

Adolescents are also at risk for motorcycle accidents. Of the individuals killed in motorcycle accidents in 1980 20% were under 20 years of age (National Safety Council, 1974). Of significance to the adolescent's involvement in motor vehicle accidents, including those on motorcycles, is their attitude about risk. Excessive speed has been found to be a major factor in almost half the vehicular accidents involving teenagers. Although shoulder and lap belts prevent serious injuries and fatalities, more than 70% of the adolescent population do not use them (Williams, 1976). Moreover, the use of helmet gear when motorcycling is significantly lower for adolescents than for any other population.

Assisting the adolescent to recognize and act positively in the prevention of these risks is a difficult task. However, reinforcement of safety education can be carried out during the health maintenance visit, in collaboration with school, through driver education classes, and through group health education seminars and workshops.

PROBLEMS SPECIFIC TO SCHOOL AGE CHILDREN

School Adjustment

Implied in the term *school age child* is the expansion of the child's world into the school sphere. Starting school creates a situation that will require adjustment on the part of the child and parent. No longer are the influences on the child's growth and development limited to the home, and both parent and child must now "let go" of some degree of security and comfort to allow the child to develop as an individual (Damon, 1977). Conflict often arises and home becomes a testing ground for new behaviors. Children must learn to cope with new challenges presented by school and peers, e.g. learning to be a productive group member, performing and mastering knowledge gained in school and assimilating the beliefs and values of others. Parents must allow their children to make decisions, accept responsibility, and learn from both positive and negative life experiences. Parents and children will need support and guidance to successfully adjust to the school experience.

Nurse's Role

The implications of nursing's involvement in facilitating parent and child adjustment are numerous. Nurses can promote adjustment to school by assisting individuals to identify potential stresses and by collaborating with parent, child, and teacher to prevent or minimize reaction. Primary areas of intervention include assisting parents to allow the freedom necessary for their child's development, assisting the child to cope with the social and cognitive demands of the school setting, and assisting teachers in dealing with problem or crisis situations involving the children and parent. Table 25-5 provides a plan of nursing intervention that facilitates school adjustment.

School Phobia

A problem unique to the school adjustment situation is school phobia, the persistent and abnormal fear of going to school. It occurs across all ethnic and socioeconomic groups with a slightly higher incidence in girls than in boys. The principal age groups affected are 7- to 9-year-olds and 12- to 14-year-olds. The initial complaints are generally a variety of somatic symptoms and conditions that prevent attendance. Occurrence of these symptoms is greater during the week and rare on weekends, holidays, or vacations. Generally more illness occurs in the fall, following holidays, and near times when tests or projects are due. The cause of this school anxiety behavior may be related to circumstances at home, at school, or both. Frequently identified factors include pressure to achieve, stressful relationships at school, fear of leaving home, and recent occurrence of a traumatic event associated with death, loss, or abandonment (Brosnan and Fond, 1980).

Nurse's Role

Assessment of the child with suspected school phobia includes a thorough history and physical examination with appropriate diagnostic and laboratory tests to rule out organic causes. Additional assessment tools that may be useful in determining the extent of the problem include the maintenance of a diary describing the child's daily activities and the administration of intellectual and emotional assessment tests such as the Wechsler Intelligence Scale for Children and the Goodenough-Harris Drawing Test.

The goal of management is to return the child to school. The approach to achieving this goal may involve the immediate return to school, home tutoring for a while, or permission for the child to return voluntarily (Brosnan and Fond, 1980). The choice of approach is based on the individual child and the circumstances that created the fear of school.

Further nursing interventions include supporting the child and family throughout the problem identification and school reentry process; assisting child and family to follow the management plan; assisting the child to de-

Table 25-5. Tasks of children, parents, teachers, and nurses in facilitating school adjustment

Statement of adjustment	Child's tasks	Parents' and teacher's role in facilitating task achievement	Nurse's role in assisting parents, teachers, child
Diffusion into larger world (5 or 6-8 yr)	1. Must adapt to differences in teacher's and parents' disciplinary approach and behavioral expectations.	1. Parents and teacher should communicate their respective expectations for the child to identify extreme differences and to work out compromises that permit him to meet expectations of each and so that parents and teachers can mutually reinforce their expectations.	1. School nurse can help organize parent-teacher interaction (e.g., preschool round-ups; parent-teacher-nurse conferences) or mediate in conflicts. a. During preschool roundup or school physical, learn what child's and parents' expectations for school are.
	2. Must compete with peers for teacher's attention and approval as teacher replaces parent for large portion of day.	2. Teachers should avoid obvious favoritism in classroom, give individual attention and praise to each child, avoid comparisons of achievement.	2. School nurse can offer guidance to teachers and intervene in unhealthy child-teacher relationships. a. During preschool registration or school physical, evaluate parent-child relationship for problems as these often carry over to teacher-child relationships.
	3. Must learn to handle blatant, hurtful honesty and downright rudeness of peers without damage to self-concept.	3. Peer activities and behaviors need close adult supervision.	3. Nurse in well-child facilities or schools can provide this guidance to parents and teachers.
	4. Needs to test out new ideas and behaviors in security of home environment.	4. Parents need to recognize developmental function of "trying on" ideas and behaviors incongruent with family's but set reasonable limits on how much and what type of "trying on" is to be allowed.	4. Nurse in well-child facilities or schools may offer this anticipatory guidance.
Disorganization created by disparities between home and school or peers (8-10 yr)	1. Must learn to concentrate on cognitive achievements as he settles into school life.	1. Parents and teachers need open communication about cognitive tasks that are being focused on at any one time and skills the child finds difficult so that both parties can support his mastery of those skills.	1. School nurse observations in classroom will help identify children having difficulty with this task. Investigation of state of health, sensory organ function, and neurological, physical, and emotional function should follow to determine source of problem in achieving task.
	2. Must learn to integrate peer values in a manner that does not deny family values and to transfer family values into larger world in socially acceptable ways.	2. Parents and teachers must understand that just as a child falls as he learns to walk, so will he fall as he learns to think. These falls during school age are typically boasting, teasing, fighting, lying, cheating, sassing and whining.	2. School nurses should regularly monitor playground and classroom activities to identify extricated children and then set the task force (parents, teachers, nurses, other pertinent school or health personnel) in motion to uncover source of problem and offer help.

From McElroy, E., and Tackett, J.J., Growth and development needs of the family with school age children: maintaining wellness. In Tackett, J.J., and Hunsberger, M., editors: Family centered care of children and adolescents, Philadelphia, 1981, W.B. Saunders Co., pp. 1044-1045; as adapted from Laige, J.: The school-aged child and his family. In Hymovich, D., and Barnard, M.: Family health care: developmental and situational crises, New York, 1973, McGraw-Hill Book Co.

Continued.

Table 25-5. Tasks of children, parents, teachers, and nurses in facilitating school adjustment

Statement of adjustment	Child's tasks	Parents' and teacher's role in facilitating task achievement	Nurse's role in assisting parents, teachers, child
		3. Teachers and parents need to develop the art of overlooking minor falls and feel comfortable seeking help for more serious or persistent falls. Children left alone with their peer group often overcome problems with peer assistance rather than adult intervention.	3. Well-child facility and school nurse should evaluate child's behavior patterns and self-concept at each contact to pick up clues that all is not well in his emotional and social relationships. Nurse in clinic or school should offer parental/teacher anticipatory guidance regarding handling of behavior problems.
Disposition of compromise between home and larger world (10-12 yr).	1. Must take increasing responsibility for initiating and carrying out own learning activities at school and home; find internal satisfaction in performance.	1. Family and teacher must acknowledge child's ability to manage responsibility and allocate responsibilities in which child can take pride and feel success.	1. Nurse in any setting in contact with parents and teachers may offer this anticipatory guidance. Nurse may be role model of such interactions in her dealings with child.
	2. Must take interest in organized school and peer activities to be accepted as a group member.	2. Parents need to see developmental advantage of child's involvement in organized activities and plan with child how he can get to these, financially handle the expenses involved, and still manage home and school responsibilities. Teachers should understand the need for such involvement and appropriate homework reasonably.	2. Same as 1 above. Nurse may help family learn about community activities available to children this age and of financial assistance available through schools, community clubs, churches.
	3. Must become capable of maintaining appropriate personal conduct (control impulses, resist temptation) with little or no adult supervision.	3. Child should be given increasing opportunity to go to school, religious, and peer functions unattended by parents and be praised for reports of good conduct. Digression from appropriate conduct should be dealt with in accordance with the seriousness of digression. Parents need to communicate faith in child's ability to handle himself adequately.	3. Same as 1 above.

velop coping behaviors that will positively affect self-concept and esteem; assisting parents and child to identify other potential support or professional services; and facilitating interaction and relationships between child and parents and school.

Other Behavior-related Problems

Enuresis and encopresis are two common behavioral problems that have a high incidence in school age chil-

dren. *Enuresis* is defined as involuntary urination in a child whose age and development are indicative of control. *Encopresis* is defined as fecal incontinence without an organic cause (Tackett and Hunsberger, 1981). When dealing with these problems as well as other behavioral-related problems, nurses must be cognizant of the following principles:

Prevention of these problems through early identification of children at risk is the primary approach

Each behavioral problem is the result of multiple causes that require assessment and management

The severity and extent of the symptoms vary from child to child

Nursing interventions require participation of the child and parents

Enuresis

Enuresis generally occurs in girls beyond 5 years of age and in boys 6 years or older. Males are generally more affected than females. Enuresis can occur during the daytime (diurnal) or at night (nocturnal) or at both times. In children who have never achieved bladder control the problem is referred to as *primary enuresis*. *Secondary enuresis* refers to loss of previously achieved bladder control for at least 3 to 6 months (Green and Haggerty, 1977; Vaughan et al., 1979).

Up to 25% of children will experience some bed-wetting, which generally occurs at times of illness or stress. These relapses are usually self-limiting and require minimal supportive therapy. More problematic relapses can be attributed to a variety of complex factors (Chow et al., 1979; Green and Haggerty, 1977):

Developmental delay in neuromuscular control or small functional bladder

Organic causes such as urinary tract infection or genitourinary tract obstruction

Deep sleep characterized by a high threshold for nocturnal arousal

Psychological-emotional factors such as loss, stress, or pressures

Before a management plan can be established, a detailed history recounting the enuretic episodes is essential (Brown and Murphy, 1975; Chow et al., 1979; Tackett and Hunsberger, 1981). See the box on this page for a list of pertinent history information. Organic cause must be ruled out as well, and it is appropriate to obtain a routine urinalysis, specific gravity, and functional bladder capacity data to determine the presence of an underlying problem.

Enuresis is a highly manageable and treatable condition. Management is most successful when carried out by the health professional with whom the child and family have developed a trusting rapport. The approach used must be agreeable to the child as well as the parents and varies for each situation. Potential management is discussed in the first box on p. 596 (Tackett and Hunsberger, 1981; Vaughan et al., 1979).

Encopresis

Encopresis generally occurs in children over 5 years and is more frequent in males. Bowel movements are usually constipated and some children actually experience fecal impaction and have a "soiling" problem. Pri-

---

Pertinent History Information for the Enuretic Child

- Amount and times of fluid intake
- Number of enuretic episodes per week or month
- Sleeping patterns
- Voiding patterns
- Any recent stressful events
- Occurrence at home and/or away from home or both
- Child's response to enuresis
- Emotional atmosphere of home
- Details of toilet training
- Family history of enuresis
- Past medical history

---

mary encopresis occurs in children who have never been toilet trained and secondary encopresis occurs in children who had at one time complete bowel control (Chow et al., 1979; Green and Haggerty, 1977).

Frequent causes of encopresis are chronic constipation or psychogenic problems associated with attention-gaining or regressive behaviors. Children who are encopretic may display compulsive behaviors and frequently have large amounts of stress in their lives. They express an unawareness of having a bowel movement and are generally quite distressed about the problem, as are parents (Vaughan et al., 1979).

A complete history must be obtained from the parents or child focusing on patterns of occurrence, bowel habits, and toilet training. The child's psychosocial development should also be explored through a history for significant loss or changes that pose threats to self-esteem. The establishment of a bowel routine is essential. Impactions require removal by use of enemas and a high-residue diet. Generally stool softeners are used.

Counseling and support are essential for the child and family, particularly if psychological problems have been identified. Education regarding nutrition, diet modifications, and fluid intake is also a necessary nursing responsibility. In addition, assisting parents and the child to deal with the anxiety created by this problem and identifying practical solutions (e.g. wearing extra underwear, skin care measures) are appropriate nursing interventions.

Physical Health Problems

Several health problems can increase in incidence during the school age years. Although some of these problems are acute in nature (e.g. bacterial and parasitic infections), others may be ongoing or chronic, reaching an intervention point when the child is older (e.g. den-

---

Management Approaches for Enuresis

Initial measures

Fluids are restricted after supper

Child voids before bedtime

Before retiring for night, parents should wake child to void

A night light is provided

Conditioning

Enuretone, a moisture-sensitive device that rings an alarm bell upon initiation of wetting, can be used

Imipramine (Tofranil), which exerts an anticholinergic effect on bladder muscle and/or an antidepressant effect on central nervous system, can be used

Bladder training (a behavior modification procedure)

Child drinks large fluid amount during day and retains urine as long as possible

When child must void, urine is measured and recorded in a daily log

Dry nights are recorded

Wall charts are maintained

Positive reinforcers such as stars or points are maintained for advances (e.g., two dry nights, dry all day, breaking record of previous voiding volume)

Counseling

Family and child should be encouraged to express feelings about enuresis

Parents and child should be informed that enuresis is not intentional and is no one's fault

Punitive or shaming techniques should be avoided

Explanation of the many variables involved in enuresis is essential for parents and child

Nurse should assist parents and child to accept problem

Nurse should help provide support for child

Nurse should maintain a positive attitude and assist parents and child to do the same

When organicity is ruled out, nurse should reassure parents and child that it is not the cause

---

Assessment for Child with Learning Disability

History

Complete history with emphasis on the following:

- Parental and child concern and perceptions
- School behaviors and performance
- Family history
- Pregnancy, birth, and infancy history
- Developmental history
- Past medical history

Physical examination

Complete physical assessment with emphasis on the following:

- Neurological examination for "soft" signs (i.e., perceptual or cognitive behaviors that persist beyond normal range)
- Evaluation of fine motor coordination
- Evaluation of sensory skills
- Evaluation of laterality and space orientation
- Evaluation of perceptual-motor function (visual-motor, auditory-motor, gross-motor)

Special studies and assessments

- Electroencephalogram
- School readiness screening tests
- Speech/hearing/language screening tests
- Educational/academic evaluation
- Psychological evaluation
- Perceptual motor function screening tests

Learning Disabilities

Approximately 10% to 30% of all school age children experience some degree of learning difficulty in school. The causes are complex, multifaceted, and often unidentifiable (Meier, 1976). In addition, many types of problems are frequently lumped under the labels of *learning disability* or *minimal brain dysfunction*. Table 25-6 identifies problems associated with learning disabilities, their probable causes and appropriate intervention (Chow et al., 1979; Meier, 1976).

Assessment of a child with learning difficulties involves a comprehensive evaluation involving specialists in language, education, psychology, and medicine (Rogers, 1976). Components of such an assessment are outlined in the above boxed material (Meier, 1976; Rogers, 1976). A management plan directed toward increasing the child's self-esteem and continuation with education is indicated.

Nurse's Role

Nursing activities can be implemented through the assessment and management. Participation in the early

tal caries or obesity). The nurse's responsibility is to provide intervention measures aimed at resolving the problem and to reinforce preventive measures that will abate reoccurrence. Appendix J discusses these health problems and appropriate nursing interventions. (American Academy of Pediatrics, 1982; American Dental Association, 1971; Krugman & Katz, 1981; Vaughan et al., 1979).

Table 25-6. Learning disabilities

Health problem definition	Etiology	Clinical signs	Interventions
Minimal Brain Dysfunction (MBD) Descriptive term for a child of average intelligence who has difficulty learning; a disorder in understanding or using language or adapting behavior	Associated with possible minimal insult to the central nervous system May result from infection, injury, chronic lead poisoning, or the slow maturation of brain function	Normal or above average intelligence May appear as learning, motor coordination, speech, or auditory difficulty, or combination of these Of children affected, 50% demonstrate ''soft signs'': they have short attention spans and mild speech impairment and are clumsy, impulsive, awkward, talkative, destructive, distractable, hyperactive, and socially immature	Management plan is provided by team and designed for individual child. Appropriate nursing interventions may include the following: Administrating screening tests Assisting parents to be consistent and to design a workable day-to-day schedule Supporting family when evaluating and venting their feelings Assisting parents to design a schedule that keeps frustrations and obstacles at a minimum Assisting parents to identify ways to positively reinforce desirable behaviors of child Teaching parents to keep directions and tasks simple Assisting parents to work with school, physician, and other therapists to implement plan Assisting family to identify useful community resources
Hyperactivity A behavior disorder with characteristic clinical manifestations resulting in non-goal-directed activity in inappropriate amounts	Most common of minimal brain dysfunction disorders, occurring more frequently in boys than girls Appears to involve a delay in the maturation of cerebral inhibitory function Dietary factors may be a contributing factor	Demonstration of characteristic behaviors of increased motor activity, short attention span, poor concentration, emotionally labile, easily distracted, prone to mood swings, and temper outbursts May be accompanied by learning difficulties and ''soft'' neurological signs	Medical management may include the following: Use of stimulant drugs (Ritalin and Dexedrine), which stimulate release of norepinephrine, thus producing a calming effect Salicylate-free diet that eliminates all artificial colors, flavors and salicylates Nursing interventions may include facilitating provision of the following (also see interventions for MBD): Structured external stimuli environment at home and school Special education classes Outlets for family feelings of frustration, inadequacy, guilt, tension, stress Avoidance of labeling child Support and encouragement
Dyslexia Inability to read or understand visual or oral printed symbols	May be primary dyslexia, which is usually familial and may be due to weakness of learning process or immaturity of brain May be developmental dyslexia resulting from cerebral dysfunction About 15% of children have reading skill difficulty and of these 3% are due to primary or developmental dyslexia; developmental dyslexia is more frequent in boys than girls	Demonstrates ability to hear and understand statement but cannot read Usually average or above-average intelligence Demonstrates difficulty distinguishing similar letters (*b* and *d*); may reverse letters when reading (*saw* for *was*); sees letter upside down or mirror image	Measures include the following (also see nursing interventions for MBD and hyperactivity): Early identification thorough screening at health assessment visits Assistance with reading instruction School and family working together Use of repetition and reinforcement Positive, relaxed home and school environment Provision of informal learning at home Games to improve reading and hand eye coordination Avoidance of negative reinforcement; praise and reassurance for child

identification, observation, and data collection is a nursing responsibility, as well as insuring appropriate referral and follow-up. Coordinating the activities of all disciplines involved in the evaluation and management frequently is the role for nursing. In addition, the nurse can best explain the problem to the parents and child and provide the support and encouragement needed for a successful outcome.

HEALTH PROBLEMS SPECIFIC TO THE ADOLESCENT

Physical Problems

Acne is a common clinical entity affecting an estimated 90% of the adolescent male and 80% of the adolescent female populations. Approximately one third of the female population experience an increase in papules or pustules in the week preceding menses. Acne is considered a disease of adolescence because of its onset at puberty and increased incidence during the teenage years. Although acne is self-limiting, it is a source of persistent embarrassment, disgust, and stress for the adolescent (Stone, 1982).

Presentation. Acne vulgaris is an inflammatory disease in which sebaceous glands overproduce sebum when stimulated by androgenic hormones. The sebaceous glands become plugged by sebum, debris, and skin scales, forming a hard plug in the opening or forming comedones along the canal of the oil gland. The oiliness of the skin is a productive environment for bacteria and frequently the skin bacterias *Corynebacterium acnes* and *Staphylococcus albus* become trapped in the comedones, creating a secondary inflammatory infection.

The presentation of this problem is seen as noninflamed comedones and/or inflamed papules, pustules, and nodulocystic lesions. The usual site is the face, but the neck, upper chest, back, and shoulders can be affected. The skin and hair are often oily. The initial assessment and data collection can be facilitated by using a questionnaire that focuses on the pertinent history, hygiene, medical, and social aspects of acne (Stone, 1982). In addition, the data can serve as an initiation point for discussion regarding this sometimes emotional problem. Appendix J includes an assessment tool useful in gathering data regarding adolescent acne.

Management. The treatment of acne involves medical management but client education and counseling are most influential to success. Management generally includes the following measures (Vaughan et al., 1979):

Thorough cleansing of the skin two to three times a day using warm water and a mild soap.

Drying and peeling lotions may be used overnight

Exposure to sun and wind

Frequent shampooing of the scalp

Proper diet with added liquids—no diet restrictions are indicated, but should the adolescent feel a certain food aggravates the acne, it should be avoided

Comedone removal by using extractor exerting gentle pressure

When indicated, systemic antibiotics (tetracycline), corticosteroids, injections, and minor surgery.

A multitude of topical medications are available for the treatment of acne. The most useful are the exfoliants. Preparations do vary in effectiveness, and their recommended use needs to be individualized to the client and severity of problem.

Education. Client education is most important for compliance with and success of therapy. Acne affects young persons at a time when they are struggling to create their own identity and are concerned about bodily image and peer opinion. The feedback adolescents receive from peers about themselves will influence their self-image and self-esteem. The presence of acne can disrupt receipt of positive peer feedback, affecting the adolescent's self-esteem. The first step in counseling a teenager about acne is to thoroughly explain its cause, its course, and the ways the adolescent can effectively manage and control it (Stone, 1982). The client must understand and be willing to accept responsibility for treatment. The social aspects of acne need to be discussed with clients as well as their feelings about the problem. In addition, clients must be aware of the realistic time frame for outcome and improvement. Acne is a chronic problem and the nurse must deal with the adolescent's expectations of treatment. Finally, follow-up is essential to the successful treatment of acne. Nurses can provide supportive care and reassurance during this time as well as assist the adolescent with other aspects of management.

Abnormal Spinal Curvatures

Abnormalities of the spinal curvature are most frequently detected during the adolescent growth spurt between the ages of 10 and 15 (Chow et al., 1979). These aberrations are exaggerations of the normal spinal curvature, which may result from organic or structural changes or as the consequence of persistent poor posture. Of particular concern is the incidence of kyphosis, lordosis, and scoliosis, which are illustrated in Fig. 25-1.

Kyphosis. Kyphosis is an exaggerated convex curve in the thoracic region resulting in a hump or hunchback appearance. Backache and pain generally accompany kyphosis, which may occur as a developmental lesion or secondary to a congenital deformity. Management of kyphosis will require immediate referral. Deformities that are minimal can be treated with Milwaukee braces. However, severe or congenital anomalies need surgical intervention.

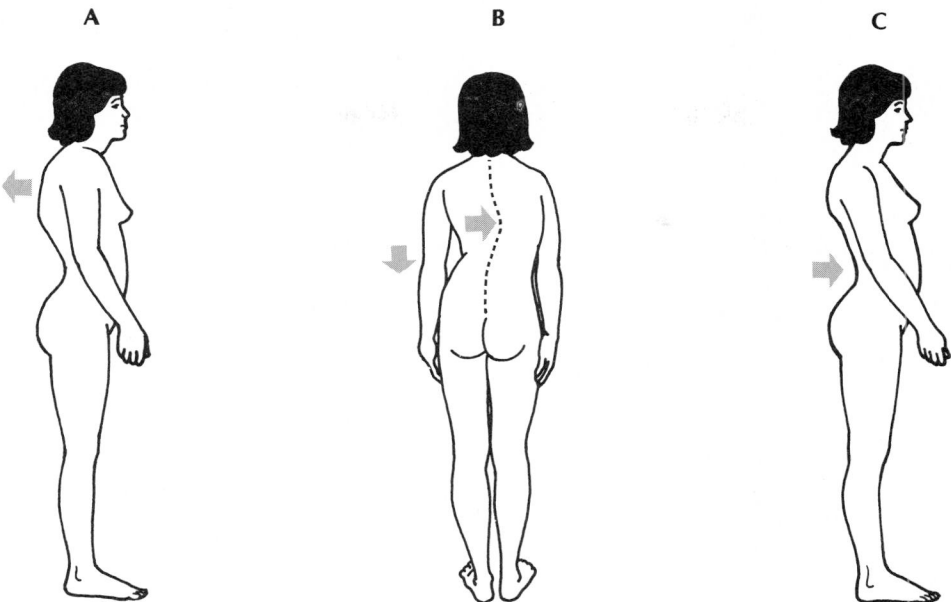

Fig. 25-1. Skeletal abnormalities of adolescence. **A**, Kyphosis: **B**, scoliosis; and **C**, lordosis. (From Tackett, J.J.: Potential stresses during adolescence; reversible alterations in health status. In Tackett, J.J., and Hunsberger, M., editors: Family centered care of children and adolescents, Philadelphia, 1981, W.B. Saunders Co.

Lordosis. Lordosis is an exaggerated concave curve in the lumbar region of the spine resulting in a sway-back appearance. A limp and pain are created by lordosis, which is largely caused by failure of hip flexors to stretch and elongate. Referral is indicated and treatment is similar to kyphosis.

Nurse's role. Since both kyphosis and lordosis are related to poor posture, nursing actions indicated should focus on assisting adolescents to develop an exercise program and learn proper sitting and standing. To achieve maximal success, a detailed explanation of the problem and its cause should precede development of a program. Incorporating activities of interest to the individual teenager further facilitates compliance and success (Dunn, 1975).

Scoliosis. Scoliosis is an S-shaped lateral curvature of the spine with rotation of vertical bodies. Scoliosis is classified as structural, indicating the curve is less flexible and not completely corrected by postural change, or functional/nonstructural, indicating no specific structural change. Further classification of structural scoliosis includes congenital curves associated with failure of vertebrae to form or segment; paralytic curves associated with polio or other neuromuscular disorders; and idiopathic curves associated with a high familial incidence. Immediate referral is indicated upon recognition of scoliosis. Treatment is aimed toward prevention of increasing deformity and may include use of a Milwaukee brace, traction, and surgery.

Nurse's role. The nurse's role lies in the early recognition of scoliosis and the provision of resources and support during the diagnosis, treatment, and follow-up stages. Early detection and implementation of a plan of care are essential to prevent the secondary complications of lung pathology and future back ailments. Thus screening for scoliosis is a necessary component of health assessment for school age children and adolescents (Dunn, 1975). Siblings of clients diagnosed with scoliosis particularly need screening because of the potential genetic etiology. Screening procedures are easily implemented in the school setting as well as in special clinics or in home. The procedure for screening requires complete exposure of back, chest, and hips and is based on observing the child when walking, standing erect, and bending forward.

Screening is implemented as follows:

1. Ask the child to bend forward in a 50% flexing position with shoulders drooping forward, arms and head dangling. Observe the spine from above the head and inspect for any lateral curvature or prominent projection of the rib cage on one side (Fig. 25-2).

2. While the child is standing erect with weight equal on both feet, observe for

    Difference in levels of shoulders, scapula, and hips

    Differences in the size of the spaces between the arms and the trunk

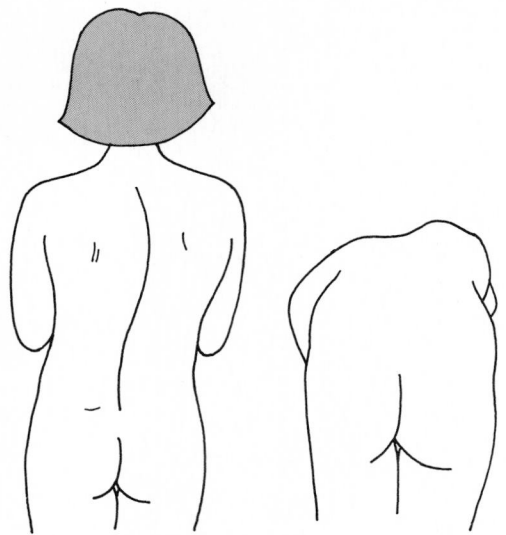

Fig. 25-2. Examination for scoliosis. Structural scoliosis is best demonstrated observing the child bending over. (From Common orthopedic conditions in childhood, Report of the Third Ross Roundtable on Critical Approaches to Common Pediatric Problems, in collaboration with the Ambulatory Pediatric Association, Seattle, Aug. 20, 1972.)

Prominence of either scapula or hip

A curve in the vertebral spinous process alignment

3. Ask the child to walk and make observations discussed in No. 2 and observe for the presence of a waddle, limp, or tilt.

Once problems are identified, nurses can act as advocates and liaisons for children with scoliosis. It is important to support and encourage as well as reassure the child and parents during the time of diagnosis and treatment. Whether the treatment is medical or surgical, child and parents need assistance in coping with the feelings created by the deformity and the ensuing treatment. Self-esteem, body image, and identity are disrupted for the teen. Parents may feel guilty and respond in an overprotective fashion. Both groups develop stress, anger, and worries about leading a normal life in the future. Nurses can facilitate the adjustment necessary to ensure such a normal life.

Each client and family must be dealt with in an individual manner. However, specific areas of intervention are indicated, particularly in the self-care of and adaptation to selected treatment methods. Table 25-7 provides guidelines by which an effective plan of nursing care can be implemented. (Anderson, 1979; Armstrong and Dickenson, 1975).

Menstrual Disorders

Disturbances in menstruation are common in adolescence, since the necessary hormonal balance can easily be disrupted. The stresses created by adolescence can delay, temporarily halt, or create uncomfortable menstrual cycles (Kreutner and Hollingsworth, 1978). In addition, being different from peers can create embarrassment and anxiety for the teenager experiencing menstrual difficulties. Seeking help for these problems is difficult, and once counsel has been sought, the teenager needs to receive reassurance, information about normal menstrual function, details about the difficulties she is experiencing, and information regarding the gynecological examination if such is indicated (Wells, 1977).

Menstrual variants frequently encountered in teenage girls are amenorrhea, dysmenorrhea, irregular cycles, and premenstrual tension.

Amenorrhea

Amenorrhea is a delay in the onset of menses. Primary amenorrhea is a temporary delay in girls over 17 years of age, generally accompanied by delays in other pubertal characteristics. Secondary amenorrhea is a delay between menstrual periods of 12 months or more during the 2 years after onset of menses or the absence of three or more periods (Vaughan et al., 1979). The goal of diagnostic procedure is to identify the cause of amenorrhea. To differentiate between primary and secondary amenorrhea, congenital malformation, hormonal insufficiency, pregnancy, and emotional or stress factors must be ruled out. Treatment is based on this differentiation and identification of causative factors. Primary amenorrhea created by delayed puberty requires no treatment, although hormonal supplementation may be used to initiate menses. Secondary amenorrhea created by pregnancy requires counseling regarding options for maintaining or terminating the pregnancy as well as referral. If emotional distress is the causative factor, counseling and possibly referral is necessary.

Nurse's Role. The nurse's primary role in the management of amenorrhea is to provide information regarding the cause and to assist the teenager to identify resources for further treatment and follow-up. A supportive empathetic approach facilitates acceptance of management.

Dysmenorrhea

Dysmenorrhea is menses associated with pain. The cause has not been identified definitively although the progesterone level, which causes forceful uterine contractions, has been associated with dysmenorrhea. Mental tension and anxiety may also serve to increase the discomforts. Primary dysmenorrhea is character-

Table 25-7. A nursing approach to scoliosis

Areas of intervention	Guidelines
Client knowledge and understanding	Discuss normal anatomy and function of spine Define problem as it relates to client and discuss causes of scoliosis Discuss potential management methods in relation to how problem will be treated Discuss management method for individual client and why chosen and the purpose Discuss management course: what will occur, when, how long, how often Provide opportunity for questions; second visit may facilitate this
Client self-care	*Devices* Discuss application of device to be worn Discuss skin care Review care and cleaning of device Discuss comfortable clothing to wear Review appropriate exercise, diet, and safety measures Discuss management of activities Discuss recognition and prevention of potential problems Request return demonstration of appropriate activities *Casting* Discuss cast application and drying techniques Review care of cast Discuss skin care and personal hygiene Review safety, diet, and elimination factors Discuss impact of immobilization Review management of activities Discuss recognition and prevention of potential problems including cast syndrome Discuss cast removal, care, and appearance (of skin) after removal
Client psychological well-being	Discuss feelings about management plan (fear, anxiety, lack of control, rejection) Discuss impact of body image and self-esteem Discuss peer and family acceptance and relationships Discuss interaction with general public Discuss ways of dressing that disguise cast or device Discuss ways to explain cast or device to others
Family support	Discuss preceding client factors with family Emphasize self-care activities Encourage understanding Discuss family feelings, perceptions, and attitudes Discuss changes in household routines and physical environment Discuss financial responsibilities

ized by cramping, abdominal pain, and back or leg aches that are intolerable. No evidence of pelvic pathological conditions is present. Secondary dysmenorrhea is associated with pelvic disease (Vaughan et al., 1979).

As in amenorrhea, differentiating the cause is essential to the treatment of dysmenorrhea. This requires a careful history, especially menstrual history, a thorough examination, and appropriate laboratory tests.

Nurse's Role. Most adolescents experience primary dysmenorrhea and nurses can be most helpful in providing education and counseling in the management phase. Appropriate nursing interventions include the following:

Verification of the client's understanding of the physiology of normal menses

Provision of information regarding causes of discomfort

Provision of support and reassurance regarding discomfort

Development of discomfort alleviation plan: use of analgesics, warmth to lower abdomen, exercises, relaxation techniques

Irregularities in the timing and amount of flow are common in teenagers. Inconsistencies may exist in the length of periods, the time between periods, or the amount of flow. Generally these inconsistencies resolve by the third year after the onset of menses. A familial tendency does exist for these irregularities and should be ruled out by taking the history. In addition, abnormalities in structure or hormonal responses will need to be ruled out through physical examination or laboratory studies or both.

Since the inconsistencies are generally self-limiting in nature, appropriate nursing interventions are similar to those discussed under dysmenorrhea. In addition, the nurse needs to explore client feelings and fears regarding the problem.

Premenstrual Tension

The phenomenon of premenstrual tension has received much attention in the past few years. Although the cause is unknown and therapies remain experimental, it is well known that women may suffer a series of symptoms preceding the onset of menstruation. Once menstruation has begun, these symptoms of headache, abdominal distention, weight gain, changes in mood, and breast discomfort subside. Assisting the adolescent to minimize these symptoms is appropriate nursing action. Counseling the teen to exercise regularly, to wear a well-fitted bra, to follow a nutritious diet avoiding salt and salt-retentive foods, to increase sleep and periods of relaxation before onset of period, and to maintain a positive attitude and appearance will assist in reducing symptoms (Tackett and Hundberger, 1981).

Mononucleosis

Infectious mononucleosis is an acute infectious disease occurring primarily in the 12- to 25-year-old range and caused by the Epstein-Barr virus (EBV). EBV is only mildly contagious; it is primarily transmitted through oropharyngeal secretions and intimate contact such as kissing. The average incubation period is 11 days, and the period of communicability is considered to be during the acute illness.

The initial symptoms of infectious mononucleosis are rather benign. Generally, the client has complaints of headache, malaise, and fatigue. A sore throat occurs by the end of the first week; the tonsils are red, enlarged, and covered with a membrane that peels off in 5 to 7 days. Lymphadenopathy and splenomegaly are common at this stage. Most symptoms subside in 3 weeks, but weakness and fatigue may persist for several weeks (Sapala and Sheldon, 1978). Laboratory studies are indicated and potentially reveal the following:

Blood smear showing 10% atypical lymphocytes
Elevated leukocyte count
Heterophile antibodies in serum by end of first week
Positive mononucleosis spot test (detects antibodies)

Nurse's Role

Treatment involves alleviation of symptoms (see Table 23-12). Additional appropriate nursing interventions include the following (Sapala and Sheldon, 1978):

Nutrition counseling that emphasizes high caloric diet
Bed rest for first 2 weeks with gradual return to activity
Reduced exposure to noninfected persons
No strenuous physical activity if splenomegaly is present
Provision of support and reassurance regarding disease process and confinement

Social Health Problems

Adolescence is a time of discovery of self, of feelings, and of the complexities of society. Complicating these discoveries are enormous pressures from multiple external and internal sources. Teenagers must behaviorally adapt to achieve an equilibrium between these pressures and their sense of self as related to the world. Often adolescents are unable to cope, resulting in health-related problems.

Nurse's Role

The nurse's role in assisting families and adolescents to adapt to socially related problems includes the following:

- Prevention by providing anticipatory guidance
- Early problem identification (i.e., case-finding)
- Problem intervention through education, resource identification, and referral
- Provision of support, nurture, and reassurance

Relevant to prevention and case-finding is the ability to recognize adolescents at risk for social problems. Table 25-8 identifies characteristics indicating an at-risk client and family situations that may place normal development in jeopardy. Assessing for the presence of these behaviors or situations facilitates the early recognition of problems, enabling the nurse to seek early intervention for the client.

Suicide

Suicide is the third leading cause of death among teenagers. Males have a higher rate (up to four times more) than girls, and it is estimated that the actual suicide rate is probably three times the reported rate (Hart and Prophit, 1979; Healthy People, 1979).

The causative factors for suicide or for attempting to take one's life are not definitive. Among these factors are developmental, social, cultural, psychological, biological, and situational variables. Generally, multiple factors combine to cause adolescents to consider suicide the only solution to their problems (Child et al., 1980; Cohen, 1978).

Most suicidal persons give verbal or behavioral warning, and 80% of those who take their own lives have made previous attempts (Hart et al., 1979).

Table 25-8. Characteristics of adolescents and families at risk for social problems

Adolescent behaviors	Family situation
Poor self-concept	Divorce
Severe mood changes	Death of one parent
School problems	Frequent family relocation
Antisocial behavior	Insufficient parental guidance
Substance abuse	Frequent absences of one parent
Decreased verbal communication	Drug or alcohol abuse
Sleep disturbances	Step-parent
Prolonged grief reaction following divorce, death, or severing of a romance	Poor relationships between family members
Communication problems at home	Mental illness
"Loner"	Economic deprivation
Friends of questionable reputation	Faulty communication patterns
Premature "growing up"	

Adapted from Bond, L.: Potential stresses during adolescence: managing behavior. In Tackett, J.J., Hunsberger, M., editors: Family centered care of children and adolescents. Philadelphia, 1980, W.B. Saunders Co., p. 1250.

Nurses have a responsibility to be cognizant of behaviors that are considered danger signs (see following box and to implement immediate intervention.

Nurse's Role. Nursing assessment and intervention, directed toward the depressed or suicidal child, are needed in the community, in the school, and in the ambulatory care setting. Nurses, particularly those in the school and community setting, are potentially the first persons the suicidal adolescent encounters. Frequently a physical complaint is the initial factor precipitating an encounter between the nurse and the adolescent. Masked in the physical complaint is the major problem or concern that is prompting suicidal thoughts. Nurses facilitate the identification of such a troubled teenager by being observant of adolescent behaviors, by encouraging adolescents to discuss their feelings, and by being an available source of support (Child et al., 1980; Hart and Prophit, 1979; Nelms and Brady, 1980).

Community resources are also essential to prevention. Crisis intervention centers and telephone hot lines provide professional help and resource referral. Educational programs directed toward the variables that create problems for adolescents facilitate early identification as well as provide a support group. Such programs should involve adolescents not only in participation but planning as well. (Hart and Prophit, 1980; Nelms and Brady, 1980).

Substance Abuse

The use of alcohol and drugs has been increasing among adolescents; 80% of the 12- to 17-year-olds report having had a drink, more than half drink at least once a month, and nearly 3% drink daily. Drug use, which was virtually unknown in the 1950s, now ac-

Behavioral Danger Signs

1. Giving away prized possessions.
2. Becoming increasingly isolated.
3. Recent loss, especially a parent, boyfriend, or girlfriend.
4. Statements such as, "No one cares about me. It would be better for everyone if I were dead." "How many aspirins do you have to take to kill yourself?"
5. A sudden elevation of mood following a depression. This could be misconstrued to mean that improvement when actually the teenager may be experiencing a sense of relief that the decision to die has been made.

From Hart, N. A., and Prophit, S.P., Adolescent suicide, Pediatr. Nurs. **5:**22-28, Nov.-Dec. 1979, p. 25.

counts for a major health problem among adolescents. By 1977, 60% of the adolescent population had tried marijuana and 20% had tried harder substances such as cocaine and hallucinogens. Beyond the experimentation phase, adolescents are also increasing the frequency and regularity of use of tobacco, marijuana, and stimulants.

Cause. The cause for increased substance experimentation and use is not definitive. As in the case of other socially related problems, many factors contribute to this behavioral expression. Among these factors are need for peer acceptance or approval, succumbing to peer pressure, curiosity, availability of substances, poor self-concept, a deteriorated parent-teen relationship, and boredom (Chow et al., 1979).

Effect. The physical and psychological effects of substance use are highly variable and will differ among individuals. However, chronic use that leads to dependency and addiction can create devastating effects such as change of life-style to accommodate drug need, malnutrition, emotional stress, and alienation by family and friends.

Nurse's Role in Prevention. Much substance abuse can be prevented, but assisting adolescents to stop or avoid misuse is not easy. Prevention will require a change in social acceptability as well as individual acceptability (Schonberg, 1978). Strategies for intervention will differ, and nurses have a vital role in these preventive efforts. Appropriate interventions include the following:

Educational programs on substance abuse for adolescents emphasizing their decision-making capabilities

Educational programs for parents in preventing abuse or recognizing early symptoms

Early identification and referral of adolescents with a substance abuse problem

Provision of support and acting as a role model

Assistance for adolescents in identifying stressors in their lives and in developing appropriate coping strategies

Use of youth organizations (such as 4-H and Scouts) and media to reinforce substance abuse education

Anorexia Nervosa

Anorexia nervosa is a psychosomatic disorder primarily affecting adolescent girls. It frequently begins with a voluntary weight reduction diet, because the client feels overweight, even though weight is within normal range. Weight loss and refusal of food become excessive and are accompanied by denial of any experience of hunger (Boyle et al., 1981; Vaughan et al., 1979). Definitive diagnostic criteria include (1) loss of at least 25% of original body weight; (2) delay or cessation of menstruation for at least 3 months; and (3) distorted body image (Bruch, 1965).

Nurse's Role. The community health nurse's assessment and intervention in the school, clinic, or home setting are essential to the early recognition and management of the anorexic adolescent. Awareness of behavioral indicators can facilitate the nurse's assessment. Personality characteristics of the adolescent which have been identified as behavioral indicators include obsessive-compulsive traits; setting of perfectionistic standards for self; neat, clean, well-behaved manner; a general immaturity and difficulty with peer and social relationships (Vaughan et al., 1979). Additionally, family dynamics and characteristics and habits require the nurse's assessment (Boyle et al., 1981). Al-

though treatment and management of the anorexic adolescent must frequently require hospitalization, the community health nurse is pivotal in facilitating early referral for treatment and in providing continuity of care during hospitalization and follow-up. Such nursing activities include (1) liaison contacts with the client, family, and tertiary care management team; (2) provision of support and reassurance; and (3) facilitation of home management and follow-up care (Boyle et al., 1981).

Sexual Activity

Sexual experimentation is common in the adolescent years. Recent statistics reveal that one half of the adolescent population is sexually active, that one million teenage pregnancies occur annually, and that an additional 30,000 pregnancies occur in girls under age 15 (Healthy People, 1979; Tackett and Hunsberger, 1981). Peer pressures, physiological and emotional changes, and societal expectations are all contributing factors in early heterosexual relations among adolescents.

Homosexuality. Homosexual experimentation may occur as well, particularly in early adolescent years. Boys specifically may pass through a stage of sexual activity with a same sex counterpart. Early homosexual experiences are not necessarily an indication of later sexual preference but rather are spurred by curiosity and the need to explore. As adolescents satisfy their need to explore various life-styles, they make a sexual preference, generally heterosexual (Hyde, 1979; Sorenson, 1973).

Sex Education. Because adolescents are more sexually active, they and their families need sex education and counseling. Counseling is based on an understanding of the adolescent's need for intimacy and the fact that involvement is a means to fulfilling this need (Hyde, 1979; Sorenson, 1973). Society accepts this behavioral expression, even though an adolescent's parent may not. Hence, while prevention of sexual activity is not entirely realistic, educational efforts can be useful tools in assisting the adolescent to make informed decisions. Nurses can provide this education, focusing on (1) the physical and emotional sexuality of adolescents and their options for expression; (2) their attitude regarding sexual activity; (3) their awareness of the potential consequences of sexual activity, e.g., pregnancy, venereal disease, emotional distress; and (4) their available resource or support persons or groups should problems arise.

The nurse can also assist parents to (1) recognize and deal with the present-day realities of increased sexual activity among adolescents; (2) express their feelings about sex positively to their teenagers; (3) handle sex education and discuss sexual issues at home; (4) be a positive role model; and (5) identify support and resources if a problem arises (Chow et al., 1979; Sapala and Sheldon, 1981; Tackett and Hunsberger, 1981).

Two prominent consequences of adolescent sexual activity are veneral disease and teenage pregnancy. Both of these health problems have experienced an increased incidence over the past decade, and each poses significant alterations to health.

Venereal Disease. Sexually transmissible diseases have become the leading type of communicable disease in our nation. Gonorrhea, syphilis, and genital herpes simplex account for an estimated 8 to 12 million cases of venereal disease a year (Healthy People, 1979). Table 25-9 outlines the clinical characteristics and accepted management of these diseases.

Similarly, the transmission of trichomoniasis and *Candida albicans,* most frequently creating vaginal infection, have become widespread health problems. Trichomoniasis is a protozoan that is generally carried in the vaginal tract, is transmitted by contact with infected perianal discharge, and has a foamy, yellow, foul-smelling discharge as the primary symptom. *Candida* is a normal vaginal fungus, usually kept in balance by normal vaginal flora. The symptoms of infection, itching, and white, cheesy discharge tend to appear during pregnancy or hormonal or antibiotic therapy, or as a result of factors that alter vaginal pH or flora levels. Microscopic examination or culture is indicated for both conditions. Trichomoniasis is treated with oral medication (Flagyl) and *Candida* is treated with an antifungal vaginal preparation.

Nurse's Role. Nurses have a vital responsibility in the prevention, identification, and encouragement of prompt treatment of the venereal diseases. Appropriate nursing interventions can be carried out effectively in group or individual counseling sessions, need to be presented in a nonjudgmental manner, and should facilitate adolescent knowledge and understanding about their sexuality. Nursing activities include the following:

Sex education (written information)

Venereal disease education (written information)

Screening of at-risk groups

Identification and treatment of infected person and their contacts

Teaching of preventive practices such as using a condom, washing well after sexual contact, urinating after intercourse, improving personal hygiene, avoiding contact with persons known to be infected

Pregnancy

Childbearing during adolescence is a high-risk experience for mother and child. One fourth of the teenage girls in the United States have had at least one pregnancy by age 19. Annually 10% of all teenage girls become pregnant and two thirds of them are unmarried. At least 3 of every 10 elect to terminate the pregnancy (Healthy People, 1979).

Response to Pregnancy. The teenager responds to the fact of her pregnancy with a wide range of emotion. Initial feelings may include denial, fear, guilt, anger, depression, or happiness. In some instances there may be a motivating factor on the part of the adolescent girl in becoming pregnant. Among the factors contributing to an adolescent's desire to become pregnant are rebellion against parents, viewing it as a means to leave a stressful home situation or to keep a boyfriend, or unrealistic desires and fantasies about motherhood and having a baby who will love her (Abbott, 1978).

Frequently the pregnant adolescent is unable to prepare adequately for the pregnancy, labor and delivery, and care of the infant. Because concrete thinking processes are still developing, the realities of the effects of pregnancy are not always understood. In addition, the pregnant teenager still needs association with her peers, and many find this difficult because of the gap pregnancy creates in life-styles. Similarly, because of the pregnancy, relationships with family may become strained at a time when support persons are most needed.

Nurse's Role. The nurse can assist the pregnant teenager in many ways. The initial nursing assessment should focus on identifying the adolescent's feeling about being pregnant; her feelings about options, i.e., termination versus continuation; her support persons and role model; and her short-term goals, e.g., medical care, school continuation, relationships with baby's father, her family, and peers (Abbott, 1978). A nonjudgmental yet supportive attitude is essential during the assessment and management phases. The pregnancy of a teenager affects many people as well as society in general. Handling the implications of the effects of her pregnancy is frequently difficult for the adolescent. Hence the goals of nursing interventions should be short term and directed at definition of the most appropriate way for the individual teenager to handle the pregnancy (Tackett and Hunsberger, 1981). Appropriate nursing activities include the following:

Providing pregnancy counseling, explaining fully the teenager's choices in regard to termination or continuation

Assisting the teenager to identify support persons in the family or among friends

Providing support and encouragement

Making appropriate referrals for medical care and school placement

Assisting the teenager to manage her altered life-style

Providing appropriate health education

Table 25-9. Characteristics of venereal disease

Venereal disease (pathogen)	Transmission	Incubation	Symptoms	Diagnostic tests	Treatment
Gonorrhea (*Neisseria gono*)	Direct contact, usually sexual; fomite contact up to 24 hours after fomite contaminated.	2-14 days (average 3-5)	*Early signs:* copious mucopurulent discharge from phagocytosis, vaginal in female and urethral in male. Pharyngeal if oral sex. Pain and frequency of urination from urethritis. 90% of females and 10% of males are asymptomatic. *Other possible signs:* cervicitis, salpingitis, peritonitis, pelvic inflammatory disease, and abscesses of Skene's or Bartholin glands in females. Epididymitis and abscess of prostate glands in males. *Late signs:* arthritis, endocarditis, sterility.	Culture of discharge for gonococcal growth (GC smear) positive. Visualization of discharge in infection on physical exam.	Simultaneous treatment of infected individual and all identified sexual partners with oral (probenecid) or intramuscular (procaine penicillin G, Trobicin) penicillin. The National Institute of Health is currently developing a gonorrheal vaccine. No permanent immunity.
Syphilis (*Treponema pallidum*)	Direct contact, usually sexual, during infective stage. Transfusion.	Primary stage 10-90 days (average 3 weeks)	*Primary*—infectious: chancre (painless, indurated ulcer) that heals spontaneously in 2-3 weeks. Located at site where pathogen entered.	Reactive STS (presence of spirochete in blood produces reaction to certain animal antigens); VDRL most common test. STS negative at this stage. Visualization of chancre on physical exam.	*Primary/secondary stages:* 2,400,000 units benzathine penicillin G IM or 4,800,000 units procaine
		6-24 weeks	*Secondary*—very infectious: Skin and mucous membrane rash, lymphadenitis, fever, headaches, sore throat that disappears spontaneously. Lasts few months to several years.	STS reactive; becomes nonreactive if treated now.	Penicillin G (half of dose in each buttock) followed by 1,200,000 units of either type penicillin G at 3 days and 6 days after initial dose.
		2-4 years	*Early latent*—may be infectious: no physical symptoms.	STS reactive.	*Latent stages:* 3,000,000 units penicillin G given IM (half of dose in each buttock to be repeated at 7 and 14 days after 1st dose).

From Tackett, J.J.: Potential stresses during adolescence: reversible alterations in health status. In Tackett, J.J., and Hunsberger, M., editors: Family centered care of children and adolescents, Philadelphia, 1981, W.B. Saunders Co., pp. 1294-1295.

Table 25-9. Characteristics of venereal disease — cont'd

Venereal disease (pathogen)	Transmission	Incubation	Symptoms	Diagnostic tests	Treatment
		After 4 years	*Late latent* — blood infectious: no symptoms.	STS reactive.	VDRL repeated each month for 3 months after treatment completed to establish cure; damage done to body before treatment is not reversible.
			Late active: Gummas in skin, bones, liver, stomach.		
			CNS involvement 10% optic atrophy, deafness. General paresis. Cardiovascular involvement in 80% of cases Aortic insufficiency or aneurysm. Endarteritis. Insanity.		No immunity is developed.
Genital herpes simplex (*Herpesvirus hominis* [HSV-2])	Direct contact, usually sexual.	3-7 days	*Symptomatic phase:* contagious. Minor itching or extensive rash of genital region followed by a cluster or blister-like lesions that then rupture and ulcerate; these are pruritic and painful, especially during intercourse. Painful urination, inguinal lymphadenitis and pain, fever, malaise. Symptoms disappear spontaneously after 2-6 weeks. Many cases asymptomatic. *Dormant phase:* symptoms absent but reappear with emotional or physical stress during which person again is infectious; once a person is infected, virus is harbored for life, though recurrences are less severe and last about 2 weeks. Cervical cancer 8 times more likely in women with HSV-2 virus.	Viral culture of lesions. Scraping and staining of ulcer tissue with Papanicolaou solution demonstrates characteristic giant cells and viral inclusion bodies. Antibody blood titer of HVH-2 21 or more days after infection.	Incurable. Treatment aimed at pain relief, fostering healing of lesions and preventing other infections. Pain medication Use of condom during intercourse to prevent spread of HVH-2 or infection with other pathogens. Local application of red dye (0.1% proflavine) followed by light exposure repeated in 18 hours. This shortens course of lesions but is controversial because of increased risk of tumor formation. Antiviral agents are being developed that may be effective against HSV-2. Cesarean section in all pregnancies if active sores exist at time of birth.

Continuation of Pregnancy. The adolescent who continues her pregnancy faces a high risk for complications. The incidence of toxemia, prolonged labor, and iron deficiency anemia are increased for teenage mothers. In addition, teenage mothers give birth to a higher proportion of low birth weight infants, infants who are retarded, and infants with epilepsy, cerebral palsy, blindness, and deafness. The younger the girl, the greater this risk appears to be for mother and infant (Kreutner et al., 1978). Although some of these risk factors are created by adolescent physical and physiological immaturity, others are attributed to the adolescent psychosocial immaturity resulting in poor compliance with prenatal care and management plans. For this reason the nurse needs to assist the adolescent in understanding the importance of prenatal care and health activities before making a decision about the pregnancy. These health education activities require reinforcement throughout the pregnancy. Information and preparation for labor and delivery and infant care should be introduced into the plan of care later in the pregnancy (Dibble, 1981).

Adoption Decision. The pregnant adolescent who decides to continue her pregnancy also faces an additional choice: whether to keep the baby or give the infant up for adoption. This decision can be made at any time during the pregnancy and legally the young mother has 72 hours after delivery before she has to sign adoption papers (Abbott, 1978; Tackett and Hunsberger, 1981). The adolescent who is contemplating adoption needs nursing support and empathy in dealing with the emotions and realities created by giving up a baby for adoption. The family and the baby's father, who has legal rights, may be exerting pressure for one decision or another. Group counseling and interaction with other pregnant teens are often helpful. The final decision belongs to the teenager, and nurses must accept the role of resource people in facilitating the decision.

The Adolescent Mother

The adolescent who decides to keep her infant poses a unique challenge for nurses. The adolescent's adjustment to parenthood relies heavily on being prepared, informed, and supported (Dibble, 1981). Nurses need to be aware that adolescents are continuing to deal with developmental tasks in addition to the pregnancy and parenthood. The pregnant adolescent frequently discovers she is in a role that requires maturity and decision making but is unable to deal with these responsibilities. Nurses can assist teenage mothers to coordinate their roles and responsibilities as well as to set priorities. Appropriate nursing interventions may include the following:

Assisting teenager and family or father in distributing responsibilities of child care

Assisting teenager to identify and use support persons and groups

Assisting the teenage father to identify his feelings, role, and level of participation in pregnancy, labor, delivery, and care of child

Providing education about infant behavior and physical care

Facilitating use of appropriate health care for teenage mother and infant

Facilitating attachment and bonding

Making referrals as appropriate identifing appropriate resources (babysitters, living arrangements)

Assisting teenager to identify and meet goals (e.g., return to work or school)

Assisting teenager to use family planning

Facilitating expression of feelings about infant, motherhood, her family, and the infant's father

Acting as an emotional support person and source of reassurance

Birth Control and Sex Education

The adequacy of knowledge and the access to information on sexual behavior and family planning services constitute a major area of concern. Much controversy arises over who should provide information, how much sex education is appropriate, and in what setting it should be given. The decision regarding early sex education generally lies with parents (Bernstein, 1976). They may choose to discuss sex and sexuality with their children or may decide to leave it to the school. Generally, inquiries about sex are best answered by parents. However, parents may feel uncomfortable in discussing sexuality. Nurses can assist parents to work through their feelings of discomfort and provide them with appropriate resources and responses to their children's questions.

Nurse's Role. The nurse's goal is always to promote healthy and informed attitudes regarding sexuality. The opportunity for the community health nurse to plan and present a sex education program can occur in the school or clinic setting. Any age group of children can be the target population. An age-appropriate bibliography of materials on reproduction and sex is often a useful tool for parents and child. The nurse should recommend that both parent and child read the book or pamphlet. Following the reading, a discussion between parent and child should occur so that the child's questions or misconceptions are clarified. Additionally, nurses can assist parents to be prepared for the inevitable inquiries from their child about sexuality. Table 25-10 provides a developmental approach to information on sexuality. When providing parents with information

Table 25-10. Developmental approach to sex education

Age	Development	Approach
Toddler	Child believes babies have always existed.	"Only people can make other people. To make a baby person, you need two grown-ups, a man and a woman to be the baby's mommy and daddy. They make the baby from an egg in mommy's body and a sperm from the daddy's body."
Preschooler	Child believes babies are manufactured.	"That's interesting. That's the way you'd make a doll. You'd buy a head and hair and put it altogether. But making a real live baby is different. Mommies and daddies have special things in their bodies to make babies. Mommies have tiny eggs and daddies have tiny sperm. When an egg from a mommy and a sperm from daddy join together, they grow into a baby."
Early school age	Child questions where the baby grows, believes tummies open up.	"Can you put your hand inside your tummy? Do you think mommies and daddies can put their hands in their tummies? There must be another way. Do you want to know how the egg and sperm come together? The daddy's sperm are in his testicles and come out through his penis. The mommy's vagina is a tunnel to where her eggs are. So if daddy puts his penis into her vagina the sperm can go through the tunnel to the egg."
School age	Child has misconceptions, apprehension, and beliefs about conception, love, and physiology. Child tries to understand how all of these relate to one another.	Provide physiological explanations. Clear up misconceptions and abate apprehension. Combine all aspects into an explanation. "It's really important for a baby that mothers and fathers love each other and love the baby, so that when the baby is born they can take good care of it. But loving is a feeling and can't start the baby all by itself. A baby is a living creature and it starts growing from living material. When the mother and father make love, a sperm from the father goes through his penis into the mother's vagina. When the sperm joins with an egg from the mother, they form a new life, which grows into a baby."
Late school age	Initial stage: Children take longer to understand why genetic material must unite to produce a baby. Later stage: Children believe whole baby exists in either sperm or egg, needing the other only to grow.	Reinforce content of previous stage. Emphasize that baby has not begun to exist until sperm and egg meet and fuse; that seeds of life come from both parents, from which baby inherits its physical characteristics. Useful explanation: "Both the sperm and egg contain coded information about the baby it will grow to be. Neither the sperm nor egg has the entire code until they unite. Together, they complete the message to develop a baby that is the child of a particular set of parents."

Adapted from Bernstein, A.C., Sex stages of understanding how children learn about sex and birth, Psychology Today, Jan. 1976, pp. 31-35.

about sex education for their child or in conducting sex education, the nurse should observe the following guidelines:

Use the child's curiosity as a guide to the explicitness of the explanation

Avoid inundating the child with information

Explain what child wants to know in understandable terms

Ask questions of the child that will elicit the child's belief

Convey a positive attitude that reflects comfort with the topic of sex

Avoid belittling or making child feel foolish

Avoid myths, vague statements, or erroneous information

Contraception. Parents and adolescents need to be informed about methods of contraception, Whether this information is sought out by the adolescent or the parent or offered by the nurse, all methods require discussion, emphasizing effectiveness and appropriateness of use for the individual. In addition, the adolescent's knowledge of reproduction needs to be verified and misconceptions and misinformation corrected. Table 25-11 presents contraception information useful to the

Table 25-11. Methods of contraception

	The pill	Minipills	Intrauterine device (IUD)	Diaphragm with spermicidal jelly or cream	Spermicidal foam, jelly, or cream	Condom (rubber)	Condom and foam	Periodic abstinence (natural family planning)	Sterilization
Description	Pills with 2 hormones, an estrogen and progestin, similar to the hormones a woman makes in her own ovaries.	Pills with just 1 type of hormone: a progestin, similar to a hormone a woman makes in her own ovaries.	A small piece of plastic with nylon threads attached. Some have copper wire wrapped around them. One IUD gives off a hormone, progesterone.	A shallow rubber cup used with a sperm-killing jelly or cream.	Cream and jelly come in tubes; foam comes in aerosol cans or individual applicators and is placed into the vagina.	A sheath of rubber shaped to fit snugly over the erect penis.	Condom and foam used together.	Method to find out days each month when you are most likely to get pregnant. Intercourse is avoided at that time.	Vasectomy (male) or tubal ligation (female). Ducts carrying sperm or the egg are tied and cut surgically.
Action	Prevents egg's release from woman's ovaries; makes cervical mucus thicker and changes lining of the uterus.	May prevent egg's release from woman's ovaries; makes cervical mucus thicker and changes lining of uterus, making it harder for a fertilized egg to start growing there.	The IUD is inserted into the uterus. It is not known exactly how the IUD prevents pregnancy.	Fits inside the vagina. The rubber cup forms a barrier between the uterus and the sperm. The jelly or cream kills the sperm.	Foam, jelly, and cream contain a chemical that kills sperm and acts as a physical barrier between sperm and the uterus.	Prevents sperm from getting inside a woman's vagina during intercourse.	Prevents sperm from getting inside the uterus by killing sperm and by preventing sperm from getting out into the vagina.	Techniques include maintaining chart of basal body temperature, checking vaginal secretions, and keeping calendar of menstrual periods, all of which can help predict when an egg is most likely to be released.	Closing of tubes in male prevents sperm from reaching egg; closing tubes in female prevents egg from reaching sperm.
Problems	Must be prescribed by a doctor.	Must be prescribed by a doctor.	Must be inserted by a doctor af-	Must be fitted by a doctor after a pel-	Must be inserted just before in-	Objectionable to some men and	Requires more effort than some	Difficult to use method if menstrual	Surgical operation has some risk

(Disadvantages, continued)	Advantages	Procedure
should have a medical exam before taking "the Pill," and some women should not take it.	Convenient, extremely effective, does not interfere with sex, and may diminish menstrual cramps.	Either of two ways: 1. A pill a day for 3 wk, stop for 1 wk, then start a new pack. 2. A pill every single day with no stopping between packs.
	Convenient, effective, does not interfere with sex, and less serious side effects than with regular birth control pills.	Take 1 pill every single day as long as you want to avoid pregnancy.
examination. Cannot be used by all women. Sometimes the uterus "pushes" it out.	Effective, always there when needed, but usually not felt by either partner.	Check string at least once a month right after the period ends to make sure your IUD is still properly in place.
Some women find it difficult to insert, inconvenient, or messy.	Effective and safe.	Insert the diaphragm and jelly (or cream) before intercourse. Can be inserted up to 6 hours before intercourse. Must stay in at least 6 hours after intercourse.
Some find it inconvenient or messy.	Effective, safe, a good lubricant, and can be purchased at a drugstore.	Put foam, jelly, or cream into your vagina each time you have intercourse, not more than 30 min before. No douching for at least 8 hours after intercourse.
like. May be messy or inconvenient. Interrupts intercourse.	Effective, safe, and can be purchased at a drugstore; excellent protection against sexually transmitted infections.	The condom should be placed on the erect penis before the penis ever comes into contact with the vagina. After ejaculation, the penis should be removed from the vagina immediately.
terrupts intercourse. May be messy. Condom may break.	Safe, effective if followed carefully; little if any religious objection to method. Teaches women about their menstrual cycles.	Careful records must be maintained of several factors: basal body temperature, vaginal secretions, and onset of menstrual bleeding. Careful study of these methods will dictate when intercourse should be avoided.
regular. Sexual intercourse must be avoided for a significant part of each cycle.	The most effective method; low rate of complications; many feel that removing fear of pregnancy improves sexual relations.	After the decision to have no more children has been well thought through, a brief surgical procedure is performed on the man or the woman.
complications are rare. Sterilizations should not be done unless no more children are desired.		

Adapted from Contraception, DHEW Pub. No. (HSA) 78-5646, Washington, D.C., 1978, Public Health Services Administration, Bureau of Community Health Services, Department of Health, Education, and Welfare.

adolescent considering the various methods of birth control. (See *Contraceptive Technology** for a complete discussion of all methods.)

Follow-up of teenagers using contraceptive methods is imperative. The nurse must assess the teenager's understanding, use, and response as well as the efficacy of the method chosen. Follow-up visits are also a time for the adolescent to voice questions or concerns about contraception and sexuality and to receive support and encouragement.

Other Common Behaviors

Frequently school age children and adolescents display behaviors of concern to parents or family. Troublesome behaviors are based on expressions of conflict or a means of testing out a situation, values, or feelings. Their occurrence in most instances is normal. Nurses should encourage parents to continue effective past and current patterns of discipline to facilitate quick passage through this stage.

Of major concern in dealing with the school age child are cheating, lying, stealing, fighting, scatology, and fears. In the adolescent years concern is created by moodiness, preoccupation with self and body image, rebellion, conformity, inferiority, study habits, and dependent versus independent ambivalence. Appendix I defines these problems and discusses appropriate interventions.

Persistence of a minor problem indicates a situation more serious than a developmental deviation. If a child or adolescent repeatedly demonstrates antisocial behavior, a more extensive management plan is indicated, including referral of child and family for counseling. Troublesome behaviors may also represent warning signals of deeper difficulties even if they are not persistent in occurrence. For this reason thoughtful assessment is necessary before designating the events or behaviors as normal. The nurse can be instrumental in initiating appropriate guidance whether directed at coping with a normal phase or referring for management of a more complex problem.

Tools for Assessment

Once school age and adolescence is reached, the nursing process does not vary significantly from that used for early childhood. Although the basic methods of the nursing process remain the same, variations in tools and techniques are indicated for the older child. These variations occur because the school age child and adolescent have the ability to participate more actively in all aspects of health assessment.

*Published annually by Irvington Publishers, Inc., New York.

Summary of Health History

1. Identifying information
   Name
   Address
   Phone number
   Clinic number
2. Present concerns
3. Family profile
   Age and health status of family members
   Familial and communicable diseases
   Socioeconomic background
   Support system
4. Child profile
   Past medical history
      Gestation
      Birth history
      Neonatal period
      Immunizations and laboratory tests
      Infectious diseases
      Operations/hospitalizations
      Accidents
      Allergies
      Current medications
      Review of systems
         Head
         Skin
         Eyes, ears, nose, throat
         Dentition
         Heart and lung
         Blood
         Genitourinary
         Skeletal
         Neuromuscular
   Personality
      The child as a person
      Interaction
   Development
      Language
      Fine motor
      Gross motor
   Nutrition
   Sleep
   Elimination
   School
   Past utilization of health care
   Special concerns of the adolescent
   24-hour history

From Chow, M. P. et al: Handbook of pediatric primary care, New York, 1979, John Wiley and Sons, Inc., pp. 6-7.

The History

The history is a long term cumulative data base. The amount and type of history information obtained depend on the purpose of the visit and the expressed concerns of the client and parents. Obtaining a complete health history is essential for a first-time encounter. A summary of health history information appropriate for the school age child is presented in the box above. Supplementary information to be obtained for the adolescent in addition to the general history is summarized in the preceding boxed material (Brown and Murphy, 1975; Chow et al., 1979; Daniel, 1977).

Child as Historian. An added dimension to the interviewing of a school age child or adolescent is use of the child as the primary informant or historian. The school age child can be a reliable historian. The older the child becomes, the greater the degree of detail and accuracy becomes (Gorman, 1980). Focusing on the school age child and adolescent as the primary informant facilitates the therapeutic relationship by promoting the nurse's trust and confidence in the child's ability. This technique assists children and adolescents in becoming an integral part of their health care and provides an opportunity for expression of concerns or feelings about their own health, growth, and development. If the nurse is concerned about the accuracy of the history data, particularly in regard to early events, unsure dates, or an identified problem, validation by the parent is indicated. This verification should be done with the child or adolescent's knowledge and is best handled in a separate interview.

Setting for Adolescent Health Visit

Further consideration must also be given to the setting and tone of a healthy assessment visit for the adolescent client. Most adolescents experience some degree of discomfort in coming to a pediatric clinic. The added factor of being accompanied by parents, who possibly wish to discuss issues of concerns to them, warrants special consideration on the part of the health care provider. The following measures are useful in facilitating the adolescent health maintenance visit (Daniel, 1970; Marks, 1978):

Schedule adolescent appointments on days different than baby or younger child appointments
Provide age-appropriate reading materials in waiting area which focus on adolescent-related problems
Ask adolescent to complete any previsit history or information forms
Interview the adolescent first and then parents, unless adolescent expresses desire for parent to be present
Explain procedure for present and future visits in detail
Direct interview to adolescent; be interested in and develop a trusting relationship with adolescent
Reassure adolescent that information shared is confidential (exception being when behavior is dangerous to self or others)
Conduct interview in friendly, concerned manner
When providing health care services to the adolescent, nurses must also be aware of the constitutional rights of minors, including the right to self-consent. All

states have legislation pertinent to the aspects of obtaining health care without parental permission. Since state statutes vary, nurses need to be familiar with those within their own jurisdiction. It is important to know the age at which minors can seek health care on their own and the type of health care services that can be offered. Other aspects of legal questions pertaining to the health care of minors are as follows (Eldridge, 1979; Jellinek and Cloonan, 1981):

A. Emancipated minors
   1. Category includes individuals who are
      a. Away from home
      b. Earning own support
      c. Married
      d. Parents themselves
      e. In service
      f. 15 years or older
      g. Working and still living at home, but contributing at least one half of their support
   2. There generally are no legal penalties to the health care agency or individual
B. Unemancipated minors
   1. Category includes individuals who are
      a. Under 15 years
      b. Dependent on parents for support, housing, etc.
   2. Laws of individual states remain quite complex and variable in defining the conditions under which an unemancipated minor can be treated
C. Treatment without parental consent
   1. The minor's right to consent to minor care depends on minor's ability to give informed consent, which is demonstrated by understanding
      a. Nature of procedure
      b. Risks involved
      c. Available alternatives
   2. Minor must demonstrate sufficient intelligence and maturity
   3. Minor must have reached "age of majority"
D. Emergencies
   1. When life or health is endangered, treatment of emergency care may be instituted without parental consent
   2. Definition of what constitutes an emergency is variable from state to state
E. Confidentiality
   1. Most states do not require health care professionals to notify parents if situation warrants this
   2. Question of minor's refusal to consent to care recommended by health care professional or contracted for by parents remains an unresolved issue

The Physical Examination

The techniques of physical assessment vary little for the school age child and the adolescent (see Chapter 23). Explaining each portion of the examination is most important for individuals of these age groups, since concern about body functioning, changes, and normal-

cy is usual (Marks, 1978). Table 23-17 describes approaches to conducting the physical examination for these age groups. In addition, explaining the what and why of the examination technique, including the results of specific parts of the examination, is useful in promoting the adolescent's confidence and trust.

The Health Assessment

A complete health assessment combines the components of health history, physical assessment, and the monitoring of physical and psychosocial growth and development. Based on these data, further activities that promote health can be implemented as needed for the individual child or adolescent. Once the child has reached school age, the frequency of health assessment visits is usually extended to every 2 years, unless the health status of the client warrants more frequent assessment. The general content of these visits is discussed in Appendix A.

Physical Growth. Monitoring physical growth continues to be a major component of the health maintenance contact. Height and weight measurements need to be taken at these encounters. Similarly, vital sign measurement of heart, respiratory rate, and particularly blood pressure is indicated.

Growth charts continue to be useful tools for recording and monitoring physical measurements (Appendix J). Since growth spurts occur at varying ages and rates, the monitoring of this major phase of physical development is essential. Growth charts assist the nurse to identify normal versus atypical growth patterns.

Laboratory Studies. Laboratory studies are a means of monitoring physical health, and selected procedures are indicated for the school age child and adolescent (Appendix J). Assessing skeletal and dental age when indicated provides information regarding normal growth patterns (see Chapter 23 for detailed discussion).

Assessment of Sexual Age. An assessment of sex characteristics is specific and important to monitoring the health of older school age children and adolescents. The tool developed by Tanner is most widely used and recognized. Tanner staging categorizes sexual development according to the appearance of certain physical characteristics (Tanner, 1962). See the section on physical growth and development of the adolescent found earlier in this chapter for a detailed discussion.

Screening Procedures. Screening procedures for vision, hearing, and tuberculosis are indicated during health maintenance contacts with school age children and adolescents. Most frequently, the Snellen alphabet chart is employed for vision screening, an audiogram for hearing screening, and the Mantoux test (intradermal purified protein derivative) for tuberculin screening (see Appendix K). Additionally, the scoliosis screening previously discussed in this chapter is definitely indicated for clients in this age group. Screening for venereal disease and sickle cell disease as indicated for the individual client is appropriate during health assessment visits (Appendix A).

Monitoring Psychosocial Development. The psychosocial skills of the school age child and adolescent can be monitored in a number of ways. Generally, the therapeutic interview focusing on the aspects of the client's emotional and social development is conducted during the health maintenance visit (see boxed material on pp. 612 and 613). Knowledge of the development of social behaviors is important to this interview as are the observations and perceptions of parents and teacher. Data derived from the interview and indicating the need for further assessment prompt the nurse to implement more extensive screening. The tool used for this additional screening is dependent on the area of concern (e.g., family problem, social maturity, intelligence, perceptual ability). The psychosocial tests most commonly used in childhood and adolescence are discussed in Table 24-5. Other tools useful in monitoring psychosocial development are discussed in the following section.

Family Coping Estimate

The health of a child is largely dependent on the family's health and ability to cope. Comprehensive nursing implies implementing the nursing process for the family as well as the individual client. The Family Coping Index is an assessment tool focusing on the family's need for nursing care, their probable response to care, the plan of care to be given, and evaluation of effectiveness. This tool defines family coping as the reasonable ability of the family to be successful in dealing with problems related to health care (Freeman and Heinrich, 1981).

The Family Coping Estimate consists of a scoring profile, a care plan sheet, and a set of instructions with rationale. Although the tool was designed for use in the community setting, it is versatile and can be used by nurses in other settings as well. A prerequisite to use, however, is the nurse's knowledge of the family's interactions, health attitudes and practices, and living situation. (Freeman and Heinrich, 1981).

Home Observation for Measurement of Environment

The Home Observation for Measurement of Environment is another useful assessment tool. This tool was discussed in Chapter 23. See that discussion and Appendix B for a review of information.

The School Conference

A major part of the older child's and adolescent's world consists of the time spent at school. Experiences, attitudes, and values encountered at school affect psychosocial development (Damon, 1977). For this reason communication between the nurse and the child's teacher and the school nurse is an essential component in monitoring psychosocial development.

The communication nurses establish with the school can be initiated in several ways: (1) between the nurse in the community and the nurse in the school and/or the child's teacher; (2) between the nurse in the school and the teacher; and (3) between the nurse (in the community and/or the school), the teacher, the parent, and the child.

The dialogue established between nurse, teacher, and child can be focused in the following directions:

A. The adjustment to school (Table 25-5) can be facilitated by
  1. Providing support for teachers and intervening in crises situations
  2. Providing support for parents and offering guidance and a means of participation in child's education and adjustment to school through preschool conferences, parent-teacher-nurse conferences throughout school year, involvement with parent-teacher groups (PTA)
  3. Providing support for child and assisting to identify peer group, appropriate after-school activities, and means of coping with new situation of school
B. Preventive health measures can be provided by
  1. Screening for physical and emotional health problems (vision, hearing, scoliosis screening, conversational conferences about how school is going, etc.)
  2. Conducting health education classes geared to specific age group (how to care for teeth, taking care of a cold, sex education, venereal disease education, etc.)
C. Assistance can be offered in managing identified problems, both physical and emotional, such as
  1. Cooperating with a prescribed medication regimen
  2. Facilitating a behavior modification plan
  3. Facilitating special dietary needs or requirements

The school conference is an essential avenue for health promotion. To be productive, the nurse must facilitate (1) the mutual identification of health goals or problems brought to or created by the setting; (2) collaboration of all parties involved to meet goal or resolve problem; and (3) periodic follow-up to ensure that health is maintained.

Parent-Teacher-Child Conference

The parent-teacher-child health conference is an added dimension to the promotion of health for the school age and adolescent person. Initiating such conferences at regular intervals during the school year permits assessment of the child's health in a strongly influential setting (Laige, 1973). The nurse can influence this setting and the child's growth and development within it in a variety of ways:

Providing health education materials or classes

Intervening in crisis situations or situations requiring medical follow up

Identifying potential health problems

Providing support

Once a child has entered the school system, nursing action can facilitate adjustment to and advancement through the educational process. To do so, the nursing process must expand across many environments: home, school, and peer groups. The nurse must have the knowledge and skill to assess the multiple factors of these environments which influence a child's growth and development. It is the nurse's responsibility, therefore, to intervene, coordinate, and facilitate a positive, healthy outcome for the child.

IMMUNIZATIONS

The process of acquiring immunity continues into the school age and adolescent years. Boosters are recommended at specific intervals for maintainance of an adequate concentration level of antibodies. Between the ages of 4 to 6 years a child should receive a booster of DTP and OPV and the adolescent should receive a tetanus booster every 10 years (see Appendix E). Older school age children and adolescents (particularly females) whose immunity status to rubella is questionable should have a rubella titer (American Academy of Pediatrics, 1982). (A rubella titer is the blood determination of the concentration of circulating rubella antibodies.) Questionable circumstances of immunity include lack of vaccination, vaccination before 13 months of age, history of disease, or uncertainty of vaccination or disease.

Children who have not received immunizations need to be started on a schedule of primary immunizations. Table 23-18 gives the recommended schedule. As in the case of younger children, the older child and adolescent may experience a mild reaction to immunizations. The treatment primarily includes supportive measures, which are discussed in Appendix E.

Nurse's Role

Ensuring child and adolescent health through appropriate implementation of the immunization schedule is the nurse's responsibility. Nurses assist parents and children in following the the recommended schedule through education and counseling, record maintenance, and referral to appropriate resources or agencies for receipt of vaccine. Nurses have the further responsibilities of being knowledgeable about state law requirements for immunizations before school entry and of

Table 25-12. Foods affecting dental health

Recommended foods	Foods to be avoided
Milk	Foods with added
Cheese	sugar
Cheese products	Sticky foods: candy,
Salami	cake, cookies,
Smoked meats	pies, ice cream,
Nuts	candied popcorn,
Raw fruit and vegetables	candy-covered
Unsweetened fruit juices	fruit, honey-
Vegetable juices	covered foods,
Crackers	dried fruit
Pretzels	Hard candies, breath
Corn chips	mints, cough
Popcorn	drops
Teething biscuits	Lemons or acidic
	fruits that are
	sucked or eaten

advising parents and children under their care about the implications of these regulations.

NUTRITION

Healthy school age children are in a period of slow and steady growth, and their nutritional needs are relatively stable. The caloric intake requirement for this age group decreases slightly as do protein and water requirements. Snacks are most likely to be the primary source of nutrients for the school age child, and the older the child becomes, the more nutrition is obtained outside the home (Pipes, 1981). Therefore, the continued promotion of good eating habits and nutritious snacks is an essential part of the health maintenance visit. Additionally, implementation of a nutrition education program is indicated for the school setting. The recommended food intake for good nutrition for the school age and adolescent person is presented in Table 24-6 and the RDAs are outlined in Table 23-19. Foods affecting dental health are presented in Table 25-12.

Nurse's Role

While the school age period is generally a time of few nutritional problems, the need for continued nutritional assessment on the part of the nurse is important. The diet history continues to be a usual tool, one that will involve children in their own assessment and potentially their own promotion of sound eating habits (see Appendix A). The nurse's responsibility is to ensure that previously established healthy eating patterns are maintained and that children with deviant patterns are assisted to recognize them and to change.

The Adolescent

Preadolescent and adolescent years are a time of increased growth that is accompanied by an increase in appetite and nutritional requirements (see Tables 23-19 and 24-6). Caloric and protein requirements increase for boy ages 11 to 18. Girls have an increased protein need but a decreased caloric need during the same age span. In addition, the iron needed by the adolescent nearly doubles that needed by adults, and iodine, calcium, niacin, and thiamine requirements increase as well (Pipes, 1977; Torre, 1977).

Adolescent nutritional needs are influenced not only by the physical alterations that are occurring but also by the psychosocial adjustments. Teenagers are generally free to eat when and where they choose. It is a time when eating habits acquired from the family are dropped, snacking outside the home is a major source of nutrition, and fad foods and diets are prominent (Torre, 1977).

The factors of accelerated growth and poor eating habits make the adolescent at risk for poor nutritional health. Adolescents have been found to demonstrate the most unsatisfactory nutritional status of all age groups. Deficiencies in iron, vitamins A and C, calcium, riboflavin, and thiamin are most common.

Nurse's Role

Nursing has a responsibility to intervene and initiate activities that promote improved nutritional status. Such activities include the following:

Provision of informational material on good nutrition in group or individual encounters

Diet assessment using a comprehensive diet history or a 24-hour diet diary

Educational activities that focus on

Effects of fad foods and fad diets

Supplying of "at risk" nutrients and their sources

Provision of a daily food guide (see Table 25-13)

Suggested snacks and "on the run" foods that supply essential nutrients

Relationship of good nutritional habits to healthy appearance

Assessment for signs of nutritional deficiencies (see Table 25-14)

Supplementation
Vitamins

Adequate amounts of vitamins and minerals are necessary for the nutritional health of people of any age. Without these essential nutrients, physical and psychosocial health may be compromised. Much controversy

Table 25-13. Daily food guide for adolescents

Food group	Servings
Milk and milk products	4
Meats	3
Fruits and vegetables	4
Vitamin C source	1
Vitamin A source	1
Breads and cereals	4

From Tackett, J.J., and Hunsberger, M., editors: Family centered care of children and adolescents, Philadelphia, 1981, W.B. Saunders Co., p. 1244.

Table 25-14. Clinical signs indicative of nutritional deficiencies

	Clinical signs
General appearance	Lethargy, excessive or inadequate body fat, muscle wasting
Skin	Dryness, flakiness, scaling, roughness (follicular hyperkeratosis), pallor
Mouth	Angular fissures, redness at corners of mouth (cheilosis); redness, swelling, or atrophic papillae on tongue; red, swollen, or bleeding gums
Teeth	Severe caries
Eyes	Pale conjunctivae
Nails	Spoon-shaped, brittle or ridged
Hair	Dull, easily plucked

From Tackett, J.J., and Hunsberger, M., editors: Family centered care of children and adolescents, Philadelphia, 1981, W.B. Saunders Co., p. 1245.

arises over the question of routinely supplementing the diet with vitamins and minerals. Of particular concern is the recent fad of taking megadoses of vitamins and minerals to ensure health.

The decision to supplement a child's or adolescent's diet with vitamins or minerals should be based on (1) the nutritional adequacy of the diet for age and growth requirements as verified by diet assessment and (2) a clinically based nutritional deficiency (Chow et al., 1979).

Fluoride

An adequate fluoride supply is essential for dental health. Fluoride sources include treated drinking water, topical application, or oral tablets and rinses. Nurses should make assessments to verify whether adequate fluoride sources are available and should assist the client to secure a source if current supply is inadequate.

Special Nutritional Situations
Athletic Child

The child or adolescent who is engaged in athletic activities will require additional nursing assessment and intervention. For individuals involved in strenuous activities a minimum of 2300 to 5000 calories per day is required. Optimal distribution of calories is considered to be 10% to 15% protein, 25% to 35% fat, and 50% to 65% carbohydrate. Increases in vitamins, minerals, and water and salt may be indicated as well (Smith 1979).

Nurses have the responsibility to be knowledgeable about the potential need for added nutritional supplements of athletic children and to implement appropriate dietary assessment and management to meet these increased needs.

Vegetarian Child

The child or adolescent who follows a vegetarian diet requires special nursing assessment and management. Knowledge of the type of vegetarian diet followed is essential. Generally these types are (1) lactoovovegetarian, a diet of all vegetables supplemented by milk, eggs, and cheese; (2) lactovegetarian, a vegetable diet with only milk and cheese added; or (3) pure vegetarian, the diet of a vegan, which excludes all foods of animal origin.

Vegetarian diets can provide the essential nutrients for the growth and development of children. Diets of these types need to be based on sound nutritional principles, and the nurse who is assessing and counseling a vegetarian diet person should be aware of the following points (Williams, 1975):

Protein sources need to be varied to ensure adequate amounts of essential amino acids

Amino acids in one food can supplement those in another food

A variety of vitamin C and folacin sources must be included

A diet that excludes all animal food is deficient in vitamin B_{12}, supplementation is essential if eggs, cheese, and milk are not used

Adequate iodine can be obtained by using iodized salt

Adequate vitamins and minerals are amply supplied if protein, vegetables and fruit are adequate

Nurse's Role. Sound nutritional counseling on the part of nurses includes teaching that a vegetarian diet that includes some animal foods is nutritionally adequate if well planned. Vegans who observe pure vegetarian diets, require vitamin B_{12} supplementation. Providing sample menus for the vegetarian dieter is often helpful in promoting sound nutritional habits.

HEALTH PROMOTION ACTIVITIES

Health Assessment

Activities implemented by nurses which facilitate health continue throughout the school age and adolescent years. The health assessment visit, using the health history and physical assessment components that focus on individuals and their potential health risks and stressors, remains a focal point for nursing intervention. Development and implementation of a health plan needs to be a cooperative, collaborative effort involving the child or adolescent, parents, and the school. The specific screening techniques and tools for assessment have been previously discussed. *Noteworthy of reemphasis are screening of hearing, vision, dentition, sex characteristics (Tanner staging), nutrition, and school and social adjustment as well as screening for scoliosis, tuberculosis, common problems, venereal disease, need for birth control, and learning disabilities.*

Encouraging school age children and adolescents to assume responsibilty for their own health can be an effective health promotion activity (Daniel, 1970). But this approach requires close follow-up to ensure that health goals are being met.

The focus of anticipatory guidance is prevention of health problems. See Appendixes A, I, J, & K for examples of appropriate anticipatory guidance tools, Preventive health counseling should focus on the following aspects:

- Nutrition
- Safety
- School
- Peers
- Identified or at-risk health problems
- Sexuality (including venereal disease and birth control)
- Family and sibling relationships
- Coping strategies

Group Health Education and Child-focused Education

Promoting health in the group education setting is an effective technique. The principles for development of health maintenance classes were discussed in Chapter 23 and can be applied to classes focusing on school age and adolescent persons. An additional technique, which is useful and specific to these age groups, is to solicit participation of the child or adolescent in outlining the content of such courses. As interest evolves, participation can be increased to presentation of material in collaboration of the nurse. In some instances, adolescents may indicate interest in helping with educational classes for younger child. The primary objective, regardless of the technique, is to involve the participants and to encourage self-care responsibilities.

The setting for health education classes varies. However, use of the school setting, where large spans of time are spent, promotes greater participation. In addition, incorporating health education into the school's curriculum is a challenge nurses should undertake. Potentially such health programs could be a required component of the curriculum or be made available during student "free periods." The topics for such programs should be of interest to the participants and focus on a special interest group or an identified problem. In addition to the topics previously discussed under preventive health counseling, potential topics include sex education, participation in sports, taking care of yourself (e.g. focus on dentition, nutrition, or managing a cold), coping as a teenager, the importance of friends, and smoking.

Parent-focused Education

Parents, as well as their school age children and adolescents, are in need of educational programs. Focusing on the topics discussed in the previous section from a parental perspective potentially facilitates more effective parent skills. For example, classes in how to cope with teenage crises, how to talk to your child about sex, or how to communicate with the teenagers in your family offer parents an opportunity to learn new skills that promote their relationship with their child as well as the child's health. A similar approach can be applied to teachers by offering seminars that focus on problems or concerns they may be experiencing, e.g., how to handle an inattentive child or how to promote a positive relationship with students.

Home Intervention

Home intervention is generally based on an individual's or family's health needs. Certainly intervention at the time of a crisis is indicated. But intervention before crisis, with the goal of promoting health and preventing crises, is a significant contribution nurses can make. Assessing the home situation and environment is the nurse's responsibility. By assisting the family and child to identify problems within the home and by facilitating their resolve, nurses promote individual, family, and community health. A home that maintains health and relies on its resources is engaging in self-care and promoting wellness, both of which are nursing goals.

Additional Activities

Knowledge and understanding facilitate responsible behavior. Nurses are the catalysts who promote these experiences. Many of the activities previously discussed will enhance knowledge and understanding about health. Additional means include making resource material and services available to the child or adolescent and to parents.

Reading bibliographies directed towards specific concerns, problems, or age groups are useful tools. Printed materials on a diversity of topics are available from governmental agencies, special interest groups, and pharmaceutical companies. Nurses have a responsibility to direct their clients to these resources. Similarly, many community groups provide needed services. A few are listed in Chapter 23. Additional community resources for the school age child and adolescent include the following:

Mental health hot lines
Drug abuse centers
Planned Parenthood centers
Venereal disease clinics
Alcoholics Anonymous
Community recreation centers
Child and youth organizations
Youth athletic clubs

Nurses have the knowledge, skills, and resources to have an impact on the status of child health. The challenge lies in utilizing their full potential.

BIBLIOGRAPHY

Abbott, M.: Teens having babies, Pediatr. Nurs. **4**:23-27, May-June 1978.

American Academy of Pediatrics: Report of the Committee on Infectious Diseases, ed. 19, Evanston, Ill., 1982, AAP.

American Dental Association: Your Child's Teeth, Chicago, 1971, the Association.

Anderson, B.: The patient with scoliosis: Carole, a girl treated with bracing, Am. J. Nurs. **79**:1592-1598, Sept. 1979.

Barnard, M.U., et al.: Handbook of comprehensive pediatric nursing, New York, 1981, McGraw-Hill Book Co.

Bernstein, A.C.: Six stages of understanding how children learn about sex and birth, Psychol. Today **1**:31-35, Jan. 1976.

Boyle, M.P., Koff, E., and Guidas, L.J.: Assessment and management of anorexia nervosa, Mater. Child Nurs. **6**:412-418, Nov.-Dec., 1981.

Brosnan, J., and Fond, K.: School phobia: the student anxiety syndrome, Pediatr. Nurs. **6**:9-16, Sept.-Oct. 1980.

Brown, M.S., and Murphy, M.A.: Ambulatory pediatrics for nurses, ed.1, New York, 1975, McGraw-Hill Book Co.

Bruch, H.: Anorexia nervosa and its differential diagnosis, J. Nerv. Ment. Dis. **141**:555-566, Nov. 1965.

Child, A.A., Murphy, C.M., and Rhyne, M.C.: Depression in children: reasons and risks, Pediatr. Nurs. **6**:9-15, July-Aug. 1980.

Chow, M.P., et al.: Handbook of pediatric primary care, New York, 1979, John Wiley & Sons, Inc.

Cohen, M.I.: The process of adolescence: its psychologic and physiologic basis, Pediatr. Nurs. **4**:27-31, July-Aug. 1978.

Committee on Adolescence, Group for the Advancement of Psychiatry: Normal adolescence, New York, 1968, Charles Scribner's Sons.

Common orthopedic conditions in children, Report of the Ross Roundtable on Critical Approaches to Common Pediatric Problems, in collaboration with the Ambulatory Pediatric Association, Seattle, Aug. 20, 1972.

Contraception, Public Health Services Administration, Bureau of Community Health Services, Department of Health, Education, and Welfare Pub. No. (HSA) 78-5646, Washington, D.C., 1978.

Damon, W.: The social world of the child, New York, 1977, Jossey-Bass Inc., Publishers.

Daniel, W.A.: The adolescent patient, St. Louis, 1970, The C.V. Mosby Co.

Daniel, W.A.: Adolescents in health and disease, St. Louis, 1977, The C.V. Mosby Co.

Dibble, J.: ABC for teens—parent education after the baby comes, Pediatr. Nurs. 7:21-25, July-Aug. 1981.

Dunn, B.: Common orthopedic problems of children, Pediatr. Nurs. 1:7-10, Nov.-Dec. 1975.

Eldridge, T.M.: Adolescent health care: the legal and ethical implications, Pediatr. Nurs. 5:51-54, March-April 1979.

Erikson, E.: Childhood and society, New York, 1963, W.W. Norton & Co., Inc.

Freeman, R.B., and Heinrich, J.: Community health nursing practice, ed. 2, Philadelphia, 1981, W.B. Saunders Co.

Gorman, G.: The school age child as historian, Pediatr. Nurs. 6:39-41, Jan.-Feb. 1980.

Green, M., and Haggerty, R.J., editors: Ambulatory pediatrics, vol. 2, Philadelphia, 1977, W.B. Saunders Co.

Hart, N.A., and Prophit, S.P.: Adolescent suicide, Pediatr. Nurs. 5:22-28, Nov.-Dec. 1979.

Havinghurst, R: Developmental tasks and education, New York, 1972, David McKay Co., Inc.

Healthy People, Department of Health, Education, and Welfare Pub. No. (PHS)79-5571, Washington, D.C., 1979.

Jellinek, B., and Cloonan, P.: Adolescent consent: questions, confusion and conflicts, Pediatr. Nurs. 7:33-37, Jan.-Feb. 1981.

Kilmon, C., and Helpin, M.: Update on dentistry for children, Pediatr. Nurs. 7:41-47, Sept.-Oct. 1981.

Kreutner, A.K., and Hollingsworth, D.R.: Adolescent obstetrics and gynecology, Chicago, 1978, Yearbook Medical Publishers, Inc.

Krugman, S. and Katz, S.L.: Infectious diseases of children, ed. 7, St. Louis, 1981, The C.V. Mosby Co.

Laige, J.: The school aged child and his family. In Hymovich, D., and Barnard, M., editors: Family health care: developmental and situational crises, New York, 1978, McGraw-Hill Book Co.

Maier, H.: Three theories of child development, New York, 1969, Harper & Row, Publishers.

Marks, A.: Health screening of the adolescent, Pediatr. Nurs. 4:37-41, July-Aug. 1978.

Meier, J.H.: Development and learning disabilities: evaluation, management and prevention in children, Baltimore, 1976, University Park Press.

National Safety Council: Accident facts, Chicago, 1974, The Council.

Nelms, B.C., and Brady, M.A.: Assessment and intervention: the depressed school-age child, Pediatr. Nurs. 6:15-21, July-Aug. 1980.

Piaget, J., and Inhelder, B.: La genese do l'idee de hasard chez l'enfant, Paris, 1951, Presses Universitaires de France.

Pipes, P.L.: Nutrition in infancy and childhood, ed. 2, St. Louis, 1981, the C.V. Mosby Co.

Rogers, M.: Early identification and intervention of children with learning problems, Pediatr. Nurs. 2:21-26, Jan.-Feb. 1976.

Sapala, S., and Sheldon, S.: Infectious mononucleosis: clinical considerations for practitioners, Pediatr. Nurs. 4:16-27, Nov.-Dec. 1978.

Sapala, S. and Strokosch, G.: Adolescent sexuality: use of a questionnaire for health teaching and counseling, Pediatr. Nurs. 7:33-35, Nov.-Dec. 1981.

Schonberg, S.K.: Drug abuse counseling, Pediatr. Nurs. 4:31-33, July-Aug. 1978.

Scipien, G.: Comprehensive pediatric nursing, ed. 2, New York, 1979, McGraw Hill Book Co.

Smith, N.: Sports medicine, Pediatr. Nurs. 5:39-46, Jan.-Feb. 1979.

Sorenson, R.: Adolescent sexuality in contemporary America, New York, 1973, The World Publishing Co.

Stone, A.C.: Facing up to acne, Pediatr. Nurs. 8:229-239, July-Aug. 1982.

Sutterley, D., and Donnelly, G.: Perspectives in human development: nursing throughout the life cycle, Philadelphia, 1973, J.B. Lippincott Co.

Tackett, J.J., and Hunsberger, M., editors: Family centered care of children and adolescents, Philadelphia, 1981, W.B. Saunders Co.

Tanner, J.M.: Growth at adolescence, Oxford, England, 1962, Blackwell Scientific Publications, Inc.

Torre, C.T.: Nutritional needs of adolescents, Am. J. Matern. Child Nurs. 2:105-112, March-April 1977.

Vaughan, V.C., McKay, R.J., and Behrman, R.E., editors: Nelson textbook of pediatrics, ed. 11, Philadelphia, 1979, W.B. Saunders Co.

Waechter, E. and Blake, F.: Nursing care of children, ed. 9, Philadelphia, 1976, J.B. Lippincott Co.

Wells, G.: Reducing the threat of a first pelvic exam, Am. J. Matern. Child Nurs. 2:304-307, Sept.-Oct. 1977.

Williams, A.F.: Observed child restraint uses in automobiles, Am. J. Dis. Child. 130:1311-1317, 1976.

Williams, E.R.: Making vegetarian diets nutritious, Am. J. Nurs. 75:2168-2173, Dec. 1975.

Williams, H.A.: Screening for testicular cancer, Pediatr. Nurs. 6:38-41, Sept.-Oct. 1981.

Wolf, W.J., and Bancroft, B.: Early detection of childhood malignancies, Pediatr. Nurs. 5:43-48, Jan.-Feb. 1980.

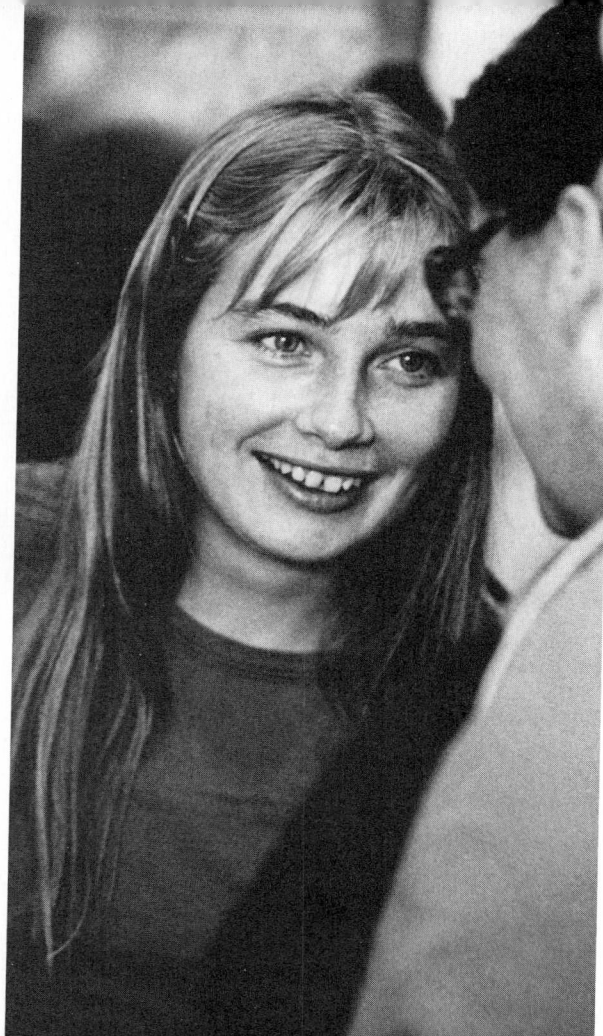

PATRICIA STARCK

MAJOR COMMUNITY HEALTH PROBLEMS OF YOUNG AND MIDDLE ADULTS

The period in life categorized as young and middle adulthood is paradoxically demanding and rewarding. Much is expected of the adult, who must support others on either end of the age continuum. Social role expectations of adults may result in stoicism about or suppression of their own needs, while they take care of the young, cope with the trials and tribulations of adolescent offspring, and take care of elderly parents. Like the middle-income strata of society, the young or middle adult may be considered the backbone of society—being responsible, accountable, and expected to take care of self as well as others.

In the health care literature, young and middle adults are a neglected, forgotten group. Other age groups are well-isolated for study and even have identifying labels such as fetus, newborns, infants, toddlers, early child-hood, adolescents, preteens, geriatric, and elderly. No such identifying terms exist for adult stages. There are no categories of adults in literature indexes. Age is used as a criterion for defining adulthood in our society. However, chronological age, maturity, and developmental task may vary. For purposes of this chapter adults are categorized as young adults and middle adults with an age range of 20 to 35 years (young) and 36 to 64 years (middle), recognizing that the dividing line is blurred. Indeed adults may move forward or backward between the young adult and the middle adult life-styles when establishing a marriage, home, and family; reentering single life; establishing a second marriage, home, and family; and developing a first and later a second career.

This chapter examines ways community health

nurses can assist young and middle adults meet health needs. Physical development and psychosocial developmental tasks are discussed, including the tasks and responsibilities characteristic of this group as well as the changes in biological functions and structures with concomitant psychosocial changes. Factors influencing progression through this stage of life including health status, resources in rural and/or urban settings, and lifestyles are explored, as are common causes of morbidity and mortality for young and middle adults. The nursing role implied by these major health problems is discussed, including tools for assessment and strategies for implementation. This chapter discusses health promotion from physical, psychosocial, and spiritual perspectives. Because a major task for the young and middle adult is career productivity, this chapter discusses careers and stress in the workplace and considers the special needs of the disabled adult. Exercises to be used by the reader to cope with health needs of this age group are also included.

PSYCHOSOCIAL DEVELOPMENT: TASKS OF ADULTHOOD

Adults progress through successive phases of stabilization and consolidation followed by change and growth in the pursuit of new goals and the confrontation of life crises at different stages.

Adulthood is a time of caring for others—children and parents. Caring for children presents challenges fluctuating with each stage of development of the child. A growing number of single parents face child rearing without partners. These years are heavy with busy events as the adults keep up with scheduled activities for many family members. The energy drain for adults with such a schedule may adversely affect health.

In addition, adults often encounter responsibilities for parent care. Reversal of the caring role (parent for child) often requires difficult decision making on behalf of a parent's welfare. Deciding on nursing home care versus living alone or with the primary family group may require professional consultation.

The primary burden of income production rests with the young and middle adult. Level of income, which determines living standards, security, and satisfaction, is often considered a measure of success. Adults feel pressure to achieve in a competitive world. During these years, an individual devotes considerable time, often in excess of the traditional 40 hours per week, to economic success.

Adults also feel pressure to fulfill societal responsibilities. Community progress is dependent on adult leadership. Much emphasis is placed on this generation's contribution to posterity.

Developmental Tasks

Adults move through various stages of psychosocial development. Common characteristics of these stages have been identified by various authors. Table 26-1 compares and contrasts viewpoints by Erikson (1950), Sheehy (1974, 1981), and Diekelmann (1976). In essence, the young adult struggles to achieve interpersonal intimacy outside the nuclear family while in the process of establishing a lifework, whereas the middle adult concentrates on making a contribution to society through work and/or family.

Psychosocial challenges may be complicated by physical changes that begin to occur in adulthood. These changes include graying hair, receding hairlines, changes in fat contours, spinal curvature changes, and skin turgor changes. The effect that these changes have varies with each individual. Exercise, nutrition, sleep, rest, play, and mental attitude affect the impact of physical changes.

The community health nurse may encounter individuals who are struggling with psychosocial tasks appropriate to the state of development or individuals who have failed to achieve normal goals. In either case, frustration impinges on the individual as well as the family system, creating barriers to achieving optimum health.

Middle adults who are single have double demands. They must revert back to the isolation versus intimacy tasks as well as deal with generativity challenges. Young or middle adults who are married may encounter problems; as Sheehy (1974) pointed out, no two people can possibly coordinate the timing and effect of their developmental crises.

Emotionally healthy adults are able to negotiate psychosocial challenges successfully. Sheehy (1981) identified 10 hallmarks of well-being in the adult.

1. Meaning and direction in life
2. Successful negotiation through transitions
3. Absence of feelings of being cheated or disappointed by life
4. Attainment of several long-term goals
5. Satisfaction with personal growth and development
6. Feelings of mutual love for partner
7. Many friends
8. Cheerful attitude
9. Not sensitive to criticism
10. No major fears

FACTORS INFLUENCING GROWTH AND DEVELOPMENT

Factors that influence growth and development of the adult include health status, a sense of responsibility

| | | | | | |

Table 26-1. Developmental tasks for young and middle adults

Stage	Erickson	Sheehy	Diekelmann
Young adult (20 to 35 years)	Intimacy versus isolation *Success:* Intimacy, facing fear of ego loss in situations of self-abandonment such as orgasm, close personal friendships, inspirational experiences *Failure:* Isolation and self-absorption	Stages: a. Pulling up roots (18-22), leaving home b. Trying 20s (23-27), establishing career and mate relationships c. Catch 30 (28-33), reassesing earlier family and or career decisions d. Rooting and extending (33-35), achieving degree of stability	Tasks: a. Achieving independence from parental controls b. Establishing intimate relationships outside the family c. Establishing a personal set of values d. Developing a sense of personal identity e. Preparing for a lifework and forming the capacity for intimacy
Middle adult (36-64 years)	Generativity versus stagnation *Success:* Generating an accomplishment — raising a family, writing a book, establishing and guiding the next generation *Failure:* Individual stagnation and interpersonal impoverishment	a. Deadline decade (35-45), recognizing urgency of achieving goals b. Comeback decade (45-55), accepting self and changes in values and life-styles	

for self-care, resources in rural and urban settings, and life-style behaviors. A unique factor for the middle adult is the challenge of "middlescence," characterized as a major turning point in life. The consummation of adult growth and development is achieving fulfillment through meaning and purpose in life.

Health Status

Health for the adult is the balanced state of well-being resulting from the harmonious interaction of body, mind, and spirit. Health care seeks to understand the human condition and to delineate the circumstances of illnesses and the underlying conflicts, hostilities, and griefs (see Chapter 18).

The panorama of health needs for adults includes prevention of health disruption, promotion of a state of high level wellness, care and/or cure services for illness states, and rehabilitation for chronic or disabling conditions. Self-care is a component of adult attempts to maintain or improve health status.

Responsibility: Self-care

Individual strivings in life are focused on efforts that life shall hold work, love, play, joy, and meaning. Diekelmann (1980) emphasized that people have the conscious power of judgment, decision, and choice to study their own circumstances and to conclude what is best and contributes to overall wellness. Participation is the essential ingredient in self-care or wellness care, and

requisite skills include self-centering, self-awareness, or self-reference (Silverman, 1980). These skills allow people to sensitize themselves to others while establishing insulation from the negativity present in the world at large. Selye (1980) emphasized the need for abilities in learning to gauge innate energies, potential weaknesses and strengths, and above all self-discipline and willpower.

Health risk appraisal as discussed in Chapter 14 is a useful technique in monitoring states of health. Though a young adult often takes good health for granted, middle adults become increasingly aware of health hazards and their contributions to these hazards. The health risk appraisal, generating a statement of probability and not a diagnosis, describes a person's chances of becoming ill or dying from selected diseases. It should not be used as a scare tactic but rather as a motivator to accentuate the positive aspects of health in the antecedent or subclinical stages of a known preexisting disease.

Perhaps the most effective means of promoting health and preventing disease is to have a comprehensive understanding of the disease process. Community health nurses must be able to anticipate and predict consequences of poor health practices. For example, community health nurses should be able to predict complications of uncontrolled diabetes such as a limb amputation and thus exert preventive measures in the young adult who is presently healthy but has a history of diabetes and tends to eat foods high in carbohydrates

Table 26-2. Predictable flow of pathophysiology of diabetes

Stages	Pathophysiology state	Symptoms
I. Antecedent	Genetic predisposition to diabetes Dietary pattern of high carbohydrate intake Smoking Sedentary work and life-style	No symptoms of illness
II. Stress-adaptation	Infection or pregnancy	Glycosuria and hyperglycemia, temporary
III. Beginning pathophysiology	Pancreas unable to meet demands for insulin	Persistent glycosuria and hyperglycemia, diagnosis of diabetes mellitus
IV. Progressive pathophysilogy	Vascular plaques, circulatory changes	Numbness in limbs, retarded healing of lower limb lesion
V. Advanced pathophysiology	Occlusion of vessel to limb, necrosis, and gangrene	Gangrene, necessitating amputation

and has a sedentary life-style. Exercises that demonstrate the predictable flow of pathophysiology from a healthy to a disabled state (Table 26-2) assist in conceptualizing the importance of prevention.

If healthy adults with particular genetic, dietary, and life-style antecedents could become aware of the predictable nature of disease conditions, perhaps self-care could be practiced with more vigor. As the stage of pathophysiology progresses, risk estimation accelerates for a crippling, permanent state of health. Personal Health Profiles are becoming popular items. Assessment data are gathered and fed into a computer, and a report is produced that predicts life expectancy and major health risks. Care should be taken that such instruments do not act as self-fulfilling prophecies.

Health Contracts

Health contracts, often used in primary health care centers, are one way individuals can exert self-discipline in self-care. The concept of participative decision making and contracting is well suited to adults who wish to maintain control over their lives. Agreement between the client and health care provider as to priorities of health problems must be reached. The purpose of a health care contract is to achieve specific health goals, with a secondary benefit of teaching clients to become more involved in health decisions. Contracts also reinforce independent rather than dependent behaviors; such participation by the client enhances the potential for improved future self-care capabilities and wellness-oriented behaviors. Hayes and Davis (1980) described the following six steps for health care contracting:

1. Identify problems
2. Rank problems in order of priority
3. Develop contract, including responsibilities and activities
4. Implement contract
5. Evaluate contract
6. Terminate contract

Contracts should include measurable criteria necessary to accomplish specific goals within an expected time frame. Responsibilities for client and clinician should be delineated, and both should sign the contract. During the implementation and evaluation phases, contracts may need to be renegotiated as situations change. Interim contracts to accomplish subgoals may be needed to supplement the major contract. Contracts should have a time limit rather than be for an indefinite period of time. For clients who are reluctant to assume self-care decision making, Hayes and Davis (1980) recommend giving concrete alternatives and facilitating a gradual process for increasing self-care responsibilities.

Nursing Centers

Nursing centers are defined as health care facilities in which the aim is to offer nursing services, including health assessment, promotion, screening, and teaching. Nursing centers offer a mechanism to promote self-care with emphasis on health assessment, promotion, and screening (Riesch et al., 1980). In addition, nursing centers often develop specialized programs such as adolescent sexuality or women's health. A multidisciplinary approach (nutrition, psychology, etc.) expands services offered at a nursing center, and established referral systems promote comprehensive care.

Resources for Health: Rural and Urban Settings

The issue of a workforce shortage in the health field in certain geographical areas has reinforced concern for health care in relation to population diversity. The total resources of the community are related to the attraction it holds for recruiting health care professionals. Mitchell and Mitchell (1980) pointed out that the health care delivery system closely parallels the basic institutional structure—pluralism—of the larger society. They identified the following six major system problems: (1) inadequate access for some, (2) overemphasis on technological care, (3) emphasis on sickness rather than wellness, (4) lack of coordination among organizations, (5) inadequate care of the elderly, and (6) continually escalating costs.

Rural areas with migrant worker populations present specific challenges to the community health nurse. Housing may be less than adequate, with such environmental hazards as rodent infestations, airborne and water-borne bacterial diseases, and poor sanitation. Community health nurses may have to adapt usual methods of teaching, since the average migrant worker over 25 years of age has completed only 3½ years of education. Illness conditions among migrant workers are appalling. Hawkins (1979) reported that the life expectancy of migrants is less than 60% that of the average U.S. citizen, and migrant infant mortality is 2.5 times the national average. Infectious diseases such as leprosy and tuberculosis are several times more prevalent than the national average. Chronic illnesses such as diabetes and hypertension are of epidemic proportions among migrants. Educational barriers and cultural differences of this population may be restraining forces in changing health practices. To be effective nurses must gain the trust of the clients and structure the plan of care according to client priorities. Only then can nurses introduce ideas for health improvement that have not been previously valued by this client population. More and more professionals are learning to blend their care with folk practices for greater compliance. That is, if clients engage in certain health rituals that do not harm, nurses can choose to be accepting as long as these individuals also improve other health practices.

Inner-city ghettos also face problems created by poverty and neglect. Although services available in the urban areas may be accessible and affordable, clients may need to be guided into active participation or may need an actual client advocate to get needed services. If such inner-city areas suffer from a shortage of health professional personnel who are discouraged by high crime rates, etc., urban services may not facilitate optimum care.

Linkage systems between rural and urban areas are the key ingredients in comprehensive, accessible care for rural citizens. Rural areas need adequate emergency services for accidents with farm machinery, etc. In addition, they need a rapid linkage mechanism with an urban medical center for continued specialized care. When the client returns to the rural area, discharge planning from the urban center must be coordinated.

Personal and Family Life-styles

Life-style, perhaps the greatest influence on health status, involves the practice of health habits and a guiding philosophy of life to promote a positive outlook. Individual and family life-styles vary according to resources, values, traditions, and family members. Like an individual, each family has its particular sources of stressors, and each adopts coping styles in attempts to maintain balance. Further stress within a family is influenced by the roles played by each member and the extent to which the tasks of family living are accomplished. For example, a family with a working mother may encounter stress from inadequate nurturing, redistribution of family living tasks, or inattention to individual needs. The working mother is likely to experience stress from such conflict. On the other hand, a second income, or in the case of the single parent the major income, may be of higher priority to the family. The boxes on pp. 626 and 627 contain tools to assist the community health nurse in assessing life-style factors that influence health.

Middlescence

Middlescence is defined as the intermediate stage of life between young adulthood and old age and is marked by physical, psychological, and social changes. The developmental task of middlescence is generativity.

The middle years are crossroads in the adult development process, and the transition is as critical as it was in adolescence. Grossman (1979) described this period as a time in the physical trajectory of life when individuals are simultaneously at a peak and yet newly vulnerable. This authenticity crisis occurs between 35 and 45 years of age. Individuals become preoccupied with signs of aging, and the inevitability of death and a last-chance urgency is noted in this period. Sheehy (1974) described the process as the end of growing up and the beginning of growing old.

The task of middlescence includes moving through a disassembling to a renewal with less concern for what society expects and attention on redesigning life according to intrinsic needs. Levinson (1978) stated that one of the major tasks for a male in the midlife transition is

---

Personal Life-style Assessment

Directions: Write your response to each of the items using a maximum of three sentences. Record your answer based on your immediate reaction; do not contemplate items for a lengthy period.

Physical dimensions

Describe your habits in a typical week as related to the following activities:

1. sleep
2. rest periods
3. exercise
4. hair care
5. dental care
6. smoking

7. alcoholic intake
8. medications
9. skin care
10. elimination
11. sex

12. foot and nail care
13. work, job
14. work, home
15. diet
16. medical checkup

How long do you expect to live?

Psychosocial and/or spiritual dimensions

Describe your habits in a typical week as related to the following activities:

1. reading for pleasure
2. reading for intellectual stimulation
3. meditation
4. interaction with friends
5. interaction with family

6. community activities for pleasure
7. community activities for service
8. recreational activities
9. hobbies
10. sports

Coping mechanisms

How do you handle stress on the job? At home?

What is your personal motto for life? (Eat, drink, and be merry: do unto others as you would have them do unto you, etc.)

What kind of actions by others make you angry? How do you handle the anger?

What goal do you have for this year? How do you plan to meet it?

What goals do you have for the next 5 years? How do you plan to meet them?

Are you satisfied with your present financial status?

What kind of things cause you the greatest anxiety?

How would you describe your relationship with your spouse or most significant other? Your children? Your in-laws and other relatives? Your parents?

What do you consider to be your life task?

On a scale from 1 to 10, how would you rate your present state of health (1–least healthy to 10–most healthy). How does your life-style contribute to or detract from your present state of health?

---

the acceptance of the feminism in himself. For example, he becomes more sensitive and capable of expressing emotions. In contrast, a woman who was been a caretaker may need to launch a career and actualize traits such as assertion and power, usually identified as master line traits. Thus both sexes become more comfortable with roles that they previously regarded as sex stereotyped.

Conflicting feelings and states of being characterize midlife crises with people experiencing paradoxical emotions, feeling wise yet confused, seeming to be independent yet dependent. This painful life dilemma is accompanied by anxiety, depression, anger, restlessness, and even physical symptoms.

Sheehy (1974) stated that individuals confront their own deaths through introspection and self-inventory. Additionally, adults in their middle years become aware of the suppressed parts of themselves. They mourn previously abandoned goals and may decide to pursue them with renewed vigor and commitment. They may experience disappointment with their marriage and wish to terminate or restructure it. They confront the reality that their children of yesterday have failed to actualize parental aspirations and sadly contemplate the effort that went into those years of raising children. Such disappointments may serve to release inhibitions and cause adoption of a life-style to please oneself, long suppressed for the sake of family convention.

Fulfillment: Meaning, Purpose in Life, and Self-Transcendence

Many adults today suffer from what Frankl* (1959, 1973, 1975) called a society-wide collective neurosis—

---

*Viktor E. Frankl is the founder of the Third School of Viennese Psychiatry—"The Will to Meaning" after Sigmund Freud's "Will to Pleasure" followed by Alfred Adler's "Will to Power."

Family Life-style Assessment

Directions: Write your responses to each of the items using a maximum of three sentences. Record your
answer based on your immediate reaction; do not contemplate items for a lengthy period.

Physical dimensions

Who in your family do you consider to be the "healthiest" member? The least healthy? How would you rate
each family member's health state?

What is your family's pattern as to:

1. mealtime
2. sleeping arrangements
3. family recreation
4. hygiene, household
5. dental care
6. sports, exercises

7. smoking
8. alcohol
9. medical checkups
10. work, household chores
11. work, jobs and schedules
12. pest control

What hereditary conditions are in your family history?

How long did your parents and grandparents live?

Directions: Contemplate each item as necessary, and record your responses as succinctly as possible.

Psychosocial and/or spiritual dimensions

Diagram your family constellation — (family tree) birth order or position, etc.

What family traditions are most important to your family? Describe a typical Christmas holiday with family.

Name three values that your family holds in high regard to complete the following statement, "One should
always . . . (tell the truth, be of service to others, etc.)."

Who fulfills or shares the following roles in your family?

1. breadwinner
2. homemaker
3. peacemaker
4. counselor

5. teacher of living skills
6. caretaker
7. financial manager
8. crisis manager

What causes stress within your family system? How does the family cope with stress?

---

increasing alcoholism, drug addiction, suicide, and aggression. Adults plunge into meaningless activities to run away from problems and at night are plagued with sleeplessness. Young adults want to be where the action is, experiencing the illusion of activity through speed. Loved ones are treated only as safety valves for tension reduction. The feeling of emptiness or of a life with no meaning is widespread among people today. This emptiness, which Frankl called an existential vacuum, is created when people feel that life has no purpose, no challenge, and it makes no difference what they do. Such adults feel hopelessly trapped by circumstances beyond their control. This existential vacuum is seen among rich and poor, young and old, the successful and the failures. Business executives try to fill the vacuum with extra work, and students try to fill it with drugs. This new type of neurosis is labeled *noo-genic neurosis,* defined as a mental health problem caused by spiritual (not religious) problems or moral conflicts; a type of mental conflict in which values are not clarified. Such a neurosis is brought about by a conflict of values and emptiness. "Nous" is the human spirit dimension of the individual.

Human life is unique; there has never been and will never be two individuals exactly alike. The meaning of life differs for each individual, and according to Frankl, the primary motivation for an individual's behavior is *not* seeking pleasure or power but searching for meaning and purpose in life. Though we cannot always control the circumstances of life, we can choose the attitude toward our fate. Each adult strives to find meaning in life experiences, and mentally healthy adults seek to lead a purposeful life. From such harmony comes a feeling of fulfillment.

According to Frankl, meaning can be found in three ways:

1. Creative values—a task or mission to complete
2. Experiential values—to experience or know the true, good, and beautiful; to lovingly encounter another human being
3. Attitudinal values—facing one's fate or choosing a positive attitude toward a fate that cannot be changed

Frankl has developed logotherapy to assist clients in finding purpose in life and meaning in life experiences. Logotherapy's aim is self-transcendence or getting outside oneself to help others. Self-transcendence involves focusing on others as contrasted with self-actualization or focusing on developing and actualizing potential within oneself. Self-transcendence is commitment to the fulfillment of life's meaning so that the joyous life comes not as a result of direct pursuit but as a by-product.

The community health nurse can use a logotherapeutic approach in working with clients who appear apathetic or otherwise lack the motivation to modify lifestyle to enhance their state of health. The key to logotherapy is attitude change. The nurse may be innovative in techniques to modify attitudes. Various intellectual exercises, such as analyzing parables, can stimulate discussion that guides the client to a broader view of a fate that cannot be changed. The nursing process may be used as a framework in logotherapy.

1. Assess—determine what is of value to the client and who are the significant others. What are immediate long-term goals? Identify the client's perception of the present state of affairs and the ways in which current health status inhibits or facilitates fulfillment. Assessment also includes comparing verbal and nonverbal behaviors for congruency in values and identifying areas of conflict. Throughout the assessment, analyze the client's abilities and disabilities for feasibility of immediate and long-range goal accomplishment. Isolate restraining and facilitating factors in the environment that influence goal accomplishment.

2. Plan—engage in mutual goal setting that combines realistic abilities with potential growth of abilities. Establish a time frame, methodologies, and criteria for evaluation.

3. Intervene—use innovative strategies to unfreeze attitudes. For example, have the parents of a child diagnosed as having cystic fibrosis discuss the following parable as it relates to their situation.

> Two frogs fell into a churn of milk. One said, "I have no chance," and he sank to the bottom and drowned. The other said, " I may not have a chance, but I won't go down without a fight." He splashed around and splashed around until lo and behold the milk turned to butter, and he was afloat on top.

4. Evaluate—measure outcomes based on previously established criteria. Make decisions regarding future action. Set new goals and evaluation criteria.

COMMON CAUSES OF MORBIDITY AND MORTALITY

Morbidity and mortality indicators for young and middle adults offer guidance to the community health nurse in planning strategies for this aggregate population. For young adults major threats to health include (1) violent death and injury, involving motor vehicle accidents, suicides, and homicides, (2) alcohol and drug abuse, (3) unwanted pregnancies, and (4) sexually transmissible diseases. The death rate for young men is three times higher than for young women. About 75% of all deaths are caused by accidents, homicides, and suicides; such deaths are often the result of the greater risk taking characteristic of this age group. Young black adults have a five times greater homicide rate than their white counterparts, with homicide the leading cause of death among black youths; accidents are a close second. Life-styles and behavior patterns that affect health are often established in this period. Health education programs with a communitywide audience should be geared to avoiding risks and practicing safety precautions. One such program involved television spots regarding the hazards involved in diving into unknown waters, a frequent cause of spinal cord injury.

Motor vehicle accidents account for a number of fatalities for adults. In 1978, 46.4 deaths per 100,000 population in the 15- to 24-year-old age group were the result of motor vehicle accidents as compared to 28.5 among young adults between 25 and 34 years; 20.2 for adults between 35 and 44 years; and 18.0 for adults in the 45- to 54-year-old age group (Health: United States, 1981). A young adult driver is twice as likely to die in an accident as a driver over 25 years of age. The risk of accidents is greater for drivers under the influence of alcohol or drugs. About one half of fatally injured drivers are found to be intoxicated (100 mg of alcohol per deciliter of blood). Motorcyclists have a seven times greater risk for fatal injury for each mile driven as compared to automobile drivers. Safety precautions such as seat belts, helmets, and enforcement of speed limits should be facilitated to reduce the morbidity and mortality in this age group.

In 1977 suicide was the third leading cause of death (5600 deaths) in the 15 to 24-year-old age group, with males having the higher rate. In 1978 there were 12.4 suicides per 100,000 population for the 15- to 24-year-old age group compared to 16.7 for the 25- to 34-year-olds; 15.8 for people between 35 and 44 years; and 17.1 and 18.1 for the 45- to 54-year-olds and the 55- to 64-year-olds, respectively (Health: United States, 1981). The modes of suicide in order of frequency include firearms, drugs, and exhaust gases. Many attempted suicides are not reported. Contrary to popular belief, most people who commit suicide give verbal and/or behavioral warnings (Healthy People, 1979).

The following box shows data regarding homicide facts. Homicide statistics for young adults are startling. Deaths of blacks are 30% and whites just under 7% as the result of homicide, with an overall rate of 10%. Of all homicides 25% are in the 15- to 24-year-old age group. Rates are also high for people between 25 and 44

Facts Regarding Homicides in Young Adults (15 to 24 years old)

- 25% of all homicides are in the 15- to 24-year-old age group
- Homicides account for 10% of deaths in this age group
  30% of deaths in black youth
  7% of deaths in white youth
- Homicide rates per 100,000 population by country
  America   10.2
  France   0.9
  Great Britain   1.0
  Sweden   1.1
  Japan   1.3
- 60% to 80% of homicides start with personal disagreements or conflicts
  Men as victims   3 to 5 times the rate for women
  Men as offenders   5 times the rate for women
- Related individual variables—homicide is associated with alcohol abuse and poverty and is more apt to occur on weekends and at night
- Related societal variables—homicide is associated with economic deprivation, family breakup, violence through the media, and easy access to firearms

From Healthy people: The Surgeon General's report on health promotion and disease prevention, DHEW Pub. No. (PHS) 79-55071, Washington, D.C., 1979, Department of Health, Education, and Welfare.

---

years, and only drops below 10 per 100,000 adults in the over 45-year-old age groups. The overall American homicide rate of 10.2 per 100,000 contrasts sharply with that of France (0.9), Great Britain (1.0), Sweden (1.1), and Japan (1.3). Societal factors thought to influence the high homicide rate are economic deprivation, family breakup, glamorizing of violence in the media, and easy access to firearms. Of American murders, 20% occur among relatives or those with a close relationship, and 40% are among acquaintances. Personal disagreements and conflict account for 60% to 80% of homicides, which are more prevalent among the poor, more frequent on weekends and at night, and often associated with alcohol abuse. Men are killed three to five times more often than women, and men are five times as likely to be the offender.

What stressors are contributing to the appalling loss of young American lives? Pressures and frustrations that lead to such violent behaviors are related to lifestyle and to conflicts experienced in developmental tasks of this generation. For the young adult, striving to establish an identity can be confused by differing role expectations between peer and family groups. Lack of success in educational pursuits and employment goals causes diminished self-esteem and loss of the approval so highly sought by the young adult. Young adults whose task is to establish intimacy find themselves in a culture in which short-term temporary relationships and social mobility are the norms. Lacking the maturity that builds patience and tolerance, young people seek a quick and easy solution (even drastic measures), to bring relief. Drugs and alcohol combined with this im-

maturity result in reckless behavior that often ends in tragedy.

What can community health nursing contribute to the resolution of this challenging problem? Using an approach that emphasizes positive mental health, nurses can provide mental health services that guide family members through stressful times and prepare them for life event changes using anticipatory guidance. Analyzing the community for healthy energy outlets such as recreational opportunities is part of the community assessment. When such resources are lacking, nurses can be instrumental in community planning. On a one-to-one basis, while working with a family in a preexplosive phase, nurses can use the therapeutic approach to help the family members discover some meaning in their circumstances, to see it as time limited, and to encourage self-transcendence (i.e., getting outside oneself and the immediate problem and focusing on a task to accomplish for others).

An additional health problem for the 15- to 24-year-olds is sexually transmittable diseases, 75% of which occur in this age group. Syphilis and gonorrhea continue to increase, as do other diseases including genital herpes and nonspecific urethritis. Each year 75,000 females become sterile as a result of sexually transmitted pelvic inflammatory disease. The incidence of these diseases decreases during the adult years after age 25.

In addition to physiological problems, the young adult faces many emotional, social, and spiritual stressors that lay the foundation for chronic ill health. Anxiety and pressure from careers, and family life interfere with optimum health and plant the seeds for illness later in life. Common causes of morbidity and mortality in middle adults are heart disease and strokes, cancer, alcohol and substance abuse, mental health problems, and periodontal disease (Healthy People, 1979).

Heart Disease and Strokes

The leading cause of death for middle adults is heart disease which affects men three times as often as premenopausal women. After menopause, heart disease in women increases and begins to approach the male rate by age 70, being equal by age 85. Coronary heart disease includes clinical syndromes of myocardial infarction, angina pectoris, and sudden death. Heart disease is also the greatest cause of permanent disability among workers under 65, responsible for more days of hospitalization than any other cause, and is the principal cause of limited activity. Stroke accounts for almost 10% of mortality. Many of those who survive are disabled by paralysis, speech difficulties, incontinence, and mental changes. Blacks in the age range of 25- to 64-years have a stroke death rate almost 2.5 times that of whites. Fortunately, however, death rates for heart disease and stroke are on the decline. Between 1968 and 1977 the heart disease death rate fell 22%, and the stroke death rate fell 32% (Healthy People, 1979).

The heart disease problem cannot be analyzed as to a singular cause and effect. Rather the combination of various predisposing conditions interact to cause disease manifestation in various individuals. Control of risk factors is the strategy most useful in community health nursing practice.

Risk Factors

Those who smoke cigarettes have twice the rate of heart disease as those who do not. Hazardous substances in cigarettes are nicotine and carbon monoxide; the risk is proportional to the amount of smoke inhaled. Risk is also related to the number of cigarettes smoked, those who smoke one pack per day are three times more likely to have a heart attack than those who do not smoke.

The World Health Organization classifies blood pressure into the following categories: (1) normal is less than 140/90 mm Hg, (2) borderline is 140/90 to 160/95 mm Hg, and (3) hypertension is 160/95+ mm Hg (O'Connor, 1981). Hypertension, the leading cause of premature disability for industry workers, costs the nation $1.7 billion annually (Lattimore et al., 1979). Hypertension increases the risks of heart disease and stroke. About 35 million Americans have hypertension, and those with systolic pressures above 160 are three times as likely to have a stroke as those with systolic pressures under 140. Lowther and Carter (1981)

cited factors involved with hypertensive control as regimentation to a medication schedule, regular follow-up appointments, sodium-restricted diets, caloric restrictions for weight control, cessation of smoking, and reduction of stress. They found that sending missed appointment reminder cards significantly increased the client's rescheduling and keeping the next appointment. Community programs can be effective in long-term treatment.

Another risk factor, cholesterol, is associated with heart disease and to a lesser extent with stroke. For the 35- to 44-year-old age group, heart attacks are five times more frequent in individuals whose cholesterol level is above 265 than among those with levels below 220. Low density lipoproteins (LDL) apparently accelerate cholesterol deposition on vessel walls. High-density lipoproteins (HDL) do not seem to have this effect and may even be protective. Dietary cholesterol is responsible for only 25% to 30% of serum cholesterol. Optimum plasma cholesterol is 200 mg; 250 mg is risky. Exercise and diet modification may increase the HDL:LDL ratio to protect against heart disease.

Individuals with diabetes have an increased risk of cardiovascular disease, with twice as many strokes and heart attacks as the nondiabetic. Women who are diabetic have a risk five times higher than other women for atherosclerotic heart disease.

Other risk factors associated with heart disease include obesity, sedentary life-style, personality patterns related to stress, genetic predisposition, and oral contraceptive use. Predisposing personality characteristics have been labeled type A behaviors in which the pattern involves high-level stress chosen to be the life-style. O'Flynn-Comiskey (1979) described the type A person as being competitive and rarely fatigued, valuing work highly, and being dominated by speed (see Chapter 38).

O'Connor (1981) classified risk factors into the following four categories:

- Major risk factors—smoking, hypertension, hypercholesterolemia
- Potentially controllable factors—smoking, hypertension, hypercholesterolemia, diet and/or obesity, lack of exercise, stress, and use of oral contraceptives
- Independent factors—diabetes mellitus and familial hyperlipidemia
- Uncontrollable factors—age, sex, race, heredity, and regional factors

Primary prevention of heart disease begins in infancy with a diet free from fats, excessive salt, and sugar as well as early regular exercise. Secondary prevention begins at the stage of arterial changes and focuses on arresting and/or retarding atherosclerosis. Tertiary prevention is used with those who already have symptoms of heart disease or actual pathological manifestations.

Cancer

One in four Americans develops cancer, making it the second leading cause of death (Healthy People, 1979). In individuals 35- to 64-years of age cancer causes more than one third of the deaths. Among the most fatal cancers in adults are those of the lung, intestine, and breast. Experts agree that cancer is not just one disease but a group of diseases with various rates of occurrence and clinical courses. A carcinogenic agent is defined as a single cancer-inducing substance that triggers the change in behavior of cells, resulting in uncontrolled growth.

Risk Factors

Various factors that increase risk for cancer include cigarette smoking, alcohol, certain dietary patterns, radiation, sunlight, occupational hazards, water and air pollutants, heredity, and certain predisposing medical conditions. As noted in Chapter 22, cigarette smoking is the greatest known agent responsible for cancer and cancer deaths; smokers have 10 times the rate of lung cancer as nonsmokers. A combination of other risks with smoking accentuates cancer probability. For example, occupational exposure to asbestos and cigarettes increases lung cancer risk 90 times. Cancer incidence is also high in uranium miners who smoke (Archer, 1973). Consumers of alcohol have higher rates of can-

cer of the esophagus, larynx, oral cavity, and liver. Although no well-established cause and effect relationship has linked diet and cancer, food additives may have carcinogenic potential. X-ray films should be kept to a minimum to avoid cumulative exposure, since low-level radiation, including natural background radiation, affects people. Individuals who spend considerable time outdoors may acquire skin cancer from overexposure to sunlight. Such cancer as well as premature wrinkling can be prevented by avoiding sunlight, wearing protective clothing, and using lotions containing paraaminobenzoic acid (PABA).

It is believed that 20% or more of cancers are occupational in origin (Moses, 1979). Though occupational health is described in Chapter 13, selected information pertinent to adults is presented. Data in Table 26-3 link occupational hazards with types of cancer. In addition to direct contact, toxic materials from industry can pollute the air, thus endangering residents in the area. A long period of latency (20 to 30 years) is characteristic of occupationally related cancers (Moses, 1979). Other work-related carcinogens include arsenic, benzene, coal tar, coke oven emissions, chromium, hematite, nickel, and petroleum distillates.

Industrial carcinogenic agents found in water supplies for drinking include chlordane, aldrin, dieldrin, and benzene. They may become concentrated in fish or shellfish. Air pollution results primarily from automobile exhausts and to a lesser extent from synthetic organic chemicals. There appears to be a clustering of

Table 26-3. Occupational hazards associated with cancers

Occupational chemical	Cancer
Asbestos	Mesothelioma (pleural and peritoneal)
	Lung
Vinyl chloride (plastics)	Liver (hemangiosarcoma) (200 times at risk)
	Brain (4 times at risk)
	Lung (2 times at risk)
Benzene	Leukemia, predominantly acute myelogenous
Bischloromethane ether	Oat cell carcinoma
Chromium	Nasal or paranasal sinus, lung, larynx
Arsenic	Lung
Coal tar pitch, coke oven emissions	Lung, larynx, skin
Iron oxide	Lung, larynx
Nickel	Lung
Petroleum distillates	Lung, larynx

From Healthy people: The Surgeon General's report on health promotion and disease prevention, DHEW Pub. No. (PHS) 79-55071, Washington, D.C., 1979, The Department of Health, Education, and Welfare; and Moses, M.: Am. J. Nurs. 79:1984-1988, 1979.
NOTE: The Toxic Substances Control Act of 1977 requires premarket testing of new chemicals.

Table 26-4. Characteristics of various cancer sites and strategies to prevent

Cancer sites	Characteristics	Prevention and/or early detection
Lung	Most common lethal malignancy Accounts for 4% of total deaths Accounts for 25% of cancer deaths 80% of victims smoked Difficult to detect early	Elimination of cigarette smoking Avoidance of occupational exposures
Breast	Affects 1 in 13 women Most common malignancy of American women	Self-examination Examination by health practitioner Mammography
Colon and rectum	Accounts for 15% of all cancers Second most common cause of cancer deaths Affects 100,000 Americans and leads to 50,000 deaths annually Most common between 50 and 70 years of age	Examination by physician, including sigmoidoscopy and colonoscopy High fiber diets (*may* help to prevent)
Prostate	80% occur after 65 years Has been increasing for the past 40 years	Rectal examination by health practitioner, especially for men over 50
Cervix	Affects 20,000 American women and causes 7500 deaths annually Incidence and deaths declined since 1950s Risks increased with multiple sex partners, early and frequent sexual activity, and multiple childbirth	Pap smear
Urinary bladder	40% of cases occur before age 65 Led to 6900 deaths in 1977 Common in heavy smokers and those exposed to occupational hazards Early sign is hematuria	Elimination of cigarette smoking Reduction of exposure to occupational carcinogens
Oral cavity	Accounts for 5% of cancers 24,000 new cases and 8000 deaths per year Associated with use of all forms of tobacco and alcohol, with synergistic effects Cancer of floor of mouth associated with poor oral hygiene Lower lip cancer associated with chronic sunshine exposure	Practice of good oral hygiene Avoidance of all forms of tobacco Avoidance of excessive alcohol intake Avoidance of excessive sun exposure

From Healthy People: The Surgeon General's report on health promotion and disease prevention, DHEW Pub. No. (PHS) 79-55071, Washington, D.C., 1979, Department of Health, Education, and Welfare; and Karman, J. and Price, J.H.: Nurs. Care 13:15-17, Aug. 1980.

cancer in some families; whether it involves heredity or environmental patterns is not known. Multiple intestinal polyps in families tend to result in cancer of the colon.

The two most effective strategies for preventing cancer and death from cancer are (1) limiting exposure to carcinogenic agents and (2) early detection and treatment before a cancer has spread. Table 26-4 presents data related to various sites of cancer.

The Cancer Client in the Community

Providing care to adults who are living at home with cancer is a challenging opportunity for the community health nurse. Such care includes (1) providing physical care, (2) teaching and counseling, and (3) giving emotional support to the client and family.

Providing physical care may include colostomy care, dressing change, or medication administration. DeMoss (1980) has had success with giving intravenous chemotheraphy in the home setting.

Teaching and counseling about the disease and its impact must be done. Sexuality counseling may be a need of the client with cancer. Lamb and Woods (1981) specified guidelines for sexual assessment, interventions to promote sexual health, and alternative ways of expressing physical love. These adults experience lifestyle changes because of their uncertain futures, often finding it difficult to plan ahead or to make decisions.

They tend to set short-term goals and focus on the present. Family relationships are disrupted, as are interactions with the community. Counseling with all family members may be needed.

Cancer clients need emotional support for the many worries and concerns such as work, financial status, relationships with the family and significant others, religious and existential concerns, fearful treatments and toxicities, prolonged hospitalizations, waiting for progress reports, pain, and death (Welch 1981). Clients may feel different or isolated, spending much time in introspection. Nurses can direct clients to focus on strengths rather than limitations and to reassess values in planning for the remaining years. Johnson and Norby (1981) described a successful weekend retreat program founded on the premise that every cancer family can actively participate in the restoration process. Many clients achieve inner joy and peace by enjoying 1 day at a time. Searle (1980) described a positive response to cancer of the breast by a woman who initiates the first step toward effective rehabilitation and continuing care to promote the quality of life; avoids psychological invalidism; accepts her diagnosis and treatment; helps her family to cope with their anxieties; and behaves in a way that prevents the family from being oversolicitous of or rejecting her. Mind, body, and emotions interact as a unit to effect recovery. The community health nurse has a responsibility to promote a hopeful attitude in the client and family.

For clients who have terminal cancer, hospice programs can provide support to the individual and family. New types of self-help groups of cancer victims enable clients to realistically prepare for impending death.

Alcohol and Substance Abuse

As discussed in Chapter 22, the statistics for alcoholism document the significance of this problem for adults. There are an estimated 10 million problem drinkers in America; 28,500 died from alcohol-related cirrhosis in 1977, and many violent and accidental deaths are indirect results of alcoholism (Healthy People, 1979). The young adult woman who consumes alcohol during pregnancy risks abnormality in the fetus, resulting in mental retardation and other defects. The community health nurse is likely to be very involved with a family who has a child with fetal alcohol syndrome. Alcohol abuse also causes many psychosocial problems in family living.

There is growing concern about substance abuse, especially in young adults. Marijuana, barbiturates, cocaine, other central nervous system drugs, and heroin are among those abused. Heroin addiction may lead to hepatitis, cardiovascular disease, chromosome damage, diabetes, gastrointestinal disorders, gynecological disease disorders, hepatic cirrhosis, infections, and trauma. Treatment centers should use the comprehensive health care approach, as basic health needs must be met if clients are to achieve the goal of remaining in the drug-free state.

Mental Health

Mental illness, as described in Chapter 18, causes much suffering among young and middle adults. It is estimated that 25% of the population suffers some form of mental anguish (Healthy People, 1979). In 1975, 7 million people (3% of the population) sought outpatient care, and 1 to 2 million were hospitalized for mental problems. In addition, many clients hospitalized for physical problems or those coping with a chronic illness suffer from mental problems. For example, psychosocial disability has been demonstrated in clients on maintenance hemodialysis (Procci, 1981). Psychiatric disorders are most frequently diagnosed among people with low levels of income, education, and occupation. City residents have a higher incidence of anxiety, mild depression, phobias, self-doubt, and personality disorders, whereas rural residents have a higher incidence of manic depressive disorders. Regardless of the disorder, early professional treatment is advisable.

The community health nurse is often concerned with support care after institutionalization. Aftercare may involve halfway house residential facilities, a private proprietary home, other innovative group homes, or a return to the family setting. Valenzuela and Hallamore (1979) described a successful "good neighbor network" using natural helpers. Every community has members who are accepted as authorities on helping and healing. They may be called *padrones* in an Italian community, *mavens* in a Jewish community, or *curanderos* in a Mexican community. This folk support system can be linked with the professional care system. This strategy may be essential in an era of legislative cutbacks for human services. The natural, neighborly helping philosophy may also promote community pride.

Cutler and Madore (1980) described an effective approach to mental health services in a rural setting with community-family network therapy. The system is designed to open lines of communication and to strengthen the supportive and adaptive qualities of the client-social network ecosystem. The network consists of family members, nuclear and extended, who relate to the identified problem. Each family member has an assigned advocate who establishes an empathic rapport, intervenes for the family member in group dialogue in a supportive manner, and helps to facilitate expression of the family members' needs or feelings. The group also has a network organizer, conductor, consultant, and monitor. A network group may contain as many as 30 to 35 people. The group motivation is to create a setting for cooperative, active problem solving. To achieve a balanced perspective from the private, public, and consumer sectors of the community for mental health aftercare services, coordinated planning and cooperation are needed.

Periodontal Disease

Diseases of gum tissues are common problems of adults. The initial causative agent is thought to be bacterial plaque, resulting in gingivitis and later periodontitis. Symptoms of gingivitis include inflammation, redness, and swelling of gums with a tendency to bleed easily. Periodontitis occurs when the supporting bones and ligaments are destroyed, resulting in loose or "drifting" teeth. Periodontitis is the leading cause of loss of teeth after age 35. In the 55- to 64-year old age group, 30% of adults lose all their natural teeth because of this disease. Proper dental care involves regular brushing and flossing of teeth and regular professional dental care.

Summary: Morbidity and Mortality

In summary, health for the young and middle adult depends to a significant degree on life-style and health practices for which the adult must assume responsibility. An individual's risk for disease development can be reduced by compliance with measures known to prevent occurrence, retard progression, and maintain a state of good health.

COMMUNITY HEALTH NURSING IMPLICATIONS

The community health nurse uses and integrates knowledge from all clinical specialty areas. Futhermore, the community health nurse has the responsibility for encouraging clients to promote their level of health, change life-styles if necessary, and confront common, inescapable life conditions of suffering and death. Several exercises for coping with conflict, stress, and future plans are given in the appendix.

Nurse's Role in Promoting Responsibility for Health

A 50-year-old man, a retired military officer, has had essential hypertension for 3 years. He is not employed and spends his days around the house. He has several projects such as repairing a fishing boat, but he paces his day as he likes. His wife is a 38-year-old professional career woman who sometimes is annoyed that he is not working or "making any worthwhile contribution to society." In discussing his health

with the nurse, the wife reveals that she suspects that he lies on the sofa all afternoon watching soap operas. He does not get any physical exercise. She puts his medicine in a dish for him every day but is not convinced that he actually takes it. She prepares a healthy lunch for him each day before she leaves for the office but frequently finds evidence that he has eaten salty foods while she is away. He also smokes one pack of cigarettes per day to the annoyance of his wife. She tells the nurse that she is at the end of her rope in trying to take care of his health.

A conference with the client reveals that he feels his wife nags him all the time. He says all he wants is to be left alone. He feels that she treats him like a naughty child and that he deserves to live his life the way he chooses. The nurse also learns that the previous nurse assigned to this case spent considerable time in teaching health to the client and his wife. She found that both comprehended information well, but that the client's attitude was one of indifference.

Who is responsible for the client's health? The thesis of this chapter is that adults are responsible for their own health. The wife in this case has been behaving as if her husband's health is her responsibility. Many who are nurturers, such as mothers, wives, and even nurses, fail to motivate the client to assume self-responsibility. After a discussion with the nurse, the wife had the following conversation with her husband.

"I realize that I have been nagging you about your diet, exercise, and medications. I also know that you are the one who is responsible for your health, and the choices are yours. From now on I won't constantly hover over you. I'll be glad to do whatever you need to help you carry out your plan." The wife stopped putting out his medicine or preparing his lunch, although she did make certain plenty of nutritious foods were available. Remarkably there was a change in the client's behavior. He purchased two exercise bicycles and began to comply with his diet and medication regimens.

What can the nurse do to promote responsibility for health? Three areas of skills are needed. *Communicate an attitude of responsibility for self.* Do not say, "You shouldn't eat sweets on a diabetic diet." Such a message presumes a superior-inferior position. It says that the nurse knows what is best, "*I* can tell *you* what *you* should do." It also creates guilt in the client who eats sweets in spite of knowing the dangers. Do say something like, "What do you (or can you) do about your craving for sweets, which would adversely affect your diabetic condition? Are there things you can do to control your desire for sweets?" Stimulate the client to think of chewing sugarless gum, brushing teeth right after meals, or using mouthwash.

Teach health information. Teaching is not telling; giving accurate information does not assure compliance. Client teaching should begin with assessment. It is important to find out what the client already knows so that time and patience are not wasted. To illustrate this point, the following example is given. A nursing student assigned to assist with discharge planning for a client recovering from a myocardial infarction set a priority goal of emphasizing the need for a gradual return to work. The night before the assignment she prepared a simplistic drawing of the heart. She used the diagram to explain to the client how his heart would be affected by overwork. Near the end of her teaching session she said, "By the way, what kind of work do you do?" He replied, "I'm a cardiologist."

After assessment of the knowledge level of the learner, objectives should be set based on mutual goals. Learning activities are designed according to the content and learning style best suited to the client. Evaluation must follow a teaching/learning session. Retention of learned material should not be taken for granted. Reinforcement of the learning is also necessary.

Use positive reinforcement of effective health behaviors. Good health has its own rewards, such as vim, vigor, and vitality. However, the first few days or weeks of losing weight may not bring such a feeling of exhilaration. Nurses must support clients who comply with healthy behaviors, and they also need to accept those who lapse back into unhealthy actions. In the latter case, the nurse can tell the client that it is not unusual to have occasional relapses. Many contracts for health behaviors allow for 1 to 2 free days per week in which jogging, for example, can be omitted. Clients should reward themselves—go to a movie to celebrate a week of adherence to the new diet.

Nurse's Role in Promoting Changes in Life-style

Life-styles like personalities are not changed easily. Personal philosophies about life have a great influence on life-style, as do economic status and peer life-styles. Philosophies about life evolve from parental influence, the educational process, and community activities. Some philosophies may be detrimental to health, such as the hedonistic life-style based on "Eat, drink, and be merry, for tomorrow you may die."

Life-style changes result from reassessed goals, changing values, and commitments to a new life pattern. These changes can be triggered suddenly through crisis or can blossom from planting a seed and nurturing ideas over a period of time. Significant others are often catalysts in the adoption of new life patterns. Nurses and/or other health professionals can also serve as facilitators of changed attitudes.

When attempting to motivate a client to change his life-style, the circuitous method of communication is often effective. Telling a story about a third party can shed insight on how the client is in the same predicament and can be suggestive of a similar solution that might work. A 19-year-old man injured in an automobile accident while speeding excessively suffered a C7 spinal cord injury. On discharge from the rehabilitation center with instructions to follow a well-defined plan of care, the community health nurse visited him in his home only to discern the following problems:

1. He had been fasting to lose weight.
2. His fluid intake was poor.
3. He decided to drop out of college.
4. He hoped to get married at the end of the year.

While discussing his fasting, the client stated that he was getting too big for his clothes, and the wheelchair was feeling tight. In an attempt to get the weight off rapidly, he seemed to discount the risk of protein depletion that could result in skin breakdown and other problems. Although aware of the need for fluids, he said he hated to ask others to get him a drink. He was apathetic about school and yet hung on to the illusion that life would go on as planned when he married his childhood sweetheart. Since he was struggling with the psychosocial task of becoming independent of parental control, the nurse decided against "teaching and preaching scare tactics" but instead told him about a client with similar problems who had made positive plans to resolve them. She gave each the other's telephone number and encouraged them to converse about mutual concerns.

Perhaps the greatest concern for modifying life-styles for the young and middle adult lies in the area of stress level. As discussed in Chapter 38, various relaxation techniques include meditation, progressive relaxation, hypnosis, and biofeedback. Relaxation should be planned and scheduled as a regular part of the day's activities. O'Flynn-Comiskey (1979) emphasized relaxation as a means for increasing efficiency and productivity, which should appeal to individuals with type A behavior.

Nurse's Role in Confronting Suffering and Death

Suffering is a common, natural life condition. Frankl (1959) stated that suffering is like gas in a chamber—no matter how much or how little—it fills the whole chamber; suffering is relative. Individuals cannot choose their fates, but they can choose the attitudes they take toward fates that cannot be changed. Suffering can be a growth experience; individuals can learn valuable lessons about life from personal suffering. Those who successfully negotiate developmental tasks grow and evolve from coping with life's challenges. Suffering can have a meaning if it changes the individual; despair is suffering without meaning.

Travelbee (1966) described two types of sufferers from a negative perspective. The *unjustly afflicteds* behave as if they should be exempt from human misfortune and human frailties. Their behavior reflects anger, annoyance, bitterness, rebellion, self-pity, depression, anguish, fear, and/or anxiety. The *punished* focus on their guilt, badness, and punishment for wrongdoing. They exhibit depression, anxiety, and self-pity. They may blame themselves, others, or God.

Frankl (1959) espoused the theory of logotherapy to help clients find meaning and purpose in life. Clients need to find meaning in suffering to cope effectively. Many clients practice hyperreflection, that is, a compulsion to self-observation that creates anticipatory anxiety. Frankl advocated the use of humor as a technique to combat phobias or fears. For example, a client who suffers from hyperhidrosis or excessive perspiration of the palms fears a situation that compels handshaking. However, fear precipitates that very symptom. The therapist in this case may encourage the client to try to perspire buckets full the next time he is in this situation—to laugh at himself for even considering taking a bucket with him. Usually the client finds that trying as hard as he can, he is no longer able to produce the state of hyperhidrosis.

Strategies the nurse could use include the following logotherapeutic techniques:

1. Dereflection—directing the focus away from the problem and focusing on assets and abilities (e.g., not focusing on paralyzed legs but rather on strong upper arms).
2. Paradoxical intention—exaggerating and wishing for the opposite; using humor. (The therapy for hyperhidrosis as just mentioned uses paradoxical intention.)
3. Socratic dialogue—engaging in thought-provoking conversation with the client. (An elderly man who has been depressed since his wife's death is asked what would have happened if he had died before his wife. He recounts how unfortunate this would have been, she would have been afraid to live alone and she had no experience managing money. The client is reminded that he has spared his wife this suffering by living past her [Frankl, 1959].)

The nurse's role in coping with death is to be supportive of the family and to assist the client in verbalizing fears and concerns. The nurse can facilitate positive progression through the grieving process as death approaches.

Conflict and Stress Level

Stress for the adult often results from speed; the urgency of getting many things done in a limited amount of time. A sense of time urgency may develop. Anything and anybody who interferes with this speeding pace causes frustration, conflict, and consequently stress. Community health nurses can help clients assess how they spend time and then evaluate whether other activities would more appropriately meet their personal goals. One way to manage stress is to immunize the body, both physically and emotionally, from stressors that are known and preventable.

BROADER VIEW OF IMMUNIZATIONS

Biological immunizations recommended for the adult are limited. A booster of tetanus toxoid should be taken at least every 10 years with repetition for an accident or injury. Polio booster doses are not recommended past age 18. Influenza vaccines are recommended for adult clients considered to be at risk.

Psychosocial immunizations may buffer the adult against stressors to be expected at this time in the life cycle. Anticipatory guidance, helping the adult know what to expect from different phases of life, may be helpful. Often an older friend or mentor eases the way, as is illustrated in the example of a 27-year-old single parent of a 10-year-old boy in fifth grade. Her neighbor has a 15-year-old son who has a motorcycle and wants very much to receive a car by his sixteenth birthday. The friendship between the two women helps the first woman to anticipate what she will face in a few short years as a parent of a teenager. The neighbor also helps by telling the woman parenting techniques she found helpful when her son was 10 years old.

NUTRITIONAL REQUIREMENTS FOR PROMOTING HEALTH

Adults have normal nutritional needs that may be slightly at variance with other periods of the life cycle. During ill health special nutritional needs may exist. The *aging process* is significantly influenced by nutritional health habits.

Normal Nutritional Needs for Young and Middle Adults

Adults, like children and the elderly, need to be counseled by community health nurses to recognize their nutritional needs and to learn how to eat wisely if poor nutritional habits exist. Several major causes of adult morbidity and mortality are related to diet. Assessment of adult dietary needs, habits, and desires often begins with a determination of nutritional myths and beliefs.

In a survey concerning the level of practical knowledge about nutrition, Poplin (1980) found that the general public holds many misconstrued or erroneous beliefs about nutrition. Some facts that Poplin determined which were often confused, are listed in the following true statements:

Drinking water is not fattening.

Synthetic vitamins are as effective in the body as natural vitamins.

Nutritionally, honey is no better than white sugar.

Body fat cannot be lost by wearing sauna suits or sweat belts.

Proper weight does not necessarily mean you are getting proper nutrition.

Foods grown with chemical fertilizers are just as nutritious as food grown with natural organic fertilizers.

Neither vinegar nor grapefruit causes the body to burn fat more rapidly.

The young adult, emerging from the adolescent period of high nutritional demand, needs slightly less calcium and protein than before (Diekelmann, 1976). Young adult men need an increase in vitamin C, E, B_6 and B_{12}. Food sources include citrus juices, whole grain products, vegetable oils, leafy vegetables, fish, and cheese. Young women have an increased need for vitamin C and for foods rich in iron, such as organ meats, eggs, fish, poultry, leafy vegetables, and dried fruit. Women need 18 mg of iron daily as compared to 10 mg needed by men. Signs of anemia include fatigue, low energy level, excess need for sleep, shortness of breath on exertion, and depression. It is safe to say that most young adults should reduce sugar consumption, including sources of hidden sugar. Recommendations for normal adult nutrition include limiting consumption of eggs to 3 per week and eating foods high in polyunsaturated rather than saturated fats. Care should be taken in consuming foods with preservatives. Foods with nitrates and nitrites—chemicals used to enhance color, flavor, and preservation of meats—may lead to the formation of nitrosamines, a known carcinogenic agent. Such foods include bacon, sausage, lunch meats, smoked fish, and hot dogs. Foods low in cholesterol should be a part of a normal diet. Small-boned fish is an excellent source of calcium. Breakfast is perhaps the most important meal of the day and should not be skipped. There is no nutritional value to meals being hot rather than cold (O'Conner, 1981).

Special Nutritional Needs During Ill Health

One of the most dreaded illnesses of adult life is cardiovascular disease, which has many nutritional implications. For primary prevention of coronary disease, Turner (1980) recommended having half the saturated fats and twice the polyunsaturated fats. This strategy has the effect of reducing total fat by 25%. Most fat is a mixture of three kinds: (1) saturated, which is not essential and is harmful in excess; (2) monosaturated, which is neutral; and (3) polyunsaturated, which is essential and protective. No intake of animal cholesterol is necessary for health, and excessive consumption is harmful. The body manufactures its own sufficient supply for daily requirements. Egg yolks have the highest concentration of cholesterol (250 mg per yolk) followed by dairy fat and meat. Frying can be replaced by other methods of cooking. A marbled meat roast can be cooked a day ahead and refrigerated. The next day the solid fat can be removed before warming. Proteins can also be obtained from mixed sources such as bread, cereals, peas, beans, and lentils. Fish, whether fresh, frozen, or canned, is equally nutritious.

Nutrition for other illnesses depends on the specific diagnosis. However, proper nutrition is necessary to promote recovery and/or stabilization of a chronic disorder.

Nutritional Influences on the Aging Process for the Middle Adult

Nutrition influences the way people age and may affect the onset or course of degenerative diseases. At this time there is no known diet, food, or food factor that can retard the aging process (Mayer, 1980). A nutritional guideline for the adult is to eat a wide variety of foods including fresh, raw, or lightly processed foods, which are high in nutrients and provide only enough calories to meet daily energy needs. In addition, adults may need one daily multivitamin/mineral capsule containing levels of nutrients according to the Recommended Daily Allowances.

As the body ages, it replaces some tissue with fat cells. As activity level declines, so should caloric intake. Loss of muscle tissue is another age-related change and may be retarded by adequate intake of high quality protein. Mayer (1980) recommended 60 to 70 g of protein per day for the adult, the same amount as required in pregnancy. (Protein (50 g) is contained in each of the following: 2 cups of milk or 4 oz of meat, poultry, or white fish.)

Osteoporosis is a common disorder related to the aging process. Post-menopausal women are susceptible to this condition. In normal bone mineralization, vitamin D and a 1:1 ratio of calcium to phosphorus exist. The typical American diet includes three times as much phosphorus as calcium. Phosphorus is found in meats, soft drinks, and processed foods. To balance the calcium : phosphorus intake, foods that may be added to the diet include leafy dark green vegetables, sesame seeds, and dark molasses. Foods containing the ideal 1:1 ratio are milk and milk products.

HEALTH PROMOTION

For the adult, promoting and maintaining a healthy state from a holistic perspective involves efforts in physical, psychosocial, and spiritual areas.

Physical Health

Good health does not just happen, it has to be worked at consistently. Promoting health requires discipline and time management skills, programming directed health behaviors into a crowded schedule. Areas for building physical health include nutrition, rest, exercise, and play. Adults may be inclined to abuse what is considered to be good nutrition in efforts to lose or control weight. A common practice counterproductive to good health and a consistent high-level energy pattern is omitting breakfast in an attempt to hold down calories. A nutritious breakfast is essential for individuals with highly demanding daily activities. Two adequate meals per day with one light meal is a good pattern to follow. Some adults tend to consume alcohol to relax after a stressful day. Drinking fruit juices instead while taking time out after a busy day to relax, talk to family members, or watch television can often accomplish the same purpose.

Rest and sleep are necessary to promote health. The amount of sleep varies with the individual, usually 6 to 8 hours for the adult. A regular bedtime preceded by relaxing activities promotes good sleep habits. Rest periods also enhance energy level and renew vitality. A 10-minute rest period at noon—reclining on a sofa, for example—can do wonders for the adult.

Exercise is also an essential part of health. The busy adult may have good intentions but fail to find time for exercise. It must be scheduled in and placed on the calendar as an appointment. Many adults get bored with routine, and therefore it is suggested that exercise routines be varied. For example, aerobics can be done in January, tennis in February, golf in March, and swimming in April.

Meeting sexual needs is also a component of health promotion. Sexuality or the totality of gender expression is more encompassing than sex, which refers to the physical act of intercourse or other physically intimate encounters. *Sexual health* according to the World Health Organization Report on Education and Treatment in Human Sexuality may be defined as "the integration of the somatic, emotional, intellectual, and social aspects of sexual beings in ways that are positively enriching and enhance personality, communication, and love" (Lamb and Woods, 1981, p. 137). A new sexual ethic emphasizing pleasure, caring, and mutual growth may be developing in Western society accord-

ing to Francoeur and Francoeur (1978). These authors suggested that in the future the nuclear family may be replaced by the multiple-adult living group, known as the intentional extended family. Such families would consist of networks of intimate friends for whom the possibility of sexual involvement with each other is open.

Frankl (1975) on the other hand stated that grasping the uniqueness of a partner understandably results in a monogamous relationship. He believed that the inflation of sex has led to a devaluation and a dehumanization of sex, which is seen as the physical expression of something metasexual, love. Frankl identified three developmental stages of sexual maturity. At an immature level, only the goal of tension reduction is sought, and masturbation will do. In the second stage the instinct centers on normal sexual intercourse regardless of partner and may lead to promiscuity. In the third stage of maturity the partner is in no way a means to an end; that person is lovingly encountered.

Psychosocial Health

Promoting psychosocial health results from balancing various roles necessary for adult activities. All work and no play is unhealthy, as is the reverse. Adults need a peer support system, but many place friends low on a priority list because of other, more pressing obligations; after the children leave home, adults may be left with few valued interpersonal relationships and find themselves feeling depressed and useless. The adult can be spurred on by new role endeavors. For some a new challenge is lively and invigorating, whereas others view change and challenge with fear or as a "necessary evil."

Psychosocial therapeutic activities promote health and are based on individual needs and desires. Hobbies, sports, and other forms of recreation and leisure are necessary to health. Adults may not feel comfortable in play, but a balanced life with laughter and light activities enhances health.

Spiritual Health

The adult has to face many struggles with the meaning of life. Confronting lost dreams, unexpected success, or unkind fate puzzles the person who is plagued with "why" and "what now" questions. Quiet periods for reflective thinking, reading, and studying help the adult resolve some of life's questions. Periods for meditation help to develop inner harmony. Adults may engage in life review processes, trying to understand how they came to where they are today.

Spiritual health may facilitate attitude change to accept conditions in life and to create positive outcomes.

Frankl (1975) promoted the philosophy that happiness or fulfillment is a side effect of living for a cause or purpose rather than as a direct pursuit of pleasure.

WORK-RELATED ISSUES

One of the primary tasks of young and middle adults is engaging in purposeful, productive life work. An individual's career, whether domestic or a highly challenging executive position, can affect health negatively or positively. The role of the nurse often involves counseling and referral for counseling regarding job problems or goals for second careers. Problems that are job related can be physical, presenting a hazard to health, or psychosocial, creating a feeling of disparity between job and worker. Although Chapter 13 discusses this subject in more detail, this section examines occupational hazards to health, overstress in the workplace, and second careers for young and middle adults.

Occupational Hazards to Health

Occupational hazards to health include musculoskeletal problems, respiratory and circulatory problems, damage to hearing organs, and accidents. Chronic misuse of one's body plus an overload of stressors result in inevitable damage.

An interesting study of 113 mine rescue workers, involved the examination of the relationship between the workers' perceived health and marital status, use of health services, nonwork physical activity, and absence from work (McKenna et al., 1981). These workers, by definition healthy and fit, averaged approximately 0.5 health problems per worker, and more than 79% of them reported no health problems at all. Of those health problems reported, 40% regarded sleep, 25% involved emotional reactions, with the fewest problems in physical mobility (8%) and social isolation (3%). There was a tendency for married respondents and those over 40 years old to perceive more health problems. Those workers who reported little physical exercise outside of work experienced three times as many health problems. The nurse working in an industrial setting may need to study the influence of different variables on absence rates and predict those who are at risk.

Overstress in the Workplace

Stress is the spice of life, but too much of the wrong kind—overstress—can lead to physical, psychosocial, and/or spiritual problems. The term *burned out* originated from a street expression of the Haight-Ashbury era and referred to hopelessly addicted drug users (Ross, 1980). Such a person experiences an energy drain that cannot be replenished with ordinary measures such as rest or a break in routine. Early signs in persons who are overstressed include the following:

1. Taking the easy way out in decision making or letting others make the decisions
2. Showing only superficial enthusiasm for the job
3. Being too willing to agree with others
4. Being unwilling to take risks
5. Directing anger at oneself and family members
6. Resisting innovations by others
7. Needing alcohol at the end of the day

Ross suggested several ways to prevent burnout.

1. Periodically take an inventory of personal strengths and weaknesses; identify both stressful and enjoyable conditions; and evaluate family life, health, and personal factors.
2. Learn to manage time more appropriately by planning according to individual rhythms.
3. Keep track of problems and projects, mixing tough tasks with easier ones.
4. Work at cultivating physical and mental health, including regular exercise.
5. Avoid the overload situation by setting decision-making priorities; ration psychic energy needed for coping.

The community health nurse should help clients identify their stressors and find solutions to their occupational problems (Chapter 38).

Second Careers: Becoming a Student Again

Many middle adults and even some young adults struggle with career identity and satisfaction and emerge with a decision to pursue another career. People often desire to explore new life experiences; many yearn for what they wish they had become. This yearning often leads to midlife career changes, many of which require further education (Best, 1978). Baer (1979) described the situation that led up to her decision to make a career change as involving feelings of boredom from routine and dissatisfaction from a lack of challenge in her job. The needs and expectations of adult learners seeking second careers are becoming a major focus of educators as they try to serve this growing population.

Best (1978) described flexible life scheduling as a concept for "recycling people." By being more flexible in the way education, work, and leisure schedules in a person's lifetime are designed, personal dreams and aspirations are more likely to become realities. Present life patterns compress work into the middle years with little activity for the young or aged. Best suggested alternative lifetime patterns, including cyclic life plans involving working hours specific to developmental tasks.

During the years of being single or having no children and the later years after raising children, individuals might work longer hours per week (45 to 50) with time-off compensations in vacations and sabbaticals. Individuals in the early child raising years and old age might work a shorter week (25 to 40 hours) with vacations moderate in length. Leaves in the middle years planned by employers, foster health as well as productivity.

PHYSICALLY DISABLED ADULTS

Approximately 35 million Americans are physically disabled to some degree, making this group the largest minority in the United States according to Tolentino (1981). Of the 17- to 44-year-old age group 55% have at least one chronic illness.

Definition of Terms

Several terms are used, often interchangeably, to describe the disability state; various definitions may be found in the literature. For purposes of discussion in this chapter, the following succinct definitions are used:

Impairment: a disturbance in structure of function resulting from anatomical, physiological, and/or psychological abnormalities. For example, a person may have impairment of flexion and extension in the right arm.

Disability: the degree of observable and measurable physical or mental impairment. For example, a person may have a 50% disability of the right arm.

Handicap: the total adjustment to disability necessitated by an impairment or disability that limits or prevents functioning at a normal or usual level. For example, a person may be handicapped in writing, driving a car, and playing tennis because of the disability of the right arm.

People may have a high degree of disability and be minimally handicapped, such as those with quadriplegia who own their own businesses, drive specially equipped vans, and maintain active family roles. Conversely, some clients with little disability may exhibit profound limitations in satisfying life patterns. In either case these clients have disabilities, but they should not be labeled according to their disabling condition. They are not quadriplegics; they have quadriplegia, just as they have blue eyes or a large frame, etc. They are not cardiacs, diabetics, or any other such label. They are human beings who have impairments that are handicapping to some extent. The nurse's role is to capitalize on the human assests or abilities and minimize and compensate for the disabilities. The nurse should also promote the rehabilitation process for optimum achievement of potential. Rehabilitation is the process by which individuals and/or families strive for the attainment and maintenance of the maximum level of need satisfaction.

A disability may be classified as congenital or acquired, visible or invisible, or stable or progressive. Regardless of the classification or the extent of the disability, individuals are entitled to the rights that anybody has for family, work, social, and sex role responsibilities. They have a right to educational opportunities, health care services, and dignity and respect from others.

Prevention

If a large group of young healthy students were asked to indicate who had a history of diabetes in their families, many would respond positively. Of that group in future years some may well develop diabetes and eventually have a leg amputated or suffer total blindness. This type of pathological disability is a predictable consequence of chronic illness. People who are able bodied may consider themselves only temporarily so, since they are susceptible to disease and/or injury. The importance of prevention and primary health care in the community is that disabling conditions can be minimized and should be approached with vigor. Table 26-5 lists the predictable consequences of certain risk factors that lead to a particular health problem, namely cardiac disability and death. In stage 1, life-style can be modified to promote health and decrease the possibility of impairment.

Impact of Disability

The community health nurse is challenged when assisting a client system with a member who has a newly acquired disability. Many rehabilitation agencies discharge clients when they have mastered the physical skills of daily living. Yet total adjustment for the individual and family involves much more. Livneh (1980) described the following 12 stages of adjustment to a disabling condition: shock, anxiety, bargaining, denial, mourning, depression, withdrawal, anger, hostility/aggression, acknowledgment, acceptance, and adjustment. These stages may overlap, and clients may skip or regress to certain stages. The community health nurse may assess the client to be in any stage after discharge from an acute care institution, but often mourning and depression set in after loss of the distracting hustle and bustle of a busy agency. These stages may be evidenced by a slowing of physiological functions such as appetite, sleep, or body movements. The client may express feelings of helplessness, hopelessness, and sadness. Withdrawal is characterized by avoidance of social contacts, increased isolation, sleeping, use of fantasy, and a general apathetic attitude. A client who is angry,

Table 26-5. Predictable consequences of cardiac risk factors

Stage		Predictable consequences
1	Risk factors and stress-adaptation Dietary pattern—high fat, high carbohydrate, high sodium Sedentary work and leisure Lack of exercise, recreation Heavy smoker	Hypertensive Obesity Artereosclerotic plaque in vessels
2	Beginning and progressive pathophysiology	Sluggish circulation Decreased oxygenation Shortness of breath Edema
3	Advanced pathophysiology	Death of tissues Dysfunction of heart and lungs Cardiac pulmonale Cardiac crippling Death

hostile, or aggressive can be particularly enigmatic to his family and the nurse. Fixing blame is often the focus of thoughts and actions. Clients in this stage may be abusive, argumentative, and even violent.

Helping professionals are no doubt eclectic in approaches used to cope with clients in various stages of adjustment. Logotherapy may be useful in helping the client acknowledge meaning in the suffering experience. As described earlier, Frankl's (1959) logotherapeutic techniques of paradoxical intention and dereflection may be useful. These techniques are illustrated in the following excerpts.

Milly was injured by a gunshot at age 15 during a domestic quarrel between her parents. The injury left her arms and legs completely paralyzed. She spent her day watching soap operas on television. While responding to the nursing history, Milly expressed surprise when the nurse asked what she did for others. Milly stated that she could not feed herself, bathe herself, write, sew, or even hold a telephone. Using *dereflection*, the nurse helped Milly to focus on her abilities—a bright mind with retentive and concentration skills, her melodious voice, and lively, expressive eyes. Over the course of nurse/client interaction, Milly learned to type with a mouthstick and wrote letters of comfort to church members who were experiencing sorrow. She began putting her inspirational messages on tape for the church library. Later she volunteered for 4 hours per week of telephone counseling.

The impact of an acquired disability on the individual varies, based on many factors. According to Maslow (1970), all people strive to meet their needs to obtain some degree of satisfaction and fulfillment. The disabled individual is entitled to no less. The Needs Satisfaction Scale found in Appendix A may serve as a useful tool in assessing current need satisfaction level as a basis for planning nursing action.

Family with a Disabled Member

Often health workers focus their entire attention on the individual client and fail to see the needs of the family, particularly the client's caretaker. Disability of one family member can have a significant impact on the entire family. As the costs of institutional care continues to spiral, many families are providing care at home for members with a disability. With these responsibilities, family members become subject to stressors that can affect their health. They may have added roles and expanded or modified patterns and life-styles. The crisis of an injury or the shock of a chronic-illness diagnosis can greatly upset the family equilibrium.

The community health nurse must be cognizant of the impact of the disability on the family system. The beginning point for assessment and planning for family needs is during the initial crisis stage when most clients are hospitalized. Hart (1981) identified the following eight categories of needs of significant others:
1. Feel adequately informed
2. Feel helpful
3. Feel able to cope with responsibilities
4. Receive emotional support
5. Express feelings, positive and negative
6. Feel that the client is getting good care
7. Compare and contrast this with past experiences in coping with crises
8. Explore the future as a result of the client's condition

Family members show grief reactions just as the client does and need to maintain hope and restore balance to family life. Concerns expressed by family members include finances, work, housing, transportation, family activities, sexual activities, social relationships, and coping with the problems (functional and emotional) caused by the disability. Open communication between the disabled persons and other family members is crucial to a healthy family pattern. Maintaining contact with extended family through telephone or letter writing is also helpful in providing an emotional support system.

In a study conducted by Davis (1980) several factors were found to be important in a family's decision about home care versus institutional care, including the nature and stage of disability; age and health status of the caretaker; social climate; beliefs about family responsibility, morality, and religion as well as the availability, adequacy, and acceptability of the caretaker role. The community health nurse needs to assess the family's patterns for tension management and conflict resolution (e.g., sudden outbursts, passive aggression, and psychosomatic ailments) as well as to assist the family in using healthy coping techniques. Referral for more intensive professional help may be warranted in some cases. Environmental stimulation and social interaction are necessary for caretakers and family members as well as clients.

The community health nurse should evaluate the client's functional ability and family health, which is complicated by the added responsibilities for a member with a disability. The effects on the major caretaker and others of providing long-term physical and emotional care must be recognized in any nursing care plan for the family. The long-term effects of unrelieved stress and frustration of needs can cause a breakdown of the caretaker as demonstrated in the following example.

Miss A. had never married, lived with her parents, and assisted with the family business. When her father died, she took on complete responsibilities for providing for herself and her mother. She worked long, hard hours at the store and then assisted her aging mother with the house and yard work. When Mrs. A. had a stroke, her daughter took care of her at home in a devoted manner. As Mrs. A's condition worsened, Miss A. found herself staying up at night yet continuing to put in a full day at the store. Mrs. A. became cranky and more demanding. She was incontinent and frequently called for help during the night. Although the doctor urged Miss A. to get help to supplement the daytime nurse, she declined, preferring to take care of her mother herself during the evening and night hours. Friends offered to relieve Miss A. for a weekend and urged her to take a relaxing trip but, she maintained her vigil. One day to the surprise and consternation of relatives, Miss A. lost all control, had her mother placed in a nursing home, and said she never wanted to see her again. At the nursing home Mrs. A. made some degree of progress, and the staff attempted to plan a visit home. However, Miss A. still refused to associate with her mother and in fact had all the locks on the doors changed to ensure that she could not return home. The mother eventually died in the nursing home. The daughter retired from the family business and became a virtual recluse.

Careers for Disabled Adults

Recent legislation has facilitated acceptance of the disabled adult into the work force. The community health nurse can be a source of support, since a newly employed disabled adult often faces many barriers, not the least of which are the attitudes of management, fellow workers, and the public.

Technology has enabled many otherwise disqualified individuals to perform satisfactorily in a job (Macleod, 1981). Products of this technology (e.g., the optophone, an electronic sensory aid that translates printed letters into vocal tones) facilitate satisfactory performance by disabled individuals. Several other examples of technology that can be used by the community health nurse are discussed. The Telesensory Sytems' Optacon is a visual to a tactile conversion system whereby an optical probe is moved across lines of a text, which converts to letters perceived tactilely and allows a reading rate of about 100 words per minute. Electronic language boards can be controlled by body actions such as eye movements and allow for nonverbal communication. Speech prostheses are also available for those with a disability. The Phonic Mirror Handi Voice contains a programmable speech synthesizer in a portable unit. The computer field promises to improve job opportunities for the disabled adult. Financial constraints often limit resourceful devices that would facilitate a self-supporting adult.

Community and National Significance

Disability influences resources and impinges on needs for services including inpatient and outpatient services, emergency care services, housing, and transportation. Today's philosophy of mainstreaming, integrating individuals who are handicapped into society rather than isolating them in a protective environment, requires planning; the community health nurse should be actively involved in this planning.

A community may need a variety of modules to provide housing options for its residents. Home as a concept is a central part of our culture, a private, independent, individual place, providing comfort and opportunity for self-expression and intimacy. Falta (1981) described four prototypes of desegregated community housing arrangements.

1. *Group homes* provide independent, semi-integrated life-styles and are often helpful after leaving a family setting or institution. A home such as a halfway or quarterway house can provide assistance without stifling protection. This type of home may be considered an extended family unit, a home shared with compatible disabled persons and able-bodied helpees in a nonprofit organization. Often this type of facility is created from a typical single-family dwelling or an apartment building. Residents contribute toward room and board with remaining costs being subsidized by government or private agencies.

2. *Apartment units with in-house staff* are apartment buildings adapted to accommodate disabled clients and/or the elderly, which provide housing with more privacy than group homes. Health care and domestic services for the building complex are provided by in-house staff, and extra security measures are an added feature.

3. *Adapted apartments* onto a private home or within an apartment complex may be adapted for a disability. Needed services can then be provided by family members or agency personnel.

4. *Modified and renovated housing* under the Homebound Program in Alabama provides that any person sustaining a spinal cord injury receives $1000 to add ramps and otherwise modify the home. Such subsidies to render a home more accessible offer suitable housing at reasonable rates.

The community health nurse should be interested in how well local health services and other aspects of the community take into consideration the needs of individuals who are disabled. For example, do emergency medical technicians receive training on how to handle the needs of a blind person who is injured and may become emotionally hypersensitive? Do restaurants provide braille menus? Do waitresses address family members of a blind person and ask, "What would he like to order?" Are churches accessible to the disabled, or do the churches prefer a ministry to "shut-ins?" Are local government buildings accessible to the disabled?

Rehabilitation following a disability is as costly to the nation as providing for special needs such as transportation or housing. However, such services may allow a disabled person and/or the caretaker to return to work. Thus the worker is contributing to the tax base instead of being dependent on government services. Rehabilitation contributes to the economic welfare of the nation as well as serves to facilitate humanitarianism.

International Significance

1981—the International Year of the Disabled Person (IYDP)—called attention to the needs as well as contributions of this segment of the population. The theme of the year was the full participation of disabled persons in the life of their society. The United Nations General Assembly adopted Resolution 34/154, a world plan of action for the IYDP. This resolution waged action to be taken at the national, regional, and international levels in prevention as well as rehabilitation. The first national task was to establish a scale of priorities, whereby each country would submit data on current problems. The General Assembly agreed to promote regional cooperation within geographical and culturally similar areas and adopted a world health plan to promote integration of disabled people into society.

Helander (1981) stated that 10% of the world population has a physical disability. Of the 250 to 300 million people in developing countries, only about 2% have any care or rehabilitation. Wilson (1981) stated that in the Middle East alone 7 million people could be saved from blindness in the next generation if eye diseases were controlled. It is estimated that in Asia 8 million people are blind from cataracts. An estimated 10 million of the world's population have trachoma, 3½ million have leprosy, and 100 million suffer from malnutrition.

Physical, Psychosocial, and Spiritual Rehabilitation

In a holistic approach to the rehabilitation process attention must be given to all component parts of human existence. Specialized centers offer a variety of services to meet these needs. Clients are usually discharged from institutions when they master certain physical tasks. The community health nurse monitors treatment plans to maintain physical achievements. Often a client who has learned to work with an artificial limb goes home and hangs it in the closet; hence nurses must constantly encourage physical conditioning. Other nursing care focuses on promoting the health of the nonpathological structures. For example, a client with diabetes who has had one leg amputated for gangrene should be taught to exercise all efforts to keep the other leg healthy.

People with a disability need psychosocial restoration as part of the broad perspective of rehabilitation. The achievement of self-care and mobility does not guarantee reintegration of social functioning. Labi (1980) found that women are slightly more likely than men to decrease their social activity in the home and in hobbies. The findings also indicate that following stroke, social reintegration outside the home is more difficult for women and for those with more education,

Major Legislation Affecting the Disabled, 1943-1977

1943   **The Barden-La Follette Act of 1943** (PL 113)
To provide comprehensive services, including federal payment for administrative guidance and placement costs; physical restoration services (i.e., hospitalization, surgery, and therapeutic treatment); maintenance for living expenses and occupational tools and equipment. Mentally handicapped (ill or retarded) became eligible for services.

1954   **Vocational Rehabilitation Amendments of 1954** (PL 565)
To assist states in rehabilitating the physically and mentally handicapped for remunerative employment to increase their social and economic well-being and the productive capacity of the nation. Provided funds to train physicians, nurses, rehabilitation counselors, physical therapists, occupational therapists, social workers, and other specialists. Provided grants for research and demonstration.

1965   **Vocational Rehabilitation Amendments of 1965**
To provide a broader financial base and to extend services to the socially handicapped (i.e., juvenile delinquents, adult public offenders). Permitted a waiver of expectation of gainful occupation. Provided grants for construction and operation of sheltered workshops.

1968   **Vocational Rehabilitation Amendments of 1968**
To increase federal funding (80:20 ratio) to basic programs, provide for new construction of facilities. Rehabilitative services rewritten to include follow-up and services to families. States were allowed to carry out a joint project. Efforts to combat poverty, included "disadvantaged" by reason of age, youth, low educational attainments, ethnic, or other factors such as prison and delinquency records.

1973   **Rehabilitation Act of 1973** (PL 112)
To provide that handicapped persons not be discriminated against in any program or activity receiving federal financial assistance. Defined handicapped solely in relation to employment.

1974   **Rehabilitation Act Amendments of 1974** (PL 516)
To amend the definition of handicapped individuals so that it is no longer limited to the dimension of employability.

1975   **Education for All Handicapped Persons** (PL 142)
To provide free and appropriate public education to all handicapped students, including special education and related services, covering persons from 3 to 21 years of age.

1976   **Educational Amendments of 1976, Title II** (PL 482)
Vocational Amendments
To specify that 10% of federal vocational funds be spent on vocational education for the handicapped and that this be matched by state and local funds to place the handicapped in regular vocational programs. Each handicapped student must have an individualized education program.

1977   **Rules and Regulations to Implement** (PL 516)
To provide explicit guidelines to implement nondiscriminatory practices. Provided new definitions of the handicapped in terms of physical or mental impairments limiting major life activities.

From Secretary of Health, Education, and Welfare: Nondiscrimination on the basis of handicaps in programs and activities receiving or benefitting from federal financial assistance, Federal Register, May 4, 1977, pp. 22676-22694.

since factors related to body image and feelings of stigma may be more intense. Many disabled persons tend to acquire new friends of lower social status than previously. Dubois (1981) used the term *socially naked* to describe humans who live with little if any human contact. The community health nurse must be innovative in individual cases to promote psychosocial restoration. Encouraging self-transcendence helps clients to focus on others. For example, a man who had been injured in a deliberate attempt on his life and left with an ileostomy and spinal cord injury, necessitating the use of a wheel chair, found meaning in volunteering in the recreational program in a nursing home. In meeting needs for others his own psychosocial health improved.

All humans have a spiritual (not synonymous with religious) dimension. The dynamic power of the human spirit can be harnessed to restore the disabled person to satisfaction and fulfillment. Logotherapeutic counseling can assist disabled persons to find meaning in their circumstances and a unique purpose in life with satisfying roles to fulfill. Life's task becomes finding an answer for the question, "Now that I am in this situation, what will I do with my life?"

Definition of Terms in Regulations for the Handicapped

Handicapped individual: any person who (1) has a physical or mental impairment that substantially limits one or more of that person's major life activities, (2) has a record of such an impairment, or (3) is regarded as having such an impairment.

Physical or mental impairment: (1) any physiological disorder or condition, cosmetic disfigurement, or anatomical loss affecting one or more of the following body systems: neurological, musculoskeletal, special sense organs, respiratory (including speech organs), cardiovascular, reproductive, digestive, genitourinary, hemic and lymphatic, skin, and endocrine or (2) any mental or psychological disorder such as mental retardation, organic brain syndrome, emotional or mental illness, and specific learning disabilities.

Major life activities: functions such as caring for oneself, performing manual tasks, walking, seeing, hearing, speaking, breathing, learning, and working.

Qualified handicapped person: with respect to employment, a handicapped person who, with reasonable accommodation, can perform the essential functions of the job in question; with respect to postsecondary and vocational education services, a handicapped person who meets the academic and technical standards requisite to admission or participation in the recipient's educational program or activity.

From Secretary of Health, Education, and Welfare: Nondiscrimination on the basis of handicaps in programs and activities receiving or benefitting from federal financial assistance, Federal Register, May 4, 1977, pp. 22676-22694.

Regulations. "Nondiscrimination on the Basis of Handicap in Programs and Activities Receiving or Benefitting from Federal Financial Assistance"—Effective June 3, 1977

Subpart A
General provisions: defines important terms, states the discriminatory acts that are prohibited, sets forth a workable system of administration (assurances of compliance, self-evaluation by recipients, establishment of grievance procedures, and notification of employees and beneficiaries of the recipient's policy of nondiscrimination on the basis of handicap).

Subpart B
Employment practices: bars discrimination in hiring, compensation, job assignment and classification, and fringe benefits. Requires employers to make reasonable accommodation.

Subpart C
Program accessibility: requires all new facilities to be constructed so as to be readily accessible and usable by handicapped persons and that existing facilities be modified so that all programs are accessible.

Subpart D
Preschool, elementary, and secondary education: closely coordinated with PL 142 to provide a free appropriate education in a normal setting. Evaluation requirements to ensure proper classification and placement as well as due process for resolving disputes.

Subpart E
Postsecondary education: requires nondiscrimination in recruitment, admission, and treatment after enrollment. Requires institutions to make reasonable adjustments and provide auxiliary aids.

Subpart F
Health, education, and social services: requires providers of services to have accessible programs.

Subpart G
Procedures: Title VI complaint and enforcement procedures to be used in implementation.

From Secretary of Health, Education, and Welfare: Nondiscrimination on the basis of handicaps in programs and activities receiving or benefitting from federal financial assistance, Federal Register, May 4, 1977, pp. 22676-22694.

Legislation

Legislation for physically disabled persons began early in this century and has grown from a focus of vocationally retraining the disabled veteran to mainstreaming handicapped individuals into every facet of American society. The box on p. 644 presents major legislation affecting the handicapped since 1943. The Rehabilitation Act of 1974 (PL 516) and the Education for All Handicapped Persons (PL 142) are the most significant legislations affecting the disabled person. The boxes on p. 645 present definitions of terms for the disabled from the Federal Register, May 4, 1977, and information describing the 1977 regulations to implement PL 516.

SUMMARY

The major health problems of young and middle adults are largely the result of life-style behaviors that are influenced by specific developmental tasks. Individuals in this age group have many stressors and pressures from social role expectations to meet not only their own needs but the needs of others who are dependent on them. The adult years are fluid, represented by growth and change in the pursuit of new life goals and coping with various life crises. The responsibilities assumed by adults range from parent to child, including primary burdens of income production.

Physical changes accompany psychosocial changes in adulthood. These changes create various effects in different individuals. However, each person needs to exert a planned effort at maintaining optimum health, including exercise, nutrition, rest, sleep, play, and mental outlook on life. Assuming responsibility for self-care is the adult health task.

The developmental tasks of young adults center around interaction with an intimate other as well as establishing a career. The middle adult's developmental task involves achieving a significant contribution for future generations and may involve stress in the workplace. Within each age category special subgroups such as single adults, adults living in rural settings, or disabled adults require the specialized attention of community health nurses who attempt to promote health and fulfillment. Morbidity and mortality of young and middle adults give direction for the community health nurse. Suicide, homicide, and accidents are serious concerns for young adults. The nurse must assess and analyze pressures and frustrations that lead to such appalling consequences if this major health problem is to be resolved. Positive mental health services are needed in a community so that families can present their problems to professionals and learn to cope with crises. Sexually transmittable diseases are also a major health problem of young adults.

Morbidity and mortality factors for the middle adult include heart disease and stroke, cancer, alcohol and substance abuse, mental health problems, and periodontal diseases. Although singular cause and effect factors cannot be demonstrated, various health practices can contribute to prevention and health promotion. Avoiding known risk factors is a constructive action to remaining healthy. The growing concern for substance abuse can be dealt with in comprehensive health centers. The community health nurse must work in a partner relationship with the adult who must assume responsibility to reduce risk for disease development and to promote a healthy life-style.

Logotherapy offers an approach for coping with pain, suffering, and illness. Strategies such as dereflection, paradoxical intention, and Socratic dialogue can be useful with the client or family. Such intervention can assist the adult to find meaning and purpose in life experiences.

Assessing the impact of a physical disability on an individual, family, or community is within the realm of the community health nurse. Today's technology has eliminated many barriers to the disabled adult's ability to function in the larger society. As the community health nurse uses this technology and coordinates community resources, attention must be given to what is often the greatest barrier—attitude toward the disabled person.

Health problems of young and middle adults relate to work, family, and community. Though major health hazards are reflected in morbidity and mortality statistics, community health nurses must be cognizant of potential problems from emerging trends of a changing society. Anticipating new health problems depends on analyzing life-styles and values of today's adult population.

BIBLIOGRAPHY

Archer, V.E., et al.: Lung cancer among uranium miners in the United States, Health Phys. **25**:351-371, 1973.

Baer, E.: A career change after twenty years, Am. J. Nurs. **79**(11): 1969-1970, Nov. 1979.

Best, F.: Recycling people: work-sharing through flexible life scheduling. In 1999 the world of tomorrow, editor: Cornish, E., Washington, D.C., 1978, World Future Society, pp. 122-123.

Cutler, D.L., and Madore, E.: Community-family network therapy in a rural setting, Community Ment. Health J. **16**:144-155, 1980.

Davis, A.J.: Disability: home care and the caretaking role in family life, J. Adv. Nurs. **5**:475-484, Sept. 1980.

DeMoss, C.J.: Giving intravenous chemotherapy at home, Am. J. Nurs. **80**:2188-2189, Dec. 1980.

Diekelmann, N.L.: The young adult: the choice is health or illness, Am. J. Nurs. **76**:1272-1277, Aug. 1976.

Diekelmann, N.L: Wellness: approaches and resources, Nurse Pract. **5**:41-42, Oct. 1980.

Dubois, R.: Celebrations of life, New York, 1981, McGraw-Hill Book Co.

Eisenberg, M.: The logotherapeutic intergenerational communications group, The International Forum for Logotherapy, vol. 2, no. 2, Summer/Fall, 1979, pp. 23-25.

Erikson, E. Childhood and society, New York, 1950, W.W. Norton & Co., Inc.

Falta, L.P.: Integration in the community: Canadian housing options for the disabled, Physiother. Can. 33:102-105, March/April 1981.

Francoeur, R.T., Francoeur, A.K.: The pleasure bond: reversing the antisex ethic. editor: Cornish, E., 1999 the world of tomorrow, Washington, D.C., 1978, World Future Society, pp. 116-120.

Frankl, V.: Man's search for meaning, New York, 1959, Simon & Schuster, Inc.

Frankl, V.: The doctor and the soul, New York, 1973, Random House.

Frankl, V.: The unconscious God, New York, 1975, Simon & Schuster, Inc.

Grossman, R.: Are you dealing with—or denying the mid-life crisis? Family Health 11:6–10, Nov.-Dec. 1979.

Hart, J.: Spinal cord injury: impact on client's significant others, Rehabil. Nurs. 6:11-15, Jan./Feb. 1981.

Hawkins, D.R., Jr.: Farmworker health: issues and perspectives. Nurs. Dimens. 7: 15-20, 1979.

Hayes, W.S., and Davis, L.L. What is a health care contract? Health Values 4:82-86, March/April 1980.

Hayne, C.: The body's reaction to noise, Occup. Health 33:75-83, Feb. 1981.

Health: United States, 1981, DHHS Pub. No. (PHS) 82-1232, Washington, D.C., 1981, Department of Health and Human Services.

Healthy People: the Surgeon General's report on health promotion and disease prevention, DHEW Pub. No. (PHS) 79-55071, Washington, D.C., 1979, Department of Health, Education and Welfare.

Helander, E.: Training the disabled in the community, World Health, 26-29, Jan. 1981.

Johnson, J.L., and Norby, P.A.: We can weekend: a program for cancer families, Cancer Nurs. 4:23-28, Feb. 1981.

Karman, J. and Price, J.H. Community organization for an oral cancer screening program, J. Nurs. Care 13:15-17, Aug. 1980.

Labi, M.L.C., et al.: Psychosocial disability in physically restored long-term stroke survivors, Arch. Phy. Med. Rehabil. 61:561-565, Dec. 1980.

Lamb, M.A., and Woods, N.F.: Sexuality and the cancer patient, Cancer Nurse 4:137-144, April 1981.

Lattimore, S., et al.: Is hypertension a problem in industry? Occup. Health Nurs. 27:19-21, Oct. 1979.

Levinson, D.J., et al.: The seasons of a man's life, New York, 1978, Ballantine Books.

Livneh, H.: The process of adjustment to disability: feelings, behaviors, and counseling strategies, Psychosoc. Rehabil. J. 4:26-35, 1980.

Lowther, N.B., and Carter, V.D.: How to increase compliance in hypertensives, Am. J. Nurs. 81(5):963, May 1981.

Macleod, I.: International Year of Disabled Persons. Information processing aids for physically handicapped people, Aust. Nurs. J. 10:46-53, Dec.-Jan. 1981.

Maslow, A.H.: Motivation and personality, New York, 1970, Harper & Row Publishers, Inc.

Mayer, J.: Eating well after 50, Fam. Health 12:52, June 1980.

McGregor, D.: The human side of enterprise, New York, 1960, McGraw-Hill Book Co.

McKenna, S.P., et al.: Mine rescue workers: their perceived health absence from work, Occup. Health 33:70-74, Feb. 1981.

Mitchell, F.H., and Mitchell, C.C.: Entering the 1980s: the health care system and primary care, Fam. Community Health 3:105-113, Aug. 1980.

Morris, C.L: Stress: relaxation therapy in a clinic, Am. J. Nurs. 79(11): 1958-1959, Nov. 1979.

Moses, M.: Cancer and the workplace, Am. J. Nurs. 79:1984-1988, Nov. 1979.

N'Kanza, Z.: Full participation and equality, World Health, Jan. 1981, pp. 3-5.

O'Connor, P.: Prevention of coronary heart disease: is there a role for the health visitor, Health Visit. 54:28-30, Jan. 1981.

O'Flynn-Comiskey, A.I.: Stress: the type A individual, Am. J. Nurs. 79(11):1956-1958, Nov. 1979.

Ouchi, W.: Theory Z: how American business can meet the Japanese challenge, Reading, Mass, 1981, Addison-Wesley Publishing Co., Inc.

Poplin, L.E.: Practical knowledge of nutrition in health science, J. Am. Diet. Assoc. 77:576-580, Nov. 1980.

Procci, W.R.: Psychosocial disability during maintenance hemodialysis, Gen. Hosp. Psychiatry 3:24-31, March 1981.

Riesch, S., et al.: Nursing centers can promote health for individuals, families and communities . . . a nursing center at the University of Wisconsin-Milwaukee School of Nursing, Nurs. Adm. Q. 4:1-8, 1980.

Rix, K.: Alcoholism and the district nurse, Community Outlook 13:275-276, Sept. 1979.

Ross, A. Managing executive stress and other related subjects, J. Ambulatory Care Manage. 3:1-10, Nov. 1980.

Searle, C.: Psychosocial aspects of mammary carcinoma: curationis, South Afr. J. Nurs. 3:12-15, Sept. 1980.

Selye, H.: Stress and holistic medicine, Fam. Community Health 3:85-88, Aug. 1980.

Sheehy, G.: Passages: predictable crises of adult life, New York, 1974, E.P. Dutton, Inc.

Sheehy, G.: Pathfinders, New York, 1981, William Morrow & Co., Inc.

Silverman, J.: On the metaphysical aspect of health care: attitudes, values, and other thoughts we use to think, Fam. Community Health 3:93-103, Aug. 1980.

Tolentino, A.: 1981: international year of the disabled person, Imprint 28:27, April 1981.

Travelbee, J.: Interpersonal aspects of nursing, Philadelphia, 1966, F.A. Davis Co.

Turner, R.: Diet and primary prevention of coronary disease, Midwife Health Visit. Community Nurse, 16:452, Nov. 1980.

Valenzuela, W.G., and Hallamore, A.G.: The "good neighbor network"—gatekeepers to a rural mental health support system . . . New Hampshire, Psychosoc. Rehabil. J. 3:20-33, 1979.

Welch, D.A.: Waiting, worry and the cancer experience, Oncology Nurs. Forum 8:14-18, 1981.

Wilson, J.: Communities re-born, World Health, Jan. 1981, pp. 22-25.

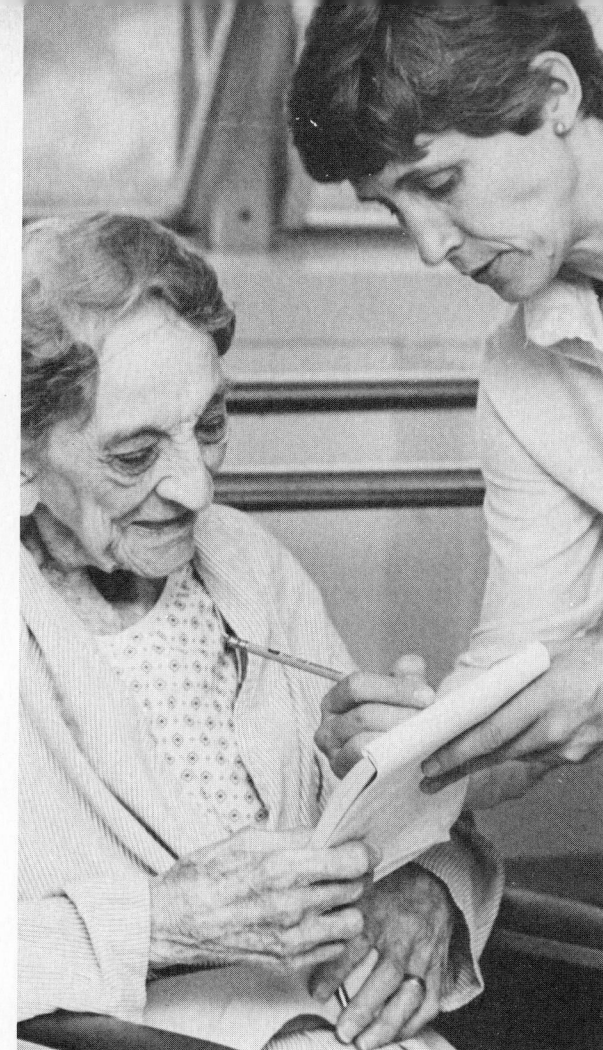

Chapter 27

DELOIS SKIPWITH

MAJOR COMMUNITY HEALTH PROBLEMS OF THE OLDER ADULT

No other American population segment is growing as rapidly as is the elderly. Health care professionals are increasingly focusing on identifying and meeting the needs of this group. Members of this age group are seeking greater participation in the definition and resolution of health and social issues affecting them. Simultaneously, increasing longevity, chronic health problems, technological advances, and twentieth century economic, social, and health issues have prompted social planners and health professionals to struggle with the issue of quality years as well as quantity years. Can they occur simultaneously? The answer must be yes if we are to care for and reward the present generation of older adults as well as establish a reason for being for future generations.

This chapter discusses the following questions: Who are the older adults? What major health problems accompany their longevity? What are appropriate community health nursing interventions in these health situations? What community programs, resources, and legislative support are available to make the older years truly golden years and not just years? The problems of the older generations must become the challenges of the current generation of health care providers.

DEMOGRAPHY

Who are the older adults? What are the age boundaries for individuals in this developmental category? Historically the decision to have age 65 as the eligible age for receipt of Social Security benefits initiated the definition of the older adult. The early 1900s saw an

Table 27-1. Older population growth and projections		
Year	**Total no.**	**% of total**
1900	3,080	4.1
1940	9,019	6.8
1980	25,544	11.3
1990	30,290	12.1
2000	32,445	12.2
2010	35,424	12.6
2020	45,669	15.4
2030	55,864	18.2

From Facts about older Americans, 1980-81, Washington, D.C., Office of Human Development Services.

older population of 1 in every 24 individuals aged 65 and over, compared to the 1980 census rate of 1 in every 9 individuals, or 25.5 million Americans. By the year 2030 it is projected that older Americans will number 56 million (Need for Long-Term Care, 1981). The increasing growth rate of the older population can be seen in Table 27-1. Blacks constitute the largest minority in this country, with 1.9 million blacks aged 65 and older. The black elderly comprise 8% of the elderly population, and this is expected to reach 11% by the year 2000 (Hill, 1978; Jackson, 1978). Asians and Pacific islanders account for 6% of the 65 and older population, with native Americans and Hispanics accounting for 4% each (Need for Long-term Care, 1981). The life expectancy at birth in 1980 has reached an all-time high of 78.7 and 70 years for women and men, respectively (Final Report, 1981). The combined effects of the increasing life expectancy and the declining birth rate figures have contributed to America becoming an aging nation, with over 11.3% of its population being 65 years old (Need for Long-term Care, 1981).

In 1980 a sex differential of 148 white women per 100 white men compared to 141 black women per 100 black men was noted (Facts About Older Americans, 1981). Since this differential is expected to continue, nursing must develop specific strategies for assisting older women to cope with the years they live alone and the concomitant problems stemming from widowhood.

Where do older adults live? Most older adults live in their own homes, near their children. Florida has the distinction of having the highest number of older adults, 17.3% of the total population, with Arkansas, Iowa, Kansas, Missouri, Nebraska, Rhode Island, and South Dakota having at least a 13% elderly population (Facts About Older Americans, 1981).

The changing demography of the elderly reveals a more educated group. The average educational attainment of the over 65 age group in 1980 was 10.2 years. Currently approximately 41% of the older adults have finished high school. However, by the year 2000, it is projected that this figure will be as high as 90% (Facts About Older Americans, 1981). Thus community health nurses will provide services to a population demanding different health education content and new teaching and learning styles. The printed pamphlet may relinquish its role to the home computer unit as a conveyor of information.

Although people are living to older ages, recent increases in Social Security and the use of Medicare have benefitted the elderly in that only 15% of older adults lived below the poverty level in 1979 and another 9.6% lived above the poverty level but below the "near poverty" level. Statistics on poverty show a racial differentiation, with 13% of elderly white, 35% of elderly blacks, and 27% of elderly Hispanics being poor (Need for Long-Term Care, 1981).

CULTURE AND AGING

The community health nurse must be knowledgeable about the impact of culture on aging and provide care congruent with the recipients' cultural affiliation and beliefs. The concepts of heterogeneity, acculturation, and assimilation can generally provide a broad framework for understanding cultural influences on health. The multiplicity of types of people in any society must be accepted and respected. Membership in a particular ethnic or cultural group may differentiate an individual from another; however, the difference is not one of less or greater societal value, it is simply an identifying characteristic. Also, ethnicity is only one variable impacting on any given state and must be taken as such and not as a causative or an explanatory factor for each and every observed phenomenon. It is necessary for the community health nurse to know and accept the fact that group membership does not mean homogeneity, with all members of the group being alike. There are differences among groups and within groups. Generalizations based on the aggregate must be examined for each individual, with emphasis on unique differences. The influences of acculturation and assimilation of the behaviors, beliefs, activities, and issue of the majority culture will usually result in persons who have combinations and blends of the primary cultural group as well as the present influences of the majority culture. The community health nurse must remember that it is the individual's as well as the group's perceptions and beliefs about health and illness which are important and must be handled with respect, care, choice, and responsibility. The community health nurse must ask such questions as the following: How does membership in a particular ethnic or cultural group predispose an individual to regard health and illness? What is significant for this individual regardless of group membership? What can I do to transcend the differences and similarities between me as provider of health care and the recipient as a consumer of that health care? Such questions may add respect and care to identity. For example, consider the community health nurse's review of a client's record that indicates a 45-year-old Southern black woman with hypertension. The community health nurse who asks the foregoing questions will arrive at answers unique for this individual situation rather than stereotyped expectations such as an obese person who likes "soul food," is noncomplaint, and is difficult to motivate.

The older adult in America lives in a culture oriented to youth, productivity, and rapid pace. This orientation has influenced the goods and services produced and marketed as well as the work, recreation, and rest options available. The youth-oriented culture implies to older adults that they may not be respected, valued, or esteemed and that certain health declines, problems, and issues are "natural" or just "old age." Some health problems therefore go undetected, are mislabeled or misdiagnosed, or are ineffectively treated or untreated. There are fewer adequately prepared health care providers for the older segment of the population than for other age groups. Additionally, the allocation of resources—type, amount, and location—imply to the older adult that their needs may go unmet. Although many demographic and social changes are beginning to alter this youth-oriented attitude, much work is needed to create an attitude of social worth for all age groups.

Knowledge of the role of the elderly in various cultural, ethnic, and cohort groups is essential to each community health nurse in providing quality care. Across cultures and ethnic groups the roles of the elderly in family relationships and as storers and transmitters of knowledge and information are evident. The black American family esteems its older members for their "adaptation" to many crises and struggles, for their strong religious affiliation, and for the life expectancy crossover phenomenon (that is, blacks aged 75 years and older live longer than whites).

The Asian-American family is viewed as one wherein the older adult man may relinquish status and responsibility to his wife and oldest son. Many older Chinese men live alone by choice and because of cultural beliefs, compared to the Japanese culture wherein the young are expected to respect and care for their elders.*

*In the Japanese culture children tend to assume responsibility for aging relatives rather than expecting them to live alone and care for themselves.

Mexican-Americans view health and illness as a balance-imbalance between the will of God and their own behavior. Additionally, children are expected to care for the aged, and there is little use of nursing homes (Ebersole and Hess, 1981).

Chapter 11 gives additional information on the influence of culture in determining the community health nursing role.

The changes in socialization, social expectations, and life-styles of each cohort of aged persons determine to some extent what will be paramount needs and issues for the group. Members of the generation of the 1960s, characterized by such issues as rebellion, rights, and freedom, at age 65 will differ greatly in character, expectation, and social participation from members of the Depression era generation who are now a part of the older population. The cohorts of the 1980s will age with an entirely different set of issues and concerns, considering the influence of education, consumerism, financial woes of inflation and unemployment, and health conscientiousness on this cohort.

MYTHS AND STEREOTYPES

Only in recent years has aging as a life process enjoyed study and research. The earlier lack of emphasis on this population group fostered the perpetuation of many myths and stereotypes, the major ones of which are discussed here. It is hoped that as knowledge expands in this area, this state of mythography will change. The public's view of old people as persons wearing glasses, who are hard of hearing, are bald or have grey hair, have wrinkled skin, and are crippled is often heard and seen. How many times have such illusions been depicted as typical of old people in dramas, drawings, and other works? What characteristics of older people are portrayed on television? Additionally, the public's conversation and jokes about older people dehumanize and stigmatize this group (Table 27-2).

A popular myth holds that most older people are institutionalized, yet only about 5% of elderly persons are actually in institutions (Health United States, 1976-1977). The second most common myth is that old people are poor. Recognizing that many are poor, the majority, 85%, of older adults live above the poverty level (Need for Long-term Care, 1981). This figure should not negate the severity of the financial as well as other problems stemming from poverty, such as living in older houses in deteriorating neighborhoods, having limited access to transportation, and receiving poor health care.

The myth of the inability of the elderly to learn has serious consequences for the health of elderly persons. Health education opportunities are often bypassed

Table 27-2. Television viewing diary: portrayal of people 65 years old and older

Program and time	Characteristics portrayed (visual and verbal)	Personal responses to portrayed characteristics	Myths, stereotypes, and cliches	Actions to alter to correct negative myths, stereotypes, and cliches

when providers believe "They can't learn." Yet investigation of the nature of learning during old age has shown that older adults are capable of learning, and when problems occur they are generally associated with other conditions. Adjustments are needed in the attitudes of the providers of information as well as the recipients.

Just as women have been characterized as "bad drivers" so have older people, regardless of sex. The automobile accident problem for people over 65 years of age is one of being injured as a pedestrian instead of as the driver of a car causing an accident. The 15- to 24-year-old group has the highest motor vehicle death rate (Healthy People, 1979).

The perception of older people as "chair rockers" is refuted by Harris' survey (The Myth and Reality of Aging in America, 1975), which revealed that people 65 years old and older are perceived as spending 42% of their time "sitting and thinking" and 27% of their time "doing nothing" in comparison to actually spending at least 20% of their time in each of the following activities: gardening, caring for others, hobbies, walking, and participating in organizations.

Additional myths center on sexuality. Sexual drive and activity are present in old age, with changes resulting from physiological and/or sociocultural perspectives. Also, health problems and medications may alter the sexual activity, as may availability of a mate, stereotypes, privacy, and living arrangements.

DEVELOPMENTAL TASKS AND THEORIES OF AGING

The developmental tasks for old age, according to Burnside (1979), Duvall (1971), and Havighurst (1953), generally include the following:

1. Adjusting to decreasing health and physical strength
2. Adjusting to retirement and reduced income
3. Adjusting to the death of a spouse
4. Acceptance of one's self as an aging person
5. Maintaining satisfactory living arrangements
6. Realigning relationships with adult children
7. Finding meaning in life

To varying degrees these tasks are incorporated into the theories of aging discussed here. In addition, key tasks and potential problems when they are not met are listed in Table 27-3.

The aging process can be described as a phenomenon beginning with conception and terminating with death, with many changes occurring during the intervening years. Psychological theories of aging have sought to describe the aging process and to explain behaviors observed during this life phase. Cummings and Henry (1961) formulated the *disengagement theory of aging.* Withdrawal is a key concept in this theory. The disengagement theory postulates that aging people withdraw from customary roles fulfilled during middle years and invest themselves in more introspective, self-focused activities. The protective mechanisms of withdrawal and introspection allow the individual to establish a new balance level, thereby adapting to the numerous changes of aging. Additionally there is withdrawal of society from the aged, thereby creating a state of mutual withdrawal.

The *activity theory,* at the opposite end of the spectrum, fosters the continuation of middle-years activities as the criterion for successful aging. The active old person who maintains social relationships, is involved in community activities, travels, and has many hobbies and activities is considered the model old person (Havighurst, 1963). Societal expectations and rewards still

Table 27-3. Developmental tasks and potential problems of the elderly

Tasks	Potential problems
Adjusting to decreasing health and physical strength	Hypochondriasis, anger, anxiety, chronicity, grief, depression, low self-esteem, loss of health
Adjusting to retirement and reduced income	Loss of status, poverty, rejection, low self-esteem
Adjusting to death of a spouse	Loss of spouse, grief, guilt, loneliness, depression
Acceptance of self as an aging person	Rejection, low self-esteem
Maintaining satisfactory living arrangements	Dependency, isolation
Realigning relationships with adult children	Conflict, hostility, rejection, loneliness, isolation
Finding meaning in life	Guilt, despair, suicide

imply support for this theory of successful aging.

The *developmental or continuity theory of aging* emphasizes a continuation of the individual's unique traits, characteristics, and habits into the later years without much change from earlier age. Interiority as a key concept in this theory emphasizes the importance of one's own system of values, introspection, and individuality (Neugarten, 1964). The developmental or continuity theory represents one balance between the extremes of the disengagement and activity theories.

The work on the *eight stages of life* (Erikson, 1963) provides even another perspective for viewing aging. Timing, sequential order of movement, and accomplishment of certain critical tasks are essential for movement from one life stage to the next. Aging is viewed as successful resolution of the conflict between the critical tasks of integrity and despair. Positive resolution results in people whose recapitulation of their lives reveals contentment over life and indicates that their relationships for life have been a blending of leading and following. The individual suffering from despair regrets that life cannot begin again and be better, for the remaining years are too few.

The *biological theories of aging,* such as free radical and immunological, rely on physiological explanations for the aging process. The free radical theory has cell oxygen use and the formation of nonusable free radical end-products as its core factors. An imbalance between production and elimination of free radical products from internal and external sources results in an accumulation of by-products, which in turn are thought to affect aging. Continuing research seeks to clarify this theory, as well as the role of vitamins A, C, and E and niacin and of the aging pigments, lipofuscins (Ebersole and Hess, 1981; Working with Older People, 1970).

With increased age, normal cells within the body are not recognized by the body as its own. Therefore the body sets off a protective mechanism, forming antibodies against the "unknown cells." The autoimmune reaction is the basis of the *autoimmunity theory of aging* (Ebersole and Hess, 1981; Working with Older People, 1970).

Although these theories provide some explanations for the aging process, no one theory explains the aging process of all older adults. The variability of individuals within the group necessitates variability in theories. Theories of aging are important to nursing inasmuch as they can provide a framework against which practice decisions can be made.

MAJOR HEALTH PROBLEMS

Although many older adults enjoy good health and freedom of activity, others do not share this distinction. Approximately 80% of the group over age 65 have at least one chronic health problem. Limitation of an activity of daily living is present in half of the elderly population, whereas 18% of this same group cannot carry on a major activity (Healthy People, 1979). Cardiovascular, arthritic, and visual problems are the three most frequently reported activity-limiting conditions experienced by this age group (Need for Long-term Care, 1981). The evidence of chronic illness makes assisting the older adult adapt to this problem a major nursing responsibility. The major health killers of those over 65 are heart disease, malignant neoplasms, and cerebrovascular diseases (Healthy People, 1979) (Table 27-4).

Hypertension

Hypertension as a type of cardiovascular disease is a common malady of aging and represents a major community health problem for this age population as well as for middle-aged adults. Risk factors such as smoking, obesity, and lack of exercise must be reduced. Blacks are more often affected by hypertension, as men are more than women. People with habits of increased salt

Table 27-4. Mortality of older adults (65 years and over), 1978

Disease	%
Heart disease	44
Malignant neoplasms	19
Cerebrovascular disease	12
Influenza and pneumonia	3

From Facts about older Americans, 1980-81, Washington, D.C., 1981, Office of Human Development Services.

intake, obesity, and cigarette smoking also are more likely to be affected by hypertension. Repeated blood pressure readings of 95 mm Hg (diastolic) and 160 mm Hg (systolic) usually indicate hypertension. Prescribed treatment regimens include antihypertensive drugs, optimum weight control, salt restriction, stress management, and a balance of rest and exercise. Nursing activities for older adults with hypertension include monitoring blood pressure and weight, giving nutrition and drug education, teaching stress management techniques, and promoting an optimal balance between rest and activity. Blood pressure measurements are important in the secondary prevention of advancement of the illness or of complications. Additionally, the person's individual normal range of blood pressure can be established. Case finding through blood pressure screening is an important primary prevention strategy.

In assisting the older adult with hypertension to achieve optimal weight, psychosociocultural factors, life-style, and overall health status must be considered. The community health nurse must assess the client's current practices and desires so that plans can be made with the client to include changes the client is willing to make. A weight reduction diet in conjunction with techniques of self-awareness, motivation, and reward will aid the older adult to substitute old eating habits with more health-promoting habits. Food selection and preparation provide the core of nutrition education. For example, canned soups and vegetables, smoked or salted meats, and condiments such as pickles, catsup, and seasoned salts are to be avoided. Lemon juice, oregano, thyme, and other spices and herbs may be substituted for salt and fat in the preparation of foods. Older adults must be taught to read labels to determine the financial as well as the nutritional value of the product. It is not enough to explain the prescribed diet to the client. Including the person with the primary responsibility for food selection and preparation and other significant family members along with the client will increase compliance with the prescribed diet, food restric-

tions, and other nutrition teaching. Chapters 21 and 38 discuss stress, exercise, and nutrition further. The activity described in the following box is one strategy the community health nurse may use to assist a client with diet modification.

Health teaching must also include information about drug and food interactions as well as interactions among drugs. The replacement of potassium via drugs and/or food may be necessary for some persons receiving diuretics as treatment for hypertension. Further, the use of cold remedies by people with hypertension can create increased blood pressure. It is essential that hypertensive individuals understand and accept the chronic nature of the illness and the need for lifelong adherence to treatment.

The interrelationship between mind and body is important in the problem of hypertension. This interrelationship can be assessed by questions such as the following: What stress or tension have you experienced during the past week (or some other time reference)? Where is the discomfort felt in your body when you are upset? What other things were going on in your life when you started to feel bad and have headaches and dizziness? The total benefits of drugs and dietary management of hypertension cannot be realized without some regard for the individual's stress level. Relaxation techniques, problem-solving skills, and exercise are all strategies for the management of stress. Chapter 38 elaborates further on stress management techniques.

Cancer

Malignant neoplasm or cancer is the second largest killer of older people in the United States (Healthy People, 1979). Early detection and treatment are still valuable for this age group, who can live many additional years. (Approximately half of the persons reaching 65 will live an additional 15 years [Healthy People, 1979].) Preventive programs for cancer must include elimination of smoking behavior; close vigilance for change in skin moles, altered bowel habits, or nonhealing sores; and regular physical examinations, including pelvic and rectal examinations. Monthly breast self-examinations and annual Pap smears are necessary for older women. Postmenopausal women should establish a consistent time each month for conducting the breast self-examination, since there is no menstrual cycle with which to pair the examination. The socio-cultural factors impacting on this age group must be dealt with so that the goals of regular breast and pelvic examinations can become realities. A health history is of immense value, and time must be allocated to focus on data that could provide the keys to early detection and diagnosis.

Older adults must be taught to get acquainted with their bodies, to attend to changes, and to reveal their

---

Dietary Modification Guide and Activity

1. Ask client to keep a dietary diary for 7 days.
2. Assist the client to compare diary to chart showing recommended dietary pattern.
3. Assist client to modify dietary intake by planning changes to include into next week's meals.
4. Keep dietary diary for 7 days. Follow with steps 2, 3, and 4 as necessary.

Food description	Amount	Time and setting	Modifications
Breakfast			
Grits	½ cup	7:00 AM, kitchen table	
Margarine	4 tb		
Toast	2 slices		
Jelly	2 tb		
Scrambled egg	1		
Coffee	2 cups		
Lunch			
Spinach	½ cup	3:00 PM, kitchen table	
Fried beef patty	1 medium		
Rolls	2		
Margarine	2 tb		
Dinner			
Tea	1 cup	8:00 PM, den	
Dry cereal	¾ cup		
Milk	½ cup		
Sugar	4 tb		

---

observations to the health care provider. Often the elderly's attitudes of "It is just old age" and "I don't want to be a bother" create a barrier to effective use of the health care system. Correction of misconceptions, provision of realistic emotional support, and quality care during diagnostic and treatment procedures are all activities within the realm of professional nursing.

Arthritis

Arthritis is a significant disease for this population, since it often limits activities and affects comfort and independence. The inflammation, swelling, stiffness, and pain combine to impair mobility and comfort. Arthritic persons comprise approximately 44% of the elderly population, with more women being affected (Healthy People, 1979). Inflammation and degenerative changes of the joints are usually involved in arthritis. Rheumatoid arthritis generally affects the peripheral joints symmetrically. Symptoms include inflammation, pain, stiffness, swelling, numbness and tingling of hands and feet, malaise, and weight loss. Treatment generally includes medication, rest-activity, heat or cold applications, and physical therapy (Luckmann and Sorenson, 1980). Education is important to help clients avoid the false hope and expense of arthritis quackery, which offers ineffective and possibly harmful "cures." Additionally, stress management is important in controlling the disease process. Persons affected by arthritis may need supportive devices and appliances

such as walkers, chairs, food utensils, and grooming aids. Human resources and mechanical aids may be needed as functional dependency increases. The community health nurse may be instrumental in counseling and assisting the family in enhancing open communication, role negotiation, and use of community resources in dealing with arthritis.

Sensory Impairments

Sensory impairments, especially of sight and hearing, contribute to limitation of activities. Reduced vision is a problem for about 22% of those over 65 years. Fewer than 20% of those over 75 years have normal vision even with correction (Healthy People, 1979). Specifically, hearing impairments are present in about 30% of older adults, increasing to 75% for those persons over 75 years, with men affected more frequently than women (Fact Book on Aging, 1978). The effects of hearing and visual problems are seen in problems of reality testing, mobility, social interaction, crime, and the recreational activities of reading and watching television. The older adult who cannot hear has a difficult time in joining the family in conversations as well as in using the telephone as a vehicle to aid with visiting. Also, hearing and visual deficits render people less aware of possible crimes against them. They may neither hear nor see intruders. Regular visual examinations and auditory evaluations are necessary and should be encouraged. Older adults with some chronic illnesses, diabetes as one example, are particularly at risk for eye problems.

Organic Brain Syndrome

Organic brain syndrome may be acute or chronic in nature. Acute disorders occur rapidly, are limited in duration, and are reversible. In contrast, chronic organic brain syndrome or dementia develops slowly, is progressive, and is irreversible. Memory impairment, disorientation, and impaired judgment characterize this disorder of older adults. The wanderer who is found on a busy street and the forgotten food left cooking on the range are familiar reports from families and neighbors of the impaired individual. As functions decline, anxiety and frustration mount in the older adult as well as in the family. Senile dementia presents a challenge to the elderly's adult children who are involved in careers, family life, and other middle-life tasks. Treatment consists of diagnosis, correction of the underlying causative disease, maintenance and use of remaining strengths and assets, and promotion of comfort and quality of life. Family support is crucial as efforts are made to keep the older adult in the community. Additionally, environmental stimuli and protection are needed by the older adult. Patience, caring, reality orientation, personal hygiene, and nutrition top the list of intervention activities. The following is a case study of organic brain syndrome.

Mrs. Hill, 80 years old, has wandered away from the home she shares with her daughter and the daughter's 10- and 15-year-old children. She is found by the local police on the expressway. Mrs. Hill is carried to the local hospital for observation and care until her family can be notified.
1. What problems would you identify?
2. What initial plan of care would you develop for Mrs. Hill and her family?
3. What community resources may be helpful to this family?

Dental Problems

Many persons aged 65 and over have some, if not all, of their natural teeth; however, the most prevalent dental health problem is tooth loss (Fact Book on Aging, 1978). The loosening of permanent teeth, periodontoclasia, may result from changes in tooth support or periodontal disease. Normal aging changes must be differentiated from pathological conditions. Diminished salivary secretion and some loss of taste sensation are considered normal changes in aging; however, these complaints still need attention. Complaints of poor dentition, dry mouth, difficult swallowing, taste changes, and sore gums may contribute to changes in eating, chewing, and utimately nutritional status. Problems of constipation, fatigue, loss of appetite, weight loss, and anemia may also occur. Medications affecting oral hygiene include antibiotics, anticonvulsants, phenothiazines, cholinergic blocking agents, and antihistamines.

Dental problems can be reduced by the early establishment of good dental health habits. Regular brushing and flossing, proper nutrition, and regular dental examinations contribute to the reduction of the incidence of dental health problems in the elderly. Vulnerability to oral health problems necessitates continuing oral assessment and care in this age group. Early recognition of problems usually can mean correction of a minor problem for minimal cost and discomfort. Oral assessment should include a thorough oral health history and inspection of color and condition of lips, gums, teeth, tongue, and mucosa. Painful swallowing and sore or bleeding gums necessitate further investigation. Caries or loose teeth should be identified as to location and presence or absence of pain. The tongue should be inspected on its upper and lower surfaces, as should the floor of the mouth, and any abnormal smoothness of the dorsal or upper surface of the tongue should be noted.

Actions such as use of mouth wash; a commercial preparation or rinsing with warm tap water; use of lubricants such as lanolin, cocoa butter, or petroleum jelly; drinking increased fluids; and eating frequent, small, nutritionally balanced meals all contribute to correcting some of the minor oral health problems. The importance of regular dental and physical examinations cannot be overemphasized. People with dentures need to be encouraged to wear and properly care for them. Complaints of malfitting dentures need to be investigated, with the necessary adjustments made to ensure proper fit. Areas for oral assessment are summarized in the following list.

Oral health history
    Health problems
    Medications
    Dentures
    Brushing and flossing practices
    Appetite
    Taste and food preferences
    Painful chewing, swallowing
    Bleeding gums
Inspection
    Structural components: lips, gums, teeth, tongue, mucosa, palate, pharnyx
    Conditions: odor, dryness-moistness, redness, soreness, color, swelling, bleeding
Caries
Loose teeth
Ulcerations
Facial grimaces

Encouragement of use of dentures and praise about appearance are strategies in the care of persons with dentures. Oral and dental health are important to digestion, speech, appearance, and body image and therefore must be stressed to older people as worthy of the time and expenditure. Efforts must be exerted to remove the dental care gap in the health care of the elderly. In addition, problems regarding financing dental care, negative stereotypes and attitudes, mistrust and fear of the dentist, and access must be acknowledged, confronted, and resolved.

Drug Uses and Abuses

Drug sensitivity, paradoxical reactions, and drug-taking behaviors are all factors contributing to elderly drug users being a population at risk for drug problems. Drug misuse includes overdoses and inadequate doses as well as inappropriate drug combinations. Many prescribed drugs are improperly self-administered in amount, frequency, and combination as well as improperly stored. The cost of medications and the frugality of the elderly combine to create a situation of saving drugs from one occasion to another and continuing to use a previously prescribed drug after a new drug has been prescribed. It is not uncommon to hear an older adult comment, "My old pill worked better than this new one so I started to take the old pill again." Comparing and sharing medicine is another common practice of this age group. The combining of prescribed medicines can be serious, as can the combining of prescribed and nonprescribed, over-the-counter (OTC) medicines.

Nursing interventions must include a drug history; directions for safe storage of drugs; cautions about drug-drug and drug-food interactions; and drug information, such as name, purpose, intended benefits, side effects, dosage, and frequency and route of administration. A checkoff system using a date and time calendar and presorting according to medication, dosage, and time are valuable techniques for persons who have difficulty preparing medications or trouble with memory. Presorting strategies include the use of egg cartons and small envelopes with the correct dosage in each labeled egg carton slot or envelope for specified time periods. The community health nurse must instruct the older adult in the proper use of the presorting technique. For example, "Mr. Yates, you are to take the medicine in the envelope marked "1" on Sunday morning at 8:00 AM, envelope "2" on Monday morning at 8:00 AM . . . and I will return on Thursday, the day you take the medicine in envelope 5." Drugs can be savers or destroyers of life, and community health nurses must help clients capitalize on the lifesaving aspects.

Substance Abuse

Although abuse of substances such as alcohol and other drugs is present in the older adult population, the exact incidence is difficult to determine because of the life-style of the elderly abuser. The older person who lives alone, drinks to avoid loneliness and boredom, and uses pills for sleep and medications for pain is in circumstances that may create an environment of substance abuse. Additionally, daily drinking of alcohol may create a greater consumption level than would be possible with less unstructured time. The problem of abuse is intensified when coupled with the effects of chronic illnesses. Alcohol abusers include those persons assuming the habit of excessive drinking during old age as well as those long-time alcoholics who have lived into old age. Other abused drugs include sedatives and tranquilizers. As discussed in Chapter 22, treatment approaches in substance abuse generally include monitored detoxification, counseling, stress management, self-help groups, and treatment of any disease stemming from the abuse practices. Community resources such as Alcoholics Anonymous and Al-Anon can be valuable agencies in the total treatment of the older adult. Education of the public continues to be a major task of the community health nurse.

PSYCHOSOCIAL ASPECTS OF AGING

Coping with Retirement

The ability to successfully adjust to retirement is affected by such factors as health status, sufficient income, number of situational changes, quality of personal relationships, ability to manage time effectively, flexibility, ability to relinquish the work routine, and anticipation and realistic expectation for retirement. The community health nurse has an important role in assisting to maximize the potentials of the retiree. The best preparation for retirement comes years before the event. Good health practices, for instance, begin in utero and continue throughout life. However, sometimes circumstances, life-style choice, and other factors combine to create health problems. In such instances the individual has to learn to adapt to illness. Chronic health problems must be dealt with through life-style adjustments and management of prescribed regimen.

The community health nurse can often provide direction and guidance to the retiree as well as the family. The provision of professional support to the family is an important nursing role benefiting retiree and family. The community health nurse may speak to a group of preretirees at a local industry, thus providing them with information about normal expectations and behaviors, time management, and other issues exclusive of the customary financial planning done with preretirees. Education regarding the normal changes of aging, health, retirement, and problems of aging will promote understanding, caring, and positive actions. Two critical aspects of adjustment to retirement relate to how effectively the retiree learns to restructure time and the quality of personal relationships.

Managing Time

Retirement, formally institutionalized in the United States by the passage of the Social Security Act in 1935, generally occurs at the age of 65 years. At the moment of retirement the worker is confronted with loss of job, reduction in income, and loss of and/or altered relations with co-workers. Time becomes available, and the individual asks "What will I do with all of this time?"

The management of time is crucial for older adults, who generally have more time than any other possession. The day must offer enough promise of being a good day that an individual is motivated to arise and meet the day's challenges and opportunities. Loneliness is one consequence of inadequate, pleasureless, interpersonal relationships, with many older adults masking loneliness with various complaints such as insomnia, indigestion, muscular aches, and general malaise. Many do not possess leisure-time skills; consequently they feel alienated, lonely, and unhappy with the increased time available in later years. Considering the present life expectancy, a person can anticipate living several years in retirement. Some realistic plans regarding the pursuit of meaningful activities during retirement must be made. Senior centers offer a social outlet as well as numerous other services.

Mrs. A, who has to take a taxi to the center, makes the trip on Monday, Wednesday, and Friday to avoid being home alone and thinking and grieving about her deceased husband. Participation in crafts, water exercise, and health education programs have proved to be effective use of her time. Other people, like Mr. J, Miss T, and Mrs. O, gain purpose and meaningful use of time by volunteering to serve juice, set the table, help in the kitchen, or do the "Thoughts for Living" at the nutrition center. Additionally, they have earned hours as Retired Senior Volunteer Program (RSVP) workers and are publicly recognized for their contribution.

The retired person should plan for ways to satisfy basic needs, to further develop the total person, and to derive happiness from living, in addition to planning for fun, entertainment, and leisure. The development of hobbies and interests during earlier years provides a pivotal point for activities during later years. A meaningful activity is one which is congruent with life-style, interests, resources, and health of the older adult.

Health-promoting leisure pursuits for older adults generally include physical fitness activities; visiting in person or via the telephone with relatives and friends; arts and crafts such as painting, sewing, and ceramics; viewing television; reading; and travel. New interests are to be encouraged by the community health nurse and other health care workers, family, and significant others. Referrals and information about available community activities can be provided by the community health nurse. Many organizations, such as nutrition centers, community schools, and multipurpose senior centers, provide places for older adults to convene for leisure pursuits and to meet other older adults.

Realignment of Relationships

Retirees often must reconsider the relationship between themselves and significant others, including spouse, family, and neighbors. Family relationships represent one of the challenges of this age period. The retired person must learn to live with or without the spouse. A man who has spent many years working away from home must now spend hours on hours at home; this requires adjustment. The woman who has been home alone must now get accustomed to having her husband underfoot all day. As families increasingly become characterized by two working adults, it will be interesting to note the adjustment impact on both persons retiring at or near the same time with many hours to spend together.

Another aspect of family relationships after retirement is the relationship realignment between aging parents and their adult children. Issues of role reversal, dependency, conflict, guilt, and loss require recognition and resolution.

The community health nurse must consider the parent who has always met the affiliative as well as the physical needs of each household member and who now needs assistance with feeding, bathing, dressing, and mobility and must rely on the adult children to accomplish such tasks daily. Such role reversal of "helper-helpee" can create a climate of kind caring and loving or one of hostile dependency. Many community health nurses hear countless expressions of "when parents grow old they are just like children experiencing second childhood." Such phrases perpetuate a decline in self-esteem, self-worth, and equalitarian relationships.

A second issue, guilt, is highlighted in adult children who feel the pangs of "if only I had 'come sooner,' made the aging adult move in with us, realized that the behaviors were symptoms of a problem rather than meanness, stubbornness, or cantankerousness." The community health nurse is in a position to assist adult children with their middle-life tasks and crises as well as be a resource for helping with the compounding problems of their parents' later-life tasks and crises. The tripling effects of the presence and influence of younger children and adolescents must be reconciled. Nursing strategies of providing knowledge about normal developmental needs throughout the life span, communication, conflict resolution, and the valuing of another person are essential in working with multigenerational families.

Living on a fixed income is another issue of importance to the retiree. Many retirees can expect to receive Social Security benefits and employment-related pensions. An additional segment may have savings or rental or other supplemental income. Thus budget planning and wise shopping can help those on a fixed income. In addition, some supplement their income with part-time work or exchange of services such as cooking, shopping, child care, or home cleaning. Other income extenders include food stamps and Supplemental Security Income (SSI) for eligible individuals.

Maintaining Self-esteem

Self-esteem is critical in the later years of life. One adaptive task associated with later years and aging is the reassessment of the criteria for evaluation of the self. Ideas used as a basis for self-concept often need to be modified to establish identity and personal worth in roles other than the work role. Planned activities and programs, satisfying interpersonal relationships, good health, quality housing, adequate income, and suitable transportation all contribute to high self-esteem (Schwartz, 1978).

Nursing activities to promote a high level of self-esteem include recognition of achievements; providing positive feedback; granting respect and courtesies; promoting choice, decision making, and control; and encouraging and facilitating interpersonal relationships. An observing community health nurse can comment on certificates, rewards, and pictures that may be visible in the living environment. Encouragement of work or volunteer services that make use of existing knowledge and skills can be valuable, for example, a retired teacher might tutor a group of schoolchildren, another might teach a special hobby to older adults at the multipurpose senior center, and a carpenter might assist in building shelves for display of the produced items. An annual bazaar and sale of crafts might be spearheaded by an older business entrepreneur. Each one can be recognized for at least one desirable trait and thereby feel needed and valued. Additionally, the community health nurse must remember the small, yet significant value of addressing older adults with the appropriate titles of Mr., Mrs., Miss, Dr., Rev., Father, etc. Policy-

makers must be made aware of the consequences of various policies for self-esteem and personhood. Implicit statements from policies can say "We care about you," "Old people are of value to this country," and "Minority producers and consumers also have clout."

Coping with Loss and Grief

Loss and grief are common companions of the elderly adult and threaten the maintenance of self-esteem. Loss of roles through retirement, declining health from chronic illnesses, and death of the spouse are just a few of the losses. Widowhood as a problem of later years occurs in addition to other problems; thereby multiple, complex issues have to be faced. Women are at higher risk of loss of a spouse because women outnumber men and live longer. Married women can expect to live some of their later years in widowhood. Additionally, remarriage following widowhood is less frequent in women inasmuch as there are fewer older men and older men generally select younger women as spouses.

Widowhood often includes identifiable behaviors. The beginning phase of grief is characterized by a person experiencing shock, disbelief, and denial that death has taken the loved one. Sadness and crying ensue as awareness of the reality of death is experienced. The survivors carry out the ritual of a funeral and other culturally meaningful practices and rites as part of grieving. The process of living alone, relinquishing the lost spouse, and reinvesting oneself in something and/or someone awaits the widow or widower. The nursing activities of providing correct information, a sense of reality, supportive listening, and caring during periods of crying and other emotional releases are essential to healthy grieving. The continuing relationship of the community health nurse provides a caring individual and provider when the family and friends have returned to their routine activities and the mourner is left alone to deal with problems of loneliness, social isolation, altered finances, changed living arrangements, and new identity.

Time is important in healing the wound and allowing for successful grieving. Self-help groups and/or counseling may be beneficial during this phase in assisting the remaining spouse to cope with loss without feeling guilty or losing self-esteem. Present practices of fewer marriages, cohabitation, more divorces, childlessness, geographic mobility, financial instability, and improved educational and health status present special challenges in planning care for future cohorts of widows or widowers. People must be educated to plan for their later years as life-style choices are made throughout life. Preparation for widowhood must be of a multifarious nature and include financial as well as psychosocial planning.

Dealing with Depression

Depression as a common health problem of the aged is often masked in and by other complaints and problems. Signs to look for when depression is suspected include complaints of sadness, insomnia, anorexia, weight loss, or constipation. Frequently these complaints are undervalued and thereby labeled as complaints of old age or hypochondriasis.

Treatment of the problem must include a thorough history, counseling, and judicious use of medication. Assessment can be made using questions such as the following: Do you awake from sleep during the early morning hours and find yourself unable to return to sleep? Is it hard to "get going" in the morning? Do you feel better as the day progresses? Have your appetite and food intake changed from its usual pattern? Do you have crying spells? Community health nurses can help older adults adjust to the changes of aging, cope with declining years and health, and view life as meaningful and valuable by aiding in arranging an activity schedule including rest periods, teaching normal expectations of aging and signs of impending health problems, and devising ways of managing financial demands with a fixed income. Nurses as sensitive listeners can be partners with older adults in the life review process. The life review process, including reminiscing and reviewing the past joys, accomplishments, and disappointments, is helpful to the older adult in resolving unresolved conflicts, in creating order to life, in relinquishing life, and in preparing for death.

After sustaining a major loss, life problems may mount so that some older adults see ending their own life as a viable option, leading to an alarming suicide rate in the elderly. Those over 65 account for one fourth of the suicides in the United States, with blacks and women committing fewer suicides (Fact Book on Aging, 1978). Thus one of America's most valuable resources is being destroyed by their own hands. Early detection of danger signs and timely interventions can decrease this problem. Cues to suicide potential include making a will, giving away possessions and valuables, and planning a funeral. Additionally, subtle and indirect clues include refusing to eat, medication misuse, and noncompliance with health-sustaining treatment regimens. During contacts with older adults community health nurses should observe suicide risks, determine lethality, recognize and compliment on areas of individual worth and esteem, and encourage meaningful activities and associations.

A sense of purpose, hope, and worth are derived from authentic encounters and experiences with a caring person. The community health nurse may determine that the client has been nonresponsive to nursing interventions and that additional care is warranted. Referral to a community mental health center, physician, or hospital may be needed. The community health nurse should maintain contact with the referral agency so the continuity of care may be provided. Additionally, a record of the care rendered by the community health nurse should be sent, with the written permission of the client, to the referral agency to avoid unnecessary delays and duplications.

Abuse of the Elderly

Abuse of the elderly can be physical, psychological, or material abuse, as well as violation of the rights of safety, security, and adequate health care. The elderly victim of abuse is generally an older woman with mental or physical impairments who lives with an adult child or other relative. Abusers are often middle-aged women, related or unrelated caretakers, often experiencing considerable stress. Other contributory factors include economics, interpersonal conflicts, life responsibilities, health, and dependency (Elder Abuse, 1980). Often out of fear, the abused person denies that abusive acts are occurring, leading to a climate of helplessness and resignation to abuse as the victim tries to protect self and the caretaker.

Using a family-oriented approach, interventions include counseling for both the abused and abusers and teaching stress management techniques. In selected instances, placement of the abused adult in a protected setting outside of the home, family vacations as respite time from the older adult, and sharing of responsibilities among children may be necessary. As described in Chapter 20, family violence continues to be a serious community problem, whether it is violence of child, spouse, or elder. Priorities in the area of prevention must be established if protection of individuals at risk is to become a reality.

Criminal Victimization

Many elderly individuals are the victims of confidence games, fraudulent consumerism, and crimes against person and property. The fear and impact of crime prevent many elderly persons from leaving their homes, thus making them prisoners in their own homes. The frail, sensory-impaired, poor, older woman who lives alone is a prime candidate for criminal victimization. Physical injury often results from the criminal activity. The popularity of confidence games or swindle tactics such as "bank examiner–crooked bank employee" and "pigeon drop–good faith money" continue to be major threats to the security of older adults. The bank examiner–crooked bank employee game consists of a stranger posing as a bank examiner, federal agent, or special police officer telling the older adult the story of trying to catch a crooked bank employee and needing the older person to withdraw a large amount of cash money from the bank to trap the employee. The pigeon drop–good faith money swindle operates on the basis of a stranger approaching an elderly person with the pretense of having found a large sum of money, which will be shared with the elderly person, but the elderly person must first withdraw some money from the bank to show good faith. The elderly person may even be given an envelope, allegedly containing the money, to hold and be instructed not to open the envelope, which in actuality contains cut-up paper.

The community health nurse can teach caution about home repair rip-offs, admitting strangers into one's residence, withdrawing large sums of money from the bank on the request of a stranger, flashing or displaying large sums of money, leaving unlocked car and/or house doors, and walking alone in dimly lighted, deserted areas. Older adults must be assisted to read and understand legal papers and transactions. Evaluation of product use, quality, and safety must be taught to older adults as part of the role of wise consumer. The slogan "Buyer Beware" can become a household watchword as law enforcement officers, health care providers, businesses, and policymakers join forces to combat the problem of criminal victimization of the elderly.

HEALTH PROMOTION

Physical as well as psychosocial or developmental changes accompany aging. The observed changes represent the cumulative and lifelong effects of heredity, environment, nutrition, rest, activity, altered health status, and aging. Both men and women experience some changes in hair color and distribution. The thinning epidermis, dehydrated dermis, lesser blood supply, and loss of elasticity, in addition to reduction and loss of subcutaneous fat, culminate in wrinkles. The skin surrounding the eye is affected by aging. Lines about the lateral canthus of the eyes form shapes resembling crow's feet. The gastrointestinal changes during aging include reduction in smelling and taste and decreased gastric and intestinal secretion and motility. These changes represent only a portion of the changes affecting each body system. Increased efforts to educate the elderly about normal changes during aging must become a priority nursing intervention.

A life-style of healthy habits during the early years contributes to the well-being of older adults, since the continuation of healthy habits and the addition of age-specific habits improve the quality and quantity of life. Aging can be healthy, and old age is not synonymous with ill health nor a pronouncement "to take it easy and retire to the rocking chair." Moderation in exercise, diet, and alcoholic beverage consumption and meaningful activities must be balanced into a day of meaningful living. Regular physical checkups, adherence to prescribed treatment regimens, and healthy life-styles must replace expressions such as "medicine won't do any good," "I haven't seen a doctor in so many years, why see a doctor now?" and "I've just got a few years left so I can eat and do what I please." Immunization and nutrition are selected health promotion issues included in this chapter.

Immunization

Immunization against influenza represents a special safeguard for older adults with chronic illnesses and respiratory problems such as emphysema. Pneumonia vaccines also are available. The older adult should discuss the advisability of individual use of influenza and pneumonia immunization with the private physician in view of the existing controversy about the use of such preventive measures.

Nutrition

As discussed in Chapter 21, a balanced diet including the four food groups is essential to good nutrition. Nutrients such as protein, minerals, calcium, and vitamins must be included in sufficient amounts, generally considered approximately the same as for younger people. A diet pattern of three meals per day is just as important now as during earlier years. Modification of caloric intake is necessary to keep off excess weight, since the physical activity of many older adults declines. Adequate hydration with sufficient amounts of water is needed as part of good nutritional practice.

Sociological, economic, and biological factors contribute to the eating habits of older persons. Some of these factors are living arrangements, transportation, limited income, dentition, sense of smell and taste, digestion, and myths about nutrition. Some typical statements of older adults are as follows: "Well it's just me and I don't feel like cooking just for myself. I just eat something light like cereal, soup, and sometimes some vegetables." "I don't like to eat alone." "I don't have an appetite; nothing tastes good." Health status, physical activity, cultural practices, individuality, and physiological changes of aging also must be considered in determining nutritional requirements. Attractive meals, companionship, and good dentition and digestion make mealtime a happy, healthy time.

HEALTH CARE

Home Health Services

Home health care services coupled with homemaker services prevent or delay institutionalization for older adults who need some assistance with self-care and other activities of daily living in addition to care for chronic health problems. Agencies providing home health care and/or homemaker services may be governmental, proprietary, or hospital based and funded accordingly. The combined professional-nonprofessional staff includes a nurse, social worker, physician, occupational therapist, and aide. Some states and agencies require some type of training program and certification for home health aides. Home health care is covered by Medicare for the person meeting an eligibility requirement for skilled care. The care is provided by a professional nurse and/or home health aide working under the direction of the professional nurse. The aide performs personal hygiene, measures vital signs, and gives technical care. In contrast to the home health aide the homemaker aide, whose services are not covered under Medicare, does light housework and cooking. The visiting nurses' association and community health nurses from local public health departments, in addition to nurses from private agencies, provide the professional nursing services to homebound persons needing skilled care.

Alternatives to Institutionalization

Day care centers, day hospitals, and respite care are other efforts aimed at delaying or preventing institutionalization. Day care centers serve the person who has some physical or mental limitations that interfere with totally independent living 24 hours per day and who needs social, nutritional, or recreational services. Day care centers also allow freedom for the permanent caretaker to have day hours away for work or other activities. The day hospital is directed toward providing day health services to a person who can live at the home during the evening. The respite care program provides care of the dependent older person while the permanent care taker has time off or relief for rest, recuperation, recreation, or an emergency. The services may be for several days to a week; however, the services are time-limited care with the goal of returning the dependent older person to a refreshed person who is better able to provide care after the respite period.

The alternatives to institutionalization are not without disadvantages. Problems of eligibility, cost, access, service limitation, and impact of long-term disability and care on the person and the family exist as challenges to the health care system. Should support for chronic care continue as a "shadow" of acute care, thus receiving only marginal support and importance? Should eligibility guidelines be such that more people are eliminated from services than receive services? Should a family that chooses to keep the older person at home be penalized with lack of assistance or reward? Is the older adult forced into a more dependent role just to obtain minimal help? The political, professional, ethical, and legal ramifications of each answer must be examined as the next decades experience a growing number of persons over 65 years old who will demand more care for and accountability to the older segment of the population.

Long-term Care

When situations of declining health; depleted physical, financial, and human resources; and increased dependency occur, institutionalization in a long-term care facility may become a reality. The time of "We have done all we can do," "I cannot look after my relative any longer," or "I have no place to go except the nursing home" signals a turning point or the crisis of relocation to a long-term care facility. A long-term care facility provides long-term or extended residential, intermediate, or skilled nursing care, medical care, and personal and psychosocial services. The level and type of services offered determine the criteria that must be met to satisfy local, state, and federal requirements. Additionally, federal Medicare and Medicaid guidelines and regulations must be met by participating agencies. Generally guidelines at each level—local, state, and federal—address type of client; staff qualifications and ratio, environment regulations; health care; client rights; and food, recreational, and social services. Individual needs and resources dictate which type of facility is most appropriate for the existing client status.

The decision to institutionalize is usually a difficult and ruminated one for the client and the family, if available. The client may experience a sense of helplessness; loss of control, independence, and love; and an overwhelming feeling of abandonment because going to a "nursing home" or an "old folk's home" is viewed as a "last resort" and "going there to die." Hope has vanished, for the client knows of no recoveries or returns by friends or relatives who have gone to nursing homes. The giving away of possessions and selling of the "home house" indicate that he is going away never to return to the familiar or the loved surroundings. The family has to cope with feelings of conflict, ambivalence, blaming, guilt, why us now, and helplessness. The community health nurse must support the family as having made the best decision for themselves at the present time and under the existing circumstances. The community health nurse can facilitate expression of feelings by such phrases as the following: "It is usually hard to place a loved one in a nursing home. I wonder what it is like for you?" "Sometimes families have second thoughts about putting a loved one in a nursing home." "I imagine this is a difficult time for you." The family and the older adult must be encouraged to talk *with* each other and not just *to* each other. Listening and hearing become important traits as the family seeks the best answer.

The community health nurse also must be an advocate for the family, a negotiator between the older adult and other family members, and a resource person. To do this, family contacts should be followed up with visits and/or telephone calls to determine what actions have been taken by the family and what additional assistance, if any, is needed. During each encounter with the family the community health nurse must remember and apply the concepts of choice, rights, responsibility, and decision making and assist the family in formulating these concepts into a practical solution. The admission of the client to the long-term care facility is not the termination of care to the family. The family needs the nurse during this period of crisis and adjustment. The community health nurse can be the link in the following chain of events: community health nurse↔family↔client↔long-term care facility↔community health nurse↔family↔client↔long-term care facility.

Long-term care facilities cannot be discussed without consideration of the image of such facilities. Many years ago these facilities were referred to as the "nursing home"; yet neither the staffing pattern nor activities denote very much "nursing" or "home." Perhaps the first effort at changing the image of these facilities is to change the name. A second factor would be to look at staffing and mechanisms for recruiting and retaining capable professional nurses for these facilities. Third, the public needs education about the different types of facilities and how to select the most appropriate facility according to the needs and preference of the individual. The public must also experience a change in values about long-term care facilities so that adequate resources are allocated to correct some of the ills of the long-term care industry. The combined forces of the population growth pattern, prevalence of chronic illnesses, and social forces such as working women, divorce rate, and declining birth rate all project a need for vitalization of the long-term care industry as well as creation of alternative resources.

Hospice

Hospice, as discussed in Chapter 2, is a community resource available for the care of the terminally ill. A hospice program has a family orientation and is concerned with the special needs and care of the terminally ill person. Quality of life and decision making, family and individual, are focal points in the delivery of medical, nursing, spiritual, and social care by an interdisciplinary team. Hospice programs may be hospital based or exist as separate entities. Many elderly persons experiencing the later stages of a terminal illness may view this community resource as an answer to the wish to live and die with comfort and dignity in addition to having the family at one's side. Additional information about hospice care is available in Chapter 2.

LEGISLATION AND COMMUNITY RESOURCES AND PROGRAMS

The legislative and political aspects of aging are pervasive of every other aspect of aging, since most health, social, and economic issues are connected to legislation and programs such as Social Security, Older American's Act, and Medicare. These programs have revamped some of the issues of later life and promise to continue to do so as the nation grapples with balancing the budget, federalism, reductions in social programs, inflation, unemployment, and an increasingly older constituency.

During the fourth decade of the nineteenth century when the Social Security Act was passed, population size, employment patterns and health problems differed. The Social Security Act became law in August, 1935, during the administration of Franklin D. Roosevelt. The Social Security Act has been amended in several significant ways. Two key amendments, Medicare in 1966 and Supplemental Security Income (SSI) in 1974, have special importance for the elderly. Eligibility for Social Security, a general public retirement pension, is based on previous work history and age. Additionally, there are survivors, disability, and health benefits. Social Security benefits constitute the only source of income for 80% of retirees (Atchley, 1977).

In 1966 Medicare was instituted as a health insurance program for older Americans with hospital and medical insurance provisions. Covered services include hospital, skilled nursing, home care, physician's services, and home health care. The services not covered by Medicare are of such magnitude that they are frequently referred to as "Medigap." Many private insurance companies have programs specifically designed to cover this gap.

The Supplemental Security Income (SSI) includes a federal supplement to the income of adults with inadequate income. Medicaid as a health care program for the poor, exclusive of age eligibility, is administered by individual states. These programs, in addition to Social

Security benefits, have meant an improved life-style, including health care, food, shelter, and clothing.

The Older American's Act of 1965 and its amendments provide for the establishment of the United States Administration on Aging, for program funding, and for training and research. The responsibility for co-ordinating and planning services for the elderly such as multipurpose senior centers, nutrition centers, employment, and transportation services at a local level is vested in the Area Agency on Aging (AAA). Multipurpose senior centers created by Title V of the Older American's Act provide the locus for a broad spectrum of services for older persons: health, social, legal, educational, and recreational. Title VII of the Older American's Act provides for nutrition programs for the elderly. Nutrition services are offered in a congregate setting or are delivered to people at home via Meals on Wheels. In addition to partially meeting individual nutritional requirements, socialization and education needs are met. The Older American's Act Amendments of 1981 provide for a state ombudsman program for long-term care facilities and boarding homes.

AGING NETWORK

The aging network reflects organizations concerned with advocacy, special populations, and volunteer services by older people. As of 1969 two components of the National Older American Volunteer Program are Retired Senior Volunteer Program and Foster Grandparents Program. Volunteer activities in hospitals, schools, nursing homes, and other settings are provided by members of the Retired Senior Volunteer Program (RSVP). Persons 60 and over may volunteer services. These volunteers are provided transportation and meals in connection with their volunteer activities. The Foster Grandparents Program offers an opportunity for older people and children to mutually share, meet needs, and experience gratification across generations. The Gray Panthers, organized by Margaret (Maggie) Kuhn, began as an advocacy group for change and social justice. Now the combined assets and forces of young and old are interested in investigative research, legislative action, monitoring of services to the aged, and organization of training for the Gray panthers network (Kuhn, 1976). The National Council of Senior Citizens (NCSC) was founded in 1961 out of the need to defeat the American Medical Association's campaign against Medicare, thereby becoming one of the first senior powers (Kleyman, 1974).

Cognizance of and sensitivity to the needs of black Americans and concern about national goals and activities to address these needs stimulated Hobart Jackson

in the organization of the National Caucus on the Black Aged (NCBA). The NCBA continues to this day as an advocacy group for the improvement of the quality of life for older persons of minority groups (Jackson, 1976). Other organizations concerned about issues of the aged include the American Association of Retired Persons and the National Retired Teachers Association.

Four White House conferences on aging have been held, one each decade beginning in 1950, to hear concerns and issues of importance to older Americans and to propose plans for national policies on aging for the next decade. The 1981 conference was centered on the theme *The Aging Society: Challenge and Opportunity.* The conference focused on more than 600 recommendations; however, the following recommendations were highlighted: strengthen the Social Security system, prohibit mandatory retirement, increase the availability of home and community-based health care, and emphasize preventive health care. A national policy on aging emerging from this fourth conference has the following goals (Final Report, 1981, p. 10):

1. To provide the elderly with the maximum opportunity to live an independent and healthy life and to encourage them to remain in the economic and social mainstream.
2. To provide economic, medical and social support to the elderly who need help.
3. To encourage serious discussion of the choices we must make as a result of the very large baby boom generation that will become elderly in the 21st century.

The gains have been many, but much work lies ahead. As the constituency of aged persons grows, so do their needs, political power, and demand for participation in the political arena.

SUMMARY

The study of older adults reflects a growing population with many assets and liabilities. The more than 25 million community-based, high school–educated older Americans are influencing the cultural orientation of this country. This influence is seen in efforts to prevent polarization between generations but yet to educate and change attitudes toward the elderly to a perception of the elderly as diverse people who are a national resource and asset. The minority groups—Blacks, Hispanics, Native Americans, and Pacific Asians—are obtaining special attention to their unique needs and assets. The myths of older adults as institutionalized, poor, unable to learn, accident prone, passive, and sexless are being replaced with new knowledge, perceptions, and attitudes. The valuing of "oldness" will possibly increase as this nation continues to grow old, with members of the great baby boom becoming 65 during the twenty-first century. The theories of aging will again be put to the test as explanations are sought for the aging phenomenon. The disengagement, activity, continuity or developmental and biological theories will all try to contribute answers to such questions as the following: Why do people age? How does aging progress? What accelerates and decelerates the process? Is quantity better than quality of life? The developmental task of adjusting to declining health, death, retirement, and changing interpersonal relationships will be researched for its contribution to healthy aging. The major health problems of this population are heart disease, malignancies, and cerebrovascular diseases. Efforts to prevent the development of hypertension are aimed at reduction of risk factors such as smoking, obesity, lack of exercise, and the dietary practice of excessive salt intake. Stress management continues to be emphasized for its value in promoting health. Additionally, regular blood pressure screening, dieting management, and drug therapy continue to save lives and prevent complications of this major disabler of older adults. Vigilance for changes in the body, regular physical examination, and elimination of smoking behavior will further the decline in the incidence of cancer for older adults.

Health problems such as arthritis, sensory impairments, and organic brain syndrome limit activity and affect comfort and independence. Decreasing functional dependency is one goal in the improvement of the health of older adults so they may function at their optimal physical, social, and psychological level. The increased years gained through advanced technology will be meaningless unless chronic, disabling conditions are controlled or eliminated and happy healthy years become a major possession during later life. Older adults' coping capacity for loss, grief, and depression must be broader so that they do not continue to terminate their lives at their own hand, a practice accounting for approximately one fourth of the suicides in the United States. Prevention, treatment, and rehabilitation must be hallmarks of the care provided within the health care and social systems. Criminal victimization, abuse at the elderly's own hands via drug misuse and at the hands of relatives and institutional care givers, and social isolation are psychosocial issues affecting the health and quality of life of this cohort of aged persons. An interdisciplinary approach to solving these problems is necessary to forestall or prevent occurrences at epidemic levels. Health, social, and political organizations must join forces and form a counterattack on the deadly forces of abuse and victimization.

Health promotion foci of adequate nutrition; a balance of exercise, rest, and activity; immunizations against influenza and pneumonia; time management; and optimum self-esteem are central to healthy older adults. The years spent dreaming of retirement and "lots of time on hand" have now become a reality. Are those years going to be the panacea and mecca dreamed or will those years become one horrible nightmare from which relief is sought? The answers begin many years before the magical turning point of age 65.

Community health nurses as care givers must assist older adults to capitalize on their assets and guide them in coping with the process of living with chronic illnesses and disability. A life theme of moderation, variety, and balance will contribute to healthy older years. Just as infectious diseases of earlier years were eliminated, the chronic diseases of the present must be conquered to ensure quality of life. The art of decision making, the privilege of choice, and the responsibility of self-discipline are the keys to solving problems of living and aging.

BIBLIOGRAPHY

Atchley, R.C.: The social forces in later life, Belmont, Calif., 1977, Wadsworth, Inc.

Burnside, I.M.: Transition to later life: developmental theories and research. In Burnside, I.M., Ebersole, P., and Monea, H.E., editors: Psychosocial caring through the life span, New York, 1979, McGraw-Hill Book Co.

Cummings, E., and Henry, W.E.: Growing old: the process of disengagement, New York, 1961, Basic Books, Inc., Publishers.

Duvall, E.M.: Family development, ed. 4, Philadelphia, 1971, J.B. Lippincott Co.

Ebersole, P., and Hess, P.: Toward healthy aging: human needs and nursing response, St. Louis, 1981, The C.V. Mosby Co.

Elder abuse, Washington, D.C., 1980, Office of Human Development Services, Department of Health and Human Services.

Erikson, E.H.: Childhood and Society, New York, 1963, W.W. Norton and Co., Inc.

Fact book on aging: a profile of America's older population, Washington, D.C., 1978, National Council on Aging.

Facts about older Americans, 1980-81, Washington, D.C., 1981, Office of Human Development Services.

Final Report: the 1981 White House Conference on Aging, Washington, D.C., 1981, Department of Health and Human Services.

Halpern, H.M.: Cutting loose, New York, 1976, Simon & Schuster, Inc.

Havighurst, R.J.: Human development and education, New York, 1953, David McKay Co., Inc.

Havighurst, R.J.: Successful aging, In Williams, R. H., Tibbilts, C., and Donahue, W., editors: Process of aging, vol. 1, New York, 1963, Atherton Press.

Health United States, 1976-77, Washington, D.C., 1976-1977, Public Health Service, Health Resources Administration, National Center for Health Statistics, Department of Health, Education, and Welfare.

Healthy people: background papers, Washington, D.C., 1979, Public Health Service, Office of the Assistant Secretary for Health and Surgeon General, Department of Health, Education, and Welfare.

Hill, R.: A demographic profile on the black elderly, Aging 287:2-9, 1978.

Jackson, H.C.: Black advocacy: techniques and trials. In Kerschner, P.A., editor: Advocacy and age, Los Angeles, 1976, The University of Southern California Press.

Jackson, H.C.: Information about the National Caucus on the Black Aged. In Seltzer, M., Corbett, S.L., and Atchley, R.C., editors: Social problems of the aging: readings, Belmont, Calif., 1978, Wadsworth, Inc.

Kleyman, P.: Senior power, San Francisco, 1974, Glide Publications.

Kuhn, M.E.: What old people want for themselves and others in society. In Kerschner, P.A., editor: Advocacy and age, Los Angeles, 1976, The University of Southern California Press.

Luckmann, J., and Sorenson, K.: Medical-surgical Nursing: a psycho-physiologic approach, ed. 2, Philadelphia, 1980, W.B. Saunders Co.

The myth and reality of aging in America, Washington, D.C., 1981, National Council on Aging.

Need for long-term care: information and issues, Washington, D.C., 1981, Office of Human Development Services.

Neugarten, B.L.: Personality in middle and late life, New York, 1964, Atherton Press.

Schwartz, A.N.: Counseling the older adult. In O'Brien, B., editor: Aging: today's research and you, Los Angeles, 1978, The University of Southern California Press.

Working with older people, vol. II: the biological, psychological, and sociological aspects of aging, Washington, D.C., 1970, Public Health Service.

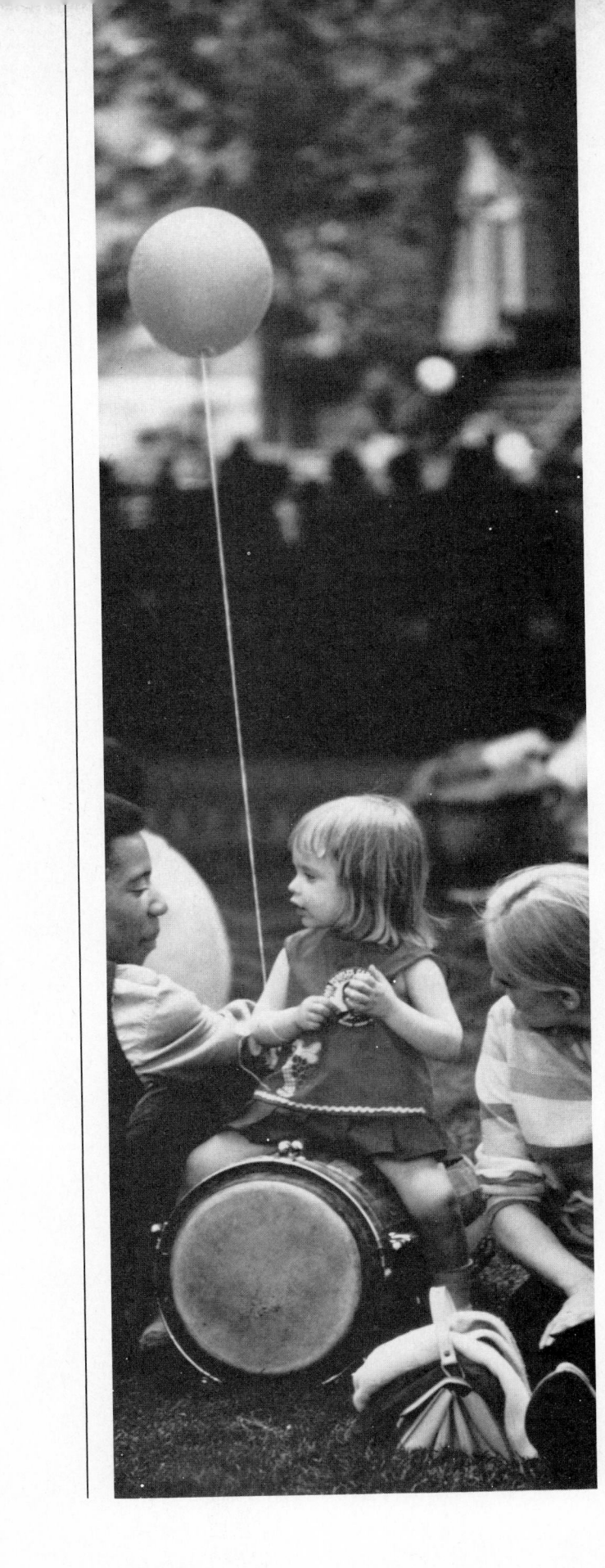

Part Five

Diversity in the Community Health Nursing Role

In the early beginnings of the health care delivery system in the United States, the community health nurse was primarily responsible for visiting the sick in the home and participating in communicable disease case finding. As the health care delivery system has evolved into a multidimensional industry, nursing education has expanded to embrace levels of preparation in university settings from the awarding of associate through doctoral degrees. Likewise, nursing practice has expanded and diversified to include multiple practice settings, functional roles such as educator, administrator, or consultant, and an assortment of clinical specialties.

As a result of these changes the community health nurse's roles, functions, client population, and practice settings have diversified and expanded. Community health nurses are found in the functional roles of administrator and consultant, as discussed in Chapters 28 and 29, as well as in the educator role. The community health nurse is also found working with identified subpopulations, as described in Chapters 30, 31, and 34.

Continued.

Part Five

In answer to the changing health care system, manpower shortages, evolving community health needs, and medically underserved rural and urban centers, a new health professional has emerged. Nursing's contribution to this category of health provider is the nurse practitioner; with a new knowledge base and set of skills, coupled with previously learned nursing principles and concepts, the nurse practitioner is able to meet primary care needs of select populations. Chapter 33 presents a discussion of the development of the family nurse practitioner role and the current status in the health care delivery system.

Regardless of the setting, the client, or the role, the community health nurse uses the techniques of collaboration and coordination (discussed in Chapter 32) to act as advocate for the client entering and progressing through the health care delivery system.

Chapter 28

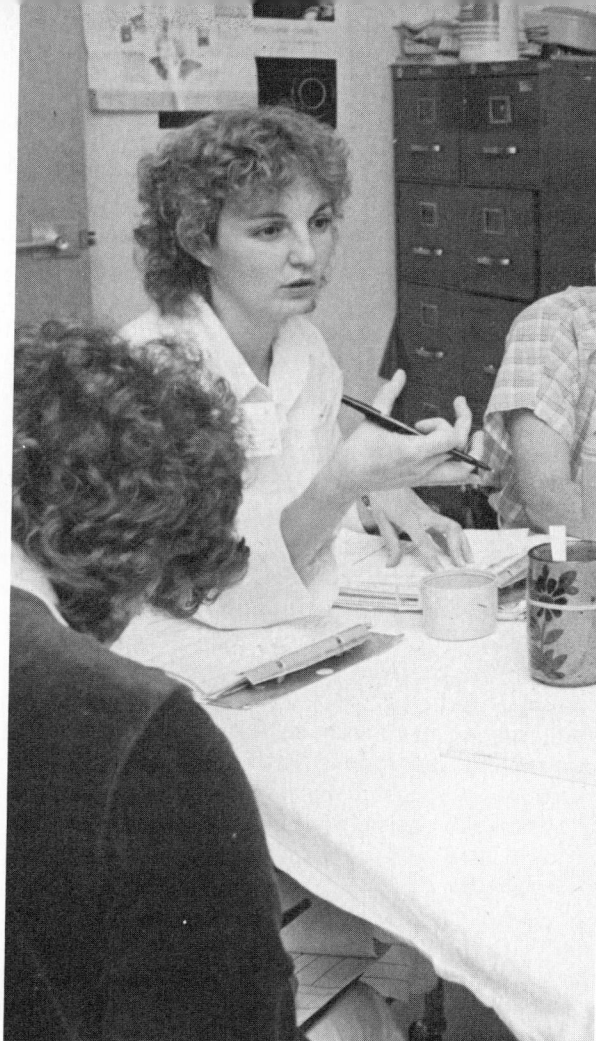

DORIS WAGNER
BOBBI LEE

THE COMMUNITY HEALTH NURSE
AS AN ADMINISTRATOR

Community health nursing services are delivered, predominantly, through community health service organizations, in which the nurse is an employee as well as a provider of services to persons. Within community health agencies the work of the nurse is directed and coordinated by the administrators of the organization, including the community health nurse administrator. The role of *administrator* can be defined as one who manages or administers a specific service or program, which may be a nursing unit of a health department or another community-based program that includes community health nursing services. The nurse administrator is responsible for directing and coordinating the work of others.

Although individual administrative nursing roles

may differ or contain different components depending on the size and purpose of the organization, all share a common conceptual framework and use common administrative processes to achieve their goal. The interface between the community health nurse and the disciplines of administration and public health results in a complex set of roles, responsibilities, and functions.

HISTORICAL PERSPECTIVE

From an historical perspective, community health nursing began with the delivery of nursing care to the ill in their homes. With the development of hospital-based nursing schools and the institution-based delivery of nursing care, community health nursing became

669

less common. Kalisch and Kalisch (1978) note that in 1891 there were only 130 community health nurses in the United States. Furthermore, these authors report that until 1907 no state recognized the community health nurse as a legitimate employee of an official health or education agency.

Since that time, growth in community health nursing has been explosive. By 1924, when the National Organization for Public Health Nursing conducted a census of community health nurses, there were 11,191 nurses employed by 3629 organizations (Kalisch and Kalisch, 1978).

By 1934 Tucker and Hilbert noted that more community health nurses were being employed by departments of health than by visiting nurse associations, although a greater number of visiting nurse associations as entities existed. It is noteworthy that of the 57 agencies surveyed in this study, only 37 employed a nurse administrator. In 15 of these 37 agencies the nurse administrator's responsibilities included hiring of the staff nurses. About half of the nurse administrators employed clerical persons as well as nurses, and 20 of the 37 nurse administrators were invited to attend agency board meetings.

Tucker and Hilbert (1934) also noted that 11 of the 57 agencies surveyed had no stated requirements for the staff nurse employee in community health. Those agencies which had requirements most often specified graduation from a school of nursing as the criterion. Some required registration in nursing while only 4 required job applicants to complete a course in community health nursing in addition to their basic training. A 2-month orientation period was considered adequate for new community health nurse employees.

The first employment criterion for community health nurse administrators appeared in the 1930s and included the following: (1) a high school diploma, (2) graduation from a fundamental nursing education program, (3) state registration, (4) a course in community health nursing, and (5) experience in community health (Tucker and Hilbert, 1934).

In a discussion of the responsibilities and relationships of community health nurse administrators, Gardner (1938) identified relationships with the following: (1) the board or agency executive (health officer), (2) the nursing staff, (3) the clients, (4) the community, and (5) the field of public health nursing. Gardner also identified five key attributes of the nurse administrator: (1) justice, (2) power to see work as a whole in which the different parts are proportionally valued, (3) orderliness, (4) power to delegate responsibility, and (5) genuine interest in people as individuals.

CONTEMPORARY PERSPECTIVE

The role of the community health nurse administrator has changed dramatically in the past 50 years. The community health nurse administrator is now clearly an administrator from a contemporary perspective. As a result of Medicare and Medicaid legislation, there has been revitalization of home health agencies, with a proliferation of certified agencies in each state. This includes primarily the increase of proprietary home health agencies. The number of official health agencies and boards of education has remained more stable, as these public agencies are defined by political and geographical boundaries versus the market.

The recommended qualifications for employment as a community health nursing administrator, the legal framework surrounding an agency's functions, and nursing care standards have also changed over time.

KNOWLEDGE BASE AND STANDARDS OF PRACTICE

Today the Commission on Nursing Services from the American Nurses' Association (ANA) and National League for Nursing (NLN) recommend the qualifications for nurse administrators at the executive level to include the following: (1) a baccalaureate in nursing and either a master's or a doctoral degree in nursing administration or in community health nursing; (2) nursing licensure in the appropriate state; and (3) progressive responsible professional nursing experience, preferably to include prior competent administration of nursing service at the middle level, or as stated in Criterion 5, Standard 5.1 of the *Criteria and Standards Manual* for NLN/APHA accreditation, to have a minimum of 5 years responsible administration experience. The background of persons who serve as nurse administrators must include clinical and administrative practice that leads to the consistent fulfillment of each responsibility inherent in the respective administrative role (ANA, 1973). Master's level education is recommended because it contains the knowledge required to function within the position. This knowledge base includes the following:

1. Knowledge of principles, practices, and methods of community health nursing and nursing administration
2. Knowledge of the health and safety codes and rules and regulations of the city, county, and state
3. Information regarding detection, evaluation, and planning to meet community public health nursing needs

4. Increased skill in establishing and maintaining effective professional relationships with community leaders, physicians, professional staffs, and others

5. Knowledge of the changing social, political, and economic influences affecting health care delivery systems

6. Knowledge of educational trends as they relate to the health care field

7. Knowledge of research methodology

8. Ability to communicate effectively both orally and in writing

9. Further development of tact, good professional judgment, emotional stability, initiative, resourcefulness, and integrity

10. Knowledge about effective use of volunteers

11. Knowledge regarding working with boards (either elected or appointed)

12. Ability to conceptualize nursing and to put nursing practice into operation

Acquisition of this knowledge and experience in applying it underlie the creation of an organizational environment that facilitates and rewards high-quality community health nursing practice.

The ANA has established standards for measuring quality for both community health nursing practice (appendix G) and for nursing administration. These two sets of national standards are established by the nursing profession. The nurse administrator also deals with two additional sets of standards: one is mandatory and one is voluntary.

The mandatory set of standards includes the laws and regulations promulgated by states which permit the organization to operate. Compliance with these laws results in a certification or a license for the organization, which is analogous to the Registered Nurse licensure of an individual. It means that minimum standards have been met.

The voluntary set of standards constitutes the criteria for agency accreditation. Evaluation of an agency for accreditation is conducted jointly by the NLN and the American Public Health Association (APHA). Accreditation implies excellence. Organizational accreditation is analogous to individual certification for excellence in nursing practice. In the past the NLN/APHA accreditation process was available to both official and voluntary community health nursing organizations. In May 1982 the National Association for Home Care was formed as the direct result of a merger of the Council of Home Health Agencies and the Community Health Services of the NLN and the National Association of Home Care. Changes in accreditation policies are currently under consideration by these national groups. To ensure quality community health nursing services, it is important to have established standards and then a process whereby an agency is measured by these standards. It is essential that nurse administrators coordinate adoption and implementation of standards of practice.

THE COMMUNITY HEALTH NURSE AS AN ADMINISTRATOR

The *key* responsibility of the community health nurse administrator is to ensure an environment in which the community health nursing personnel can function and provide quality nursing services that meet the goals and objectives of specific health care organizations. Nursing administrators are accountable to consumers, to the nursing profession, and to the agencies of which they are employees. The nurse administrator has a direct influence on how nursing is practiced within the health care organization and therefore has a direct influence on professional nursing's impact on the health care system.

The overall purpose of administration in any organization is to provide the structure or framework within which the personnel can organize goals and objectives as efficiently and effectively as possible (Tinkham and Voorhies, 1972). The nurse administrator's role is defined within the job description of the organization, by law, by precedents, and by professional standards; thus the nurse administrator has the responsibilities to design a system that augments community health nursing services that are of a high quality, are cost effective, and meet the needs of the individuals and families within the community.

The position of the nurse administrator within the organization should be such that it allows direct input as well as responsibility for setting the tone and creating the climate in which the nursing staff can practice nursing. The nurse administrator is responsible for the development of the umbrella or framework that allows nurses to provide effective and efficient nursing services in the home, school, or clinic setting (Fig. 28-1). The umbrella provides an analogy. When fully open and in an upright position, an umbrella protects as well as allows for a safe and functional area for movement. Development and maintenance of an appropriate organizational structure and administrative process is similar to the open, upright umbrella, permitting and promoting staff nurses' use of their education and expertise to the fullest extent within the confines of legal and professional standards in accordance with the mission of the organization. If the nursing administration position is placed other than at the top

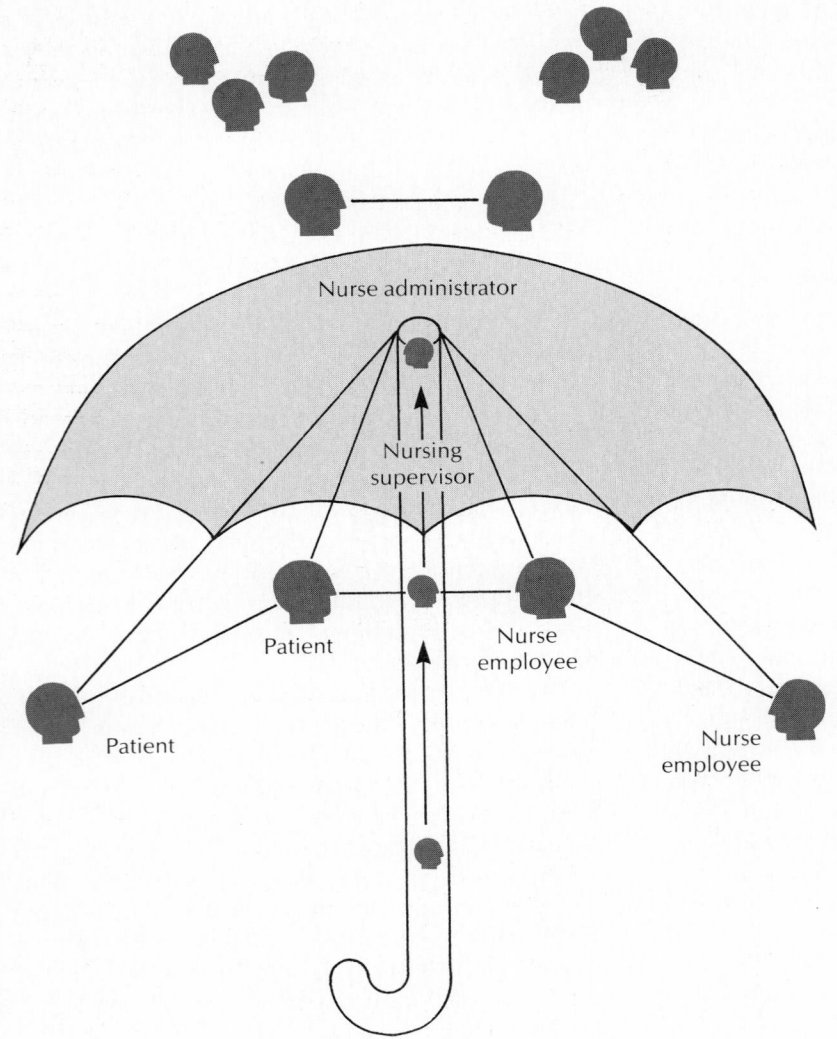

Fig. 28-1. Umbrella framework of nurse administrator.

of the organization, resulting in no umbrella for supervisors, the area for safe and effective nursing practice is reduced. If in the overall organization the nurse administrator is placed at the bottom of the administrative structure, the result is conflict, confusion, and disorganization. Staff members then tend to develop independent practices without standards. Their practice may or may not be consistent with the organization's mission. This produces fragmented and uncoordinated services.

In general terms, nurse administrators set the organizational climate and coordinate the multiple organizational factors with the external environment in a way

that allows effective and efficient delivery of nursing services to clients. The problem-solving process in nursing administration is considerably more intangible, more complex, more diffuse, and more political in nature. Nurse administrators must bring together all of the essential components necessary to create this ideal type of environment for practice. These components range from setting goals to offering input about the physical plant in which the service is to be provided and provision made for the necessary supplies and equipment. Highly developed analytical and conceptual skills are required both in administration and in nursing.

THE ADMINISTRATOR: A NURSE

One important administrative approach to coordinating community health nursing practice in an organization is adoption and use of a nursing theory. It serves to unify nursing practice within the organization. An example would be using Orem's theory. According to Orem (1980, p. 13), one characteristic of professional nursing is "the ability of nurses to creatively design adequate means for identifying and describing nursing requirements and to design, put into operation, and manage systems of nursing assistance for individuals, families, and groups." Additionally Orem notes that where nursing is provided through a health care institution, such as a community health agency, there is a contract or agreement between the client and the organization. In this arrangement the client comes in contact with nurses who are not only employees of the organization, but also practitioners of nursing (Orem, 1980).

Depending on the client's self-care needs, limitations, and potential, the relationship between the client and the organization usually involves the nurse, the nursing department, the medical care system (either directly or indirectly), and other health personnel. The nurse as an employee often uses and coordinates the plan of care for clients with these health personnel. In a health service organization, however, the mechanisms for establishing the availability of other health personnel and for selecting the types of clients who will be seen are set by the organization. For example, in a traditional public health department the nurse is likely to encounter clients whose health care deficits include inadequate immunizations, inadequate information about pregnancy, and/or inadequate information about child health. In a voluntary nursing association the nurse is more likely to encounter clients whose health care deficits are more related to medical problems and/or are long-term, such as needing instruction to prevent intensifying the client's congestive heart failure, including managing a special nutritional plan on a limited income. The organization has focused, through its mission and economic structure, on a selected client population and has directed its practice to specific sets of client and/or family self-care deficits.

The nurse administrator, through personal analysis of information about the community, which is based on data about self-care deficits at the individual and family levels, is in a position to help determine the nature and scope of nursing care within the organization. It is the responsibility of the nurse who works with the individual clients and their families to provide the nurse administrator with accurate information about nursing services provided, results of care, and observed deficits or unmet self-care needs in the community.

The community health nurse administrator must be concerned with external relationships with related agencies and must have a grasp of the health needs within the total community and know how these health needs are to be met. However, it is also the nurse administrator's role to provide the staff nurse with organizational assistance and mechanisms to facilitate the delivery of care, as previously noted.

In many ways the relationship between the nurse administrator and the staff nurse is based on the same interest but using different types of expertise. The staff nurse's expertise is developed with respect to the client and family in the community. Staff nurses implement organizational programs with clients. The nurse administrator's expertise is at the aggregate level, both internally within the organization and externally with the community. Nurse administrators focus on the needs of the community and its component parts, development of community objectives, implementation of programs to meet those needs, and evaluation.

MANAGEMENT FUNCTIONS OF THE NURSE ADMINISTRATOR

The community health nurse administrator is required to have a sound knowledge of both nursing and management. Nursing and management must fuse to allow nursing to be understood and practiced. The distinguishing characteristic of the role of the community health nurse administrator is that it emerges from a fusion of professional nurse and professional manager. Nursing goals need to be translated into management terms by integrating expertise from both disciplines. Nursing service administrators must be professional nurses who represent and interpret nursing at the organizational level for all nursing staff (AHA, 1977).

It can become overwhelming to list the many areas for which the nurse administrator is responsible, but most simply and traditionally the responsibilities fall into the following three areas: budget, personnel, and programs. Another way one can identify these areas is financial resources, human resources, and program goals and expectations. Fig. 28-2 shows how the three overlap and indeed become the responsibility of the executive person.

The nurse administrator is responsible for the development of programs. An effective method of making sure that the program will work is to go through the planning process and determine the need for the program, the cost of the program, and the personnel available to administer the program. Chapter 9 in this text discusses program planning and evaluation in greater

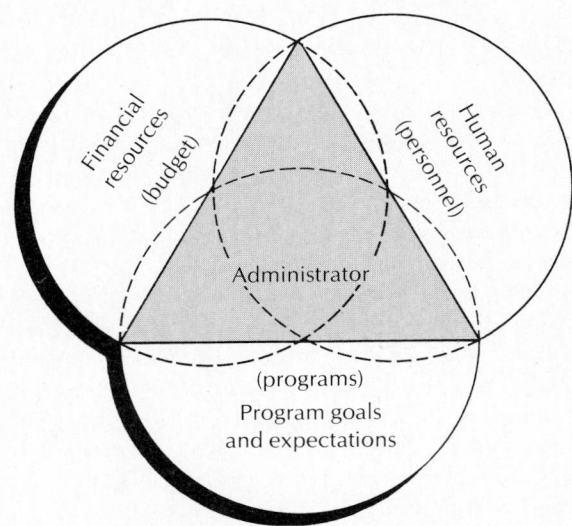

Fig. 28-2. Overlapping functions of the administrator.

detail. Any program planning must be done in concert with other units of the organization and not in isolation, especially when other disciplines are involved.

Financial Resources

Without funds one is unable to implement any type of program. In community health the funding comes from a variety of resources. In public health agencies the funds basically are from public tax funds, a limited amount coming from direct fees, and federal or state grants (for example, federal funds for the Maternal and Infant Care Project). Additionally, Miller and Moos (1981) note that all of the 15 health departments they studied received third party reimbursement from Medicare, Medicaid, and/or insurance. Several of these health departments have a combined nursing service, employing nurses for public health nursing services and nurses to provide home care nursing services.

The primary organization employing community health nurses is the official public health department in which the community health nurse renders direct personal services to individuals and families within the community. The service may be provided in the home, a clinic, or the school. Community health nurses may also be employed by local boards of education, industry, the American Red Cross, or various voluntary and proprietary health agencies, including a home care agency. The fiscal support of voluntary agencies varies.

It is important to the understanding and evaluation of voluntary agencies to know the manner in which they are financed. Agencies concerned with specific diseases like the American Cancer Society are supported by citizen donations and private contributions, whereas professional organizations like the NLN are financed by membership dues. The primary purpose of professional organizations is to improve health standards and the qualifications of health providers. Large bequests of philanthropic foundations are decreasing. The most important support comes from small contributions or donations from large numbers of individuals (Hanlon and Pickett, 1984). The United Fund/Community Chest epitomizes a joint fund-raising effort to assist many local health and social agencies. It is common that visiting nurse/home care agencies may be financed not only by fees, insurance, and reimbursement from Medicare and Medicaid but also by United Fund monies.

A budget is required by law, and regardless of the organizational structure one needs to know what monies are available and required for the nursing services. A budget is a statement of organizational goals expressed in financial terms. Budgets may be classified as program budgets or performance budgets.

In a program budget the costs are related to a specific service, the scope and nature of activities undertaken, and identifiable and measurable units of work. This type of budget has the advantage of being able to more directly relate fiscal planning and responsibility to the operating staff and forms a good base for evaluation of a specific program. Its major disadvantage is that it may foster duplication, fragmentation of services, and confusion for the consumer as well as staff. The federal grant programs are an excellent example of this.

The performance budget shows clearly and concisely the programs of work done and services to be rendered in return for the funds appropriated. The advantage of performance budgeting is that it provides more exact information on the cost-service relationship. The disadvantage may arise from the complexity of developing this type of budget and the danger of placing value on seeking measurable service units rather than an expression of valid expected outcomes.

Regardless of type of budgeting method used (and there are many more types of budgets), the manner in which the financial resources are obtained will frequently dictate the method used for budgetary purposes.

Human Resources

The heart of any organization is the human resources that have been attracted to the organization—the human knowledge and skills available that lead to the ability to implement the plans for the programs that have been designed or are expected to be accomplished. To be identified are the type, classification, availability, and mix of the personnel needed. The staff usually includes professional and nonprofessional personnel commensurate with the needs of the programs. A key to any program is the importance of knowing how to use personnel. Therefore if one has a flu clinic, it would be poor use of professional personnel to have the community health nurse set up the clinic and be responsible for intake and then for cleaning and reordering of room if technicians, volunteers, and other nonprofessional staff members are available. Another example would be the use of a community health nurse to do mass vision screening when volunteers, school health aides, or other technical personnel can be taught the procedure under the nurse's direction.

The community health nurse administrator usually is responsible for a large number of professional staff; if the nursing staff function within a local health agency, the administrator is usually responsible for the largest number of agency employees. According to the 1981 Division of Associated Health Professions, Bureau of Health Professions, Health Resource Administration, approximately 250,000 individuals in public health are in the primary work force. About 65% of this group are community health nurses working in clinics, state or local health departments, neighborhood health centers, or school systems. These community health nurses are all registered nurses. Since community health nurses are usually the largest pool of employees in a local health department, it is frequently perceived by other units within the organization that there is always manpower available for other services. The nurse administrator needs to work closely with other administrators in the deployment of personnel.

The nurse administrator needs to be assured that written job descriptions exist for personnel and all employees understand their scope of responsibility. For the most effective use of personnel, new employees need a planned orientation and in-service education must be planned for staff development. Job descriptions, classifications, and compensation are frequently handled through personnel departments, especially in larger agencies.

Program Goals and Expectations

Within each organization, programs are planned and provided in accordance with the agency's purpose, in relation to community health needs, and with respect to the total community health program. Within government agencies the nursing program component includes the programs dealing with control of infectious disease, health education, illness prevention, and disease control. Each program is identified, and objectives are written and stated in measurable client outcomes. There is need for a statement of priorities among the programs. These priorities are used to determine priority of services when the demand for services exceeds the resources available. In community health the governmental organization is frequently identified as the resource required to ensure that individuals and families are served during disaster and/or crisis. This responsibility may be shared with the local Red Cross program.

Practice policies and procedures for each program incorporate professional standards and statutory and regulatory requirements for each discipline working within the program. Program policies are prepared and closely monitored to assure that the services meet the goals and objectives of the organization. With programs there is a need to develop a service record. These records include certain basic components, namely, diagnosis, problem lists, progress notes, and level of services provided.

The nurse administrator must have a keen sense of the timeliness of administering any part of the program. The time to move, to inform, to develop, to implement, to change is *essential* to a successful operation. Frequently forces make it unwise to implement a program until other aspects of the program are in place. For example, if a nurse administrator identified a need to cut a family planning program from the list of nursing services offered through the health department and to upgrade the prenatal program, it would be critical to inform the community health nurses and the clients of the pending change before making the change. If the change is made without proper notification, employee morale and motivation could be negatively affected and embarrassing publicity may result.

COMMON PROBLEMS IN COMMUNITY HEALTH NURSING ADMINISTRATION

Blending human resources, financial resources, and programs into a cohesive unit requires effort. In many organizations, staff members perceive that the nurse administrator has the simple role of purely directing. Staff members need to understand the problems inherent to budgeting, planning, and timing. There are other major distractors for the nurse administrator, including the following:

1. Personnel problems, including problems of poor performance
2. Grievances
3. Lack of financial resources
4. Lack of administrative support
5. Staff members who are inflexible and resist any type of change
6. Assignment to projects other than those committed to perform
7. Lack of political support

8. Staff members who do not accept or support the program goals
9. Conflict within the nursing unit itself
10. Inability to proceed (for many reasons) because the timing is wrong
11. Inability to hire qualified personnel
12. Changes in program priorities

Other issues facing the nurse administrator can include anything from car rental, uniform allowance, security of the staff within the community, need for supplies and equipment, or ramifications of the nurse practice act within the state to the monitoring of duplication of services provided by another organization. The problems are numerous, but when put in the proper perspective need not be obstructive. The nurse administrator not only plans and executes the programs within the nursing unit to achieve the goals of the specific unit, but also fits those programs into the whole of the health department or health agency to meet the overall goals and objectives. Thus the administrator needs a working knowledge of the total operation of the health care organization and has the responsibility for identifying nursing's role within the organization. It is important to keep the nursing personnel informed about the organization's activities and plans.

MANAGEMENT PROCESS

To have an effective service the community health nurse administrator needs a thorough understanding of the management process. Management is a problem-solving process that includes the functions of planning, organizing, leading, and evaluating (DiVincente, 1972).

Planning

Historically planning has not been emphasized as much as it is today. Planning is viewed as that ingredient of administration that will make any decision more likely to have a positive outcome. Three factors are prerequisites for planning: (1) identification of a need, or what we would like things to be; (2) knowledge of the factors, or how things are now; and (3) development of a proposal for getting from here to there (Last, 1980). The nurse administrator should lead the nursing unit through the planning process.

As simple as this may seem, the many factors involved in planning may create departures from the norm. When an organization exists in a highly differentiated and turbulent environment marked by complex interdependencies between departments, agencies, and political units, planning is more difficult. When other factors, such as education, regulation, services available as mentioned, research applied and/or reviewed, or community needs of the various age

groups, are all taken into consideration, the planning process becomes highly complex. Rigid planning according to specific planning objectives can lead to total disaster. What is needed is flexibility that allows the plan to continually shift within the broader, ever-changing organizational system. Planning can be as complex and as difficult as putting together the Rubik's Cube. If one knows all the various factors influencing the plan, the solution or the outcome of the plan can be effective and complete. However, complete information is rarely available.

Planning can be approached from various perspectives. Planning can be classified as strategic and tactical (Levey and Loomba, 1973). Strategic planning is the process by which basic organizational goals and directions are determined. Strategic planning is long range and encompasses ends as well as means. In contrast, tactical plans look at shorter time frames, have a narrower scope, focus on more detail, and are more flexible (Arndt and Huckabay, 1975).

An example of the importance of planning can be shown in the following case.

A group of citizens, prompted by a nursing student's suggestion, requested the local health department to set up a weekly blood pressure screening clinic within their high-rise apartment. Assuming the students had validated all their findings, a district nursing supervisor assigned a staff nurse to set up such a clinic each Thursday and to notify the population of 65 or over regarding the service. The clinic was set up. Notices were sent out. After 3 weeks the total who attended number four. There had been numerous phone calls from local physicians questioning this clinic. The drug store and a neighborhood center less than five blocks away notified the administrator that they did blood pressure screening.

A plan to set up a clinic had been done; organization for the clinic was delegated to the staff nurse, who was then responsible for directing the clinic. However, evaluation of the clinic 3 weeks later pointed out it was a "failure."

This is an excellent example demonstrating that while the tactical plans to implement the clinic worked, it was the wrong strategic plan. For a discussion on the process of needs assessment and strategic program planning, see Chapter 9.

Organizing

When one knows the plan, knows the amount of monies available, and knows the type of personnel needed and available, then it is the time to organize. This is the time to gather all necessary facts, to decide on tactics, to delineate implementation specifics, and to decide how to proceed. Organizing involves arranging and defining the relationships between both personnel and other resources by establishing a structure. An examination of the structural chart on any organization will quickly reveal that it is only the formal structure. There is also an informal structure, and the nurse administrator must be conscious of both. The communication flow occurs not only within a given program or department but also within other units of the organization and between individuals and agencies outside the organization. The plan needs to be put into an organized system that allows for effective use of personnel, who have been selected and prepared, and of the resources available.

Leading

With appropriate planning and a clearly delineated organization developed, the community nurse administrator provides leadership for the implementation of the plan.

Everyone whose work involves the direction and supervision of other people is in a leadership position; however, the concept of *leadership* is a broader concept than the concept of *manager*. Managers limit choices in personal behaviors by establishing and requiring rigid adherence to policies and procedure to meet organizational goals that were never intended to prescribe all behavior for a given situation. Leaders work in the opposite direction and strive to develop fresh approaches to long-standing problems and to open issues for new options which may or may not be congruent with organizational goals. However, the effective leader projects ideas into images that excite people and only then develops choices that give the projected images substance. Leaders create excitement.

The nurse manager will see that action is taken on all referrals and will make sure that there is a systematic approach developed to carry out each request. If managers are leaders and use leadership skills, they can create an environment that allows for creativity and risk taking to meet the mandates of the organization. Leaders and managers differ in their conceptions. Leaders tend to view work as an enabling process involving some combination of people and ideas interacting to establish strategies and make decisions. In the enabling process leaders help the process along, using a range of skills, including calculating the interests in opposing situations, staging and timing the surfacing of controversial issues, and reducing tensions. The manager, on the other hand, is more concerned with the accomplishment of organizational goals.

The following is an example of a method used by one administrator to be sure that there is a built-in method of releasing tension. One can use the simple illustrations of a teakettle—without a spout the lid would come off. This nurse administrator made sure there was a qualified person on the staff that could listen to staff members regarding some of their stresses. The

stress might be related to a problem in their personal life, or with a co-worker, a physician, or their supervisor. Whatever the source, stress hampers individual performance. The staff members are allowed up to six planned conferences with either the mental health nurse or a social worker regarding the problems. If the problem is not then resolved, the employee is referred outside of the organization. These conferences are not recorded or shared unless the employee makes a special request to do so. In this organization it was a mental health nurse and a social worker who were available. This type of a program would be considered to represent leadership.

Staff members need to become aware of the management style of the nurse administrator, which, when once understood, will allow that person to function much more effectively and constructively.

Evaluating

The community health nurse administrator assumes the responsibility to see that there is an ongoing evaluation of the plan as it is implemented. The agency is accountable to the community for the quality of its care, and accountability is ensured by an effective evaluation process. Evaluation includes a reexamination of the original plan and its rationale, as well as the organization and the degree to which goals were achieved. Evaluation may determine that there is need for reorganization. Including the staff in the evaluation process assists them to develop accountability for the program's success. As previously noted, standards for evaluation of the community nursing service have been developed by the NLN and the APHA. Meaningful criteria have been developed to verify the quality of the nursing unit's performance.

The planning, organizing, leading, and evaluating process used in community health nursing administration is essentially a problem-solving process. It is similar in many respects to the nursing process. The theoretical base, however, is different. The community health nurse administrator uses a combination of theories from nursing (using conceptualizations of nursing practice such as Orem's), organization and management theory, and public health science and practice.

Separate overviews of organization and management theory and public health will be presented. Several important factors will be illustrated and applied to community health nursing administrative practice. These applications of theory are intended to introduce the conceptualization for community health nursing administration practice as a synthesis of knowledge and theory from the fields of public health nursing, and administration.

ORGANIZATION AND MANAGEMENT THEORY

Organization theory has a relatively brief history. The literature may be described in three phases: 1) scientific or classical period, (2) human relations period, and (3) contemporary period.

The *scientific period* (approximately 1900-1935) is typically characterized by a concern for understanding the relationships between administrative functions (described by Fayol (1925) as planning, organizing, directing, and controlling) and production. F. W. Taylor, an engineer, made major contributions to organization theory (Filley and House, 1969). During this period workers were seen as motivated only by economic rewards, and the organization was characterized by (1) a clearly defined division of labor with highly specialized personnel and (2) a distinct hierarchy of authority (Etzioni, 1964). Administrative duties, according to classical or scientific thinking, include study of the work, deduction of the "best" or most efficient procedure, selection of the right person(s) for the job, and training personnel in the proper method.

The scientific period made several significant contributions to the conceptualization of organizations and administration, including the delineation of management functions and the development of concepts of authority, responsibility, accountability, and viewing the organization as an entity. Limitations, however, included an incomplete understanding of worker motivations, especially in noneconomic areas, and a concept of unilateral (administrator to employee) direction for administrative functions.

The second major phase in the development of organization theory, the *human relations period,* is generally considered to begin with the writing of Barnard (1938), who described the interrelationships between the individual, the organization, and the informal organization. Barnard's work, and its extension by Simon (1947), emphasized the human dimension of organizations. This shift in the theory was strengthened by the social movement toward formal organization of labor, the emergence of labor unions (for instance, the Wagner Act of 1935), and the Hawthorne studies. These experiments suggested that productivity was affected by attitudes of individuals and the social situation in the work groups as well as mechanical efficiency in the plant (Filley and House, 1969).

The studies in organization theory that were completed following the Hawthorne findings ultimately concluded that there are limits to the belief that the happy worker and work group are necessarily productive. In the *contemporary period* theoretical perspectives regarding administration reflect a blend between the research about types of organizations and research done in organizations. Behavioral science research has contributed to contemporary thinking about administration.

General Systems Theory

General systems theory is used extensively in contemporary organization theory. This approach, as mentioned in Chapter 7, views organizations as "a complex of elements in mutual interaction" (Arndt and Huckabay, 1975). Systems theory and thinking represent a macro rather than a micro perspective in that they specify gross relationships between the components within the whole organization. According to Stevens (1979) a systems model or framework contains at least eight categories of information, one of which (describing the input-transformation-output process) is applicable to community health nursing.

Community health nursing applications

In community health nursing the input component includes the personnel, financial, environmental, and other "raw materials" resources that are needed to produce community health nursing services. In the transformation phase the organizations, personnel, information, and knowledge become community health nursing services (Fig. 28-3). This transformation is difficult to describe. From the perspective of the community health nurse administrator, the transformation process has been illustrated as follows:

There was a request for nursing to handle the growing demand for scoliosis screening in all public schools, which involved a large student population and a declining number of school nurses. An ad hoc committee was appointed to study the request and make a recommendation to the nurse administrator within a few weeks. Staff members were randomly selected to serve on this committee. The group met, and a recommendation was made to management. The plan adopted was modified; however, it included some of the recommendations. One nurse was overheard to say, "It doesn't pay to meet to assure input, for our recommendations were not followed." This was not true, for without the nurses' input, the plan of action taken for an effective program could not have been made. To assist staff members to understand how valuable their input is, the following explanation was given: If I were to ask you for an egg to bake a cake and you gave me that egg, I would thank you and use it. However, after the cake was baked, and indeed it was a fine cake, you ask, "Where is my egg?" There would be no way to identify the egg. The end product or resolution to the problem required that ingredient from the nurses, yet the staff personnel were not able to see how their suggestion was transformed.

This story, additionally, illustrates the idea of interface between the system's subcomponents, the commu-

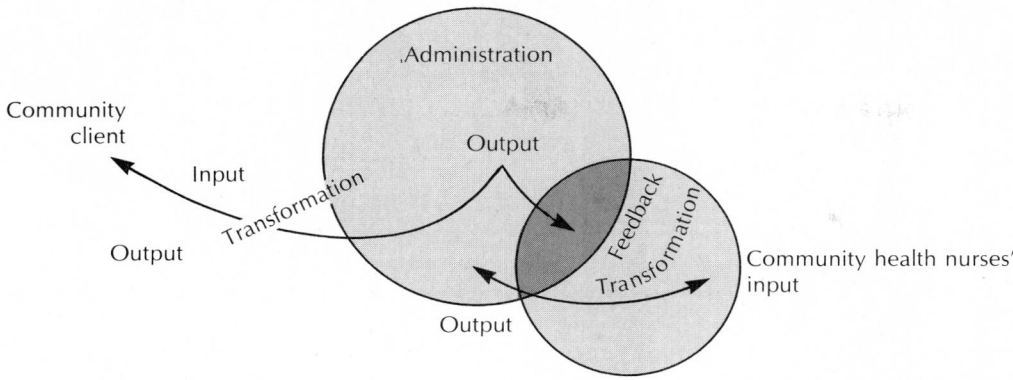

Fig. 28-3. Transformation phase.

nity health organization and the community. The community health organization considered the community's request (output) for scoliosis screening. The screening request provided input to the organization, which then requested additional information from nursing service. Nursing's information and expertise (inputs) were transformed and expressed in a recommendation. The recommendation, viewed by the nurses as a final output, was, however, an additional input to the organization. The program for the community was the organization's output.

Whether information or other resources are an output or an input depends on the level of organization under consideration (Lancaster, 1982). The nurse administrator must deal with contingencies that are different from those considered relevant by staff nurses.

The following situation illustrates the systems theory concept of input, transformation, and output with respect to the administrative process as compared to the nursing process. A community health nurse analyzes her caseload and travel schedule and notices that she is making home visits to six mothers with infants who are less than 1 year of age and who all live in the same apartment building. The nurse considers establishing a mother's group within the building for the following reasons:

1. In a group, mothers could learn from and get support from each other as well as from the nurse, who would participate in the group.
2. The nurse's productivity could be increased by seeing the six mothers together versus separately, which would create more visit time, decrease travel time, and increase time for other activities.
3. Advertising the group in the apartment building may result in involvement of other mothers who are not currently receiving community health nursing service.

The nurse discusses this idea with the supervisor, who agrees to support the idea and bring it to the nurse administrator. The administrator, knowing that there is no precedent for staff members working with community groups like this, concurs that the idea is good but requests additional considerations:

1. If the group meets at times outside of regular business hours, how will compensation for the nurse be managed?
2. Will the agency need to consider paying rent and/or housekeeping charges for a meeting room?
3. Has the nurse had education and experience in managing group process?
4. Is it necessary to establish a procedure for this situation?
5. How will this activity be evaluated?
6. How will the recording be done on the clients' records? Will changes in the format of the nurse's daily record be needed?

In this situation the nurse's concept of inputs includes information from clients, such as feeling isolated and needing to talk with other mothers, and the nurse's time and willingness to try a group approach. The administrator's concept of inputs includes those provided by the nurse and those having to do with organizational resources, staff knowledge, insurance, space, money, supervision, and security.

In addition, administrative considerations include whether the request or suggestion from the staff nurse is consistent with the organization's mission. Does the organization's structure permit supervision of the nurse if it is decided that the suggestion is approved? In the area of technologies, consideration is given as to whether the individual possesses adequate expertise to do the tasks suggested. Should the proposal be done by the organization but by another individual who possibly has the required skills? In that instance, would there be conflict between the person making the suggestion and the one assigned to do the task? Could this potential conflict be managed? Additionally, do the personnel policies adequately support this request, and is it possible to appropriately reward the individual with the idea? Consideration of these areas, obtaining information as available, and assessing whether the decision to act may be made by the nurse administrator is essential.

Information is also needed to evaluate the quality of the organization and to assess whether change is needed. Information obtained by written and verbal communication provides feedback for the nurse administrator.

Some administrators make ongoing efforts to open and maintain the lines of *communication* with staff members in numerous ways. Open and frequent communication is essential to maintain a smoothly running organization. In large organizations with decentralized offices, maintaining open lines of communication is indeed a challenge. Ideas for keeping communication open include circulating weekly newsbriefs, publishing monthly news bulletins, and holding open forums where staff members belonging to the unit, regardless of classification, can present their concerns and raise questions or share successes. The traditional suggestion box can be helpful to allow staff members freedom to make recommendations. In small offices the bulletin board is still perceived as effective. In addition to these somewhat traditional methods, administrative personnel in a large agency have made tapes and sent them to various district offices for staff members to hear. If offices have computer terminals, it is conceivable that the day will come when flash bulletins can be printed out at the site of the terminal. The prearranged conference telephone call can be another effective and economical way of communication.

Communication, however, should be a two-way process. Staff members need to develop skills in presenting their concerns. Nurses tend to place themselves in an adversary position to administration, as illustrated by the following statements: "*They* won't give us . . . "; *They* don't communicate"; "*They* don't understand"; "*They* don't include me"; "*They* don't listen"; "*They* won't tell us." "I challenge this," stated one of the nursing service administrators at a conference held several years ago on "The Role of the Director of Nursing Service." As Hassenplug once said, "We have met the enemy and it was us." (Moore, 1977, p. 4). How many nurses confront and share their feelings openly and honestly with the administrator? How often do nurses inform the administrator?

Needless to say, the administrative role in community health is a demanding position that offers unlimited challenges and is indeed complex. Furthermore, the information required to solve problems from an adminis-

trative perspective is different from the information required for planning client care. Lack of understanding about these differences and lack of appreciation for differences in information needed and available may lead to dysfunctional organizational conflict.

THE COMMUNITY HEALTH NURSE ADMINISTRATOR AND PUBLIC HEALTH

The first parts of this chapter described the blend between the disciplines of nursing and administration. The nurse administrator who works for organizations with a public health mission also needs to be aware of the values and goals of public health and to consider them in managing the nursing services.

The administrative and organizational process involves consideration of values, either overtly through direct consideration or covertly through examination of organizational behavior (Suchman, 1967). The values that underlie the practice of public health are rarely discussed in public health literature, but appear to be known primarily through a process of oral tradition or oral history. Consideration of public health values, especially as compared to medical and nursing values, is an important component to understanding community health nursing administration.

Values regarding public health stem from society's interest in the health of the persons who comprise that society and its labor force, the foundation of the economy. Health is an essential factor in human performance, and its maintenance and protection are of social importance.

Protection of the community's health is a public concern. The location of public health organizations within the public sector of health services delivery gives rise to values that differ from those arising from a free enterprise or market orientation. These values include the following:

1. The mandate for the availability of public health services comes from the community's social interest rather than the self-interest of the individual.
2. Accountability for public health services, both in terms of effectiveness and efficiency of these programs, is to the community that is served.
3. Achieving the goal of protecting the public health involves a complex, community-based, political and economic process, requiring the skills of many health and health-related disciplines.

Thus *public health work* may be defined as an interdisciplinary activity that seeks to provide the greatest good for the greatest number at the least cost for purposes of maintaining or improving the level of health in a population. Since the focus of public health is the community, it is necessary to understand and use the appropriate sciences and analytical methods. Epidemiology, demography, and biometry are appropriate because their focus is at the level of the population or community. These concepts are discussed in other chapters of the text.

In public health organizations it is desirable to specify organizational goals and objectives in terms that reflect the interest in the community's health. Miller and Moos (1981) discuss this point and note the renewed interest in using measures of community health to define organizational objectives and outcomes of programs. An example of such measures would be the use of a specific vital rate as an objective and outcome criteria. If a community has a high fertility rate among adolescents, a reduction in the rate could be stated as an objective for the public health agency. Development and implementation of a health services program for adolescents, including family planning services, might then be considered as a program strategy for achieving the objective. Because of the community-level focus and the relationship to the social policy process, selecting intervention strategies in public health has a different focus than selecting those used by clinicians, such as in medical care settings. These strategies include regulation and provision of personal health services, education and research.

Regulation

Regulation, according to Hanlon (1984), has as its purpose the protection and promotion of individual and community health by controlling factors that inhibit or reduce health. Regulations are the rules and procedures for implementing laws. According to Clute (1973, p. 140), "Law is a dynamic, functioning entity . . . not static rules . . . a type of process for restoring, creating or maintaining social order." Health departments are often involved in the process of establishing and implementing laws and regulations that pertain to health.

In general three types of regulations exist. These are (1) police powers (to protect citizens from a threat such as unsafe food or quarantines), (2) administrative rulings (to assure proper management of resources) and (3) licensing of individuals and groups. The degree of involvement of a public health agency in the regulatory process depends on the scope of the agency (local, state, or national). According to Wing (1976), federal legal authority for health is limited to regulation of goods and services purchased with federal tax money and regulation of people and activities related to interstate commerce. In comparison, state authority for regulation includes protection of individual health (even over the individual's objection) and of the community's health.

The regulatory authority of states is limited by the federal Constitution. Both state and federal authorities are limited by the Bill of Rights and the right to due process.

The overlap of authority to regulate health between state and federal levels often leads to confusing directives from multiple regulatory bodies. The many diverse constituencies in community health have been able to create differing responses from differing levels of social policymakers. (See Pickett [1980] for a more complete discussion of this problem). Additionally, appropriate management of constituencies is especially difficult for the administrator (Kaufman, 1973) because of this diversity. Thus, as Bellin (1977, p. 46) states, "Enmeshed as it is in the political process, the practice of administration becomes the art of the possible."

Legislated requirements for sanitary restaurants and restaurant inspection laws are examples of regulations to protect the public's health. Laws to assure safe, clean water and air have been enacted. They are implemented by regulating individuals and industries that have a potential to pollute water and air and by developing public treatment facilities.

Community health nurse administrators and nurses are affected by these regulations and influence their development. An example of this would be efforts to establish regulations requiring immunization of children before their enrollment in school and developing methods for nurses assigned to schools to implement these regulations.

Provision of Personal Health Services

Whether it is appropriate for public health organizations to be involved in the delivery of personal health services is often debated. However, most local or county health departments do deliver some personal health (medical) services. These services are usually targeted at specific portions of the community's population perceived as unserved, underserved, or poorly served by the medical care system (Miller and Moos, 1981). These population groups include persons who cannot afford private medical care, those who are migrants, and those whose health problems are best managed through an interdisciplinary approach. Services for crippled children provide an example of the latter. Although public health organizations receive public financial support for many of their activities, the use of fee schedules for personal services is increasing (Miller and Moos, 1981).

In contrast, medical care and medical services organizations focus on different priorities than do community health organizations. The physician functions in professional and entrepreneurial or private sector roles with respect to individuals who seek medical services and pay for them. The goal of medical care is alleviation or cure of disease in individuals through diagnosis and appropriate treatment.

Education

Client education and health education are intervention strategies used in medical services and community services organizations, respectively. In medical services organizations client education is primarily directed toward assisting clients to understand their illness, to learn how to care for themselves after discharge from the hospital, and to know how to recognize or prevent complications from their present illness.

Health education in community organizations has as its major goal the education of the community, groups, or individuals for the prevention of illness and disability, the control of disease, and the promotion of wellness.

Research

Research is an integral intervention strategy in public health and in medicine. Public health research primarily focuses on the study of causes of disease, disease patterns, proper diagnosis, and reporting of diseases; disease surveillance methods; incidence and prevalence of disease; risk factors related to the environment; and life-styles, to name a few.

Medical research focuses on improvement in knowledge about disease, its diagnosis, and its treatment. Medical researchers are also interested in finding disease cures, testing chemical agents, and trying technological methods for palliative care.

Members of the nursing profession are predominantly employed by the medical care delivery system and have tended to develop a research and practice perspective similar to that of medicine. That is, the focus has been on understanding the art and science of nursing by describing the natural course of nursing care problems in individuals and ameliorating problems by appropriate nursing interventions or treatment. In public health organizations, nurses are most often involved with personal health service delivery programs and thus tend to focus their research on service delivery or on clinical questions applicable to the individual client rather than to the entire community.

■   ■   ■

The intervention strategies of regulation, personal health services, education, and research used in medical care are predominantly directed toward service delivery to individuals. From values and operational perspectives, the practice of public health and the practice of medicine differ fundamentally in that public health is focused on the community and medicine is focused

on individuals. Although these two fields are fundamentally different, they are not necessarily in conflict with each other.

Need and Demand for Community Health Nursing Services

An important distinction for the community health nurse administrator is the difference between need and demand in community health. *Need* in community health refers to "ought-to-be" services. The definition of need in public health arises from analysis of vital statistics and health surveys and data on the use of and gaps in health services. *Demand* is a measure of the type and amount of services requested or desired by the public once they know the prices involved. Demand is frequently expressed in public action by consumers.

Analysis of need and demand for health services, whether medical nursing services or community health services, including nursing, does not differ substantially in terms of the analytical processes involved. However, there is a difference in the degree of emphasis on community-based data and the role of the public policy process in determining the nature and structure of the community health services available. In the context of the medical care system, decisions about services are most heavily influenced by the economic situations of the user.

In the public health agency, need and demand are often further broken down by consideration of vital and demographic factors that seem to influence community need and to describe it in a way that is useful for program planning from an administrative perspective.

Vital and demographic data about the community are helpful for this purpose. Table 28-1 identifies sources of data for estimating community needs. This information is routinely collected and summarized as shown in Fig. 28-4. The community health nurse administrator uses the data in considering the range of services that ought to be available in this community based on its structure.

Data such as these, when stated in terms of the community of interest, provide some method for determining whether particular problems in community health may be anticipated in this particular community. For example, in considering whether detection of sickle cell anemia might be a major effort of any particular organization it is helpful to know the proportion of blacks in the population of the community. The need for such a screening effort will vary depending on whether the proportion of blacks within the population is 1% or 20%.

The nature of a need in the community also depends on the age structure of the population. For example, the need for geriatric services will be different in a commu-

Table 28-1. Sources of data for estimating community need

	Demographic data	Vital statistics	Health statistics
Description	Specific information regarding the population, e.g., the number of inhabitants, age, sex, race, marital status, number and makeup of households, condition of housing, migration, income, education, occupation, distance traveled to and from work.	The vital events that occur over a period of time within a population — such as birth, death, marriage, divorce, adoption, annulment, and separation — often called the "bookkeeping of public health."	1. Measurements of the state of health, i.e., morbidity data that relate to the distribution of illness (incidence and prevalence), as distinct from mortality. 2. Measurement of factors closely related to health, e.g., sanitation, nutrition, poverty. 3. Measurements of health programs, services, activities.
How gathered	Nationwide census enumeration every 10 years as decreed by the Constitution — first census was taken in 1790; for each state a census report is published with four sections — the number of inhabitants, general population characteristics, general social and economic characteristics, detailed characteristics.	Facts, systematically selected and compiled in numerical form, are derived from official records; compulsory reporting of births and deaths is a function of state and local governments; standard recommended certificates are provided by the National Center for Health Statistics, but must be approved by state legislatures (the right to privacy must be standardized by international agreements through WHO (International Classification of Diseases, Injuries, and Causes of Death).	Morbidity data are gathered from official sources (such as the reports of notifiable diseases, the National Health Survey, state and local health registries, other health surveys) as well as voluntary sources (such as industry, mass screening, insurance companies); other health data are derived from surveys, agency reports, peer review groups, etc.
How applied in public health	Census data, expressed in statistical terms such as averages, percentages, and ratios, offer information relevant to public health, e.g., (1) age distribution of a population, (2) dependency ratio, related to the age distribution, (3) socioeconomic characteristics (income, education, employment); all of these factors are considered in community health planning.	Data are expressed in vital rates — a vital rate is the number of occurrences of a vital event that take place during a given period of time (usually a calendar year) divided by the average population "at risk" to the event (usually the estimated midyear population); examples of vital rates are crude birth rate, crude death rate, infant mortality, perinatal mortality, maternal mortality, and cause-specific death rate; these facts are helpful in identifying health needs, establishing priorities, determining allocation of funds, planning and evaluating health programs.	Health statistics serve as the basis for assessing specific health needs and planning public health programs; incidence and prevalence rates help in determining priorities for prevention and control of disease; health data provide information for allocation of funds, evaluation of health programs, and research.

National vital statistics needs. A report of the U.S. National Committee on Vital and Health Statistics, Washington, D.C., 1965, National Center for Vital Statistics, Department of Health, Education, and Welfare.

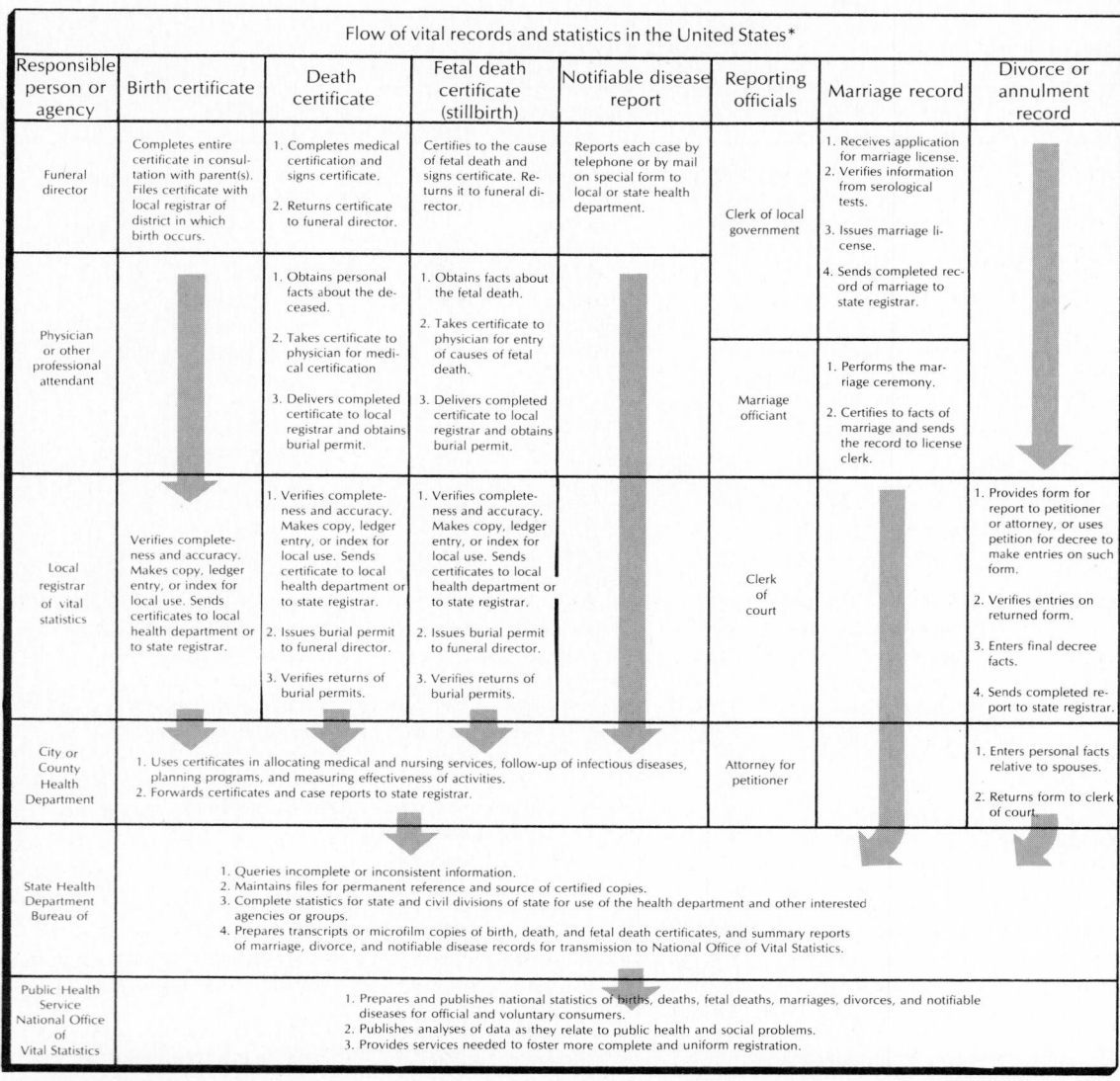

| Responsible person or agency | \multicolumn{7}{c}{Flow of vital records and statistics in the United States*} |

Responsible person or agency	Birth certificate	Death certificate	Fetal death certificate (stillbirth)	Notifiable disease report	Reporting officials	Marriage record	Divorce or annulment record
Funeral director	Completes entire certificate in consultation with parent(s). Files certificate with local registrar of district in which birth occurs.	1. Completes medical certification and signs certificate. 2. Returns certificate to funeral director.	Certifies to the cause of fetal death and signs certificate. Returns it to funeral director.	Reports each case by telephone or by mail on special form to local or state health department.	Clerk of local government	1. Receives application for marriage license. 2. Verifies information from serological tests. 3. Issues marriage license. 4. Sends completed record of marriage to state registrar.	
Physician or other professional attendant		1. Obtains personal facts about the deceased. 2. Takes certificate to physician for medical certification. 3. Delivers completed certificate to local registrar and obtains burial permit.	1. Obtains facts about the fetal death. 2. Takes certificate to physician for entry of causes of fetal death. 3. Delivers completed certificate to local registrar and obtains burial permit.		Marriage officiant	1. Performs the marriage ceremony. 2. Certifies to facts of marriage and sends the record to license clerk.	
Local registrar of vital statistics	Verifies completeness and accuracy. Makes copy, ledger entry, or index for local use. Sends certificates to local health department or to state registrar.	1. Verifies completeness and accuracy. Makes copy, ledger entry, or index for local use. Sends certificate to local health department or to state registrar. 2. Issues burial permit to funeral director. 3. Verifies returns of burial permits.	1. Verifies completeness and accuracy. Makes copy, ledger entry, or index for local use. Sends certificates to local health department or to state registrar. 2. Issues burial permit to funeral director. 3. Verifies returns of burial permits.		Clerk of court		1. Provides form for report to petitioner or attorney, or uses petition for decree to make entries on such form. 2. Verifies entries on returned form. 3. Enters final decree facts. 4. Sends completed report to state registrar.
City or County Health Department	\multicolumn{4}{l}{1. Uses certificates in allocating medical and nursing services, follow-up of infectious diseases, planning programs, and measuring effectiveness of activities. 2. Forwards certificates and case reports to state registrar.}	Attorney for petitioner		1. Enters personal facts relative to spouses. 2. Returns form to clerk of court.
State Health Department Bureau of	\multicolumn{7}{l}{1. Queries incomplete or inconsistent information. 2. Maintains files for permanent reference and source of certified copies. 3. Complete statistics for state and civil divisions of state for use of the health department and other interested agencies or groups. 4. Prepares transcripts or microfilm copies of birth, death, and fetal death certificates, and summary reports of marriage, divorce, and notifiable disease records for transmission to National Office of Vital Statistics.}
Public Health Service National Office of Vital Statistics	\multicolumn{7}{l}{1. Prepares and publishes national statistics of births, deaths, fetal deaths, marriages, divorces, and notifiable diseases for official and voluntary consumers. 2. Publishes analyses of data as they relate to public health and social problems. 3. Provides services needed to foster more complete and uniform registration.}

Fig. 28-4. Information routinely collected and summarized as illustrated in this flow chart. (From *National vital statistics needs,* a report of the U.S. National Committee on Vital and Health Statistics, Washington, D.C., 1965, National Center for Vital Statistics, Department of Health, Education, Welfare.)

nity whose proportion of elderly is very high as compared to a community in which it is low.

The occupational structure of the community is also a relevant variable to consider when defining need. That is, the health needs of a labor force in a predominantly agricultural area will be different from the health needs of a labor force in a region geared toward petrochemical production.

While this information is useful in terms of considering community needs, it is, in community health, not usually construed as meaning one service program and not another, but rather indicates the relative emphasis

of the community health effort in a particular community.

Program Strategies

In considering the nature of the programs to be available in the community, the community health nurse administrator again will find epidemiological and demographic data useful in determining the type of effort, if any, to make. This kind of analysis will assist in determining whether the problem is amenable to some type of intervention. And, when this is analyzed with information about the quality and quantity of other pro-

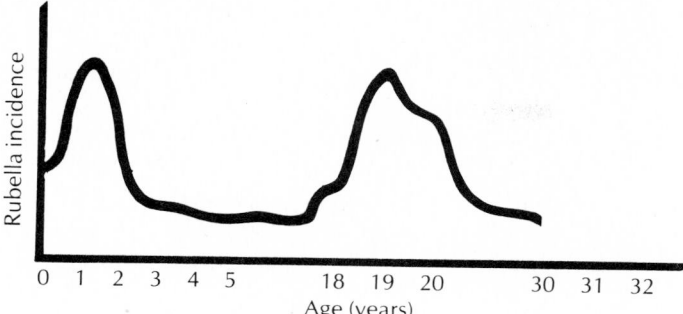

Fig. 28-5. Incidence of rubella.

grams available in the community, it will provide some guidance about the direction any program might take.

As noted previously, intervention strategies in community health organizations may include regulation, provision of services, education, and research. The community health nurse administrator is most commonly involved with service delivery efforts, but needs to be knowledgeable about and supportive of the total organizational effort.

From a service perspective, the array of possible strategies includes the following: (1) preventing, (2) giving health education, (3) screening and referring, (4) diagnosing, and (5) treating. The type of service focus will depend on both the population-based goals to be achieved and the availability of other services within the community. For example, if the program objective to be achieved is to reduce rubella incidence by 10% in this community in the coming 2 years, and since epidemiological and clinical trials research indicate that this can be done by immunizing rubella-susceptible individuals, the service strategy is likely to include immunization clinics for rubella-susceptible persons. If the rubella incidence graph looks like the one shown in Fig. 28-5, attention should be directed at both children and young adults, especially women. If, however, the objective is to decrease the incidence of herpes genitalia, the best strategy would be prevention, with health education directed at the susceptible population. According to what is known about the natural history of this disease, as discussed in Chapter 14, it is transmitted sexually, and is not treatable in its recurrent stages, although new drugs are appearing.

These examples of how program plans might be derived and what program strategies might be considered have dealt with infectious diseases. It is also important for the community health nurse administrator to develop program goals and strategies for community health problems that are chronic or known to be related to multiple causes.

In the situation of chronic health problems, such as

coronary heart disease or motor vehicle casualties, the problem of planning community interventions is somewhat more complex. For example, as noted in Chapter 14, with respect to coronary heart disease, hypertension, smoking, high-stress life-style, and possibly a high cholesterol diet appear to be related to the onset of disease. Early detection and adequate treatment of hypertension should, in the long run, reduce the prevalence of coronary heart disease. Strategies that a community health nurse administrator might consider would include hypertension detection and referral activities and smoking cessation education/intervention activities. Additionally, the community health nurse administrator may choose to be involved through the political process in supporting the activities of other organizations to deal with availability of medical care for the individual who has coronary heart disease. Or the community health administrator may seek assistance to conduct an evaluation research project to evaluate the effects of health instruction.

With the problem of motor vehicle accidents, the community health nurse administrator's program goals will vary according to the individual and the community. Goals may include reducing the number of injuries to children by making child auto restraints available through the maternal-child health program already in existence. There might be a need for preparing and disseminating instructional materials about safe driving or the hazards of driving while under the influence of alcohol to schools and other community groups. The community health nurse administrator may choose to be involved in the policy-making process that would establish better regulations having as their ultimate purpose the reduction of motor vehicle accidents. Finally, the administrator may lend support to community services designed to provide improved emergency services for the victims of such accidents.

In summary, the use of community-based data, the information from epidemiological studies about the natural course of disease-specific mortality and morbidity, and the selection of one or more program goals and intervention strategies to deal with community problems in the area of health represent a complex process. The individual who functions in the role of staff nurse in an organization that focuses on health problems in the community is likely to have direct experience with those activities which occur at the interface between the organization and the consumer. That is, the staff nurse may be the individual who takes health educational materials to the schools in the community. Or the staff nurse may be the individual who screens and refers a client with hypertension for diagnosis. These activities are essential parts of the effort to improve the level of health in the community.

Program Economics

It would be wonderful to be able to state that because the objectives of achieving community health are so clearly in the social interest, society has chosen to provide the economic resources to achieve its goal. However, such has not been the case, and financing for community health varies both in terms of sources and quantities over time.

From a public policy perspective, it would seem reasonable to suggest that if a healthy public is a societal need, there should be public financial support through taxes to meet this need. Indeed there are taxes paid by the general public to cities, counties, states, and the federal government. Taxes are usually unrestricted with respect to what public goals should be financially supported by tax dollars. The amount of financial support for public goals varies enormously over time. Additionally, the degree of public support for health as compared to education, social services, safety, and transportation (road and bridges) also varies, as discussed in Chapter 3.

From the national perspective, the federal system has been involved in financing health since 1797 (Wilson and Neuhauser, 1974). Over time there have been swings toward and away from categorical as compared to block approaches to financing services. The categorical idea includes identification of a national health priority with financial incentives to states or smaller units of government who implement plans to achieve the national objective. Programs such as the Children and Youth Projects and WIC (nutrition program for women, infants, and children) illustrates this strategy. In comparison, the block method of financing health leaves decisions about what specific objectives are to be accomplished to smaller units of government such as states and provides money to the states on a per capita formula.

Currently in the United States the federal government is moving in the direction of block-type financing to states for health programs. Robins (1977) notes that if a block grant is primarily intended to be a device for budgetary control (while also a means for increasing flexibility in funds) and contains no mechanism for reforming the health care delivery system, the result is decrease of services to target populations and/or increase in financial burdens on states, localities, and the poor. When block funding is the federal strategy, the community health nurse administrator will be highly involved in the state and local policy setting processes to enhance the chances for program maintenance.

In addition to taxation, categorical grants, and block grants, a fourth common form of financing health activities, including services to individuals, is the fee-for-service process in which the actual user of the service pays for that service. Based on analysis of the costs of providing service, a fee (usually an average cost) per service is established. In public health agencies and other community-based organizations, the fee may be adjusted or eliminated if the client is unable to pay. According to a recent survey, public health agencies also bill Medicare, Medicaid, and insurance companies when that is appropriate.

Other sources of funds include contributions from members of the community and grants from private foundations.

COMMUNITY HEALTH NURSING ADMINISTRATION: A COMPOSITE PROCESS

The responsibilities of the community health nurse administrator vary from agency to agency, from program to program, and from one community to another. The responsibilities may encompass all the activities identified in the standards given at the beginning of this chapter.

Fig. 28-6 represents three of the dimensions of community health nursing administration. These dimensions are the community's characteristics, the administrative process, and intervention strategies used in public health. Any three-dimensional model is, by definition, complex. In reality, this diagram underrepresents the complexities of functioning in top-level administration in public health. Another dimension that should be considered, for example, involves the other community social systems, including the legislative system, the jurisprudence system, and the "scientific" community. The Rubik's model presented could also be labeled "a matrix of loose ends." In many ways the role of the community health nurse administrator is not unlike solving the Rubik's Cube puzzle.

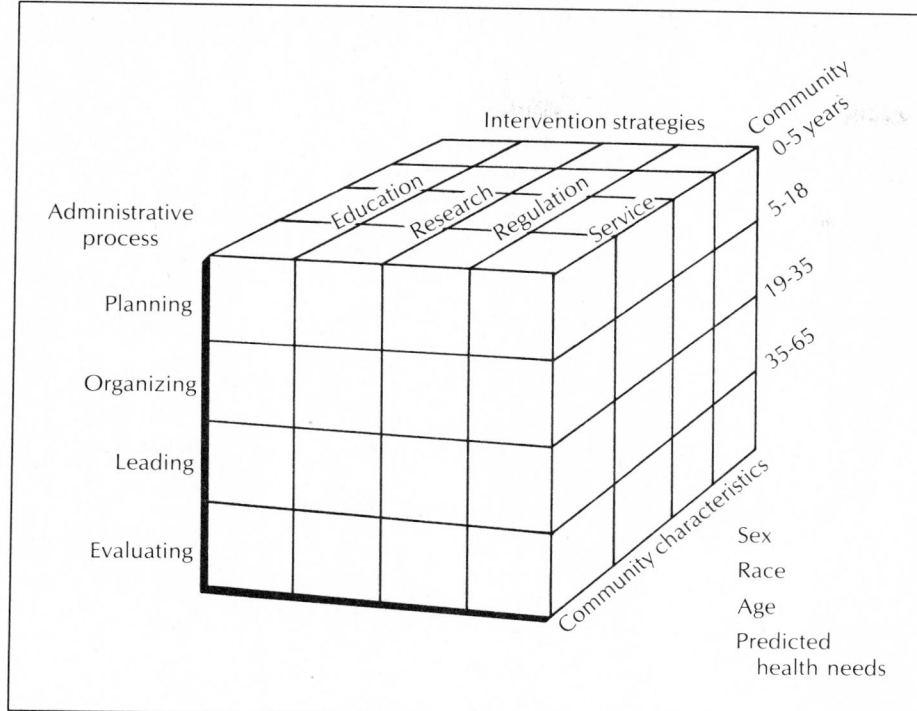

Administrative process

Planning

Organizing

Leading

Evaluating

Intervention strategies

Education   Research   Regulation   Service

Community

0-5 years

5-18

19-35

35-65

Community characteristics

Sex

Race

Age

Predicted
health needs

Fig. 28-6. The Rubik's Cube
of administrative process.

SUMMARY

The community health nurse administrator has what can be perceived by many as an awesome responsibility. Administrative practice challenges the nurse to create an organization from which the mission to create a safe environment in which to live can be accomplished. As David Brewer stated, "Moving waters are full of life and health. Only in still waters is there stagnation and death" (Simmons, 1977, p. 170). Administration is exciting. Nurses who understand the practice of nursing administration will join as members of a drama team, helping see that the stage is properly set and, despite economic risk and turbulence of plans, the production is positively reviewed. The total cast—all actors, staff, students, managers, and community support personnel—along with the manager can enjoy the applause as plans are implemented and health care needs for the community are met.

BIBLIOGRAPHY

American Hospital Association: The role of the nursing service in a health care institution, Chicago, 1977, The Association.

American Nurses' Association: Roles, responsibilities, and qualifications for nurse administrators. Commission on Nursing Service, Kansas City, 1973, The Association.

American Nurses' Association: Standards for community health nursing practice, Kansas City, 1973, The Association.

American Nurses' Association: Standards for organized nursing services, Kansas City, 1982, The Association.

Arndt, C., and Huckabay, L.: Nursing Administration: Theory for practice with a systems approach, St. Louis, 1975, The C.V. Mosby Co.

Barnard, C.: The functions of the executive, Cambridge, 1938, Harvard University Press.

Bellin, L.E.: Local health departments: A prescription against obsolescence. In Levin, A., editor: Health services: the local perspective, New York, 1977, Academy of Political Science.

Clute, K.: Law and health. In McKinlay, J.B., editor: Politics and the law in health care policy, New York, 1973, Prodist.

DiVincente, M.: Administering nursing service, Boston, 1972, Little, Brown, & Co.

Etzioni, A.: Modern organizations, Englewood Cliffs, N.J., 1964, Prentice-Hall, Inc.

Fayol, H.: Industrial and general administration, Paris, 1925, Dunod.

Fiedler, F.E., and Chemers, M.M.: Leadership and effective management, Glenview, Ill., 1974, Scott, Foresman & Co.

Filley, A., and House, R.J.: Managerial process and organizational behavior, Glenview, Ill., 1969, Scott, Foresman & Co.

Folwinkle, E.: The state's role in the delivery of local health services. In Levin, A., editor: Health services: the local perspective, New York, 1977, Academy of Political Science.

Gardner, M.: Public health nursing, New York, 1938, Macmillan Publishing Co., Inc.

Hanlon, J.J., and Pickett, G.E.: Public health: administration and practice, ed. 8, St. Louis, 1984, The C.V. Mosby Co.

Kalisch, P.A., and Kalisch, B., The advance of american nursing, Boston, 1978, Little, Brown & Co.

Kaufman, H.: The political ingredient of public health services. In McKinlay, J.B., editor: Politics and the law in health care policy, New York, 1973, Prodist.

Lancaster, J.: Systems theory and the process of change. In Lancaster, J., and Lancaster, W., editors: Concepts for advanced nursing practice: The nurse as a change agent, St. Louis, 1982, The C.V. Mosby Co.

Last, J.M., editor: Public health and preventive medicine, New York, 1980, Appleton-Century-Crofts.

Levey, S., and Loomba, N.P.: Health care administration: a managerial perspective, Philadelphia, 1973, J.B. Lippincott Co.

McIver, P.: An analysis of first level public health nursing in ten selected health organizations, unpublished master's thesis, New York, 1934, Teachers College, Columbia University.

Miller, C.A., and Moos, M.D.: Local health departments, Washington, D.C., 1981, American Public Health Association.

Moore, J.: The role of the nurse administrator, Pub. No. 20-1646, New York, 1977, National League for Nursing.

Mustard, H.S., and Stebbins, E.L.: An introduction to public health. New York, 1959, Macmillan Publishing Co., Inc.

National league for nursing: Criteria and guide for preparing reports, accreditation of home health agencies and community nursing services, Pub. No. 21-1306, New York, 1980, The League.

National vital statistics needs. A report of the U.S. National Committee on Vital and Health Statistics, Washington, D.C., 1965, National Center for Vital Statistics, Department of Health, Education and Welfare.

Orem, D.E.: Nursing: concepts of practice, New York, 1980, McGraw-Hill Book Co.

Pickett, G.: The future of health departments: the governmental presence, Annu. Rev. Public Health 1:297, 1980.

Robins, L.: Health care costs. In Levine, A., editor: Health services: the local perspective, New York, 1977, Academy of Political Science.

Sackett, D.L.: Evaluation of health services. In Last, J.M., editor: Public health and preventive medicine, New York, 1980, Appleton-Century-Crofts.

Schaefer, M.: Managing complexity, J. Nurs. Adm. 5:13-16, 1975.

Simmons, D.: Nursing administration: issues for the '80s—solutions for the '70s, conference proceedings, Minneapolis, 1977, University of Minnesota.

Simon, H.: Administrative behavior, New York, 1947, Macmillan Publishing Co., Inc.

Stevens, B.: Nursing theory: analysis, application, and evaluation, Boston, 1979, Little, Brown & Co.

Suchman, E.: Evaluation research: principles and practice in public service and social action programs, New York, 1967, Russell Sage Foundation.

Tinkham, C.W., and Voorhies, E.F.: Community health nursing: evolution and process, New York, 1972, Appleton-Century-Crofts.

Tucker, K., and Hilbert, H.: Survey of public health nursing, New York, 1934, Oxford University Press, Inc.

Wilson, F., and Neuhauser, D.: Health services in the United States, Cambridge, Mass., 1974, Ballinger Publishing Co.

Wing, K.: The law and the public's health, St. Louis, 1976, The C.V. Mosby Co.

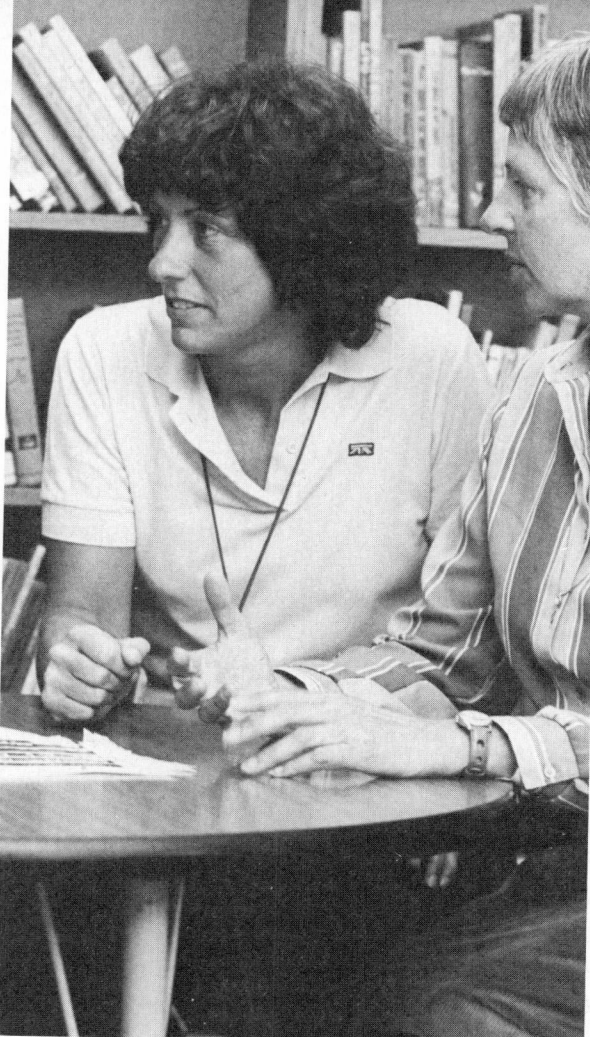

Chapter 29

MARCIA STANHOPE
RENA ALFORD

THE COMMUNITY HEALTH NURSE CONSULTANT ROLE

Nurses bring to the community a set of skills which allows them to be valuable contributing members in their work setting and in the community-at-large. The specific skills helpful in the community are the nurses' preparation for comprehensively assessing all variables that have an influence on individual, family, group, and community health status; the nurses' abilities to plan, implement, and evaluate goals and programs for individuals, groups, families, and communities as units of service; and the nurses' extensive knowledge of community resources and the referral process. These skills provide the nurse with the expertise and information to function as a consultant to the individual, family, group, or community client as well as to others working with a variety of clients.

This chapter focuses on the definition and goals of consultation, consultative theories pertinent to community health nursing, principles relative to process consultation, and the scope of the nurse consultant role. The purpose of the discussion will be to acquaint the reader with consultation as a role function of community health nursing.

DEFINITIONS AND GOALS

Consultation, like many other concepts, has a variety of definitions. Caplan (1970) defined *consultation* as a process in which the help of a specialist is sought to identify ways to handle work problems involving either the management of clients or the planning and implementation of programs. Lippitt and Lippitt (1977) described *consultation* as a general label for many varia-

689

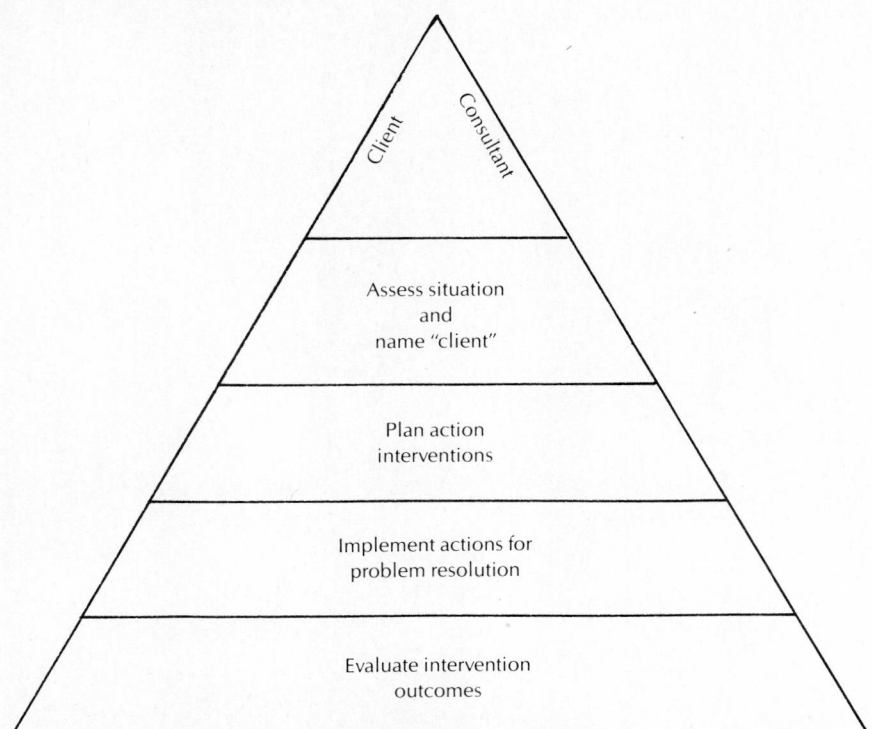

Fig. 29-1. The process model.

tions of relationships whereas Schein (1969) stated that *consultation* is a process involving a set of activities on the part of the helper which assists the client to perceive, understand, and act on events occurring in the client's environment.

The *goal* of consultation is to stimulate clients to take more responsibility, feel more secure, deal constructively with their feelings and with others in interaction, and internalize skills of a flexible and creative nature. The functions of the consultant differ from the role functions of administrator, supervisor, coordinator, planner, educator, researcher, and client advocate in that consultation typically is a temporary and a voluntary relationship between a professional helper and a client who has perceived a need for assistance. The relationship is a cooperative effort between consultant and client, established to share equally in the resolution of a problem.

Although Lippitt and Lippitt (1977) indicated that a consultant is an "outsider," not part of the power system in the work setting, this statement may not apply to the community health nurse consultant. The community health nurse finds position expectations to include both internal and external consultation. For example, the community health nurse may be employed to consult with other nurses in the agency about client care problems, or the community heath nurse as an employee of the health department may serve as a consultant to a local health planning agency about the public health care needs of the community.

"*Internal consultants* are persons employed on a full-time salaried basis by the organization with which they consult" (Blake and Mouton, 1976, p. 442; Walton, 1969). Clients of the internal nurse consultants range from staff members to departments to consumers of agency service. *External consultants* are employed on a contractual basis within a time period by the client with whom they consult. The client of the external nurse consultant may be a colleague, another health provider, or a community group or organization. The nature of the consultative relationship, internal or external, should not change the goal of consultation.

THEORIES OF CONSULTATION

Although nursing's involvement in consultation has expanded through the decades, few data are found in the literature about the impact of the nurse consultant on health care delivery. Selected theories of consultation are discussed to provide a basic understanding of approaches for establishing the consultation relationship.

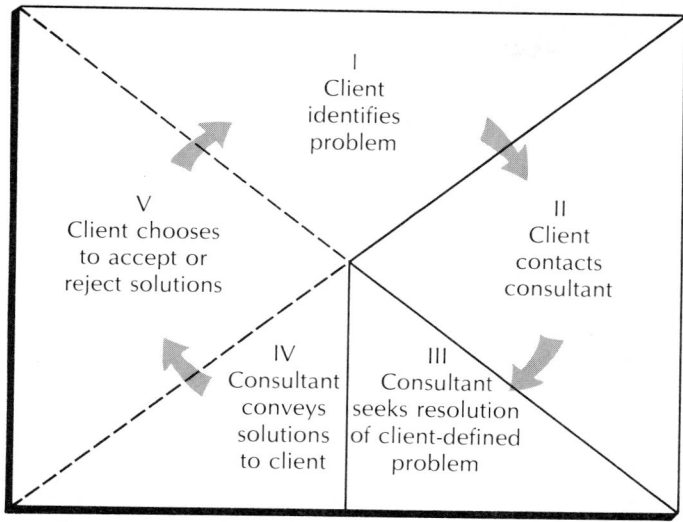

Fig. 29-2. The purchase model.

——— Actual interaction
- - - - - Potential interaction

The Process Model

Schein's definition of consultation (1969) describes process consultation and will not be redefined in this section. The major goals of the process model, as seen in Fig. 29-1, are to assist the client to assess the problem as well as the kind of help needed to resolve the problem. Problem solving is a key tool used in process consultation. Both the consultant and the consultee engage in the problem-solving steps that lead to situation changes or to action programs for problem resolution (Keithley et al., 1979).

The assumptions underlying process consultation are as follows:

1. Clients often do not know what the problem is and need assistance in problem diagnosis.
2. Clients are not aware of the services a consultant may offer and need assistance in finding proper help.
3. Clients want to improve situations and need guidance in identifying appropriate methods to reach goals.
4. Clients can be more effective if they learn to diagnose their own strengths and limitations.
5. Consultants usually cannot spend enough time learning all variables that may help or hinder suggested courses of action, so they need to work with the client who has intimate knowledge of the effects of proposed courses of action.
6. The client who learns to diagnose situation problems and who engages in decision making about alternative courses of action will be actively involved in implementing actions for problems resolution.

7. The consultant who is an expert in problem diagnosis and in establishing an effective helping relationship will be able to pass these skills to the client.

Since process consultation emphasizes human interactions, the consultant must be an expert in individual, group, and community interaction processes (Schein, 1969). Because of the similarity between the focus of process consultation, the skills of the community health nurse, and the emphasis on problem solving, process consultation forms the basis of discussion for this chapter. However, other theories are introduced to show alternative methods used in the consultant-consultee relationship. Because process consultation closely parallels the nursing process, this model is viewed as the most appropriate model to apply in nursing.

The Purchase Model

Purchase model consultation, Fig. 29-2, is defined as the purchase (hiring) of a professional helper by a client for the purpose of providing expert information or expert service (Schein, 1969). Buyers may be individuals, groups, or organizations. In this model the client predetermines the need for the consultant. The need is defined as something the client wants to know or some activity the client wants implemented.

The purchase model assumes the following:

1. The client will correctly diagnose the problem.
2. The client will be able to correctly communicate the needs to the consultant.
3. The client will correctly assess the consultant's expertise to provide the information or perform the service.

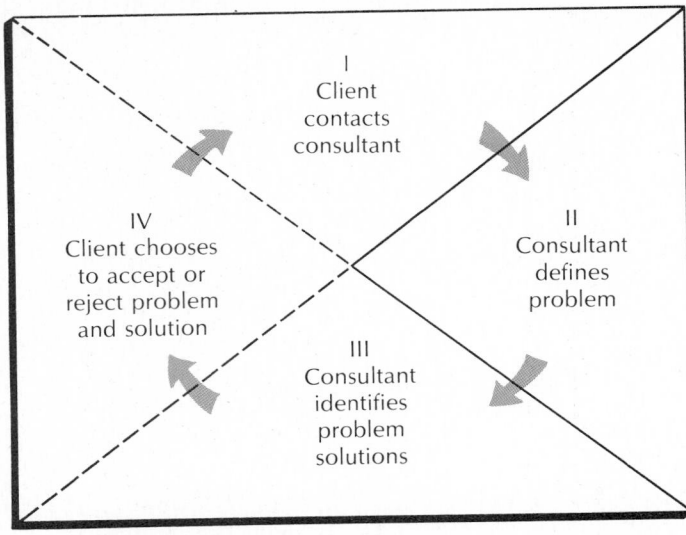

Fig. 29-3. The doctor-patient model.

—————— Actual interaction
- - - - - - Potential interaction

Diagram labels:
I
Client
contacts
consultant

II
Consultant
defines
problem

III
Consultant
identifies
problem
solutions

IV
Client chooses
to accept or
reject problem
and solution

4. The client knows the consequences of having the consultant provide the information or the consequences of implementing services suggested by the consultant.

The advantage of using the popular purchase model is that the client does not have to spend time or energy in solving the identified problem. The disadvantage of the model is that the quality of the consultation may be questioned by the client if the client has identified the wrong problem (Schein, 1969).

Examples of use of the purchase model *when information is being sought* by the buyer are varied. For example, the executive director of a home health agency may employ a consultant to provide direction for a survey of client satisfaction with nursing services. The public health department supervisors may employ a consultant to instruct them in designing a method for improving nurse productivity. Similarly, a clinic administrator may request information about how to design an accounting system to highlight the costs of nursing services. In all instances the client has defined the problem before employing the consultant.

Examples of consultant services *purchased to provide services* are as follows: (1) The district nursing supervisor requests the state health department's maternal-child health nursing consultant to come to the district health department and reorganize the family planning clinic for efficient operation. The consultant may need to survey client scheduling procedures, numbers of staff available to implement the clinic, client compliance, absenteeism, and clinic demand as well as available facilities and equipment in order to make recommendations about clinic reorganization. (2) The community

health nursing staff members request a consultant to analyze their caseloads to establish client mix guidelines for future client assignments. To do so, the nurse consultant may need to review records for age, sex, diagnosis, physical activity, and client service demands to arrive at a client classification system to be used for distributing equitable caseloads.

Although the purchase model is often used by consultants and consultees, the consultant enters the picture at the point of implementation for problem resolution. This model may be unsatisfactory in effectively and efficiently identifying and resolving client problems. Thus it is not viewed as the best model to apply in community health nursing.

The Doctor-Patient Model

Another popular consultative model in use is the *doctor-patient model* (Fig. 29-3), in which the consultant is employed by the client to find the problem and offer solutions without background data or assistance from the client (Schein, 1969). This model assumes the following:

1. The client is willing to reveal information needed by the consultant to make an appropriate diagnosis.
2. The consultant, through observations, will be able to get an accurate picture of the problem situation.
3. The client will accept the diagnosis and the prescriptions offered by the consultant.

Again, the major advantage of this model from the client's viewpoint is the limited time and energy expenditure required of the client. However, disadvantages

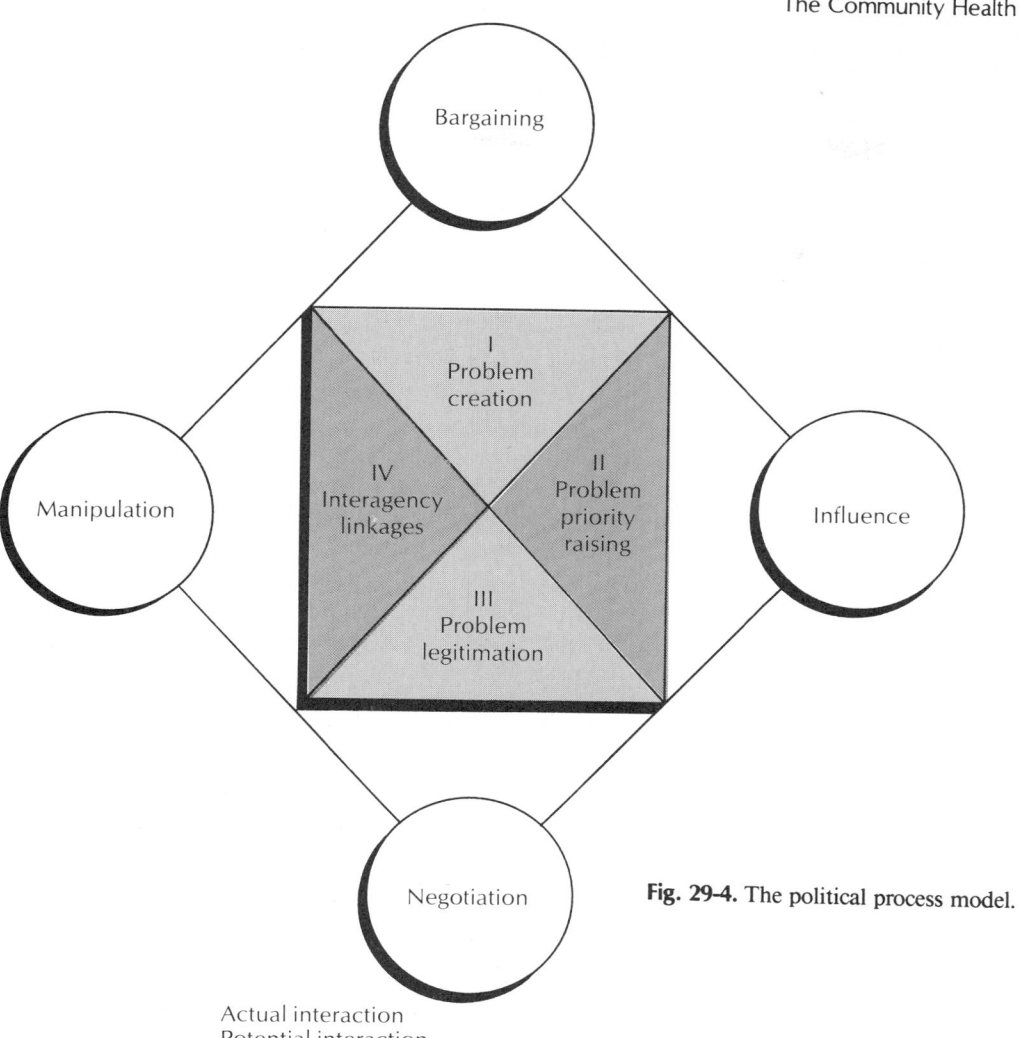

Fig. 29-4. The political process model.

outweigh any advantage that may exist in using this model. The patient (the problem identified by the employing client) may be uncooperative and reluctant to share information the consultant needs to arrive at a fair diagnosis. Given the diagnosis, the patient and the client may be unwilling to believe and to accept suggestions for change. Also, the consultant-client-patient communication relationship is not well established, and the ensuing communication gap, resulting from lack of involvement in the diagnosis process, may make the prescriptions seem irrelevant or untenable to the client and the patient (Schein, 1969).

This model is often applied in nursing situations requiring consultative services. The director of nursing at the public health department calls in a nurse consultant from the local university. Nurse performance is poor, according to the director, and the nurse consultant is asked to diagnose what is wrong with the department. In this example the nursing director is the client and the staff nurses are the *patient.* The staff nurses must pro-

vide the data that will identify the problem for the consultant (doctor). If the problem is found to be poor administrative organization and direction rather than lack of quality of performance among the staff, the administrator may be reluctant to accept the diagnosis. Since the client and the patient are reluctant to be a part of the assessment of the problem, the goals of consultation cannot be met. This model, therefore, is seen as an ineffective model to apply in community health nursing.

The Political Process Model

Consultation has been described as a political process (Baizerman and Hall, 1977; Hendrix and La-Godna, 1982). The definition offered for the political process model (Fig. 29-4) is "consultation is a political bargaining process in which expertise, organizational position, personal and organizational reputation are the currency of the bargaining between consultant and consultee; and in which each actor attempts to maximize his currency at a minimum cost" (Baizerman and Hall, 1977, p. 143).

This model assumes the following:

1. A persistent pattern of human relationships exist in consultation which are influenced by power and authority.
2. The consultant is an agent acting on behalf of or for another.
3. Manipulation, influence, and negotiation are acceptable ways to control differences, reach settlement, and exchange expertise.
4. Participants in the bargaining system will benefit from the system.
5. Open and closed issues exist in the bargaining situation.

The political process model assumes that the consultant has four major functions:

1. Defining and legitimizing the problem—*problem creation*
2. Raising the problem as a priority to get action within the consultee agency—*priority raising*
3. Legitimating or redefining the problem to arrive at problem resolution or continued bargaining—*legitimation*
4. Creating and sustaining interagency linkage—*interagency linkages*

For example, a staff nurse in the local public health department may have noticed a number of alcoholics among her caseload. She requests and is given permission to call in a member of the local alcoholism council to assist her in finding data that will show alcoholism to be a major local problem (problem creation). The consultant is asked by the staff nurse (consultee) to present the facts and alternative actions to the agency administration (priority raising). The administration has ignored the need for an alcohol abuse program for years because the administration's philosophy is that alcoholism is a social problem and not a health problem. The consultant presents data to indicate the nature of alcoholism and the health-related problems (legitimation) and suggests a joint program to be sponsored by the health department and the alcoholism council (interagency linkage). The political process model is viewed as a process more applicable to the community client than to the individual or family client where interagency linkage may not be an issue. The process model and the political process model are similar in scope, and each may be equally applicable in community health nursing depending on the nature of the client.

Four models have been reviewed to offer an overview of consultation: the process consultation model, the purchase model, the doctor-patient model, and the political process model. The remaining discussion will focus on the process consultation model and its application in community health nursing.

PRINCIPLES OF PROCESS CONSULTATION

Process consultation involves "a set of activities on the part of the consultant which assists the client (consultee) to perceive, understand, and act on events occurring in the clients' environment" (Schein, 1969, p. 9). The process consultation model parallels the nursing process by requiring the assessing, planning, implementing, and evaluating of a problem through mutual interaction between client and consultant. The application of this model requires appropriate identification of the client, definition of the problem by client and consultant, and the choice of a technique to be employed by the consultant for the attainment of problem resolution. The analysis and synthesis of the process consultation model by Blake and Mouton (1976) serves as the basis for discussion and application of this model.

Client Population

One of the most important decisions a consultant makes before accepting or writing a consultative contract is to identify the client in the situation. Clients of the community health nurse consultant may be individuals, a family, a group within the agency, a community group, or a community organization. The client is determined by identifying who in the situation has the problem and needs to change. For example, the staff nurse at the district health department is resistant to working in the family planning clinic because of religious beliefs about abortion and contraception. The state community health nurse consultant may negotiate a consultative contract with the staff nurse to deal with her feelings and to arrive at alternative methods for problem resolution. It would not serve any purpose for the consultant to contract with the director of nursing or the nursing supervisor to solve a staff nurse's personal problem. Contracts with management may serve to make the staff nurse more resistant to her assigned duties.

As a second example, a school health nurse consultant receives an inquiry from the school board about ways to get parents to support the visual and hearing screening programs of the schools. The nurse consultant decides that the consultative contract needs to include representatives of the school board and representatives of the parent group to find effective answers to the issue question. The nurse consultant realizes that time would be wasted and resistance to change would still be present if she focuses on only one group at a time. For example, if the nurse meets separately with the parent group, they may decide the school board should employ someone to do the screening. At the school board meeting the consultant may find that the school board does not have the money to employ persons to do all of the screening but may be willing to employ one person to coordinate the parents' efforts. Although expending much energy meeting with both groups separately, the nurse consultant finds that by becoming a messenger between the two factions rather than a facilitator for problem resolution, the consultant role has been diluted.

Intervention Modes

Blake and Mouton (1976) describe five basic intervention modes or techniques that can be applied to the process consultation model: acceptant, catalytic, confrontation, prescriptive, and theory-principles. The *acceptant intervention mode* is defined as a process of catharsis intended to clear emotional blockages in order to engage in more objective problem solving. The use of this intervention mode to solve problems benefits the client by improving self-acceptance, spontaniety, emotional health, appropriate situational emotional responses, and the ability to objectively define and deal with problem situations. The disadvantages of the intervention mode are described as twofold. The cathartic process may assist the client in accepting the circumstances leading to the problem rather than in taking actions to correct the problem, and the emotional catharsis may be viewed by others as a hostile and aggressive act (Blake and Mouton, 1976). For example, Jane, the staff nurse, in interaction with the consultant, may realize that she is not motivated to increase her output because she never gets positive reinforcement from her supervisor. However, she may not wish to change the situation because of reluctance to discuss the problem with the supervisor. Conversely, Jane may learn to be assertive and show the supervisor evidence of quality client care during the supervisor-nurse evaluation conference. The supervisor may interpret Jane's behavior as aggressive and out of character and may penalize the nurse further with a poor evaluation.

When the acceptant intervention mode is being used, the consultant will engage in the following activities:

1. Attempt to understand the client's feelings about the situation.
2. Listen actively.
3. Encourage the client to talk.
4. Try to clarify the client's feelings and help the client to accept the feelings.
5. Refrain from agreeing or disagreeing with the client's situation.
6. Encourage the client to explore ways of dealing with the problem.
7. Listen for more data to reveal the total scope of the problem.

The *catalytic intervention mode* is described as a situation whereby the consultant assists clients to broaden their view of an existing situation by gaining additional information or by unifying existing data (Blake and Mouton, 1976). The consultant assists clients to (1) strengthen perceptions about problems by improving available information, (2) break down barriers to communication by identifying inadequate communication process and procedures, and (3) raise the awareness level of all involved regarding the problem issue. In the catalytic intervention mode the consultant is viewed as a facilitator moving the client toward improving information needed to solve a problem. The lack of information, however, may be the symptom and not the problem, and the resultant disadvantage of having the consultant improve information flow is that the client may rely on the facilitator for the data rather than becoming efficient in finding solutions to future problems (Caplan, 1970; Blake and Mouton, 1976).

In the local public health department the director of nurses received resignations from all of the nursing staff members on the home health care team. The director called the state health department and requested that the home health nurse consultant be sent to provide assistance in problem identification and resolution. The nurse consultant planned interviews with the staff nurses to determine the cause of the resignations. After sharing the information with the director, a staff meeting was called so the director could discuss problems with the staff and suggest solutions to the problems. The consultant served as a facilitator in the meeting to promote discussion between the staff and the director. After the meeting the consultant assisted the director in analyzing the content of the meeting. Three months later a related communication problem occurred with the same group. Rather than seek causes of the problem, the director phoned for the consultant to return to find the causes and solutions.

When the catalytic intervention mode is employed, the consultant will take the following actions:

1. Set a nonauthoritarian tone for the interaction by beginning the intervention with social conversation.
2. Ask the client to describe the situation and use the description as the basis for the interaction.
3. Suggest data-gathering techniques that may provide new information of interest to the client.
4. Provide support to the client as the client attempts to accurately perceive the problem.
5. Avoid specific suggestions for problem solving or resolution.
6. Encourage the client to make decisions about problem resolution.

The *confrontation intervention mode* serves to "present the client with facts that reveal the client's values and assumptions in ways that are undeniable and indisputable" (Blake and Mouton, 1976, p. 288). This intervention mode provides clients with an objective look at how their values and beliefs control their behavior. By looking at present behavior, the consultant can examine, with the client, alternative values to redirect behavior towards more conducive methods of problem solving. The disadvantage to this mode is the client may not wish to participate in interactions that may be interpreted as criticism (Blake and Mouton, 1976).

In the previous example the consultant may have found that the staff nurses were all going to resign from their positions because they viewed all of the director's decisions as autocratic and uncompromising. On the second visit to the agency the consultant may confront the director with these observations of the director's behavior. The director may deny the existence of the behavior and point out evidence of having been democratic. As a result of the confrontation the director may either regard the consultant's observations as a personal affront or be willing to examine and analyze the discrepancies between the perceived and the actual behavior.

Activities of consultants engaged in confrontation interventions will include the following:

1. Continually question clients about their description of the situation.
2. Present data and logic to test clients' objectivity.
3. Challenge clients' chosen courses of action.
4. Probe for motives and causes of present situation.
5. Provide own thoughts about situations without personally attacking clients' values.

The *prescriptive intervention mode* requires less collaboration between consultant and client because in this mode the consultant explicitly tells the client how to solve the problem (Blake and Mouton, 1976). To adhere to the interaction goal of process consultation, the prescriptive mode is best used in conjunction with other intervention modes such as acceptant or catalytic. If clients do not participate in problem resolution, they will not be able to solve future problems and may not adhere to the prescriptions offered. The advantage of the prescriptive intervention mode is its applicability in situations where clients have lost confidence in their ability to solve problems or have given up in despair (Blake and Mouton, 1976).

The nurse consultant has decided the best method of dealing with the problems between the home health staff and the director is to present a prescription for behavioral conduct to be implemented by the director and the staff. The consultant tells the group when and how follow-up evaluation will be conducted to look at the progress of both parties in resolving their differences.

When prescriptive interventions are necessary, the consultant will take the following steps:

1. Probe for data about the client's situation.
2. Act authoritatively.
3. Control by telling the client how the problem is to be perceived.
4. Tell the client the best solutions.
5. Remind the client if the client procrastinates in implementing actions.
6. Offer praise if client does exactly what the consultant wants done.

Use of the *theory-principles intervention mode* requires the client to be taught theories, such as behavioral theory, and the application to problem solving. This intervention mode allows for the introduction of the theories after clients have shared their usual methods of problem solving. It also provides for the application of the theories to problem situations by the client and for opportunities to develop client skills in problem diagnosis and resolution through theory application. The major problem with this intervention mode is determining how to help the client internalize use of the theory for practical application, thus removing the abstract connotation that theories usually hold (Blake and Mouton, 1976).

Before using prescriptions with the home health staff and director, the consultant may present a conference on leadership theories and principles as well as a discussion of the inherent responsibilities in administrative decision making. The consultant may be able to show both parties that leadership styles should vary with the type of decisions to be made and with the people who are to be affected by the decision.

The consultant using theory-principles intervention will proceed as follows:

1. Introduce theories for problem solving to the client.
2. Use techniques to assist the client to internalize theories.
3. Provide strategies for practical application of theories, such as simulated problem situations or critiques of applications.
4. Offer support when the theory is applied in the actual problem situation.

Determinants of Intervention Modes

The use of a particular intervention mode is decided by two factors: (1) the client and (2) the problem. Blake and Mouton (1976) have identified four categories of problem issues: *power/authority, morale/cohesion, norms/standards,* and *goals/objectives.* Several of the intervention modes may be used with each of the problem issues.

The power/authority issue becomes a question of who has the right to be in charge (boss) and who has the right to make decisions. The morale/cohesion problem occurs when the client has lost confidence in ability to solve problems and feels powerless to institute corrective action. The norms/standards problems occur when group norms, professional or organizational standards, are violated or changed. Problems related to goals/objectives usually involve the establishing of new goals, changing of goals, or the inability to meet goals/objectives.

Several of the intervention modes may be used with each of the problem issues. When the consultant is trying to decide which intervention mode to use, the client and the nature of the problem must be considered. Although there are exceptions, when the problem with a client is identified as a morale/cohesion problem or a power/authority issue the most common intervention may be the acceptant mode because the issue generally elicits feelings that block action in decision making; when a norms/standards or goals/objectives problem is the issue, the *catalytic mode* may be the choice to strengthen the client's perceptions of the most effective decision-making methods. The theory-principles intervention mode may be helpful regardless of the problem, especially when additional insights are needed. However, the prescriptive mode may not be helpful unless the client is unable to cope with the situation and needs immediate direction or answers to solve the problem.

The Consultative Contract

By nature the consultative relationship is based on expectations. The consultant has expectations concerning time, reimbursement, resources, and the participation of the client in the process. Clients have expectations about what they will gain from the consultant relationship. Although nurses do not usually contract for their services, it is becoming commonplace for consultants to have written contracts. The discussion of the terms of the contract makes expectations more explicit, reduces the likelihood of violations of contract terms, and reduces the risk of additional demands being made on either party. Kolb & Frohmen (1970) and Sedgwick (1973) have identified areas that should be included in the written consultative contract: (1) the goals of client and consultant; (2) the identified problem; (3) the consultant's resources; (4) the time commitment; (5) limitations of the contract; (6) cost; (7) conditions under which the contract may be broken or renegotiated; (8) intervention mode to be used; (9) expected benefits for the client; (10) methods of data collection to be used; (11) client resources; (12) potential interventions; and (13) methods of evaluation of the interaction. Appendix F contains an example of a consultation contract that may be used to establish a consultant-consultee relationship.

Writing a contract for consultative relationships has a number of advantages. The contract terms assist the consultant in determining the number of hours that must be devoted to the interaction and assist the consultant in identifying needed resources and out-of-pocket expenses required to complete the interaction. Negotiation of the contract assists the client in identifying realistic expectations of the consultant and firmly establishes what the consultant will and will not do. The client has the opportunity during the negotiation to place limits on what the consultant can do, and the contract allows for future renegotiation of terms.

Consultation Phases

The process of consultation involves seven basic phases:

1. Initial contact with the client
2. Definition of the relationship
3. Selection of a setting and approach
4. Collection of data and problem diagnoses
5. Intervention
6. Reduction of involvement and evaluation
7. Termination

The initial contact is made when the client or someone in a family, group, or community communicates with the consultant about a potential problem that requires intervention. The communication may be person to person during a home visit, may be written, or may occur by telephone. On initial contact the client and the consultant have an exploratory meeting to define the problem, assess the consultant's ability to help, assess the consultant's interest, and formulate future actions.

If the consultant decides at the initial meeting that the real client has been identified, the terms of the relationship will be discussed. The consultant will be interested in finding out what the client expects to gain from the relationship, and the consultant will establish terms for the interaction.

Finally, in the initial exploratory meeting the setting for the consultation will be decided on, the time schedule will be set, the goals of the interaction will be established, and the mode of intervention will be chosen.

When the terms of the contract are agreed on, the data gathering methods will be a part of the agreement. The consultant may find it essential to gather more data before finalizing the diagnosis of the problem. Data gathering methods used by consultants include direct observation, individual and group interviews, use of questionnaires or surveys, and tape recordings.

While data are being gathered as well as after the diagnosis has been finalized, the consultant will be actively engaged in the intervention mode chosen for the interaction.

Upon fulfillment of the terms of the contract, the consultant must be concerned with disengagement or reducing the amount of involvement of the consultant with the client. The disengagement process requires mutual agreement between consultant and consultee that involvement should be reduced. The amount of continuing involvement desired should be checked at varying intervals during the consultative relationship. It is at these points that contract renegotiation may take place. Determinants of continued involvement include, but are not limited to, the client's willingness to continue, value of the interaction for client and consultant, and situational changes that have resulted. Before termination the number of contacts between consultant and consultee should be decreased. The continued but decreased contacts will allow each party to evaluate the effectiveness of the intervention. During the disengagement period the consultant reassures the client that future interactions are possible at the client's discretion. When the agreed-on time for disengagement has passed, the relationship is terminated (Blake and Mouton, 1976; Schein, 1969; Sedgwick, 1973). As a component of the disengagement and termination phases of the consultative process, the consultant typically provides the consultee with a written summary of the findings and recommendations resulting from the interaction.

As with any formal interaction, there are three stages of consultation which encompass the several phases previously described. The three stages are trust-building, which includes the initial contact, definition of the relationship, and selection of the setting and intervention approach; problem solving, which involves gathering data, formalizing the problem, and intervening; and closure, which involves disengagement and termination (Stevens, 1978; Norris, 1977).

Examples of Consultation

Five examples of consultative interactions modes are outlined as follows:

Intervention: prescriptive
Client: Director of Nursing
Consultant: internal
Problem: norms/standards

The client telephones the state nursing consultant and requests a meeting in the local health unit. The purpose of the meeting is to review the serious problems the local nursing staff is having in meeting program goals and requirements as identified in a recent program audit. The consultant, Elizabeth, met with the client, Maggie, and reviewed her findings, sharing her analysis of problems and causative factors. The central problem issue was defined as inconsistent supervision of staff with a need for definitive role clarification of supervisory responsibilities. Maggie was immobilized by the situa-

tion. Elizabeth directed Maggie to restructure the supervisory job descriptions to clearly reflect supervisory roles and expectations and to give supervisors written performance evaluations and guidelines for improving staff performance.

Elizabeth maintained contact with Maggie until termination of the consultation occurred as corrective action was completed.

Intervention: acceptant
Client: staff nurse
Consultant: internal
Problem: morale/cohesion

Elizabeth received a phone call from staff nurse Susan requesting a meeting to discuss problems that Susan was experiencing in her job situation. Susan was obviously under stress as evidenced by the immediacy of the requested need for the meeting. Susan talked about her perceived inability to communicate with administration, the impact of her feelings on her ability to function, and her feelings of being out of control in the job situation. Susan had decided that resignation was her only alternative. Elizabeth listened and provided a nonthreatening opportunity for Susan to verbalize freely. Elizabeth did not agree or disagree with Susan's perceptions of the job situation or respond to her direct question about resignation. Elizabeth focused on Susan's perceived problems with the job and her feelings about her performance. She then attempted to clarify events described by Susan and keep events in perspective. Finally, Elizabeth explored with Susan ways in which she might facilitate communication with administration. Ultimately Susan decided to choose resignation as the problem solution.

Intervention: theory-principles
Client: community group
Consultant: external
Problem: goals/objectives

Josie was contacted as a consultant by a representative of a local community hospital. The hospital staff and the pediatrician had expressed concern about child neglect problems the hospital was seeing and about the lack of information many mothers seemingly had about basic child care. Josie, acting as a facilitator, recognized that the problem involved not only the single community hospital but the two other community hospitals, and the county department of social services, the health department, and the county home extension office. These groups were identified by Josie as having the potential to influence the identified health issue.

Josie contacted and requested a representative from each of the involved agencies to be present at a planning meeting. At the initial meeting Josie, acting as a resource, presented the magnitude of the infant morbidity and mortality problem of the local county, presented data for 3 years regarding the causes of infant mortality, and raised the issue of preventive intervention through a hospital discharge system. Hospitalization and discharge of the newborn were identified as prime times to provide parents with information on basic child care and local resources. The client group believed that educational materials currently provided to hospitals for use with new parents was not designed for the level of understanding of many parents in a rural multi-income-level area.

The decision was made by the group to develop a county-specific, newborn hospital discharge packet that was easily understandable and provided county-specific resource information. Through a series of five or six meetings the group reviewed and selected the most significant principles from an extensive literature review and applied them to their identified local health issue. They subsequently developed a discharge planning model with community-wide applicability. During disengagement the group renegotiated with Josie to evaluate the application of the model at the end of a 3-month period.

Intervention: confrontation
Client: departmental group
Consultant: internal
Problem: power/authority

The Director of Nursing solicited consultation for assisting the health department program supervisors to assume management-supervisory responsibility for their staff. The lack of management responsibility was having a domino effect on program standards, fiscal accountability, and nursing practice standards. In an initial meeting with the director, the consultant determined that the client was the supervisory group, not the Director of Nursing.

The consultant then met individually with supervisors to ascertain their perceptions of administration's expectations in the area of program management. The consultant through the use of client care findings on a record audit and an audit of staff evaluations revealed the managerial problems related to each supervisor. Reasons offered by the supervisors for lack of involvement in management functions were excessive caseload, lack of clear understanding of their management functions, the expectations of administration, and insecurity in management techniques.

The consultant met with the supervisors as a group. At this point the consultant reviewed specifically the management tasks for which the supervisors would be held responsible by administration and reviewed the organizational structure and the line authority held by each supervisor. The consultant also reviewed their caseloads and the amount of projected time they needed to perform managerial functions. The consultant-client relationship was to be continued monthly for a minimum period of 6 months at which time the contract would be renegotiated or terminated.

Intervention: catalytic
Client: community agency
Consultant: external
Problem: goals/objectives

The consultant was contacted by the Family Practice Center to discuss the issue of adolescent pregnancy problems in the county and the Family Practice Center's involvement in providing an adolescent maternity service clinic within a residency training program. A meeting was scheduled at which time the nurse consultant presented adolescent pregnancy data for the county, outlined the local health department's role in adolescent prenatal services and the current adolescent prenatal caseload, and provided data by which to project the caseload and service demands the adolescent clinic would be expected to meet. The center staff, health department staff, and consultant made a site visit to observe an adolescent prenatal clinic at another medical center.

As a result of several additional meetings the consultant was able to negotiate a collaborative arrangement between the health department and the Family Practice Center. The services to be provided included short-term nursing education, social work, and nutrition support services. The consultant assumed the facilitator role and continually clarified the ongoing developmental and agency commitments (goals) in this collaborative effort. The adolescent prenatal clinic was initiated with the aid of the short-term commitments that grew out of the interagency relationships. After the clinic was established, health department services were withdrawn and replaced by the Family Practice Center staff as scheduled. The consultant's relationship continued for approximately 6 months and was terminated after meeting a request from the center staff for evaluation.

THE NURSE CONSULTANT

As previously indicated, nurse consultants in the community health setting may function as internal consultants employed on a full-time basis by an organization for the purpose of facilitating the staff in problem solving; or nurses may be employed as external consultants with a contractual arrangement to assist an individual, group, or community organization to find solutions to existing problems. Nurses may provide consultation for a wide range of issues related to community health nursing or they may narrow their scope of expertise and provide consultation only in an identified area of specialty. The following discussion focuses on the differences in the internal and external consultant, the generalist versus the specialist, the sources of conflict in the role, and the effect funding sources have on the availability of consultation.

The Internal Nurse Consultant Generalist

The delivery system of a health agency will determine the specific framework in which a consultant functions. An agency whose delivery system is structured along the lines of an official generalized community health service will more likely employ a consultant who provides traditional or comprehensive community health nursing consultation within a broad range of community health activities.

A study of generalist nurse consultants by Stetler and Downs (1974) showed that official community agencies often require nurse consultants to function in dual roles, such as supervisor-consultant. The dual role functions of the consultant result in ambiguity for the staff nurse and the consultant. Role strain may result when neither the staff nurse nor the consultant knows which hat the consultant should wear in a given situation. Role stress occurs from conflict in defining role expectations and because the consultant may be experiencing *role overload* or may lack time to carry out all *role obligations*.

The generalist consultant tends to experience role conflict when the agency moves into the provision of more specialized areas of primary care. The conflict occurs when the demands of agency staff in specialized skill areas, like pediatrics, exceed the expertise of the generalized consultant. Conflicts also evolve from different role expectations between the administrator and the nurse consultant.

Specialist

A community health agency which provides a programmatic approach or specialized approach to the delivery of community health services, such as family planning, maternity, child health, crippled children services, school health, and home health, to name a few, will tend to employ specialized consultants who may, in addition to broad community health expertise, have skills and specialized training in a primary clinical area, e.g.,the clinical nurse specialist in pediatrics.

The degree to which the agency is involved in specific primary care areas influences the use of the specialized consultant. Agencies providing primary health care require a consultant with a broad knowledge of community health practice as well as specialized knowledge in a clinical area. This is also a requirement in agencies involved in long-term and home health care. The specialist nurse consultant functioning within a programmatic framework, by virtue of the agency's expectations and the consultant's functional expertise, generally tends to be less involved in the administrative aspects of the program. This factor offers the potential for conflict. The consultant is expected to provide the clinical expertise to community health nursing staff and to have nursing input into administrative and programmatic development of policies, guidelines, and procedures. The conflict arises when administrative priorities differ from community health nursing practice priorities.

Despite the conflict potential existing within this delivery framework, a nurse consultant with management and administrative preparation and/or background is able to function effectively while also representing community health nursing practice. The sources for role stress and strain for the specialist are similar to those of the generalist consultant. Role ambiguity and role overload are often the results of the role expectations, as defined for the consultant, by the administration and the nursing staff.

Role Functions and Expectations

The community health nurse consultant employed within an official health agency functions as an internal consultant to the employing agency and provides nursing and community health consultation to nurses at all levels, other disciplines, agency administration, and other health and human service agencies and/or community groups as a representative of the agency.

Two primary roles of the internal consultant are resource person and facilitator (Pati, 1980). Both roles emerge from the accessibility of the consultant to all aspects of the agency and community. The degree of accessibility is enhanced or diminished by the place the consultant fits in the organizational structure of the agency. For example, the consultant may hold a line position with responsibility to the nursing director and authority over staff nurses; or the consultant may hold an advisory position to the nursing director without direct authority over the staff.

The resource role has traditionally been associated with the community health nurse consultant both within and outside of the official health agency. With the advent in the last decade of new and varied health delivery models within communities, the resource role has assumed increased significance. The community health consultant with knowledge of available resources can identify deficiencies and gaps in service, identify the critical components provided by the myriad of health delivery systems, and promote the interface of these systems in meeting health or social needs of the population.

With the shrinking health dollars of the 1980s, the facilitator role of the community health consultant has assumed renewed significance. The facilitator role of the consultant has been described at length throughout this chapter. The nurse consultant as a facilitator assists staff nurses, administration, groups, and organizations to solve problems relating to the needs of clients, staff, or the organization. Performing the facilitator function, the consultant will guide the staff nurse in solving problems about individual client and family health needs, health needs of a group of clients, or professional concerns and attitudes. The consultant may assist supervisors, managers, directors, and administrators to solve problems about personnel matters, program needs, organizational goals, community relationships, and client population needs. The consultant may also facilitate communications between the employing agency and facilities or other health providers in the community.

Conflict Sources

The internal consultant as a representative of the employing agency has implied authority that may present conflict between the consultant and consultee. The degree of conflict may be determined by centralization or decentralization of the health agency and the degree of autonomy of the individual units in the organizational structure. The administrative or managerial strength of the individual unit can also determine the role the consultant may assume and, to a large measure, determine the involvement of the consultant in an implementation role. One means of negating potential conflict is to clearly define the role the consultant is to assume. A consultant functioning within an agency that is strongly controlled by a central unit will tend to be more actively involved in an implementation role, such as supervisor. For example, in one state the state health department has jurisdiction over all county health departments throughout the state (centralized). The state has decided to make each county health department autonomous in their delivery of health services to the county (decentralized). The state health department will continue to provide advice to the county units about delivery of services but will not supervise the delivery of care. Nursing in the county units will have its own directors and the nursing consultants at the state level will be utilized as resource persons and facilitators offering information and advice to the county units in matters requiring problem solving. While the state health department was centralized and provided direct supervision to the counties for delivery of health care, the state family planning consultant was also responsible for supervising the county health department staff members who were responsible for delivery of family planning services.

Role Relationships

The consultant's role with nursing administration and staff is determined by the organizational structure. The internal consultant is generally responsible to and strongly influenced by nursing administration and agency administration. The nursing administration's framework for nursing practice, goals for nursing service, and the role the consultant is to assume should be clearly defined before employment. Who is responsible for nursing practice with commensurate authority should be clearly defined for the consultant, the supervising staff, and the staff nurses. The internal consultant by virtue of staff level alignment has no formal authority but informally will have inherent responsibility for making changes in nursing practice (Kohnke, 1978). The perception of the staff regarding the consultant's alignment to administration, as "eyes and ears" of administration, no doubt is a factor in the staff's relationship to the consultant. The degree to which this is true is dependent upon the consultant/consultee relationship developed and established by the consultant.

Kohnke suggested that as the bureaucracy has ex-

panded since the 1960s, the supervising framework of nursing practice has shifted from clinical supervisor to administrator. This shift of the supervisor's functional responsibilities toward the administrative role has resulted in a diminution or void in clinical nursing supervision (Kohnke, 1978).

A similar situation can be described for the consultant. The dual supervisor-consultant role with its inherent problems were described by Stetler and Downs (1975) in a research project conducted in a state public health system. *Supervision* denotes line responsibility (authority) with active involvement in decision making and implementation activities in an ongoing relationship, which is the very antithesis of consultation. It can be seen that the supervising role functions could usurp the consultative role parameters and the staff could perceive the supervisor/consultant as being directly aligned with administration. Stetler and Downs (1975) stated that communication is vital in this dual role.

A plethora of allied health professionals are functioning within community health practice: clinical social workers, nutritionists, occupational therapists, physical therapists, health educators, home economists, and home health aides. The community health nurse and the allied health providers share mutual skills and commitment to community health practice and provide specific professional skills to mutual clients, to families, and to each other. The nurse consultant provides consultation to the allied health provider and serves as a resource and content person to these professionals in the areas of community health nursing practice. The nurse consultant, in a facilitator role, can enhance the efficient use of other health providers and often circumvent "turf" issues. The consultant's broad knowledge base and multidisciplinary approach to health care helps to determine the effective use of allied health providers and also promotes more efficient use of nursing manpower.

Funding Implications

Categorical funding mechanisms within the last decade have promoted in some agencies the position of specialist consultant within community health departments. Title X of the *Social Security Act* included provisions for funding of family planning services. This funding mechanism is one example of how a federally funded community health service promoted the use of specialist consultants within a specific area of community health care. The funding mechanism gave rise to use of the family planning nurse practitioner. To meet the agency needs, consultants with special skills and expertise in reproductive health were employed by official health agencies. Similarly, Title V of the *Social Security Act* provided funding that traditionally focused on more generalized services to mothers and children and has brought about use of the crippled children nurse consultant and the school health nurse consultant. The Medicare funding for home health care in 1965 gave rise to the home health services consultant with community skills in medical and surgical nursing practice.

The impact of state block grant funding and the move of some health agencies from programmatic to a more integrated service delivery framework will effect the role and use of nursing consultants in official community health agencies. The competition for limited health dollars, the increasing focus on the at-risk population, and the anticipated surplus of physician manpower are going to affect, with a potential emphasis on hiring generalist consultants, the specialist versus generalist consultant role in official health agencies.

The External Nurse Consultant
Role Functions and Expectations

When the community health nurse consultant is contacted by an agency or organization other than the employing agency, the consultant is considered an outsider to the organization and as such an external consultant. Again, the external nurse consultant acts as a facilitator or a resource person using one or a combination of the approaches described throughout the chapter. The external nurse consultant may serve as a representative of the employing agency and provide information to the consultee for the planning of interagency programs to meet population needs. The external nurse consultant may serve as a resource to health educators, health planners, school personnel, psychologists, audiologists, counselors, dentists, social workers, physicians, legislators, and probation officers providing data about individual client, group, or community needs.

The external consultant may be asked to serve as a facilitator to an agency board, such as a health planning board, to solve problems about community health priorities. Similarly the consultant may be asked to serve as a facilitator or resource person to a voluntary agency, such as the American Red Cross or the American Heart Association.

Consultants from federal agencies are often used in community health as external nurse consultants. The nurse consultant from the federal agency may come to the local or state agency, on request, to serve as facilitator or resource person relative to program planning, development, and implementation. The primary role function of this consultant is to serve as a resource person although the consultant may facilitate movement toward identifying actual program parameters.

Conflict Sources

The external consultant, an outsider to the client agency, has only assumed authority that may present conflict for the consultant and the consultee (Polk, 1980). Since the consultant is external to the consultee situation, upon exit from the agency the consultee may not feel impelled to implement actions agreed on by consultant and consultee. In many instances the consultant may hold a role complementary to the consultee, such as community health nurse consultant to the school health nurse.

Although equal sharing and input should be the motto of a consultant-consultee relationship, conflict may arise if the school nurse interprets the community nurse consultant's involvement as an invasion of space. One means of preventing potential conflicts is to clearly establish the terms of the contract for the consultant-consultee interaction. For example, the community health nurse consultant is called by the school health nurse. The school nurse needs input from the consultant regarding development and implementation of a health education program for sexually transmitted diseases. The terms of the contract stipulate that the consultant will provide input on *how* to develop and implement the program and the school health nurse will actually *do* the work for the program. Thus the consultant is not involved in the program and the school nurse's turf is protected. The consultative relationship is also on a time-limited basis. The consultant may not have enough time to identify all variables in the situation to arrive at a diagnosis of the real problem. The consultee may be frustrated in attempts to make changes suggested by the consultant and may meet resistance because the real problem did not surface during the consultant-consultee interaction.

Role Relationships

The role relationships of the external consultant with groups or individuals are determined by the client (individual or group). The principles and process of consultation are the same for either the internal or external consultative functional framework. The external consultant was previously defined in this chapter, and the roles are the same as the roles of the internal consultant, that is, facilitator and resource.

One of the principal differences between the internal and the external consultant is the time constraint for the consultant to assimilate data for problem identification.

Funding Implications

As federal, state, local, and private funding becomes more competitive, fewer external nurse consultants will be available. If an external consultant is used, costs for the consulting services must be built into the consultee's budget. Such future limited funds may be reserved for program implementation rather than for the luxury of contracting with consultants. Although all external nurse consultants do not receive direct reimbursement for their services, such as the consultants acting as agency representatives, the needs of the employing agency for internal consultation may become greater and the agency may not be willing to pay, either in time or travel, for the consultant to be away from the organization.

EDUCATIONAL REQUIREMENTS

The educational requirements for the community health nurse consultant are primarily determined by two factors: the practice setting and the client population. The community health nurse with undergraduate preparation may serve as a generalist nurse consultant to individuals, families, and groups of clients with an identified health problem like hypertension or diabetes. The consultant serves either as a facilitator to seek problem resolution or as a resource to provide for community referral. This nurse may also consult with other health provider agencies involved with client groups such as the hospital, the ambulatory hypertensive clinic, the private physician, and the physical therapist.

The community health nurse consultant described in the preceding pages, however, has graduate preparation with a generalist or specialist clinical and functional focus and has expert knowledge in the application of theories of change, group, systems, interaction, motivation, communications, behavior, management, and epidemiology. In-depth knowledge is needed in family and individual development, advocacy, and health and nursing issues (Kohnke, 1978). This nurse may be an internal or external consultant serving as an expert resource person or as a facilitator to the client groups previously identified.

PRACTICE ARENAS

The nurse who wishes to become a consultant will find employment opportunities with governmental agencies: federal, state, and local; with private enterprise and philanthropic organizations; and with voluntary and professional organizations.

The federal government employs nurse consultants in many branches of the Public Health Service. The Division of Nursing of the Health Resources Administration employs a group of nurse consultants to serve as resource persons for education. The Health Care Financing Administration employs nurse consultants to serve as resource persons for programs such as home

health. Many state health departments employ clinical specialist consultants who serve as facilitators and resource persons to local health departments regarding program needs, such as child health. State health departments also employ clinical nurse consultants to serve as resource persons to such agencies as schools and rehabilitation centers. Local city, county, or district health departments employ nurse consultants, usually generalists, who facilitate staff members in meeting client and program needs.

Private organizations use the expertise of nurses in consultation with clients (purchasers of services) of the organization (Koch, 1979). Publishing and audiovisual equipment companies often employ nurses who serve as resources and facilitators for persons who are interested in writing or developing audiovisuals for sale or for persons who require assistance in the use of goods purchased from the companies. Pharmaceutical companies and health care supply and equipment companies employ nurse consultants for similar purposes.

Private philanthropic organizations, such as the Robert Wood Johnson Foundation, may use nurse consultants to serve as resource persons for health care or education programs funded by the organizations; professional organizations, such as ANA and NLN, offer nurse consulting services to clinical agencies, for example, home health, and to educational institutions who require assistance in setting program standards or in readying themselves for accreditation review.

An employment arena that is becoming more popular to nurse consultants is the private consulting firm. The private health care consulting firms, numbering over 200 in the nation's capital alone, exist to offer assistance to individuals, groups, institutions, and government organizations in such matters as setting health care priorities; writing goals, standards, policies, and procedures; developing better managerial solutions for program efficiency; and planning health care programs. Nurses may even incorporate for the purpose of providing services directed toward nursing issues (Rafferty and Carner, 1973; Wright, 1981).

Similarly, voluntary organizations, for example, the American Red Cross, may employ nurses to serve as resource persons in the development of local programs such as blood banks, and the World Health Organization may employ nurses to serve as resource and facilitator to third world countries in the development of health care programs. Community health nurses are prepared to meet the challenges of these employment arenas because of their expertise in comprehensive client assessment and in program development and evaluation and their extensive knowledge of the use of available resources.

SUMMARY

This chapter has outlined and discussed the definition of consultation, consultation theory, principles of process consultation, intervention modes, determinants of intervention modes, client populations, various frameworks for nurse consultation, academic preparation, and practice arenas for nurse consultants. The practical application of the consultative process in community health is reflected in the varied practice situations inherent in this chapter with consultative intervention reflected in community health practice outcomes.

Kohnke (1978) described the availability of nursing consultation as a serious issue. Nursing administration's acceptance of this concept is a critical component of nursing practice. With continually diminishing health dollars and the focus on fiscal accountability, the cost effectiveness of nursing consultation will no doubt be studied and become an added dimension to the acceptance and use of nurse consultation.

BIBLIOGRAPHY

Anders, R.: Program consultation by a clinical specialist, Nur. Adm. **8**(11):34-38, Nov. 1978.

Baizerman, M., and Hall, W.: Consultation as a political process, Community Ment. Health J. **13**(2):142-149, 1977.

Blake, R., and Mouton, J.: Consultation, Reading, Mass., 1976, Addison-Wesley Publishing Co., Inc.

Caplan, G.: The theory and practice of mental health consultation, New York, 1970, Basic Books, Inc., Publishers.

Covent, A.B.: Community mental health nursing: the role of the consultant in the nursing home, J. Psychiatr. Nur. **17**(7):15-19, July 1979.

Dean, L.P.: The change from functional to primary nursing, Nur. Clin. North Am. **14**(2):357-364, June 1979.

Everly, G.S., Jr., and Girdano, D.A.: The health educator as industrial health consultant, Health Educ. **10**(4):11-13, July/Aug. 1979.

Hendrix, M. and LaGodna, G.: Consultation: a political process aimed at change. In Lancaster, J., and Lancaster, W., Concepts for advanced nursing practice: the nurse as a change agent, St. Louis, 1982, the C.V. Mosby Co.

Keithley, J.E., Shelley, S., and Benner, J.A.: Help at hand: using the nurse consultant, Nursing '79. **9**(11):105-112, Nov. 1979.

Koch, M.: Moving ahead, Nursing '79. 72-73, July 1979.

Kohnke, M.: The case for consultation in nursing: design for professional practice, New York, 1978, John Wiley & Sons.

Kolb, D., and Frohman, A.: An organization development approach to consulting, Sloan Management Rev. **12**(1):51-65, 1970.

Lippitt, R., and Lippitt, G.: Consulting process in action. In Jones, I., and Pfeiffer, J., The 1977 annual handbook for group facilitators, San Diego, Calif., 1977, University Associates, Inc.

Martin, F.A.: The state consultant, Occup. Health Nurs. **23**(2):14-15, Feb. 1975.

Norris, C.: A few notes on consultation, Nurs. Outlook **25**(12):756-761, Dec. 1977.

Pati, B.: Nursing consultation: a collaborative process, J. Nurs. Adm. **10**(11):33-36, Nov. 1980.

Polk, G.: The socialization and utilization of nurse consultants, J. Psychiatr. Nurs. **18**(2):33-36, Feb. 1980.

Rafferty, R., and Carner, J.: Nursing consultants, Inc.: a corporation, Nurs. Outlook, **21**(4):233-235, April 1973.

Sanders, L., Chesley, D., and Kishi, A.: Curriculum consultant, would you help us out? Nurs. Outlook **11**(6):315-321, June 1981.

Schein, E.: Process consultation: its role in organization development, Reading, Mass., 1969, Addison-Wesley Publishing Co., Inc.

Sedgwick, R.: The role of the process consultant, Nurs. Outlook **21**(12):773-774, Dec. 1973.

Slack, P.: Aspects of clinical practice and management, Nurs. Times **76**(11):468-469, March 13, 1980.

Stetler, C. and Downs, C.: The supervisor/consultant: a difficult role, Community Health Adm., Wakefield, Mass., 1975, Contemporary Publishing, Inc.

Stevens, B.: The use of consultants in nursing service, J. Nurs. Adm. **8**(8):7-15, Aug. 1978.

Wallace, S.: Some aspects of consultation and management by objectives, Occup. Health Nurs. **28**:26-30, Oct. 1980.

Walton, R.: Interpersonal peacemaking: confrontation and third party consultation, Reading, Mass., 1969, Addison-Wesley Publishing Co., Inc.

Wright, B.L.: The nurse consultant, Can. Nurse **77**(2):34-36, Feb. 1981.

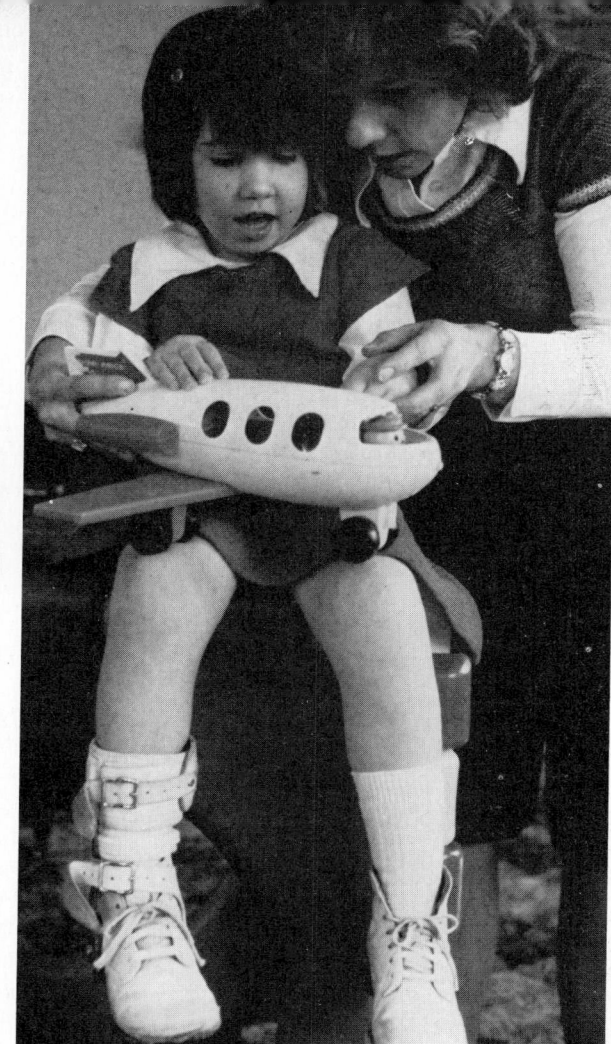

MARGARET MILLSAP

THE DEVELOPMENTALLY DISABLED CHILD AS A COMMUNITY HEALTH TARGET

Providing care for those who are developmentally disabled in our society is a goal that has been emphasized by the federal government for many years. It is a broad goal that encompasses the work of many people in a variety of professions. Only in the last 20 years have we as a people recognized that all individuals, regardless of condition, have all the rights of other individuals. This implies that all people will be treated with dignity and afforded the opportunity of growing, learning, and enjoying the pleasures of a healthy, rewarding life.

Nurses have a responsibility to provide to these people services that have positive impact on communities. The proper use of their knowledge, skill, and concern can provide the leadership needed to improve the quality of life for this population.

The term *developmental disability* refers to a variety of conditions, mental and physical, that interfere with the ability of an individual to function in an acceptable manner in society. Public Law (PL) 95-602 (Comprehensive Rehabilitation Service Amendments of 1978) gives the following definition:

A developmental disability is a severe, chronic disability of a person which:
A. is attributable to a mental or physical impairment or combination of mental and physical impairments;
B. is manifested before the person attains age twenty two;
C. is likely to continue indefinitely;
D. results in substantial limitations in three or more of the following areas of major life activity:
1. self-care
2. receptive and expressive language

3. learning
4. mobility
5. self-direction
6. capacity for independent living
7. economic sufficiency

E. reflects the person's need for a combination and sequence of special, interdisciplinary or generic care, treatment, or the services which are of lifelong or extended duration and are individually planned and coordinated.

This definition has considerably changed the focus of the one previously used by governmental agencies, which specified conditions such as cerebral palsy, mental retardation, autism, and epilepsy. The definition also expanded the age from 18 to 22. This allows for a longer period of help for this population.

Most people who fall within this category are classified as being mentally retarded. A more recent definition of mental retardation approved by the American Association on Mental Deficiency has eliminated those previously diagnosed as having borderline intelligence. This definition has thereby reduced the number of mentally retarded individuals and consequently reduced the total number of the developmentally disabled.

A special report on the impact of the change in the definition of developmental disabilities was prepared by the Office of Human Development Services Administration (May 1981). This report states

There has been a 27% decrease in the estimated total developmental disabilities population, as defined in the 1978 amendments, based on an analysis of the 1980 Developmental Disabilities State Plans. Whereas in FY* 1978 the estimated number of individuals defined as developmentally disabled in the United States was 5,265,846, in FY 1980 the estimated figure was 3,906,913. . . . . .Mental retardation in FY 1980 represented 54.8% of those defined as developmentally disabled, compared with 65.5% in FY 1978. During the same time period, the estimated number of individuals considered developmentally disabled with cerebral palsy increased, with epilepsy decreased, and with autism remaining essentially the same. In addition, individuals with other conditions who are now included within the developmentally disabled target population currently account for almost 12% of the population. There continue to be differences in the population considered to be developmentally disabled. Although the total population estimate in the State plans was almost 4 million developmentally disabled individuals, a study utilizing the developmental disabilities definition in conjunction with the 1976 Survey of Income and Education estimated 2.5 million developmentally disabled individuals.

There is another group referred to as the developmentally disadvantaged, as yet not clearly identified,

* Fiscal year.

but victimized by society. These are the children growing up in deprived homes where they are neglected, abused, and offered little stimulation or encouragement to learn. Many of these children have been placed in programs such as Head Start. The innate ability to learn seems to be there, but the opportunity is lacking. These children are often exploited by their families and peers and erroneously referred to as mentally retarded. Through the interest of private and public programs there is much more hope that these children will develop into productive, well-adjusted adults.

SCOPE OF THE PROBLEM

The problems associated with developmental disabilities are complex, far-reaching, and profound. Despite all the technological and humanistic knowledge abundant today, we do not have the answers. This situation is described by Wallace et al. (1973, p. 931).

In spite of—and in part because of—advances in medical care, the task of meeting the needs of the handicapped is growing larger, not smaller. Reasons for this include the increasing size of the population, our continued inability to control the incidence of many kinds of disabling conditions, the lengthening survival time of disabled newborn infants (even those with catastrophic disabilities), and the increasing expectations coupled with increasing demands for care.

CAUSES OF DEVELOPMENTAL DISABILITIES

Definitive causes for developmental disabilities are difficult to identify in the majority of cases. Etiology is known in only about 25% of the cases. Of this small percentage, the causes are usually categorized as central nervous system damage occurring during the prenatal, perinatal, or postnatal period (spina bifida); intoxication from maternal infection, drugs, or alcohol; chromosomal aberrations (Down's syndrome); metabolic disorders (phenylketonuria); or infections of the newborn (meningitis).

Down's syndrome is the most commonly found chromosomal abnormality. This condition occurs approximately once in every 600 to 650 live births (Whaley and Wong, 1982). Maternal age has been demonstrated to be closely related to the incidence of this condition, which increases remarkably when the woman is past the age of 35.

Spina bifida is the second most common birth defect affecting 1 to 2 infants per 1000 births (Stark, 1977). These children usually have many serious physical and mental problems. Early surgical intervention and infant stimulation programs have improved the outlook for these children. However, treatment is expensive,

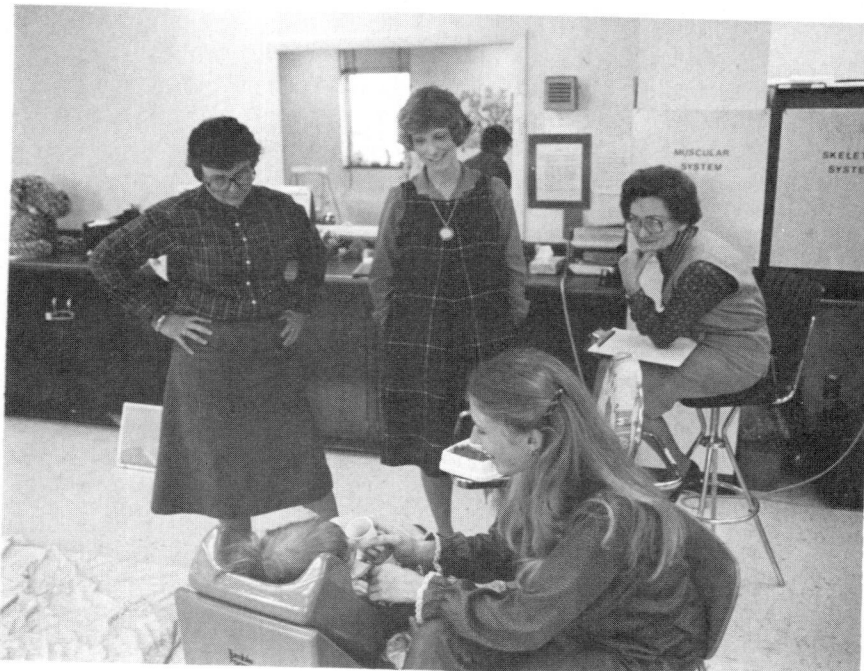

Fig. 30-1. Interdisciplinary team evaluation.

difficult for some families to obtain, and emotionally stressful for the entire family. The constant care, prolonged grief, and financial burden create a tremendous problem for the child and family.

Most children who have spina bifida have normal intelligence, but because of severe physical problems, it is most difficult to find suitable educational programs for them. Consequently, many test out with lower intelligence quotient scores simply because they lacked the opportunity to learn or cannot participate in the educational activities as a result of physical limitations.

Children with minimal brain dysfunction may also fall into the classification of being developmentally disabled because the problems they have affect their ability to function normally in society. Prevalence of this condition is not well documented, but the statistic most frequently quoted is 5% to 10% of the population (Wender, 1973). These children display a variety of symptoms that vary with age and severity of the condition. Wender listed the following symptoms: (1) short attention span, (2) subject to distraction, (3) hyperactivity, (4) impulsiveness, (5) emotional lability, (6) difficulties in coordination, (7) perceptual problems, and (8) impairments of language and symbols.

PRIMARY PREVENTION
Role of Professionals

If effective, preventive measures must begin with education before conception. This is a tremendous task that concerned professionals have been attempting for years. Social behavior, environmental factors, family mores, and moral issues are parts of this complex problem. Technological advances, research, and improved standards of living have contributed to the survival of many and to a longer life span for all of us, yet we continue to have a large number of children who have developmental disabilities.

Application of knowledge and techniques known to be effective would have a great impact on our society. Family planning services, genetic counseling, comprehensive prenatal care, immunizations, decreasing use of drugs and alcohol, and continuing research are all preventive means that need to be used to the fullest extent. It has been predicted that we could reduce the number of developmentally disabled children by one half in the next decade if we applied all the knowledge we have now.

"The aim of professionals who deal with handicapped children and their families is to lessen the susceptibility of such children at risk and to increase their sense of mastery and competence" (Waechter, 1975, p. 110). This aim may be reached by recognizing the areas of vulnerability of families through rejection or overprotection of the child. Early assessment of the child and family should help the nurse plan effective intervention. To support the child in the normal development of independence and autonomous living and to increase his self-esteem, a complete assessment should be made early in his life. This includes (1) complete physical examination; (2) developmental assessment; (3) psychological testing; (4) evaluation of the quality, quantity, and consistency of environmental support; and (5) determination of the ego capacities of the parents (Waechter, 1975). Fig. 30-1 shows an interdisciplinary team in action.

Nurses play a vital role in preventive measures before conception. Family planning and counseling with high risk parents such as teenagers, women over 35, and families known to have histories of developmental disabilities are essential activities that must be carried out.

Prenatal care that begins early and continues throughout pregnancy has long been recognized as a vital factor in the prevention of problematic pregnancies and births. Included in this care is identification of mothers-at-risk for having a child with a developmental disability. This list includes women age 35 and older; women who have had a child with a congenital abnormality such as Down's syndrome, spina bifida, or other genetic problems; and those how have a history of drug abuse, alcoholism, infectious diseases, or environmental exposure to toxic substances.

These families need support from the nurse. They may need information, referral, and/or encouragement to seek and follow through with services that are provided. Amniocentesis is frequently suggested to these mothers. Both parents need to understand the procedure, its purpose, and its value. They need counseling to assist them in understanding this procedure.

The possibility of aborting the pregnancy presents a difficult decision for most parents. The nurse must be skilled in supporting the parents in the decision they make concerning this question. Referral to another professional is quite often useful to the nurse and family.

Prevention of Further Handicaps

Prevention of further handicapping conditions is a sound reason for recommending early intervention programs. Although much controversy still exists about the value of early stimulation for the child with a developmental disability, its importance has been recognized by many nurses working with these children and their families. Fig. 30-2 depicts an early infant stimulation program.

A 10-month-old child was brought to a university-affiliated program by the mother through a referral from a community health nurse. When examined by the nurse, this child, Amy, could not lift her head, did not attend well to voice commands, and had a weak sucking reflex. The mother was distraught, discouraged, and physically exhausted. She had accepted the physician's diagnosis that Amy had severe brain damage and had been giving the medications as ordered for her child. She had continued to care for her like a newborn infant but expressed the need to know what she could do to help her child.

A team of experts evaluated the child, and a program was designed with the participation of the mother. The program involved some visits to the center for demonstration and reinforcement, but most of the activities prescribed were carried out in the home by the parents. The nurse at the center coordi-

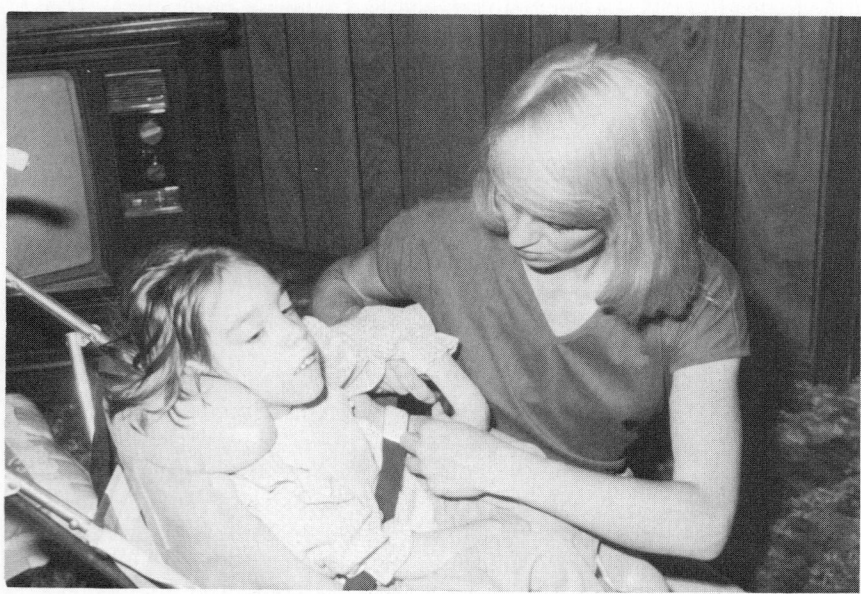

Fig. 30-2. Early infant stimulation program.

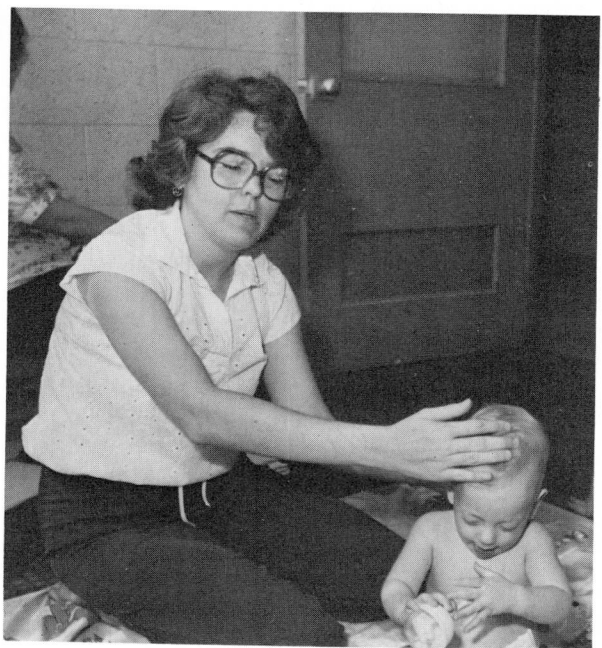

Fig. 30-3. Assessment of motor function.

nated the program with the community health nurse, family, and the center.

Progress was slow for Amy, but it did occur. Within 3 months she was lifting and turning her head in response to sound. Moreover, socialization was seen as she began to respond positively to the parents with some eye contact and facial expressions.

Experiences such as this have demonstrated that many of these children can be helped through early stimulation programs. The value to the family is inestimable. This young mother took on the appearance of one having a new lease on life as a result of the progress made by her child.

Early and continuous assessment of these children aids in identifying other problems, such as hearing or visual deficits. Recognition and treatment should enhance the learning ability of the child. Physical stimulation helps to prevent contractures and to strengthen the muscular development of the child. Fig. 30-3 illustrates the assessment of motor function. Encouraging the parents to keep the child under medical supervision prevents the development of further physical problems. Nutritional counseling, intellectual stimulation, and

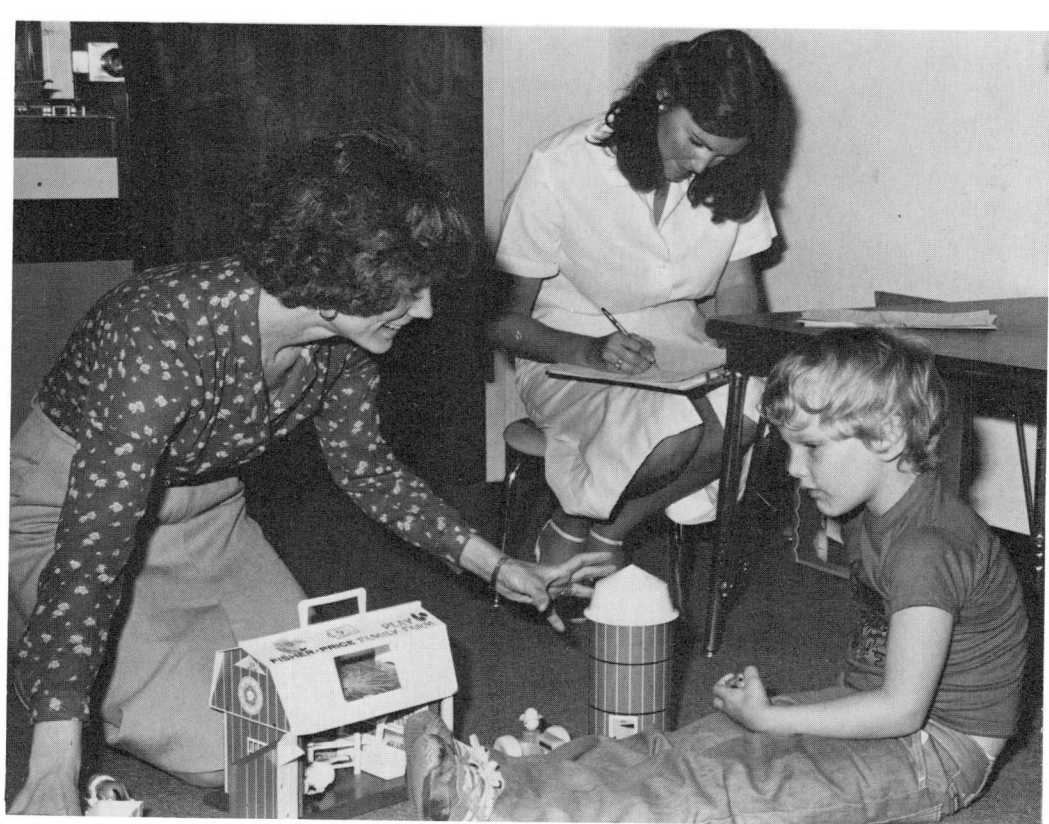

Fig. 30-4. Speech evaluation.

up-to-date immunizations are also valuable components of a preventive program for these children.

Screening Procedures

Screening procedures for early detection of children with learning problems have been difficult, but some studies indicate that such predictions may be possible. Environmental factors, dental enamel defects, physical anomalies, and family histories may be used effectively to identify high risk children at an early age and begin appropriate intervention earlier. Further research in this area is needed for validation of the procedures suggested as well as refinement of the instrument proposed (Mercer and Trifiletti, 1977). Though many of the children who have learning problems fit the definition of developmentally disabled, others may not. However, in attempting to meet the total needs of the child, his intellectual achievement is just as important as his physical status. Speech evaluation of a developmentally disabled child is seen in Fig. 30-4.

ROLE OF THE COMMUNITY HEALTH NURSE

The role of the community health nurse in the care of the child must be built on a sincere concern for the child and his family. The child with a problem must first be viewed as an individual worthy of dignity and capable of living for a purpose. The attitude of the nurse is reflected in all that is done with, to, and by the nurse. Unless that attitude conveys concern for the child and understanding of the grief and frustration of the family, the therapy will be ineffective.

The nurse must help the parents and siblings see the potential in the child and build a program around his assets. Dealing with the reaction of the family to the child who has a developmental disability is the first step in working with the child. Sensitivity to this need and acceptance of the family's reaction should provide the opportunity to make an adequate assessment of the child and family.

Ideally, physicians and hospital personnel are working more closely with the community nurse today so that referral of the child from hospital to home is made early in the child's life. The community health nurse should visit the child and mother while they are in the hospital. This would provide an opportunity to meet the medical team and nursing staff as well as the parents. The community health nurse should have access to all the medical information and the medical plan for the child so that steps for the child's care within the community can be coordinated.

Meeting the mother at this stage is an excellent way to let her know she has a friend in the community. Understanding the stages of grief helps the nurse to be supportive rather than intrusive. Plans can be made to visit in the home at a later time. It is essential that a feeling of trust be established between the nurse and the family.

Unfortunately, not all children with developmental disabilities are referred to the community health nurse during the immediate neonatal period. Often the nurse learns from neighbors, the kindergarten teacher, the church, or the clinic that there is a child with a problem in the community. Care for these children must be planned and implemented at a highly professional level.

Assessment

Nurses are taught to make the first assessment of the child 1 minute after birth. From this initial quick evaluation the skills assessed become more comprehensive as the child continues throughout life. Several conditions that cause a child to be categorized as developmentally disabled can be identified at birth, but many do not become apparent until the child is much older.

Physical examinations, developmental assessments, and adaptive behavior judgments are made by nurses. As for as physical examinations are concerned, the nurse executes only basic procedures to determine normal characteristics. If findings suggest any abnormality or need for a more comprehensive examination, the child is referred to a physician.

Developmental assessments and adaptive behavior judgments are made by observing the child in the home, office, or clinic. One or several tools may be used by the nurse to validate observations.

A number of instruments have been used to assist the nurse with this. The Denver Developmental Screening Test (DDST) is one of the simplest, more economical measures to use for the child from birth to 6 years. The test can be administered in less than 30 minutes and identifies many of the strengths and weaknesses of the child.

Four areas of evaluation included in the DDST are personal/social, fine motor/adaptive, language, and gross motor development. The test may be used repeatedly on the individual child to plot his development over a period of time. Instructions for using the test are written on the back of each form.

This test must be administered by the examiner to one child at a time. Some items require observation of performance, and some may be reported by the parent. It yields reliable information that can be most helpful as a screening tool. The test may be administered by nonprofessionals with very little training and is relatively inexpensive.

The DDST is used effectively to identify developmental delays or for follow-up assessments. The test does not measure intelligence quotient, and those who use the DDST should explain its purpose clearly to the parents to lessen the tension associated with any examination. (See Appendix C for source.)

The *Denver Pre-screening Developmental Questionnaire* (PDQ) is a short test designed to identify children who need more testing with the DDST. It is designed for children 3 months to 6 years of age and is a series of questions designed to be answered with a "yes" or "no" by the parent or caretaker. The test requires less than 10 minutes to complete. Referral is recommended for any child with six or fewer "yes" answers. (See Appendix C, and use source for DDST.)

The *Developmental Profile* is another instrument that is based on the responses of the mother or care taker to questions posed by the nurse. This standardized test can be used for measurement of children from birth to preadolescence. The test provides developmental age scores in the following five categories: physical/motor, self-help, social, academic, and communication skills.

The test can be used after a short training period and is relatively inexpensive. The evaluation is made in an interview and can be completed in approximately 30 minutes. Responses to the questions asked the parent can yield valuable information that can be used in developing a program for the child.

Referrals for further evaluation or placement into programs for children can be made using this instrument if agreeable to those involved. It is a single test that has been used effectively for a number of years with purposes of screening and has been found to be a reliable and valid tool. (See Appendix C for source.)

The American Association on Mental Deficiency has two instruments that can be used easily by the community health nurse to assess the development of children or adults. Both instruments are called the AAMD Adaptive Behavior Scale. One has been designed to be used by staff members who work with clients in institutions, and this is the first that was developed. The later version is called the *Public School Version* and was designed to be used by schoolteachers or school nurses. Either test yields valuable information that can be used to develop appropriate care plans for children or adults. (See Appendix C for source.)

The following is a list of guides that can be used easily to help the nurse develop a program for a child. Sources for these guides are in Appendix C.

Portage Guide
Washington Guide for Promoting Development in the Young Child
San Juan Development Progression Chart

Each of these guides gives very specific steps that may be followed by the parent or teacher to help a child learn a particular skill or advance his development. No one guide meets every need, so that the nurse requires a repertoire of tools that can be used. Most are easy to understand and simple to use. The slow progress that most developmentally disabled children make requires repetition and a great deal of patience for the parents, nurse, or therapist.

Many screening tests have been developed by professionals in many disciplines and can be used effectively be nurses and other health workers to plan and give care to children and their families. A useful book by Stangler et al. (1980) provides a comprehensive guide for test selection of instruments that can be used in evaluating preschool children as well as developmentally disabled children.

Information acquired from observation, interview, and test results is used to develop care plans for the child. Often the community health nurse is the health care coordinator for the child and his family. Assessment skills, knowledge of community resources, familiarity with the medical plan, and effective communication abilities are essential assets for such a coordinator.

Family Support

Sharing information with the family and including them in the plan of care is essential for successful implementation. The impact of the diagnosis of a developmentally disabled child tends to envelop most parents with a paralyzing grief that often lessens their ability to cope. Lacking the medical knowledge to understand the cause, treatment procedures, and prognosis, they are frightened, grief stricken, and easily confused.

Parents' Reactions

Parents of developmentally disabled children react to the knowledge of having such a child in a fairly predictive manner according to Rosen (1955). These stages are

1. Awareness of a problem
2. Recognition of the basic problem
3. Search for a cause
4. Search for a cure
5. Acceptance of the problem

The time involved in moving from one stage to another varies with each family. Unfortunately, there are some parents who never accept the problem and therefore never progress beyond the first stage. Awareness may come early in the life of the child, particularly if he has a physical handicap. It may be as late as the beginning of school if it is a mental problem.

Recognition of the basic problem, the second stage, helps the parents gain insight and motivates most to

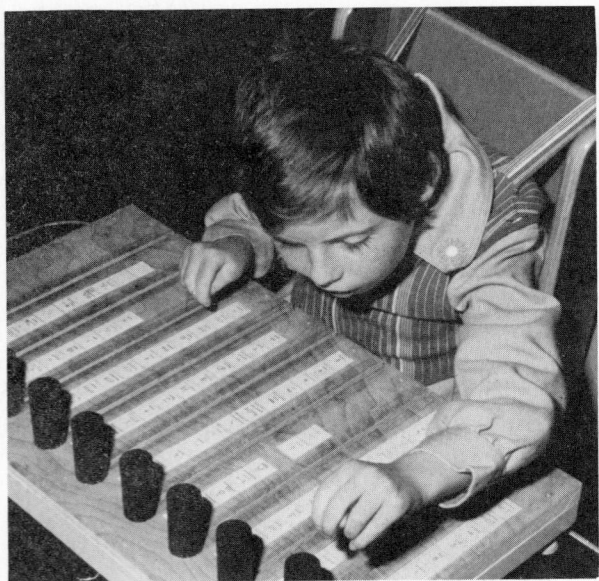

Fig. 30-5. Coordination training.

seek a cause, the third and perhaps most difficult stage in the parents' reactions. Mothers tend to blame themselves, and inability to cope with an unknown cause leads to poor adjustment, which is often manifested in misplaced hostility, anger, or self-pity. Many parents exhaust all their financial, physical, and emotional resources in attempting to find a reason for the child's problem.

Searching for a cure, the fourth stage, can also lead to destruction of a family. Hoping that each new drug, therapy, or published bit of research will help their child, many families travel from one physician to another, city to city, and school to school find little real help. The despair and grief are overwhelming for many. These families need support from the social worker, nurse, or other professionals.

The final stage, acceptance of the problem, takes much time. Often it is years before the parents can accept the reality of the problem of the child. It is only when they have accepted the problem that they can begin to actively participate in the therapeutic plan of care. Until that time, their grief interferes with their ability to completely understand what information is

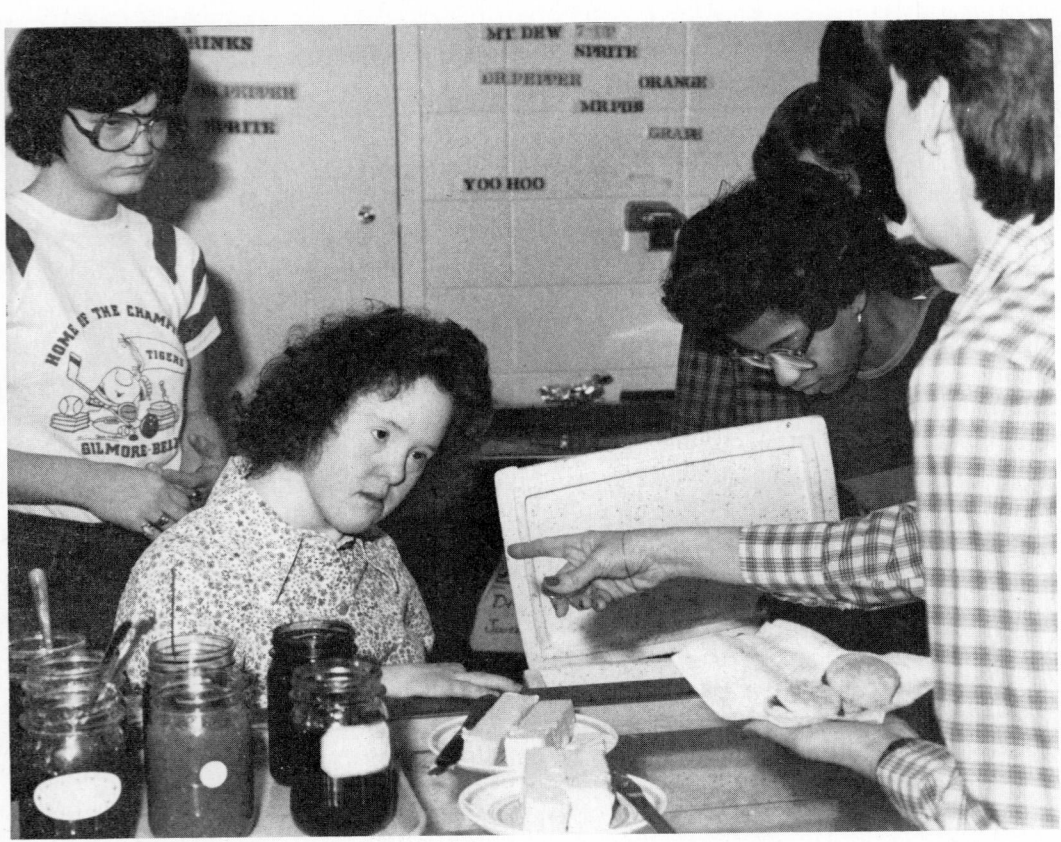

Fig. 30-6. Activities of daily living laboratory.

being shared with them. Their participation in the care of the child is essential, and professionals must be aware of the personal struggle the parents face every day as they live and work with the child.

Many nurses and other professionals seem to be unaware of the fact that grief over a child with a developmental disability moves in cycles. Parents appear to be accepting the problem and coping well for a while, and then a seemingly insignificant act may completely disrupt their stability. As the child grows older and parents are associated with other children of the same age, the sorrow is often intensified when they view the accomplishments of the other children. Sharing with other parents and professionals can provide a great deal of support during these periods.

Intervention

Responding to the needs of families who have children with developmental disabilities begins with an understanding of the deep pain experienced by these families. It is important that professionals recognize, appreciate, and validate the pain families experience (Tudor, 1981). From the moment the family members learn that they have a "less than perfect" child they need a nurse who is sensitive to their grief.

Planning strategies that support the child and family should be based on the development and abilities the child has with less attention to his deficiencies. Projecting the image of the child first, rather than planning for

a handicapped child, is one concept that can be shared with the family.

Recognition that the child does have a problem aids the nurse in assisting the family to set realistic goals. Working with the family in the home affords the nurse the opportunity to appraise the coping ability of the family and give support and encouragement as needed (Tudor, 1981).

Intervention programs for the child with a handicap must be planned cooperatively with the family and other professionals as needs arise. The parents are the first teachers the child knows; they are the caretakers, and they are the ones to meet the emotional needs of the child as well. They must be taught parenting skills that they can accept and practice within the limits of their abilities. Nurses must be careful not to increase the burden of the family members by asking them to become the teacher, therapist, mother, and homemaker. Fig. 30-5 depicts coordination-training activities.

Nurses must identify interventions that assist the child to develop to his highest level of health, independence, and growth, It is sometimes difficult for parents to encourage independence in children who have problems. In Fig. 30-6 a child is being taught activities of daily living.

These children also have a need to be accepted by their family and the community as individuals with the same rights and privileges as those with no handicaps. Encouraging the capabilities the child has and provid-

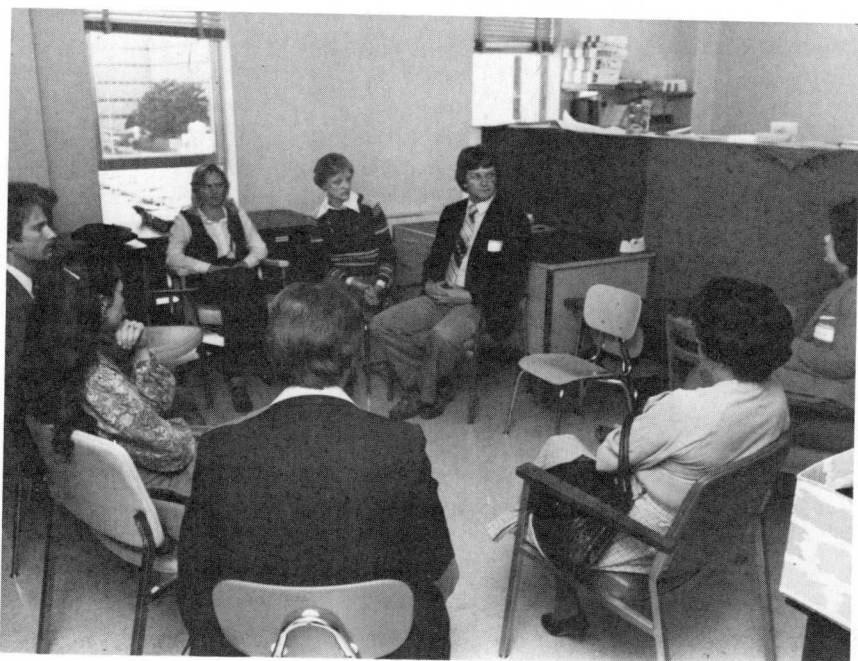

Fig. 30-7. Parent group.

ing opportunities for enrichment in his life through participation in family and community activities can strengthen self-image of the child.

Support groups

As the child grows, his needs change. Parents need to be supported by their extended families, friends, and others who have experienced similar problems. Small groups of parents who can share their problems and their joys with others are very supportive. Voluntary groups such as those sponsored by the Association for Retarded Citizens groups, the Spina Bifida Association, and the Cerebral Palsy Organizations provide a mechanism for communication. As seen in Fig. 30-7, parent groups are vital in working with developmentally disabled children. The nurse should encourage the parents to join these groups and share their experiences with others. Frequently these groups can help solve problems by identifying with the family. This is rewarding to both groups.

Parents are also helped by continuing to participate in the normal day-to-day activities of the community. They need to be encouraged to find responsible baby-sitters and respite care services so that they have time to spend with other children, their spouse, and community members.

THE ROLE OF FEDERAL PROGRAMS

Federal programs for the care of children with handicaps were initiated by legislative mandate of Title V of the Social Security Act. This act required states to identify and provide services to crippled children. Through the years federal programs have been expanded to provide screening and service to many more children. Over 300 categorical programs have ben authorized by congress in recent years (Norris, 1975).

The Social Security Act has been amended many times in the last 20 years to provide services for the developmentally disabled. Title XIX was amended in 1967 to require early and periodic screening, diagnosis, and treatment (EPSDT) of children eligible for Medicaid. These services were designed to provide a program of prevention, early detection, and treatment for our indigent population. This program is financed by federal and state funds and has provided a much needed service. Included in this program are the following elements (Norris, 1975, p. 314):

History
Physical growth assessment
Developmental assessment
Physical inspection of unclothed child
Ear, nose, mouth, teeth, and throat inspections
Vision screening
Hearing screening
Screening tests for anemia, sickle-cell anemia, tuberculosis, urinary tract problems, and lead-based paint poisoning
Nutritional status
Immunization status with boosters
Other individually determined screenings such as chest x-ray films, throat cultures, pinworm slides, blood pressure, serological tests, drug-dependency screening, and stool specimens for parasites, ova, and blood

In 1974 the Office for the Handicapped was created as a result of the Rehabilitation as the result of the Rehabilitation Act of 1973 (93-112). The following are five needed functions related to the many and varied federally funded programs and are the responsibility of the Office of the Handicapped (Norris, 1975, pp. 315-316):

1. Prepare a long-range projection for the provision of comprehensive services.
2. Continually analyze the operation of the Health and Human Services programs and evaluate their effectiveness.
3. Encourage coordination and cooperative planning among the Health and Human Services' programs.
4. Develop ways to promote the use of research findings and the adoption of exemplary practices.
5. Provide for a central clearinghouse for information and resources available for handicapped persons.

A landmark act was passed by Congress with enactment of the Education for All Handicapped Children Act (94-142) in 1975. This act provides "education for every child, regardless of handicaps, in the least restrictive environment possible." Implementation of this act had created blessings and problems for the state and children served in the public schools.

Only a few of the many federal acts have been listed to note the input that federal intervention had had on the care of developmentally disabled children and their families. This population needed federal and public support to be able to meet the problems of everyday living.

Nurses and nursing have benefited from this federal legislation as well as the families. Nursing skills have been refined and expanded to be able to meet the demands in a professional manner. Support through grants to states, schools, scholars, and handicapped individuals has been a great boon to advancing knowledge, concern, and methods of assisting the developmentally disabled population and their families.

These monies have enable states to fund nursing positions in community health departments, crippled children's services, developmental diagnostic centers, and genetic laboratories. Educational grants have provided the funds needed to update the knowledge and skill of nurses working with this population.

Nurses like all other professionals need the opportunity to learn new techniques and add to their knowledge base. Nursing skills needed to care for the developmentally disabled are being addressed by a program that was developed by the School of Nursing at the University of Colorado Health Science Center. A grant was funded from the Office of the Bureau of Education for the Handicapped to organize, implement, and evaluate a national educational program for school nurses. This program, called the *School Nurse Achievement Program (SNAP),* is an 8-week course designed to enable school nurses to deliver health care to children with developmental disabilities during the school day. The program was piloted in Colorado in 1981, implemented in four other states in 1982, and will be offered in four more states in 1983. It will be offered to all the remaining states in 1984. Since many community health nurses also serves as school nurses, they will be invited to participate in these classes. All of these programs should assist the nurse in further developing the expertise needed to plan and implement quality care to developmentally disabled children.

FOLLOW-UP CARE

With early and more comprehensive evaluation of infants and young children, many are receiving better care than a few years ago. It is imperative that children who have been diagnosed as having a developmental disability be assigned to some responsible professional in the community who will maintain contact with the child and document his care and program.

It is far more economical for families as well as professional health providers to develop such plans cooperatively. When this is done, community health nurses are the most logical people in the community to assume the role of coordinator. Their expertise in working with individuals, families, and agencies is usually well-known and accepted in the community. In addition to serving as the coordinator, the nurse also acts as an advocate for the child and his family. Often it is the nurse who initiates activities that lead to more and better services for this group of people. Knowledge of the conditions, therapy, and need should motivate the community health nurse to be active in promoting local, state, and federal legislation to assist these people. Participation in civic and professional groups also provides an avenue for sharing knowledge and concern. Many professionals have little insight into the overwhelming problems faced by individuals who have handicapping conditions. Community health nurses have an obligation to demonstrate an attitude of concern to facilitate continuing care for this group.

A well-documented record that follows the child can be a valuable tool in planning for ongoing care. Such a record prevents repetitive evaluations and provides evidence of therapy that assists with the periodic evaluation of care and progress of the child. Ideally computerization of records will assist individuals and agencies in keeping tabs on our mobile society.

ABILITIES AND INDEPENDENT LIVING

The goal of care for all the developmentally disabled people in our society is to assist the individual in living a productive life. All are not able to achieve the goal of living independently, but many are capable of accomplishing this with the help from the community. Fig. 30-8 depicts developmentally disabled teenagers practicing sales skills.

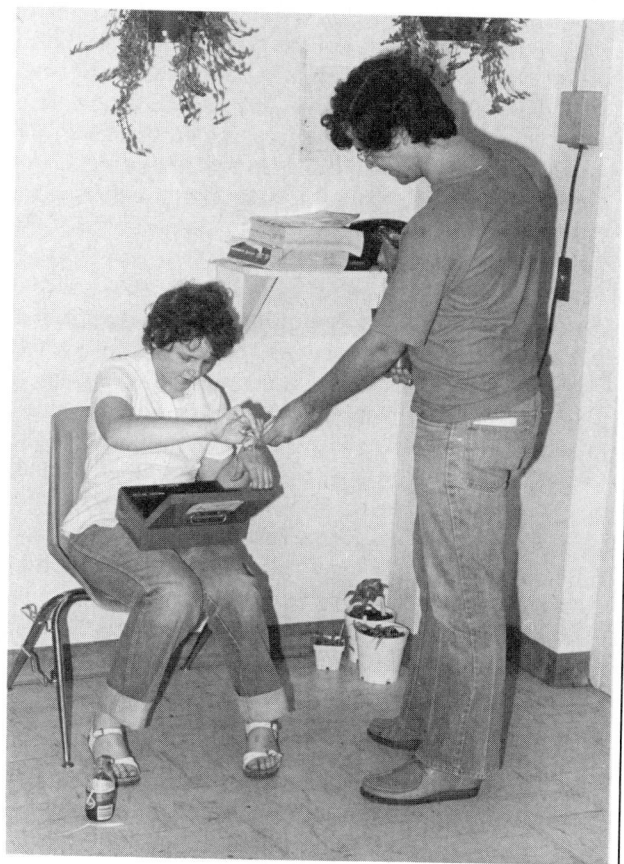

Fig. 30-8. Teenagers practicing sales skills.

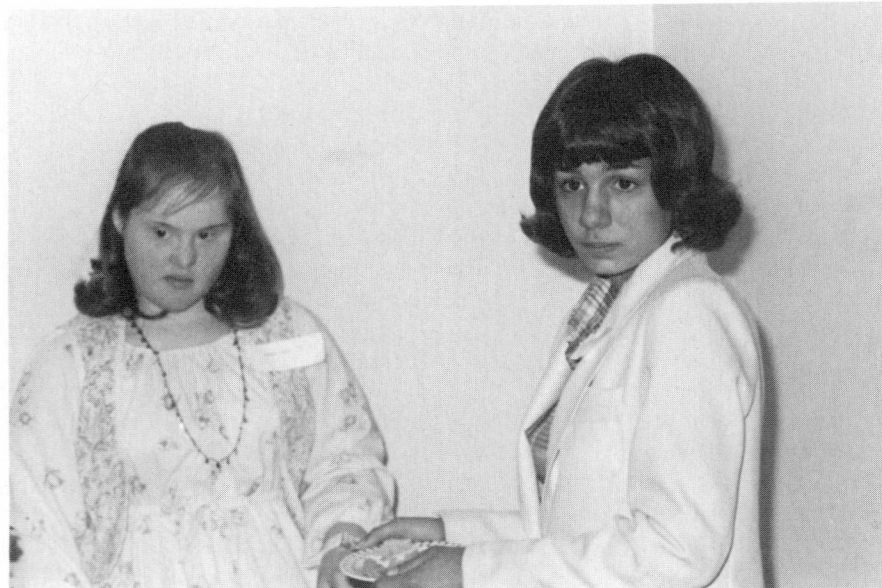

Fig. 30-9. Development of social skills.

In the last 10 years emphasis has been placed on early training, recognition of the rights of all people, and public support for programs that provide services for the developmentally disabled. Ideally public attitudes can be changed to offer encouragement to the people and support of programs that are geared toward helping this population achieve independent living. Many avenues are open today, but all require public support. Fig. 30-9 illustrates the development of social skills.

Since the implementation of PL 94-142, provision has been made for these people to have an opportunity to be included in the public school system. Adoption of such a program is expensive and requires a great deal of interpretation to the public as well as constant surveillance of the program. Many children and young adults have had an opportunity to learn that was never offered to them before this time.

The inclusion of these children into the public school has intensified their need for health supervision. School nurses need additional preparation in the care of developmentally disabled children to assist the schools in providing this attention.

In addition to academic opportunity, these children are increasingly being taught how to manage activities of daily living. Learning social, self-help, and communication skills requires personnel who have an interest in and an understanding of many disciplines. Often it is the nurse who must learn from a speech therapist, physical therapist, or nutritionist the procedures to be taught to the individual child. In turn, the nurse must

then teach these techniques to the aides or parents because most school systems cannot support all the specialists that a child might need.

In planning for the child's care at home, his emotional, social, and spiritual needs should also be a part of the care program. Again it is the public health nurse who would provide the leadership for such planning. Recognition of the totality of needs for the child and his family is a realistic goal, one that should be a part of basic preparation of community health nurses.

THE FUTURE

Planning in the health field must include children and adults who have developmental disabilities. Increasingly they are living in the community and are cared for by their families and local agencies. Support of families through adequate funding for community services, provision of respite care to relieve families from the ongoing burden of constant care, continuation of research into causes and preventative measures, and increased recognition of the rights of this population are the concerns that must be addressed by any group that is involved in planning care for the large number of people with developmental disabilities. The community as a whole must not lose sight of the needs of these individuals as they grow from childhood to adulthood and from adulthood into senility. Far too often in the past, recognition has been given to the child, but as he ages, less and less attention is given to him.Community health nurses can help add meaning to the life of these individuals and their families.

SUMMARY

Recognition of the need for community health nurses to become more skilled in meeting the requirements of the developmentally disabled child and his family has led to greater interest and desire to learn more about this population. Concern and commitment to care can be augmented through use of techniques and study of the problems that have become increasingly apparent in communities today. With emphasis on care of the child at home and in the community, nurses must pursue the resources available through study and planned experiences to enhance their ability to provide more professional service for this group. This can be accomplished through the cooperative efforts of the service and educational groups found in all the states. Nurses working in harmony with professionals in other fields can help provide a brighter future for our developmentally disabled population and their families.

BIBLIOGRAPHY

American Association on Mental Deficiency: Manual on terminology and classification in mental retardation, Washington, D.C., 1977, The Association.

Barnard, K.E., and Erickson, M.L.: Teaching children with developmental problems: a family care approach, ed. 2, 1976, The C.V. Mosby Co.

Better health for our children: a national strategy, Report of the Select Panel for the Promotion of Child Health vols. 1, 2, 3, and 55, DHHS Pub. No. 79-55071, Washington, D.C., 1981. Department of Health and Human Sciences.

Blackwell, M.W., Care of the mentally retarded, Boston, 1979, Little, Brown & Co.

Brazelton, T.B.: The Neonatal Behavioral Assessment Scale, Philadelphia and London, 1973, J.B. Lippincott Co., and William Heinemann Ltd.

Bumbalo, J.A. and Seikel, M.A. Identifying and serving a multiply handicapped population. Deaf-blind children and their families, Nurs. Clin. North Am. **10**(2):341-352, 1975.

Buser, B.N.: The evaluation of school health services, J. Sch. Health, **50**:475-477, 1980.

Caldwell, B.M.: Home Observation for Measurement of Environment (birth to three) and (three to six), Little Rock, 1970 and 1976, University of Arkansas.

Caldwell, B.M.: Instructors manual inventory for infants (Home Observation for Measurement of the Environment), University of Arkansas, Little Rock, 1970.

Chinn, P.C., Drew, C.S., and Logan, D.R.: Mental retardation, a life cycle approach, St. Louis, 1975, The C.V. Mosby Co.

Curry, M.F.: Where are we with education of the handicapped: new approaches to screening, J. Sch. Health **51**:442-442, 1981.

Erickson, M.L.: Assessment and management of developmental changes in children, St. Louis, 1976, The C.V. Mosby Co.

Fleming, J.W.: Care and management of exceptional children, New York, 1973, Appleton-Century-Crofts.

Groninga, S.: Emotional/behavioral disorders: assessment and management, J. Sch. Health **50**:228-229, 1980.

Haynes, U.: A developmental approach to case finding among infants and children, Washington, D.C., 1979, DHEW, Pub. N. (HSA) 79-5210, U.S. Government Printing Office.

Holmberg, N.J.: Serving the child with MBD and his family, Nurs. Clin. North Am. **10**:301-391, 1975.

House of Representatives Conference Committee: Conference report: Comprehensive Rehabilitation Services Amendments of 1978, Rep. No., 95-1780, Washington, D.C., 1978, pp. 51-52.

Jarvis, L.L.: Community health nursing: keeping the public healthy, Philadelphia, 1981, F.A. Davis Co.

Johnston, R.B., and Magrab, P.R.: Developmental disorder, assessment, treatment, education, Baltimore, 1976, University Park Press.

Mercer, C.D., and Trifiletti, J.: The development of screening procedures for the early detection of children with learning problems, J. Sch. Health **47**:526-532, 1977.

Miller, L.G.: Towards a greater understanding of parents of the mentally retarded child, J. Pediatr. **73**:699-705, 1968.

Norris, G.J.: National concerns for children with handicaps, Nurs. Clin. North Am. **10**:309-317, 1975.

Office of Human Development Services Administration on Developmental Disabilities: Special report on the impact of the change in the definition of developmental disabilities, Washington, D.C., May 1981. Department of Health and Human Services.

Passo, S.: Symposium on CNS disorders in children. Malformation of the neural tube, Nurs. Clin. North Am. **15**:5-21, 1980.

Porter, P.: The role of the independent community nurse practitioner in providing services to the developmentally disabled children and their families, Nur. Clin. North Am. **15**:419-428, 1980.

Robinson, T.: Clinics for children with handicaps, J. Sch. Health **50**:541-542, 1982.

Rodgers, B.M.: Comprehensive care for the child with a chronic disability, Am. J. Nurs. 1106-1108, 1979.

Rose, T.L.: The education of all handicapped children act (PL 94-142): new responsibilities and opportunities for the school nurse, J. Sch. Health **50**: 30-31, 1980.

Rosen, L.: Selected aspects in the development of the mother's understanding of her mentally retarded child, Am. J. Ment. Defic. **59**:522, 1955.

Stangler, S.R., Huber, C.J., and Routh, D.K.: Screening growth and development of preschool children.: a guide for test selection, New York, 1980, McGraw-Hill Book Co.

Stark, G.D.: Spina bifida: problems and management, Oxford, Eng. 1977, Blackwell Scientific Publications.

Tudor, M.: Child development, New York, 1981, McGraw Hill Book Co.

Waechter, E.H.: Developmental consequences of congenital abnormalities, Nurs. Forum, **14**: 108-129, 1975.

Wallace, H.M., Gold, E.M., and Lis, E.: Maternal and child practices; problems, resources and methods, Springfield, Ill., 1973, Charles C. Thomas, Publisher.

Wender, P.H.: Minimal brain dysfunction in children, New York, 1971, Wiley Interscience.

Whaley, L.F., and Wong, D.L.: Essentials of pediatric nursing, St. Louis, 1982, The C.V. Mosby Co.

Whaley, L.F., and Wong, D.L.: Nursing care of infants and children, ed. 2, St. Louis, 1983, The C.V. Mosby Co.

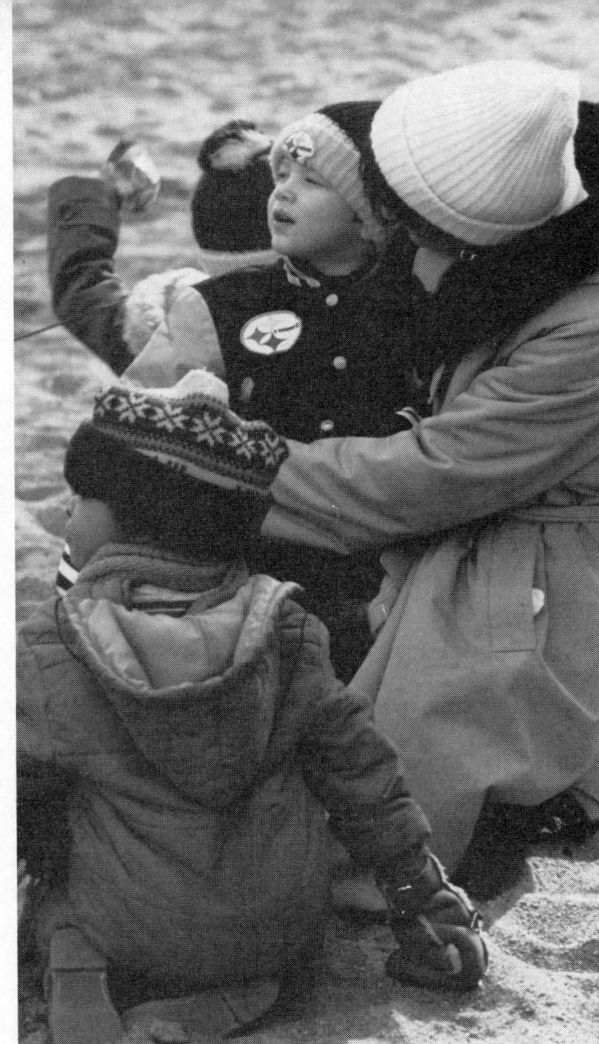

Chapter 31

CORA WITHROW

SCHOOL NURSING

School nursing practice is easier to describe than to define. Wide diversities exist in professional training, the roles nurses play in school health programs, the programs themselves, and the legal and bureaucratic constraints within which school health goals must be pursued. Size of the school district, local characteristics and values, availability of resources, and the abilities of the individual nurse explain this variation in part. But the diversity can also be understood by looking at trends in school health delivery.

The overall trend has been for school health, and consequently school nursing, to become more comprehensive. In fact, the American Nurses' Association characterizes school nursing as both comprehensive and complex. This can be seen in a variety of ways. School nurses now try to work with children holistically: to help them grow emotionally and socially as well as physically. Individuality and cultural variation are

recognized and appreciated, even though health programs often involve working with large groups of children. Nurses practicing in schools have adopted community health concepts and approaches such as the three levels of prevention, control of communicable diseases, identification of children at risk for chronic disease and possible premature death, referral, follow-up, and family health care from a nursing perspective (Dagg, 1981).

The promotion of these enlarged health goals had led to a more complex interpenetration of school health programs within the total school system. Nurses have taken on new roles and adopted new strategies to fulfill their growing responsibilities. They are becoming more astute politically, organizing networks, using marketing concepts, and pursuing higher education, thus learning to work more effectively within the system. These new roles and strategies have also necessitated the acquisition of new skills, both technical and conceptual. School nursing has become as versatile as the nurse practicing, as varied as the differing school health needs.

This fluid situation, while providing challenging opportunities for professional growth, has also posed dilemmas for both the individual nurse and for the profession as a whole. At a time when important issues affecting the well-being of children are being confronted, school nurses must struggle to define their domain. They must cope not only with the demands made by their multiple roles in a changing health care field, but also with the external forces that impinge on school nursing. As a result, there are calls for clarification of nursing's domain and responsibilities, more relevant research, changes in the nursing profession's organization, and increased involvement in activities that affect health education and health care for children and youths.

This chapter will outline the changes that have occurred in school nursing and describe the range of contemporary school nursing practices. The description will not be exhaustive—full description of all activities engaged in by school nurses would take more than a chapter. Instead, a selection of roles school nurses fill, arenas in which they work, and important services they provide will be presented to illustrate the comprehensiveness and complexity of this nursing field. Finally, the issues now facing those who work in this area will be presented to the student, and potential school nurse, for consideration.

TRADITIONAL SCHOOL NURSING

The first school health services in the United States were medical inspections begun in 1894 in the Boston schools. These cursory inspections were made for the purpose of keeping away from schools those children with communicable diseases such as mumps, chickenpox, diphtheria, pertussis, and scarlet fever (Means, 1975; Wold and Dagg, 1981). Children with other health problems were ignored. But Lillian Wald, a community health nurse working among the immigrants and other poor on New York's Lower East Side, believed that much could be done by the schools to keep children healthy. Through a campaign for the rights of children to receive health care and health services in school settings, she was able to convince officials that "a sick child cannot learn." In 1902 in New York City, Wald organized the first nursing program for school children, creating a pattern that rapidly spread across the county (Means, 1975).

Traditionally, school health programs have focused on acute episodic care and devoted limited attention to

prevention (Better Health for Our Children, 1981). School nurses provided health-centered direct and indirect nursing services, direct supervision of children's health problems, and a minimum of counseling.

The direct nursing services consisted of inspecting throats, removing head lice, checking for impetigo, screening for vision and hearing, and monitoring students who were consistently absent. Although children with communicable problems were still sent home, attempts were made to assist parents and child in getting appropriate medical assistance, either through referral or recommendations. Indirect services consisted mainly of paper work.

Direct supervision involved nurses in a variety of health services designed to serve individual children with specific health problems. Helping asthmatic children cope in school by teaching them relaxation techniques is one example; supervising overweight children with diet and exercise is another.

Immunization was the major preventive measure. Most school boards, however, required only smallpox vaccination; a few more required typhoid or diphtheria shots or both. Massive immunization programs, although tried in the 1960s (polio), were not successful until the 1970s when, in many states, school jurisdictions were expanded to allow schools to require immunization series and to exclude from school those children who were in need of additional immunizations.

CONTEMPORARY SCHOOL NURSING

School nursing today, according to the American School Health Association (1975), should enhance the child's or youth's individual ability to use his or her intellectual potential and to make worthwhile decisions affecting present and future physical, social, and emotional health. This view illustrates something of the increasingly comprehensive and complex nature of contemporary school nursing. Emphasis now is on disease prevention and health promotion from a holistic point of view. School health programs are seen as ideal mechanisms for transmitting health knowledge and developing health competencies. Associated with these developments has been the incorporation of community health concepts and approaches into school health nursing.

Disease Prevention and Health Promotion

A concern with disease prevention and health promotion is not surprising. Most states require students to attend school until they are 16 years old, thus creating a large captive population—which is generally a well population. What better place than a school for making an impact on the nation's health? Now, schools are receiving renewed attention as sites for disease prevention and health promotion (Better Health for Our Children, 1981). This trend reflects a growing awareness of the complexity of disease processes and the development of educational methods that allow for more effective intervention in these areas.

Disease prevention and health promotion can be pursued in a number of ways: screening, immunizing, creating a healthful school environment, finding ways to supplement inadequate diets, and making health care and services more accessible. But health instruction is also essential. The goal of health instruction is to provide students and their families with the knowledge and skills that will permit them to make decisions about their health care, to recognize health problems, and to use health promotion practices. Unfortunately, providing knowledge is not enough: mechanisms must be incorporated into health instruction which help students translate what they have learned into appropriate behavior patterns. For example, a major goal of a safety program might be to get children to fasten their seat belts as soon as they enter a car.

The need to focus on behavior has long been recognized, and the growing body of knowledge about the interrelationships between behavior and health has underlined its importance. Nevertheless, nurses and teachers are still being called on to use health promotion techniques that can influence student behavior (Nader et al., 1977; Pigg, 1976), suggesting the difficulties of effecting behavior change by health instruction alone. As methods of behavior modification and motivation have been developed, however, health instruction in this larger sense has become more feasible.

Whether in the classroom or in more traditional arenas, school nurses try to promote healthy behaviors. Sometimes there is a fortuitous relationship between behavior and health: for example, there are those who regularly engage in exercise and eat well-balanced meals because they are so inclined or have grown up that way. But often, positive health-promoting behaviors must be adopted through conscious choice because of knowledge of their benefits. By integrating their health knowledge with educational concepts, school nurses can hope to make an impact on the health of children and youths by encouraging these behaviors.

The discouragement of dysfunctional behaviors are equally important, however, especially for disease prevention. They, rather than diseases, cause many chronic illnesses and premature deaths (Healthy People, 1979). Efforts to discourage such habits as smoking, considered a risk factor for cardiovascular disease, are important elements in health programs.

Health promotion in schools implies the need to affect the behavior of parents as well as students. It may be sufficient to reach only children with some health programs such as toothbrushing, smoking, or safety practices, but for the most part children must have at least the support and often the active assistance of their parents to make significant behavioral changes. Consider, for example, nutrition, weight control, or immunization. Most young people are limited by what parents provide in the way of food and health care. Unless parents are willing to make adjustments, children may be unable to manage changes on their own. As a consequence, school nurses have had to consider ways to reach parents as a part of school health promotion.

Holistic Approach

From a holistic perspective, health is a multidimensional concept based on the interactions of psychological, social, and cultural factors as well as physiological and environmental ones (Langlie, 1978). This point of view, although present in school nursing, was not pervasive until the 1970s. Since them, it has led to an expansion of the domain of school nursing. To understand the directions this expansion has taken, it is helpful to look at the implications of this way of thinking applied to school health situations.

The holistic perspective implies a concern for all aspects of health, not just physical fitness. Nurses are concerned with emotional state and social functioning as well as with physical well-being. Screening programs include psychological as well as physiological tests. Observations are made of social functioning and relationships, and educational programs cover a wide range of topics related to personal and social coping strategies as well as more traditional health-related topics. The following list of common topics for health programs—expanded from McCamy and Presley (1975)—illustrates the breadth of the holistic approach to health.

Health practices: dental health, active exercise, nutrition, immunizations, substance abuse, safety, weight control, smoking, sexually transmitted disease, self-care

Coping strategies: developing and maintaining interpersonal relationships, values clarification, decision making, stress reduction, relaxation, enrichment of one's self-esteem, identity, independence, school phobia, school dropouts, depression

Family life: dating, courtship, marriage, parenthood, older adults, single parents, singles, homosexuals, reproduction and family planning, role relationships, role functions

Furthermore, the approach to a single topic will tend to be multidimensional. For example, the program of reproduction and family planning will be covered from emotional and social as well as physiological perspectives.

This perspective also encourages the search for the interrelated attitudes, behaviors, social relationships, physiological factors, and environmental agents underlying particular health problems. Consider, for example, obesity. In addition to the physiological factors that predispose people to obesity, it is recognized that there are many possible psychological (loneliness, depression), sociological (income, living situation, food offered at family meals), cultural (ethnic affiliation, equation of food with love), and environmental (adequacy of places to prepare food, local variation in availability of certain foods) factors that interact to produce individual eating patterns. These relationships may be more complex than they seem on the surface. Thus familiarity with the state of knowledge about these factors and a sensitivity to clues about the significant factors in a particular school population are prerequisites of effective school nursing.

For example, a nurse conducting a program on birth control would, before planning the presentation, consider the ethnic and social composition of the targeted student body. If students were largely from a urban, low-income area, the discussion might include many of the social and psychological consequences of early pregnancy. In a school with a large black population, the nurse would probably want to include genetic counseling for sickle-cell anemia. With a suburban Jewish group, the nurse might want to discuss the prevalence Tay-Sachs disease and the stresses of intermarriage. In a rural, southern school, religious sensitivities and reticence about discussing sexual topics might have to be considered to an extent that would not be necessary in the urban context.

This awareness of the wide range of factors affecting health problems also affects the way nurses look at and deal with individual children. School nurses must recognize the necessity for appreciating the individuality of each student. Listening, observing, and responding to the individual will guide the nurse in providing appropriate counseling.

Community Health Orientation

As early as 1970 community health nursing leaders urged that community health concepts be used in school nursing. The incorporation of school nursing into general community health programs was supported, the advantages being provision of both in-school and out-of-school care and economies in the allocation of nursing time. Similarity of goals between community health and school health, such as the concern with communicable disease, or similarity in the problems faced in working with large population groups, has been cited (Dagg, 1981). Some school health programs are now affiliated with community health programs, but

many more are using the approaches and concepts of community health.

School health services now often encompass control of communicable disease, family health care, early identification of high-risk groups, case finding, risk reduction, monitoring of chronic conditions, referral, and follow-up. Health promotion and maintenance efforts have been reinforced. Also, the three levels of prevention have been adopted, thus providing one way to conceptualize and organize school health practice (Dagg, 1981). For these reason school nursing can be seen as community health nursing or as a component of community health practice. But community health has also affected school nursing in other ways.

A community health orientation involves a concern for a healthy, safe environment. A safe environment is one that is free from exposure to hazardous chemicals, fire, communicable diseases, and accidents in both classroom and playground. It is the responsibility of the school nurse to help assure safety in the school. For example, laboratory inspections may be part of the school nurse's regular duties. If chemicals and equipment are not safely stored and handled, the nurse must try to change the dangerous conditions, first by discussion or persuasion, but eventually by calling in state environmental authorities if necessary.

A community health orientation means that nurses "work with" students and their families. Students are clients, not patients, and are actively involved in the services they receive and the decision making process.

Finally, a community health orientation implies an awareness of the value of *mortality* and *morbidity* information and of epidemiological studies in dealing with the health of groups. The question often needs to be asked: "What is the probability of x happening in these particular conditions?" With morbidity and mortality data available, questions about incidence and prevalence of many physiological conditions can be answered. Epidemiological studies take their orientation even further. Epidemiology is the study of the distribution of a disease or other physiological condition in a population, or subgroup of that population, and *factors affecting its distribution*. Epidemiological studies provide clues to the causes of morbidity, mortality, prevalence, incidence, and severity of diseases. They also allow us to compare patterns among the various subgroups of a society and suggest factors affecting those patterns.

Epidemiological studies are important to anyone working in a school—which is not only an important subgroup of our society but often a cross-section of a local population (both culturally and socially). Consider a study of substance abuse (drugs) among 13-years-old in a middle school. Results should suggest which students tend to use drugs; the amounts, frequency, and types of drugs used; and the conditions under which drugs are used. Depending on the degree to which results can be generalized, they might be invaluable for designing effective drug abuse programs for middle school or junior high school students.

SCHOOL NURSE ROLES

School nurses have responded to the changes in school health by assuming a wide variety of roles, often more than one at a time. A number of recognized roles have emerged, some of which will be discussed, but first, the concept of *role* will be explained.

Stated simply, the holder of any one school nursing position may occupy a cluster of roles, some of them more important and some of them less important. Associated with each role is a cluster of *functions*. If a function has a clearly enough defined set of expectations surrounding it, it may be considered a secondary role.

A distinguishing characteristic of a role is that it can be visualized. *Assistant,* for example, is not a satisfactory role description: it is too vague. The terms *dental assistant, laboratory assistant,* and *administrative assistant* are role designations because they offer certain expectations about the behavior of people filling these roles. We have a fairly clear idea of their responsibilities and the tasks they are likely to perform. We can visualize aspects of their relationships with superiors, clients, or patients. We can make statements about the skill they might be expected to have or the education they would need. We might even predict dress and demeanor in specified circumstances.

Both nurses and others in the school community or the community-at-large may have perceptions or appropriate roles for school nurses and the attendant role expectations (Nadar, et. al., 1977). These expectations may or may not be clearly defined, and often there are differences of opinion about expectations or appropriate roles. Such situations can give rise to role conflict or role incongruity. Role conflict occurs when roles occupied by different individuals overlap or do not mesh; for example, a nurse and a teacher might differ over who is best qualified to teach safety or substance abuse. Role incongruity occurs when the occupier of a role does not find the role (as defined by others) to the individuals's own expectations. Sometimes school nurse practitioners hired as primary care providers find themselves responsible only for truancy. Alternately, nurses may be expected to discharge functions, such as teaching or public relations, for which they are unprepared.

Each nurse comes to a role with a set of expectations

an an array of *skills,* which have been built up through training, experience, and talent. On the basis of these skills, the nurse will select *tools* and *strategies* to carry out the functions associated with the role. If the skill base is large enough to allow choice in the selection of strategies and tools, role performance is likely to be more satisfactory and less stressful than if the skill base is merely adequate. When inadequately prepared, nurses must work to develop skills while using them in discharging role obligations.

Roles, functions, strategies, and sometimes tools are defined by context; that is, at one time a designation may be a role, at another time a strategy or function. Advocacy illustrates this variability. Consider a nurse serving on a curriculum committee. One of her roles may be that of *advocate* for student health needs. Publicly pleading for a particular cause and fighting for time and resources may be seen as major responsibilities. For nurses who work with mainstreamed children, advocacy may be perceived as a function. When necessary, they will act as advocates for these children when dealing with teachers, administration, and parents. In a third case, nurses who are actively campaigning to get junk food banned from school lunchrooms might use any one of a number of strategies (i.e., teaching, negotiating with the food service director or principal, networking) in pursuing their cause. When they present a petition to the school board, however, they are using advocacy as a strategy. In spite of the apparent arbitrariness in applying these terms, the concepts are helpful. They provide a scheme, not for categorizing, but for looking at relationships and priorities.

Another aspect of roles which is relevant to school nursing is *territory.* A territory refers to knowledge and expertise, but it also implies control over physical space (Hayter, 1981; Leininger, 1979). Lack of control over physical space can be a problem for school nurses, since in many instances they have little to say about the space allocated to nursing. Often they are assigned to a gymnasium, coatroom, or reception room. This lack of permanent and private space assignment interferes with the nurse's self-identity and perhaps conveys the message to the recipients of care that nurses are not in control (Hayter, 1981).

Types of Roles

The roles a school nurse assumes are conditioned by training, experience, job description, and the problems and opportunities arising in the particular school health program. But they will also be affected by the philosophies of school administrators and the local populace about appropriate school nursing activities, by the constraints placed on the nurse by law and the regulatory mechanisms imposed by professional associations, and by the working relationships with colleagues within the health care delivery system and within the school system. Commonalities in these factors have led to the emergence of identifiable school nursing roles. Seven of them—five primary roles (functional role, primary nurse, team member, nurse practitioner, and nurse teacher) and two secondary roles (consultant and advocate)—will be discussed here.

Functional Role

Nurses in a functional role may be responsible only for screening, follow-up, immunizations, or responding to calls when a school makes a request. Usually, such nurses are assigned to a group of schools.

Primary Nurse

Primary nurses are responsible for all direct health services (within the scope of their expertise) to students within a school or school system. In short, primary nurses are generalists: all health care in school comes from or is channeled through them. They make initial contact with the client population and provide continuity and coordination for all those who need individual attention. At different times these nurses may act as advocates, as consultants, or as educators.

Team Member

A school nurse, as a member of an interdisciplinary team, is usually part of a core group consisting of the school doctor and possibly the school counselor. Health teams are generally problem oriented, have variable membership, and are activated when a problem arises. At those times others, such as school psychologists, social workers, or teachers will be pulled into the team if the problem requires their expertise. The nurse's primary role within the team is usually to coordinate or act as advocate or *consultant*. Responsibility for health promotion and disease prevention practices are often the focus of the nurse who works on a community or school health care team.

Members of such teams rely on each other for expertise in the execution of health services; they share information and collaborate. In the team process the members' behaviors each other's role performance, and interpersonal relationships develop. In these ways the effectiveness and efficiency of the team can either be enhanced or diminished. Chen (1975) found in her study of role relationships on a school health team that professionals each took the major responsibility for their own role definition and role performance. Such a situation can be productive but can also lead to role conflict if areas of expertise are not clearly distinguished and accepted by all members of the team (Hardy and Conway, 1978).

Nurse Practitioner

The school nurse practitioner program originated in Colorado in 1970 and was developed "to assure that schools, especially in poverty areas, could serve as the principal means of bringing comprehensive and continuing care to these children" (Igoe, 1975, p. 381). Program goals have been to train school nurses to extend their capabilities beyond the traditional role of inspection to a broader and more comprehensive approach (Igoe, 1975). School nurse practitioners are particularly concerned with identification of children at risk for specific health problems such as substance abuse and the management of certain chronic conditions, such as diabetes, cardiac and kidney disease, and orthopedic problems. They are able to manage these problems under *protocol* with far more autonomy than other nurses because of their specialized training in *health assessment* and physical examination techniques. They are trained to carry out some functions that would normally require referral and, as a consequence, also have more tools at their command in case finding than do primary nurses.

Nurse Teacher

The nurse teacher's primary job is to educate. These individuals are responsible for teaching health concepts and identifying ways of transmitting knowledge that supports changes in health behavior. Persons in this position may sit on curriculum committees and are often required to have education credentials. This requirement, however, varies with each state.

Consultant

Nurses act as consultants when giving professional advice to school personnel, parent-teacher associations, health committees, or external groups that are concerned about the health needs of school children. The role of consultant may be secondary to their roles as team member, primary nurse, nurse teacher, or functional nurse.

Advocate

A most important role is that of advocate, especially for clients such as the handicapped or abused, who are unable to speak for themselves. Nurses work to assure that such children are not discriminated against by their placement within the school system and that their learning and health needs are met. Furthermore, nurses may teach these students and their families how to act as advocates for their own needs (Doster, 1979)

Advocates may represent individual students, special needs groups, or all school children. Arenas for operating vary: they may be within the school system or in the larger community; they may be in a bureaucratic or a political context. Even the school nurse who speaks to a civic organization about the special health needs of children in the community may be playing the role of advocate.

Advocacy in the political arena provides opportunities for those nurses who wish to affect changes in school health. The concern over funding sources for social services is an issue that calls for nurses to assume this role. Block grants, rather than categorical funding sources, are currently being used to pay for these services. When these grants are discussed in the community, nurses can be present to speak for those programs that support and provide health services for children and youths. They can also be present when these and other health care issues are being debated at the state or national levels.

Functions

The primary function of school nurses 80 years ago was early detection of communicable diseases (Pigg, 1976). Detection and prevention of communicable diseases remain functions of school nurses today; however, now nurses are responsible for much more (Wold, 1981). Commonly, nursing responsibilities include health assessment and management of the school population through observation, communication, and examination (physical, psychological, and social); monitoring the safety of the school environment; coordinating and conducting screening programs; health education; counseling; referral; and follow-up. A selection of these services, which are the important, primary functions of school nurses, will be discussed later in the section on health services.

Some secondary functions are frequently part of the role expectations for school nurses. These functions are liaison, leadership and management, and program planning; they are secondary only in the sense that they are supportive, that is, they enable the nurse to carry out major functions more effectively.

Liaison

Liaison involves acting as the school's and the student's communication link with others. The person with liaison responsibilities is expected to be able to deal skillfully and expeditiously with health departments, police departments, the medical community, detention homes, hospitals, churches, families, social service agencies, and any others within the larger community whose services or cooperation may affect the welfare of students. Discharging this function requires not only skill in communication and human relations but a knowledge of the correct channels, procedures, and language to use in the various situations.

Leadership and Management

All school nursing roles involve leadership and management. Leadership implies influencing the behavior of others; management implies getting a job done through others. Both require high levels of skill in human relations. Management requires considerable conceptual and organizational skill as well.

Nurses accept leadership responsibilities by simply sitting on committees within parent-teacher associations, parent organizations, community groups, or professional organizations. As a committee member nurses can influence decision making. The behavior of other committee members by offering their expertise about school health needs. They become involved in management as soon as they accept responsibility for running any activity that involves others, for example, a screening program, a health education class, or a team project. Although conceptually distinct, leadership and management are discussed together because in practice they are often intertwined.

There are four aspects of management—planning, organizing, motivating, and controlling (Hersey and Blanchard, 1982)—each of which can be considered a function in its own right.

Planning is a necessary component of all school nursing activity. If nothing else, a nurse must plan each day because school nursing does not take place in the structured environment of a hospital, clinic, or office. The nurse must usually impose her own structure. But also, nurses must plan at higher levels. If, for example, a visual screening program has been planned, the nurse must decide the following: (1) whether to use volunteers and in what manner, (2) how to train volunteers, (3) the flow of children to and from the testing site, (4) rescheduling procedures for a second screening, and (5) referral and follow-up procedures. At even higher levels, the nurse may be involved in planning a complete school health program.

Planning at any level involves several steps. First, goals must be set and objectives defined. Second, resources (personnel, space, material, and equipment) must be allocated to the specific objectives. Finally, tools and strategies for accomplishing the goals must be selected or devised.

Organizing involves integrating and coordinating all resources and activities so they run smoothly. Running meetings, scheduling, making arrangements with cooperating services or individuals, assigning tasks, or delegating authority are all tasks connected with organizing.

Motivating means getting school personnel (teachers, principals, secretaries, dietary and housekeeping staff), families, or others more active or committed to the project in hand. For nurses, health promotion requires that they spend time advising, encouraging, reinforcing, and

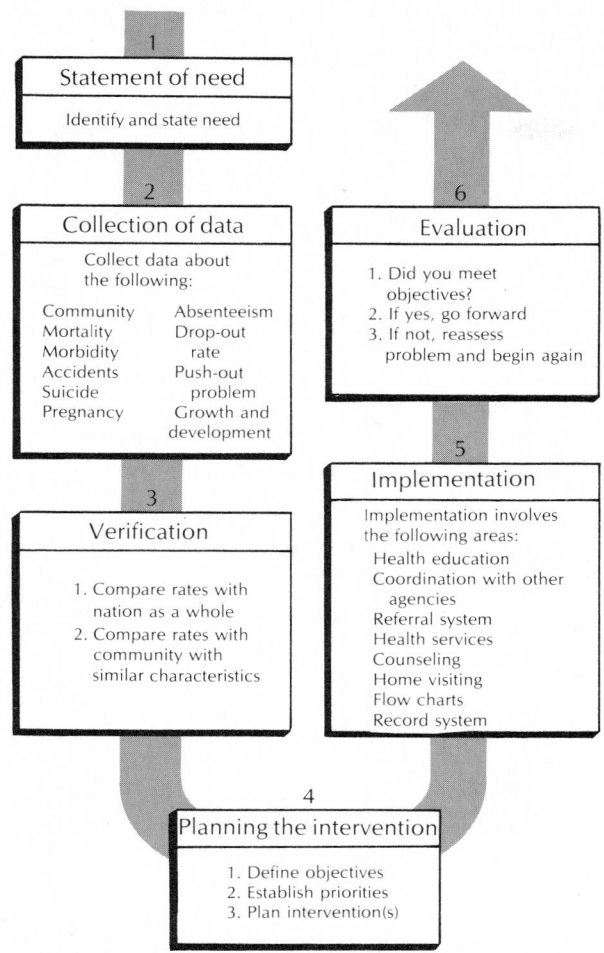

Fig. 31-1. Steps in the design of a school health program.

supporting students, their families, and school personnel.

Controlling is essentially monitoring and evaluating. Responsibility for any project or activity requires that attention be given to seeing that goals are actually being met and that progress is as planned. This usually requires that arrangements be made for measurement, feedback, and adjustments in the procedures, personnel, or material resources when necessary.

Program Planning

School nurses may be expected to do more formal planning for specific health programs or even for the total school health program for a school or community. This type of planning requires documentation and a presentation in writing. Fig. 31-1 outlines the steps in this process. A discussion of each of these steps follows.

1. The *statement of need* should be a concise statement identifying a need that the proposed health program is to fill. The statement should include

several other elements. First, there should be a description of the cultural and socioeconomic characteristics of the children for whom the services are planned. Second, the reasons for developing the program should be given. Frequently, this is done by referring to national and local trends in school health.

2. The *collection of data* should reflect the nature of the proposed program and be designed to support the statements made in the statement of need. At this stage in the planning process, any relevant information that would document (or dispute) the asserted need and the description of target population characteristics should be gathered and organized so it can be examined and compared. These data may also serve to guide planners in subsequent steps.

3. *Verification* is an evaluative process, which is necessary to determine whether the assertion of need is supported by the data collected and examined. By definition a statement of need reflects judgment. The comparisons suggested allow for an assessment of that judgment. At this point, any inconsistencies in the reasoning or any potential problems because of unusually high or low rates or some other anomaly in the data can be identified.

4. There are three steps in planning the *intervention*. First, specific objectives—as opposed to overall goals expressed in the statement of need—must be defined. Second, priorities for these objectives must be established. Finally, in light of the specific objectives and priorities, major decisions, especially as they relate to the allocation of resources, must be made. For example, if there are going to be large-scale interventions, will hospital outpatient clinics, private physicians, health departments, or school nurses provide the personal health services? Will protocols be part of the service? How will school social workers and school counselors fit into the program? What type of record system is needed to facilitate services?

5. Details of the *implementation* must be outlined, that is, the specific methods, tools, and techniques for accomplishing the tasks must be selected or devised. Detailed plans for the procedures must be worked out. These plans will be for such things as follow-up, referral, and reexamination. Decisions must be made about the ways clients will be monitored, counseled, and educated. This is also the point at which problems should be anticipated and contingency plans made.

6. For an *evaluation* of how well goals are being met, it is helpful to have as much information as possi-

Table 31-1. Guide to organizing a program evaluation

Aspect of program	Questions to ask
Structure	Do policies facilitate or impede program
	Are the objectives measurable?
	Are there standards for measurement of the staff?
	Which standards are being used (ANA, ASHA, local school district)?
	Are they measurable?
	How do staff members rate?
	Is the assigned space adequate?
	If not, how can it be improved?
	Have the following factors in the organization of delivery been assessed?
	Method of delivery
	Flowchart's effectiveness
	Adequacy of equipment
	Role of management
Process	Having adequate records of the following been kept?
	Number of cases found
	Screening results
	Treatments given
	Observations of process
	Has a specified percentage of randomly selected records been audited?
	Have teachers, parents, and students been asked for input?
Outcome	Have the following factors decreased or increased?
	Social functioning of children as a result of contact with nurse or other team member
	Morbidity
	School absenteeism
	Accidents
	Communicable diseases
	Number of children seen
	Number of children excluded from school
	Did program meet its objectives?

ble on how the program is working and what results it is getting. Therefore, thought should be given during the planning process to some of the following questions: What will tell us if the program is working or not working? How do we measure it? What will tell us if the procedures we are using are effective? How do we assess effectiveness? What about the organizational structure, personnel, and policies; do they promote or interfere with the functioning of the program? Ways must be found to measure and provide feedback about the structure, process, and results of the project so that, where necessary, adjustments can be made to better achieve the goals (Shortell and Richardson, 1978). Table 31-1 suggests a number of items that might be examined in the evaluation of a school health program.

The design of any health program must integrate children's health needs, available and accessible services, available resources (money, people, support services, equipment, space) and a set of philosophical beliefs and orientations. Since all those elements will vary

from situation to situation, discriminative judgment is crucial for this task. A program designed to fit the needs of a particular school community might have to include plans for meeting the needs of many types of children: depressed groups, special population groups such as adolescent parents, ethnic groups, the developmentally disabled, and younger siblings who need referral to preschool programs for early stimulation. In weighing the potential value of any program, reference to the literature is helpful. In trying to decide on the value of a preschool program, it would be necessary to consult the Surgeon General's report (Healthy People, 1979), which speaks to a new morbidity (i.e., learning disorders) and a 1979 General Accounting Office's report (cited in Healthy People, 1979) that indicates children benefit from early stimulation programs.

Tools

Nurses who work in schools use a wide array of tools in discharging the obligations connected with their roles. Generally, a tool is a mechanism for getting a specific job done or for dealing with a particular problem.

For convenience, they have been categorized as technical tools, educational tools, interpersonal tools, and forms.

Technical Tools

The technical tools are, in general, more closely associated with nursing than are the other types of tools. These are, for the most part, screening or assessment tools. Some are technological; others are written or drawn tests related to sociological or psychological variables. This list is not exhaustive; it is designed only to illustrate the wide range of tools and tests used in school nursing.

Audiometers
Blood pressure equipment
Stethoscope
Opthalmoscope
Pin light
Visual screening equipment
Weight scale
Sample urinalysis (by tape)
Height chart
Vineland Maturity Scale
Peabody Vocabulary Test
Health Locus of Control Scale
Health-Seeking Behavior Scale (adolescents)
Developmental Profile II
General Anxiety Scale for School Children
Children's Illness Anxiety Scale
Social Profile (sociometrics)
Goodenough Draw-a-Man Test
Denver Developmental Screening test (5 to 6 year olds)
Self-concept Scale

It is good to remember, however, that technical screening tools are not diagnostic tools; their purpose is to alert the examiner to the need for further diagnostic study (Haynes, 1979).

Educational Tools

Most of the educational tools have been adopted by nurses to get their health messages across when they are discharging their educational functions. Common educational tools are films, manuals, and games. Some of the techniques developed in education for leading discussions, asking questions, role playing, giving demonstrations, and devising test questions have also been incorporated into the repertoire of the school nurse.

Interpersonal Tools

The use of a number of interpersonal tools has become common in school nursing. The interview, the conference, and the workshop will be discussed here. All provide the context for specific kinds of interpersonal exchange, and guidelines for using all of them are available.

Collecting and organizing information is often the first step in assessment or counseling. Nurses must frequently gather information from interviews with students, teachers, and others. For these reasons a knowledge of interviewing techniques is valuable to assure not only that information is as unambiguous as possible but that it can be gathered without hostility or discomfort from the respondent.

Conferences are meetings set up to promote interchange of views and ideas about a specific topic with the expectation that the discussion will lead to purposeful actions. School nurses regularly confer with teachers, children, and parents. These conferences may be formal or informal, but in either case, they should be planned. Any materials that must be handled or examined during the interview should be organized ahead of time as well. An example of a tool that is helpful in guiding nurse-teacher conferences is the Classroom Observation Sheet (Appendix A). The purpose of the observation form is to help the teacher separate those children with potential problems from children without identifiable problems. This form can also be used in case finding.

Workshops are seminars emphasizing free discussion, exchange of ideas, and development of practical methods and skills. School nurses will participate in workshops and may conduct workshops with teachers, other nurses, or students. Unlike interviews or conferences, workshops are usually arranged through negotiation with the school principal, teachers, and in some instances, the superintendant. The best time to schedule a teacher workshop is the beginning of the academic year, since it provides opportunities for introducing classroom teachers to the methods of tools of the school nurse.

Forms

Any bureaucracy, including a school, requires the use of forms. They are helpful in organizing information that must be used in dealing with the many individuals or agencies with whom a nurse is in contact, in organizing observations for later use, and in record keeping.

The Classroom Observation Sheet (Appendix A) is a tool used by classroom teachers to list children in their classroom who may have health problems or symptoms that need the school nurse's attention. This tool provides nurses with data for compiling a composite picture of the total health problems existing within the school. The data can be used to develop a health program for the school, and program plans can be shared with teachers in workshops or conferences.

The School and Classroom Assessment Guide (Appendix I) guides the nurse's observations of children's behaviors. The purposes of this observation are to identify behavior patterns, identify developmental lags and other specific health or social problems, and discover any environmental behavioral relationships.

The Case Presentation Guide for Agency Communication (Appendix F) is used to facilitate and organize data collection and sharing of information with other agencies.

The Sample Note to Parents (Appendix F) is used to communicate with parents about their children's health needs. This sample note is not a consent form; therefore, it cannot be considered an authorization. Consent is an authorization by the individual or person authorized by law to consent on the person's behalf (Cazalas, 1978). Consent forms must be designed to conform to the Family Right's and Privacy Act of 1978.

The Referral Form (Appendix F) is used to share information when collaborating with other service agencies or to obtain for students those services that are not available in school. Referrals, for whatever purpose, cannot be made without the consent of the legal guardian of the student. There is one exception—the youth who is classified as *emancipated*. States and individual school districts define emancipation differently, but emancipated youths are often those who maintain separate residence—outside of their parents' home—and have their own income. It is advisable when confronted with a possible emancipated student to consult with the school attorney to clarify the meaning of emancipation in that particular school district.

The School Record (Appendix F) is an example of a tool used to record all information gathered and all actions taken in regard to a single student. Accurate record keeping and documentation are nursing responsibilities that require some such system for keeping information accessible.

Strategies

The strategies referred to here are ways of dealing with people that are commonly called for in the discharge of nursing functions, including those of the school nurse. Unlike interpersonal tools, which are more formalized and provide a context for a particular type of interaction,—that is, they are usually scheduled for an explicit purpose and may have leaders and use special materials,—these interpersonal strategies may be used as needed whenever people must deal with one another. A nurse who is able to identify what is occurring in an exchange and make adjustments is more likely to be effective.

Cooperation

Cooperation involves mutually beneficial exchanges of information, assistance, or accommoda-

tion which allow each party to achieve its goals more effectively. No conflict of interest is inherent in the situation. Cooperation may simply involve being aware of or sensitive to the needs of others and communicating your needs to them so that mutual adjustments can occur.

Cooperation might be illustrated by a situation in a high school in which the administration is pushing for programs with vocational emphasis. A nurse who believes it important that adolescents know of the many career possibilities in counseling open to them might agree to work on a school committee for bringing various professionals in to talk about their fields. The speaking program would provide a platform and unpressured atmosphere for the clinical psychologist and psychiatric social worker brought in to pass on the needed information. The committee and the administration, on the other hand, would have help in implementing the program and providing the students with professional role models.

Collaboration. Collaboration is a special form of cooperation characterized by two or more individuals applying their efforts to a common endeavor. The implication is that each party comes to the collaboration with different skills and perspectives.

Collaboration is often used when complex problems arise for which no solution is clearly superior. Children who are bed wetters or who are handicapped and must be taught some skill such as feeding themselves present such problems. Because of the complexity of the problems, their causes, and the techniques that may have to be used to deal with them, a health team may be activated. Each member has seen the children under different conditions, has a distinct area of expertise, and is probably more sensitive to different aspects of the situation. When they get together to analyze the problem and work out a treatment plan, they are collaborating. All have the same goal: to help the children with their problems. Each member brings unique insight and skills to bear on it.

Negotiation

Negotiation also involves mutual exchange, but implies a balancing of the good and the bad in a conflict of interest so that each party can accept the solution. The keys to negotiation are to know (1) when to compromise and (2) how not to place the other party in a losing situation (Nierenberg, 1978).

As an example, consider the speaking program described earlier. There are a limited number of speaking spots, and the other staff member on the committee have their own priorities for selecting speakers. As a consequence, the members may negotiate for the number of speaking spots each will be allowed to fill. Negotiation is not argument to see who wins or loses; it is a search for a plan (or alternatives) that will allow all parties to win to some extent.

Role bargaining is a special type of negotiation common to interdisciplinary health teams. When role conflict or role incongruity arises, role bargaining is one way of trying to resolve the problem. It may take place between nurse and school physician, principal, or classroom teacher. They meet, discuss alternatives, and try to reach a mutually acceptable agreement on appropriate role behaviors. For example, the physician and school nurse practitioner are both capable of performing physical examinations on school children. The two people will meet and decide which health provider could appropriately perform the physical examinations on the school children. Routine screening physical exams may be performed by the school nurse practitioner while children with an acute illness problem may be referred directly to the physician for examination.

Networking

Networking is the process of establishing and maintaining relationships with others outside one's immediate reference group. These relationships are based on common interest but also imply an establishment of mutual trust, respect, and reciprocity. People establish their own individual networks to meet their own individual needs, or groups may be organized for the purpose of networking. School nurses in Ohio, for example, may form a loosely organized group with school nurses in California, and they will all interact at meetings and telephone conferences around a specific issue.

A network can be activated. Professional networks may include individuals in various agencies, professional organizations, or positions of authority who can be relied on to respond to requests for information, advice, or help in facilitating a procedure or for some other kind of assistance. These personal links with people in constituent groups help to ensure that the best possible health services and information will be secured for the students.

School nurses form networks to exchange and share information and to plan strategies with classroom teachers, school administrators, counselors, and other school personnel. These networks provide a medium for identifying and presenting positions and concerns. They are also helpful in anticipating problems or disagreements and in providing feedback and support to one another. With the help of school nurses, students also form peer networks to reinforce desired behavior changes.

Skills

Ultimately, role performance rests on the skills brought to a position and skills developed on the job. A skill has two components: knowledge and the abilty to apply that knowledge. When an individual practices applying a skill (or a group of skills) to a specific task and reaches an acceptable level of performance at the task, the individual can be said to have a *competency*. Fig. 31-2 lists some competencies necessary for adequate performance as a school nurse and others that are merely desirable. This list is not exhaustive, but it is representative of the many different skills a school nurse must command to perform competently.

Examination of these competencies uncovers several things about the skills a nurse working in a school needs. First, there are different types of skills. Here they have been designated as technical, human, conceptual, educational, and research. These skills will be explained later. Furthermore, most competencies require a combination of skills. The nurse who is proficient at carrying out the technical skills associated with nursing but has difficulty taking initiative in human relations, is only moderately perceptive, does not like thinking and planning, or needs a relatively structured situation might find school nursing frustrating. The nurse who enjoys working in a wide variety of situations, is a problem solver, and does not mind flux or ambiguity may be more willing to develop the breadth needed to meet the challenges encountered in this field.

Technical Skills

Technical skills include the ability to use procedures, techniques, and technology (equipment) to perform specific tasks such as taking blood pressure, using audiometers and visual screening equipment, or administering the various social or psychological tests.

Human Skills

Human skills involve the exercise of judgment and the application of human relations concepts in working with people. Sensitivity and skill in dealing with others may be honed by training and supported by knowledge of interpersonal relationships, group behavior, value systems, and cultural variation (e.g., dealing with a student who may be pregnant).

Conceptual Skills

Conceptual skills revolve around the ability to understand, manipulate, and integrate complex concepts and knowledge. Especially important is an understanding of the ways school health programs and school nursing mesh within the total school system. Conceptual skills permit nurses to plan and act according to overall program goals rather than individual or group goals.

Educational Skills

Educational skills relate to the ability to handle the various educational methods and concepts in classroom presentations, in workshops or in-service pro-

COMPETENCY	T*	H*	C*	E*	R*
Necessary					
Carry out nursing tasks (including health assessment based on the nursing process).					
Understand and use public/community health concepts (primary, secondary, and tertiary prevention; health promotion; control of communicable diseases, etc.).					
Have knowledge of growth and development in children and youths.					
Understand cultural and ethnic differences and ways these differences affect compliance and use of health services.					
Recognize individual factors operating in each individual in a heterogenous group.					
Identify interferences with basic human needs.					
Conduct casefinding activities.					
Provide anticipatory guidance.					
Counsel students and parents.					
Assume leadership and management obligations.					
Desirable					
Devise and use a theoretical or conceptual gramework to guide practice.					
Plan, organize, and use a referral system.					
Use community resources knowledgeably.					
Transmit health knowledge that affects or produces changes in behavior.					
Extend nursing influence to the students' families.					
Identify researchable problems.					
Form coalitions and networks.					
Develop political awareness and astuteness.					

*T=Technical, H=Human, C=Conceptual, E=Educational, R=Research.

Fig. 31-2. School nursing competencies. Checklist enables prospective school nurse to check off the types of skills that must be combined to achieve competency at any one of the tasks listed. *T,* technical; *H,* human; *C,* conceptual; *E,* educational; *R,* research.

grams, or in individual encounters with students. The ability to integrate concepts and methods is an essential aspect of the process. Educational skills include such things as formal teaching, demonstration, laboratory teaching, team teaching and leading seminars.

Research Skills

Research skills useful to a school nurse would involve understanding the methods and methodology of science—at least as far as looking at problems systematically, learning how to ask scientific questions, knowing how to use the professional literature (knowledge of major journals and indexing, abstracting, and computer accessing systems). Nurses armed with such research skills may help gather useful data, participate in research, and suggest researchable topics. They may also be equipped to answer some of their own questions, for example, Which health-promoting practices are 9-year-old children currently using?

Requirements

Requirements for school nurses vary. As a consequence, there are licensed practical nurses, diploma nurses, and associate degree nurses working in schools along side of nurses with baccalaureate and master's degrees. Furthermore, neither baccalaureate nor master's degrees of nurses are necessarily in nursing: some states allow a bachelor of arts degree, which does not assist those nurses to assume primary care role responsibilities but does meet requirements for a teaching certificate.

As would be expected, some states (e.g., Ohio) have certification requirements and others do not. Johnson represents the views of many in the profession when she suggests that this question must be decided for all school nurses and should not vary from state to state (1979).

The trend, however, for first-level entry into school nursing is to require both the baccalaureate degree and certification. The American Nurses' Association and the American Association for School Health support this requirement (ANA, 1979; AASH, 1975). The American Association for Health, Physical Education, Recreation and Dance goes even further and recommends that nurses have graduate degrees in school health.

Accountability

In most respects, accountability in school nursing does not differ from other nursing specialties. School nurses are accountable for conforming to their practice acts (Thompson, 1979). Accountability also includes the responsibility for meeting practice competencies, which are defined by the professional association (American Nurses' Association, 1973). These standards, which focus on practice, provide a means for determining the quality of nursing a client receives. The standards are given in Appendix G.

Accountability in school nursing, as measured by these standards of practice, speaks to the scope of nursing practice and the current state of the art, provides a definition of the professional, and prescribes the maintenance of health records to document nursing interventions and dispositions.

SCHOOL HEALTH PROGRAMS

School nurses do not perform their roles autonomously within the school system. Usually, they must work in the context of a school health program. Programs vary from state to state and from location to location depending on a number of factors. First, state laws or policies may govern the scope of health care provided within a school and the nature of the organizational structure that provides it. Second, programs will be strongly influenced by the local factors such as nature and composition of the target population (i.e., urban or rural, racial and ethnic mix, socioeconomic characteristics); the philosophical beliefs and commitments of the general populace, the school board, and the administration; the accessibility of support or supplementary community services; and, of course, the resources.

The number of nurses also varies from state to state. Alabama, for example, has about 50 nurses for the entire state, whereas some states legislate the placement of a nurse in every school (e.g., Ohio). Kentucky, among others, assigns its nurses to a cluster of schools. Of course, this variation affects the range and quality of services provided in school health programs.

Furthermore, there is a continuum of organizational complexity. Toward one end are a number of districts in Ohio, among other places, where organizational structure consists of a supervisor of school nurses with a number of nurses working under the supervisor. Each nurse works with from one to three schools and has clearly defined responsibilities. At the other end of the continuum, some school districts only sporadically have school health programs. When funding becomes available for a specific purpose, a temporary program will be set up; it will be closed down when funds run out.

Bureaucratic Organization

In spite of this variability in programs, authority for and administration of school health programs are usually established in one of several ways. The delivery of school health programs may be administered under the

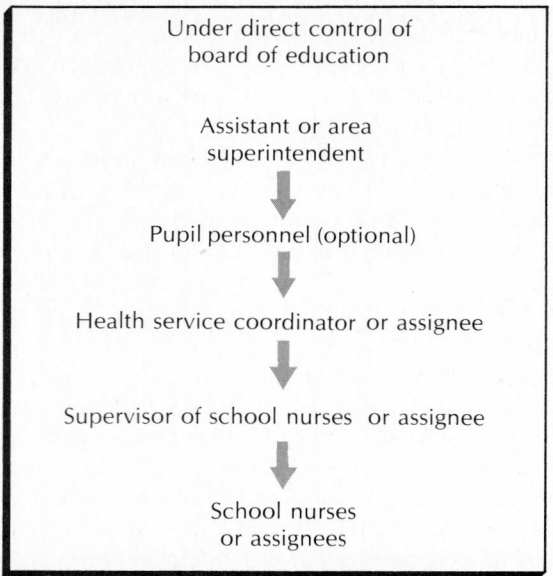

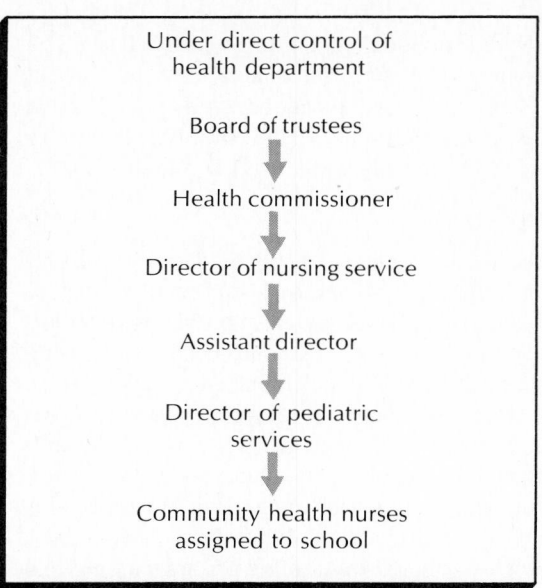

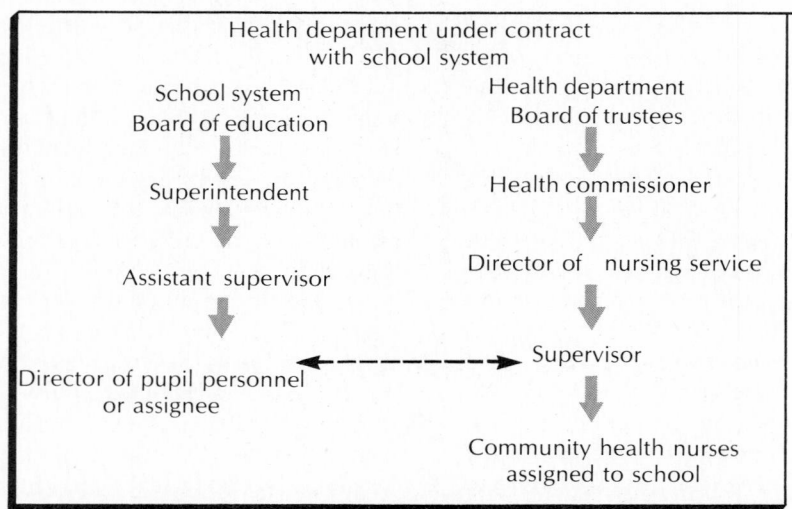

Fig. 31-3. Bureaucratic organization of school health programs and decision-making process.

direct control of a board of education or, alternately, under the direct control of a local health department (Fig. 31-3). There are advantages to both structures. Nurses in community health departments are backed by public health law and the power of the health department. Thus they have more flexibility in carrying out their functions, and they are in stronger negotiating positions when faced with conflicts. Nurses working for the school system do not have this firm backing from a medical structure and law, but they may encounter less resistance and more cooperation in carrying out their responsibilities. As in-group members, even though peripheral, they have a more effective base for dealing with school personnel and are less likely to be caught in the middle of a conflict.

Another possible structure is for a board of education to contract for services from a local health department (Humes, 1975). In this case, although the delivery of health services may be by community health nurses, planning and coordination are assigned to a team consisting of representatives from both the health department and the school system.

Decision making tends to be centralized regardless of the system of administration. This means that major decisions, such as sex education, are made by central authorities. If policy dictates some decentralization, the

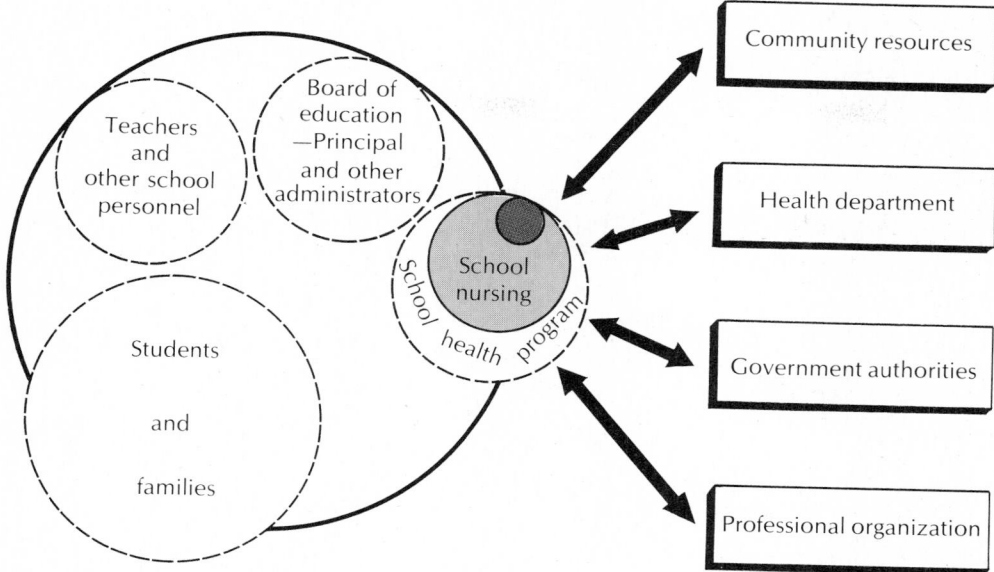

Fig. 31-4. Systemic organization of a school health program. The cross-hatched and lined circles represent the two ends of the continuum of school nursing involvement in school health programs: the cross-hatched circle indicates those where nurses work within a collaborative interdisciplinary structure, and the lined circle where nurses dominate the school health program. The circle representing the school health program extends beyond the school system boundary to indicate the possibility of health department affiliation.

principal tends to be the lowest policy-making level. In practice, this means that the school nurse rarely has the autonomy of the classroom teacher, and many more of the nurse's decisions and plans must be cleared through the administrative hierarchy.

Place of School Nursing in School Health and Total School Programs

School health programs are not synonymous with school nursing programs because many different types of people may occupy positions as health providers in schools. According to Nader (1978), school health is a cooperative effort that encourages the involvement of health personnel, school personnel, and other community people. Without input from all of these representatives, he claims, school health might not progress. In addition to nurses, there may be teachers (physical education, health, or home economics), social workers, counselors, school physicians and psychologists, secretaries, parents, and other volunteers. Some of these individuals perform complementary functions; others perform functions that overlap with nursing functions. Thus, school nurses operate as only one component of a school health team, although they may be the dominant one.

Fig. 31-4 provides a graphic illustration of the place of school nursing within the larger school system. School nursing may be visualized as an open subsystem within the larger health and total school systems. There are many points of articulation (or contact) with other subsystems within the total school: with students, and by extension, their families; with the school authority structure represented by the principal, school administrators, and board of education; and with teachers and other school personnel. School nursing, however, is also open to many influences from outside the system. The many direct interactions nurses have with the various social service agencies, the local medical delivery system, community organizations, local and state authority structure, and the nursing organizations distinguish this subsystem from others such as teachers. Other subsystems are also open to external influences, but they are more often mediated through the administration.

When operating effectively, school nursing contributes to the balance (equilibrium) of the entire school system. In short, when health related activities, values, and concepts are successfully introduced into the system (input) through health promotion, case finding, education, referral, shaping, modeling, counseling, or follow-up, the outcome (output) will generally be increased levels of wellness, new, more functional health behaviors among students, and students who are prepared to become more effective learners and better adapted members of this subgroup.

If there is a disruption in the relationships between

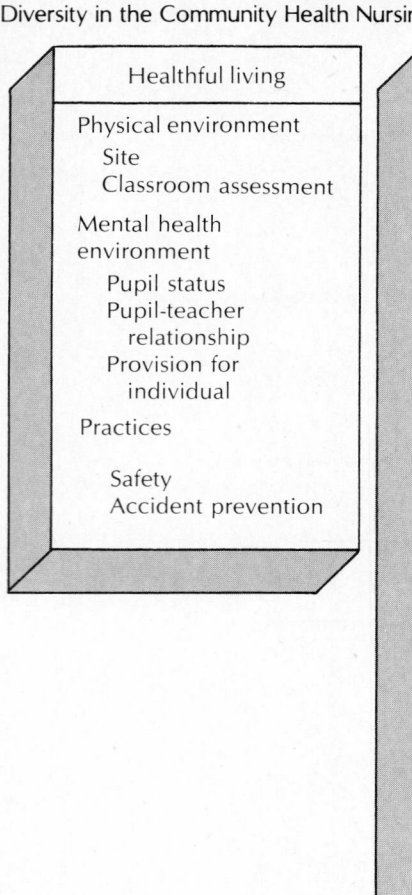

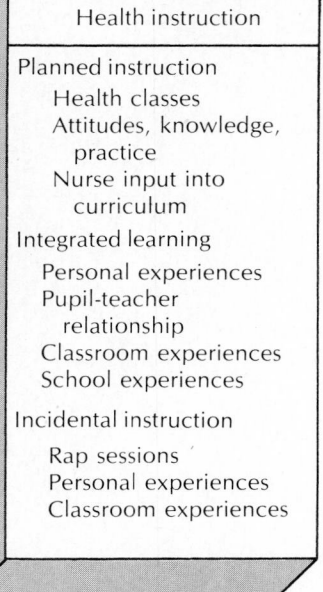

Fig. 31-5. School health program based on Bryan's three perspectives. (Modified from Bryan, D.: School nursing in transition, 1974.)

the nursing subsystem and other subsystems, school nursing can contribute to an imbalance in the system. Disruptions come from misunderstandings, conflicts over goals or domain, or insensitivity in carrying out nursing functions. Teachers of home economics, for example, may consider instruction in family life, safety, or coping strategies to be in their realm rather than in that of the school nurse. Likewise, the chemistry instructor may consider his domain invaded when the school nurse makes a safety inspection. Tact, consideration, knowing when to acquiese or when to compromise are invaluable when confronting this situations.

Disruption may also occur when health providers attempt to make health services the central focus in the education system when in fact they are supportive (Means, 1975). It is important to remember that the values of parents, educators, and health providers often

conflict over such things as the need to discuss sexuality.

Another way nurses may introduce disruption is through the use of tools that are designed to bring change: to change unhealthy behaviors to healthy ones. The School and Assessment Guide (Appendix H) provides an excellent example of such a tool. Teachers may see these assessments as invasion of their domain, and a threat to established time commitments and priorities as well as their self-images of values. Very few teachers would quickly accept evaluations of their classrooms and their relationships with their students without extensive preliminary preparation and, probably, the role of collaborator in the process. In any case, the introduction of one of several of these tools may lead to disruption and should be planned with caution and sensitivity so as to minimize disruptions.

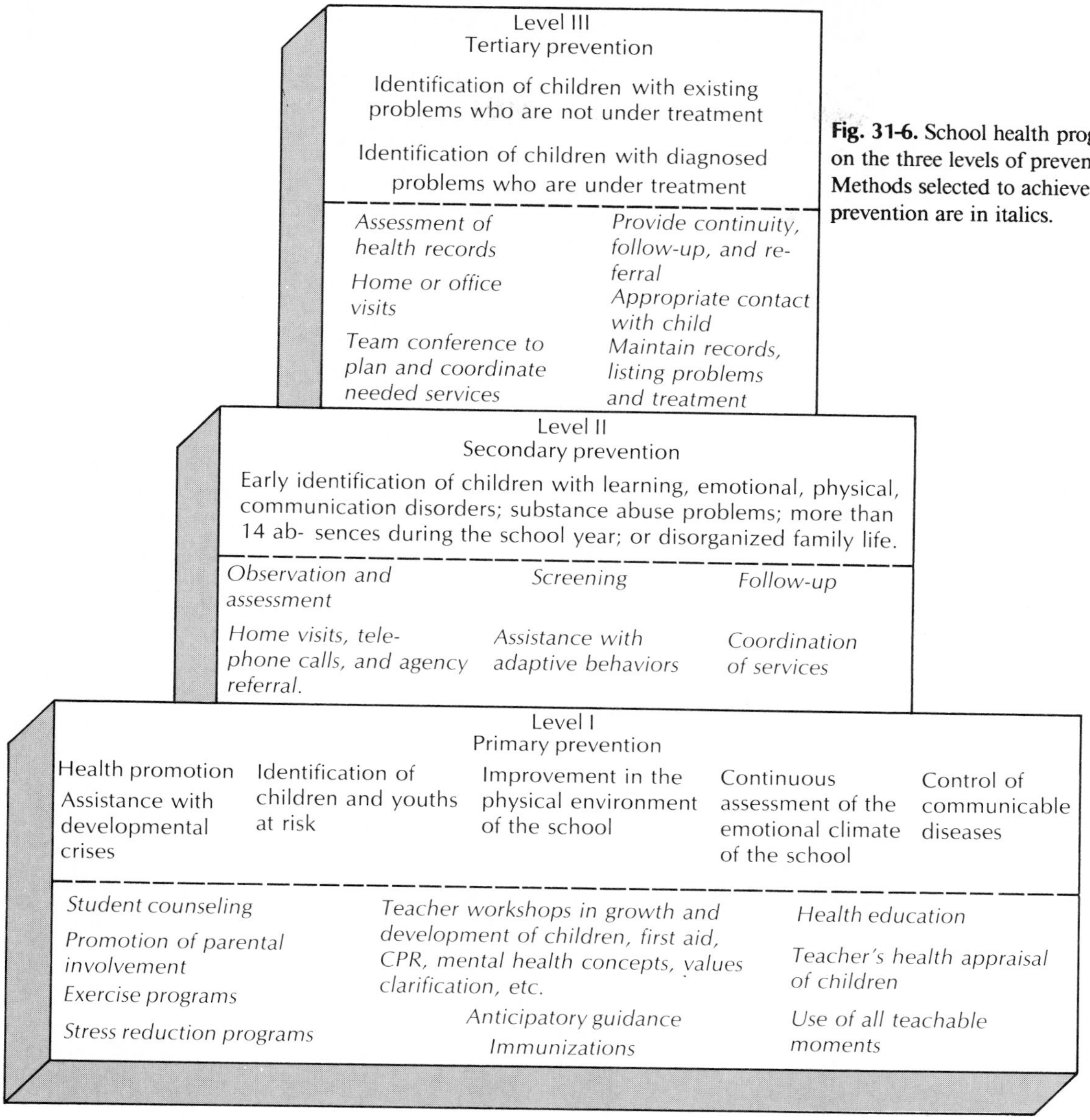

Level III
Tertiary prevention

Identification of children with existing
problems who are not under treatment

Identification of children with diagnosed
problems who are under treatment

*Assessment of
health records*

*Home or office
visits*

*Team conference to
plan and coordinate
needed services*

*Provide continuity,
follow-up, and re-
ferral*

*Appropriate contact
with child*

*Maintain records,
listing problems
and treatment*

Level II
Secondary prevention

Early identification of children with learning, emotional, physical,
communication disorders; substance abuse problems; more than
14 ab- sences during the school year; or disorganized family life.

*Observation and
assessment*

*Home visits, tele-
phone calls, and agency
referral.*

Screening

*Assistance with
adaptive behaviors*

Follow-up

*Coordination
of services*

Level I
Primary prevention

Health promotion

Assistance with
developmental
crises

Identification of
children and youths
at risk

Improvement in the
physical environment
of the school

Continuous
assessment of the
emotional climate
of the school

Control of
communicable
diseases

Student counseling

*Promotion of parental
involvement*

Exercise programs

Stress reduction programs

*Teacher workshops in growth and
development of children, first aid,
CPR, mental health concepts, values
clarification, etc.*

*Anticipatory guidance
Immunizations*

Health education

*Teacher's health appraisal
of children*

*Use of all teachable
moments*

Fig. 31-6. School health program based
on the three levels of prevention.
Methods selected to achieve levels of
prevention are in italics.

Methods selected to achieve levels of prevention are in italics.

Theoretical Framework

It is helpful to have a theoretical framework to guide a school health program for a number of reasons. First, it provides a basis for making decisions and establishing priorities. Second, it is a way to look at programs systematically, that is, to see if there are any gaps or overemphasis, to look for continuity, and to uncover problems (real or potential). Third, it provides a framework for explaining to others who need to know, such as colleagues, teachers, and superiors, what the nurse is doing and why it is being done.

If no such framework exists, one can be designed using a number of different schemes to provide the basic perspective. Fig. 31-5 shows one possible program based on the three perspectives suggested by Bryan (1974). The three perspectives have been modified to meet contemporary needs. There is no one answer to the organization of a viable school health program. Leavell's and Clark's three levels of prevention (1965) could just as easily be used. Fig. 31-6 is a school health program based on that scheme.

In either program nurses would perform many of the same services, and major health problems could be attacked using either scheme. Differences would lie in the way the nurse approached the program planning. Consider obesity as an example. Using a framework based on the three perspectives, the nurse would first consider what services could be offered to help combat obesity.

A decision might be made to provide exercise groups for all children and examinations, counseling, and instruction in keeping nutrition logs for overweight children. Attention could then be turned to instruction; classes in nutrition might get most of the effort here. Efforts could then be expended in promoting healthful living by trying to involve the family, getting low-calorie lunches offered in the lunchroom at school, and helping to organize support groups. Using a framework based on the three levels of prevention, the questions asked would be, which activities and services would be most appropriate for prevention of obesity? Which would identify those children who are likely to become obese and help to prevent it? Which would help obese children deal with this problem? The program might end up with the same activities either way.

HEALTH SERVICES

The range of health services offered in schools has been stressed throughout this chapter. A selection of commonly provided health services will be discussed here. But first, it should be noted that it is no longer economically feasible, realistic, or fair to students to have an open door policy for those who need health services. How students arrive for service should be planned and organized in the form of appointments and referrals. They are essential to the smooth functioning of a health service: they help with organization and planning of the service, enable the nurse to provide in-depth rather than cursory inspections, and allow sufficient time with each student who needs counseling, teaching, or follow-up. Fig. 31-7 is an example of a flowchart for students entering a school health service for the first time.

Referrals

Referrals are used to provide access to health care for students in need. The object of a referral service is to identify contact people within agencies and to facilitate easy movement of referred clients so they are not lost in the system. The school nurse's responsibility is to act as liaison, dealing with the proper community or medical resources on behalf of the child. The following is a list of some of the guidelines used in handling clients referred for special education.

A. School nurse works cooperatively with the principal, speech teacher for the educationally handicapped, and other staff members in the school.

B. School nurse assists in appraising (both developmentally and functionally) the health status of pupils considered for admission to these classes. Nurse also interprets findings and any other pertinent data.

C. Some additional nursing functions are as follows:
   1. Contact parents, after-school counselor or social worker, or school designee.
   2. Obtain developmental history.
   3. Obtain medical reports.
   4. Obtain signed authorizations.
   5. Collect data for and from source of medical care.
   6. Reevaluate pupils (if needed).
   7. Refer students (if needed).
   8. Provide nursing follow-up.

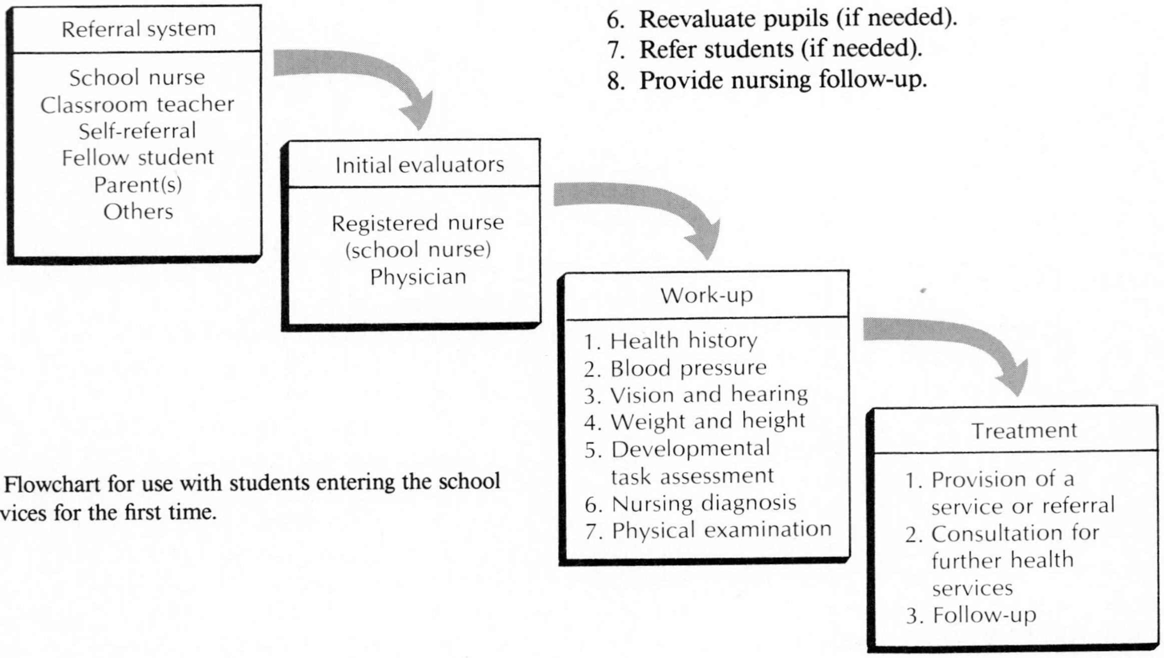

Fig. 31-7. Flowchart for use with students entering the school health services for the first time.

Referral system

School nurse
Classroom teacher
Self-referral
Fellow student
Parent(s)
Others

Initial evaluators

Registered nurse
(school nurse)
Physician

Work-up

1. Health history
2. Blood pressure
3. Vision and hearing
4. Weight and height
5. Developmental task assessment
6. Nursing diagnosis
7. Physical examination

Treatment

1. Provision of a service or referral
2. Consultation for further health services
3. Follow-up

Agency conferences are also a part of a referral service. Before a nurse can participate in an agency conference, parental consent must be obtained. Parental input is also necessary and may come by attending the conference, sending a written statement, or talking to the nurse before the conference. The family's involvement promotes compliance. Appendix F includes an example of a referral form that can be used for sharing information and keeping record of the dispositions.

An effective referral service is based on networking relationships built up through meetings, informal gatherings, and telephone conversations. Also, it is essential that all teachers, students, principals, secretaries, and school counselors be instructed in the use of the referral system. Appendix H contains an example of the guidelines for using a referral system that might be circulated among faculty and staff members in the school system.

Screening

Basic screening tests determine whether children can hear, see, speak, and communicate and whether their coordination, motor development, and anthropometric measurements are appropriate for their stages of development. The list of technical tools given earlier give a good idea of the types of screening frequently carried out in schools. Added to these, however, would be scoliosis screening and instruction in self-examination of breast and testicles.

The nurse's responsibility in the screening process is to determine, with families and other team members, the appropriate resources for additional diagnostic workup for children with symptoms. The nurse who has screened for scoliosis and found some children who are symptomatic may, for example, decide in conjunction with the families to refer one student to a private physician and another to a scoliosis clinic sponsored by Crippled Children's Services for confirmation and treatment.

The nurse must be cautious of one problem that frequently arises because of screening—although it can also arise for other reasons. This is labeling. To label is to describe, designate, or identify with a word or phrase. Frequently, the label *slow learner* is carelessly and inaccurately applied. If children are inaccurately labeled, they may be deprived of some educational opportunities and potential. Even when the label is accurate, its use as a designation is usually insensitive and a gross oversimplification of a human being.

Case Finding

School nurses can help to alleviate problems such as those just described by using case finding techniques. The purpose of case finding is to identify those children who have special problems so that they can be helped

to uncover the sources and resolve them. Case finding techniques are designed to uncover those cases that do not surface in the screening programs. Basically, nurses practice careful, systematic observation of all children they come in contact with, looking for anomalies or suspect symptoms. It is also wise to check the following categories regularly:

1. Absentee list
2. Students sent more than twice to principal's office for illness.
3. Students sent more than twice to principal's office for "acting out in classroom"
4. Students who appear ill
5. Students with subtle as well as obvious physical defects
6. Students who independently seek out nurse for services
7. Incidental survey yields

Perhaps the most likely places to begin, however, are with observations of children who are physically and mentally different; children who have been bused out of their neighborhood or who have moved from rural, mountain, urban, or suburban settings into a totally different social environment; and children from stressful situations where parental expectations may, at times, seem unreasonable for the child's stage of cognitive development. School nurses are especially concerned about uncovering cases of children who are neglected or abused. The nurse's responsibility in working with children who are suspected of being abused is to provide them with a nonthreatening environment and to report the problem to appropriate authorities such as the children's protective services.

Health Education

Health education programs provide an ideal opportunity to help students develop health practices and life-style behaviors that will aid them in developing coping strategies for confronting the societal and environmental stresses specific to future developmental stages (Daniel, 1970; Miliar, 1974). Educational programs are central to health promotion and preparation for screening, and they aid in maintaining or restoring one's health, that is, they are useful at all levels of prevention.

School nurses are involved in educational activities in both direct and indirect ways as they teach, act as consultant, plan programs, and take advantage of every "teachable moment." Nurses may even be guest speakers in classes and in the community.

School nurses are responsible for the planning, organizing, and implementing, and controlling of any health program or class they conduct. When cooperating with faculty in planning health education, the nurse

---

Safety Lesson Plan

Objective

To demonstrate how to cross the street safely.

Content

1. What does safety mean?
2. How should I cross the street?

Materials

Comic books, pamphlets, puppets, movies.

Learning activities

1. Ask children to tell how they cross the street.
2. Discuss the ways to cross the street.
3. Demonstrate how to cross the street.
4. Discuss the dangers of crossing the street between cars, unsupervised, or against the red light.
5. Design a game; include in the design a means whereby children can earn points or a reward (good reinforcers).

---

is responsible for some of these activities. Whether involved only in the planning or in both planning and teaching, a knowledge of teaching techniques and curriculum design is extremely useful to the school nurse. It is also important to be able to formulate educational programs according to the developmental stages of the different age groups.

The boxed material gives a sample lesson plan for a safety program for elementary school children. This plan illustrates some of the guidelines for this age group. In the early years of a child's school experience, special emphasis should be placed on the total approach to health—especially as it relates to changes in behaviors. These are the formative years for the attitude development; the critical period for developing health attitudes in children is 8 years of age (Palmer and Lewis, 1976). Self-motivation must be encouraged and supported, and health behaviors reinforced.

The essential elements of educational planning are the integration of community health, educational, and management concepts. This means that the nurse must be able to understand the topic content (factors involved, relationships, desirable behaviors), select and use educational methods appropriate for the particular subject and target population, and finally, plan and coordinate activities, personnel, and resources.

As a consultant the nurse provides assistance and acts as a resource person for the individual who is responsible for the health education. A nurse is also performing an educational function when providing stu-

dents with health information on request; the request may have been for counseling, but what was wanted was information from the school health expert.

Counseling

The ability to counsel students or others skillfully is an art. The counselor's responsibility is to provide information, listen objectively, and be supportive, caring, and trustworthy. Counselors do not make decisions; they help the client arrive at the decisions that best suits them. As such, counseling differs from both teaching and interviewing. Teaching is giving information; interviewing is obtaining information from someone; counseling is helping people arrive at workable solutions to their problems or conflicts.

Students usually request counseling when they are unable to make decisions about personal concerns that affect their lives, for example, birth control methods. If the nurse does not have the ability to counsel or to recognize that counseling is needed, the student may never be able to fully comprehend the depth of the problem or find possible alternatives to resolve the problems.

Peers of students can be used as counselors, especially in sensitive areas such as substance abuse and birth control. Students who are used as counselors must be trained for the role. It is often effective, after providing students with technical information, to encourage them to use their personal experiences, to role play, and to be available and accessible to other students.

Serving Special Needs

A number of problems can pull a child out of the group and make him or her a subject for special attention. Through screening and case finding, nurses may uncover children who have, or are likely to have, the following problems: overweight; underweight; sedentary life-style; stress caused by family, peers, or school pressure; accident; smoking; substance abuse; early pregnancy; sexually transmitted diseases; poor self-concept or self-image. All of these problems represent common risk factors for school age children (Healthy People, 1979). Each of these children has special needs, and school nurses try to help in finding solutions to the problems faced in each case.

There are two categories of students with special needs whose needs are so pressing that laws have been passed to protect them and programs have been designed to meet their special needs. These are the handicapped and the abused.

The Handicapped

In 1975 Public Law 94-142, the Education for All Handicapped Children Act, was passed to protect the right of all handicapped children to an education and special services. PL 94-142 encouraged every state to make public education available to every handicapped child (Moorehead, 1982).

Handicapped children are classified as visually impaired, having communication disorders, deaf, emotionally disturbed, mentally retarded, physically impaired (that is, orthopedically or neurologically), or having other health related impairments or learning disabilities.

Encompassed in this law is the concept of *mainstreaming,* which is defined as the inclusion of handicapped children into nonhandicapped or regular school situations (Moorehead, 1982). When working with children who are mainstreamed, the school nurse has the responsibility of identifying children who need help in the following areas:

A. Social skills (interpersonal skills and job training)
B. Personal skills (self-dressing, bathing, feeding, toileting)
C. Health education (appropriate material for this group such as hygiene, sexuality, daily life skills)
   1. State objectives for session.
   2. List objectives to be used in evaluation
   3. List aids and facilities to be used
   4. Develop methods for collecting baseline data and post-program data
   5. Organize manpower, technology, and monies for implementation.
   6. Outline methodology for meeting program objectives and list skills to be learned
D. Health problems (vision, hearing, communication, orthopedic, language, nutrition, cognitive, and physical)

The Abused

Child abuse is considered by some to have reached epidemic proportions (Justin and Justin, 1976). Not until 1975, however, was national concern sufficient to mobilize resources to eliminate this problem, even though the Child Abuse Prevention and Treatment Act had been signed into law in 1973 (PL 93-247). Before 1973 states specified methods and responsibilities for reporting. Alabama, Florida, Hawaii, and Idaho, for example, specifically identified nurses and school teachers as reporters. Illinois and the District of Columbia, on the other hand, referred only to physicians.

There are several types of child abuse: (1) physical abuse, (2) emotional abuse, (3) sexual abuse, and (4) medical neglect. According to Newberge (1977), child abuse is a preventable community health problem that is environmentally influenced. Child abuse is a family problem created by tension, anger, and fears; therefore, it must be resolved by the family with the help of supportive services (see Chapter 20).

LEGAL INFLUENCES

PL 94-142 and PL 93-247 are examples of the types of federal legal constraint which regulate school nurses when dealing with school age children. There are also legal constraints regulating their professional behavior as nurses. Together, they reflect the web of legal constraints which is part of the context within which school nurses must work.

The Nurse Practice Act of the 50 states defines nursing practice and controls what the nurse is able to do according to the law. The definitions of nursing vary from state to state; however, each of the 50 nurse practice acts identify specific independent and dependent functions of the nurse. In most instances nurses may have input into the writing of regulations relative to the independent and dependent functions that govern their practice.

The quality of nursing a client population receives is determined by the professional organizations' standards of nursing practice (ANA, 1973).

School nurses are judged, as are other professional nurses, according to their standards of practice and what other nurses would do in the same or "similar circumstances" (ANA, 1973; Creighton, 1974, p. 469). On these bases, school nurses are liable for their own acts when their acts are less than prudent.

The mechanisms through which nurses obtain their credentials *(licensure, registration,* and *certification)* help to assure that the definition of the nurse and the standards for practice can be met.

There are also legal restrictions on the ways school nurses deal with their clients. Because these also vary from place to place, the school system attorney should be asked to clarify the following points.:

   1. For how long are signed consent forms for screening procedures valid?
   2. How binding is a school system's code book? (Code is defined as a systematic statement of a body of law or a system of principles or rules. In Kentucky, for example, there is a school code book that governs what health services are to be provided.)
   3. When are consent forms not necessary?
   4. Are emancipated youths recognized as responsible individuals who are able to make their own decisions in school systems?

It is also recommended that school nurses evaluate both federal and state laws regarding treatment for sexually transmitted diseases and information on birth control methods, since state laws do not always conform to federal guidelines. According to the law, youths have a right to receive treatment for sexually transmitted diseases, to receive information about birth control, and to obtain birth control methods. At the federal level, however, it is now being suggested that personnel working in birth control clinics which are receiving federal support must inform parents when their minor children (under 18) are receiving birth control services. In addition, states such as Kentucky now require that parental consent be obtained before minor children can receive an abortion. The term *minor children* is defined by age and varies from state to state.

ISSUES AND CONCERNS

Nurses are confronted with a number of serious issues and concerns which directly or indirectly affect their practice in the 1980s: President Reagan's New Federalism, social illness, budgetary cutbacks, mainstreaming, child abuse, decline in school enrollment, and the nationally recognized need for health education (Haro, 1974; Wold and Dagg, 1981). Other concerns center around the professional rank-and-file membership's lack of political awareness and their poor information and communication mechanisms for identifying and presenting positions and demands.

President Reagan's New Federalism has affected school nursing practice directly, especially as it relates to state control and direction of social programs. The consequences of the *transfer of program management from national to state control* have been devastating for health care of poor, near poor, and middle class Americans. There have been cutbacks on, and sometimes elimination of, school lunch and breakfast programs which, especially for the near poor, supplemented and, in some cases, took the place of meals that families were unable to provide.

More *research* on social illnesses and risk-taking behaviors among adolescents is needed to design more effective intervention programs to reduce substance abuse, deaths by accident, smoking, and early pregnancies. We need to know why, at this stage in life, adolescents are often so willing to take risks without considering the consequences.

Other questions need to be answered, and much could be done by nurses to fill this gap. A review of the literature shows a paucity of research by school nurses, yet nurses, especially those with graduate degrees, are going into the school system with education in research methodologies. Whether or not they are equipped by education and position to direct research projects, they are often in ideal situations to help enlarge the body of nursing knowledge. They can participate in research projects, especially in the clinical setting (schools). They can direct attention to problems or situations that need attention and may elude to the less involved researcher. As the consumer of the research results, they can pro-

vide the judgment, criticism, and feedback necessary for ongoing research in any field.

A number of researchable areas in school nursing can be suggested. (1) How many nurses are necessary to provide a quality health service for x number of students? Although the Western Interstate Council on Higher Education in Nursing (WICHEN) suggests a ratio of 1 registered nurse for every 1000 students, does this include schools in depressed areas where health problems may be overwhelming? (2) What are the long-term effects of risk factors on children, and what are the necessary nursing interventions? How effective is the external environmental influence of risk reduction factors on the families of children who have received care (Stevens, 1980)? (3) What are the critical steps in adolescent decision making? (4) What methods are necessary to assess competency levels of school nurses?

The *use of scientific methods* in accounting for their practice is a new dimension of accountability in nursing (Gornter, 1974). In the past, school nurses have not consistently used scientific rationales in accounting for their goals, decisions, behaviors, use of time and resources, and proposed programs. Such methods of accountability appear, from the literature, to be more frequently used (Ode, 1979).

Issues related to the profession and its practice are many. One relates to the *delivery of nursing care* within the school system. There is, seemingly, a consensus on the need for nursing services but little agreement on the scope of these services. Primary care, for example, is supported in the literature as one mode of delivery (Doster, 1979; Switzer and Kelly, 1981). Primary care, by definition, means continuous coverage 24 hours a day, 7 days a week, by coordinated comprehensive services, which are accessible and acceptable to people (Doster, 1979). If primary care is the goal for school health, can health providers in school systems live up to the definition? Many decisions about education of school nurses and program planning are contingent on some agreement about this issue.

Another issue is the need for more *school nurse representation* on national, state, and local committees where decisions can facilitate or impede nursing services in school health and health services for children. It is especially important that nurses belong to local committees since federal funding is provided through block grants, which are federal funds not earmarked for specific social programs. An example is the Maternal Health Program and the Child Health Program. These grants are issued by the federal government to the states, and local groups can influence the decisions on who gets funded. This is an arena for political involvement and the use of marketing skills to assure that young people get their share of help.

In general, school nurses lack the organized power and influence needed to bring about change. This lack is, partially, a consequence of school nurses' isolation from each other and from nursing colleagues in other specialties. As an organized group, school nurses must continue to form coalitions and networks with other professional and consumer groups. Without *organization and communication with others,* it is difficult even to identify common concerns (Hamilton, 1982).

As leaders, school nurses must develop *analytical and managerial skills* to deal with organizations, program planning, and conflict of interest or goals. It is especially important to be able to analyze a situation before attempting to arrive at alternative actions (French and Bell, 1978).

There are a number of *ethical issues* in school nursing as well. One revolves around the need of nurses to understand why they are helping (Leitch, 1978). School nurses do not differ from other professionals in the range of their empathetic understanding, acceptance of clients, responsibility, and caring behaviors, but these abilities and activities need to be directed by an underlying purpose and meaning.

Another issue relates to accountability. To whom and for what are school nurses accountable. The position of the school nurse in the hierarchy of health care makes answering this question difficult. There are four interrelated publics which the nurse must respond to; which has priority? Yura e al. (1976) suggests the nurses are first accountable to their clients and then to the administration of the organization, their colleagues, and other members of the health team.

There are also ethical issues relating to student rights. All children and youths have a right to receive a school health service and they have a right to refuse these services. They also have a right to expect confidentiality when they share information, and they have a right to know when a confidence has to be broken. These rights can conflict with some of the nurse's reporting responsibilities, however. What does the nurse do in these situations?

Under public law, children and youths have the right to be protected from undue harm from abusers such as parents, other relatives, teachers, and nurses. Ethically school nurses are bound to report suspected cases as well as identified cases of abuse, but cases are not always clear cut.

The nurse must also be concerned about what is being taught and the possible effects on behavior. Subjects such as abortion, values clarification, and euthanasia must be handled with possible consequences carefully thought out and in mind (Fulton, 1977).

SUMMARY

The goal of helping young people develop into competent, coping, and healthy adults presents a heady challenge to the nurse whose personal philosophy is based on the belief that all people are entitled to health care. It is with this group that the nurse can have the greatest effect on the nation's health.

Nevertheless, the problems are dismaying. School nurses must be prepared to respond to diverse situations and work with many different kinds of people at a wide variety of tasks. Completing these tasks will demand that the nurse develop a host of new skills, some of which will be poorly related to nursing experience and training. Much of this work will be done while isolated from nursing colleagues and with little direction and no clear guidelines.

However, the nurse who does elect the role of school nurse will have an opportunity for professional development and personal growth. That nurse can help to clarify the school nurse's role, define the domain of school nursing, and participate in finding solutions to the many dilemmas and issues facing those nurses who work in schools. Having enough of these qualified nurses in schools as primary care providers will help to assure that future generations will be oriented to self-care responsibilities, will maintain high levels of wellness, and will develop into productive adult members of society.

BIBLIOGRAPHY

American Nurses' Association: Nursing practice, Kansas City, Mo., 1973, The Association.

American Nurses' Association: The study of credentialing in nursing: a new approach, vol. I, Kansas City, Mo., 1979, The Association.

American School Health Association: Philosophy and goals for school nurse educational preparation, Position paper by Subcommittee on Educational Preparation for School Nurses of the Committee on School Nursing, J. Sch. Health **45**:409, 1975.

American School Health Association: Teaching about drugs: a curriculum Guide, K-12, Cuyahoga Falls, Ohio, 1978, Probst Printing Services, Inc.

Bandura, A.: Principles of behavior modification, New York, 1969, Holt, Rinehart and Winston, Inc.

Bandura, A., and Walters, R.H.: Social learning and personality development, New York, 1963, Holt, Rinehart and Winston, Inc.

Barlet, H., et al.: Assessing the quality of care, Nurs. Outlook **23**(3), 153-159, 1975.

Bennis, W.G., Benne, K.W., and Chin, R.: The planning of change, ed. 2, North Scituate, Mass., 1969, Duxbury Press.

Better health for our children: a national strategy, Report of the Select Panel for the Promotion of Child Health DHHS Pub. No. 79-55071, Washington, D.C., 1981, Department of Health and Human Services.

Bryan, D.S.: School nursing in transition, St. Louis, 1973, The C.V. Mosby Co.

Castile, A.S., and Jerrick, S.J.: School health in America: summary report of a survey of state school health programs, J. Sch. Health **46**:216-221, 1976.

Cazalas, M.W.: Nursing and the law, Germantown, M., 1978, Aspen Systems Corp.

Chen, S.P.C.: Role relationships in a school health interdisciplinary team, J. Sch. Health 65:3, 1975.

Chilman, C.S.: Adolescent sexuality in a changing American society: social and psychological perspectives, Washington, D.C., 1980, Department of Health, Education, and Welfare.

Creighton, H., and Squaires, G.M.: School nurses: legal aspects of their work, Nurs. Clin. North Am. 9:467-474, 1974.

Dagg, N.V.: Primary prevention: health promotion and specific protection. In Wold, S.J.: School nursing: a framework for practice, St. Louis, 1981, The C.V. Mosby Co.

Daniel, W.: The adolescent patient, St. Louis, 1970, The C.V. Mosby Company.

Doster, M.: The role of the school in primary health care, J. Sch. Health 79:113-114, 1979.

Duvall, E.M.: Family development, ed. 4, New York, 1971, J.B. Lippincott Co.

Elkind, D.: Child development and education, Oxford England, 1976, Oxford University Press, Ltd.

Farquhar, J.W.: The American way of life need not be hazardous to your health, New York, 1978, W.W. Norton & Co., Inc.

Fraser, B.G.: A summary of child abuse legislation. in Helfer, R.E., and Kempe, C.H., editors: The battered child, Chicago, 1974, The University of Chicago Press.

French, W.L., and Bell, C.H.: Organizational development behavior science interventions for organizational improvement, Englewood Cliffs, N.J., 1978, Prentice-Hall, Inc.

Fulton, G.B.: Bioethics and health education: some issues of the biological revolution, J. Sch. Health 47:205-211, 1977.

Gornter, S.R.: Scientific accountability in nursing, 1974, Nurs. Outlook 22(2):764-768, 1974.

Gross, D., and O'Rourke, T.W.: Research and the future of health education, J. Sch. Health 45:30-32, 1975.

Hamilton, P.A.: Health care consumerism, St. Louis, 1982, The C.V. Mosby Co.

Hardy, M.E., and Conway, M.E.: Role theory perspectives for health professionals, New York, 1978, Appleton-Century-Crofts.

Haro, M.S.: School health revisited, J. Sch. Health 44:363-368, 1974.

Haynes, U.: A developmental approach to casefinding among infants and children, Review edition, Rockville, M., 1979, Department of Health, Education, and Welfare, Public Health Services.

Hayter, J.: Territoriality as a universal need, J. Adv. Nurs. 6(2):79-85, 1981.

Healthy People: the Surgeon General's report on health promotion and disease prevention, Pub. No. 79-55071, Washington, D.C., Dec. 1979, Department of Health, Education, and Welfare.

Hersey, P., and Blanchard, K.: Management of organizational behavior utilizing human resources, Englewood Cliffs, N.J., 1982, Prentice-Hall, Inc.

Humes, C.W.: Who should administer school nursing services? Am. J. Pub. Health 65:394-396, 1975.

Igoe, J.B.: The school nurse practitioner, Nurs. Outlook 23:381-384, 1975.

Igoe, J.B.: Project health PACT in action, Am. J. Nurs. 80(11):2016-2021, 1980.

Igoe, J.B., and Silver, H.H.: Improving health care in the school setting, Nurse Pract. 2(7):7-9, 1977.

Justin, B., and Justin, R.: The abusing family, New York, 1976, Human Services Press.

Kovar, M.G.: Some indicators of health related behaviors among adolescents in the United States, Report No. 21979, Washington, D.C., 1978, Public Health Service, Department of Health, Education, and Welfare.

Langlie, J.K.: Interrelationships among preventive health behaviors: a test of competing hypotheses, Report No. 21979, Washington, D.C., 1978, Public Health Report 94:216-225, 1979.

Leavell, H., and Clark, E.G.: Preventive medicine for the doctor in the community, ed. 3, New York, 1965, McGraw-Hill Book Co.

Leininger, M.: Territoriality, power, and creative leadership in administrative nursing contexts, Nurs. Dimens. 7:33-42, 1979.

Leitch, C.J.: Helping and human relationships. In Leitch, C.J., and Tinker, R.V., editors: Philadelphia, 1978, F.A. Davis Co.

Lipstiz, J.: Adolescent development: myths and realities, Child Today 8:2-7, 1979.

MacDonough, G.P.: School health—1977, J. Sch. Health, 47:427-428, 1977.

Marram, G.D., Barrett, M.W., and Bevis E.O.: Primary nursing, ed. 2, St. Louis, 1979, The C.V. Mosby Co.

McCamy, J.C., and Presley, J.: Human life styling, New York, 1975, Harper & Row, Publishers.

Means, R.K.: Historical perspectives on school health, Thorofare, N.Y., 1975, Charles B. Slack, Inc.

Miliar, W.: Adolescent perspectives, Washington, D.C., 1974, Department of Health, Education, and Welfare.

Minuchin, S.: Families and family therapy, Cambridge, Mass., 1974, Harvard University Press.

Moorehead, Y.: The year of the disabled: everybody counts, New York Spring 1982, Ivy Leaf, Inc.

Morgan, W., and Engel, G.L.: Interviewing the patient, Philadelphia, 1973, W.B. Saunders Company.

Murray, R.B., and Zentner, J.P.: Nursing concepts for health promotion, ed. 2, Englewood Cliffs, N.J., 1979, Prentice-Hall, Inc.

Nader, P.R.: Options for school health: meeting community needs, Germantown, M., 1978, Aspen Systems Corp.

Newberger, E.H.: Pediatric social illness: toward an etiologic classification, Pediatrics 60:178-184, 1977.

Nierenberg, G.I.: The art of negotiating, New York, 1978, Cornerstone Library Publications.

Ode, D.S.: Community health nursing in schools: developing a specialized role. In Archer, S.E., and Fleshman, R.P., editors: Community health nursing patterns and practice, North Scituate, Mass., 1979, Duxbury Press.

Orem, D.: Nursing: concepts of practice, ed. 2, New York, 1980, McGraw-Hill Book Co.

Palmer, B., and Lewis, L.: Development of health attitudes and behaviors, J. Sch. Health 46(7):401, 1976.

Parcel, G., Nadar, P.R., and Meyer, M.P.: Assessing adolescent health concerns: problems and patterns of utilization in a triethnic urban population, Pediatrics 60 (2):146-157, 1977.

Perry, C.L.: Enhancing the transition years: the challenge of adolescent health promotion, Speech presented at meeting of the American Association of School Health Education, Washington, D.C., Oct. 1981.

Perry, C.L.: Health promotion, Speech presented at meeting of the American School Health Association, Washington, D.C., Oct. 14-17, 1981.

Perry, C.L., and Murray, D.M.: Enhancing the transition years: the challenge of adolescent health promotion, J. Sch. Health 52:307-311, 1982.

Pesznecker, M.I.: The process of adolescence: its psychological and physiological basis, Adolescent Med., pp. 9-12, 1979.

Pigg, R.M.: A history of school health program evaluation in the United States, J. Sch. Health 46:583-589, 1976.

Redman, B.K.: The process of patient teaching in nursing, St. Louis, 1972, The C.V. Mosby Co.

Report on Licensure and Related Health Personnel Credentialing, Pub. No. (HMS)72-11, Washington, D.C., 1971, Office of Assistant

Secretary for Health and Science Affairs, Department of Health, Education, and Welfare.

Roberts, S.L.: Behavioral concepts and nursing throughout the life span, Englewood Cliffs, N.J., 1978, Prentice-Hall, Inc.

Rosenstock, H.: The health belief model and preventive health behavior, vol. 2, Thorofare, N.J., 1974, Charles B. Slack, Inc.

Rowan, F.P.: The chronically distressed client, St. Louis, 1980, The C.V. Mosby Company.

Seybold, S., and Klisch, M.R.: Preparing the grade school faculty to teach family life education, Matern. Child Nurs. J. 7:50-54, 1982.

Shortell, S.M., and Richardson, W.C.: Health program evaluation, St. Louis, 1978, The C.V. Mosby Company.

Simonds, S.K.: Health education today: issues and challenges, J. Sch. Health 47:584-593, 1977.

Stevens, B.J.: The nurse as an executive, Wakefield, Mass., 1980, Nursing Resources, Inc.

Switzer, K., and Kelly, J.T.: The nurse: a member of the school team, Matern. Child Nurs. J. 6:189-193, 1981.

Thompson, V.M.: Accountability in school health, J. Sch. Health 49:40-42, 1979.

Wieczorek, R.r., and Natapoff, J.N.: A conceptual approach to the nursing of children: health care from birth through adolescence, Philadelphia, 1981, J.B. Lippincott Co.

Withrow, C.: The school nurse takes a look at her charges, Nursing, 9:48-51, 1979.

Wold, S.J.: School nursing: a framework for practice, St. Louis, 1981, The C.V. Mosby Co.

Wold, S.J., and Dagg, N.V.: A framework for practice, J. Sch. Health 48:111-114, 1978.

Wold, S.J., and Dagg, N.V.: A framework for practice. In Wold, S.J.: School nursing: a framework for practice, St. Louis, 1981, The C.V. Mosby Co.

Yura, H., Ozimek, D., and Walsh, M.B.: Nursing leadership theory and process, New York, 1976, Appleton-Century-Crofts.

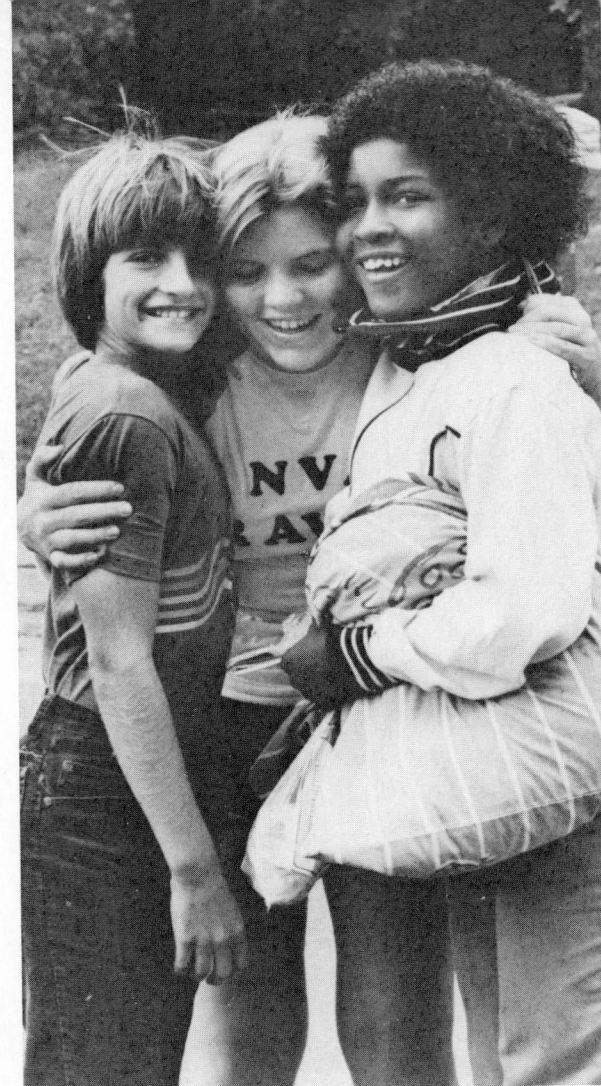

Chapter
32

MARCIA STANHOPE
SHARON SHEAHAN
ELLEN KENT

THE COMMUNITY HEALTH NURSE
AS CLIENT CARE
COORDINATOR-COLLABORATOR

Sue Jones, thirty five years old and mother of two small children, discovered that her family had many unmet needs after their husband and father deserted them. She knew that money for food, clothing, and shelter would be her greatest priority, but how was she to work and also provide a safe environment for her children?

Being an innovative person, she looked in the local phone directory reference section and found that the community services and health services categories listed many agencies who could assist her in this time of

need. Through these resources she identified social services for aid to mothers with dependent children; Medicaid, Head Start, and low-income day care services for the children; the health department for all their health care needs; and several volunteer organizations for food, clothing, and financial aid. By the end of the first year as a single parent, Sue had managed to accumulate a tidy income from several sources plus additional assistance with food, clothing, and health care needs. By chance, at a multiagency meeting Sue's name was mentioned by the community health nurse to a social worker friend. A chain reaction of events occurred as each agency present realized they were all contributing to the care of this mother and her family, without their knowledge of other assistance being received by Sue. The agency representatives were astonished to realize that Sue was receiving financial and other assistance from 50 community agencies, with multiple examples of duplication of service efforts. Sue's initiative in helping herself and her family is a commendable attribute, and such behavior should be rewarded by health providers. However, in this instance, the community health nurse could have been helpful by facilitating Sue's efforts to seek assistance from only the most appropriate agencies.

This example demonstrates what can happen in a community where there is little or no coordination of effort and collaboration among community services agencies. An example with opposite results is often encountered in the community. Members of a family or group have needs for which the community is capable of providing, but they lack the direction and knowledge of available resources and their needs continue unassisted.

Coordination among community services and collaboration about alternative ways of providing comprehensive community services can rectify these situations. This chapter focuses on the community health nurse's role functions as client care coordinator and collaborator. Advocacy, discharge planning, and referral are discussed as well as communication techniques useful to the community health nurse in fulfilling these role functions.

DEFINITIONS AND GOALS

Coordination is the conscious activity of assembling and directing the work efforts of a group of health providers so they function harmoniously in the attainment of the objectives of client care (Haimann and Scott, 1974; Rakich et al., 1977). The *goal* of coordination is to maximize the collaborative effort of health providers while minimizing friction among the providers in the attainment of the client care objectives. Coordination efforts require leadership skills, which are applied to achieve unity of effort among the group of providers to accomplish their objectives (Rakich et al., 1977).

Whereas the goal of coordination is to maximize collaborative effort, *collaboration* requires health providers to work together as a team of equals toward a common goal. The community health nurse's goal in collaboration is to contribute to a comprehensive effort that provides continuity of services to clients whether they be individuals, groups, families, or communities.

Effective collaboration requires assertive persons with varied ideas and expertise as well as a commitment to seeking goals that lead to the best alternatives to meet client needs. Collaboration involves setting mutual goals, clarifying each team member's role, identifying all possible resources, delineating alternative approaches to attain goals, selecting specific interventions, mobilizing resources, and putting a plan into operation (Friedman, 1981).

The responsibilities of the community health nurse as coordinator-collaborator include advocacy and discharge planning activities. The community health nurse as *client advocate* acts on behalf of the client to attain two goals: health care delivery system responsiveness to clients and client independence. *Discharge planning activities* are planned events which prepare for clients' ongoing and future needs for health care resources as they move long the health-illness continuum toward their maximum potential. Referral is a significant function of the discharge planning process. *Referral* involves actions that guide clients toward and assists them to use resources available to resolve their problems. Referrals can be made for clients by the community health nurse and can be directed toward illness prevention, health promotion, health maintenance, or restoration.

Effective communication is the key to quality coordinating and collaborating activities. Communication has two major components: formal and informal. *Communication* is an interactive process of sharing or transmitting thoughts and feelings (Travelbee, 1974). *Formal communication* involves an organization of channels for transmitting and receiving information within a network—social, professional, political, and economic—whereas *informal communication* consists of interaction channels that arise out of the interpersonal relationships of network participants (Rakich et al., 1977). The interactive process of communication involves the sending and receiving of written or oral and nonverbal or verbal messages.

ROLE OF CLIENT CARE COORDINATOR-COLLABORATOR

Role Functions

The community health nurse has two specific role functions relative to coordination: (1) coordination of client care and (2) coordination of resources. A third function that may be assigned to the nurse is coordination of an interagency program such as a family planning program. Additionally, there are two levels of coordination in which the nurse may engage to fulfill these role functions: (1) horizontal coordination and (2) vertical coordination. In *horizontal coordination* the nurse, a member of the health department, acts as an agent for the client in assembling and directing the work efforts of a group of resource agencies, who are external to the employing agency and who have common goals for the identified client. For example, Helen Smith, the home health nurse, has been notified by Dr. Doe that Mary Jones has had a cerebral vascular accident resulting in hemiplegia and has been hospitalized. By visiting Mary in the hospital and attending multidisciplinary staff conferences, Helen finds that Mary's prognosis is good and she is progressing rapidly. Helen describes Mary's home situation and family to the hospital staff and the staff agrees that Mary should be discharged to home care at the earliest possible date. Helen discusses plans for discharge with Mary and her family, asking for their input into the plans for Mary's discharge.

As plans develop for Mary's discharge, Helen contacts the agencies who can appropriately continue Mary's care regimen at home. Helen contacts the hospital supply house to arrange for a bed, walker, bedside commode, and essential supplies to make Mary's transition easier from hospital to home. She also arranges for a speech therapist, a physical therapist, and a home health aide for personal care.

After initial plans are made for Mary's discharge, Helen calls a meeting with Mary, the other members of the health team, and the family to arrange for scheduling of activities and to discuss the group's goals for Mary's care. The meeting provides an opportunity for each person to know the roles of others in Mary's care, reduces the likelihood of duplication of services, allows Mary and the family to have input into the planned goals, and provides goal information to Helen which she can follow up on and reinforce during her home visits.

In *vertical coordination* community health nurses serve as links between their level in the organization and those above and below them. They also serve as links between the agency and the client population. The following is an example of vertical coordination within the agency. Connie Cole, the community health nurse supervisor, has been asked by the Director of Nursing to coordinate activities for the establishment of a prenatal clinic at the health department. Connie collects information about the need for prenatal care in the area, explores cost and funding sources, projects the number of staff needed and the staff availability, and projects client use of the clinic. Connie arranges a meeting with the nursing staff, the director of nursing, the nurse practitioners, and the medical officer to present her findings, to answer questions, to allow input into the planning of the clinic, and to assist the group to work collaboratively toward the development of the clinic.

Vertical coordination between a client group and the agency is depicted in the following example. The local consumer board for the high-rise apartment complex for the elderly has noted that a number of their residents have health needs. One day Connie is visiting a resident of the high-rise complex and is approached by the manager about the health needs of these elderly residents. The consumer board is interested in developing a health screening and referral program with the health department. Connie returns to the health department to discuss the issue with her supervisor and the agency administration. After careful deliberation about costs, availability of resources, and the anticipated input from the high-rise board and residents, the administration directs Connie to implement the screening program for the client group.

Role Expectations

Community health nurses who serve as a client care coordinator-collaborator expect their functions to include (1) facilitating of continuous client care between health care resources; (2) optimizing client use of and access to health care services; and (3) assisting health care professionals to recognize and plan for individual, group, and community client needs. The goal of these functions is to alleviate clients' anxieties about their needs.

Clients expect the community health nurse to make available and accessible the services necessary to resolve their problems; to offer assistance in the use of available services; and to avoid duplication of service so they are not subjected to unnecessary and repetitive services that tend to increase risk of harm and cost to clients. In addition, clients expect high-quality service and a reasonable effort on the part of practitioners to care for their needs with skill, knowledge, and sound judgment (Williams and Torrens, 1980).

The *community agency* for whom the nurse works expects clients' needs to be recognized, assessed, and met by the nurse; expects the nurse to follow agency policy and procedures in meeting client needs and to serve as an agency representative; expects clients to be satisfied with the services received; and expects services to be rendered at an efficient cost to the agency. The agency also expects the nurse to have expertise as a coordinator-collaborator of client care services.

Role Relationships

As client care coordinator, the community health nurse establishes relationships with many persons to synchronize activities directed toward meeting clients' needs. As client advocate, the nurse establishes communication networks with citizen's groups, local government officials, social services agencies, media personnel (such as the local newspaper or radio station), school personnel, community leaders, and self-help groups, to name a few.

As a collaborator, the community health nurse is involved with multidisciplinary relationships in working with the health team to help meet client needs. The multidisciplinary team may involve nurses representing other agencies, physicians, social workers, physical therapists, nutritionists, speech therapists, attorneys, clerical personnel, environmental engineers, mental health personnel such as psychologists, other health professionals, and clients.

The nurse is also involved in intraagency collaboration: nurse to nurse, nurse to supervisor, nurse to aide, nurse to other health professionals. In the agency using team assignments, the nurse must collaborate with team members to assure continuity of care and must coordinate case conferences for communicating clients health care needs. The case conference keeps health personnel and community aides informed of the progress and needs of their assigned clients.

Spradley (1981) points out that planning and implementing activities to meet client needs should not be done in isolation. Such activities lead to service fragmentation, duplications and gaps that are costly both to clients and health care systems. Coordination and collaboration efforts are essential to reduce the occurrence of such isolated activities.

Barriers to Coordination and Collaboration

Role ambiguity often occurs when management does not designate a primary provider who will serve as coordinator of client care. In agency team assignments, if one nurse is not designated as primary provider for a group of clients, often no nurse will assume the responsibility of coordinator; if someone attempts to assume responsibility, a problem with conflict may occur and questions of territorialism arise among the members of the team.

Problems of territorialism and lack of coordination and collaboration arise in the multidisciplinary team if members' roles are not clarified during the planning activities. This is a common problem occurring, for example, in the home health arena where a person may be the client of the home health agency, the attending private physician, and the private practice physical therapists. If special efforts are not made to plan client services as a multidisciplinary team, then services may overlap, may be duplicated, or may not be offered because of the lack of an effective method of communication about client-related activities among the providers of service.

In the presence of these barriers clients become dissatisfied with both providers and services offered; communication breaks down among providers and between providers and clients; referral patterns may

change; and feelings of frustration, insecurity, and failure may occur in providers and clients. Client noncompliance may result, leading clients to seek health care elsewhere.

Educational Requirements

The nurse as coordinator-collaborator of client care and health care resources is prepared at the baccalaureate level. The community health nurse often coordinates activities for individual clients and for families to provide for comprehensive personal care services. The community health nurse makes continuing efforts to improve referral systems between all agencies working with the client, shares knowledge about client needs and progress, and functions as a bridge between individual and family as well as between the family and community resources.

At the graduate level, the nurse is prepared to coordinate program development and implementation within the agency and to serve as a collaborator for the development of services to meet community needs. In this role the community health clinical nurse specialist functions as a supervisor or administrator and supports the staff nurse acting as client care and resource coordinator. The clinical specialist documents client and referral problems and uses these data in intraagency meetings to communicate established patterns of dysfunction within the system as well as problems with resource use. The clinical specialist may also work with another community agency to establish a community-based health program like the Early and Periodic Developmental Screening and Testing Program. The clinical specialist has the necessary skills and expertise to make community contacts, arrange and plan meetings, identify funding sources, tap community leaders, and direct the planning focus toward the main objectives.

Knowledge and Skills

Effective communication is the key ingredient to the role functions of coordination and collaboration. Knowledge of the theories of management, decision making, perception, motivation, and change are essential when guiding the work of others toward a common goal (see Chapter 6 for a brief discussion of these theories).

Management

The managerial functions of planning, organizing, and controlling are necessary tools for getting things done with and through people. As a coordinator the community health nurse is involved in *planning* goals and objectives. Once the planning has been done, the community health nurse is responsible for *organizing* or integrating the resources—people, supplies, equipment, and facilities—in the most effective way to accomplish the goals. The community health nurse *controls* the flow of work by providing feedback (evaluation) about movement toward goals and by following up the workers' accomplishments. The information is then compared with initial plans so adjustments can be made in directing future activities toward desired outcomes.

Decision Making

Inherent in successfully accomplishing the managerial functions of planning, organizing, and controlling is the involvement of the total group, including the client, in the decision-making process. The functions of coordinator and collaborator are integrated throughout the nursing process, which is the decision-making framework. First, the client situation is *assessed* and the problem is defined. The group involved in meeting the client's needs engages in problem analysis, listing all possible alternative solutions for *planning* to meet client needs. The choice of solutions for meeting client needs is made by the group and the group organizes to *implement* the chosen solutions. A schedule of periodic *evaluation* is established during the planning phase so the group can make adjustments in their plans during implementation. When initial goals are met, the group evaluates the total plan to determine the need for continuing involvement with the client. At this point termination may occur for one or all members of the multidisciplinary team, including the community health nurse.

Motivation

As client care coordinator, the community health nurse must recognize and understand the motives and needs that are most important to the other people—client or team member. The amount of energy the players (client or team member) will expend in moving toward the established goals depends on the motivating forces directing the person. The motivating forces may be tangible and easily recognized such as the need for food, clothing, shelter, and health care; or the forces may be intangible such as needs for recognition, achievement, or competence. It is important for the coordinator to note that commitment to attain a goal increases when individuals are involved in their own goal setting. If the community health nurse sets goals for the client or the multidisciplinary team, more frustration and less goal-directed activity will be evidenced than if a collaborative goal-setting process occurs.

Perception

Another important factor for the community health nurse to recognize is the influence of perception on goal-directed behavior. Perceptions are influenced by previous experiences with successes and failures that have occurred when engaging in goal-related activity. If a client attempting to learn to walk again after an accident is faced with persisting failure on a day-to-day basis, frustration will occur and goal-directed activity will decrease. The speech therapist who is planning activities for the aphasic client will find that past successes and failures with similar clients will influence the goals set for the new client.

Change

All coordinating and collaborating activities are change oriented. The activities of the community health nurse are directed toward changing the client's health status or changing the client's *risk ratio,* that is, assisting the client to change life style habits to reduce the future risk of illness.

The community health nurse as client coordinator assumes two leadership styles in achieving change (moving a group toward a common goal). The community health nurse may be a *situational leader,* one recognized by the group as the person with the leadership skills to help the group achieve their goals, or a *functional leader,* one who performs certain functions for attaining the group's goals with the client.

Throughout the discussion in this chapter the level of change promoted has been *participative change,* or involvement of all parties in helping to formalize and implement methods for attaining client goals. There may be instances where a more effective strategy is *directive change,* or forced change whereby a new behavior is engaged in, new knowledge is acquired, a commitment to the change develops, and the reinforced behavior becomes voluntary (Hersey and Blanchard, 1977). For example, the client who continually fails at crutch walking is forced by the physical therapist to continue to practice. As muscles are strengthened and techniques are learned, the client voluntarily begins to walk with crutches and directive change has been effective. Similarly, when the health department administration recognizes a need for a prenatal clinic, the nursing staff is directed to operate the clinic. As client population increases and neonatal, infant, and maternal mortality decreases, nurses recognize the need for the clinic and begin to identify with and internalize the need for it. Again, directive change has been successfully used.

Communication Models

For the role functions of coordination and collaboration there are basically two communication models that depict the interaction between the community health nurse and multidisciplinary team or family members. These models are described by Hersey and Blanchard (1977) as the star and circle.

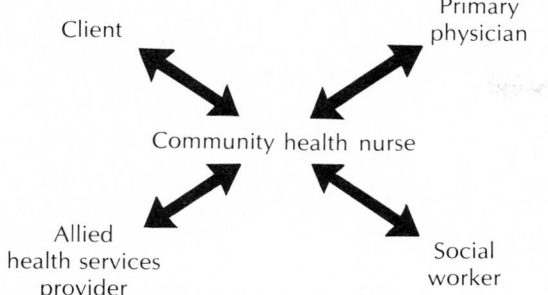

Fig. 32-1. Star coordinative communication model. (From Hersey, P., and Blanchard, K.: Management of organization behavior: utilizing human resources, Englewood Cliffs, N.J., 1977, Prentice-Hall, Inc.)

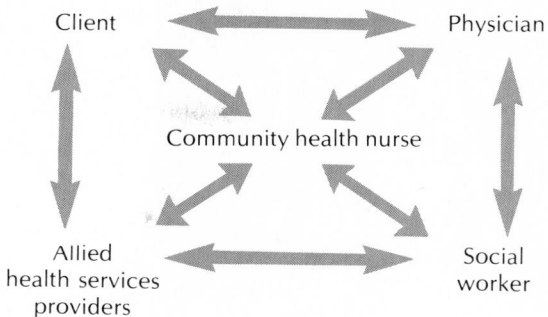

Fig. 32-2. Interactive communication model with community heath nurse as coordinator. (Adapted from Hersey, P., and Blanchard, K.: Management of organization behavior: utilizing human resources, Englewood Cliffs, N.J., 1977, Prentice-Hall, Inc.)

The star model provides a schema of the communication pattern that primarily exists when the community health nurse serves as the coordinator of client care and coordinator of resources (Fig. 32-1). In this model the nurse is identified in the leadership position with responsibility for communicating with the client and other members of the team. Unless the community health nurse calls a meeting of the group to discuss the efforts of the group in meeting the client goals, there may or may not be direct interaction between the other team members (Fig. 32-2).

The circle model depicts a schema of the communication pattern that primarily exists when the community health nurse is involved in collaboration with others on behalf of the clients (Fig. 32-3). For this model each person interacts with the two colleagues in either direction, and the group is free to communicate all around the circle.

The star communication model presents a picture of the directive change pattern, since one person is identified in the leadership role and a clear organizational network to solve problems is apparent. The adapted star and circle models show more of a participative change pattern in that all members have an opportunity for equal input in the solving of problems and in assuming leadership in the situation.

Communication Components

Hein (1973) describes a communication framework consisting of six elements: referent, source-encoder, message, channel, receiver-decoder, and feedback. Whether communication is formal or informal, spontaneous or deliberate, there is a purpose for engaging in

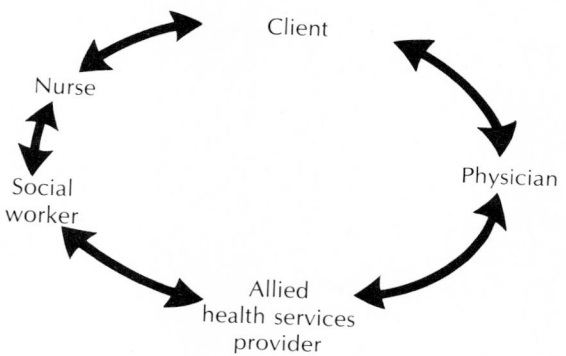

Fig. 32-3. Circle collaborative communication model. (Adapted from Hersey, P., and Blanchard, K.: Management of organization behavior: utilizing human resources, Englewood Cliffs, N.J., 1977, Prentice-Hall, Inc.)

interaction with others. The purpose for the interaction is called a *referent*. For the community health nurse's functions of coordinating and collaborating, the referent is the client situation. The community health nurse is the *source-encoder*, or the person responsible for verbally or nonverbally communicating with others about the client situation. The *message*, the expression or content of the client situation, is conveyed to others by phone or written referral through one-to-one or group interaction. The methods of conveyance are called the communication *channels*. The message is directed to a *receiver-decoder*, who is a member of the family, the client, or a multidisciplinary team member.

Just as the source-encoders' messages are influenced by communication skill, attitudes, knowledge, and a sociocultural system, the receiver-decoders' interpretations of the messages are affected by their perception of the message. The decoders' perceptions are also related to skills, attitudes, knowledge, a sociocultural system.

With the communication framework the *feedback,* or translation of the message into action (movement toward the client goal) by the decoder, shows the success or failure of the communication efforts.

Communication Techniques

As previously indicated, communication is the key ingredient in effective coordination and collaboration. The two role functions often require the community health nurse to be the facilitator of movement toward client goals. In the facilitative situation, initially the community health nurse can listen to the client's and family's description of the client situation. The community health nurse can clarify the perceptions, ideas, and feelings of the client and elaborate on the perceptions of the client. The nurse can validate and substantiate facts and feelings through observations of the client situation and can assess the reliability of the information received from the client by comparing it to previously recorded data and to family interpretations of the situation.

After gathering data from the client through interview and observation, the community health nurse may present and interpret the client situation to the multidisciplinary team. The community health nurse must be ready to listen to the team's perceptions and interpretations of the situation, to move the group toward agreement on solutions, to restate team input for accuracy, to check for goal consensus among the team, to allow all team members to evaluate new ideas introduced, and to evaluate the outcome of the team's plan of action.

CLIENT ADVOCACY

Advocacy as a Function of Coordination and Collaboration

Advocacy as an issue has come to the forefront of public attention in recent years as a result of society's increased emphasis on basic human needs and concomitant freedom to strive for actualization of human potential. Advocacy becomes inexorably entwined with human rights when people are unable to fully defend their rights or meet basic human needs without assistance. When the right or freedom of self-determination is threatened, the advocate assumes the role of the defender. *Advocacy* is defined as pleading the cause of another. Various professional and lay persons have assumed the advocate role, including lawyers, educators, social workers, family, and friends. Nurses too

have embraced advocacy and many consider it the cornerstone of the profession.

Advocacy in Nursing

Curtin (1979), Director of the National Center for Nursing Ethics, Cincinnati, Ohio, maintains that advocacy is the very philosophical foundation of nursing with the end purpose being the welfare of other human beings. She postulates that nursing is a moral art that incorporates the unique nurse-client relationship and shared humanity into a process that acknowledges what illness does to the physical and psychological limits of a person's being. Curtin further delineates how illness damages one's humanity through loss of independence, freedom of action, and interference with the ability to make choices.

The *nurse as advocate* is one who acts in the client's best interest; recalling that advocacy is based on self-determination, it is the client who defines the boundaries (Mauksch, 1980). There is a fine line between being a decision maker on behalf of another and being one who informs the client of available options and subsequently supports the client's decision. The nurse is a resource person who gathers information to assist clients and families in their efforts to become informed about their rights, who encourages self-help, and who contributes to the data base that enhances rational decision making. This is done with an appreciation of the individual as a unique human being who is particularly vulnerable because of the stress associated with injury or illness (Gadow, 1979). The advocate supports the individual's right to fully participate in the decision-making process and acts as a buffer to prevent others from undermining that process (Kohnke, 1980). Once the decision is implemented, the nurse serves as gatekeeper, maintaining responsibility for monitoring the quality and continuity of care on the client's behalf (Abrams, 1978).

It is conceivable that conflicts in values between the client and nurse may arise. Thus it may be helpful for the nurse to try to see the situation through the client's eyes. Advocacy does not mean imposing one's values on another even though the advocate may view the situation as being detrimental to the client's health (Mauksch, 1980). In dealing with such a dilemma, Aroskar (1980) believes that the choice is usually between two or more equally unsatisfactory solutions.

As an example of a values conflict between the client and the provider, Kohnke (1980) describes the situation of an 80-year-old woman who has diabetic complications and develops gangrene of the foot. The physician recommends amputation, but the woman wants to die "whole." The dilemma of death versus mutilation does not offer a pleasant choice. Philosophy and values are extremely subjective, with no two people viewing a given situation from exactly the same perspective. This may be a point of conflict for nurses who feel they know what is best.

Conflict Sources of the Advocacy Role

Since the advocate is not chosen by the client, the paternalistic attitude of knowing what is best should be avoided by the professional. Conflict may arise because of the nature of the nurse-client relationship and the dependency that altered health status tends to foster. Nurses are obligated to interpret their role as representative and act as spokesperson for the client's interests (Abrams, 1978).

Nurses often put themselves in a position, either willingly or innocently, of being rescuers. Rescuers often make decisions for others and therefore are put in a position of jeopardy if the decision does not turn out as well as expected. The backlash of being blamed for an action, carried out for the purpose of doing good, creates an awkward position for the well-intended advocate (Kohnke, 1980).

Other conflict sources of the advocacy role for nurses working in the community become apparent as clients become informed and begin to assert themselves. A ripple effect is created by the client's assertion, which impinges on administrators and other health professionals. Nurses who take a position and stick to it may draw criticism and be labeled as troublemaker or informer. Nurses advocating for individuals or groups have occasionally encountered enough pressure to force them to resign their positions to prevent compromising their beliefs (Smith, 1980).

Lamb (1981) distinguishes between responsible and irresponsible advocacy and suggests in-depth training for advocates. In addition, he proposes setting up advocacy review boards to monitor activities. Lamb's remarks are not directed toward nurses per se, but toward activists who have power without clinical responsibility. However, those embarking on the advocacy venture might do well to be aware of the prevailing general attitude of a few in the health care sector toward advocacy. Some of the pitfalls of advocacy can be avoided by being aware of possible problems, clarifying one's position with the client and others, being knowledgeable about the system, and planning carefully.

Characteristics of the Advocate

Individuals engaged in positive, assertive action on behalf of others share some of the following characteristics (Donahue, 1978; Spradley, 1981):

1. Understanding—of the issues of human rights
2. Accountability—thinking and acting in a rational manner; assuming the responsibility for one's actions

3. Risk taking—willingness to step forward and take a chance
4. Communication—presenting the client's concerns in a succinct and convincing manner
5. Resourcefulness—identifying resources to be tapped for the client's benefit

In the health care delivery system the community health nurse and the client are continually faced with several concerns: (1) the frustrations of interacting with several public agencies, each providing different and sometimes conflicting information; (2) existing rules and regulations that often interfere with access to needed resources; and (3) communication barriers in a system that is often insensitive to providing essential services to its clients. The community health nurse client advocate must possess these characteristics and, in addition, be motivated to seek the best possible care for clients. The nurse must have the skill and expertise to perform the tasks required in advocacy and must have the necessary knowledge to know how, why, where, and when to intervene for the client.

Advocacy in Community Health Nursing

The discussion thus far has been directed toward defining advocacy and its role in nursing as well as exploring some of the conflicts associated with advocacy. Characteristics of the nurse as advocate have also been noted. The following discussion will focus on the client-consumer in the community and the problems associated with the complexity of the health care system. Attention is given to the community health nurse's planned intervention to increase consumer independence and to make the system more responsive to expressed grievances.

Inexperienced health care consumers may face two problems when they need services. First, they often lack knowledge of available resources, and second, they may lack a visible entry point into the health care system. With the myriad of medical specialties, agencies, and institutions, the chance of making the correct connection with the appropriate service without meeting one or more barriers is as unpredictable as a game of roulette. Consumers find themselves caught in a complex maze without knowledge of the rules of the game and consequently find many dead ends with little more than guesswork to determine which turn to take next. They may find that physicians are not taking new patients, that they do not qualify financially for a particular service, or that the hours of facility operation coincide with their hours of employment. Frustration and discouragement are inevitable outcomes and are compounded if the search for assistance is made in the urgency of a crisis situation.

Many barriers to admittance to the health care system exist. Resource and economic categories are prime barriers. Resource barriers are caused either by lack of specific services in the community or by insufficient services resulting from increased demand for those services by the public. Economic barriers, created because of skyrocketing health care costs, affect uninsured individuals who do not qualify for medical assistance and also the insured who are hard hit by sizable deductibles and exempt services. Consumers relying on medical assistance have to search for providers who accept their form of payment.

Use of Community Resources

The community health nurse uses a variety of community resources to aid the client's plight. Sources of information include service directories that list agencies in the community with a brief description of each service, times of availability, terms of qualification, fees required, and the agency contact person. This source of information is helpful in spelling out the population for whom the services are directed.

When making inquiries about services, it is frustrating to deal with numerous public agencies and their conflicting information, rules, and regulations. The community health nurse can better empathize with a client after a tedious session of information seeking. Communications are often hampered when attempting to make connections with the appropriate person within an agency. Clients may have difficulty articulating questions to receptionists and translating them into the bureaucratic framework. Knowledge of the system and persistence of the community health nurse can help to educate the client as to the nature of the resources available to meet specific needs and how to use them. For example, clients seeking information about a Medicare statement for home health services may call the Social Security general information number only to find that clients must know whether the home health services were covered under Part A or Part B of Medicare to receive the correct phone number to call. The community health nurse can assist the client in interpreting the Medicare handbook and in seeking the correct source to contact for billing information.

Follow-up Activities

Once resources have been identified, the next step is sharing the acquired information with the client. The process to that point may well have been a joint effort with the client playing an active part in gathering information. When the client understands what outcomes can reasonably be expected from identified resources, the stage is set for positive planning and gives the client a sense of renewed hope. The community health nurse acts as gatekeeper during the action phase to see that the best possible services are provided in a continuous

and comprehensive manner. Monitoring selected services through home visits and observation is a vital follow-up activity performed by the nurse and includes discussing the client's care with the family members and professionals as a safety measure to prevent backsliding.

Community Health Nurse's Role in Manipulation of the Health Care Delivery System

Nurses can participate in a number of activities associated with increasing the visibility of issues through advocacy. They can cut through red tape and make the health care delivery system more responsive to clients needs. If one door is closed, others can be opened to achieve the same end. Writing and speaking skills, mentioned earlier, come to play in building a coalition of support. Letters to the editor, articles in professional journals, and news spots on radio or television help to gain support for a cause. For example, a community health nurse is concerned that the street people of Anytown, U.S.A., do not have facilities for shelter during cold winter months. The community health nurse elicits support from key community organizations, the Chamber of Commerce, and professional organizations to raise monies to support the shelter concept. The nurse then speaks to the local television station and is offered a spot on the local news to plead for a location to house the shelter. The presentation is effective and the shelter coalition is offered a lease on an old nursing home site.

Working through political systems at the local, state, and even national levels helps to establish credibility. The community health nurse continues the drive for the shelter by seeking matching funds from the local government to support the shelter.

Other options for nurses include appearing at public hearings with prepared statements and arranging appointments to speak with key legislators about issues, such as the maternal and child health block grants to see that prenatal care has continued funding in the state. Advocates should seek membership on committees and policy-making boards in order to influence the system through established channels. Presenting public education programs to local service organizations also spreads the message about client needs at the grass roots level. These advocacy activities are but a few of the many that can be developed to bring about greater awareness of the issues affecting consumers today (Brower, 1982).

Identifying Community Patterns and Potentials

Community analysis is an effective method for the community health nurse to use in collecting data about community resources available to the consumer. Lancaster (1982) approaches community analysis by looking at four component parts: (1) community attitudes, (2) assessment of community resources, (3) constraints, and (4) identification of target market.

Community attitudes. Information gathered from professionals and lay people who work with health-related services in the community is helpful in developing attitudes regarding the community's potential to solve specific consumer problems. Input from special interest groups such as the Parent-Teacher Association or the target groups to be served balances consumer and provider positions on the community issues.

Assessment of community resources is a procedure similar to the process used on behalf of the individual client. The scope of investigation, however, is more detailed and includes examination of data from health planning groups including numbers of public health facilities, availability of health personnel, availability of funds, and a multitude of other statistics such as mortality and morbidity data.

Constraints. Investigation of services, resources, and facilities may highlight problems that may potentially impede the planning of programs to meet consumer needs. Economic constraints, for example, would necessitate altering the recommendations for problem solution and require development of new alternatives. See Chapter 9 for further discussion of constraints related to program planning.

Identification of target market involves the identification of a specific geographic area and the boundaries that define the market area comprising a selected group of residents. Defining the area to be served makes the approach to planning more manageable. Examining demographic variables provides a starting point and validates consumers' perceived need for service expansion.

Planning Change

Once the community analysis is complete, steps can be taken to proceed to program planning. Alternatives are explored in light of the defined goals. The values of the planning group are incorporated into the operational philosophy and become actualized in the form of objectives, policies, and procedures. The outcome of the planning process must be agreed on and consensus reached. The planning process is influenced by such factors as the characteristics of the people involved as well as general morale and motivation. Group interaction is crucial to the planning process, with any obstruction affecting the outcome (Lancaster and Lancaster, 1982). See Chapter 16 for further discussion of the group process.

Community health nurse advocates who work with consumer groups and plan for change may find themselves assuming an initial functional leadership role, but as the group establishes its own identity and cohesiveness, others may assume more of the leadership tasks (situational). At that point the community health nurse's role may revert to that of collaborator and resource person.

Further insight into the modus operandi of the nurse as a participant in the group effort to promote change comes from examining the strategies of change. Kurt Lewin's theory of force-field analysis is described as "a dynamic balance of forces working in opposite directions . . ." (Benne and Birnbaum, 1969, p. 328). The forces in balance tend to equalize each other most of the time. Change occurs when the driving forces and the restraining forces become imbalanced; when forces lose their equilibrium and the driving forces are increased, tension is generated. The tension tends to be sustained until new ideas are accepted and equilibrium is reestablished, with simultaneous reduction in tension (Benne and Birnbaum, 1969). Understanding of change theory and its application to group process gives the nurse, as participant, some insight into the dynamics of the situation. Anticipating events as they progress helps the nurse appreciate the importance of timing and may foster a greater tolerance for the frustrations involved in the process.

Promoting Activities for Illness Prevention and Health Promotion

Health is both a social and an individual responsibility. Pender (1982) state that personal health practices are only one determinant of health. To develop a comprehensive approach to health promotion, careful attention must be given to the environment, culture, and social constraints imposed on clients seeking maximal health states. The community health nurse can serve as client advocate by assisting clients toward assertive behavior in personal health practices. Personal health services must be coordinated with national, state, and local community health services to effectively address problems that result in illness or slow movement toward maximal health states. As priority for enhanced health status emerges, even more innovative approaches to health promotion will be developed, and the community health nurse can provide input into planning for health promotion activities by identifying and asserting the needs of the client population.

Currently there are many programs directed toward prevention and promotion activities. These include the following (Pender, 1982, p. 370):

- Accident prevention
- Early detection of disabilities among children
- Immunization
- Case finding and contact investigation (communicable disease)

- Substance abuse control
- Suicide prevention
- Family planning
- Industrial hygiene and occupational health
- Environmental sanitation and pollution control

In addition, health programs for reduction of health-damaging behaviors have been on the rise in recent years. These include programs designed for such health maintenance activities as diet instruction for reducing weight, decreasing lipid intake, and increasing the amount of high-fiber foods consumed. Exercise has been an integral part of health instruction and, coupled with smoking cessation classes, is designed to minimize risks of cardiovascular disease. Health promotion activities are delivered by various means including group classes at ambulatory care centers, individualized instruction, and programs designed by industry for their employees. Health information is also disseminated through mass media via television, radio, and newspapers (Pender, 1982).

Changing health behaviors is difficult because of the need to overcome long-standing life habits. Individuals act out of habit or feel "powerless" in controlling their environment, thus they will continue to limit personal options even though knowledge is available about risk of illness resulting from existing life-styles (Pender, 1982).

Igoe (1980, p. 2016) reports on a project entitled PACT (Participatory and Assertive Consumer Training), which is designed to teach responsible, assertive health behaviors and self-advocacy to school age children. Three stated objectives for PACT are the following:

1. To prepare students for assertive, participatory health consumer roles so they can communicate and negotiate more effectively with health professionals
2. To develop reciprocal relationships between consumers and providers so that health care plans may be mutually developed and approved
3. To tailor the delivery of professional health services to the consumers' needs for participation and health education at the time the care is provided

Evaluation of the project has shown a statistically significantly increase in knowledge about health and altered consumer behaviors as compared with control groups. The theoretical basis for the project is that the attitudes about behavior for most health consumers begins early in life. Igoe (1980) notes that, consumer activists, social scientists, and health professionals are advocating more assertive client behavior. These behaviors include the acknowledgment of one's own expectations during a client-provider encounter, more discrimina-

tion in selecting professional services, more negotiation with providers of services, and more self-care activity.

■ ■ ■

Advocacy, set within the larger framework of human rights, is a vital role for contemporary nursing. Assisting individuals and groups to become informed about health, without controlling the process, is paramount. The nurse serves as a guide through the maze of health delivery services and monitors the quality of care once clients are established with the appropriate resources.

Advocacy occurs on both the individual and community levels. Community assessment and participation in the group process for planned change allows nursing to maximize its creative potential. The future for consumerism lies in prevention and promotion activities and in adoption of more assertive behaviors by individuals in dealing with health issues facing themselves, their families, and communities. Finally, responding to the call of advocacy for health consumers is a challenge for nurses to meet rather than a dilemma to avoid.

THE NURSE AS DISCHARGE PLANNER

Discharge Planning as a Function of Coordination and Collaboration

With the greater influx of clients to hospitals and the shorter length of hospital stay, more emphasis must be placed on helping clients better understand their illness or health state and on preparing them to care for themselves after discharge to the community. The present health care system might well be described as an illness system. Providers wait until clients are sick and then give them sophisticated, expensive, expert technical care. Clients are then discharged from the system, and in many instances complications develop because of a client's or family's lack of understanding of the client's health state, thus resulting in a need for readmission. For example, an incident occurred in which a client had to be rehospitalized for acute congestive heart failure with pulmonary edema 1 month after discharge because the client stopped taking the prescribed digoxin and diuretic each day. Explanation and understanding of the medication regimen had been omitted in the discharge process. Neither the client nor the spouse understood the purpose of the medications or the consequences of omitting them.

A similar incident occurred when a client was given a prescription for a different strength of digoxin upon discharge. The client was not told to discontinue the existing dosage. The result of taking the combined amounts of digoxin was a second-degree heart block with severe digoxin toxicity. In addition to the severity of the physiological condition, which caused much discomfort, these clients and their families were subjected to a great amount of stress, anxiety, and financial strain.

These two incidents might have been prevented by a systematic discharge care plan implemented on the date of admission, periodically reevaluated, and emphasized throughout the hospital stay.

Definition

Discharge planning can be defined as an event often planned by a multidisciplinary team within a given setting which enhances the client's ability to return to an optimal life-style. It is part of a continuum of care in which those responsible for a client's treatment collaborate in a multidisciplinary team approach to assist the client and family to move from one phase of care to the next. It incorporates the concept of holistic health planning, which includes preventive, primary, therapeutic, rehabilitative, and custodial care. Inherent in the concept of discharge planning is the need for client and family to work with the health care team in arranging a suitable plan of care.

Continuity of care, which is a series of client care activities rendered to the client in three situations (before hospital entry, during hospital stay, and after discharge) is a basic objective of discharge planning. Comprehensive health care is an additional objective of discharge planning. Four essential components of comprehensive health care are (1) health education, (2) personal preventive services, (3) diagnostic and therapeutic services, and (4) rehabilitative and restorative services (Bristow et al., 1976).

Legislation

In 1972 discharge planning was recognized as one of the 12 essential items in the American Hospital Association's "Statement on a Patient's Bill of Rights." The eighth right states the following (Annas, 1975, p. 35):

The patient has the right to expect reasonable continuity of care. He has the right to know in advance what appointment time and physicians are available and where. The patient has the right to expect that the hospital will provide a mechanism whereby he is informed by his physician or a delegate of the physician of the patient's continuing health care requirement following discharge."

Many other governmental agencies and professional organizations have issued statements and declarations on discharge planning. The following statement appears in the Joint Commission Accreditation Manual for Hospitals: "The nursing care plan should be initiated upon admission of the patient and, as part of the long term goal, should include discharge plans" (JCAH, 1977 p. 124).

Medicare regulations require hospitals and nursing homes to provide discharge planning. Standard H, which deals with discharge planning, states that a facility should maintain a centralized coordinated program to ensure that each patient has a planned program of continuing care and follow-up which meets individual post-discharge needs (HCFA, 1978). The Social Security amendments enacted in 1972 instituted Professional Standards Review Organizations (PSRO) and included a section on discharge planning. The Department of Health, Education, and Welfare PSRO guidelines state, "Where problems in post-discharge care or discharge placement are anticipated, discharge planning should be initiated as soon as possible after admission to the short stay hospital. Discharge planning should include both preparation of the patient for the next level of care and arrangement for placement in the appropriate care setting" (Public Law 92-603, 1972).

Discharge Planning Coordinator

Who should coordinate the discharge planning activities: a nurse, social worker, or physician? Many institutions are adding a variety of health professionals such as pharmacists, chaplains, physical therapists, social workers, and nutritionists to the discharge planning team. However, there should be one person to coordinate the activities of the team. Nurses have in the past proven to be effective discharge planning coordinators. A recent survey of 27 facilities in the Greater Boston area showed that over 50% of discharge planning departments are based within nursing departments. This seems logical when nurses are responsible for clients 24 hours a day (McKeehan, 1981).

The position of a discharge planner requires an individual to possess (1) tact; (2) resourcefulness; (3) initiative; (4) ability to communicate effectively with agency staff, clients, and families; and (5) a knowledge of community resources. The nurse must be assertive enough to initiate the discharge process if the client's condition and resources deem it advisable. In large institutions there may be a nurse to coordinate discharge planning for each major unit. These nurses are very knowledgeable regarding community resources and skilled in assisting clients and families to make the transition from one facility to another. The agency staff nurse functions in an independent and collaborative manner to ensure continuity of care for clients after discharge.

Programs and Settings

There are four basic options to consider in the planning of care following discharge: (1) home health care programs; (2) after-care programs; (3) outpatient visits; and (4) nursing home and day care centers. All options provide services outside the hospital, are considerably more economical, and strive to provide and enhance the health of the client and family. Home health care programs provide services of a physician, nurse, social worker, physical therapist, or occupational therapist in the client's home. Home health aides are also frequently used for the chronically ill client. Use of their services frees up hospital beds and assists family members in the continued care of chronically ill relatives. Home health care teams may serve a particular population group. For example, an oncology team consisting of a doctor, nurse, and social worker may assist cancer victims to maintain themselves outside the hospital. Likewise, pediatric teams may work exclusively with high-risk parents such as those in abused child or premature infant situations.

After-care programs provide services by ensuring transportation and continuity of care for clients when they return to the hospital for treatment and then go home again. Fewer hospital visits are required if all health care needs and appointments can be coordinated in a 1-day visit. This program is especially helpful for those clients who must travel long distances.

Outpatient follow-up is the most common method of providing care after discharge and medical treatment for clients receiving home health care. Clients are given an appointment to a clinic or service. This is the least expensive type of care, since clients arrange their own transportation. Clients with especially troublesome illnesses, such as those having difficulty getting around or those having severe discomfort and unable to endure continuous care on an outpatient basis, find that home health care is the best option for them in reducing the number of outpatient visits that are required.

Use of day care centers for the chronically ill is an innovative program to assist families by caring for a relative throughout the day and thus permitting family members to continue working. These centers are more economical than home or institutional care. Most clients are ambulatory, but some centers provide weekend services for the bedridden client. The family can have a weekend respite from the daily care of a chronically ill relative (Burston, 1973).

Long-term convalescent or nursing home care is used for persons requiring round-the-clock supervision. Nursing homes also provide care for clients who are psychologically or physically handicapped and are unable to cope outside an institutional setting. Many elderly clients view nursing homes as the least desirable option for them. Nursing home care is expensive and often there are rigorous admission requirements and long waiting lists (Ratliff, 1981).

The Community Health Nurse as Discharge Planner

In some areas, such as California, the community health nurse is used for discharge planning with increasing frequency. Institutions contract with the health department or Visiting Nurse Association to place nurses in their facility. The nurse remains an employee of the Visiting Nurse Association, although the hospital pays for the time the nurse spends there. The community health nurse is adept in making a home and community assessment that enhances the effectiveness of the discharge plan (Bristow et al., 1976).

A typical day for a discharge planning nurse would include the following:

1. Meet all admissions and screen for potential discharge problems
2. Attend morning report and rounds at the institution
3. Give high priority to planning for clients whose discharge is imminent
4. Complete pending referrals
5. Contact physicians for completion of forms and contact the appropriate referral agency
6. Interview the client and family immediately before discharge
7. Make home visits to assess the resource and liability of the home environment

Discharge planning nurses practice not only in the secondary or tertiary care setting but also in the primary care setting. Many outpatient clinics and emergency departments employ a nurse to coordinate discharge plans for clients and families (O'Boyle, 1972). Basically the activities of this nurse are the same as those of the nurse practicing in the institutional setting but with minor variation. The nurse in the primary care setting does not make rounds, since the clients are usually referred to the nurse by other staff members. This nurse may, however, review and screen the daily appointment schedules for potential clients. The nurse is often involved in extensive client education and referral to community agencies.

Whether the setting is an inpatient facility such as a secondary or tertiary care hospital, a nursing home, or a primary care outpatient clinic or emergency facility, the nurse works closely with other health care providers, especially social work services. Social workers have traditionally participated in discharge planning services for clients and families. In addition to a vast knowledge of community resources, social workers can assist with financial arrangements. They usually have knowledge of private and governmental programs that offer assistance.

The nutritionist or dietician can also provide information on community resources for food purchases, food substitutes, and adaptions for food preparations used in the home. Information on available programs in the community which provide nutrition, education, and weight loss plans are being used on a more frequent basis in the overall therapeutic plan.

The clinical pharmacist can provide information on community resources for reduced drug costs and valuable client education information literature. The hospital chaplain can promote access to a community pastor for the client if contact has not been established. Chaplains also have knowledge of various church-related resources such as therapy groups, clothing, food banks, and health-related clinics. Physical therapists can assist in planning for a home care adaptation program. Many of the larger institutions providing long-term care also employ a vocational rehabilitation counselor and a recreational therapist. All of these individuals are excellent resources to assist in the discharge planning process.

Referrals

All clients need some form of discharge teaching and preparation, but not all clients will need extensive discharge planning. In the hospital the discharge planning nurse screens all admissions for a specific unit and assigns a rating scale for specific groups of clients identified as having a greater need for more intensive planning. This need may be the result of the nature of the clients' health problems, financial and family situations, or availability of existing community resources.

Some pediatric or maternity clients who require discharge planning and follow-up are the following:

1. Baby weighing 4½ pounds or less or weighing over 10 pounds at birth
2. Baby with an Apgar score at 5 minutes of 7 or lower
3. Baby with major congenital anomaly such as cleft palate or spina bifida
4. Infant with positive PKU test result
5. New teenage mother
6. Mother discharged after delivery in past 48 hours
7. Family with indication of dysfunction, parental rejection, or child abuse
8. Baby failing to thrive and with poor feeding prognosis
9. Family with a crisis such as having a child with a newly diagnosed serious illness (e.g., leukemia) or traumatic injuries
10. Child of a mother with a serious medical or mental problem, such as a maternity client with depression

The client who is admitted to the hospital to have radical or mutilating surgery may require follow-up, especially if the surgery is of such a nature that marked changes in life-style or family relations may result. Examples include the following:

1. Nephrectomy
2. Ostomy
3. Radical neck or face reconstruction
4. Extremity amputation
5. Surgery for weight reduction
6. Cardiovascular reconstruction

Adult or pediatric clients with an acute or chronic illness would also benefit from follow-up, for example, clients with diabetes, arthritis, or heart disease who require the following:

1. Medication injections
2. Special diets or treatments
3. Exercises or physical therapy

Many of these clients can benefit psychologically and economically from an early discharge. The cost of coordinated home care is approximately one fourth of the cost of inpatient hospital care (Bristow et al., 1976). Clients with chronic illnesses who have multiple hospitalizations soon exhaust their financial resources. Clients are usually happier in their own homes, because their identity and sense of stability are maintained and they are not exposed to hospital-borne infections.

The geriatric client often presents a different set of problems to consider. Many do not have homes or relatives to assist with their care. Because of physical impairments, many cannot be discharged to go home alone, and special arrangements must often be made on a permanent basis. Facilities for placement of these cases are foster homes, custodial care facilities, or the client's own home with frequent periodic home visits by a community health nurse. Many communities have resources such as Meals on Wheels and home health aides, making it possible for the elderly client to stay in their home. Special apartment complexes for the elderly are often staffed on certain days with a nurse to look in on clients who are recuperating or who need assistance.

The client who has an emotional problem will also need discharge planning. As in the case of the elderly, establishment of a food service and a resocialization program is often necessary. In a halfway house, both of these can be met along with a structured vocational rehabilitative program. Unfortunately, communities often have too few of these resources available.

The Process

Discharge planning begins on the date of admission. The predicted date of discharge is entered on the hospital chart at the time of admission and altered if necessary (Fenwick, 1979, Tilburg, 1971). An assessment of the clients' problems, their resources, and family support are indicators as to how much discharge preparation will be necessary. The nurse will meet with the client, family, and physician periodically throughout the hospitalization. Essential information to obtain for effective discharge planning includes current level of care needed, projected level of care needed, projected time frame for moving client to next level of care, therapies and teaching that must be accomplished before hospital discharge, available resources for care after discharge, and mechanisms for facilitating the transfer.

The concept of client readiness must be considered by a multidisciplinary team. This readiness includes physiological, psychological, and social phenomena. All too often only the physiological needs are considered, and the psychological resources for the family and client are neglected. This is especially true of families who are coping with long debilitating or terminal problems (Fenwick, 1979). A visit to the home by a nurse to assess family and environmental resources will enhance discharge planning effectiveness. Dietary and nutritional resources as well as assets or impairments in the home to ambulation are particularly assessed.

Optimally, a formal discharge conference will be conducted with unit nurses, the physician, and possibly the dietician, chaplain, and physical therapists if they are involved. The discharge nurse as the coordinator of the team will in most cases make the necessary follow-up referrals.

A written discharge summary note is entered in the nursing notations and some type of formal discharge instruction form is sent home with the client. The form can be tailored to a particular unit, outlining specific needs of the client, or be very general in format. All forms should contain information regarding basic needs: follow-up appointments, diet, medications, treatments, bathing, and activity instructions, including when to drive and when to resume sexual relations.

An example of a discharge planning form for an orthopedic client is shown in the boxed material (Sheahan, 1974). This form encourages periodic discharge teaching with documentation of progress throughout the hospitalization. The client and family should be given explicit written instructions on discharge. The discharge planning nurse should be accessible if a problem does arise within a short time after returning to the home. All too often the client or family will have questions that arise after discharge when the physician is unavailable. These questions will go unanswered until the next day, or in desperation, the client will contact the local emergency department. All discharged clients need to have an emergency phone number and access to the discharge planning nurse or agency department,

which would provide a resource in an emergency. The primary care nurses may also assume responsibility for follow-up telephone inquiries of their discharge clients.

Barriers to Discharge Planning

Lack of communication and knowledge of community resources are the two major barriers to effective discharge planning. A team approach with regularly scheduled meetings has proven successful in reviewing discharge needs of clients on a specific unit. As the coordinator of the team, the discharge planning nurse assures that communication lines are established between staff, client, family, and physicians. Most communities have a compiled list or book that contains available community resources. Usually eligibility criteria are listed as well as the individual to contact. Optimally the discharge planning nurse has an opportunity to meet the various agency contact persons and thus can talk to them on a more personal basis when a telephone referral is made. Some institutions have found that inviting resource agency representatives to speak with staff members facilitates the referral process.

It is desirable for the discharge planning nurse to provide feedback to the unit nurses. Information about the client's progress and receptiveness to the new environment and results of past nursing care are needed for the unit nurse's growth and evaluation. This information will assist the nurse to modify future nursing care where indicated. Also, administrative support is essential to the provision of adequate nursing staff for a unit so that quality discharge planning can be implemented. Frequently discharge planning is subordinate to maintenance of basic needs when an agency unit is understaffed.

Health care providers need to understand Medicare and Medicaid resources that can be used in discharge planning for the growing population over 65 years. The Medicare and Medicaid programs are limited in the types of services covered and are restricted to covering clients who meet eligibility criteria. The Medicare handbook lists the services that are covered for hospital care after discharge and the conditions that must be met for the person to qualify for home health visits (Health Care Financing Administration, 1982). Clients can qualify for home visits under Medicare's medical insurance program by meeting certain conditions. Currently, home health visits are covered after a yearly deductible is met.

Discharge planning nurses should routinely counsel clients and families on the availability of Medicaid services. A person may qualify for Medicaid if their income is low, if they have high medical costs in relation to their income, or if they are aged, blind, or disabled and living on a limited income. To apply for Medicaid,

Discharge Planning Form

Admission date

Diagnosis

	Date	Comments

1. Client's understanding of disease
   Condition
   Prevention
   Symptoms of complications
2. Medications
   Name
   Purpose
   Correct administration
   Toxic reaction
   Side effects
   Length of time to be taken
   Where purchased
3. Treatments
   Checking urine
   Soaks and compresses
   Exercises and positions
   Irrigations
   Dressings, bandages,
      and cast care
   Other
4. Diet
   Reason for diet
   Special preparation
   Substitutions
   General diet teaching
5. General physical care
   Skin, hair, and nails
   Mode of bathing
6. Amount of activity
   Daily rest
   Limitations
   Recreation
   Ability to drive
   Resuming work
   Sexual relations
7. Referrals and follow-up
   Name of agency or clinic
   Physician
   Date and time
   Address and directions
   Preparation (if any)
   Reason for referral
8. Discharge notes: ambulatory_____ wheelchair_____ stretcher_____ date_____

a client goes to a local welfare and Social Security office with proof of income level, proof of United States citizenship, and medical records proving disability or large medical bills. Aged persons may qualify for Medicare and medicaid and there are certain children's services that are provided by Medicaid under Early Periodic Screening, Diagnosis and Treatment programs (EPSDT). These services include screening examinations, immunizations, and diagnostic and treatment programs to prevent and correct health problems in children.

Some state Medicaid programs provide additional services not required by federal guideline. The local Social Security or State Human Resource office would have information as to Medicaid benefits for that locality. Many clients think they cannot qualify for Medicaid programs if they own property or an automobile. This is not necessarily true, thus benefit eligibility should always be explored by the discharge planner. Because the eligibility requirements and services offered by Medicare and Medicaid change frequently, the community health nurse discharge planner should seek annual up-to-date information on Medicare and Medicaid from the Social Security Administration.

Benefits of Discharge Planning

Several rewards for clients, families, health providers, and the community can be realized when an effective discharge planning program is implemented. Among these are (1) money is saved to finance comprehensive service for a greater number of clients; (2) hospital beds are freed up; (3) relapses, needless hospital stays, and unnecessary emergency visits are decreased; and (4) client and families become involved in the planning and participate actively in the education process. This involvement encourages a sense of responsibility for their own care. They develop trust in themselves to make future health care decisions and in the health provider to assist them with relevant information. Nurses in all settings can experience the rewarding feeling of observing a client and family make the transition from one phase of health status to another if they take the opportunity to participate collaboratively and creatively in the discharge plan.

SUMMARY

The community health nurse coordinator-collaborator has two major role functions: coordinating client care and coordinating resources. The nurse may also be assigned to coordinate and collaborate in the development of programs. The key ingredient to effective coordination and collaboration is communication. Communication may be formal, with interaction occurring through organized channels, or it may be informal, with interaction occurring primarily between active participants.

There are two levels of coordination: horizontal, which occurs across agencies, and vertical, which occurs within an agency. The nurse acting as client advocate may engage in either coordinating level, whereas the nurse acting as discharge planner primarily uses horizontal coordination. The major goals of the nurse advocate and the nurse discharge planner are to make the health care system more responsive to the client's needs and to move the client toward independence.

The community health nurse with knowledge about the community and its resources is the ideal provider to serve as discharge planner and client advocate. To be effective in fulfilling these functions the nurse must be an assertive, facilitative, responsible, resourceful, and understanding risk taker. Better coordination and collaboration through discharge planning and advocacy will benefit the consumer, the health care provider, and the system by providing greater efficiency and effectiveness of services while reducing the likelihood of costly duplication of health care services.

BIBLIOGRAPHY

Abdellah, F., Forest, H., and Chow, R.: PACE: an approach to improving care of the elderly, Am. J. Nurs. **79**:1109, 1979.

Abrams, N.: A contrary view of the nurse as patient advocate, Nurs. Forum **8**(3):258-267, 1978.

American Nurses' Association: Standards of nursing practice, Kansas City, Mo., 1973, The Association.

Annas, G.: The right of hospital patients, New York, 1975, E.P. Dutton & Co., Inc. p. 35.

Aroskar, M.A.: Anatomy of an ethical dilemma. I. The theory, II. The practice, Am. J. Nurs. **80**:658-663, 1980.

Benne, K.D., and Birnbaum, M.: Principles of changing. In Bennis, W.G., et al., editors: Dynamics of planned change, New York, 1969, Holt, Rinehart & Winston, Inc.

Bristow, O., Stickney, C., and Thompson, S.: Discharge planning for continuity of care, NLN Pub. No. 21-1604, 1976.

Brower, T.H.: Advocacy: what it is, J. Gerontol. Nurs. **8**(3): 141-143, 1982.

Burston, G.R.: A holiday relief service for elderly patients normally cared for at home, Practitioner **211**(263):345-350, 1973.

Channing, L.: Medicaid and you, Greenfield, Mass., 1979, Bet Co., Inc.

Clemen, S.A., Eigsti, D.G., and McGuire, S.L.: Comprehensive family and community health nursing, New York, 1981, McGraw-Hill Book Co.

Coe, R.M., and Andrews, K.R.: Effects of medicare on the provision of community health resources, Am. J. Public Health, **62**(6):854-856, 1972.

Curtin, L.L.: The nurse as advocate: a philosophical foundation for nursing, ANS Adv. nurs. sci. **1**(3):1-10, 1979.

Donahue, P.M.: The nurse: a patient advocate? Nurs. Forum, **12**(2):143-151, 1978.

Fenwick, A.: An interdisciplinary tool for assessing patients' readiness for discharge in the rehabilitation setting, J. Adv. Nurs., **4**:9-21, 1979.

Friedman, M.: Family nursing theory and assessment, New York, 1981, Appleton-Century-Crofts.

Gadow, S.: Advocacy nursing and new meanings of aging, Nurs Clin. North Am. **14**(1):81-91, 1979.

Haimann, T., and Scott, W.G.: Management in the modern organization, Boston, 1974, Houghton Mifflin Co.

Health Care Financing Administration: Medicaid regulations, Washington, D.C., 1978, Department of Health, Education, and Welfare.

Health Care Financing Administration: Your medicare handbook, SSA Pub. No. 05-10050, Washington, D.C., 1982, Department of Health and Human services.

Hein, E.C.: Communication in nursing practice, Boston, 1973, Little, Brown & Co.

Hersey, P., and Blanchard, K.: Management of organization behavior: utilizing human resources, Englewood Cliffs, N.J., 1977, Prentice-Hall, Inc.

Hicks, A.P., and Ashby, D.J.: Teaching discharge planning, Nurs. Outlook **26**(5):306.

Hollingsworth, C.E., and Sokal, B.: Predischarge family conference, JAMA, **239**(8):740-741, 1978.

Huey, R.: Discharge planning: good planning means fewer hospitalizations for the chronically ill, Grand rounds, Nurs. 81, p. 70-75. 1981.

Hushower, G., Gamberg,D., and Smith, N.: The nursing process in discharge planning, Superv. Nurse **9**:55-58, 1978.

Igoe, J.B.: Project health PACT in action, Am. J. Nurs. **80**(11):2016-2021, 1980.

Inui, T., et al.: Identifying hospital patients who need early discharge planning for special dispositions: a comparison of alternative techniques, Med. Care **19**(9):922-929, 1981.

Joint Commission on Accreditation of Hospitals: Accreditation manual for hospitals, Chicago, 1977, JCAH.

Kohnke, M.F.: The nurse as advocate, Am. J. Nurs. **80**(11):2038-2040, 1980.

Lamb, H.R.: Securing patient's rights-responsibility, Hosp. Community Psychiatry **32**(6):393-397, 1981.

Lancaster, J., and Lancaster, W., editors: Concepts for advanced nursing practice: the nurse as a change agent, St. Louis, 1982, The C.V. Mosby Co.

Mauksch, I.G.: Advocacy or control: which do we offer the elderly? Geriatric Nurs. **1**(4): 278, 1980.

McDonnell, D.: An evaluation of day care center care, Int. J. Soc. Psychiatry **23**(2):110-119, 1977.

McKeehan, K.: Continuing care, St. Louis, 1981, The C.V. Mosby Co.

O'Boyle,C.: A new era in emergency services, AJN. **72**:1392-1397, Aug. 1972.

Pender, N.J.: Health promotion in nursing practice, New York, 1982, Appleton-Century-Crofts.

Previte, V.: Continuing care in a primary nursing setting: role of a clinical specialist, Int. Nurs. Rev. **26**(2):53-6, 1979.

Public Law 92-603, Social Security Amendments of 1972, 92nd Congress, Oct. 30, 1972.

Rakich, J.S., Longest, B.B., and O'Donovan, T.R.: Managing health care organizations, Philadelphia, 1977, W.B. Saunders Co.

Ratliff, B.: Leaving the hospital: discharge planning for total patient care, Springfield, Ill., 1981, Charles C Thomas, Publisher.

Savedra, M.: Moving from hospital to home, Am. J. Maternal Child Nurs. **6**:220-222, 1977.

Sheahan, S.L.: A discharge planning guide: an aid to discharge teaching, unpublished master's project, Lexington, Ky., 1974. University of Kentucky College of Nursing.

Smith, C.S.: Outrageous or outraged: a nurse advocate story, Nurs. Outlook **28**(10):624-625, 1980.

Smith, J., Buchaler, J., and Rosales, S.: Coordinating a workable system, Am. J. Nurs. **79**:1439, 1978.

Spradley, B.W.: Community health nursing concepts and practice, Boston, 1981, Little, Brown & Co.

Stone, M.: Discharge planning guide, Am. J. Nurs. **79**:1446, 1979.

Travelbee, J.: Interpersonal aspects of nursing, Philadelphia, 1974, F.A. Davis Co.

Thoms, F.L., and Mott, R.: A new role for the R.N.: discharge coordinator, Hosp. Prog. **59**(2):38-40, 1978.

Tilburg, V.: How one hospital increased the effectiveness of its bed and service utilization, Canadian Hospital, Feb. 1971, pp. 49-51.

Williams, S.F., and Torrens, P.R.: Introduction to health services, New York, 1980, John Wiley & Sons, Inc.

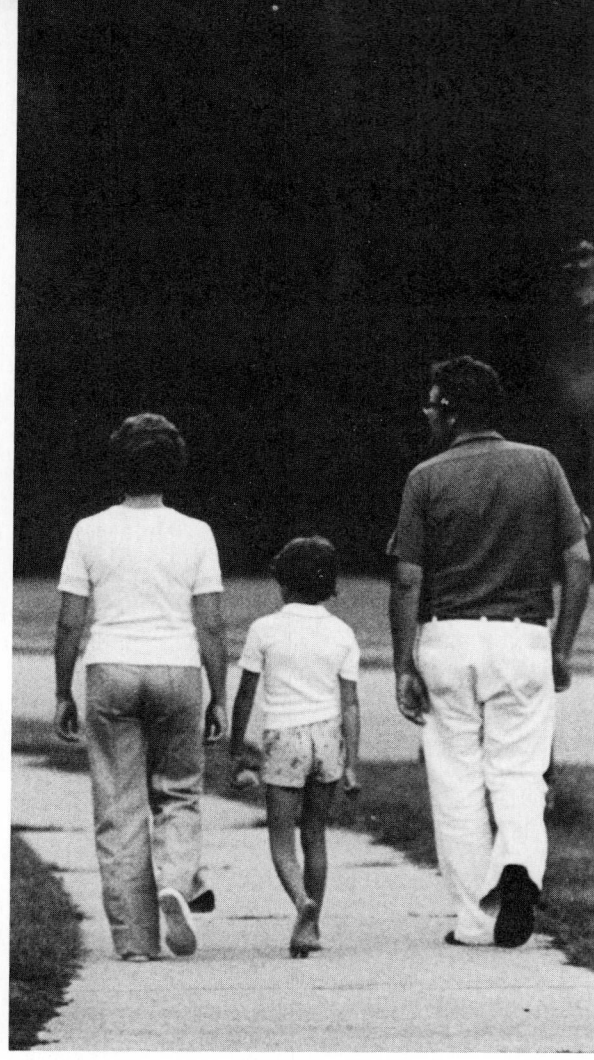

Chapter
33

CYNTHIA SELLECK HENSON
ANN SIRLES
REBECCA SLOAN

THE COMMUNITY HEALTH NURSE AS FAMILY NURSE PRACTITIONER

Several social phenomena and a shift in health problems over the past century have combined to redefine the pattern of health care in this country. Among these changes, and in part because of them, came the introduction of primary care. Although there have been many definitions of primary care, it is most often described as accessible, comprehensive, coordinated, and continuous care provided by accountable care givers (Institute of Medicine, 1978).

The philosophy inherent in primary care is similar to that of primary nursing, which has become a popular modality for delivering nursing care to clients in a variety of settings, particularly the hospital. The client contributes to as well as receives care, and the provider is not only available, but has authority, autonomy, and accountability.

It has been estimated that most of the nation's health care could be managed at the primary care level. However, only 25% of physicians today practice in primary care fields (Andrus and Mitchell, 1980). This and similar data indicate that one profession alone cannot provide primary care for the combined health and illness needs of the population.

In looking at the demands of the primary care system and in analyzing the needs of clients who have access to this system, it became evident to health care planners that nurses, by expanding their existing skills, would be uniquely qualified to provide a major portion of primary care, using the physicians as consultants (Rogers, 1977).

This chapter provides historical perspectives of the nurse practitioner (NP) movement as well as information regarding the current status of NPs, particularly family nurse practitioners (FNPs) who are primary health care providers directing their services toward all age groups. Role functions assumed by FNPs are addressed as are the arenas for FNP practice. Finally, the legal implications and areas of role stress relative to the practice of NPs are discussed.

HISTORICAL PERSPECTIVE

The evolution and use of nonphysician providers of direct primary care services are not unique to the United States. Other parts of the world have used nonphysicians in primary care who have functioned successfully with varying degrees of autonomy. Historically the development of these roles occurred as a response to the health needs of a population and the insufficient numbers of physicians to meet these needs (Nichols, 1980).

In the United States the 1960s witnessed not only a physician shortage but the increasing tendency among physicians to specialize. The number of physicians who might have provided medical care to communities and families across the nation was thus reduced. As this trend continued, a serious gap in primary care services developed (Bullough, 1980).

Demographic factors also influenced the evolution of nonphysician providers. Though the number of medical personnel in primary care was decreasing, the population was increasing. The lower socioeconomic groups that tended to cluster in the inner cities and rural areas were most affected by these changes. Additionally, the median age of the population was steadily rising, resulting in an increasingly higher proportion of aged persons. Many of these people live for long periods with chronic disease or the infirmities of old age coupled with dwindling financial resources and other social problems. Access to primary care for these two groups in particular was becoming a nationally recognized problem (Bullough, 1980).

Nursing and medicine responded to these inadequacies of the health care system. In 1965 at the University of Colorado School of Nursing, Loretta Ford determined that the morbidity among medically deprived children could be decreased by educating community health nurses to provide well care to children of all ages. Their scope of nursing practice included the identification, assessment, and management of common acute and chronic conditions with the appropriate referral of more complex problems (Silver et al., 1967). These nurses were referred to as pediatric nurse associates or pediatric NPs. That same year the physician assistant (PA) role was initiated at Duke University. This program was intended to attract ex-military corpsmen for training as medical extenders (Fisher and Horowitz, 1977).

These innovative programs, directed at alleviating the problems of physician shortage and access to primary care for rural and other medically underserved populations, attracted the interest of the federal government. A report issued by the Department of Health, Education, and Welfare on *Extending the Scope of Nursing Practice* (1971) helped convince Congress of the value of NPs as primary care providers. The Nurse Training Act of 1971 (PL 92-150) and the Comprehensive Health Manpower Act of 1971 (PL 92-157) provided educational funding for many NP and PA programs. Although nonphysician providers are often lumped together into a single category, there are more differences than similarities in the backgrounds, education, and practice of NPs and PAs.

PRIMARY HEALTH CARE TEAM

The primary health care team may consist of a variety of members. Such members usually have specialized and complementary skills that help to strengthen the team. Table 33-1 lists possible primary health care team members along with their educational backgrounds and role functions.

FNPs must practice as colleagues with physicians and other health care professionals. Physicians and FNPs need to continue to develop strategies for combining their expertise so that they can be integrated in a complementary fashion, which would provide a team approach in addressing the health needs of the client.

Physicians, NPs, and PAs may all have roles on the primary health care team. It is important to recognize that the role of the PA is defined entirely by medicine, and the role of the NP is defined entirely by nursing. Fig. 33-1 illustrates the functional areas of these three roles. As is shown by the model, all three roles have overlapping functions.

The use of FNPs as primary health care providers goes beyond that of physician extender or physician substitute. In a study done by Kweskin (1979) on the use of FNPs in a team approach, four positive outcomes were demonstrated. First, the FNP facilitates access to primary care by increasing the number of qualified providers. The consumer generally seeks primary care in response to a perceived health problem. Because a significant number of health problems are of a minor or health maintenance nature and do not require specialized medical skills, FNPs are well equipped to effectively manage such problems.

Table 33-1. Possible primary health care team members

Role	Education	Qualification	Function
Physician (MD)	Baccalaureate degree (4 years) plus graduation from medical school (4 years), plus an internship and residency of variable years, depending on specialtay area	May be certified by examination in a specialty area, however, not mandatory	Elicits histories and performs physical examinations; performs appropriate diagnostic and therapeutic procedures; provides counseling and guidance; performs other procedures, including surgery, depending on specialty area
Family nurse practitioner (FNP)	Continuing education programs: must be RN with diploma, AD, or BSN preparation, granted a certificate on completion of program, usually 9-12 months Degree programs: must be RN with BSN preparation to enter master's level FNP program, usually 18-24 months	Successful completion of state board of nursing examination; licensure by state; state certification mandatory in some states; national certification not mandatory; physician supervision not mandatory	Elicit histories and perform physical examinations; assess health and illness status; provide health screening, education, and counseling; assist with health maintenance and promotion activities; initiate appropriate diagnostic and therapeutic procedures with physician consultation
Physician's assistant (PA)	Baccalaureate degree preparation as PA, usually 4 years	Variable; licensure by some states; physician supervision mandatory	Elicits histories and performs physical examinations; initiates appropriate diagnostic and therapeutic procedures under physician supervision
Registered nurse (RN)	Diploma through a hospital school of nursing (3 years); associate degree through a community college (2 years) or baccalaureate degree through a college or university (4 years); master's and doctoral (DSN, PhD, EdD) preparation available	Successful completion of state board of nursing examination; licensure by state	Use the nursing process in supervising and providing total client care; carry out physician's orders for medications and therapeutic measures; carry out nursing procedures; provide health education and counseling
Licensed practical (vocational) nurse (LPN or LVN)	Course of study, usually 9-12 months through a vocational school	Variable; usually state licensed; RN or physician supervision mandatory	Assist with physical examinations; perform simple laboratory tests; carry out nursing and medically prescribed procedures; provide health education and counseling
Social worker	Master's level preparation usually required for unsupervised clinical practice; doctoral preparation (DSW, PhD) available	Variable; licensed by some states; membership in national association of social workers and academy of certified social workers and 2 years of supervised practice desirable	Provide counseling and guidance; assist client and family in locating appropriate community resources
Dietitian	Baccalaureate degree (4 years) plus a 1-year internship required; master's preparation available	Registered through the American Dietetic Association	Assess nutritional status and counsel clients and families on nutritional needs for specific situations
Medical assistant/receptionist	Course of study offered through a vocational school or community college teaches first aid and simple laboratory tests as well as office managerial skills	No registration or licensure	Serve as receptionist; make appointments; work with billing; assist with laboratory procedures

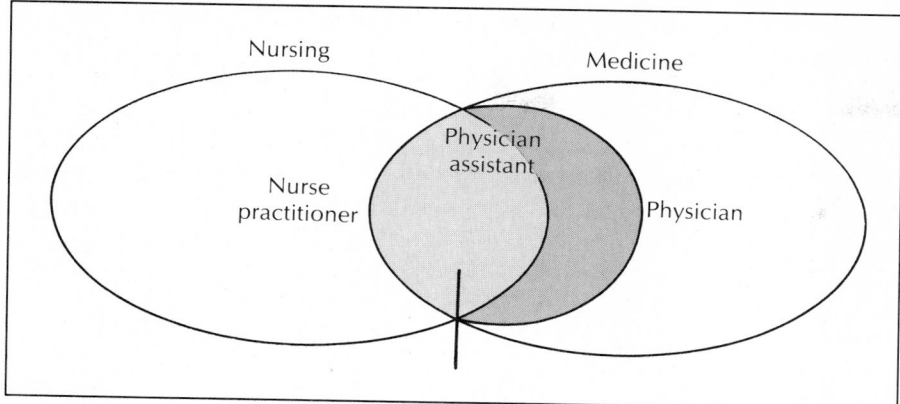

Fig. 33-1. Nurse practitioner and physician assistant roles in relation to nursing and medicine in primary care. (Adapted from Graduate Medical Education National Advisory Committee: Nonphysician health care provider technical panel, vol. 7, DHHS, Washington, D.C., 1980, U.S. Government Printing Office.)

Second, the FNP provides prompt screening and referral. FNPs are taught to recognize the subjective and objective signs and symptoms of potentially serious medical problems that require referral to a physician. Conversely, physicians should recognize that when clients' health problems are more amenable to care than cure, the specialized skills of self-care health counseling and guidance provided by FNPs may be the best treatment (Kweskin, 1979).

Third, the FNP improves the health records by establishing baseline health profiles. FNPs assure through the practice of nursing that a client's record reflects the consideration of personal, family, and community health and illness variables. Such records also contribute to continuity of care and health maintenance (Kweskin, 1979).

Fourth, the FNP contributes to increased quality and comprehensiveness of health care, which is also cost effective (Kweskin, 1979). Three arguments are offered, which are relative to FNPs' contributions to reduction in the costs of health care:

1. The total cost of educating FNPs is only one third to one fifth that of educating primary care physicians (Sadler, 1975).
2. The average earnings of an FNP are about 40% those of a physician (Scheffler, 1975).
3. FNPs have been found to provide care at about half the cost prevailing in the community (Tennant et al, 1980).

Adding the dimension of nursing to the health care team increases primary care services in diversity and quality. The use of such providers becomes cost effective when the needs of the client seeking services are matched with the provider who, by virtue of professional education and specialized skills, is best able to meet those needs.

EDUCATION OF FNPs

FNPs are currently educated in master's level programs in nursing or in nondegree, continuing education programs. Most programs preparing FNPs in 1979 were in departments of continuing education in nursing, and the baccalaureate degree was not a uniform admission criterion (Golden, 1979). Early FNP programs relied heavily on physician faculty for didactic and clinical teaching as few nurse faculty members in the 1960s and early 1970s were clinically prepared to provide direct primary care. When physicians dominated content and practice, students were not strongly socialized into the nursing role, and the physician extender concept of the FNP was likely to be fostered (Spicer, 1978).

As FNPs increased their knowledge and clinical expertise, the realization of the complex knowledge and skills necessary to provide accountable primary care services became apparent. Such skills are most effectively built on a professional nursing base. Out of such realizations came the trend toward master's degree FNP educational programs in which nurse faculty members take major responsibility for the didactic content and clinical preceptorships.

A 1977 nationwide survey of 356 FNPs revealed that primary care FNPs manage a variety of health problems (Draye and Pesznecker, 1979). The five top diagnostic categories seen by FNPs were prevention and health supervision, respiratory problems (primarily of an acute nature), cardiovascular problems (primarily hypertension), genitourinary problems, and ear problems. These five categories accounted for 64% of the visits to the FNPs in the survey. The remaining 36% were dispersed over many diagnostic categories, none of which accounted for more than 2% of the visits. Table 33-2 summarizes these data.

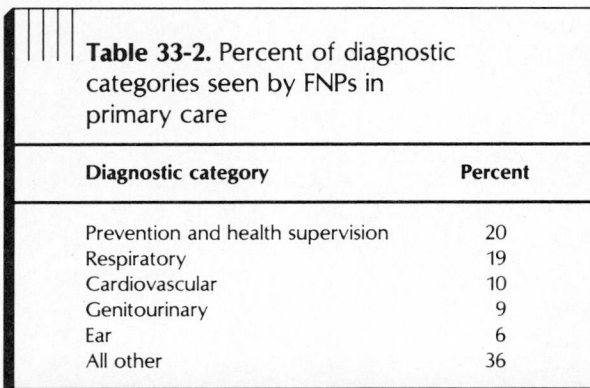

Table 33-2. Percent of diagnostic categories seen by FNPs in primary care

Diagnostic category	Percent
Prevention and health supervision	20
Respiratory	19
Cardiovascular	10
Genitourinary	9
Ear	6
All other	36

Adapted from Draye, M.A., and Pesznecker, B.L.: Nurse Pract. **4**(1):15, Jan.-Feb. 1979.

Although some master's programs have retained the term *practitioner* for graduates of their expanded role programs, others have adopted the term *clinician*, believing the latter to be consistent with graduate education and the former with continuing education programs. In 1979 the National League for Nursing issued its statement on education of the nurse practitioner/clinician (p.2):

... the nurse practitioner should hold a master's degree in nursing in order to ensure competence and quality care ... where emphasis in graduate nursing study would be placed on an expanded specialized nursing function, rather than on the performance of certain medical tasks ... to prepare them for independent decision-making and provide them with a specialized in-depth knowledge base.

Length of programs to prepare FNPs varies from an academic year (9 months) to 2 years. Shorter programs are generally continuing education nondegree programs. Most master's level programs are 18 months to 2 years in length.

It is important to recognize that the NP movement has created several types of NPs. Currently, in the United States there are programs preparing adult nurse practitioners (ANP), pediatric nurse practitioners (PNP), school nurse practitioners (SNP), geriatric nurse practitioners (GNP), obstetric and gynecological nurse practitioners (OGNP), family planning nurse practitioners (FPNP), emergency nurse practitioners (ENP), and nurse midwives (NM). Whereas the FNP is prepared as a specialist in the primary care area of family practice with the ability to provide care to people of all ages and both sexes, NPs from these other programs are prepared as specialists in providing primary care to a select group of individuals (adults, children, the aged, or women).

CREDENTIALS FOR FNPs

Nursing's diversified primary care roles have influenced the need for credentials beyond basic licensure. Primarily, giving credentials in the health professions serves to protect the public from educationally unqualified providers.

There are four credential mechanisms in nursing: licensure, certification, accreditation, and academic degrees. Degrees are static credentials having no mechanism within to assure continued growth and competency in practice. Accreditation assesses the quality of educational programs (ANA, 1979). Both the academic degree and accreditation are of importance to FNPs; however, it is licensure and certification that affect their practice most directly.

Individual state nurse practice acts set forth qualifications for licensure and legally define the practice of nursing within the state. The purpose of certification on the other hand is to complement other credential mechanisms in assuring that the public receives care from qualified nurses. Certification is the profession's way to assure itself and the public it serves that an individual's skill and knowledge in a speciality area are current. Where there is diversity of programs and educational criteria, as presently exist in FNP education, certification also serves to facilitate mobility of qualified nursing specialists across geographical boundaries (ANA, 1979).

FNPs are certified by the American Nurses' Association (ANA) through the Division of Community Health Nursing. Presently, successful completion of a formal FNP educational program is a basic criterion to qualify for the certification examination. Beginning in 1985, the basic qualification for certification will be successful completion of a formal FNP program and a baccalaureate degree in nursing.

Certification in a speciality area is for 5 years. Recertification mechanisms vary among specialties and include written examinations, presentation of written case studies, evidence of continuing education in topics applicable to the specialty area, or combinations of these.

ROLE FUNCTIONS OF THE FNP

FNPs emerged as an answer to a population's need for primary care. To provide this primary care FNPs have practiced an expanded nursing role, taking on an array of functions, some of which had not previously been considered part of nursing's domain. Unfortunately, because of taking on some of these functions, FNPs have been and continue to be considered by some as extenders of medical care without offering an otherwise valuable and unique service. Because of their nursing background, diagnosis and treatment should be only a part of the functions an FNP performs. Though physicians deal mainly with illness, nurses' main concerns are in preventing illness and providing care that is aimed at the total individual.

Health Practitioner

As health practitioners, nurses have long been assessing and evaluating their clients' health status by both "hands off" and "hands on" means. In other words, nurses have been listening and questioning and using limited physical assessment techniques for years. The acquisition by FNPs of additional skills in taking histories and assessing physical status has helped to facilitate nurses in their transition to providing primary care.

Though nursing and medical histories are similar, nurses place more emphasis on the emotional, social, cultural, economic, and environmental aspects of the client—areas in which nursing care can impact heavily—assisting the client toward a more healthful existence (Mundinger, 1980).

As with taking histories, systematic physical assessment by FNPs has proven to be quite successful. Though nurses are not as well equipped as physicians to diagnose specific pathology, they are certainly able to discriminate normal from abnormal findings and identify changes or conditions that may necessitate the need for medical assistance or referral to other health providers or agencies. Also, nurses can use the data gathered from the physical assessment in counseling and assisting clients with health maintenance and promotion toward a higher level of functioning.

It is quite useful for health care providers to use health maintenance flow sheets, such as the one shown in Appendix I, which help to guide the practitioner in the health maintenance procedures that are recommended for different ages. A flow sheet also serves as a simple, easy-to-read summary of the client's health maintenance status (Hoole, et al., 1982).

Health care services are the third largest industry in the United States today with over $200 billion expended annually. For decades health care has concentrated largely on detecting and curing disease rather than on preventing illness and promoting health. In fact, more than 90% of the annual health care expenditure in the United States goes toward efforts to control and cure disease; less than 3% goes toward prevention, and less than 1% goes toward education (Mundinger, 1980).

The average life expectancy has risen from 47 years in 1900 to 72 years today, but the American Medical Association's Council on Medical Services believes that with our existing knowledge all people should live to be 90 to 100 years or older (Dangott, 1978). However, this can be the case only when society and the health care system place value on wellness and encourage programs oriented toward prevention, which is not happening. Society does not typically reward a person for staying well and continues to promote behaviors, such as smoking and drinking, known to be associated with illness. The prevailing attitude has been one of taking health for granted until ill health develops.

There has been a growing concern in the United States for at least the last 20 years that the most effective way of dealing with the nation's major health problems is through prevention, and efforts have begun to move in that direction, though slowly. This means refocusing the health care system, teaching people that they control their own health, and encouraging health promotion and health maintenance activities.

Nursing's major focus is on health, and with the advent of disease prevention and health promotion nurses can and should have a great impact. In fact, counseling people on ways to improve their health and prevent disease and assisting and supporting them in this process is a major function of FNPs in primary care. It is also the service that makes FNPs most valuable whether they practice independently or jointly.

FNPs may use various tools in assisting people with health maintenance and promotion. Their psychosocial and behavioral background assists them in listening to and counseling clients, and a good knowledge of health as well as disease helps them to educate clients on the necessity of promoting the discouraging certain health behaviors in striving toward wellness.

Health appraisal techniques such as health histories, physical examinations, and various screening procedures (vision and hearing screening; cancer screening through Pap smear, breast and rectal examination; developmental screening; sickle cell and hematocrit blood tests to screen for anemia; blood pressure and urine screening to detect hypertension and diabetes mellitus; tuberculosis and sexually transmitted disease screening) are also performed by FNPs to detect potential problems before symptoms develop. Education of clients on the importance of health screening and responsibility for self-care is also part of the health maintenance efforts of FNPs.

Health hazard appraisal tools such as the one shown in Appendix C can be used by FNPs to determine the client's personal health risks. These health hazard appraisal tools can be brief so that the client completes them, or they can be quite lengthy and necessitate assistance from the FNP to complete. In either case the tool alerts the practitioner to the risk factors for that particular client and provides an entree for the discus-

Otitis Externa (Pediatric and Adult)

I. Definition: Inflammation of the external canal and auricle caused by infectious agents that may be initiated by trauma from scratching, earplugs, bobby pins, and other foreign objects. Water from swimming or bathing may be absorbed by cerumen, forming a culture medium for infection

II. Etiology
   A. Bacteria: *Pseudomonas, Proteus,* staphylococci, streptococci
   B. Fungi

III. Clinical features
   A. Symptoms
      1. Pain in ear
      2. Occasionally, decreased hearing or sensation of obstruction
   B. Signs
      1. Pain aggravated by movement of auricle or pressure on tragus
      2. External canal partially occluded by edema or discharge
      3. External canal tender to otoscopy; erythema and exudate seen
      4. TM may be normal, injected, or covered with flecks of exudate; does *not* show signs of OM (i.e., bulging, disappearance of bony landmarks)
      5. Preauricular or postauricular lymphadenopathy may be present
      6. *No* swelling or pain over mastoid

IV. Laboratory studies: None

V. Differential diagnosis
   A. Otitis media: Pus may be present in the external canal, disappearance of bony landmarks, bulging, and exudate in middle ear
   B. Mastoiditis: Swelling and pain over mastoid area associated with an abnormal TM
   C. Chronic dermatitides: Usually not painful, may itch chronically, may be associated with cracking and scaling of auricle, and in some cases have discharge; pain may occur with secondary infection; types of chronic dermatitides include
      1. Seborrhea
      2. Eczema
      3. Psoriasis

VI. Promotion of self-care and prevention
   A. Instruments, including cotton swabs, should be kept out of ears; counsel that ear canal does not need cleaning — cleans itself
   B. Keep head out of water when bathing to avoid filling ear canals with water and irritating dirt and soap (common cause of external otitis in children)
   C. For swimmers or infection prone, use 2-3 drops of vinegar in ear canal after swimming or bathing to restore normal pH (acid)
   D. Persistent itching of the external canal should prompt consultation with health professional

sion of health maintenance and promotion methods. In turn the FNP can begin to screen the client for the most prominent risks. Health hazard appraisal tools provide clients with information on paper about their health risks and therefore are often strong motivational tools for changing behavior patterns.

Diagnosis and treatment are two functions of FNPs that were once considered to be solely the responsibility of the physician. FNPs learn to diagnose and treat a variety of common, acute, self-limiting diseases as well as monitor chronic, stabilized conditions. The nurse may gather the pertinent history, perform the necessary physical examination, diagnose the problem, and confer with the physician for validation and to jointly decide on the plan of management. Or the FNP may use protocols or algorithms (see box) that have been previously agreed on by the physician and FNP. These documents serve as standing orders for the management of

certain illnesses. Protocols enable the FNP to diagnose and treat clients without the physician personally seeing each one.

The ability of FNPs to diagnose and treat has been a boost to the provision of primary care and to client compliance. It means that the FNP can provide total care to many individuals. Though physician input may be necessary at times, the nurse can usually carry out the treatment regimen and establish the relationship of primary care giver.

Studies have shown that clients tend to be more compliant when they see the same provider regularly. Many illnesses, particularly those chronic conditions requiring a great deal of teaching and counseling, may be better managed by FNPs than physicians, with physician consultation as conditions change. When medical care is the primary need, the client is more appropriately managed by either the physician alone or jointly

Otitis Externa (Pediatric and Adult)—cont'd

VII. Specific therapy (check about any allergies)
    A. Gentle and thorough removal of debris in office to facilitate topical treatment
    B. Control of pain
        1. Heat to ear by compress, water bottle, or heating pad
        2. OTC acetaminophen (Tylenol, Datril), or aspirin
          a. Adults and children over 12 years of age
            Acetaminophen (325 mg/tab) 1 or 2 tab q 6h
            Aspirin (325 mg/tab) 1 or 2 tab q 4h
          b. Children under 12 years of age

Acetaminophen

Age	Prep	Dosage	Frequency
3 mo-1 yr	Drops	0.6 ml	
1-3 yr	Drops	1.2 ml	
3-6 yr	Elixir	1 tsp	q 6h
over 6	Elixir	2 tsp	

Aspirin (1¼ gr tab)

Kg	(lb)	Dosage	Frequency
7-11	(14-24)	1 tab	
11-16	(24-35)	2 "	
16-23	(35-50)	3 "	q 4h
23+	(50+)	4 "	

    C. Antibiotic treatment

Rx: Neo Cort Dome otic drops or Cortisporin otic drops

Disp: 5 ml   Refill × 1
Sig: 4 gtts in affected ear qid × 7d
    Lie with affected ear up for 5 min p tx

Instruct: Keep ear dry during tx
          Keep dropper tip out of ear
          Reinforce method of instilling gtts
VIII. Complications—requires consultation/referral to physician
    A. Severe otitis externa associated with
        1. Swelling of canal to complete closure so that wick is required
        2. Severe pain or fever
        3. Cellulitis
        4. Failure to respond to tx in 1 wk
    B. Allergy to neomycin
    C. Recurrent otitis externa
  IX. Follow-up: Return visit with physician if condition persists after 1 wk of tx

with the FNP providing the necessary education and/or counseling.

Health Educator

Health education of clients is a function nurses have been performing since nursing began. As the population grows more conscious of health and fitness, educating people about good health habits becomes increasingly important. FNPs are in an excellent position to provide health education to clients, and as previously discussed, this is a major function of their role. The FNP intervenes while the client is still well and assists with health maintenance and promotion by teaching the importance of good nutrition, physical exercise, stress management, and life-style. During illness the FNP educates the client about the disease process, what can be expected, and the importance of adhering to the treatment regimen. FNPs provide anticipatory guidance and educate clients on the use of medications, diet, birth control methods, and other therapeutic procedures. They also counsel clients and their families on the importance of assuming responsibility for their own health.

In the community the FNP often serves as a resource person for educating community groups and organizations on different aspects of health and self-care.

Health Administrator

Because of advanced knowledge and skills and often the setting where they choose to practice, FNPs may function in administrative roles. As health administrator, the FNP may be in a position to assume ultimate responsibility for all administrative matters within the setting. The FNP may be responsible and have direct or indirect authority and supervision over the clinic staff as well as client care. In this capacity the FNP serves as decision maker and problem solver and may also be involved in other business and management aspects of the organization such as policy making, finances, public relations, evaluation, and future planning (Jacox and Norris, 1977). Remember, however, that administrative responsibilities are time-consuming. The FNP who functions as health practitioner and administrator may find that certain tasks need to be delegated to others for both roles to be performed effectively.

Health Consultant

Another function of the FNP is that of health consultant. Physicians can use FNPs as consultants on nursing care, such as counseling and health promotion efforts, for their clients just as FNPs use physicians as consultants on medical care. This exchange of professional expertise should be encouraged. Consultation is more common between physicians and FNPs who practice jointly. It is important that FNPs educate physicians to the fact that they have expertise in an area different from medicine but which is essential to the total care of the client.

FNPs may serve as health consultants to other nurses or NPs on a formal or informal basis, providing them with information to be used in improving client care. They may also consult with other health care providers or with organizations, schools, or programs educating FNPs.

Health Researcher

Nursing research is a necessity. It is important that FNPs use research knowledge and skills to answer questions relevant to nursing practice and primary care. Identifying, defining, and investigating clinical nursing problems and reporting findings foster collegial relationships with other professions and contribute to health care policy and decision making.

ARENAS FOR PRACTICE

Private Practice
Joint Practice

Because of their additional educational preparation and subsequent expansion of traditional nursing roles and responsibilities, FNPs are well suited for practice in a variety of employment settings. One setting, that of practicing jointly with a physician in a private practice, has aroused much interest.

In 1972 the National Joint Practice Commission (NJPC), was established by the ANA and the AMA to promote collaborative efforts between medicine and nursing for the purpose of improving client care. The NJPC which consisted of an equal number of practicing nurses and physicians, held to the philosophy that neither the nurse nor physician alone can adequately provide total primary care. They believed that although there is some shared knowledge base and overlap of functions, each professional has additional information and expertise that the other alone is unable to provide.

The NJPC stated

> although both nurses and physicians concern themselves with diagnosis, treatment, disease prevention, and the maintenance of health, physicians tend to bring a diagnostic and therapeutic perspective to the medical needs of patients, while nurses tend increasingly to bring health-oriented and educational perspectives to the physical, emotional, and social needs of patients (1977, p. 3).

The NJPC, which has since been disbanded, recommended that primary care is best accomplished by physicians and nurses practicing jointly.

Though many physicians are beginning to realize the advantages of joint practice with FNPs, practice with nonphysicians is a new concept, and it is the responsibility of practitioners to market themselves. The joint practice model becomes increasingly popular as physicians, nurses, and clients become aware of the advantages the relationship offers.

Independent Practice

Another type of private practice chosen by a smaller number of FNPs is that of independent practice. Many reasons motivate nurses to go into independent practice, including a personal or professional desire to forge ahead and break new ground for nursing and to meet health care needs within a given community.

FNPs have a great deal to offer in an independent nursing practice, but it is important to investigate the particular state's nurse practice act to determine the limitations and legal ramifications of such an arrangement. FNPs functioning without medical backup may perform nursing activities (histories, physical examinations, education, counseling) and expanded activities as defined by state nursing laws.

Aside from the legality of functioning independently in an expanded role, there are other areas of concern to the FNP setting up a private practice. These include defining the role to clients and other health care providers as well as dealing with whether third party reimbursement will be available for FNPs. There are also the considerations of setting up the practice, such as the financial aspects (office space, telephone, furniture, and supplies), making appointments, keeping records, billing, and secretarial or clerical support (Webster-Stratton, 1978). Despite the problems and the barriers imposed, some FNPs find the gratification they receive from practicing nursing care independently to be worth the problems.

Institutional Settings
Hospital Outpatient Clinics

The FNP may choose to practice in an institution such as the outpatient clinic or emergency room. Hospital outpatient clinics are the fastest growing service within our health care system. Generally, these clinics provide follow-up care after hospitalization, and clients can be seen for nonemergency problems. The FNP who practices in an outpatient clinic typically does so jointly with a physician to provide primary care services to a wide range of clients. The FNP may have a role in one or more of the various outpatient clinics offered by the hospital (e.g., medicine, family practice, pediatric, well-child, obstetric-gynecological).

The functions of the FNP in the hospital outpatient setting typically depend on the hospital's job description for FNPs, though this may be negotiable. These functions generally include histories, physical examinations, health education and counseling, and diagnosis and illness management in collaboration with a physician. FNPs in outpatient clinics may be granted institutional privileges to follow their clients through hospitalizations if they occur.

Emergency Rooms

Because some people feel a lack of access to health care and because others do without health care services until illness strikes, the emergency room in many cases is being used for nonemergency, episodic problems. Though this may be considered inappropriate use of the emergency room, it is a reality resulting from the current system.

Some FNPs practicing in emergency rooms perform triage of clients (deciding who needs the most immediate attention and by whom), perform the initial workup (history and physical examination), assist the individual and/or family with crisis intervention, and manage the less acute problems. Emergency rooms are notorious for long waits and rapid treatment with little or no counseling and guidance given. FNPs can remedy this inadequacy by seeing clients with nonemergency problems and providing counseling. They may also help to educate clients on the importance of health care and how to gain access to the health care system.

Satellite Clinics

Satellite clinics are operated under the auspices of a larger institution like a hospital or health department but are situated in a location away from the larger facility. The purpose of a satellite clinic is to provide accessible, high-quality health care to a population in need. These clinics often offer a range of preventive and primary care services, though some offer only skeleton services and rely heavily on referral to the larger institution.

FNPs in satellite clinics may practice alone, with physician backup from the larger institution available by telephone, or the physician may practice jointly with the FNP during some or all of the clinic hours. Practitioners may work with other support staff in the satellite clinic, or they may function alone, taking on the administrative and clerical functions as well as the health provider functions.

Long-Term Care Facilities

One out of every 20 Americans age 65 and older lives in some type of long-term care facility or nursing home for the elderly. Currently, in the United States there are approximately 20,000 of these long-term care facilities (Clemen et al., 1981).

Those FNPs with an interest in geriatrics may choose a practice within a nursing home setting. In this capacity the FNP may have an office within the facility where ambulatory clients are seen for health maintenance and nursing care with off-the-premises physician backup. In less ambulatory long-term nursing facilities, the FNP may make regular nursing home rounds, assessing the health status of clients and providing care and counseling as appropriate. The FNP is an asset to the long-term care facility by serving as a role model and consultant to the nursing staff; providing continuity of care; counseling with the client and family; and promoting health, activity, self-care, a positive view of aging, and when appropriate a dignified death.

Industry

The National Safety Council estimates that annually 14,000 deaths and 2.2 million disabling injuries can be attributed to on-the-job accidents. Similarly, the Department of Health and Human Services estimates 390,000 new cases of disease and 100,000 deaths from occupational exposures each year (Silberstein, 1981).

For decades the industrial or occupational health setting has been recognized as an area that benefits from nursing practice, but only recently has occupational health nursing been viewed as a nursing specialty. The number of continuing education and advanced educational programs in occupational health nursing is steadily increasing. The ANA recommends that nurses, and this holds true for FNPs, planning to practice in an occupational setting have previous courses in industrial and social law, industrial psychology, industrial health, statistics, research, and business management to effectively deal with the special concerns of the occupational setting (Clemen et al., 1981).

FNPs in occupational settings generally practice independently without direct physician supervision. As described in Chapter 13, a major concern is with the health and welfare of the worker; therefore concentration is on health maintenance, health promotion, and health education activities. Responsibilities include direct nursing care for on-the-job injuries and accidents and, in some cases, care of nonoccupationally related illnesses (such as follow-up of workers with hypertension and diabetes). The FNP in this role would also function administratively in the operation and management of the occupational health service (supply ordering, careful keeping of records, collecting of data on environmental hazards, cooperating with federal and state regulations regarding occupational health and safety, planning, and evaluating). The practitioner would also be responsible for developing educational programs on health and safety for the employees and keeping abreast of the community services available for both consultation and referral.

National Government
National Health Service Corps

The National Health Service Corps, a program sponsored by the Public Health Service, was established in 1970 to recruit health providers (physicians, NPs, PAs) to health manpower shortage areas. The first NPs were used by the Corps in 1972, and since that time over 450 practitioners have been placed by the National Health Service Corps. Though the National Health Service Corps has employed some pediatric and adult nurse practitioners, the majority of those employed are FNPs or certified nurse midwives.

In the past the National Health Service Corps employed NPs who had completed their practitioner education and provided scholarships to nurses interested in becoming NPs. The latter had a 2-year commitment to the Corps following their graduation. Currently the Corps is employing only those FNPs who are in the National Health Service Corps scholarship program. These nurses are used in clinic sites in health manpower shortage areas to provide primary care services to the local population. Depending on the needs of the area, the FNP may be the only health care provider in the clinic with physician backup available by telephone, or the practitioner and a Corps physician may practice jointly. It is anticipated and encouraged that at the end of the 2-year commitment the local community will be able to provide financial support for maintaining the health care provider in the clinic setting.

Armed Services

The role of the FNP in the armed services (army, navy, air force) was significant during the 1970s. Because of the physician shortage at that time, FNPs as well as other types of NPs were used in outpatient clinics to perform the bulk of duties that had previously been performed by physicians. In fact, all three branches of the armed services developed their own NP training programs to educate nurses to take on expanded functions. Currently, however, because of the increasing number of physicians, the role of the NP in the armed services has diminished. At present there is little active recruitment of NPs for the armed forces.

Indian Health Service

Many Indians still live in environments with limited health care facilities, inadequate waste disposal, and inadequate water supply systems. There is significantly higher morbidity and mortality among these people than among the general population.

The Indian Health Service, a bureau of the Public Health Service since 1954, is the primary health resource for approximately 800,000 Indians and Alaskan natives. It is the mission of the Indian Health Service to provide high-quality, comprehensive primary health care to Indian people. In so doing the Indian Health Service employs FNPs in hospital ambulatory clinics, health centers, and smaller outlying facilities. The FNP may practice directly with a physician or indirectly via telephone consultation (Indian Health Program, 1980).

Rural Health Initiative

Rural Health Initiative (RHI) clinics, in accordance with the Rural Health Clinic Services Act of 1977, are federally funded clinics that are situated in rural areas. The purpose of these clinics, similar to that of satellite and National Health Service Corps clinics, is to provide easily accessible, quality primary care health services to a needy population. As with other clinics, RHIs may be staffed by FNPs alone or jointly with a physician to provide these primary care services.

Health Maintenance Organizations

As mentioned in Chapter 2, health maintenance organizations (HMOs) are organized systems of health care that provide comprehensive services to a voluntarily enrolled population for a per capita fee. Comprehensive services include primary care, emergency care, acute inpatient care, and rehabilitation for chronic problems. Current HMO practices are aimed at holding down the increasing cost of health care by instituting incentives for providers of care to keep people well. Health maintenance and disease prevention activities are emphasized to reduce health risks and avoid expensive medical care. It is common for FNPs to be employed in HMOs for their provision of cost effective basic health care services.

Public Health Departments

"The majority of the nurses who consider themselves to be public health/community health nurses are those who are giving direct care in communities as a major focus of their work" (Barkauskas, 1982, p. 387). Community health nurses were among the first to expand their roles. During the 1960s and 1970s the majority of nurses entering NP programs were community health nurses. Public health departments seeking to provide preventive services and chronic care to increasing populations viewed employment of NPs as a cost effective strategy to meet the community's health needs. For example, well-child clinics, family planning clinics, and prenatal clinics have commonly and efficiently used FNPs. Home health care, another expanded area within community health nursing, has also used FNPs. Efforts to reduce health care expenditures have resulted in earlier hospital discharge with an increasing need for discharge follow-up. The extent to which a public health department uses FNPs is dependent on the community's health priorities and the fiscal restraints under which the agency functions (Ervin, 1982).

Schools

The school nurse practitioner concept evolved from the pediatric nurse practitioner model. The school nurse practitioner role revolves around the concepts that relate to comprehensive assessment and management of care with particular emphasis on health education as a mechanism for changing health behavior in children and families (Igoe, 1975).

FNPs functioning in the school system assume a direct role in securing health care for the school age child through collaboration with educators and other health professionals. In addition to health maintenance and management functions, the FNP within the school system has the responsibility for planning a health education curriculum. In some states this may require that the nurse be eligible for teacher certification.

The ANA currently offers a certification examination for school nurse practitioners. Beginning in 1985, all applicants desiring certification as school nurse prac-

titioners must submit evidence that they have completed a baccalaureate in a nursing program and an additional formal program preparing them as school nurse practitioners. For further information on school nursing see Chapter 31.

ISSUES AND CONCERNS

Legal Status

The 1970s witnessed increasing numbers of FNPs and other NPs and the performance by these nurses of acts that traditionally had been considered within the province of medicine. It was in the performance of acts of diagnosis and treatment that the role of the NP assumed legal significance. It was not just that FNPs performed these acts, but rather it was the environment in which the tasks were performed. FNPs as licensed professionals functioned primarily in collaboration with physicians rather than under their supervision. Many state nursing laws were vague on the functions and responsibilities of nurses, and the legal status of NPs was being questioned.

Since 1971, states have amended their nurse practice acts or revised their definition of nursing to reflect the professional developments within nursing. The functions of nursing must be recognized and legally sanctioned if the health and illness needs of the public are to be met. An option to revise the definition of nursing was to amend the nurse practice act. This approach to legislation was the "additional acts" amendments. The wordings of additional acts amendments used by various states are similar, they legally sanction expanded roles and assure public safety. The following additional acts amendment was adopted by the Alabama legislature:

Additional acts requiring appropriate education and training designed to maintain access to a level of health care for the consumer may be performed under emergency or other conditions which are recognized by the nursing and medical professions as proper to be performed by a registered nurse. (Alabama, Act No. 867 as amended by Act No. 427, Regular Session, 1975).

The additional acts amendment served a purpose but was open to a variety of interpretations. Rules and regulations for specific expanded roles (NP, nurse anesthetist, nurse midwife) have been used in some states to supplement and clarify the amendment (Hall, 1977). Promulgation of rules and regulations is allowed at the discretion of boards of nursing in most states. A notable exception is a bill passed in 1981 by the Nebraska legislature stipulating that legislative approval is required for each NP and other expanded role category and that these roles may not be defined by rules and regulations (Nebraska Legislature, 1981). It is likely that when state boards of nursing review and revise their nurse practice acts, definitions of professional nursing will allow for growth and development of practice in accordance with current nursing education.

The lack of precise legislation has been cited by FNPs as a barrier to practice. FNPs have been charged with practicing medicine without a license (Adler, 1979; Bursic, 1977; Johnson, 1980). Potential employers have hesitated to hire FNPs because of the uncertain legal and liable status. During 1981 the *American Journal of Nursing* published news that the boards of medicine in Arkansas, Florida, Kansas, Louisiana, and Oregon were making efforts to curtail the use and practice of NPs by either declaring their practice illegal, limiting physicians in their employment of NPs, denying liability insurance to physicians who employed NPs or sponsoring bills to repeal legislation that allowed qualified NPs to practice and prescribe under their own license. These recent attempts by medicine to exert control over the practice of nurses are attributed in part to a potential client shortage as physicians increase in number (Gardner and Fiske, 1981)

Reimbursement

The lack of third party reimbursement for nursing services has long been a concern among nurses. When FNPs provide services that are categorized as reimbursable but are unable to collect from insurers unless the claim is filed by a physician, it is viewed by the nurses as exploitation of themselves and the public. Exploitation of nurses occurs when fees are collected by one professional (physician) for services performed by another (FNP). Exploitation of the public occurs because financial constraints force clients to seek care from providers whose fees will be honored by insurers. Since over half of all personal health care services are financed by third party payers, providers must have access to third party reimbursement to be economically solvent. This effectively limits alternatives in health care, which could be available to the client, by discouraging independent practice by nurses (Griffith, 1982).

The Rural Health Clinic Services Act of 1977 (PL 95-210) was the first major breakthrough in third party reimbursement for nurses in primary care roles. However, the act applies only to FNPs and PAs providing care as physician extenders in federally recognized, medically underserved areas. Under the provisions of the act, Medicare and Medicaid funds are made available for reimbursement of clinics operated or owned by qualified non physician providers. Under this act, a physician is not required to see the clients or be physically present for the clinic or providers to be reimbursed. A physician, however, is required to provide medical direction and be available for consultation, emergency assistance, and client referral (Silver and McAtee, 1978).

Lobbying efforts by state nurses' associations have been successful in passing reimbursement legislation that is not limited to particular sites or consumer categories. Griffith (1982) and Goldwater (1982) documented the lobbying, legislative, and negotiation efforts in Maryland where legislation was passed providing that reimbursement by any insurance company is not contingent on the NP being employed by a physician or acting according to a physician's orders. Washington state law places the requirement to reimburse nurses for services only on Blue Cross and Blue Shield (Washington Law, 1981). A prerequisite for such legislation is for nurse practice acts and rules and regulations to legally sanction nurses' diagnostic, treatment, and prescriptive authority. Both Maryland and Washington have such rules and regulations which incorporate a requirement for a collaborative and consultative relationship with a physician in place of physician direction or supervision.

Institutional Privileges

It is often difficult for FNPs to obtain hospital privileges through the department of nursing within institutions where their clients are admitted. The traditional hospital nurse is automatically responsible to and governed by the department of nursing as a condition of employment. However, if an FNP is employed, for example, in a private, joint practice with a physician, there is rarely a mechanism for clinical privileges to be granted by the department of nursing because the nurse is not employed by the hospital.

There are two purposes for providing a mechanism for community-based FNPs to gain access to their hospitalized clients. First, if people are allowed to choose or purchase direct nursing care, access to hospitalized clients is a necessity. Second, nursing must be accountable for and regulate the practice of its practitioners. No other group can knowledgeably review or set forth the standards for nursing practice (Manley, 1981).

Many institutions do grant clinical privileges to nonphysicians, including nurses, through the department of medicine. The *Accreditation Manual for Hospitals* published in 1976 by the Joint Commission on the Accreditation of Hospitals states that hospitals will, within their bylaws and rules and regulations, have their medical staffs delineate privileges for nonphysician practitioners as well as identify the roles and responsibilities of the medical staff in relation to the nonphysician practitioners.

This mechanism fails to recognize that nurses as professionals are accountable for their own actions. Such policies limit nursing's autonomy and professional responsibility within the hospital setting. Further, it leaves a gap in the institution's ability to monitor the nursing care that is provided by nurses who have been granted clinical privileges under medical authority.

Since departments of nursing should be responsible for establishing and maintaining standards of nursing care within institutions, nurses should have the authority to grant or deny nursing privileges for all nurses within the setting whether or not they are employed by the institution (Manley, 1981).

ROLE NEGOTIATION

If the FNP is going to collaboratively provide comprehensive primary care, negotiation skills must be thoroughly understood and developed. Positive working relationships with health professionals, organizations, and clients do not happen by virtue of proximity alone.

Job opportunities for nurses traditionally have been easily identified and clearly defined. However, as nurses expand their education and responsibilities, roles become less clear. This is particularly true for FNPs who often find themselves considering pioneer positions in which few if any guidelines exist or the position is new and underdeveloped. In this instance, though it may be difficult for the FNP to informally assess the internal politics of the organization, it is a necessary skill that should be developed.

Another potential obstacle is that FNPs often seek employment rather than being sought by the employer. Assertiveness is desirable in exploring and developing potential job opportunities. It is important for FNPs to feel comfortable and confident in marketing their skills. Creative approaches and innovative ways of implementing their new role require negotiation skills.

It is necessary for the FNP to prepare for a job interview by doing homework that not only includes writing a description of capabilities that address the needs of the potential employer but also finding out as much as possible about the job. This allows a sufficient exchange of information to occur during the interview so that uncertainty on the part of the FNP and the potential employer is reduced to a minimum. When job expectations and goals are shared and there is commitment to them by those involved, the expectations potentially govern behavior and provide stability (Sherwood and Glidewell, 1973).

Renegotiation of expectations and goals may need to take place as disruptions in the work environment occur. Examples of disruptions might include employment of additional physicians and/or NPs, additional training or education by either party, budgetary cuts, or reallocation of resources. Renegotiation of expectations potentially allows for growth, which is more likely if disruptions are anticipated and used to introduce controlled change. This anticipatory approach to change requires astuteness and organizational sensitivity on the part of the FNP. Planned renegotiation means that when any signal of an impending disruption is identified, it should be defined and shared, thereby decreasing uncertainty and anxiety and promoting a planned change that produces a return to stability and productivity (Sherwood and Glidewell, 1973).

Following negotiation for position and functions, salary discussions begin. Individual salary is generally determined by education, experience, availability of qualified applicants, and the FNP's assertiveness in negotiating for money and a fringe benefit package. Fringe benefits generally represent 25% of the salary. Benefits for which the FNP should negotiate include but are not limited to health insurance, retirement, sick leave, holidays, vacation, personal days, professional organization dues and journals, license and certification fees, malpractice insurance, mileage reimbursement, and military (if applicable) and continuing education time and fee reimbursement. Also to be negotiated are substitute coverage while away from clinical facilities, physician backup, and a written job description. A letter or contract indicating mutual understanding of these items by the FNP and employer should be on file.

Tools that may facilitate the FNP negotiating process include a job description written beforehand, resume or curriculum vitae, copies of credential documents, and samples of professional accomplishments such as audiovisual materials, client education packets, or history and physical tools that the FNP has developed.

The FNP should keep a folder containing examples of all professional activities that may be used for prospective employment. However, it is important to be realistic and practical in choosing examples of work and activities to be used during the interview process so as not to oversell. Names, addresses, and telephone numbers of professional and personal references should be furnished only after permission has been obtained. A business card left at the conclusion of the interview is another way of increasing visibility.

ROLE STRESS

There exist a number of stressors that have a direct bearing on the nurse in an expanded role. In addition to the legal issues that have previously been addressed, stressors include professional isolation, liability, collaborative practice, conflicting expectations, and professional responsibilities.

Professional Isolation

Professional isolation has become a source of considerable conflict for FNPs. Practicing as they do across all age groups, FNPs more than any other expanded role category are most likely to be sought for remote practice employment sites. Rural communities that are unable to support a physician find the FNP an affordable and logical alternative to answer their need for primary care services. The autonomy of practice in such sites attracts many FNPs who may fail to consider the liabilities of an isolated practice. Long drives, long hours, lack of social life and cultural activities, and lack of opportunity for professional development are often experienced by these rural practitioners. Such sources of stress that lead to job dissatisfaction can be reduced or eliminated by negotiating the employment contract at the outset to include periodic educational and personal leaves with provision of backup providers. Such anticipatory planning assures that health services are not compromised (Sirles, 1981). FNPs who choose isolated employment settings should consider their own needs as well as those of the community and negotiate accordingly.

Liability

All nurses are liable for their actions. With liability becoming more public today and more legal action specifically concerning NPs appearing in the judicial system, the importance of liability and/or malpractice insurance cannot be overemphasized. Although malpractice insurance is not a prerequisite to functioning as an FNP, most do carry their own liability insurance. It is in the best interest of FNPs to thoroughly investigate the coverage offered by different companies rather than assuming that the coverage is adequate. Particularly vulnerable are those practitioners who function without a physician on site (Daughterty and Buchanan, 1981).

NPs who have been successful in defense of illegal practice charges against them emphasize the importance of clear, objective documentation of findings, therapy, counseling, and when appropriate, physician consultation when charting client visits. Such charting should be habitual practice for nurses in expanded roles (Adler, 1979; Johnson, 1980).

Collaborative Practice

The future of FNPs depends on whether they make a recognizable difference in the health of families and communities and on their ability to practice collaboratively with physicians. Collaborative practice denotes a collegial relationship with mutual trust and respect of coprofessionals. The working out of a collaborative practice takes a considerable amount of time, and the FNP and physician may be convinced that they do not have this time available to them. However, until time and energy are spent to achieve the mutual understanding of role relationships and responsibilities, collaborative practice will continue to remain more theory than practice. Until such practice relationships evolve within joint practice situations, the quality health care that nursing and medicine collaboratively can provide will not be achieved. In addition to the professional maturity required to work together without feeling the need to be protective of one's own territory, the organizational structure and philosophy of the practice must support joint practice as a mechanism for health care delivery. The growing pains of establishing such a practice produce stress for the FNP and physician: however, the results and benefits to professionals and clients are worth the effort (Steel, 1981).

Conflicting Expectations

Nursing services provided by the FNP in health promotion and maintenance are often more time-consuming and complex than the management of the client's current health problem. FNPs frequently experience conflict between their practice goals in health promotion and the need to see the number of clients required to maintain a clinic's economic goals. This is particularly true in clinics where the FNP is the sole provider. The problem is compounded when the clinic administrator or physician views the FNP as a medical extender only, and third party reimbursement is limited to medical services (Sirles, 1981).

The FNP may easily take the path of least resistance to decrease conflict and stress in such situations by adopting the medical extender role. To avoid such a situation a practice model using flexible scheduling, health maintenance flow sheets, and problem-oriented recording with nursing goals and plans prominently displayed in the client's health record assists the FNP to integrate health promotion and maintenance activities into each client visit.

Professional Responsibilities

Professional responsibilities contribute to role stress. The majority of states currently require NPs to become nationally certified and to maintain that certification for approval to practice. Recertification for FNPs requires documentation of continuing education hours in primary care topics. Considering that the practitioner role is a minority role in nursing, continuing education in primary care topics may not be locally available. Continuing education offerings may necessitate significant travel and lodging expenses in addition to time away from practice. Anticipating professional responsibilities and attendant expenses in financial planning decreases these concerns. As previously mentioned, negotiating with the employer for educational leave and expenses should be part of any FNP's contract. Certification and recertification are predictable expenses and necessitate the FNP continually identifying and meeting learning needs to maintain current knowledge and skills. Quality of client care, however, cannot be measured or assured by the hours of continuing education or the FNP's credentials. Professional responsibility includes monitoring one's own practice in relation to standards specified in advance.

A quality assurance process with peer review is becoming recognized as a professional responsibility among NPs. Such a process should evaluate need, cost, and effectiveness of care in relation to client outcomes. In 1977 a group of FNPs in Tennessee determined the need for an evaluation method that recognized the responsibility of nurses in monitoring their own practices, included characteristics of the provider that influenced care, and could be easily implemented in a rural setting. A number of factors that influenced the quality of health care were identified and developed into a peer review process that encompassed multiple components. An unexpected benefit was the sharing of knowledge and experience among NPs working in isolated, rural settings (Hiserote et al., 1980).

The difficulties encountered in the peer review quality assurance process included the time and distance involved in traveling to widely separated clinics and planning the reviews so that there was a minimum of interference with individual schedules. Although peer review can be stressful, the Tennessee nurses came away from the review of their FNP colleagues with new ideas for their own practices and agreed that the benefits compensated for the difficulties encountered (Hiserote et al., 1980). In addition to peer review, there is self-review that can also serve as a quality assurance process.

Chart audit using protocols as standards with which care can be measured is a mechanism for self-review. Many states require protocols for practicing in an expanded role. Although there are numerous published protocols to guide practice, the FNP and physician who work together must agree on the protocols' diagnostic scope and treatment regimens. This involves selecting and adapting from among published protocols or writing them to fit the particular needs of the practitioners and the practice.

Protocols may be used as quality assurance tools for peer or self-review through chart audit. Using protocols as standards of care for quality assurance through chart review requires that key elements for client history, positive and negative diagnostic findings, indications for consultation and referral, treatment regimen, and client education relative to treatment, prevention, and follow-up be clearly defined within each protocol. An example of such a protocol adapted from several sources (Hoole et al., 1982; Komaroff, 1977; Leitch and Tinker, 1978) is shown in the box on p. 768-769. Such protocols take considerable time to develop, but they do provide a mechanism for establishing a standard against which client care may be objectively measured by the FNP or others.

Establishing mechanisms for quality assurance is a professional responsibility that FNPs must employ within their practice. By accepting the responsibility for monitoring their client care, FNPs assume the challenge of directing their future and defining their potential within the primary health care system.

SUMMARY

The shortage of physicians that transpired during the 1960s, along with their maldistribution, created problems of access to primary care services. NPs and PAs were viewed as an answer to these medical manpower shortage and distribution problems. As nurses became knowledgeable and comfortable with the assessment and management skills of their role in primary care, it became apparent that their major contribution was not in the acute care management functions they performed but in the nursing skills that they brought to primary care.

The FNP role is one of the most comprehensive roles in primary care. FNPs specialize in the ambulatory health management of the family unit. Family dynamics, family assessment, growth and development, and management aspects of minor acute and stabilized chronic health problems provide the framework for the primary care nursing practice of FNPs. Within this framework are the components of health maintenance and management, which focus on problems in child health, women's health, adult health, and health problems of the aged.

NPs remain a controversial issue. Are they practicing medicine or nursing? Should they practice independently? How should they be educated? What is their legal relationship to the physician? Do they make a difference in the health of the people to whom they provide services? In the 15 years since the introduction of the role, these questions have yet to be fully answered.

There is a limited amount of nursing research with implications relative to the roles and functions of NPs. Studies directed toward outcome as well as the process of care are greatly needed. Further, a long-range follow-up evaluation of the impact of NPs is also necessary. Nursing practice and research must continue to demonstrate the quality of the trends within the profession, which are acceptable to the clients of primary care services. To remain a viable entity in the health care system FNPs must be perceived and valued by clients for meeting health care needs not addressed by other providers.

BIBLIOGRAPHY

Adler, J.: You are charged with . . . , Nurse Pract. **4**(1):6, Jan.-Feb. 1979.

American Nurses' Association: The study of credentialing in nursing: a new approach, vol. 1, Report of the committee, Kansas City, Mo., Jan. 1979, The Association.

Andrus, L.H., and Mitchell, F.H..: Change processes in primary care. In Renihardt, A.M., and Quinn, M.D., editors: Family-centered community nursing: a sociocultural framework, St. Louis, 1980, The C.V. Mosby Co.

Arkansas MDs charged with attempts to restrain nurse practitioners, Am. J. Nurs. **81**:908, May 1981.

Barkauskas, V.H.: Public health nursing: an educator's view, Nurs. Outlook, **30**(7):384, July 1982.

Bullough, B., editor: The law and the expanding nursing role, ed. 2, New York, 1980, Appleton-Century-Crofts.

Bursic, E.: Problems of PAs and Medex from their own perspective. In Bliss, A.A., and Cohen, E.D., editors: The new health professionals, Germantown, MD., 1977, Aspen Systems Corp.

Clemen, S.A., Eigsti, D.G., and McGuire, S.L.: Comprehensive family and community health nursing, New York, 1981, McGraw-Hill Book Co.

Dangott, L.: Aging and a high level of wellness, Health Values: Achieving High Level Wellness, **2**(1):40 Jan.-Feb. 1978.

Daugherty, L.G., and Buchanan, G.J.: Nursing role in ambulatory care. In Jarvis, L.L., editor: Community health nursing: keeping the public healthy, Philadelphia, 1981, F.A. Davis Co.

Draye, M.A., and Pesznecker, B.L.: Diagnostic scope and certainty: an analysis of FNP practice, Nurse Pract. **4**(1):15, Jan-Feb. 1979.

Ervin, N.: Public health nursing: an administrator's view, Nurs. Outlook **30**(7):370, July 1982.

Extending the scope of nursing practice, Department of Health, Education, and Welfare, Washington, D.C., 1971, U.S. Government Printing Office.

Fisher, D.W., and Horowitz, S.M.:The physician's assistant: profile of a new health profession. In Bliss, A.A., and Cohen, E.D., editors: The new health professionals, Germantown, Md., 1977, Aspen Systems Corp.

FNA fights moves to limit nurse practitioners and control practice, Am. J. Nurs. **81**:1784, Oct. 1981.

Gardener, H.H., and Fishe, M.: Pluralism and competition: a possibility for primary care, Am. J. Nurs. **81**:2152, Dec. 1981.

Golden, A.S.: The impact of health professionals. In National League for Nursing: health care in the 1980s: who provides? who plans? who pays? New York, 1979, National League for Nursing.

Goldwater, M.: From a legislator: views on third-party reimbursement for nurses, Am. J. Nurs. **82**:411, March 1982.

Graduate Medical Education National Advisory Committee: Non-physician health care provider technical panel, vol. 7, DHHS, Washington, D.C., 1980, U.S. Government Printing Office.

Griffith, H.M.: Strategies for direct third-party reimbursement for nurses, Am. J. Nurs **82**:408, March 1982.

Hall, V.C.: The legal scope of nurse practitioners under nurse practice and medical practice acts. In Bliss, A.A., and Cohen E.D., editors: The new health professionals, Germantown, MD., 1977, Aspen Systems Corp.

Hiserote, J.L., et al.: Peer review among rural clinics, Nurse Pract. **5**(1):30, Jan-Feb. 1980.

Hoole, A.J., Greenberg, R.A., and Pickard, C.G.: Patient care guidelines for nurse practitioners, ed. 2, Boston, 1982, Little, Brown, & Co.

Igoe, J.B.: The school nurse practitioner, Nurs. Outlook **23**:381, 1975.

Indian health program 1955-1980, (HSA) Pub. No. 80-12005, DHHS, Washington, D.C., 1980, Indian Health Service.

Institute of Medicine: A manpower policy for primary health care, Washington, D.C., 1978, National Academy of Sciences.

Jacox, A.K., and Norris, C.M.: Organizing for independent nursing practice, New York, 1977, Appleton-Century-Crofts.

Johnson, M.L.: I don't want to be a test case . . . , Nurse Pract. **5**(3):7, May-June, 1980.

Joint Commission on Accreditation of Hospitals: Accreditation manual for hospitals, Chicago, 1976, The Commission.

Komaroff, A., editor: Common acute illnesses: a problems-oriented textbook with protocols, Boston, 1977, Little, Brown, & Co.

Kweskin, S., and Taller, S.L.: Where nurse practitioners expand good care . . . , Kaiser-Permanente Medical Center in Oakland, Calif., Patient Care **13**:194-195, Oct. 15, 1979.

Letich, C.J., and Tinker, R.V., editors: Primary care, Philadelphia, 1978, F.A. Davis Co.

Manley, M.V.: Clinical privileges for nonhospital-based nurses, Am. J. Nurs. **81**:1822-1825, 1981.

Maryland nursing, medical Boards agree on nurse practitioner regulations, Am. J. Nurs. **81**:910, May 1981.

Mundinger, M.O.: Autonomy in nursing, Germantown, Md., 1980, Aspen Systems Corp.

National Joint Practice Commission: Statement on joint practice in primary care: definition and guidelines, Chicago, Sept. 1977, The Commission.

National League for Nursing: Position statement on the education of nurse practitioners, Pub. No. 11-1808, New York, 1979, The League.

Nebraska legislature says nurse practitioner roles must be set by law, not regulations, Am. J. Nurs. **81**:1446, Aug. 1981.

Nichols, A.W.: Physician extenders: the law and the future, J. Fam. Pract. **11**(1):101, 1980.

Nurse practitioner prescribing privileges attacked in Oregon, Am. J. Nurs. **81**:653, April 1981.

Rogers, D.: The challenge of primary care. In Knowles, J.H., editor: Doing better and feeling worse, New York, 1977, W.W. Norton & Co.

Sadler, A.M.: New health practitioner education: problems and issues, part 2, J. Med. Educ. **50**:67, 1975.

Scheffler, R.M.: Estimating the private rate of return to training the physician's assistant, Industrial Relations, **14**:178, 1975.

Sherwood, J.J., and Glidewell, J.C.: Planned renegotiation: a norm-setting O.D. intervention. In Bennis, W.G.. et at., editors: Interpersonal dynamics: essays and readings on human interaction, ed. 3, Homewood, Ill., 1973, Dorsey Press.

Silberstein, C.A.: Nursing role in occupational health. In Jarvis, L.L., editor: Community health nursing: keeping the public healthy, Philadelphia, 1981, F.A. Davis Co.

Silver, H., and McAtee, P.: The rural health clinic services act of 1977, Nurse Pract. **3**(5):30, Sept.-Oct. 1978.

Silver, H.K., Ford, L.C., and Stearly, S.A.: A program to increase health care for children: the pediatric nurse practitioner program, Pediatrics **39**:756-760, May 1967.

Sirles, A.: The potential for the family nurse practitioner in the community, Ala. J. Med. Sci. **11**(3):229, July 1981.

Spicer, W.S.: Joint practice: conceptualization and implementation, part 2. In Johnson, R.W.: First annual symposium on nurse faculty fellowships in primary care, 1978.

State board regulations for nurse practitioners become legal issue in two states, Am. J. Nurs. **81**:1432, Aug. 1981.

Steel, J.E.: Putting joint practice into practice, Am. J. Nurs. **81**(5):964, May 1981.

Tennant, F.S., et al.: A study of the economic viability of low-cost, fee-for-service clinics staffed by nurse practitioners, Public Health Rep. **95**:321, July-Aug. 1980.

Washington law requires Blue Cross, Shield to pay RNs directly for own services, Am. J. Nurs. **81**:1557, Sept. 1981.

Webster-Stratton, C.: The nurse practitioner in private practice, Pediatr. Nurs. **4**:24-30, Jan.-Feb. 1978.

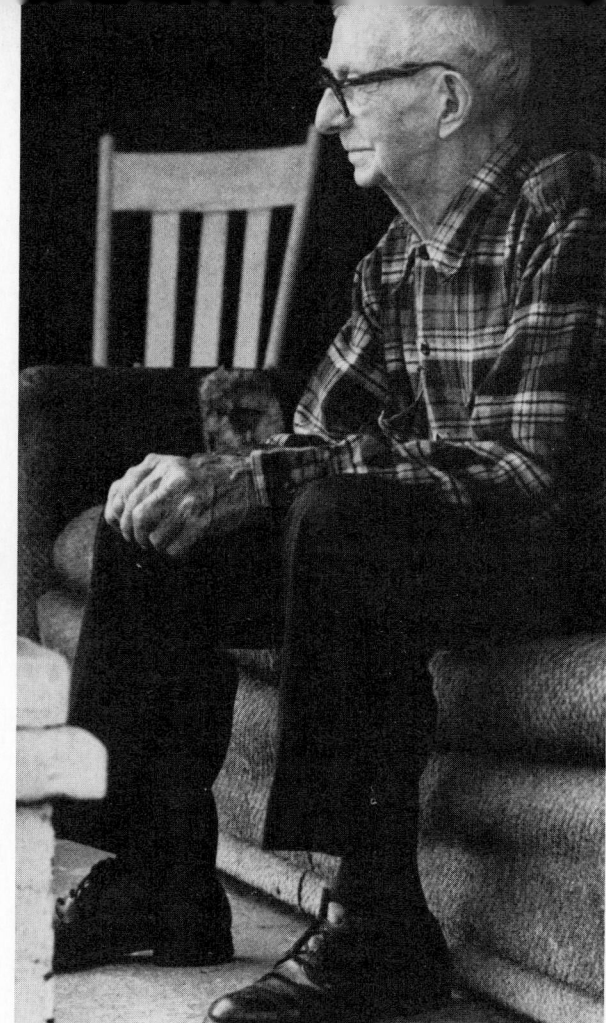

Chapter 34

EILEEN WILES

HOME HEALTH CARE NURSING

This chapter presents another aspect of community health nursing: home health care. Home health care is different from other areas of health care—it is the only health care setting in which the health care providers practice on the client's turf. There are several components that directly affect the nurse who is practicing in the home care setting. These elements will be discussed to acquaint the nurse with the roles, functions, and responsibilities of practice.

Home health care is often viewed incorrectly by not only consumers but also health care professionals. It can incorrectly be used or viewed as an alternative to hospitalization or viewed as the best and only means of cutting health care costs.

Home health care as a component of the health care system should be provided only when it is deemed appropriate for the individual. It should not be provided for those people who need intensive, full-time care but rather should be provided for those who need intermittent, short-term care. Home health care can either follow or precede institutionalization based on the client's needs.

DEFINITION OF HOME HEALTH CARE

Home health care in today's society cannot be simply defined as "care at home." It includes an arrangement of health-related services that are provided to people in their place of residence. A more comprehensive definition of home health care has been prepared by a Department of Health and Human Services interdepartmental work group with the assistance of materials provided by the Assembly of Ambulatory and Home Care Services of the American Hospital Association, the National Association of Home Health Agencies, the National Council for Homemaker–Home Health Aide

Services, Inc., the Council of Home Health Agencies and Community Health Services of the National League for Nursing (NLN), the American Nurses' Association (ANA), the National Health Council, and the American Medical Association (Warhola, 1980):

> *Home health care* is that component of a continuum of comprehensive health care whereby health services are provided to individuals and families in their places of residence for the purpose of promoting, maintaining or restoring health, or of maximizing the level of independence, while minimizing the effects of disability and illness, including terminal illness. Services appropriate to the needs of the individual patient and family are planned, coordinated, and made available by providers organized for the delivery of home health care through the use of employed staff, contractual arrangements, or a combination of the two patterns.

Another definition, prepared by the American Medical Association (1979), described home health care as follows:

> The provision of nursing care, social work, therapies (such as diet, occupational, physical, psychological and speech), vocational and social services, and homemaker–home health aide services may be included as basic components of home health care. The provision of these needed services to the patient at home constitutes a logical extension of the physician's therapeutic responsibility. At the physician's request and under his medical direction, personnel who provide these home health care services operate as a team in assessing and developing the home care plan.

Home health care as defined by Medicare includes the following items and services (Home Health Services, 1982):

1. Part-time or intermittent nursing care provided by or under the supervision of a registered professional nurse
2. Physical, occupational, or speech therapy
3. Medical social services under the direction of a physician
4. Part-time or intermittent services of a home health aide as permitted by the regulations
5. Medical supplies (other than drugs and biologicals such as serum and vaccinations) and the use of medical appliances
6. Medical services provided by an intern or resident enrolled in a teaching program in hospitals affiliated or under contract with a home health agency

Furthermore, Trager (1972) has interpreted *home health care* as follows:

> . . . an array of services which may be brought into the home singly or in combination in order to achieve and sustain the optimum state of health, activity and independence for individuals of all ages who require such services because of acute illness, exacerbations of chronic illness, or long term permanent limitations due to chronic illness and disability.

All of these definitions integrate the components of home health care—the client, family, health care professionals (multidisciplinary) and goals to assist the client to return to an optimum level of health and independence. The differences rest on the fact that interpretation and actual deliverance of home health care vary according to not only the client, but also the provider and reimburser of these services.

Family is an integral part of home health care. The term *family* can be loosely defined to include any caretaker or significant person who takes the responsibility to assist the client in need of care at home. Roles of the caretaker include supervising clients by assuring their basic needs are being met and providing direct care such as personal hygiene, meal preparation, and administering medications. This person is valuable in providing the needed maintenance care between the skilled visits of the professional provider.

A person's *place of residence* has its own uniqueness in terms of the location for providing care. Home health care clients are located in trailers, apartments, houses, or even in boarding homes, depending on what the person calls home.

The client *goals* are related to the principles of health promotion, maintenance, and restoration regardless of the primary health care provider. By maximizing the level of independence, home health care nurses can assist the clients to function at the best possible level for preventing dependency. This assistance can take the form of teaching or linking the client up with community services that provide limited assistance for enabling the client to stay at home. In addition, prevention of complications of chronically ill persons can help to minimize the effects of disability and illness. Countless complications of long-term illness seen in the form of disability are preventable with adequate home health care intervention. Terminal illness, as seen by the development of hospice home care programs, can be handled at home instead of in the hospital if there is acceptance of this concept on the part of client and family. Alleviation of pain and suffering is possible in the home care setting. Pain control through the use of medications is closely supervised by nurses in the home. They assess the client's response to the medication and report these findings to the client's physician, who then modifies the medication as needed.

Services that are provided can be tailored to any client need or problem. They can be delivered in a flexible nature based on the need, type, and frequency of service required. When the client's level of independence increases, then the need for services decreases. The services are coordinated as an agency obligation to maintain quality care and provide for continuity. Thus the range of services provided in home health care is extensive. The challenge of home health care to community health nurses can be more fully appreciated by briefly tracing the history of this nursing role.

HISTORY OF HOME HEALTH CARE

As mentioned in Chapter 1, home health care began in the United States around the 1800s. The Boston Dispensary served as one of the initial providers of home care, dating back to 1796. During this era few hospitals were available. In the 1800s people did not always go to the hospital for illnesses. Public health nursing began in the United States as in England when philanthropic organizations sponsored visiting nurses, who gave care to individuals in their homes and taught families how to take care of the sick. In 1877 the New York City Mission and the New York Society for Ethical Culture had visiting nurses. The idea grew slowly, with nurses being paid by the client or by a philanthropic society. Eventually the community became more involved and developed projects and funds to support the cause of home care. In 1890 there were 21 visiting nurses associations in the United States, most of them employing only one nurse. After 1894 the use of visiting nurses grew more rapidly with the advent of growing social consciousness on the part of the nation.

The Waltham (Massachusetts) Training school was established in 1885 by Dr. Alfred Worcester after he conferred with Florence Nightingale and designed a course to train nurses for private duty. The course included experience in the home. Later public health nursing with field experience was added to the program. The school was criticized for sending students into homes to earn money for the hospital and for overworking and not supervising the students (Dolan, 1958). In 1842 a nurse society was established in Philadelphia to supply nurses to the independent sick and to those individuals who could pay. American communities established similar organizations primarily because visiting nursing in England had developed into a viable social service.

In the 1940s hospitals began to take a more serious interest in home care as a result of the increased number of chronically ill clients being hospitalized. The Montefiore Hospital Home Care Program in New York began in 1947 and offered comprehensive home care services such as medical nursing and social services. Before enactment of Medicare in 1966, most agencies relied on charity and public contributions for survival.

In 1967, 1 year after Medicare was enacted, there were 1,753 Medicare-participating home health agencies in the United states with the majority being either visiting nursing associations or programs in public health departments. By 1974 the number of home health agencies was 2,237—an increase of about 48 percent (Callender, 1975).

Home care as it is today reached a turning point with the arrival of Medicare, thereby forming regulations for home care practice as well as for reimbursement mechanisms. For an in-depth account of the history of public health nursing, refer to Chapter 1.

TYPES OF HOME HEALTH CARE AGENCIES

Since the beginning of organized home care, many types of organizations have established programs to meet the home care needs of people in the community. Home health agencies are divided into the following five general types based on the administrative and organizational structure:

1. Official
2. Private and voluntary
3. Combination
4. Hospital-based
5. Proprietary

These types differ in organization and administration but are similar in terms of the standards they must meet for licensure, certification, and accreditation. Fig. 34-1 shows the types of home health agencies.

Official Agencies

Official, or public, agencies include those agencies operated by the state or by local governments (county, city) such as health departments. They are financed primarily by tax funds and are nonprofit entities. Most official agencies, in addition to having a home care component in the agency, also provide health education and disease prevention programs to people in the community.

Community health nurses employed in this setting may provide not only general home health care but also well-child clinics, well-child home visits, immunization, health education programs, and home visits for preventive health care. Official agencies, in addition to being funded for services with local monies, are reimbursed for home care services as are the other types of home health care agencies. Medicare, Medicaid, and private insurance companies reimburse for home health care but not equally or totally in all cases. The reimbursement system is complicated and standard-

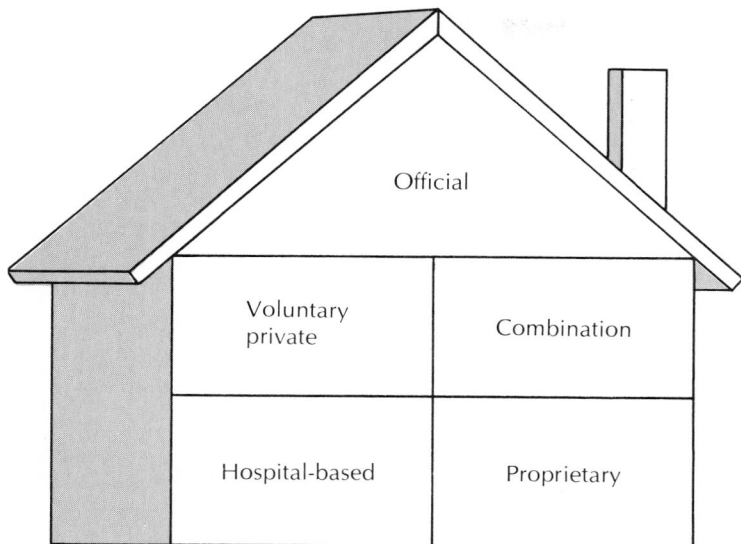

Fig. 34-1. Types of home health care agencies.

ized. Medicare has the most standardized payment system of all third party payers.

Official agencies can offer more comprehensive types of community health service than other kinds of agencies because of their objectives of health promotion and disease prevention and also because of the additional public funding often available.

Voluntary and Private Nonprofit Agencies

Voluntary and private agencies are grouped together as the nonprofit type of home health agency. Voluntary agencies are supported by charities such as the United Way as well as by Medicare, Medicaid, and other third party payers and the client payments. The amount of financial assistance the voluntary agency receives depends on the community it serves. Traditionally, visiting nurses associations were the principal voluntary type of home health agency. With the advent of Medicare in 1965, the private nonprofit agency emerged as a viable establishment.

Voluntary and private nonprofit agencies are governed by boards of directors, which are representative of the community they serve. These agencies are nongovernmental organizations and are exempt from federal income tax. Historically, voluntary agencies were responsible for the initial development of nursing in the home, based on the client's need for service rather than ability to pay.

Combination Agencies

In some communities, to decrease cost and prevent duplication of services, home health agencies of the official and voluntary type have merged to provide home health care. The services remain the same with the administration members being from either one of the two existing sources or a new board. In this case the nurse may serve in several community health nursing roles as does the nurse in the official type of agency.

Hospital-based Agencies

Hospitals have long been a pivotal point for health care services. In the 1970s hospital-based home health agencies developed in response to the need for continuity of care from the acute care setting and also in response to the high cost of institutionalization.

Hospital-based agencies differ from other home health care agencies in that the already-established hospital board of directors is responsible for governing the agency. Moreover, existing inpatient services are accessible to the recipients of hospital-based home health care. Whether the agencies are official, voluntary, private nonprofit, or proprietary depends on the hospital structure. These agencies are a source of revenue for the hospital and may compete with community-based agencies.

Proprietary Agencies

Agencies that are ineligible for tax exemption are called proprietary or profit-making agencies. Proprietary agencies can be licensed and certified for Medicare by the state licensing agency. The owner of the agency is responsible for the governing. Reimbursement is primarily from third party payers and individual clients if agencies are ineligible for Medicare.

Opponents of this type of agency claim that proprietary agencies offer substandard quality of care and are involved only for monetary gains. There is little evidence to support this claim because agencies that are Medicare certified must comply with the same conditions of participation that the other types of agencies do.

Summary

Regardless of the type of home health agency existing in a community, the primary goal should be to provide quality home health care to the community based on the health needs of people. The development of additional agencies can be an emotional issue to already-established home health agencies in a community. Competition in home health care is on the rise. Traditionally, most agencies have maintained a noncompetitive countenance because of the humanitarian aspect of the service. The competitive thrust is the result of the federal government's move to deregulate and deinstitutionalize areas of health care. Competition can be a positive force in developing and maintaining quality home health care programs. Nevertheless, there is profit to be made in home health care, which necessitates utilization review and quality assurance mechanisms.

This direction has several implications for the community health nurse. Clients are being discharged at earlier stages of treatment, thereby needing a highly skilled level of care. The community health nurse must be "equipped" to care for these clients with a storehouse of knowledge and experience. To survive in the competitive arena one must continue to provide quality care and also be cost effective without compromising accountability.

EDUCATIONAL REQUIREMENTS FOR PRACTICE

Demonstration of professional competency is the foremost requirement for home health care nurses. Home health care nurses evolve from a variety of educational and experiential settings. Differences in both experience and educational preparation influence the contributions the nurse makes to home health care.

The NLN and the ANA advocate that a baccalaureate degree be the minimum level of professional preparation for a community health nurse. Nurses are prepared at the baccalaureate level to be generalists who are capable of practicing in community health settings, provided that the following curricula is included along with clinical materials (ANA, 1980): general systems theory, introductory epidemiology, statistics, community assessment (structure patterns, resources), history, principles and practices of public and community

health, knowledge of public health laws, and environmental health and safety. By blending theory into actual clinical practice, the care nurse can effectively care for individual clients and families.

The specialist in home care is prepared at the master's level with in-depth knowledge and ability to apply this knowledge to problems in community health. Such preparation requires advanced study in community health nursing theory, advanced clinical skills, public health science, leadership, management, interdisciplinary collaboration, research process, health policy and planning, community organization, dynamics of health politics, and health economics (ANA, 1980).

Home health care nurses should be trained and educated to function at a high level of competency, so they can be relied on not only by their professional colleagues but also by the community. In today's society it is a foregone conclusion that a baccalaureate degree in nursing should be the minimum requirement for entry into professional practice, particularly in the community health care setting. Nursing education has the responsibility of producing competent, skillful practitioners. A baccalaureate degree does not assure that a qualified, mature professional nurse will be produced, but a quality education does lay the foundation for the development of such important characteristics. Life experience, compassion, and awareness of self are factors that are inherent in the delivery of quality client care and professionalism.

In home health care the nurse with a baccalaureate degree usually functions in the role of a staff nurse or home health care nurse. The nurse with a master's degree is better prepared for the practitioner, administrator, or teacher role.

SCOPE OF PRACTICE OF THE COMMUNITY HEALTH NURSE IN HOME HEALTH CARE

Objectives in Home Health Care

A common misconception of home health care is that it is a "custodial" type of nursing. It is important to remember that home health care nursing is a *division* of community health nursing. Thus health promotion activities are a fundamental component of practice.

According to Orem (1971), "Self care is the practice of activities that individuals personally initiate and perform in their own behalf in maintaining life, health, and well-being." This definition falls into line with the practice of community health nursing activities and notably of home health care nursing. Home health care nurses use this concept for all clients no matter what their abilities are. As an example, a client may be recuperating at home after suffering a stroke and unable to perform activities of daily living (ADL) without assistance. Such

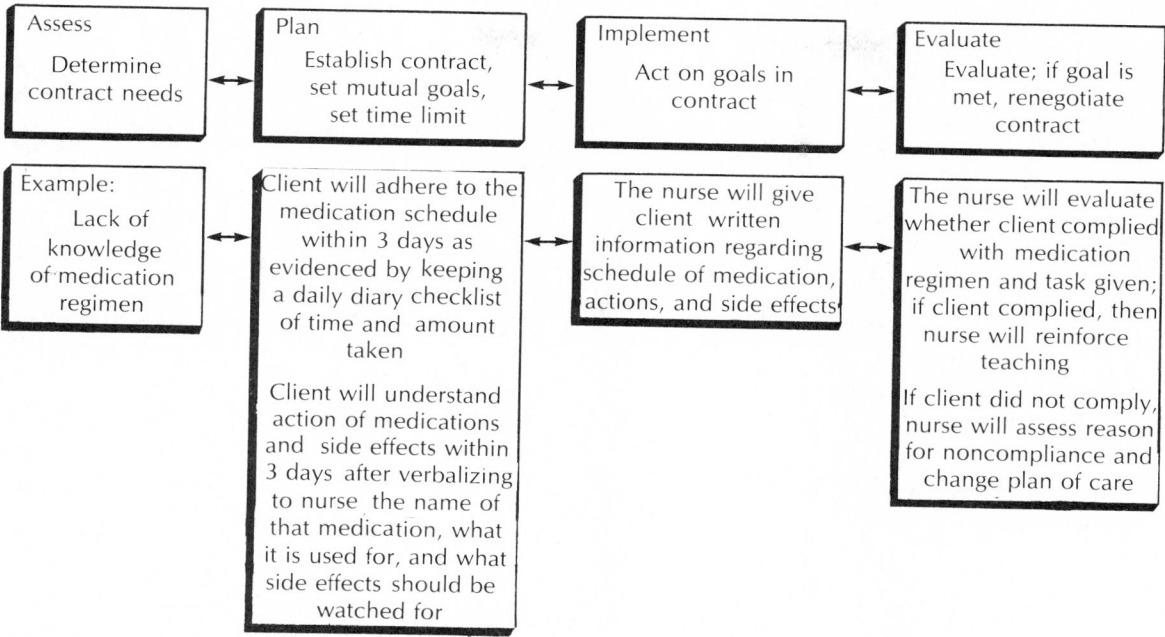

Fig. 34-2. Process of contracting in relation to nursing process.

clients are unable to perform self-care activities as formerly but can be instructed in the performance of ADLs in a modified form. In this way they have some control over their life and self-care activities, and they can be taught to prevent possible losses in other self-care areas. This example also supports another definition, which is even more specific to the home health care population. *Self-care* is "an action taken by the consumer or client, to reduce, to the degree possible, incremental debilitation resulting from chronic disease (Funkhouser, 1976)."

A primary goal in the home setting is to help prevent the occurrence of illness and to promote the client's well-being. With the aid of basic tools such as a nursing history, physical examination, medication, and diet teaching guides, the home care nurse can use the nursing process to assess the client's needs, establish a plan of care, implement nursing actions, and then evaluate the effectiveness of nursing actions with plans for modification or resolution as needed.

In the home care setting the clients possess more control and ability for determining their own health care needs. The "client" role is an active one in that continuance of service depends a great deal on their understanding of plans established jointly by the client and community health nurse. The nurse serves as a *facilitator* for development of positive health behaviors for the individual who has had an episode of illness. Goals can be met by using contracting as a tool.

The process of contracting in home care involves not only the client and the nurse but the family as well. *Contracting* refers to any working agreement, continuously renegotiable, between the nurse, client, and family (Sloan and Schummer, 1975). The process of contracting can be reflected in the client's care plan and clinical notes. Contracting allows the client and family to set their own goals and alleviates the problem of nurses who set unrealistic expectations of themselves or of the client and family.

Contracting is directly related to use of the nursing process (Fig. 34-2). During each phase of the nursing process the contract is operational. As an example, during an initial home visit the nurses gather data for establishing the client/home health care nurse/family contract. They determine the components of the agreement and plan for subsequent actions by establishing the contract with the client and family. During that visit, if appropriate, portions of the contract may be implemented. If not, subsequent visits will afford the opportunities.

Contracts can be formal (written) or informal (verbal), depending on the client's needs. In either case, the process is recorded in the client's chart. The most important aspect is not the type of contract but rather it is the actual collaborative participation in the establishment, implementation, and evaluation of the process.

To avoid what Mayers (1973) refers to as the "home visit—ritual or therapy," the home care nurse must establish not only short-term but also long-term goals with the clients and families. The purpose of this is not only for continuity of care but also for the evaluation of the client's condition and progress towards an optimum level of self-care. Mayers found in her study of community health nurses who made home visits that half of the purposes of the visits were unknown to the clients, since the nurses in the study did not share the purposes for the visits with them. Much of the dialogue failed to show any *development* of the interrelationship between the client and nurse.

Practice Functions of the Home Health Care Nurse

Nursing launched home health care by providing the first home health service, which still is the service most often used. Home health care nursing involves both direct and indirect functions. In performing these functions, the home health care nurse assumes a variety of roles.

Direct care refers to the actual "laying on of hands." In home health care, direct care activities include performing a physical assessment on the patient, dressing changes of wounds, injections, insertion of an indwelling catheter, and so on. Direct care also involves teaching clients and family caretakers how to do a certain procedure or duty. By serving as a role model, the nurse can assist the client and family to develop positive health care behaviors. Technical skill competency must be demonstrated by the nurse to receive reimbursement by Medicare and Medicaid. Nursing care is covered by Medicare and other third party payers as long as the care being delivered is "skilled." In determining whether a service performed by the nurse is skilled, several factors are evaluated and also must be adequately documented (refer to reimbursement section later in chapter):

1. Is the service complex, thereby requiring the knowledge and skill of a registered nurse?
2. Does the client's condition warrant skilled intervention?
3. Can this service be performed by a nonmedical person?
4. Does the instruction of a service to a client involve knowledge, instructions, and demonstrations by a registered nurse?

To adequately answer these questions, the home health care nurse must have a sufficient knowledge base of regulatory mechanisms and also must be competent and experienced to know how to interpret "skilled." These interpretations can be subjective, therefore objective data is necessary to account for the service.

Some examples of skilled nursing services include the following:

1. Observing and evaluating of client's condition, both physical and emotional
2. Providing direct care in administering treatments, rehabilitative exercises and medications, catheter insertion, colostomy irrigation, and wound care
3. Assisting client and family toward developing positive coping behavior
4. Teaching client and/or family to give these treatments and medications when indicated
5. Teaching client and family to carry out physician's orders such as use of a special diet, remembering to consider cultural background, financial status, and personal preferences
6. Reporting to physician any new signs and symptoms relative to client's status and arranging for medical follow-up as indicated.
7. Assisting client and family to identify resources that will help client attain state of optimal functioning

Indirect care occurs when a client does not have personal contact with the nurse. This type of care is seen when home health care nurses serve as consultants to other health personnel who provide home care or even to those who provide in-hospital care. Clients often have their own patterns for care (such as colostomy care) and, when hospitalized, need assistance from hospital nurses to continue this program. Hospital nurses frequently contact the home health care nurse for advice on how to accomplish the client's usual method of care.

Team conferences are a means of providing indirect care in home health care. It is a choice time for increasing coordination and continuity of services for optimal client care and use of resources and services. Advice on how to manage clients with particular problems can be shared with various members of the team. Supervision of home health aides is a direct and indirect function because the home health care nurse may not always see the home health aide performing but can evaluate the care given to the client. Regular supervision of the aide by the nurse for at least 2-week intervals is mandated. There is much indirect care in the home health care setting. It may not be directly visible to the client, but it does exist and assures quality home health care.

Although Medicare places an emphasis on episodic or acute care because of its limitations on benefits and requirements for skilled care, the home health care nurse cannot separate episodic and distributive nursing practice entirely because of the interrelationship. According to Hall and Weaver (1977), distributive nursing practice is "the application of knowledge of the life process in human systems with consideration for their health maintenance requirements, contextual variables influencing their functioning, and the strategies and tactics of intervention.

Episodic care refers to the curative and restorative aspect of practice, and *distributive care* refers to health maintenance and disease prevention. A clinical example can best illustrate the application of these two aspects in home health care:

Mr. Jones, a 70-year-old white male discharged from the hospital the previous day, was admitted to home health care services for skilled nursing to assess his cardiovascular status following heart surgery for coronary artery disease. The episodic care involves teaching Mr. and Mrs. Jones about medications, exercise, and the signs and symptoms of possible heart problems postoperatively. In addition, the home health care nurse will provide direct care in assessing his cardiovascular status and helping Mr. Jones return to his optimum state of functioning.

Mr. Jones' psychosocial adaptation and needs will also be addressed in addition to assessing his level of self-care and adjustment relative to post-cardiac-surgery status. In regard to the distributive aspect, the home health care nurse will do additional teaching about ways Mr. Jones can possibly prevent exacerbation of his condition by maintaining medical follow-up and adhering to the programs set up for him.

The *roles* of clinician, educator, researcher, administrator, and consultant are seen in home health care. They can be demonstrated by the experienced home health care nurse, the nursing supervisor, the director of nursing, or the administrator.

Home health care nurses in a staff position are clinicians because thy provide direct nursing care to clients and families. The educator role is inherent to home health care nurses because they are always teaching clients and families the "how to's" and "why's" of self-care. Formally, they may teach classes to community groups regarding health education topics. The researcher role in home health care has been relatively dormant, even though the home health care nurses often provide the data required for clinical or administrative changes to occur within the agency they are employed. The home health care setting abounds with areas to study and serve as sites for research. This role needs to take priority in the future if the quality and cost effectiveness are to be maintained. A home health care administrator can be a nurse who has had advanced education with community health experience. Requirements are set by both federal and state rules and regulations. Consultants may provide advice and counsel to staff as well as clients. Refer to specific chapters for content relative to the specific roles in community health nursing.

Confusion exists in some health care circles regarding role differentiation between the private duty nurse and the home health care nurse. Even registered nurses who have not been directly exposed to home health care in either their educational or clinical experiences do not know that private duty nursing and home health care are two different entities of nursing practice. The only similarity is that both types are provided to a client in the home. Table 34-1 clarifies the different components of private duty nursing and home health care nursing.

Integration of Standards of Community Health Nursing Practice into Home Health Care

The home health care nurse practices in accordance with the Standards of Community Health Nursing Practice developed by the American Nurses' Associa-

---

Table 34-1. Components of private duty and home health care nursing

	Private duty	Home health care
Role and function	One-to-one client care assignment Maintenance Custodial Episodic	Distributive Skilled care Rehabilitative Episodic
Reimbursement	Payment to nurse Paid by some third party insurances	Payment to agency Medicare and Medicaid Third party insurance
Cost	Daily or hourly rate charge	Per visit charge
Frequency	Full-time and shift duty	Intermittent visits based on frequency and need of clients

The Nursing Process and Standards of Community Health Nursing

Nursing process	Standard	Description
Assess	I	The collection of data about the health status of the consumer is systematic and continuous. The data are accessible, communicated, and recorded.
	II	Nursing diagnoses are derived from health status data.
Plan	III	Plans for nursing service include goals derived from nursing diagnoses.
	IV	Plans for nursing service include priorities and nursing approaches or measures to achieve the goals derived from nursing diagnoses.
Implement	V	Nursing actions provide for consumer participation in health promotion, maintenance, and restoration.
	VI	Nursing actions assist consumers to maximize health potential.
Evaluate	VII	The consumer's progress toward goal achievement is determined by the consumer and the nurse.
	VIII	Nursing actions involve ongoing reassessment, reordering of priorities, new goal setting, and revision of the nursing plan.

tion, Division of Community Health Nursing (ANA, 1973). The boxed material represents the relationship between the nursing process and the Standards of Practice.* The use of the nursing process in the home care setting is well represented as evidenced by the legal requirement of documentation of all nursing actions.

Assess—Standards I and II

Standard I: The collection of data about the health status of the consumer is systematic and continuous. The data are accessible, communicated, and recorded.

Standard II: Nursing diagnoses are derived from health status data.

The home care nurse is responsible for assessing the client and family during the initial home visit as well as during all subsequent visits. The home health nurse acquires *data base* information from the client and family by obtaining subjective and objective data. Examples of *subjective* data include information that the client, family, and physician relate to the nurse by means of verbal communication. This information is obtained from direct questioning of these sources. Information necessary to obtain a thorough data base for the information of nursing diagnoses include the following:

Diagnosis
Present health status
Family history
Review of systems (health/illness history of cardiovascular, pulmonary, musculoskeletal, gastrointestinal, genitourinary, endocrine, neurological, integumentary systems)
Socioeconomic status (source of income, amount, religion, education level, number of dependents, oc-

cupation, support systems, environmental safety)
Daily patterns (diet, meal pattern, elimination, rest and sleep, exercise, activity, recreation, interests, hygiene)

Objective data are also obtained by directly assessing the client's physical status, using a review of systems approach and physical assessment skills.

These data are recorded in the client's clinical home care record in the form of a flow sheet, or assessment chart. From these baseline data the home health nurse develops *nursing diagnoses* relative to the problems identified. It is during the assessment phase that the home health nurse determines that other resources are needed (such as physical therapy, occupational therapy, speech therapy, home health aide, medical social services, Meals on Wheels, transportation assistance, nutritional counseling). The family is included throughout the entire nursing process because it is they who will assist with the implementation and evaluation of the plan of care.

Plan—Standards III and IV

Standard III: Plans for nursing service include goals derived from nursing diagnoses.

Standard IV: Plans for nursing service include priorities and nursing approaches or measures to achieve the goals derived from nursing diagnoses.

Nursing diagnoses give the home health nurse the necessary information to develop *short-term* and *long-term* goals for the client and family in addition to formulating a *plan* for direct actions. This plan based on nursing diagnoses must have some indications of the expected or anticipated outcomes for each identified problem or nursing diagnosis. The information is documented on the developed client care plan, which serves

*Reprinted with permission of ANA.

as a continuous resource for the health care providers. This not only represents accountability for actions but also serves as a means to promote continuity of care. The plan is individualized for each client and family based on their special needs. The goals focus on health promotion, maintenance, and restoration of the client's condition and prevention of complications.

Implement—Standards V and VI

Standard V: Nursing actions provide for consumer participation in health promotion, maintenance, and restoration.

Standard VI: Nursing actions assist consumers to maximize health potential.

Implementation of the plan occurs in three phases: before the home visit, during the home visit, and after the visit has been made, depending on what the plan requires. The client and family are active participants in home care because it is they who must follow through with the plans for promotion of maintenance and restoration. It is the home health nurse's responsibility to assist the client to return to an optimal level of functioning and health. Instruction, supervision of mediations, diet teaching, and evaluation of diabetic management are examples of such actions.

Evaluate—Standards VII and VIII

Standard VII: The consumer's progress toward goal achievement is determined by the consumer and the nurse.

Standard VIII: Nursing actions involve ongoing reassessment, reordering of priorities, new goal setting, and revision of the nursing plan.

Together the client, family, and home health nurse evaluate the client's status on a continual basis. The home health nurse shares an assessment with the client and family. During subsequent visits previous goals may be met with new ones being developed based on the changing status of the client. The home health nurse prepares the client and family for the client's discharge as early as the initial visit because this will enable the client to reach the measurable goals designed for the client.

The decision for discharge is a collaborative one. The client, family, home health nurse, and physician evaluate the client's status and progress toward goal achievement. The home health nurse during the initial evaluation visit explains to the client and family the short-term nature of the services. The frequency of visits and the duration of the service are decreased when the client is able to assume self-care and the client and family have learned how to care for the client. Discharge must include provisions for aftercare on a periodic basis in those cases where the illness episode is not resolved.

INTERDISCIPLINARY APPROACH TO HOME HEALTH CARE

Interdisciplinary collaboration is a required and expected process in the home health care setting. A vast amount of literature has been published in the last decade on interdisciplinary collaboration in health care. For example, Aradine and Pridham (1973) offer the following explanation:

> Collaboration implies a process of working together, with shared goals and philosophy and understanding the professional and individual skills, knowledge and characteristics of one's self and one's partner. It requires the willingness and maturity to share, to adapt, to listen, to communicate directly and openly about one's feelings, thoughts and differences, and to be sensitive and responsive to one another's expectations.

Collaboration is an integral part of home care. Without effective collaboration there would be no continuity of care provided and the client's and family's understanding of the home care program would be fragmented. Each client has an individualized care plan even though the client may have problems similar to others in a specific disease category classification.

In home care, as in other health care settings, professionals experience stress associated with changing roles and overlapping boundaries. In collaborating, each health care provider in the home should carefully analyze each other's role to determine if overlapping occurs.

As an example, the home care physical therapist and the home care nurse would confer to discuss the plan of treatment and avoid overlapping of functions for a client requiring both services.

In terms of legal accountability and compliance with federal regulatory mechanisms, it is the physician who must certify the plan of treatment for the client. However, in most instances, it is the health care professional who reevaluates the client's status in the home, reports the findings to the physician, and then collaboratively with the physician modifies the plan of treatment for the client in the home.

Home health care affords the client and family opportunity and responsibility to be an active component of the interdisciplinary process. In home care, *interdisciplinary* is the name of the game. Medicare conditions of participation (to be discussed later in the chapter) require that interdisciplinary services be documented. This requirement allows for accountability of each professional and fosters continuity of care. Documentation in the client's chart reflects interdisciplinary collaboration as evidence by case conferences and contracts made between the care givers. Documentation is the evidence or means, not the end product of care.

Successful interdisciplinary functioning depends on numerous factors of knowledge, skills, and attitudes with the foremost characteristic being that the team members must be competent practitioners in their own field (Kane, 1977). The interdisciplinary team member should observe the following:

Knowledge
1. Understand how the group process can be used to achieve group goals
2. Understand problem-solving process
3. Understand role theory
4. Understand what other professionals do and how they see their roles
5. Understand the conceptual differences between home care and practice and institutional care and practices

Skill
1. Use principles of group process effectively
2. Communicate clearly and accurately
3. Communicate without using own profession's jargon
4. Express self clearly and concisely in writing

Attitude
1. Feel confident in role as a professional
2. Trust and respect other professionals with whom they work
3. Share task with other professionals
4. Work toward conflict resolution effectively
5. Be flexible
6. Be "research-minded"
7. Be timely

These factors offer a successful operational approach to working in the interdisciplinary home care setting. It would be unrealistic to assume that there is a clear-cut panacea for avoidance of role stress, ambiguity, or overlapping. Professionals in home care are in a unique setting in which they can function interdependently and truly work together to accomplish the client's care goals since the clients and their families are the focus of the program. Again, regulations require that appropriate resources are used with documentation of collaboration with other disciplines. Care plans and treatments by each discipline are to be built on by other health care providers involved. As an example, nurses must reinforce the teaching by the physical therapist of exercise regimens and gait training.

Responsibilities of the Disciplines

In home health care the responsibilities and functions of the disciplines are dictated by Medicare regulations, professional organizations, and state licensing boards. The home health care providers' roles discussed in the following sections are different from providers' roles in other health care settings. Other professional services (not discussed below) can be provided in the home such as podiatry, pharmacology follow-up nutrition counseling, respiratory therapy, and psychiatric or mental health nursing when indicated. Much of these contributions can be provided on a consultant basis in the form of in-service training or direct referral information.

Physician

Each client in the home care program must be under the current care of a physician to certify that the client does have a medical problem. *Physician* refers to a doctor of medicine or osteopathy legally authorized to practice by a state in which the doctor performs the function. A nurse can make an assessment visit without physician approval but must have the physician's certification if a plan of care with follow-up is developed. The physician must *certify* a plan of treatment for the home health agency before care is provided to the client. This plan must be reviewed at least every 60 days to modify or continue the client's plan of care.

The plan of treatment must include the following information: diagnosis, functional limitations, anticipated length of care, type and frequency of services needed (nursing, physical therapy, occupational therapy, speech therapy, home health aide, medical social services), medications, diet, activities permitted, medical supplies, and appliances. Additionally, the plan of treatment needs to be reviewed by the physician in collaboration with home care professionals at least every 60 days the client is under care but more often if the person's condition warrants more frequent assessment and alternation of care. This is called *recertification.*

Physicians in the community also serve in an advisory capacity to the home health agency by assisting in the development of home care policies and procedures relative to client care. Physician involvement in and acceptance of home health care is necessary if the benefits of this form of health care are to be recognized. The American Medical Association in the early 1960s urged physicians to "participate in organized home health care programs for any patient who can benefit from the program and to promote such programs in their communities." The Physician Guide to Home Health Care (AMA, 1979) explains the important role of the home health care and and the benefits that clients can receive from this service. Examples cited include a more rapid client recovery, improved client emotional well-being, early discharge from the hospital, reduction in readmissions, and a savings over costs of institutional care.

Physical Therapist

Physical therapists provide maintenance, preventive, and restorative treatment for clients in the home.

Services enable clients to improve or maintain their level of functioning, prevent loss of functional ability, and restore clients to their optimal level of functioning. Physical therapists accomplish these goals by evaluating the client's neuromuscular and functional abilities, conferring with the client's physician and home health care nurse. The treatment modalities include therapeutic exercise, massage, transcutaneous electrical nerve stimulation, heat, water, ultraviolet light, ultrasound, postural drainage, and pulmonary exercises. Physical therapists must be licensed by the state in which they practice and are graduates of a baccalaureate or master's level physical therapy program.

Physical therapy assistants provide some therapy under the direction of a registered physical therapist. Assistants are high school graduates who have completed an approved assistant's program and have been licensed.

Physical therapist roles and function are similar to the home health care nurse in that a physical therapist provides direct and indirect care. Direct care activities include strengthening muscles, restoring mobility, controlling spasticity, gait training, and teaching active-passive resistive exercises. The therapist is also responsible for teaching the client and family the treatment regimen to promote self-care and responsibility. Regarding indirect care, the physical therapist serves as a consultant to the staff and also contributes to client care conferences as does the home health care nurse by sharing skills and area of expertise.

Occupational Therapist

Occupational therapists (OT) help clients to achieve their optimal level of functioning by teaching them to develop and maintain the abilities to perform activities of daily living in their home. Occupational therapists focus must of their treatment on the client's upper extremities by assisting to restore muscle strength and mobility for functional skills. Occupational therapists or OTs, receive their basic educational preparation at the baccalaureate level. When the OT becomes registered by the National Occupational Therapy Association, they are subsequently referred to as OTRs.

Certified occupational therapy assistants (COTAs) are high school graduates with an approved continuing education certificate from an occupational therapy program. The COTA works under the supervision of the OTR.

Direct functions of the OTR include evaluating the client's level of function and ability by testing muscles and joints. The OTR teaches self-care activities, assesses the client's home for safety with possible modifications for removing barriers, and provides adaptive equipment when needed. Indirect care is similar to the other home care professional's roles of serving as a consultant for special client needs regarding self-care activities and adapting the home for the client. Occupational therapy has not been used to its full potential in the home because of the lack of knowledge of health care providers. This discipline is a valuable resource in assisting the client to become independent in self-care again—a mutual goal of all home health care professionals.

Speech Therapist

Speech therapists or pathologists are certified by the American Speech and Hearing Association and are educated at the master's level. People with a communication problem related to speech, language, or hearing are served in the home health care setting. Most clients receive direct care services, such as evaluation of speech and language ability, with specific plans being taught to the client and family for follow-up. The goal of speech therapy is to assist the individuals to develop and maintain maximum speech and language ability so that they can use these abilities to their optimal level. Speech pathologists also work with swallowing and eating problems. By serving as a consultant to other home care staff members, the speech pathologist can teach other providers of care and families how to encourage development of the best method of communication for clients.

Social Worker

The social worker in home health care holds a master's degree in social work (M.S.W.) and is prepared to help clients and families deal with social, emotional, and environmental factors that affect their well-being. Social workers assist directly by intervening or referring clients to appropriate community resources. Often after an episode in the hospital the clients return home unable to cope with their present state of functioning and need assistance in getting their lives reorganized. Many indirect care duties are performed by the social worker, since consultation and referral constitute the major focus of their practice. Other functions include resource identification and application, crisis intervention, and equipment procurement when payment is a problem.

Social work assistants are prepared at the baccalaureate level and function similarly to the social worker, who directly supervises the activities of the assistant.

Homemaker Home Health Aide

With the advent of Medicare, the home health aide, (sometimes referred to as the homemaker) became an important member of the home health care team because Medicare reimburses provided that a skilled service is furnished to clients in their home. The home health aide (HHA) is directly supervised by the home health care nurse or physical therapist. The role of the HHA is to assist clients to reach their level of independence by temporarily assisting with personal hygiene. Additional duties include light housekeeping and other homemaking skills. The HHA must be experienced as an aide and be trained to provide home care services. The HHA follows through with the plan of care established by the nurse or other professionals to reinforce teaching that has been done.

The role of the homemaker, as distinct from the HHA, emphasizes housekeeping chores.

ACCOUNTABILITY AND QUALITY ASSURANCE

Quality Control Mechanisms

Accountability, a contemporary buzzword, is not a new term to home health care. Since the advent of Medicare, home health agencies have monitored the quality of care to their clients as a mandatory requirement for certification as a home health agency. All agencies are accountable to the clients and families, to their reimbursement sources, to themselves as a health care provider, and to professional standards. Quality is demonstrated through evaluations reflecting that appropriate and needed care has been given to clients in a professional manner.

Clinical records are the basis for documentation of all the care and services the client receives and of any communication between the physicians and other home health providers. It is in the clinical record that nurses must *prove* that they are delivering quality care and also identify means to *improve* the quality care. Documentation of actions is of paramount importance in home health care, because it is a legal method by which quality care can be assessed. This documentation also demonstrates the client's ongoing need for services and shows how the multiple disciplines arrange for continuity and comprehensive care. Phaneuf (1972) says that "if it isn't recorded, it probably didn't happen!"

Evaluation of the agency is required to monitor the control of cost and quality of care. Two standards serve as requirements for the evaluation (Health Care Financing Administration, 1982):

A. Policy and administrative review. The home care program is evaluated to determine that the administrative policies and practices are appropriate, adequate, effective and efficient is promoting patient care.

B. Clinical record review. An interdisciplinary quarterly review is needed of both active and closed clinical records to assure that policies are followed in the provision of patient care services. In addition, there is a continuing review of clinical records for every 60-day period that the patient is under home care services. This determines the adequacy of the plan of treatment and appropriateness of the continuation of home care.

These standards are viewed as an external means of evaluating each agency because individuals from "outside" the agency evaluate the records. Representatives from appropriate disciplines such as nursing, physical therapy, occupational therapy, speech therapy, and medicine as well as consumers objectively report the findings of the review. It is the responsibility of the agency to plan and implement goals for the revision, modification, and correction of the deficiencies noted. The evaluative process is a valuable one to the home health agency. From these reviews the agency can maintain and promote better client care for the consumers in the community. Devising the method of implementing the process of clinical review is the responsibility of the individual agency.

Furthermore, agencies also institute internal auditing processes such as peer review or nursing audit. The Phaneuf audit (1972) is used by many home health agencies and serves as a peer review mechanism. The National League for Nursing also published review methods to assist agencies to meet the Medicare requirement, (NLN, 1971) and criteria to measure quality of care in home health agencies (NLN, 1980). Each publication deals with developing standards of care, outcome criteria, and the evaluation process. Two other noteworthy contributions to quality assurance are the Quality Assurance Manual (1980), developed by the Florida Association of Home Health Agency, Inc. (FAHHA), and Quality Assurance for Community Health Agencies (1980), developed by the Massachusetts Association of Community Health Agencies.

Paperwork in home health is the malady of the home care nurse. It affects the home care nurse more than the nurse in any other setting. As an example, during the initial evaluation visit, the home care nurse or other health care professional assesses the client's and family's status. Factors to be assessed include history, physical, psychological, and environmental characteristics. This information becomes a permanent part of the clinical record. Subsequent integration of health services must be noted. Besides clinical notes of all home visits, progress notes are required to be sent to the client's physician, including the assessment of the client to see if the plan of care is still applicable.

Home health care offers the unique opportunity to be able not only to assess, plan, implement, and evaluate but also to document in writing what is being done. These tasks are satisfying to home health care nurses who enjoy using the nursing process in delivering client care. Home health care nurses know that performance evaluation is based not only on the direct care delivered but also on how well one can communicate in writing what has been done.

Accreditation

Another means of evaluating quality assurance in home health care is accreditation. In 1975 the National League for Nursing and American Public Health Association developed criteria to evaluate home health agencies and community nursing services. The committee represented all personnel who delivered community and home health services. In 1980, the criteria were revised and standards for measurement of quality were added.

The purpose of the accreditation process is to evaluate the administrative practices of the agency and conditions based on the major assumption that there is a relationship between the quality of administration and the quality of services delivered to the community. The following list gives the components of an evaluation.

1. Community assessment
2. Organization and administration
3. Program
4. Staff
5. Evaluation
6. Future plans

The process of self-study is an educational experience for all involved with the home health agency. The board of directors, executive director, professional advisory committee, and the entire staff participate in the ongoing process of evaluation, since it is they who make up the home care program. Refer to Appendix G for criteria used to measure the quality of care.

Self-study is a monitoring tool that is voluntarily imposed on the agency at the agency's discretion. The accreditation decision is based on the data in the self-study, the report of the site visit team, and any additional information. A noteworthy trend for the future may be the requirement of accreditation for certification for licensure of all home health agencies. As of October 1982, 105 home health agencies were accredited by the NLN.

Regulatory Mechanisms

Regulation in home health care is an important concern to the home health nurse. The home health nurse is responsible on a day-to-day basis for assuring that the clinical practice is being performed within the guidelines set up by the regulatory agencies. In view of this, the home health nurse must interpret not only to colleagues but also to clients, families, and community what the regulations say is allowable in the performance of nursing care. According to Krause (1975), regulation is defined as "a process which is meant, in theory, to protect the public in vulnerable areas." In terms of home health care, the vulnerable areas are the target population of the elderly, the disabled, and the poor.

The Health Care Financing Administration (HCFA) is accountable for the overseeing of the Medicare program, federal participation in the Medicaid program, Professional Standards Review Organization Program (PSRO), and other health care quality assurance programs. HCFA is responsible for the combination of two administrative functions—health financing and quality assurance.

The purpose of the HCFA (1980) is to accomplish the following:

1. Promote timely delivery of appropriate quality health care to its beneficiaries who represent approximately 47 million of the nation's aged, disabled, and poor
2. Ensure that beneficiaries are aware of the services for which they are eligible
3. Ensure that those services are accessible and of high quality
4. Establish policies and determine actions that promote efficiency and quality in the health care delivery system

Home health regulation is carried out mainly at the state level with state health departments certifying home health agencies according to the HCFA Conditions of Participation for Home Health Agencies (1982). The Conditions of Participation serve as the basis to evaluate each aspect of home health agencies. The criteria used for evaluation cover the following conditions:

1. Definitions (of home health agency terminology)
2. Compliance with federal, state, and local laws
3. Organization, services, and administration
4. Group of professional personnel with advisory and evaluation function
5. Acceptance of patients, plan of treatment, and medical supervision
6. Services—skilled nursing, therapy, medical social worker, home health aide
7. Establishment and maintenance of clinical records
8. Evaluation of the agency's total program and behavior (Krause, 1975)

The state agencies responsible for licensure and certification of home health agencies use these criteria in evaluating whether the agencies are conforming with federal regulations. Each criterion has minimum standards to which the program should be adhering. Failure to meet these conditions can result in loss of licensure and the closing of the agency. Refer to Chapters 5 and 10 for further discussion of quality assurance and regulatory control.

FINANCIAL ASPECTS OF HOME HEALTH CARE

Reimbursement Mechanisms

Before federal intervention, home health care was reimbursed by clients who could pay for the service and by donations that subsidized the care provided to those who could pay a portion or not pay at all. Even now, Medicare and Medicaid are the principal funding sources with third party health insurance as another major source.

Medicare

Reimbursement of home health services is handled through fiscal intermediaries under contract to the federal government. A fiscal intermediary is an insurance company under contract to the Social Security Administration to pay home care agencies for Medicare-covered services rendered to beneficiaries. To qualify for home health services, a beneficiary must be over 65 years of age or disabled and

1. Under the care of a physician
2. Confined to the home (homebound)
3. In need of skilled nursing services, physical therapy, occupational therapy, or speech therapy on an intermittent basis

The person's attending physician establishes the plan of treatment and also certifies to the necessity of home health services. The plan must specify the following:

1. Types of services required
2. Frequency of visits
3. Anticipated length of care
4. Diagnosis
5. Description of the client's functional limitations
6. Medications
7. Diet
8. Activities permitted
9. Medical supplies and appliances needed
10. Safety of home environment

This plan must be reviewed at least every 60 days and continuance of care requires recertification of the plan by the physician.

A beneficiary is considered eligible for home health services provided that a physician certifies that the client is confined at home. Clients do not have to be bedridden but must be unable to leave their residence without assistance because of illness or injury. Feebleness and insecurity brought on by advanced age do not qualify the person to receive home health care.

Skilled services refer to those services required by an individual that are reasonable and necessary for treatment of the individual's illness or injury. The following factors are evaluated in determining the degree of skill:

1. Complexity of service and condition of client
2. service must be performed or directly supervised by a registered nurse or registered physical therapist
3. teaching of service must be performed by skilled professional
4. type of service can be accomplished by nonmedical person

Services that are directed toward the prevention of illness or injury are not covered by Medicare. This does not mean, however, that these activities cannot be performed. They must be done in conjunction with a "skilled" service. The following are examples of services that are reimbursable and covered under Medicare because they require skill, knowledge, and judgment on the part of the practitioner:

1. Observation and evaluation of physical status
2. Teaching and training activities to client, family, or caretaker
3. Therapeutic exercises (for restoration of loss of function)
4. Insertion and irrigation of catheter
5. Administration of medications (intravenous and intramuscular injections and teaching of medication regimen)
6. Skin care (extensive decubitus ulcer)

Unlike the general population, Medicare beneficiaries usually suffer from chronic conditions with multiple disease processes. Medicare beneficiaries rely on federal reimbursement criteria which definitely influence the provision of care. Medicare places an emphasis on episodic care because of its limitations in benefits and requirements for skilled care. One of the shortcomings of Medicare is the limited protection it gives against medical expenses as a result of the limitations and restrictions in the benefit package. Medicare usually reimburses 80% of "usual, customary, and reasonable charges" in Part B. The remaining 20% must be "coinsured" for protection against excessive expense. It is beneficial to encourage the elderly to acquire supplemental health insurance to cover the cost of charges that Medicare does not pay. The use of home health services under Medicare has increased significantly since the passage of the 1972 amendments. New rules and regulations are being written for Medicare and intermediaries from time to time. These changes are published in bulletins sent to agencies.

Medicaid

Authorized by Title XIX of the Social Security Act, Medicaid provides health services to low-income persons. It is a medical assistance program for eligible people under Title IV (Aid to Families with Dependent Children) or Title XVI (Supplemental Security In-

Table 34-2. Comparison of the two major federally supported programs for home health care

Medicare (Title XVIII)	Medicaid (Title XVIX)
Federal *insurance* program administered by Social Security Administration	Federal and state *assistance* program administered by the state
Age 65 and over or disabled	Income-based eligibility
Conditions of participation	Conditions of participation
Homebound status	Not necessarily homebound status
Intermittent service	Intermittent service
Skilled service	Not necessarily skilled service
Restorative program	Custodial and maintenance program
Physician certification	Physician certification
Therapies, medical social service	State option — therapist, medical social service
Pays rental and purchase	Pays purchase
Reimbursement — "reasonable cost"	Reimbursement — maximum allowed at state level

come) of the Social Security Act and also is available for those individuals whose income is insufficient to cover medical services and also for disability coverage. Medicaid is administered by the states but is state and federally subsidized. Providers are directly reimbursed by the state, which is also responsible for monitoring the operations and enforcing the regulations. Medicaid covers home health services including skilled and unskilled services such as personal care. Needy children are eligible under Medicaid whereas the elderly usually receive Medicare.

A comparison of Medicare and Medicaid is depicted in Table 34-2. If a client has both Medicare and Medicaid or a private insurance plan, Medicare is used as the primary payment source provided the services being delivered to the client are "skilled." When the client is no longer eligible for home care under Medicare, the Medicaid benefits can be used.

Private Insurance

Third party payers are represented by private health insurance companies in which the person subscribes in-

dividually or with a group such as an employer. Some states (e.g., Connecticut) have laws that require home health care to be a provision in health insurance coverage. Individuals who most often use this benefit are those under 65 years who need home care follow-up after surgery or prolonged hospitalization. This benefit can decrease a client's length of stay in the hospital, thereby assisting clients to return to their former level of functioning. Some third party payers have incentive programs such as the Blue Cross/Blue Shield Direct Admission Program, planned as a cost-containment effort, which bypasses the hospitalization of an eligible case.

Payment by Individual

Some individuals who do not have health insurance and require home health services may pay the home health agency directly. Individuals who do not meet their insurance coverage requirements and still want the services pay the established charge or may be offered the service on a sliding scale or established fee based on their financial status. An example of this is illustrated by clients who no longer require skilled nursing service for assessment of their condition but need the help of a home health aide to assist with personal hygiene needs. Some persons may pay for home health services that are needed or desired above and beyond the home health services the Medicare program offers.

Nursing Visit Charges

The National League for Nursing prepares an annual review of the costs and charges for home care of all official, nonofficial, and combination agencies that elect to participate in the study. In 1981, 96% (245) of the responding agencies gave sufficient information to determine the cost and charge. Of the official agencies, 88% reported cost and charge data.

Table 34-3 reflects the median cost and charge per nursing visit by type of agency, region, and size of nursing staff (NLN, 1981). The official agencies are more costly than nonofficial agencies except in regions VIII, IX, and X. Several factors influence the cost and charge data: (1) type of service provided, (2) geographical location of the agency, (3) current community salaries, (4) population characteristics, (5) type of agency, and (6) staffing patterns.

The term *cost* refers to the dollar amount agencies spend to provide the service. The term *charge* is the dollar amount expected or billed for rendering of the service. In the official agencies, cost may be calculated on a statewide basis, whereas in other agencies (nonofficial or combination agencies) one cost may be apportioned for all types of service such as nursing, therapy, and home health aide.

Table 34-3. Median cost and charge per nursing visit by type of agency, region, and size of nursing staff, 1981

	Nonofficial and combination agencies (245)		Official agencies (115)	
	Cost	Charge	Cost	Charge
Region*				
All regions	$28.06	$31.65	$37.78	$35.84
I, II, III	25.45	28.75	37.50	37.19
IV, V, VI, VII	33.05	39.17	34.65	35.17
VIII, IX, X	38.93	42.75	33.75	35.65
Size of nursing staff				
Under 5	$27.92	$29.17	$33.50	$38.57
5-14	26.70	30.16	35.84	35.46
15-24	27.84	32.29	34.00	35.84
25-49	28.89	32.00	37.50	36.67
50 and over	33.00	36.67	38.75	37.50

From National League of Nursing: Cost and charge for home care of sick services — 1981, New York, 1981, NLN.
*I: Conn., Me., Mass., N.H., R.I., Vt.; II: N.J., N.Y.; III: Del., D.C., Md., Pa., Va., W.Va.; IV: Ala., Fla., Ga., Ky., Miss., N.C., S.C., Tenn.; V: Ill., Ind., Mich., Minn., Ohio, Wis.; VI: Ark., La., N.M., Okla., Tex.; VII: Iowa, Kan., Mo., Neb.; VIII: Colo., Mont., N.D., S.D., Utah, Wyo.; IX: Ariz., Calif., Hawaii, Nev.; X: Alaska, Idaho, Ore., Wash.

The Health Care Financing Administration continuously gathers data regarding use of home care services by analyzing such factors as cost, frequency, duration of services, number of visits, and so on. The federal government is interested in cost containment and also in quality of care.

Cost Effectiveness

Refer to Chapter 3 for an in-depth discussion of the economics of health care and its impact on community health nursing. Updated published data are lacking regarding the cost effectiveness of home health care. Public attention is now being focused on home health care as a cost-effective alternative to institutionalization.

In 1981 President Reagan introduced home health care to public discussion by relating an occurrence "of overregulation and expensive institutionalization" in the case of a young girl who needed skilled care that home health could provide but who instead was institutionalized at greater expense to the state's Medicaid program (Home Health Line, 1981).

The growth of home care agencies has historically been slow because home care services were not covered by many third party reimbursement sources until recently. Rising institutional costs and a growing concern over institutionalization has now helped to focus on home health care.

Nurses are usually not directly exposed to the financial aspects of health care in their clinical setting. In home health, nurses are "cost conscious" because of

their responsibility to interpret to clients what Medicare *will* or *will not* pay. It is difficult for the elderly to understand why Medicare will not pay for the nurse to make home visits to take their blood pressures if they continue to be stable. Medicare pays for services only if the client's condition remains unstable. The key words to remember for Medicare home health coverage are *skilled, homebound, intermittent,* and *unstable.*

IMPACT OF LEGISLATION ON HOME HEALTH CARE SERVICES

The federal government plays a significant role, described in this section, in the delivery of home health care services. The information is organized to present an overview of the historical development of the laws and their direct impact on home health. Some of the material presented in this section on legislation and in the following section on trends and issues may be altered by the occurrence of changing events. Congressional activity can change federal legislation with regard to home health care. For updated information concerning new amendments or bills presented in Congress, consult the *Federal Register.*

The Social Security Act of 1935 served as an important piece of legislation because it signaled the major entrance of the federal government into the area of social insurance. It significantly expanded assistance to the states and formed the foundation for the two major health programs—Medicare and Medicaid.

Amendments of the original Social Security Act which have impacted indirectly on home health include the following (Wilson and Newhauser, 1974):

1939—Benefits for dependents and survivors were added to the old age program.

1950—The program of federal aid to state public assistance programs was extended to disabled persons (Title XIV). Federal participation in state payments to providers of medical services (vendor payments) to persons on public assistance was also added.

1956—A federal program of disability benefits was added to OASI. The program was now known as Old Age, Survivors and Disability Insurance (OASDI).

1960—The Kerr-Mills Act established a program of medical assistance to the needy aged, providing payments for medical care for needy elderly persons not receiving public assistance ("medically indigent aged"). This was the forerunner of the Medicaid program.

1965—Two new sections were added: Health Insurance for the Aged (Title XVIII, Medicare) and Grants to the States for Medical Assistance Programs (Title XIX, Medicaid).

1966 and 1967—Several adjustments were made in the Medicare and Medicaid programs including provision for limitation of federal participation in Medicaid and other benefit changes.

1972—Many amendments were made to the Medicare and Medicaid programs, including the inclusion of persons receiving federal disability benefits in Medicare and the establishment of Professional Standards Review Organizations (PSRO): a new federal minimum income program, Supplemental Security Income (SSI) replaced the federally aided adult public assistance programs.

1980—PL 96-499, the Onnibus Reconciliation Act of 1980, carried provisions to modify existing programs of Medicare and Medicaid (see following discussion of changes).

The Medicare program was enacted on July 30, 1965, as Title XVIII of the Social Security Act and became effective July 1, 1966. The program offers two coordinated insurance coverages—hospital insurance, referred to as Part A; and supplemental medical insurance, referred to as Part B. Each provides reimbursement for home health agency services. This legislation established requirements for client eligibility, reimbursable costs, physician participation, and agency eligibility (for specific details see the section of this chapter dealing with financial aspects of home care).

The Social Security Amendments of 1972 made the following changes in home health coverage to provide incentives for greater use of the benefit:

1. In the supplementary insurance section (Part B) the 20% coinsurance requirement was eliminated for services furnished on or after January 1, 1973.
2. The Secretary of Health, Education, and Welfare was authorized to establish by diagnoses the permissible periods of coverage of home health care under Part A for clients with specified conditions.
3. Payments for services that neither the home health agency or beneficiary knew were not covered.
4. Medicare coverage (including home health care) was extended to individuals receiving Social Security benefits based on disability or end-stage renal disease. This coverage began in July 1973.

The early 1980s have brought substantial changes in the area of home health care services. Effective May 4, 1980, the Department of Health, Education, and Welfare (DHEW) was redesignated the Department of Health and Human Services (DHHS). During December 1980 in the lame duck session of the 96th Congress, a law was passed that modified the existing programs of Medicare and Medicaid—the Medicare and Medicaid Amendments of 1980, Title IX of the Omnibus Reconciliation Act of 1980 (Public Law 96-499). Public Law 96-499 carries provisions relating not only to home health but also to hospital services, skilled nursing facilities, intermediate care facilities, and physicians who are involved with reimbursement from Medicare and Medicaid.

The Omnibus Reconciliation Act of 1980 broadened Medicare coverage for home health services by instituting the following changes effective July 1, 1981:

1. Unlimited visits. There is no limit to the number of medically necessary home health visits that Medicare will cover under Part A or Part B.
2. Elimination of 3-day hospital stay. There is no longer a prior hospitalization requirement of 3 days before Part A will pay for home health care.
3. Part B deductible. The $60 deductible charge for home health benefits under Part B is eliminated. The charge is required, however, for other health services provided under Part B and was increased on January 1, 1982, to $75. This was the first increase since 1972.
4. Occupational therapy. Occupational therapy qualifies as a skilled qualifying criterion to receive home care services. (Effective December 1, 1981, it does not qualify as an admitting criterion for home care but can remain as the only skilled service after other disciplines no longer need to see the patient.)

5. Proprietary agency involvement. In states without licensure laws, proprietary home health agencies can participate in the Medicare program.

6. Other important features of the Omnibus Reconciliation Act include the establishment of regional intermediaries for home health agencies by the Department of Health and Human Services and the achievement of more effective administration of the home health benefits. (Law, Paragraph 924,097; Committee reports, Paragraph 24,347).

The Medicaid Community Care Act—Section 2176 of the Omnibus Reconciliation Act—recognizes and supports the concept of community care as a viable alternative for clients requiring long-term care. The states and providers of home health services are being afforded the opportunity to develop their own plan and implement their own ideas without the burden of excessive federal regulation. Some individuals feel, however, that the decrease in federal involvement will foster fraud and abuse in Medicare home care use by some not-so-honest entrepreneurs.

TRENDS AND ISSUES IN HOME HEALTH CARE

Legal and Ethical Issues Confronting the Home Health Nurse

In any health care subsystem there is a potential for illegal and unethical actions. Much publicity has been given to medicare fraud and abuse within the last decade. This avenue for exploitation has been partially caused by the increase in available federal monies. Examples of such practices include overuse of home health services when the client does not need them, inaccurate billing for services, excessive administrative staff, "kickbacks" for referrals, and billing of noncovered medical supplies. In 1977, the Medicare-Medicaid Anti-Fraud and Abuse Amendments (PL 95-142) were passed to deter such practices.

Home health care nurses can be confronted with multiple issues in everyday practice. The definition of skilled care can be judgmental, and its interpretation can vary. The home health care nurse must abide by the federal regulations established when delivering care to clients. Frequency of visiting poses another issue. Home health care clients require only intermittent visits for evaluation of status. If the frequency increases, then the need for full-time skilled services may be required. Reevaluation of the client and family needs are imperative so that overuse and inappropriate use of services can be avoided. Home health care nurses must be knowledgeable about what medical supplies are covered. This information is readily available to home health care nurses, and as professionals, nurses must work within the regulatory guideline framework and educate the community as to what home health care is and should be.

Stressors in home health care impinge on practicing nurses. Paperwork, while often overwhelming, is necessary to document accountability. Being accountable can be a stressor because the home health care nurse must demonstrate that all actions are valid and that each can be justified. The expanded role of the home health care nurse can be complex, since the assumption of nontraditional responsibilities can be viewed as a threat by other health team members. Physician support may be lacking and home health care underused because of hospital orientation and a view of home care as second rate and bothersome because of the excess paperwork it entails. Others view home health care as service for the poorer classes and therefore find little appeal in this mode of care. *Cost effective* is another negative phrase to some health care professionals because it is difficult to link cost effectiveness with quality in all situations. But to exist in the competitive health care arena today, home health care must be competitive. By properly organizing and using decision-making principles, home health care nurses do not have to sacrifice quality for cost effectiveness.

Issues in the 1980s

The 1970s brought an era of regulation primarily since the government played an important part in financing health care. Regulations have now been accused of jeopardizing the quality of care that clients received. Thus with the onset of the 1980s, we see a different trend—that of deregulation. We will also see a more comprehensive restructuring of the health care system. Appropriate questions about roles and control are being proposed.

Health care providers and consumers are concerned about high quality and cost-effective alternatives to institutional care. Home health nurses can play a vital role in providing the leadership to see that this realistic dream can come true. Quality care can be provided in the home setting as evidenced by review of the literature (Hall et al., 1982). The benefit of home health care is measurable in terms of evaluating client outcomes, as described in the quality assurance section of this chapter. Unfortunately, most of the information published is based on subjective data acquired from clients and providers of home health. Data regarding actual benefits are limited at this time.

Maintenance of well-being and return to a semi-independent state can be documented and seen in the home. Rehabilitation occurs faster at home in some instances because the clients have greater control and are able to assume their former roles at home. In an institution, however, the sick role is promoted, thereby eliminating much of the client's previous responsibility and control.

In terms of cost, the per diem cost of home health care is less than the per diem cost of hospital care (Harris, 1982). It is assumed that greater self-care is a means to cutting health care costs. Home health care encourages promotion of self-care. If home health care is to exist as a viable alternative to institutionalization, then nurses must not only continue to provide quality care but participate in research to clarify the contribution of home health care to cost effectiveness in the health care delivery system. Home health care need not be referred to only as an alternative to institutionalization. It should be the first choice with institutionalization being an alternative when appropriate.

In relation to continuity of care and appropriateness of home health care, Gikow (1981) has developed a decision model for individuals responsible for referring clients to community resources to assist them in matching clients up with the appropriate resource. The tool depends on an accurate and complete client assessment so that either skilled or supportive care can be appropriately and adequately provided.

In January 1982 a single national association for home health care was formed, the National Association for Home Care (NAHC). The National Association of Home Health Agencies (NAHHA) and the Council of Home Health Agencies/Community Health Services (CHHA/CHS) agreed to dissolve their respective groups and merge to form a more unified organization. The purpose and definition for the new organization were developed by a National Task Force for Home Health Services. Some of the areas that will influence home health in the 1980s include increasing political awareness of home health services, participating in legislative and regulatory processes, focusing on the positive aspects of home health care services with not only the governmental but also the private sector agencies, compiling data, and distributing educational information to the public regarding home health care (Rak, 1982).

Competition in home health care is on the rise. This factor is based primarily on the slant of federal programs to deinstitutionalize and deregulate areas of health care. Administrators of home health agencies are being faced with "selling" home health care to consumers. This task, although seemingly difficult, can be easy if accountability and quality assurance exist in the agencies. Clients are being discharged in a more "acute" condition than previously. The level of care requires a highly skilled practitioner in community health nursing.

Family Responsibility, Roles, and Functions

The family plays an important part in the delivery of home health care. The term *family*, as discussed previously, refers to a caretaker responsible for the client's well-being. An issue being discussed at this time is whether home health care services should be used as a respite or relief type of care. There are some instances when a family member is debilitated and is unable to help the client without assistance. Should supportive services be paid by the federal government? On the other hand, some family members are capable of providing the needed care but are unwilling to do so. Who should pay for the service and who should provide the needed care? Family responsibility is an issue that may not be resolved. The situations vary from one family to another. Assistance from social support systems facilitates coping with the stress of caring for an ill family member. The goal to keep in mind, however, is to assist in maintaining the client at home for as long as possible and to provide a high quality of life. To do this, resources must be used appropriately and effectively. Determining this use, however, poses a problem.

Population Trends and Their Effects on Home Health Care Services

The growing need for home health care services is supported by official data regarding our older American population (Healthy People, 1979):

> Despite a common misconception, most elderly Americans can and do remain in their own homes. In 1975, 77 percent had their own households—51 percent living with a spouse, 27 percent living alone—and 18 percent lived with someone other than a spouse. Only 5 percent lived in institutions.

> Although the majority of the elderly are vigorous and completely independent, there are 45 percent with certain activity limitations—some associated with mental disabilities, but most due to physical handicaps caused by heart conditions, arthritis, hearing and visual impairments.

> Up to 20 percent of older people—from one-third to one-half of those with any activity limitations—are handicapped in ability to move freely, compared with two or three percent of the 17 to 64 year old population.

The Medicare program provides coverage for approximately 24 million elderly people and approximately 3 million people under age 65 with long-term disabilities or chronic renal disease (Link, et al. 1980).

Presently there is no federal program mandated to provide long-term in-home services for the elderly. Restrictions limit in-home services for Medicare and Medicaid recipients. There is lack of information regarding the cost and benefits of home care services. According to a recent report, various studies support the belief that in-home services prolong life and maintain or increase the elderly person's independence. However, little is known about the costs and benefits of increasing the availability of long-term, in-home care (Improved Knowledge Base, 1981).

As most literature has pointed out, the elderly do constitute a large portion of the population (Improved Knowledge Base, 1981):

> The number of elderly persons in the United States is large and is rapidly increasing. The Nation's elderly population increased from about 9 million in 1940 to about 24 million in 1978 and is projected to reach 45 million by the year 2020. For instance, in 1940 the elderly represented about 7 percent of the population. By 1978, their representation had increased to about 11 percent. Also increasing is the percentage of the elderly who are over age 75. The Commissioner on Aging, in the annual report for fiscal year 1979, stated that about 40 percent of the elderly population was over age 75 and that this percentage was expected to increase to 45 by the year 2020.

Hospice Home Care

The historical meaning of the word *hospice* referred to a place of refuge for travelers. The contemporary meaning now refers to "a way of caring for people nearing the end of their journey through life, faced with dying and in need of refuge (Vines and Hartzell, 1981). Terminal care in the home is a familiar aspect of home care, even before the advent of the hospice movement in the United States. People with terminal disease now are offered the opportunity to die at home, if it is their choice, with the supportive services that home care can provide. There are a variety of hospice care models in the United States using either institutional and home care service or both. Those that use an existing hospital in conjunction with an established home health agency are probably the most cost efficient because each organization can contribute a portion of its resources to this concept of care (Meyer, 1980).

In any case, hospice care requires a team of professionals and para-professionals with experience in caring for the terminally ill. Interdisciplinary coordination is imperative for a smooth flow of transfer of clients to the home care setting from the hospital. In keeping clients at home, the prime goal is to help both the client and family in maintaining the client's integrity and comfort. This goal is met by nursing actions such as alleviating symptoms and meeting the special needs of the dying client and the client's family.

Health care providers who work with the dying often experience stress, which must be identified and appropriately dealt with so that quality client care continues to be delivered. Stress factors include the following:

1. Difficulty accepting the fact that a patient's physi-

cal and psychosocial problems cannot always be controlled
2. Frustration because of investing large amounts of energy for people who then die
3. Anger at being subjected to "higher-than-standard" performance expectations
4. Difficulty deciding when to set limits on involvement with patients and family
5. Difficulty establishing realistic limitations as to what can be provided by hospice (Vachon, 1979).

One of the major issues confronting hospice care is the present reimbursement structures in the health care delivery system. The federal government as well as private third party payers are actively studying reimbursement for hospice care through established demonstration projects (Home Health Line, 1982). The apparent lack of data regarding hospice programs presents a difficult situation for community planners who have assessed the need for hospice programs in their community and do not have the resources to fund such programs. Much hospice care can be covered under home care for terminally ill if the nurse is cognizant of the system. It takes cooperation and innovation to use the existing available resources.

SUMMARY

Home health care is a component of health care delivery which is continuing to develop and grow. This subsystem is receiving increasing interest by governments as reflected in the recent changes in Medicare and Medicaid regulations. These changes are beginning to eliminate past barriers to home health care delivery and are encouraging more flexibility in the delivery of services to eligible beneficiaries.

Three recent changes in home health care criteria are (1) the allowance of unlimited visits to those who qualify, making it possible to receive care until a change in client status occurs; (2) the elimination of the 3-day hospital stay, making it possible to use home health care as a posthospital service or "instead of" hospitalization; and (3) the discontinuation of the deductible, thereby removing cost barriers for those in need of service.

The major issues surrounding the delivery of home health care are many. Fraud and abuse in the system have largely been linked to the amount of federal monies available to promote home health care services. One wonders what may happen now that regulations have opened home health care reimbursement to "for profit" agencies as well as to nonprofit agencies now providing care. The definition of skilled care is judgmental and may continue to eliminate persons in need of services from qualifying for such services; moreover, the growing elderly population may play an increasing demand on the delivery system to provide a broader range of services to more categories of persons.

Home health care continues to be the only service offered to clients on their own turf. This service, above all, has more potential for a multidisciplinary approach to health care involving all provider disciplines in serving the client. Nurses play a vital role in home health care because they continue to be the mechanism for coordinating care and for collaborating with other health team members, the client, and the family to delivery quality care to the client.

BIBLIOGRAPHY

American Medical Association: Physician guide to home health care, Monroe, Wis., 1979, The Association, pp. 1-3.

American Nurses Association: Standards of community health nursing practice, Kansas City, Mo., 1973, The Association.

American Nurses' Association, Division of Community Health Nursing: A Conceptual Model of Community Health Nursing, Pub. No. CH-102M, Kansas City, Mo., 1980, The Association, p. 9.

Aradine, C.R., and Pridham, K.F.: A model for collaboration, Nurs. Outlook 21:655-657, 1973.

Callender, M., and LaVor, J.: Home health care: Development, problems and potential, Washington, D.C., 1975, Office of the Assistant Secretary for Planning and Evaluation, Social Services and Human Development, Department of Health, Education, and Welfare.

Corwin, R.G.: A society of education, New York, 1965, Appleton-Century-Crofts, pp. 222-231.

Dolan, J.; Goodnow's history of nursing, Philadelphia, 1958, W.B. Saunders Co., p. 264.

Funkhouser, R.: Quality of care, Part I, Nurs. 76 16:11, 1976.

Gikow, F.F.: How to determine appropriate community services for the elderly, Nurs. Health Care 2(6):322-326, June 1981.

Hall, A.D., Baud, W.R., and Elliston, E.B.: Comparing staff attitudes and patient satisfactions in a home health agency, Home Health Rev. 4(1):4-11, June 1982.

Hall, J., and Weaver, B.: Distributive nursing practice: a systems approach to community health, New York, 1977, J.B. Lippincott Co., p. 6.

Harris, M.: Evaluating home care: compare viewpoints, Nurs. Health Care 2(4):207, April 1982.

Health Care Financing Administration: Conditions of participation for home health agencies, Subpart 1, Section 405.1229, Evaluation, Washington, D.C., 1982a, Department of Health and Human Services.

Health Care Financing Administration: Conditions of participation, Subpart L, Reg. 8, Section 405.1201, Washington, D.C., 1982b, Department of Health and Human Services.

Health Care Financing Administration: Health care financing review, vol. II, no. 2, Washington, D.C., HCFA office of Research, Demonstration, and Statistics.

Healthy people, The surgeon general's report on health promotion and disease prevention, Pub. No. 79-55071, Washington, D.C., 1979, Department of Health, Education and Welfare.

Home Health Line, Nov. 13, 1981, p. 186.

Home Health Line, April 2, 1982, p. 41.

Home Health Services: Commerce Clearinghouse Medicare and Medicaid Guide, Paragraph 1401, Washington, D.C., 1982, Department of Health and Human Services.

Improved knowledge base would be helpful in reaching policy decisions on providing long-term in-home services for the elderly, Report to the Honorable Pete V. Domenici, U.S. Senate, Washington, D.C., 1981, U.S. General Accounting Office, pp. 1 and 24.

Kane, R.: Competency for collaboration. In Reinhardt, A., and Quinn, M., editors: Current practice in family-centered community nursing, Vol. 1, St. Louis, 1977, The C.V. Mosby Co.

Krause, F.: The political contest of health service regulation, Int. J. Health Serv., 5(4):593-607, 1975.

Link, D., Long, S., and Settle, R.: Cost sharing supplementary insurance and health services utilization among the Medicare elderly, Health Care Financing Rev., 2(2):25, Fall 1980.

Mayers, M.: Home visit—ritual or therapy, Nurs. Outlook 21(5):328, 1973.

Meyer, K.A.: Hospice concept integrated with existing community health care, Nurs. Adm. Q. 4(3):49-54, Spring 1980.

National League for Nursing: Utilization review—guidelines for home health agencies, New York, 1971, NLN.

National League for Nursing: Criteria and standards manual for National League for Nursing/American Public Health Association accreditation of home health agencies and community nursing services, Pub. No. 21-1306, New York, 1980, NLN.

National League for Nursing: Cost and charge for home care of sick service—1981, New York, 1981, NLN.

Orem, D.E.: Nursing: concepts of practice, New York, 1971, McGraw-Hill Book Co.

Phaneuf, M.C.: The nursing audit; profile for excellence, New York, 1972, Appleton-Century-Crofts.

Quality assurance for community health agencies, Waltham, Mass., 1980, Massachusetts Association of Home Health and Community Health Agencies.

Quality assurance manual, 1980, Florida Association of Home Health Agencies.

Rak, K.: Home Health Line, Jan. 15, 1982, p. 5.

Sloan, M.R., and Schummer, B.T.: The process of contracting in community nursing. In Spradley, B.W., editor: Contemporary community nursing, Boston, 1975, Little, Brown & Co.

Trager, B.: Home health services in the United States: a report to the Special Committee on Aging, 92nd Congress, 2nd Session, Washington, D.C., 1972, U.S. Government Printing Office, p. 5.

Vachon, M.L.: Staff stress in care of the terminally ill, Q. Rev. Bull. 5(5):13-17, May 1979.

Vines, E., and Hartzell, D.H.:The hospice movement in the United States, National Health Standards and Quality Information Clearinghouse Information Bulletin, Baltimore, March 1981, p. 3.

Warhola, C.: Planning for home health services: a resource handbook, Pub. No. (HRA) 80-14017, Washington, D.C., August, 1980, Public Health Service, Department of Health and human Services.

Wilson, F., and Newhauser, F.: Health services in the United States, Cambridge, Mass., 1974, Ballinger Publishing Co., p. 123.

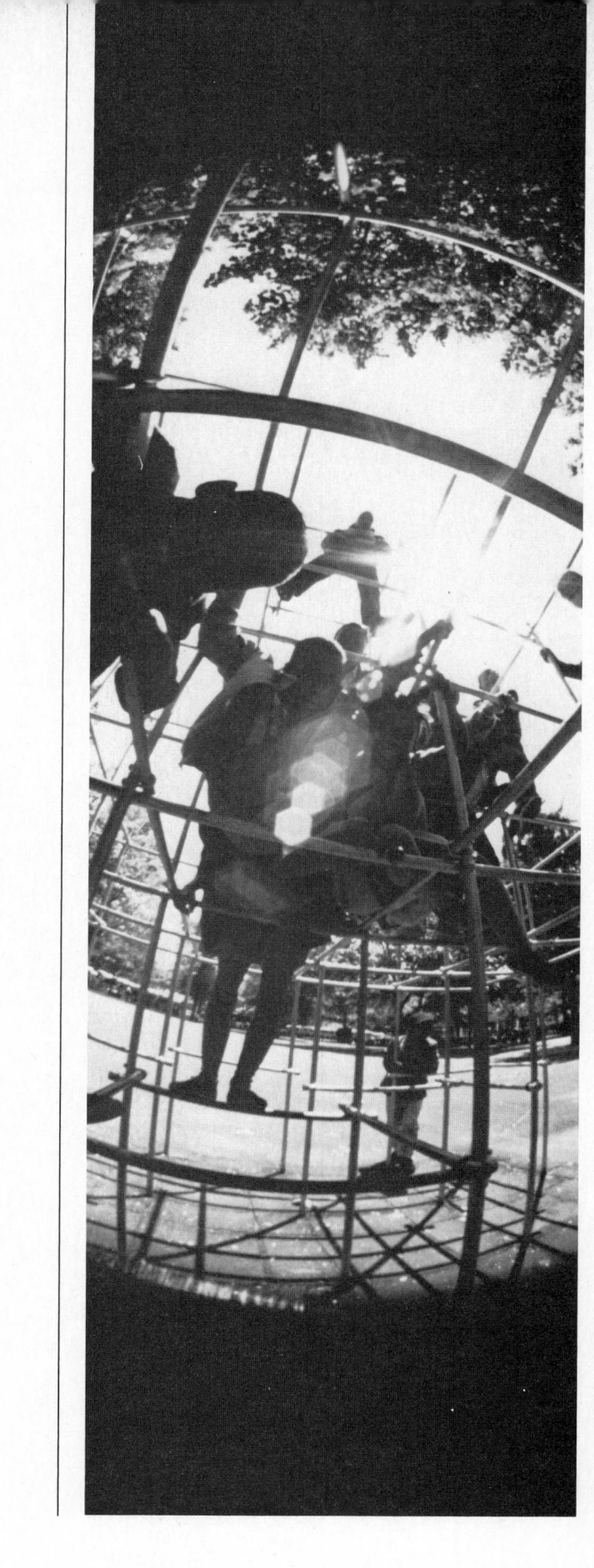

Part Six

COMMUNITY HEALTH NURSING FOR TODAY AND TOMORROW

It has been estimated that the medical care system affects about 10% of the usual indexes for measuring health. The remaining 90% are determined by factors over which health care providers have little or no direct control, such as life-style and social and physical environmental conditions. The focus of this text is on the processes and practices for promoting health, and the community health nurse is considered an ideal person to personally demonstrate and teach others how to promote health. To be effective, health promotion necessitates that people cease focusing on how to "fix" themselves and others when they detect physical and/ or emotional disequilibrium but rather that people acknowledge and accept personal responsibility for health. Such a change in emphasis requires that all health care providers shift from a "we will make you well" approach to a "let us work together as partners for better individual, family, and community health."

Such a shift cannot be expected to come easily, since health may not be consistently highly valued in the United States. It is often easy to verbally acknowledge an orientation toward health promotion, but the actual implementation and continuance has many associated costs in terms of time, energy, and to some extent a reorientation of firmly held habits like diet, sleep, exercise, smoking, and drinking, as well as management of emotions and attitudes.

If personal expenditures are any indication of a given society's values, tobacco, alcohol, and cigarettes are more highly valued by Americans than is health. Responsibility for health must be returned from health care providers to communities, families, and individuals. Such a renewal of interest in health promotion is not new; people have known for decades that what they eat, drink, do, and think largely determines their well-being.

Continued.

Part Six

What is the community health nurse's role in health promotion for today and tomorrow? As pointed out in Chapter 35, there are many arenas for practice in community health nursing. However, this chapter makes clear the belief that the community as a focus of care and attention should be a major priority in community health nursing. No longer is community health based on a site for practice, but rather it reflects an orientation to health care delivery, which blends nursing and community health ideology to focus on the overall well-being of the total community.

Chapter 36 describes the importance of research as a basis for community health nursing practice. Nursing, including community health, has been trying for several years to derive a knowledge base to become a separate entity within the health care field. Scientific research in nursing did not begin until the 1950s, and only in the 1970s did nurses begin to concentrate on defining a scientific knowledge base for practice. Before that time nurses focused on the study of educational and administrative practices. Research in community health nursing is essential to the future development of this area of nursing.

Chapters 37 and 38 provide practical guidelines for community health nurses to use both in personally implementing and in teaching health promotion to others. In a rapidly changing world nurses must learn ways in which they can practice and teach others to stand up for themselves and to deal effectively with the multiple demands and stressors facing them. These chapters present techniques that are easy to understand and apply for personal health promotion.

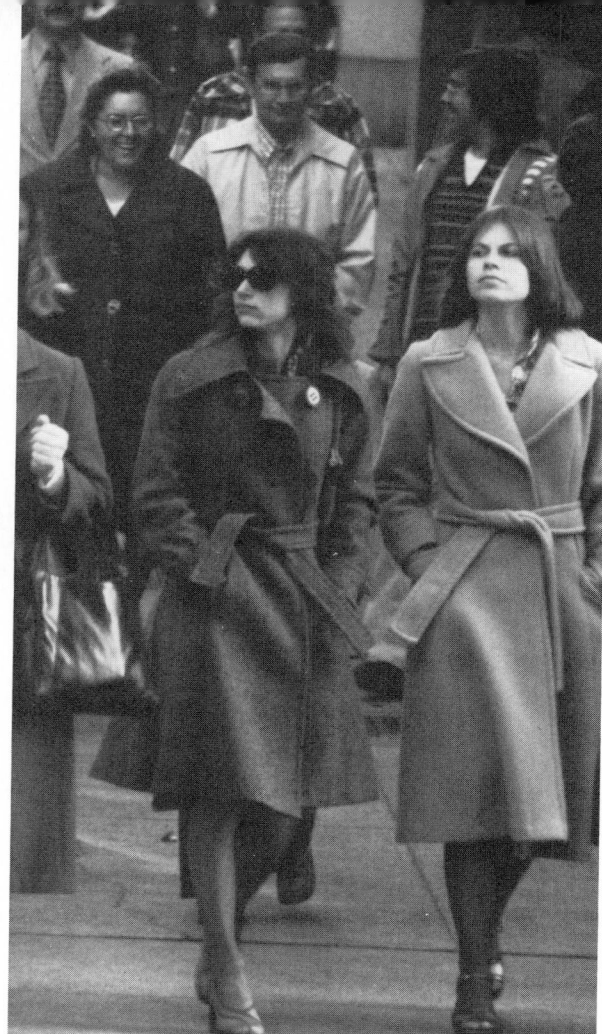

Chapter 35

CAROLYN A. WILLIAMS

POPULATION-FOCUSED PRACTICE

In this chapter issues of concern to those interested in the specialty of community health nursing are discussed. The chapter begins with an overview of the nature of community health nursing through a discussion of contemporary conceptualizations of community health nursing practice, characteristics frequently used to distinguish community health nursing from other speciality areas of nursing, and unique aspects of the specialty. The second part of the chapter examines the importance of population-focused practice, suggesting that the population focus is what distinguishes community health nursing from other specialties. Further, it is argued that population-focused community health nursing is consistent with a public health philosophy and is scientifically desirable. Barriers that mitigate against such practices are also considered.

The chapter concludes with a discussion of three dilemmas that occur as a result of the adoption of popula-

tion-focused practice. Questions considered in this section include the following: What is the arena for community health nursing practice? Is it limited to populations outside of institutions? Is it useful to talk about the role of the community health nurse? How does one prepare for population-focused practice?

COMMUNITY HEALTH NURSING TODAY: VIEWS AND PROBLEMS

The answer to the question, "What is community health nursing?" is not a straightforward one. Diverse opinions abound as to the answer. However, it is important to distinguish between population-focused nursing and clinical nursing delivered in community settings. In so doing, major conceptual difficulties in the field may be clarified and further thinking and discussion encouraged.

805

Conceptualizations of Community Health Nursing

As an introduction to the topic of the nature of community health nursing, two contemporary but different conceptualizations of community health nursing are described.

Provision of Personal Nursing Services in Community Settings

The notion that the focus of community health nursing is ". . . the provision of health services among people of the community and the encouragement of health promoting behavior" is one held by many nurses and was recently articulated in a paper by de Tornyay (1980, p. 85). de Tornyay emphasized that community health nursing places particular attention on the maintenance of health, the provision of service extending over time as opposed to episodic services, and the prevention of disease. She described the responsibilities of community health nurses in the area of long-term care, in primary care, in work with certain population groups, and in provision of a range of services for people living in a specific area. In each of the descriptions the emphasis is on the direct care services provided by the nurse. Although population groups variously defined are mentioned, the basic message is that a community health nurse is primarily a direct care clinician, providing services to the members of various groups in the community. In de Tornyay's discussion only brief mention was made of the administrative and supervisory responsibilities of community health nurses.

The paper by de Tornyay was selected because it presents a prevalent conceptualization of community health nursing in the United States. Much of the material in current textbooks reflects a perspective similar to that of de Tornyay's. The emphasis on providing clinical services in community settings is also the predominant focus of the American Nurses' Association's statement, A Conceptual Model of Community Health Nursing, developed by the Division of Community Health Nursing (1980).

Several distinctions are set forth in the Conceptual Model, which are relevant to this discussion. First, the statement identifies two categories of nurses in community health—generalists prepared at the baccalaureate level who practice in community health settings and specialists in community health nursing who have master's level preparation or beyond. The statement does not refer to the generalist as a specialist or even as a community health nurse, although the latter is implied. The practice of the generalist is described as follows (ANA, 1980, p. 9):

The nursing process is applied to the client, who may be an individual, family, group, or community. While working with individual clients, the nurse keeps the community perspective in mind.

In describing the scope of practice for community health nursing, the major objectives of the community health nurse are stated as "the preservation and improvement of the health of a community"(ANA, 1980, p. 11). These are accomplished through what are referred to as "two major modes or roles" (ANA, 1980, p. 11). The first mode is the direct care of individuals, families, and groups in a specified community; in the second mode the community is the client. It is interesting that the direct care mode is discussed first as opposed to the second mode, which is more consistent with historical understanding of public health practice.

A contribution of the conceptual model is the attempt to distinguish between nurses who function in community settings (generalists) and specialists in community health nursing. However, serious limitations include the emphasis given the clinical focus, the lack of an in-depth treatment of the second mode (which it could be argued should have been the focus of the statement), and the resultant failure to clearly identify what differentiates community health nursing from other specialty areas. The statement's declaration that "the distinguishing characteristic of community health nursing is primary health care, with emphasis on prevention of illness and promotion in maintaining and restoring maximum health" (ANA, 1980, p. 13) does little to set community health nursing apart from other nursing specialty areas.

Community Nurse Practitioner

A different conceptualization of community health nursing is reflected in descriptions of the community health nurse practitioner. The term *community nurse practitioner* is sometimes used to refer to nurses who work with individuals and families in providing direct care services outside of institutional settings, as was the case in the paper by de Tornyay (1980) cited earlier. Use of the term in the present discussion is different and refers to a role first developed in the early 1970s by faculty members associated with the School of Public Health at the University of Texas (Skrovan et al., 1974). The intent of the master's level program at the University of Texas was to develop a nursing role in which the nurse would focus on the community as the client. The approach was innovative and had a number of positive features.

A major strength was the serious effort to translate into practice terms the community component of community health nursing that was so seriously neglected in many other programs during that period. As stated by the program's originators, "it is the emphasis upon community self-help and the focusing upon the health of the total community as one's caresphere which differentiates the CNP role from others today" (Skrovan et al, 1974, p. 849). Much attention was placed on determining health care needs and priorities from the perspective of the community and working with the community to develop acceptable and effective approaches to the problem. Philosophically, the approach to make operational the community component was based on understanding community development processes as a foundation for working with communities. Students were prepared to assess communities through observation, participation in various action groups, and use of secondary data sources; work with community members as facilitators and collaborators in the formulation of health-related goals and plans for implementation; and monitor and evaluate progress with appropriate feedback to the community (Skrovan et al., 1974).

At the end of the grant period the community nurse practitioner training program at the School of Public Health was phased out; however, the key idea of developing a master's level practitioner with a clear focus on working with communities to improve health status did not die and has been adopted in varying degrees by several other graduate programs (Flynn et al., 1978; Goeppinger, 1979, Woods and Ohlson, 1977).

CONFUSION AND FERMENT REGARDING THE FOCUS OF COMMUNITY HEALTH NURSING PRACTICE

The central distinguishing feature of the two conceptualizations of community health nursing just discussed is the clear effort on the part of those who worked with the community health nurse practitioner role to focus on making operational what it means to have the community as a client. Such an effort is clearly differentiated from simply providing nursing service in a community setting. A commonality of both conceptualizations is that emphasis is placed on a practitioner orientation as opposed to considering managerial and administrative components.

The effort to develop a community nurse practitioner program, to facilitate such practice, and to see the outcomes that have followed from that original endeavor represents some of the most interesting and refreshing developments in the field of community health nursing. Yet the attempt to implement the community focus in practice has been extraordinarily difficult for many who have adopted such an agenda. In struggling with the basic idea of community as client, which underlies the community nurse practitioner role, the following questions have been repeatedly asked by faculty members associated with the program, other faculty members in the schools who may have serious doubts about the program, students, and service personnel:

To what extent should the community nurse practitioner have a direct care clinical role?

Should preparation for the role include those direct care assessment and management skills associated with other practitioner roles, such as the family nurse practitioner or the pediatric nurse practitioner?

If advanced preparation in the direct care role is to be provided, will there be sufficient time in a master's curriculum for the development of the community skills?

Is a conceptualization of community health nursing with emphasis on skills such as community development a focus that nursing should adopt?

Can other groups provide such services?

Where does a community nurse practitioner fit into the present delivery system?

These questions and others that accompany efforts to develop roles similar to the community nurse practitioner can be seen as reflective of the present ferment and confusion surrounding community health nursing. This confusion has a number of facets, such as perplexity regarding how this specialty is distinct from other areas of nursing practice, the lack of clarity regarding what it means to have a community focus for practice, and the ambivalence many nurses who identify with community nursing have about moving from a direct care orientation to dealing with the concept of population groups or aggregates.*

Ferment in the field of community health nursing is evident from the meetings in which community health nursing is a topic for discussion and by the fact that two national organizations, the American Public Health Association (1981) and the Community Health Nursing Division of the American Nurses' Association (1980), have felt it necessary to develop position statements to clarify the scope of the specialty. However, the lack of consistency in the content of the two statements has led to further debate. Although there is confusion about the nature of community health nursing, both of the statements and many leaders in the field agree that community health nursing is a synthesis of public health and nursing. This agreement, however, does not greatly further our understanding because there is considerable variability about what the area of overlap means in conceptual and practice terms. In other words, there seems to be little agreement on what counts as an example of the synthesis.

*The terms *population, population groups,* and *aggregates* are used interchangeably.

Population-focused Community Health Nursing

What is special about the speciality of community health nursing? A review of current community health nursing textbooks, the content of community health nursing program meetings, discussions with colleagues, and observations of those defined as community health nursing specialists might lead to the conclusion that the synthesis is represented by the setting in which nursing care is provided. Such settings are predominantly outside the hospital, but not all settings outside hospitals are considered (e.g., not usually included are the private offices of physicians). Thus the characteristic of location has been frequently used as a distinguishing feature, as have family focus, preventive orientation, and concern with the environment (social, cultural, biological, and physical) of the client (individual or family). Not only do such characteristics fail to distinguish community health nursing from other specializations in nursing, as other nursing groups are increasingly encompassing such factors in their definitions of practice, but most importantly such distinctions also ignore the essence of community health practice, a focus on the health of population groups.

Elsewhere it has been argued that the primary focus of community health nursing practice should be on defining problems (assessment) and proposing solutions (treatment) for population groups or aggregates (Williams, 1981). Such a focus entails decision making that is categorically different from the decisions nurses and other direct care providers have been prepared to make in the process of giving direct care to individuals or families. In other words, basic professional education in nursing, medicine, and other clinical disciplines focuses primarily on developing competence in decision making at the level of the individual client—assessing health status, making management decision (ideally with the client), and evaluating the effects of care. This is at the level of the individual X's, O's, and Y's in Fig. 35-1. Little attention is given to defining problems and proposing solutions at the population or subpopulation level, the groups of X's, O's, and Y's in Fig. 35-1. Population level decision making is different from that which occurs in clinical care. For example, in a clinical direct care situation the clinician may determine if a client is hypertensive and if so explore with the person options for intervention. At the population level the questions are different and might include the following:

What is the prevalence of hypertension among various age, race, and sex groups?

Which subpopulations have the highest rates of untreated hypertension?

What programmatic options are there for reducing the problem of untreated hypertension and thereby lowering the risk of further cardiovascular morbidity and mortality?

It is suggested that the fundamental factor that should distinguish community health nursing from other specialties in nursing is a population focus. Not only is a population focus historically consistent with community health philosophy but it is necessary if one is to deal with community nursing needs in a scientific manner. It is therefore gratifying that the population focus is in accord with the definition of community health nursing developed by the Public Health Nursing Section and officially adopted by the American Public

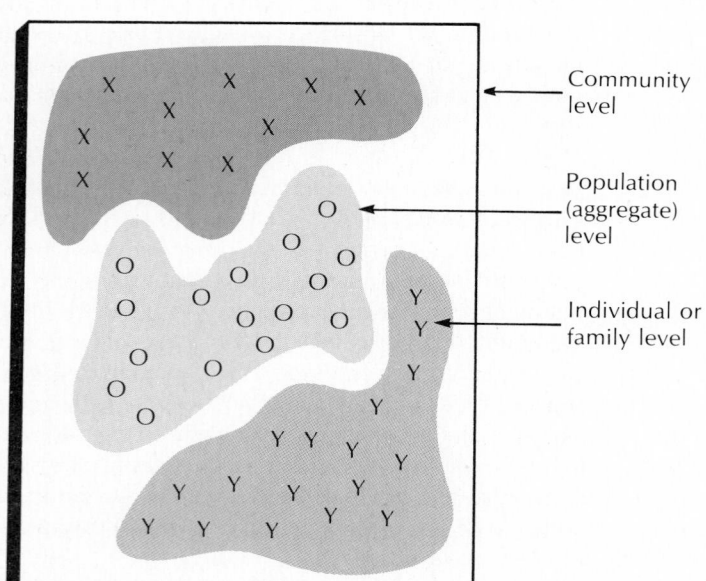

Community level

Population (aggregate) level

Individual or family level

Fig. 35-1. Levels of practice.

Health Association (APHA) (1981). That statement defines the goal of community health nursing as "improving the health of the entire community" (p. 4). Of particular significance to this discussion is the following quote from the APHA statement: "Identifying subgroups (aggregates) within the population which are at high risk of illness, disability, or premature death and directing resources toward these groups is the most effective approach for accomplishing the goal of public health nursing" (p. 4).

Meaning of a Population Focus

At this point it may be useful to elaborate on the meaning of the term *population*. A basic definition of population is a collection of individuals who share in common one or more personal or environmental characteristics. Thus those who are members of a community defined either in terms of geography or special interests can be seen as constituting a population or an aggregate. Frequently it is useful to move beyond a broad understanding of population and identify subpopulations within the larger group. Examples include high risk infants under 1 year, unmarried pregnant adolescents, and school age children. The groups of X's, O's, and Y's in Fig. 35-1 are meant to denote such subpopulations.

It is important to recognize that the specialty of community health nursing involves more than a focus on one subpopulation. Although individual professionals and some agencies or other health organizations may limit their attention to one subpopulation, those concerned with the health of a given community must ultimately give attention to the health of many subpopulations. Therefore specialization in community health nursing necessitates attention to multiple and sometimes overlapping subpopulations. Further, in contrast to the usual clinical approach, a population focus requires that community health specialists not limit their concern to individuals who seek care but extend attention to those who may need particular services and who are not in the care system (e.g., untreated hypertensive patients [Williams and Highriter, 1978]).

Population-focused Practice: a Must for Scientific Community Health Nursing

No one would want to have as a primary care provider an individual (e.g., a family nurse practitioner) who makes recommendations regarding therapy without first obtaining information from the client. A minimum assessment should include data on health status, characteristics of life-style, and preferences regarding the management of identified problems. No less should be expected when the client is the community. To obtain information, that is valued and provides a clear picture of the status of the community, one must take a population focus. For example, looking only at the health status of those clients who happen to come to a particular clinic is likely to produce a biased, unrepresentative picture of the community's health status.

A systematic process analogous to what is referred to in clinical nursing as the *nursing process* should be used in making assessment and management (programming) decisions regarding the community's health status. However, the process has two major differences. First, rather than an individual (an X, O, or Y in Fig. 35-1), the unit of analysis is a population or perhaps several subpopulations (a group of X's, O's, and Y's as in Fig. 35-1). Second, the type of data obtained and the sources are different. In other words, rather than directly obtaining information through one's own assessment of a client, the nurse may have to use data gathered by others. Examples include the use of vital statistics and data gathered in surveys. Or if the nurse does actually gather data, they are not only obtained on one individual but from all people in the population on a representative sample, and the data are obtained in a systematic and consistent manner.

A scientific approach to community health nursing practice requires that assessment and management decisions be based on solid data obtained through the use of objective techniques. Two types of information are necessary. One type is generally referred to as the *body of knowledge* or the epidemiology of a given problem and represents what is know about specified health problems and potential solutions. Included in this body of knowledge is information on etiological factors, groups at highest risk, and treatment methods and their relative effectiveness. This type of information, usually obtained from the literature, has been generated by basic epidemiological studies; community health nursing research; and research in clinical nursing, clinical medicine, and other fields.

The second type of information must be obtained from the populations in the community of interest and is usually more difficult to obtain than the first type. Information on the community should include demographic data, the health status of various subpopulations, the services given to defined subpopulations, and the effectiveness of the services. Ideally, for community health nursing to be scientific, there should be ongoing mechanisms for assessment at the population level, which are systematic, objective, and would allow a continuing surveillance of both the population's health status and the services given. Such surveillance would be analogous to the monitoring of an individual client but should include the entire population and not be limited to those who seek care (Williams and Highriter, 1978). An excellent example of such an approach to surveillance, developed by community nursing specialists, is the computerized monitoring information system for high-risk infants in the Gaston County Health Department, in North Carolina. Through the use of birth certificates of infants possessing a selected group of high-risk characteristics, the nursing unit of the health department defines a target population. All infants who meet the criteria for high risk are entered into the system and monitored for information about health status and services rendered. The system is set up to expect information on each infant at ages 3, 6, 12, and 24 months, and if data are not submitted at the appropriate times, the names of those infants who may need to be located are printed out. In addition to providing for the tracking of individual infants who are members of the target population, this system allows for the generation of population-level data. Examples of the latter include the proportion of infants born in a specified time period who are receiving care from the health department and the proportion receiving care from private physicians; the proportion of infants cared for by the health department who received initial DPT injections by 3 months of age; and the proportion (and names) of infants who have a specified deviation from the norm (e.g., low hemoglobin or underweight). A fuller description of this pacesetting project can be found in Highriter (1981).

If a population focus is taken seriously and strategies for implementing assessment, intervention, and evaluation activities at the population level are considered carefully, the nurse must think of organized approaches. The one-to-one care of individual clients by clinicians is a necessary part of any care system that deals with a population or subpopulation. However, with a population focus the emphasis should be on the interrelationship between the health status of the population, factors that influence health status, and the responses and effectiveness of the care system in dealing with the population's health. Therefore community health nursing specialists who adopt a population focus should have the following as priority practice responsibilities: developing and maintaining organized mechanisms for the provision of care to defined populations; collaborating with clients in the identification of needs and the development of solutions; participating actively in system-level decisions; and influencing other decision makers to enable such development.

Adoption of this understanding of community health nursing has an important implication for the specialty. For such practice to take firm root it is necessary for more community health nurses to be at high level positions in structures within the community that have the authority and funding to provide such ser-

vices. Though roles like the community nurse practitioner may be viable ones, additional attention must be given to the development of nurses with high-level management skills—nurses who can be involved in the decisions associated with top echelon leadership—"developing policy, setting priorities, allocating resources, and modifying and manipulating organizational structure" (Milbank, 1976, p. 39). Many of the roles nurses currently occupy in organizations are at lower levels at which policy making is limited and carrying out policy is emphasized.

BARRIERS, DILEMMAS, AND CHALLENGES

Barriers to Acceptance of Population-focused Community Health Nursing

There are several barriers that mitigate against the fuller development of population-focused community health nursing. Perhaps one of the most serious is the "mind set" of many nurses that the proper role for a nurse is at the bedside or at the client's side, the direct care role. Clearly, the heart of nursing is the direct care provided in personal contacts with clients. On the other hand, two things should be clear to the observant nurse. The first is that whether a nurse is able to provide direct care services to a given client is contingent on a number of decisions on the part of individuals within and without the care system, and second, nursing needs to be involved in those fundamental decisions. Perhaps the one-to-one focus of nursing and the cultural expectation of the "proper role" of women has influenced nursing's hesitancy in viewing positively more indirect modes of contributing, such as administration, consultation, and research. Unfortunately, this mind set on the part of many nurses is reinforced and adopted by others.

A case in point is a recent discussion of the roles of the community nurse and the community physician presented in a monograph by Kark (1981) on community-oriented primary health care. In that discussion community nurses were described as having major clinical roles in a unified practice of community medicine and primary health care. Not only were comments made about their direct care roles in the community setting but it was mentioned also that their roles should go beyond the nurse-client relationship to include skills in community diagnosis and action directed to meeting community health problems. All the comments were positive; however, it was interesting that in the discussion of community physicians there was a clear indication that community physicians would assume a major responsibility for community diagnosis and evaluation of health care. Because of this major responsibility, it was stated that physicians would need to have preparation in the principles and methods of epidemiology and its use in primary care. There was absolutely no comment about the need for nurses to have such preparation. The clear implication is that physicians would assume leadership in the scientific aspects of making operational the community-oriented primary care being described.

What Kark stated I observed in a World Health Organization sponsored tour of selected service and educational settings in Great Britain. In the British system the practice of community medicine has developed into a specialty for physicians with specific training programs that include strong components in biostatistics/epidemiology (Acheson, 1976). In contrast, community nursing is conceptualized in direct care terms (i.e., health visitors, district nurses, and nurses attached to general practitioners' practices). The distinction between what nurses do in relation to community diagnosis, programming, and evaluation and what the community physicians do is quite apparent.

In 1972 the Royal Colleges of Physicians of London, Glasgow, and Edinburgh established a Faculty of Community Medicine that defined community medicine as "that branch of medicine which deals with populations or groups rather than individual patients" (Jagdish, 1978, p. 54). Further, the faculty identified that this specialty required specific knowledge in the following areas: epidemiology, ". . . the organization and evaluation of medical care systems . . . the medical aspects of the administration of health services," and health education and rehabilitation techniques from ". . . the field of social and preventive medicine" (Jagdish, 1978, p. 54).

In the reorganized National Health Service of Great Britain, physicians have key leadership roles at each administrative level (regional health authorities and districts), and they receive formal preparation in the scientific aspects of practice at the population level. Nurses also have leadership roles at each organizational level, but there is no comparable effort to prepare them for practice at the population level.

Another barrier to the type of practice implied in population-focused community health nursing is the structures within which nurses work and the process of role socialization that occurs within those structures. The fact that a particular role might not exist within the nursing unit may suggest that it is undesirable or impossible for nurses. For example, nurses interested in using political strategies to effect changes in health-related policy, an activity clearly within the practice domain of community health nursing, may run into a number of barriers if their goals disrupt the agendas of other groups within the health care arena. Such groups may use subtle but effective maneuvers to lead nurses to conclude that involvement takes them from the client and is not in their own or the client's best interests.

There is also the barrier of relatively few nurses receiving graduate level preparation in the concepts and strategies of disciplines basic to community health (e.g., epidemiology, biostatistics, community development, service administration, and policy formation). One of the problems mentioned earlier in the discussion on the community health nurse practitioner, which continues to be a problem in master's level preparation for community health nursing, is that in many programs the skills necessary for population assessment and management are not given the in-depth treatment accorded other components of the curriculum, particularly the direct care aspects. In short, with few exceptions within the graduate programs in community health nursing there is no aggressive effort to develop population-focused skills commensurate with the need. The bias of many nurses seems to be that these skills are less important than clinical skills. However, these skills are as essential as direct care skills; they are just as difficult to develop and they should be given more attention in community health nursing graduate programs.

In discussing population-focused skills, selected analytical and measurement skills from the disciplines of epidemiology and biostatistics as they relate to population surveillance and programming for the delivery of personal health services are especially important. It must be clarified that epidemiological and biostatistical skills represent only two of many important skills for population-focused community health practice. A 1976 report of the Milbank Memorial Fund Commission on Higher Education for Public Health suggested that there were three elements that were central and generic to public health: ". . . the measurement and *analytical* sciences of epidemiology and biostatistics; social policy and the history and philosophy of public health; and the principles of management and organization for public health" (Milbank, 1976, p. 74-75). Noticeably absent from this general list is a clear identification of community development processes cited in the discussion of the community nurse practitioner. The issue is not to enumerate all of the areas that might be important to population-focused practice but rather to focus attention on the reality that those concerned about the future of community health should place more effort on developing community health nursing specialists with advanced skills in one or more of these arenas. Unless such attention is given, the lack of knowledge and skills represents a serious barrier to further development of the specialty.

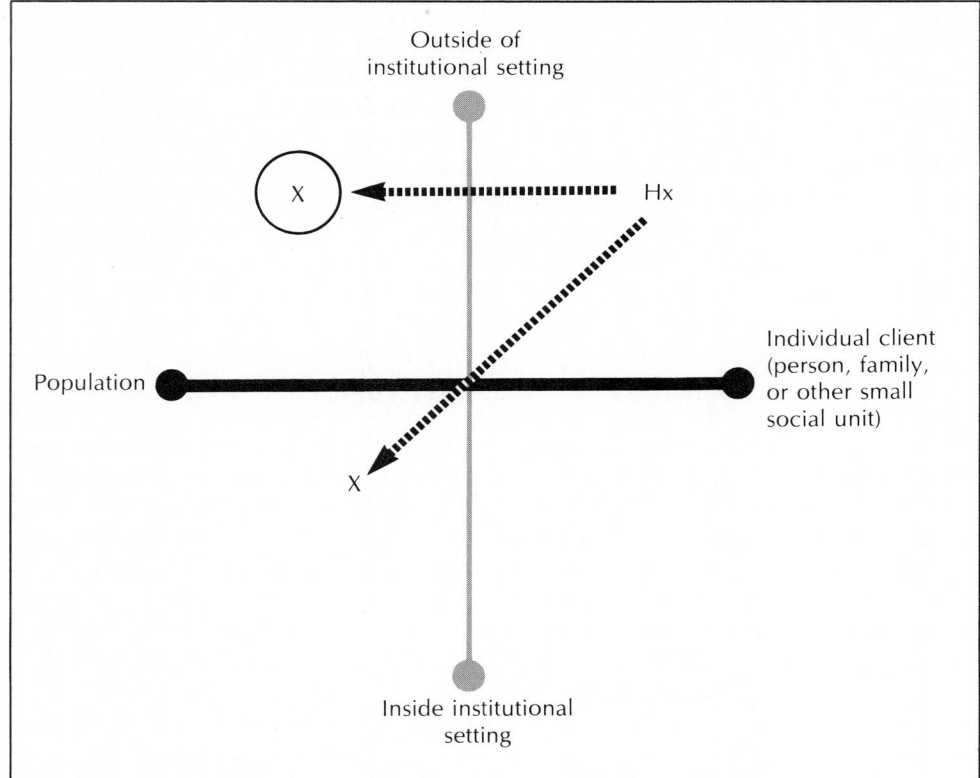

Fig. 35-2. Arenas for practice.

Dilemmas and Challenges from Acceptance of Population-focused Community Health Nursing
What is the Arena for Practice?

If the premise is accepted that the distinctive feature of community health nursing is a focus on populations and the interplay between the health status of populations and other characteristics of the community, an important question is whether the only populations that should be considered are those outside of institutional settings. To answer "no" to this question implies that all of nursing practice can be subsumed under community health nursing practice. Although this might not appear to be a satisfactory conclusion for those who do not define themselves as community health nursing specialists, a broad understanding of community health should include all populations within the community. Further, a broad approach should also consider the match between the health needs of the population and the health care resources in the community, including services offered in institutional settings. Such an understanding was adopted by the British Health System with the 1974 reorganization.

However, to say that all populations and health-related services within a geographically defined community should be of concern to community health specialists is not to say that everybody who provides direct care services within a community is a community health specialist. All direct care providers may contribute in their individual ways to the community's health in the broad sense, but not all are primarily concerned with the population focus, the big picture. Thus all nurses in a given community, including those in hospitals, physicians' offices, and health clinics, should theoretically be contributing positively to the health of the community. However, the special contribution of the community health specialists is to look at the community as a whole and raise questions about its overall health status and factors associated with that status.

The prevalent view of community health nursing at present and historically has been to provide direct care services, including health education, to persons or family units outside of institutional settings. Such practice falls into the upper right quadrant in Fig. 35-2, where the Hx appears. To adopt the arguments made earlier for population-focused practice would mean at least that community health nursing should be moving toward the upper left quadrant, a population focus outside of institutional settings. What about populations within institutional settings? Should population approaches be considered there? Would the nursing services of a given hospital be more appropriately developed if systematic mechanisms were in place to identify clinical subpopulations with particular nursing needs and target services to those subpopulations? Are some of the assessment and management decisions analogous to those necessary in dealing with subpopulations outside of institutional settings? Clearly, there are important conceptual, analytical, and methodological commonalities between noninstitutional populations and those within institutions. A key example is the common need for computerized information systems.

Within the field of epidemiology there is an emerging subdiscipline that attracts mainly physicians who identify themselves as clinical epidemiologists and who concentrate on subpopulations within clinical settings. In working with these clinical populations, the same epidemiological strategies are applied as are used with free-living populations more traditionally associated with epidemiology, the difference is in the questions being pursued.

Should the specialty of community health nursing claim as its arena for practice a population focus regardless of where the population is located? An affirmative response makes more sense than a negative one particularly in terms of the knowledge and skills needed for decision-making versus the way health services are currently organized within the United States. Thus the argument could be made that when responsibilty for population-focused decisions regarding nursing needs is assumed, the nurse is practicing in the arena of community health nursing. In Fig. 35-2 this is represented by the upper and lower left quadrants. There are, however, three reasons the upper left quadrant should be the most important practice arena for community health nursing.

First, in dealing with noninstitutionalized populations, which represent the majority of a community most of the time, preventive strategies can have the greatest impact. Second, the major interface between health status and the environment (physical, biological, sociocultural) occurs in the noninstitutional population. Third, for philosophical, historical, and economic reasons it is in organizational structures that serve noninstitutionalized populations (health departments, health maintenance organizations, health centers, etc.) that population-focused practice is most likely to flourish.

Is It Useful to Talk about the "Role" of the Community Health Nurse?

Within community nursing circles there has been quite a tendency to talk about community health nursing from the point of view of a role, such as the public health nursing role or the community health nursing specialist. This is viewed as limiting for two reasons. First, in discussing such roles there is an enormous preoccupation with a provider orientation. Even in discussions about how a population perspective can be made operational in practice, it is most interesting that the focus is frequently on how an individual practitioner, such as a staff nurse in an agency, can adopt such a practice focus. Rarely is attention given to how nurse administrators might reorient their practice to be concerned with a population focus, which is more critical, useful, and possible for an administrator than for the staff nurse. This is because in many agencies nursing administrators, supervisors, or others (sometimes program directors who are not nurses) make the key decisions about how staff nurses will spend their time—what types of clients will be seen and under what circumstances. It can be asked to what extent such decisions are based on the types of data described earlier.

With regard to administrators it is suggested that those who are prepared to practice in a population-focused manner are more effective than those who are not prepared. Further, staff nurses would benefit from having a clear understanding of population-focused practice for three reasons. First, it would give them professional satisfaction in being able to put their own clinical activities into perspective, to see how what they do clinically contributes at the population level. Second, it would help them understand and appreciate the practice of their associates who are population-focused specialists. Third, it would give them a firmer basis for providing clinical input to decision making at the programmatic or agency level, necessary contribution to effective and efficient population-focused practice. Clearly it is desirable that staff nurses have a population focus, but the reality is that their ability to make decisions at that level is more limited than that of the nurse with some administrative responsibility.

Another problem with thinking in terms of roles, particularly in terms of those occupied by nurses, is that present role conceptualizations are frequently too limited to allow for population-focused practice. Also, roles that might include the type of decision making being suggested may not be defined as nursing roles. Examples of the latter include directorships of health departments, state or regional programs, and units of health planning and evaluation. If population-focused community health nursing is to be taken seriously and strategies for its implementation (assessment, intervention, and evaluation) at the population level are to be applied, more consideration must be given to organized systems for assessing population needs and managing care. Such a view of community health nursing clearly places those who specialize in this area in the position of dealing with health care policy. In other words, community health nurses must move into situations in which policy formation is a recognized component, but to do so some may have to assume positions outside of what is usually thought of as a nursing position or a nursing role. This is true because at present much of the policy making that directly affects whether nursing services are provided to certain populations and what services are rendered occurs outside of the range of what are normally referred to as *nursing roles.*

Too much attention on defining nursing roles, particularly defining them in such a manner that they would fit into the present way of structuring nursing services, may have unfortunate limitations. For the immediate future it may be more useful to concentrate on the identification of skills and knowledge necessary for the type of decision making suggested as being inherent in population-focused practice. The question can be raised of where in the broader community and health care system such decisions are made and given the answers, the strategy should be to develop nurses with the substantive knowledge, skills, and political finesse necessary for success in such positions. Some of these positions are within nursing settings, particularly roles such as the administrator of the nursing service and top level staff nurse administrators, but as suggested earlier, other such positions may be outside of what are traditionally viewed as nursing roles.

Can a Viable Balance Be Achieved between Clinical and Population-focused Skills in Graduate Preparation?

Whether or not a balance between clinical and population-focused skills can be achieved is a question that community health nursing educators and service people have asked in contemplating a more serious effort in developing aggregate and community skills, as was undertaken in the community nurse practitioner program discussed earlier. There are several issues that need to be considered in dealing with this question. First, there is the issue of appropriate preparation. Second, there is the question of what is possible in the practice world following preparation, discussed in part earlier.

To date most of the discussion regarding preparation for community health nursing has been limited to thinking in terms of baccalaureate and master's level presentation. One of the definite problems with present-day master's preparation is the fact that there is not sufficient emphasis in most curricula to lead to an in-depth understanding and reasonable level of skill in those areas basic to population-focused practice. Much of this has been the result of the fact that master's programs in community health nursing have tried to include a component of direct care. In only a few exceptions has there been a strong emphasis on population-focused skills. If master's level programming concentrated on such a perspective, and started with students who were well prepared at the undergraduate level and experienced in direct care, it would be possible to go further in the development of population skills. Clearly master's programs might be profitably strengthened by refocusing objectives, but such developments should not detract from the serious attention that must be given to doctoral study as a basis for the further development of community health nursing practice.

Doctoral work could be concentrated in one of the areas identified by the Milbank report (1976) cited earlier. With regard to the health assessment of populations and the evaluation of outcomes, there is a high level of congruence between the skills necessary for such functions and research skills, for which there is wide consensus that doctoral study is essential. This should not be taken to mean that all assessment and evaluation activities of community health nursing specialists should be viewed as research; the objectives are different, but the knowledge and skills necessarily overlap to a high degree, particularly in the use of content from epidemiology and biostatistics. It is important to remember that the use of such skills in population-focused practice has as its primary objective obtaining a sound knowledge base of the population being served as opposed to a primary concern of developing generalized knowledge, the goal of research. There are some circumstances in which both goals can be met, and a challenge for the future is to work toward creating more of them.

Achievement of a balance between preparation, advanced clinical skills, and population-focused skills should not be an objective of a graduate program in community health nursing. At the graduate level a choice needs to be made so that advanced preparation in one area does not suffer at the expense of the other. Those who want graduate preparation in both areas should consider two separate programs of study. For example, a sequence that may become increasingly familiar is a clinical master's (direct care–focused) and a population-focused doctorate.

SUMMARY

Arguments for population-focused community health nursing have been offered, and it has been suggested that preparation for practice would include graduate study in areas such as epidemiology, biostatistics, community development, policy formation, and administration. Further, the relationship between the type of position held in an organizational structure and the potential to practice with a population focus has been discussed. The central point is that those in administrative roles in settings providing personal care services make decisions affecting aggregates or populations; thus population-focused community health nursing is more directly relevant and applicable to their situation. Such administrators would profit from being prepared to practice in a population-focused manner and from having staff associates who are also prepared (e.g., specialists in planning, evaluation, and community development).

In view of the previous comments, the question of how baccalaureate level preparation fits in can be raised, and there are various opinions on this topic. One is that at the baccalaureate level there ought to be two types of learning objectives. First, undergraduate students ought to be introduced to the earlier mentioned key concepts and strategies of the disciplines basic to community health. Second, baccalaureate students ought to be provided opportunities to understand how (a) decision making on the part of those responsible for population-level decisions differs from clinical decisions made by individual providers but (b) influences the latter in a variety of ways (i.e., population-focused decisions determine what kinds of providers are hired, nurse practitioner or physician, what patients can be seen; what range of services are offered; and in what type of settings).

A key distinction between the focus of preparation at the baccalaureate level as opposed to the intent of master's and doctoral preparation is that preparation at the baccalaureate level should be directed to providing beginning insight into what population-focused practice is—its benefits and some understanding of the knowledge and skills necessary for such practice. Preparing graduates to assume primary responsibilities as community health nursing specialists should be left to graduate programs.

For several reasons it is important to emphasize that undergraduate programs introduce students to population-focused practice. First, as professionals, all baccalaureate graduates entering first-level staff positions should have an appreciation of the context of their practice—how what they do as clinicians relates to the populations served by the settings in which they work. Second, such preparation should facilitate a better understanding of the reciprocal relationship that is desirable between direct care clinicians and population-focused specialists. Such reciprocity might lead to better collaboration and more effective and efficient nursing services. Finally, a good foundation in community health nursing at the undergraduate level can be extremely important in attracting students to this practice specialty. Without such preparation they might be lost to other areas of specialization.

BIBLIOGRAPHY

Acheson, R.M.: Epidemiology: the training of community physicians in Great Britain. In White, K.L., and Henderson, M.M., editor: Epidemiology as a fundamental science, New York, 1976, Oxford University Press, Inc.

American Nurses' Association, Division on Community Health Nursing: Conceptual model of community health nursing, Pub. No. CH-10, Kansas City, Mo., 1980, The Association.

American Public Health Association: The definition and role of public health nursing in the delivery of health care: a statement of the public health nursing section, Washington, D.C., 1981, The Association.

deTornyay, R.: Public health nursing: the nurse's role in community-based practice, Annu. Rev. Public Health 1:83, 1980.

Flynn, B.C., et al.: One master's curriculum in community health nursing, Nurs. Outlook 26:633, 1978.

Goeppinger, J.: Community health nursing: primary nursing care in society. In Flynn, B.C., and Miller, M.H., editor: Current perspectives in nursing, II, St. Louis, 1979, The C.V. Mosby Co.

Highriter, M.E.: A computerized nursing management information system for identification and community follow-up of high-risk infants. In Werley, H.H. and Grier M.R. editors: Nursing information systems, New York, 1981, Springer Publishing Co., Inc.

Jagdish, V.: Community medicine in the British National Health Service, Am. J. Public health 68:54, 1978.

Kark, S.L.: The practice of community-oriented primary health care, New York, 1981, Appleton-Century-Crofts.

Milbank Memorial Fund: Commission on higher education for public health, (Cecil G. Sheps, Chairman), New York, 1976, Prodist.

Skrovan, C., Anderson, E.T., and Gottschalk, J.: Community nurse practitioner, an emerging role, Am. J. Public Health 64:847, 1974.

Williams, C.A.: Nursing leadership in community health: a neglected issue. In McCloskey, J.C., and Grace, H.K., editors: Current issues in nursing, Oxford, England, 1981, Blackwell Scientific Publications, Ltd.

Williams, C. A., and Highriter, M.E.: Community health nursing: population focus and evaluation, Public health Reviews 7:197, 1978.

Woods, J., and Ohlson, V.: Graduate preparation for community nursing practice. In Flynn, B.C., and Miller, M.H., editors: Current perspectives in nursing: social issues and trends, St. Louis, 1977, The C.V. Mosby Co.

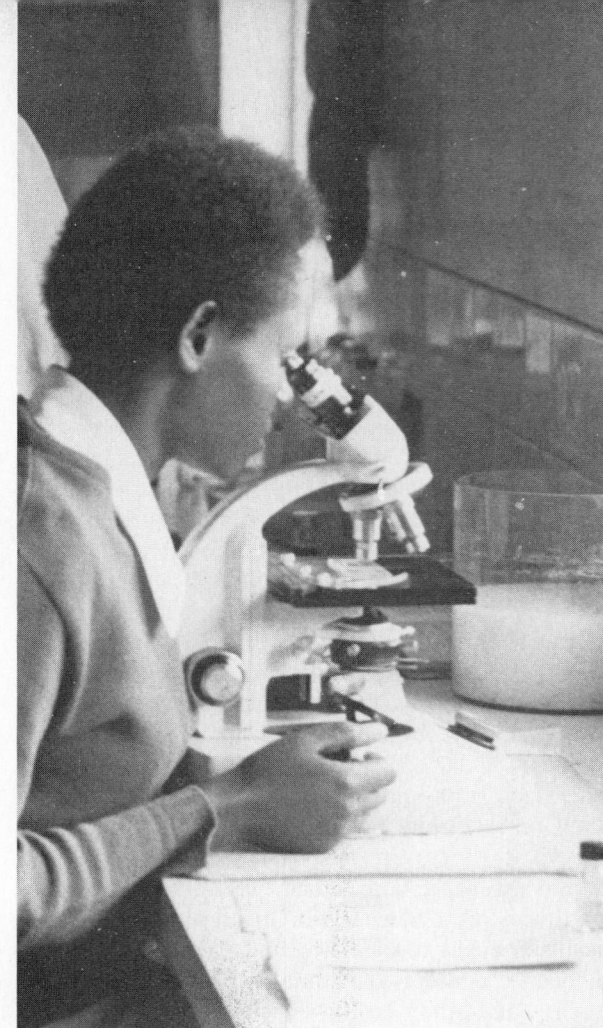

Chapter 36

BEVERLY FLYNN

RESEARCH AS A GUIDE TO COMMUNITY HEALTH NURSING PRACTICE

The need for research in nursing has been clearly documented for over 30 years (Taylor, 1975). Although increasing efforts are devoted to nursing research, only recently have nurses tried to examine the applicability of research findings to practice. Many studies in nursing do not meet the criteria for scientific research. Furthermore, the findings of relatively few studies have actually been used in clinical practice (Highriter, 1977, Horsley and Pelz, 1979). Barriers to involvement by nurses in research-related activities have been cited, for example, heavy work loads, lack of access to research expertise, and lack of funding to support these activities (Horsley and Pelz, 1979). In addition, many studies in community health nursing research have been found to lack a community-oriented approach (Highriter, 1977). It is no wonder that much practice in nursing, let alone community health nursing practice, remains largely intuitive, based on tradition rather than on a search for creative, scientifically oriented solutions to health and nursing problems facing the population today.

This chapter focuses on selected issues surrounding community health nursing research and offers possible solutions to many of the problems identified. The author proposes that primary health care as defined by the World Health Organization (WHO and UNICEF, 1978) is an appropriate approach that can guide research in community health nursing. An examination of the major concepts of primary health care suggests to the investigator key research questions relevant to practice. Selected conceptual and methodological considerations will be presented here as well as the roles and functions of the researcher and others.

DEFINITIONS

Over the last several years considerable attention has been given to the definitions of community health nursing and primary health care. Since there are varied approaches to these terms, their use in this chapter will need to be clarified.

Community Health Nursing

In 1980 three separate nursing organizations prepared statements on the definition of community health nursing or public health nursing (American Nurses' Association, 1980; American Public Health Association, 1980; Association of State and Territorial Directors of Nursing, 1980). Although important differences exist among the definitions (discussion of which is beyond the scope of this chapter), they contain a common core of elements. Community health nursing is focused on improving the health of the entire community. Primary prevention and health promotion are the foundations of practice that is directed at working with groups, families, and individuals within the context of the total population or community. Integral to the practice is the involvement of community residents and health and health-related professionals from varied disciplines in jointly seeking solutions to complex health concerns facing communities today. Health is viewed broadly, incorporating environmental, social, political and other factors affecting health status. The problem-solving approach is applied to the community in assessing community strengths and problems, planning strategies of intervention, and implementing and evaluating these strategies.

Primary Health Care

The concept of primary health case is not new. However, it has greatly different meanings in different contexts. (Refer to Chapter 2 for a discussion of the relationship between primary, secondary, and tertiary

The work presented in this paper was conducted under an American Nurses' Foundation Competitive grant, entitled "Primary Health Care: A Research Framework," in which the author was an American Journal of Nursing Company Scholar for 1981-1982. The author wishes to thank Eugene Selmanoff, Associate Professor, Department of Community Health Nursing, Indiana University School of Nursing, Indianapolis, for his helpful comments and suggestions on the final draft of this paper.

health care for individuals.) The meaning that is presented here is the approach to achieving the WHO goal of "health for all by the year 2000," endorsed by all member states and given in a joint report by WHO and UNICEF (1978, p. 16):

> Primary health care is essential health care based on practical, scientifically sound and socially acceptable methods and technology made universally accessible to individuals and families in the community through their full participation and at a cost that the community and country can afford to maintain at every stage of their development in the spirit of self-reliance and self-determination. It forms an integral part both of the country's health system, of which it is the central function and main focus, and of the overall social and economic development of the community. It is the first level of contact of individuals, the family and community with the national health system bringing health care as close as possible to where people live and work, and constitutes the first element of a continuing health care process.

Primary health care is a strategy that focuses on the community and individuals and families within it. Health is integrated with community development. There are five key concepts that distinguish this definition from other definitions of primary health care: (1) care is accessible, (2) it involves the community, (3) it focuses on disease prevention and health promotion, (4) it uses appropriate technology, and (5) it uses a multisectoral approach (Walt and Vaughan, 1981).

Relationship of Community Health Nursing to Primary Health Care

The contribution of nursing to the primary health care approach is currently being considered within countries supporting the goal of health for all. In addition, the International Council of Nurses (ICN) and the World Health Organization have taken leadership roles in supporting national nursing associations in their exploration of contributions nursing can make in primary health care (ICN and WHO, 1979; PAHO, 1977; WHO, 1974; WHO, 1982).

There is a link between the view of community health nursing delineated in this chapter and primary health care. Both concepts incorporate community-based practice, involvement of the community in health care decisions, a focus on disease prevention and health promotion, and use of an interdisciplinary approach in planning and implementing appropriate solutions to health problems.

However, the role of nursing in research relevant to primary health care, is a topic that has only been touched on by the world organizations noted earlier. It is suggested here that community health nursing and primary health care are mutually supportive. Based on this premise, it is proposed that community health nursing can also make a significant contribution to research in primary health care.

RESEARCH FOR PRACTICE

Significant research questions can be generated from the key concepts of primary health care. These concepts are useful as a means for classification and generalization, as a beginning conceptual framework. It should be noted that although primary health care is deemed applicable in developed and developing nations, the questions generated here are applicable to the United States, an industrialized country. Similar questions could be generated for the developing world countries, but such examples, although relevant, are beyond the scope of this chapter. Several documents were found useful in the preparation of this discussion (WHO, 1981a; WHO, 1981b, WHO and UNICEF, 1978).

Accessible Health Care

This particular concept is concerned with the accessibility of health services, particularly to those persons who might be considered at the social periphery, e.g., rural, urban, and isolated population groups who are at greatest risk to health problems. The issue here is whether or not the health services are reaching the people who need them the most or whether they are equitably distributed throughout the population.

Research questions that evolve from this concept relate to whether the health services are accessible to those in need. For example, are community health nursing services available in both urban and rural areas? Are these services available to groups of people most in need of the services, in terms of time, location, and personnel? Other questions that could be studied relate to the use of services. For example, who uses and who does not use the community health nursing services? What are their characteristics? What are the health care needs of the people who use the service compared to those who do not? What are the barriers to the use of services, e.g., costs, irrelevance of services to the needs perceived by consumers, or indifference from health professionals to the concerns of consumers?

Community Involvement

This concept of primary health care is concerned with the level of citizen or community resident participation in health decision-making. In promoting the development of the community and, in turn, the community's self-reliance, citizens themselves need to participate in decisions about the health of the community. In primary health care citizens and health and health-re-

lated providers need to work together in a partnership. They each have their own area and level of expertise that are needed in seeking solutions to the complex problems facing communities today.

This concept guides research in attempting to answer questions that relate to the level and mechanism of community involvement in health decision making. For example, to what extent is the community involved in the various stages of assessing health care needs, planning, management, and monitoring community health nursing services? What mechanisms and processes exist to enable people to be actively involved and to take joint responsibility, along with health professionals, for decisions? In particular, what decisions involving the community have been implemented? And are the community health nursing services better utilized as a result?

Focus on Disease Prevention and Health Promotion

Emphasis in primary health care is directed toward health promotion and prevention of disease rather than being focused on curative services. However, in primary health care the curative or therapeutic aspects must often be addressed before health promotion and preventive services can be instituted. People need to have their illness attended to before they can focus their attention on such future-oriented concerns as prevention of further disease or health promotion activities. However, the latter is the major focus in primary health care, according to WHO.

Priority questions for research include the following: Are the major local health problems being addressed by prevention of disease and health promotion measures? What are the major problems in the community that are preventable? What measures are being taken to ameliorate or control these problems? Have these measures reduced the incidence of health problems? How can community health nursing services be reorganized or strengthened to promote health and prevent disease in the population?

Appropriate Technology

Appropriate technology refers to health care that is relevant to people's health needs and concerns as well as being acceptable to them. It includes issues of costs and affordability of services within the context of existing resources, such as the number and type of health professionals and workers, equipment, and supplies and their pattern of distribution throughout the community. The National Science Foundations's definition of appropriate technology (1979, p. 1) summarizes these considerations: ". . . appropriate technologies are defined as those which are decentralized, require low capital investment, conserve natural resources, are managed by their users, and are in harmony with the environment."

The following are the overriding questions to be answered by research: Are the community health nursing services appropriate? Do they address the major local diseases? Do the services use the simplest and cheapest technology necessary? Are the services acceptable to the community? Are they affordable? What is the cost effectiveness of alternative approaches or strategies for community health nursing services? Are nonprofessionals effective in providing some aspects of community health nursing services? What is the most effective management for nonprofessionals and professionals within a primary health care program?

Multisectoral Approach

In primary health care it is recognized that the health of a community cannot be improved by intervention within just the health sector. Other sectors are equally important, and in some cases more so, in promoting the community's health and self-reliance. For example, education, environment, industry, housing, and nutrition are interrelated with health. Therefore, these sectors need to work together in coordinating their goals, plans, and activities to assure that they contribute to the health of the community and to avoid conflicting or duplicating efforts.

Research questions that are relevant here include the following: What mechanisms exist that promote and/or hinder intersectoral collaboration? What are examples of intersectoral efforts in seeking solutions to community problems? Of the successful solutions, how were these decisions arrived at? How are conflicting activities across the various sectors resolved? What are the gaps in efforts across the various sectors in solving community health problems? What can community health nursing do to facilitate joint collaboration in seeking solutions to these problems?

Examples

Selected examples of research studies are presented here to clarify the types of research proposed in this chapter. These studies were selected because they represent the basic concepts of primary health care, involve a community health nurse as an investigator, or have implications for the use of research findings in community health nursing practice.

The first study is a good example of research relevant to questions of accessibility of health care services and appropriate technology. The nursing division of the DuPage County Health Department in Illinois undertook a survey of noninstitutionalized older adults to determine their needs for services (Managan et al., 1974). The study described the elderly in terms of their health condition, physical functioning, accessibility of medical care, social isolation, and service needs. The major problems found were functional impairment, lack of a family physician, and social isolation. The results indicated that there was a 10.8% increase in services needed by the elderly population. The services needed were for intensive case finding, well-adult conferences, and programs providing friendly visitors. The findings were also beneficial in that they provided baseline information for evaluation and planning of future services.

A study by Thompson (1980) addressed research questions related to consumer or citizen involvement, prevention of disease, and appropriate technology. In this investigation the consumer participation process in health care decision was studied. Consumers from three community health centers were interviewed to determine their opinions, attitudes, and perceived knowledge of the consumer participation process in their respective centers. Consumers with a high knowledge level of the participation process were more satisfied with the health centers and reported carrying out more preventive health practices. The findings supported the notation that health is related to what consumers do for themselves rather than to what is done by providers.

The last study was interesting because it related to all the major concepts of primary health care. This was an international survey conducted to determine the relationship between nursing and primary health care (Jaeger-Burns, 1981). Chief nurses from 54 countries participated in the survey. It was found that except for their collaboration with the sanitation sector, nurses did not cooperate with other sectors in promoting improved community health. Nursing faculties were found to be inexperienced in primary health care, and students received little experience in the community. Yet it was also found that nurses were involved in primary health care management and relayed information about community health problems to their health agencies. Also noteworthy was an association between the presence of primary health care nursing in a country and improved health status. These latter findings suggest the relevance of nursing in primary health care and warrant further study.

RESEARCH APPROACH

Two aspects of the research process having implications for primary health care and community health nursing will be highlighted here. One is related to the conceptual underpinnings of research and the other is a type of research—action research.

Conceptual Base for Practice

In addressing many of the research questions noted previously, there is a need to have a clear understanding of the community as a whole. One might reply that it is difficult enough to try to study these complex research questions without giving consideration to the complicated features of the community. However, the primary health care approach emphasizes the conducting of research within the context of the community. Some time ago Diers (1970, p. 52) challenged the profession by claiming such research was possible. She stated that "It is possible to do quite good clinical research if one is deeply enough involved in practice to know what can be controlled and how." Research can assist the practitioner in finding answers to practice issues and in the process help in developing a conceptual base for professional practice.

There is considerable agreement in the nursing literature as to the need for developing a body of knowledge through research relevant to nursing. Dickoff and James (1975) have criticized nursing research for leaving nursing practice virtually untouched. One of the reasons given has been a lack of conceptual clarity and consistency on which research is based.

Some of the difficulties may stem from the approaches used in generating conceptual formulations for research. The favored approach in nursing research has been deductive testing of hypotheses with data that can be quantified. This focus has been dictated by predetermined, logical theoretical considerations rather than by empirical questions or experiences. It may be that the deductive approach is too constraining at this stage of the profession's development.

The alternative approach is the inductive one, focusing on practice problems examined within their own context rather than from some predetermined theoretical or conceptual basis and typically using only qualitative data. In other words, because concepts and theories often have not been generated from the data collected, the conceptual relevance of the data is sometimes missed. In using an inductive approach to begin with, an understanding of the real world more relevant to nursing practice may result. For example, the study of community participation in health care decision making could be appropriately investigated using participant observation and interview data. The concepts generated from the inductive approach would come from the data collected rather that having the results reinterpreted from other theoretical perspectives. In this way new theoretical formulations that are more appropriate to the problem under study may result.

The argument made here is not to abandon one approach in favor of another but to emphasize the benefits of the inductive approach which have not been given adequate attention in nursing research, especially in relation to community health nursing.

The application of the grounded theory methodology has been suggested as a useful inductive approach (Muller and Reynolds, 1978). This method uses empirical data comparisons to generate concepts and hypotheses. It is purported to generate middle-range theory, which can provide a link between more general theory and situations faced by health practitioners. Stern (1980) also has noted the relevance of grounded theory in nursing research.

Action Research

The primary health care approach is based on the premise that desired changes in health are rooted in the community and must involve citizens themselves in the creation of their own future. Research suitable for this approach to health care has been pretty much neglected by the social sciences. However, arising from the community development, health education, and adult education disciplines, action research has been promoted as an appropriate methodology for research relevant to community action. Since primary health care is a form of community action toward achieving the goal of "health for all by the year 2000," the relevance of action research to primary health care will be explored.

Stinson (1979) makes a distinction between research *for* action and research *about* action. He claims that only the latter is action research because action research is about the change in a group rather than research into information areas that can be used by the group for its planned activities. Action research focuses on the process of change in a group or community. Futhermore, in action research, information is fed back into the group and plays an important role in the growth of the group.

Some investigators may challenge this concept of research as contrary to the emphasis on scientific rigor that is stressed in nursing research or social science research in general. However, Diers (1970 p. 52) notes that "research in controlled laboratories has low generality for clinical settings, no matter how rigorous it is."

Participatory Research

Stinson (1979) reviews a number of types of action research; one type, participatory research, has gained the most attention in primary health care. Participatory research stems from the field of adult education, which has been influenced by Freire (1970) and his concern for liberation of people, particularly the oppressed. Freire's efforts are directed at increasing people's ability to participate and gain some degree of control over their own lives. Involving people in all stages of the research process, in itself supports his goal of consciousness raising.

Rahman (1978) sees participatory research as action research directed toward self-reliance. He contends that scholars and scientists also need to be integrated with the rural poor to introduce a consciousness-raising process into research and development. These links will not only advance collective knowledge but also stimulate local effort that relates to a broader movement.

Hall (1975) delineates a number of key principles of participatory research. First of all, the community is involved in all phases of the research process. Second, the research team includes persons representing all components involved in the charge. Third, the research process is part of the educational experience and involves a dialogue over time. Finally, participatory research is aimed at liberating people so that they can creatively reach solutions to social problems.

A good example of participatory research is Feuerstein's report (1978) on the evaluation of health services by the people of Honduras. In this research the people themselves collaborated in all phases of the evaluation. They were able not only to identify the strengths and weaknesses of the program but also to increase these strengths and remedy the weaknesses.

ROLES AND FUNCTIONS IN RESEARCH

Although some of the roles and functions of the researcher are implied in other sections of this chapter, additional aspects are worthy of consideration.

Relationships

The practicing community health nurse may conduct research or more commonly work within an organization with a researcher in carrying out a study. The relationship of the practicing community health nurse, the administrator of these nursing services, and the researcher is one of partnership in a joint endeavor. Partners have their own areas of expertise, yet will benefit from the expertise of the others. The community health nurse is an expert in practice and can identify problems needing to be researched in community work as well as the feasibility of research from this perspective. The administrator is an expert in organizational functioning and can help identify policy issues related to the research and can render organizational support, which is often needed. The researcher, on the other hand, is an expert in the research process and, for example, can help develop practice problems into researchable questions.

In conducting community research relevant to community health nursing practice, another relationship is also important. It pertains to a partnership with the community group concerned with the research problems, that is, participatory research. Citizens, professionals, and other persons interested in the health of the community may identify a priority problem needing research. In this case, persons in the group have expertise about the community, and the researcher and the community health nurse have to work as resources to the group in conducting the research.

Involving others in the research process is not without its problems. Perhaps the most difficult for researchers is the sharing of activities that are usually under their domain. Since primary health care research is occurring in a dynamic setting in which the chief responsibility is often health care (e.g., a neighborhood clinic), priority may not always be given to the research. For example, access to records and files may be controlled by others, and information may be withheld. As a result the research itself may become part of the politics of the situation. Researchers will need to be aware of these dynamics and use their expertise to ensure the research is conducted with proper attention to sound principles of research, yet allow for citizen involvement that will foster use of the results. A clear understanding of the different roles of researcher and citizen will need to be made.

Communication

Whether research involves the community or not, other issues arise which influence the roles and functions in research. One reason often given for the lack of use of research findings in practice is the practitioner's lack of receptivity. This is suggestive of "victim blaming" rather than addressing a constructive approach to this complex problem. One approach is to ensure good two-way communication between the researcher and the people in the field involved in the research, namely, the subjects or users of the research.

This communication can take many forms and the researcher needs to consider the appropriateness of verbal, written, and visual aids in clarifying information being presented. Information needs to be disseminated about the research early in the study and then throughout the project. Often the researcher has an academic background and appointment and has been educated quite differently than practitioners and community citizens. The fact that researchers in nursing are often practitioners first may help close this gap. Even so, the researcher must give careful consideration to the way in which information is presented, including the level of the reader or listener, and must ensure that issues of concern to the audience are being addressed. Careful attention to the presentation of negative findings as well as positive results also must be made. A focus on concepts rather than on the specific program being studied may facilitate the acceptance of negative findings. Certainly a different presentation would be given to a group of academic researchers than to a group of practicing community health nurses, policy makers, or community citizens even if some of the same material is common for all groups.

Ethics

Ethical issues need careful attention when research of any type is conducted. Examination of these issues begin for researchers with the problem identified for study and whether or not it is a priority question for practice. Other considerations occur in planning and implementing the various stages of the research. There may be dilemmas over assuring the confidentiality of responses, disclosing the actual purpose of the research to the respondents, or even over disseminating results of the research to the respondents. For further discussion of ethical issues in community health nursing, see Chapter 4.

Research plans are under close scrutiny by human-subject review committees in most institutions today. Human-subject review committees are groups of representatives of various disciplines or departments brought together for the purpose of reviewing research proposals. Their major concern is the protection of the rights of the human participants in the research project.

The role of the researcher here is to communicate clearly in writing to the review committee what is planned, how subjects will be used in the research, and whether or not they are at risk as a result of participating in the research. The researcher is responsible for carrying out these plans as directed or approved by the committee. Changes that occur in the plans need to be reported to the committee for further sanctioning.

Position of Researcher in Employment Setting

The issue of who employs the researcher and potential uncertainties about the authority structure is often a major source of role strain. In an academic setting the researcher may be a faculty member who also has responsibilities for classroom teaching, clinical supervision of students, academic advising, and committee work. To be involved in a major research effort, the faculty member typically will need to be relieved of some of these responsibilities. Consideration can be given to a semester of full-time research, a reduction in teaching responsibilities and committee work, or some combination of these for the duration of the project.

It may be possible to establish more innovative employment opportunities in research, such as status as visiting scholar or visiting researcher within a community organization or university, shared positions between universities and other organizations, or the promotion of sabbatical leave opportunities between service and university institutions. Whether researchers are hired by community organizations as part-time or full-time workers, questions to be asked in considering their functioning in research include the following: What are the other expectations for this position, for example, service, administration, or other research? Also, how will the results be disseminated if they reflect negative features of a service program or a professional group? In any case, researchers should have a clear understanding with their employers and administrators about the organization and expectations for their work.

Funding of Research

A final issue relates to obtaining funds for research, especially when federal monies for research are being cut. Researchers and others need to explore alternative funding sources and use creative financing options in the future. For example, employers could grant released time so that educators, administrators, consultants, and practitioners can be involved in conducting the research; or joint financing could be arranged between the community group, the service agency and university for the research. The pursuit of funding from voluntary foundations and organizations should not be overlooked. Likewise, state and local funding, such as block grants should be considered.

In addition to funding for specific research projects, mechanisms for collaborative research need to be established and similarly funded. Research institutes and centers with joint connections between community groups, health care organizations, and universities can facilitate research in primary health care. Such institutes should promote interdisciplinary collaboration dedicated to the study of community health problems and practice issues. Responsible persons in these institutes need to publicize potential funding sources for research relevant to primary health care. The institutes also provide a unique environment for the delineation and articulation of the various roles in research and afford collaborative opportunities for community residents, students, educators, and service personnel in seeking solutions to community health problems.

SUMMARY

This chapter has highlighted selected issues surrounding community health nursing research and offered potential solutions to many of the problems identified. Primary health care was described as an approach to achieving the WHO goal of "health for all by the year 2000." Nursing practice, particularly community health nursing, plays an integral role in primary health care. The key concepts of primary health care provide a framework in which research questions relevant to practice may be generated. Examples of research findings were cited that supported the role of community health nursing in primary health care. Grounded theory and action research, especially participatory research, were suggested as relevant to primary health care. Roles and functions within research have also been discussed in an attempt to identify possible sources of role strain.

Several challenges for the future come to mind in concluding this chapter. One challenge is to establish the necessary linkages between practitioners, researchers, and communities so that research relevant to community-based practice becomes a reality. Community health nurses need not view their practice or research in a narrow perspective but instead within the broader context of community health and health care. It is the primary health care approach that supports this view. The challenge of obtaining funding for research becomes increasingly problematical, and researchers and others need to be creative in financing their research endeavors. Along with scarce resources comes the challenge of increased accountability in research, especially in relation to the utilization of research findings in practice.

BIBLIOGRAPHY

American Nurses' Association, Division on Community Health Nursing: A conceptual model of community health nursing, Kansas City, Mo., 1980, The Association.

American Public Health Association, Public Health Nursing Section; The definition and role of public health nursing in the delivery of health care, Washington, D.C., Nov. 1980, The Association.

Association of State and Territorial Directors of Nursing: Statements of competencies—public health/community health nursing, Unpublished paper, May, 1980.

Dickoff, J., and James, P.: Research. I. A stance for nursing research—tenacity or inquiry, Nurs. Res. 24:84-88, 1975.

Diers, D.: This I believe about nursing research, Nurs. Outlook 18(11):50-54, 1970.

Feuerstein, M.: Evaluation—by the people, Int. Nurs. Rev. 25(5):146-153, 1978.

Freire, P.: Cultural action for freedom, Cambridge, Mass. 1970, Center for the Study of Development and Social Change.

Hall, B.: Participatory research: an approach for change, convergence 8(2):24-32, 1975.

Highriter, M.E.: The status of CHN research, Nurs. Res. 26(3):183-192, May-June 1977.

Horsley, J.A., and Pelz, D.C.: Conduct and utilization of clinical nursing research, Kansas City, Mo., 1979, ANA Pub. (D-67):13, American Nurses' Association.

ICN and WHO, Report of the Workshop on the Role of Nursing in Primary Health Care, Geneva, 1979, World Health Organization.

Jaeger-Burns, J.: The relationship of nursing to primary health care internationally, Int. Nurs. Rev. 28(6):167-175, 1981.

Managan, D. et al.: Older adults: a community survey of health needs, Nurs. Res. 23(5): 426-432, Sept.-Oct. 1974.

Muller, P.D., and Reynolds, R.: The potential of grounded theory for health education research: linking theory and practice, Health Educ. Monogr. 6(3): 280-293, Fall 1978.

National Science Foundation: NSF announcements for December, NSF bulletin, Washington D.C., Dec. 1979, p. 1.

Pan American Health Organization: The role of the nurse in primary health care, Washington, D.C., 1977, PAHO, World Health Organization.

Rahman, A.: A methodology for participatory research with the rural poor, Assignment Children 41:110-124, Jan.-March 1978.

Stern, P.N., Grounded theory methodology: its uses and processes, Image 7(1):20-23, Feb. 1980.

Stinson, A.: Action research for community action. In Chekki, D.A. editor: Community development: theory and method or planned change, New Delhi, 1979, Vikas Publishing House, pp. 137-153, 234-235.

Taylor, S.D., Bibliography on nursing research 1950-1974, Nurs, Res. 24(3):207-229, May-June 1975.

Thompson, T.: An ordinal evaluation of the consumer participation process, Nurs. Res. 29(1):50-54, Jan.-Feb. 1980.

Walt, G., and Vaughan, P.: An introduction to the primary health care approach in developing countries, London, 1981, Ross Institute of Tropical Hugiene, London School of Hygiene and Tropical Medicine.

WHO and UNICEF: Primary health care: a joint report, Geneva, 1978, World Health Organization.

World Health Organization: Community health nursing, Report of a WHO Expert Committee, Geneva, 1974, WHO.

World Health Organization: Development of indicators for monitoring progress towards health for all by the year 2000, Geneva, 1981a, WHO.

World Health Organization: Health programme evaluation, Geneva, 1981b, WHO.

World Health Organization: Nursing in support of the goal health for all by the year 2000, Geneva, 1982, Division of Manpower Development, WHO.

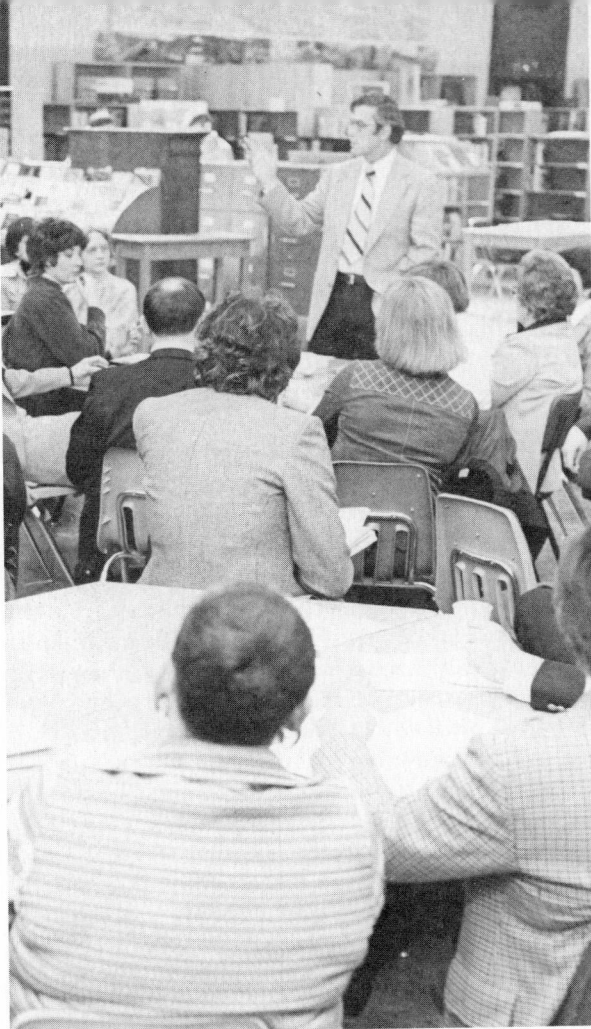

Chapter
37

PAULA POINTER
JEANETTE LANCASTER

ASSERTIVENESS IN COMMUNITY HEALTH NURSING

This chapter and the following one on stress management are included in this text because the practice of health promotion within personal and professional roles is a part of community health nursing. Nurses as well as clients need to use assertiveness skills, since neither have assumed their full positions of responsibility within the health care system. Both groups have much to gain by doing so; both have a great deal to lose by being passive and noneffectual in their roles. Certainly not all community health nurses lack assertiveness skills, but many have difficulty applying these techniques either in their own best interests or in the best interests of their clients.

Assertiveness, like stress management, is a skill that nurses can use to promote their own health, and they can teach clients to use the same skills and techniques. Assertiveness means standing up for one's own rights without violating the rights of others. Assertiveness techniques assist people to meet their own needs while respecting the needs of others.

This chapter discusses assertiveness by reviewing selected theories regarding socialization in nursing, followed by an exploration of basic assumptions of assertive behavior and description of techniques for evaluating personal actions and making informed choices about future behaviors. The final section discusses conflict as a part of human interaction and describes the use of confrontation and negotiation as assertive techniques for dealing with conflict.

SELF-CONCEPT AS A BASIS FOR BEHAVIOR

A person's attitude and self-view continuously affect behavior. People hold attitudes reflecting what they think and feel about themselves, which have been acquired throughout life and have been influenced by the way others have responded to them. These attitudes form an abstraction known as the *self-concept* and are represented by the symbol *me*. According to Coopersmith (1967, p. 5) self-esteem refers to the "evaluation which the individual makes and customarily maintains with regard to himself; it expresses an attitude of approval or disapproval, and indicates the extent to which the individual believes himself to be capable, significant, successful, and worthy." The terms *self-esteem* and *self-concept* are used interchangeably in this discussion.

Cooley (1902, p.152) described the "looking-glass" self in which an individual imagines the reactions of others to this image and is satisfied or ashamed as a result. The following are the three principal elements of the self:

1. The imagination of one's appearance to others
2. The imagination of the other person's judgment of that appearance
3. Some sort of self-feeling

For example, nurses who were obese as children often continue to think of themselves in this way even though as adults they have attained through diet control and exercise an average physique. Imagining that others see them as overweight, the nurses feel unattractive and ashamed of their appearance.

William James, one of the early theorists about the concept of self held that aspirations and values have an essential role in determining whether people regard themselves favorably. When achievement approximates aspirations in a value area, high self-esteem develops; low self-esteem results from a discrepancy between aspirations and achievement. James (1890) also described a ratio between a person's actualities and supposed potentialities as being the determining factor in the development of self-perception. In this ratio, success is the numerator and pretensions the denominator: success/pretension. James also proposed the notion of a social self, which referred to the recognition people received from peers.

Similarly, Mead (1934) elaborated on James' social self by addressing the process by which people become compatible and integrated members of their social group. In this process, people internalize the ideas and attitudes expressed by the key figures in their lives through observing their actions and attitudes and often unknowingly adopting them as their own. Mead's formulations led to the notion that self-esteem largely derives from the reflected appraisals of others.

Current Theories on the Origins of Self-Esteem

Horney (1950), focusing on the interpersonal processes influential in the development of self-esteem, postulated that feelings of helplessness and isolation constituted key determinants of self-esteem and sources of "basic anxiety." According to Horney, anxiety occurs in situations characterized by domination, indifference, lack of respect, disparagement, lack of admiration and warmth, as well as in situations of isolation and discrimination.

In many families, parents dominate children, fail to acknowledge their accomplishments, and find fault rather than praise for their actions. If they earn a B, the parents question why it was not an A. These children grow up questioning their competency. Their lack of faith in their abilities and diminished self-regard generate considerable anxiety in adulthood in that they frequently question whether they are adequate and as capable as others. In a later section, methods for dealing with such anxiety are discussed, since nurses are by no means immune to such feelings.

Sullivan (1953) accepted Mead's interpretation of the social origins of personality and emphasized the interpersonal relationships influencing self-esteem. According to Sullivan, other people play a significant role in the development of self-esteem for each person.

Based on a review of many early views of self-esteem, Coopersmith (1967) described four major factors contributing to the development of self-esteem. First, stating that the most significant factor in the enhancement of self-esteem was respectful, accepting, and concerned treatment from significant others, Coopersmith concluded that people view and value themselves in accordance with how others view and value them. Second, a history of previous successes, position, and status contribute to self-esteem. Third, a person's values and aspirations influence the interpretation and modification of experiences. Thus the degree of felt success influences status in the community. Success and status achievements for one person may seem totally insignificant to another. Fourth, a person's manner of responding to devaluation also affects self-esteem; some people defend themselves against negative responses more effectively than others.

Branden (1969) said that no other value judgment is more important to people than their self-estimates, since self-esteem has a profound effect on thinking processes, emotions, desires, values, and goals. Combs (1965) extended Branden's emphasis on the significance of self-esteem to say that what people believe about themselves affects every aspect of functioning.

Clinard (1971, p.174) provided a synthesis of the concept of self when he stated, "The self, then, in interactionist terms, is a set of discrete roles and identities which require both the responses of others and the acceptance of such designations by the actor himself." When interpreting events around them, people must sort out the meaning of an occurrence in terms of their individual self-perceptions. People, then, build unique identities in an interactive context, mediating their experiences with those of others and interpreting and responding to them in a unique way. People perceive, interpret, and respond to labeling reactions based on multiple sources including self-view, state of health and energy, supports available, and quality and quantity of stimuli at a given time.

How a person responds to the statement by the wife of a prominent physician "Oh, you're a nurse?" depends on the state of mind and current self-view of the listener. If the nurse, Ms. Jones, is feeling good about her work as a home health care nurse, she might interpret the comment as one of respect and admiration and respond with "Yes, and it is a challenging profession." However, if Ms. Jones is upset about her handling of a nurse-client situation and questioning her own ability, she might interpret the remark as condescending and feel even worse about herself, since "I am only a nurse."

SOCIALIZATION AND SOCIAL ROLES

Social behavior must be acquired; it is not present at birth but rather develops through socialization with others. Almost all behavior results from social interaction and is modified in response to the demands and expectations of others (Clinard, 1971). People acquire social roles linked to status and position and with a set of role prescriptions that influence actions. In addition, each person plays a number of roles depending on age, sex, social class, occupation, and family constellation. While considerable socialization occurs in childhood, it continues into later life as people encounter new situations.

Perception influences the development of social roles. Social behavior develops not only as people actually respond to one another, but also in accordance with their perceptions of the responses of others. For example, people respond to one another in different ways when they perceive the reaction of the others to be anger rather than joy. A frown can represent anger in some people, while others frown when in deep contemplation.

Socialization, then, represents the learning of roles and refers to the "process by which the individual acquires the skills, knowledge, attitudes, values, and motives necessary for performance of social roles (Sewell, 1963, p. 163). According to Clinard (1971, p. 176), "the required behaviors (habits, beliefs, attitudes and motives) are an individual's prescribed roles; the requirements themselves are the role prescriptions." Interactions as well as specific positions affect role *prescriptions,* or the script that occupants of a position enact. In addition, because of the complexity of life situations, some people play more roles than others. Hence, *role strain* results from situations requiring complex role demands and the fulfillment of multiple roles. Whether or not a new role or a change in self takes place depends on several factors including the following:

1. Whether the proposed new role enhances the person's self-perception or fulfills a basic need
2. Whether the new role is compatible with the person's other roles
3. How clearly defined the new role expectation is
4. Whether a transitional procedure is available in the acquisition of the new role

How Roles Are Learned

Never static, roles are constantly changing as a result of maturation processes, external stressors, and unique life situations. The earliest learnings about roles occur in families where children are taught the expected ways to behave in social situations. The next significant form of intentional instruction regarding roles occurs in schools when children are rapidly and clearly apprised of the expected behaviors. At this point, children learn that others hold expectations about what their actions should encompass.

Behavior that is rewarded is repeated, and both boys and girls are rewarded for sex-specific behaviors. In childhood, girls have a greater range of behaviors available to them in that they can be both feminine and tomboyish without causing consternation. In contrast, society expects young boys to rapidly develop masculine behaviors and avoid any sign of femininity.

Stereotypes also affect the roles members of different groups hold. The media typically portrays women as consumers and housewives, often depicted as nurturing, emotionally unstable, weak, intuitive, inconsistent, dependent, passive, sensitive, and interpersonally oriented creatures (Dean, 1982, p. 251). In contrast, media characterizes men as aggressive, independent, competitive, task-oriented, stoic, analytical, rational, self-disciplined, objective, and confident. The traits attributed to men tend to be more highly valued by society. These stereotypes influence behavior because roles do not exist in isolation, but rather role behavior results from interactions in which one individual (or group) responds to the behavior of another.

Society specifies behaviors for people in specific roles. According to Biddle (1979, p. 5), the most common notion in role theory associates roles with social positions or an "identity" that designates a commonly recognized set of persons." The terms *nurse, physician, mother, sister,* and *brother* all refer to recognized sets of people. Members of a given social position exhibit a common role because of expectations attached to that role.

Socialization in the Nursing Role

Several unique features in the nurse-physician relationship influence the socialization of nurses and the subsequent role of the community health nurse. Historically, nurses have tended to be obedient to physicians. Although the demands for subservient behaviors have diminished in recent years, the behavior of nurses still reflects deference to physicians. This theme of deference has been attributed to a variety of factors including that physicians tend to be older, to come from a higher socioeconomic class, and to be recognized as experts requiring greater rewards and prestige than other health providers.

Speaking on the United States health care industry from a social policy perspective, Ehrenreich (1975) described the development of nursing in health care from the women's view. In contrast to the previously well-established European system of medical education, there was nothing in the United States that could be called a medical profession until late in the nineteenth century. She claimed that "while most European countries had established, university trained, medical professions for centuries, the United States had only a large number of competing healers representing various degrees of training and diverse philosophies of healing" (Ehrenreich, 175, p. 6).

In the early days of American medicine, "regular doctors" were not highly paid and faced severe competition from a variety of healing groups; women constituted most of these groups. Ehrenreich (1975, p. 6) noted that "the struggle to establish the medical profession as an occupational monopoly and the struggle to oust women from healing roles were in this country, completely intertwined." The implication is not that nursing in European countries has a higher status or more autonomy than in the United States; however, interrelationship of the medical profession and nursing is different in Europe, although nursing remains of lower status.

As the medical profession tried to establish itself in a position of considerable power and authority, nursing was in its infancy. The fledgling nursing profession of the late nineteenth century often felt that its existence would only be tolerated in a role subservient to medicine. The threat that medicine perceived to come from nursing's gains is reflected in a 1901 report of the Journal of the American Medical Association which stated that many physicians found the new nurse "often conceited and too unconscious of the due subordination she owes to the medical profession of which she is a sort of useful parasite" (Ehrenreich, 1975, p. 33).

Thus, nursing and medicine developed as complementary disciplines with one focusing on caring and the other on curing. The immediate economic ramifications of this division are clear: people prefer to reward cure rather than care! Ehrenreich observed that over the decades the medical profession made deliberate and calculated efforts to limit their practitioners primarily to white, upper–middle class males. She cited several examples in the medical literature reflecting negative attitudes toward women. For example, the following statement was found in a 1948 obstetrics text: "She (woman) has a heart almost too small for intellect but just big enough for love" (Ehrenreich, 1975, p. 7). Even as late as 1971, an obstetrics and gynecology textbook stated: "The traits that compose the core of the female personality are feminine narcissism, masochism, and passivity" (Ehrenreich, 1975, p. 11).

Kalisch and Kalisch (1977) identified sources of conflict between nurses and physicians which are influential in the socialization of nurses. One source of difference leading toward conflict is the physician's propensity to evidence dominance in contrast to the nurse's deferent role. Although people do tend to solicit second opinions from other physicians, there continues to be a tendency by patients to reinforce physician dominance by depending heavily on the physician's judgment and actions to determine their fate. Lacking knowledge about health and holding an attitude of the "doctor knows best," many otherwise responsible, rational decisions makers negate their ability to be part of the health care team. Instead, they assume little, if any, responsibility for decisions concerning their most precious possession, their life.

Most patients reinforce the exalted view physicians often hold of themselves. In contrast, neither physicians nor nurses nor patients hold nurses in such unerringly positive regard. Until recently, many nurses have not behaved in ways that conveyed a belief in personal rights. Self-depreciation simultaneously coupled with a deference to physicians has been partially due to male-female role development and increased by socialization practices in schools of nursing.

Schools of nursing have not traditionally generated bold and and fearless thinkers (Kalisch and Kalisch, 1977). In some instances the creative, questioning student with the highly stimulated mind has been called a "troublemaker." The history of nursing education as being gleaned in exchange for services rendered at an institution has tended to subjugate nurses to control by more powerful members of the health care system.

Becoming a Role Breaker in Nursing

Grissum (1976) suggested nurses should consider whether they are risk takers or role breakers. She contended that nurses must risk the professional commitment required to try out new roles and break the stereotypic image of the nurse as the physician's helpmate. She warned that the risk of doing so may be high, since society still rewards conformity. According to Grissum (1976, p.89), "when you accept accountability and responsibility for your patients—you'll have greater self-esteem, your patients will get better care, and our health care systems will be better for it."

Becoming a risk taker and role breaker begins by recognizing that pleasing others will not always be possible. The qualities of compassion, tenderness, and nurturance characteristic of many nurses often become handicaps to developing an assertive role when they fail to be carefully integrated into an assertive stance. For example, assertiveness necessitates that people be honest and clear in their messages and may include telling others about their unacceptable behavior. Hence, such openness, although stated in a kindly manner, may not be consistent with a self-view of compassion and nurturing of others. Role breakers must not only be competent, skilled nurses but must also be accountable and responsible for their actions. Assertive risk requires nurses who are forthright, genuinely individual, and willing to take the risk of being different. Seemingly risk takers have a clear view of themselves; they know who they are, what they really want to be, and also how to meet their needs without jeopardizing the need fulfillment of others. It takes a lot of hard work and maturity.

The remainder of this chapter looks at ways in which community health nurses can promote their own health as well as the health of their clients by becoming role breakers. The traditional health care system does not consistently focus on promoting the health of providers or clients! However, several skills can be learned and taught to clients which will both enable providers to take more self-responsibility and teach their clients to do likewise.

THE ASSERTIVE STYLE OF BEHAVIOR

The way people behave gives observers some indication of the actor's self-concept. As mentioned, self-concept and perception influence the professional development of nurses.

The assertive behavioral style develops most readily from healthy self-esteem and projects confidence and assurance. Assertive behavior may be defined as "standing up for personal rights and expressing thoughts, feelings, and beliefs in direct, honest and appropriate ways which do not violate another person's rights" (Lange and Jakubowski, 1976, p.7). Basically, assertive communication declares to the world, "This is how I perceive and interpret the situation; this is what I see, think, and feel." Such messages do not degrade or humiliate others. Assertive actions tend to decrease anxiety and increase self-esteem, thereby creating a positive cycle.

A recent Ziggy cartoon showed Ziggy approaching a door with a sign "Assertiveness Training Center, Don't Bother to Knock, Barge Right In." This reflects a common misconception that being assertive has a "barging" quality. Not so; assertive behavior at its best takes into account the rights and needs of all persons involved in the interaction. Assertiveness means standing up for one's rights, but *not* at the expense of other people's rights. An assertive community health nurse might say to a client, "I can't schedule a routine visit on Tuesday unless it is an emergency—I can come Wednesday or Friday."

Contrasting Styles

In contrast to being assertive, nurses' behavior may be either nonassertive or aggressive. Nonassertive actions generally deny self by failing to express thoughts, beliefs, and emotions honestly. The nonassertive style implies, "My thoughts and feelings don't count. I am not as important as you. Take advantage of me. I aim to please others and avoid conflict." Nonassertive people often let others make choices for them. By forfeiting their rights to make their own choices and decisions, nonassertive people elicit responses of disgust or pity from those whom they seek to please. For example, because of inability to say "no" a nurse may schedule so many home visits that she is frazzled at the end of the day, thereby doing a disservice to herself and her clients. Nonassertive behavior does not help nurses develop or maintain good relationships with patients, physicians or colleagues.

Aggressive behavior, diametrically opposite to non-assertiveness, occurs when people infringe on the rights of others while standing up for their own rights. Aggressiveness implies, "My thoughts and feelings are more important than yours. You have no right to be different from me. I plan to dominate and win even if you lose in the process." While aggressive behavior may help people meet short-term goals or have their way temporarily through intimidation, it generally prevents the development of optimal relationships. An aggressive nurse might say in an angry tone, "You're not my only patient, nor my sickest patient. I'll get to you when I can." Although aggressive behavior may seem strong and powerful, it, like nonassertive behavior, develops from feelings of low self-esteem.

Assertive Rights

Assertiveness purports that people have basic interpersonal rights. Specifically, people have a basic right to be respected as unique persons of worth and to express who they are in ways judged to be appropriate. Each one has the right to express thoughts, feelings, opinions, doubts, and preferences without feeling guilty as well as the right to decide how best to use resources—time, property, and one's body—to help meet personal goals. Responsibility to be fair and reasonable and to accept the consequences of one's behavior accompanies these rights. The responsibilities to the profession and to the team influence the behavior of nurses.

Recognizing Choices

Assertive behavior creates an atmosphere of openness where people can engage in mutual goal setting and action toward reaching their goals while recognizing the uniqueness, strengths, and limitations of others. A key element in developing skills of assertive behavior includes the recognition of the choices available to participants in every situation. Often, nurses limit themselves when they fail to recognize their ever-present range of choices. Assertiveness training helps participants recognize, evaluate, and act on their choices. An assertive philosophy recognizes that although circumstances and the behavior of others may be beyond nurses' control, they can control their own responses.

On occasion, people may choose not to be assertive. Choosing to remain silent is not the same as remaining silent because of anxiety or failure to see other choices. People may choose not to be assertive when the other person would profit from learning and practicing assertiveness. Nurturing nurses may want to do more than is best for the client. People benefit from doing for themselves; however, nurses often do for clients what they could do for themselves with instruction and practice. There may also be situations when the perceived penalty for being assertive may outweigh the benefits gained. For instance, an opinion may be withheld when it is unnecessary or when it may distract persons or a team from moving toward common goals. This risk must be estimated and taken into account. In reality, people choose daily which opinions, ideas, and feelings to assert and which to refrain from asserting.

Self-Assessment

Where can nurses begin? Assertiveness starts wherever people are in their personal development through a program of small, systematic, gradually learned, and practiced steps. The first step includes a personal assessment. Self-assessment may be done individually or in a group or class where the interaction serves as a catalyst for each nurse. Increasing self-awareness usually accompanies assertiveness. As people become aware of how their thoughts, emotions, and intentions influence their behavior as well as how others respond to their behavior, they become better able to modify behavior and more effective in interpersonal relationships. Just because assertiveness can be simply described in a sentence does not mean it is a simple process! It takes persistence and patience to develop new, more satisfying ways of behaving—persistence in the practice of the skills and patience with oneself in a slow, but rewarding process of growth. Just as patterns of behaving in a certain way do not develop overnight, major shifts from either nonassertiveness or aggressiveness to assertiveness will not occur instantly. Furthermore, setbacks do occur. Remember, though, each assertive action is a step forward in promoting health by exercising the full range of rights and privileges. As nurses learn to be assertive, they can teach these behaviors to others including clients, families, students, and colleagues.

Assertiveness is really a style of living and interacting in the broadest sense. For purposes of learning, the style may be characterized as having a number of facets or aspects that can be discussed separately though each facet is always part of the whole person's style.

SKILLS FOR BEING ASSERTIVE

Nonverbal Components of Assertive Behavior

Body language communicates more than words about self-image and confidence, as Fig. 37-1 illustrates. As the old saying goes, "A picture is worth a thousand words." Thus the picture or image nurses present conveys a great deal both about the individual nurse and the profession. Assertive nurses convey with their entire bodies through erect posture and with feet firmly on the ground, "I am a person of value, worth paying attention to." Level, steady eye contact also communicates willingness and readiness to see and be seen and inspires self-confidence as well as the confidence of patients and professional colleagues. Eyes cast downward often accompany nonassertive behavior and communicate insecurity.

Appropriate voice tone and loudness, facial expressions, and hand gestures emphasize an assertive message. For example, a whispered message with eyes

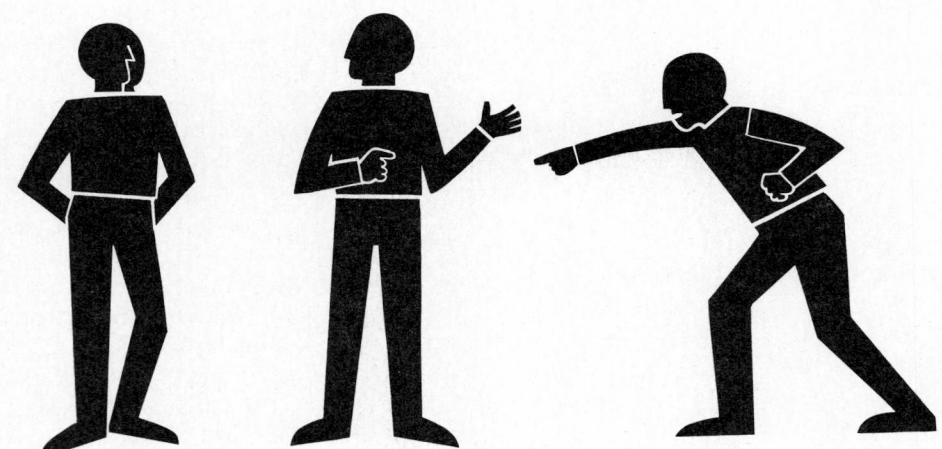

Fig. 37-1. Body language makes a difference. (Examples of passive, assertive and aggressive stances)

downcast conveys different information about the nurse than a message delivered in a clear, carefully modulated tone of voice with the nurse looking directly into the eyes of the listener. A nurse's view of self and others is communicated by the total person—body language as well as the way of speaking the chosen words. Behavior that says to others "I have a right to take up space in the world" increases the individual nurse's self-esteem and invites others to believe and affirm the person's worthiness. Assertive behavior actually stimulates assertive behavior in others and teaches others the necessity for fair, professional treatment.

Speaking Clearly

The core of assertive behavior is taking responsibility for self. Nurses, like other people, verbalize self-responsibility primarily by using "I" messages—"I think," "I feel," "I want" rather than the commonly used "You should" or "You did." The use of "I" messages minimizes the likelihood that the other person will feel defensive and simultaneously creates an atmosphere of trust. Such messages do not eliminate conflict, which is always possible when people interact. However, the messages foster problem-solving and give the listener an opportunity to know the speaker through self-disclosure. What people disclose of themselves gives others information about their self-image, values, and goals; they reveal who they are and what makes them tick. Self-disclosure is always risky, for others may not like what one reveals, but the potential reward is liking and respect from others. Action always involves risk; the alternative is to be passive and safe.

Steady, nonhesitant speech has the best chance of

communicating confidence. Elimination of "uhs" and "ahs" is a step toward assertive speaking. Good eye contact, voice of appropriate loudness, suitable hand and arm gestures, and erect but relaxed posture constitute assertive speaking. When speaking, nurses should make their messages complete and specific and should include all the information the other person needs to understand the message.

Incomplete message
Nurse: "Your recovery depends on proper eating."
Patient to herself: "I wonder if that means I have to give up chocolate bars?"
More complete message
Nurse: "If you are to recover, your diet should contain foods from each of the four groups listed on this page and a limited amount of refined sugar."

Similarly, the verbal and nonverbal aspects of the message must be congruent to avoid the confusion that typically results from mixed messages. When the voice says one thing and the body another, most people hear the nonverbal message. Gentle words accompanied by rough and hurtful handling convey a message of anger or apathy or both.

A facet of clear speech is behavior description that leaves no doubt about what is being discussed. Describing behavior means reporting specific, observable actions of others without placing a value judgment on them as good or bad and without making accusations or generalizations about the other's motives, attitudes, or personality traits. Such objective descriptions enable participants to hear what is being said with the least chance of the listener's becoming defensive.

Examples of behavior description

Supervisor to nurse: "Mrs. Brown, you have been late to work three times in the last 2 weeks."

Administrator to nurse: "Mary, I've noticed that you haven't said anything in staff meeting today and you look unhappy."

After a behavior description, a statement of feeling can be added, using "I" messages that are honest and direct without carrying the threat of judgment.

Examples of statements of feeling

Supervisor to nurse: "When you are late, Mrs. Brown, I'm frustrated because I have the responsibility for seeing that every job is covered. I like your work and wonder what we can do about the situation."

Administrator to nurse: "I'm afraid the proposal we just discussed doesn't suit you and that you are hesitant to say so. I would like to have your opinion before we reach a final decision."

In both examples, the speaker assumes a problem-solving attitude and invites a collaborative effort for mutual benefit. The message is honest, clear, and non-defensive. Such messages make no value judgments or inferences about the nurse as a person or about other unrelated characteristics of the person. Clear, direct, descriptive messages should also be given to clients. For example, in the following material it is much more supportive of health promotion to discuss lack of compliance with a systematic diet by using the first approach rather than the second.

Nurse: "Mr. Brown, I am concerned that your blood sugar is high and you have been eating quite a few sweets. Can we reexamine your diet plan and determine how you can use natural sugars rather than refined sugar to satisfy your cravings?"

Nurse: "Mr. Brown, you received an hour and a half of instruction last week about excluding refined sugar from your diet. Don't you want to try to help yourself?"

Note the use of "I" messages in the first example as well as the focus on mutual problem solving. This markedly contrasts with the accusing nature of the second example in which the blame is placed on the client for not adhering to prior nutrition counseling.

Active Listening

Although volumes have been written on the art of listening, many people need to improve this skill. Assertive behavior recognizes the needs and rights of all participants in an interaction; active listening is the key to discovering the other person's needs and values.

Communicating the desire to hear and understand is the first step in listening. That desire is communicated largely through body language, such as by facing the speaker, establishing eye contact, and showing with the whole body that listening is the goal.

One can let another know the message is heard by paraphrasing what was said and by affirming the speaker's feelings before making comments. Frequently nurses fail to hear what clients say because they are busy with their own thoughts and needs, including lining up their arguments, before carefully listening to the message. When Mrs. Smith says, "The new medicine is not working," a response such as "You're feeling discouraged that you aren't getting better" affirms her as a valuable person and sets the stage for her to say, "Well, I guess it will take more time." A brusque "It's too soon to tell" may be true but does not deal with Mrs. Smith's present experience.

Nurses may think that because they are busy and often feel harried and overworked, they don't have time for such amenities. The actual time used in active listening is minimal compared to the value to the client. Actually time may be saved in the long run by hearing the message before responding. Frequently we answer what seems to be the question asked or the concern expressed only to learn later that we were 90 degrees off target. The client may not have been worried about the surgery when she said, "I guess the operation will take a long time," but rather she may have been worried about who would stay with her retarded son if she had to remain in the hospital more than 2 or 3 days.

In taking instructions from a physician or supervisor, the time spent in clarifying and understanding is well spent if the job is done with more competence and understanding. Nurses often think that asking clarifying questions indicates inadequacy or is insulting to the one giving the instructions. Not so! All people are so influenced by their own interpretations of what they hear that they should not assume they understand. This truth is reflected in the epigram, "I know you believe you understand what you think I said but I'm not sure you realize that what you heard is not what I meant."

Dealing with Manipulation

According to Phelps and Austin (1975), manipulation is the conscious or unconscious use of indirect and dishonest means to achieve a desired goal. All nurses need attitudes and techniques that allow them to protect themselves from being "used" by others.

Saying "No"

Nurses have the right to set priorities on the use of their time and energy in order to meet their goals. To be able to say "yes" to the priorities, they must say "no" to other things. This presents a dilemma to a profession that has traditionally been "at your service" and to each professional nurse who wants to please everyone (whether consciously or unconsciously). If nurses try to say "yes" to every possibility or request they become fatigued and overstressed and feel inadequate for the high-priority activities in their life and work. Hence, nurses must be vigilant in the use of their time and energy and direct these resources toward the accomplishment of their goals.

Learning to say "no" is the primary tool to use against manipulation. No one wants to feel or be manipulated. Nurses do not want to be manipulated by other staff members, physicians, clients, friends, spouses, or children. Likewise, clients do not want to feel used by people in their personal life or by health care providers. However, the way "no" is said is of prime importance. "I" messages delivered firmly and kindly make one's position clear without offending the other person.

"I won't be able to get to that today. I'll be glad to do it tomorrow." Or "Today I was planning to make visits in the community. Is this job more important? If I do your work today, my community visits will have to be delayed. Which takes priority?" The latter example adopts a problem-solving stance and invites negotiation toward resolving conflicting demands on time.

Generally the person making the request will stop asking when the "no" is decisively heard. Hesitant, vague responses say to the asker, "Persuade me." In some situations the most assertive response to a request is to say, "I'll have to check my schedule and let you know if I have some time to do that" or "I'll need to think about that and let you know." Such actions give you time to gather your thoughts carefully and decide on a response without feeling pressured or threatened by the presence of the person making the request. Few requests cannot be delayed a few minutes or even longer if schedules and other factors need to be checked. Nurses often fail to exercise the option of "I'll check and let you know in 10 minutes (tomorrow)." Such reluctance reflects lack of respect for one's rights and privileges as a person of worth. Likewise, clients should be afforded time to consider the alternatives and make careful and thoughtful choices.

Negotiating compromises is an assertive skill worth cultivating. It is appropriate to compromise except when one's integrity is at stake. If a visiting nurse is asked to make a home visit every day and determines that twice a week would be sufficient for the patient's needs, the answer to the original request may be "no" but a workable compromise will be offered. Negotiation as an assertive skill is discussed in depth in a later section.

In the case of a request to obtain drugs or perform a service not within one's professional scope, no compromise should be offered because the nurse's integrity would become an issue. Refusal of such a request might provoke a response of anger and create temporary distance in the relationship, but in the long run the nurse's self-esteem will be increased by such an action. Furthermore, on occasion nurses would be legally jeopardizing their role by not saying "no." To provide services not within the realm of either nursing or appropriate health care is, of course, inadvisable. For example, just because a physician orders an excessive dosage of medication for a home health care client does not mean that the nurse should give it. To do so would make the nurse legally liable for this erroneous action should complications arise.

Manipulative Ploys

It is particularly distressing to feel manipulated and perceive that you have no power to do anything about it. In their efforts to meet personal goals many people use other people's time and talent and energy. However, such actions cannot happen without one's own participation in the manipulation—good news indeed! So the question becomes: How can nurses protect themselves from manipulation in their professional roles as well as in their personal lives?

The first step, as always, begins with self-awareness about what promotes or allows manipulation to take place. What are the vulnerable areas that a manipulator can touch to get what is desired? Most people, including nurses, respond to various ploys, and several are discussed in the following paragraphs.

Flattery. How many people are unresponsive to flattery? Each person has one or more areas vulnerable to "buttering-up" efforts. An assertive nurse certainly wants to be able to accept a genuine compliment graciously and yet resist the urge to comply with a request from a flatterer simply because that person's regard is highly valued. Therefore, one must learn to differentiate between flattery and an honest and sincerely delivered compliment. For example, two nurses at a home health care agency have equal client loads yet Ms. Jones seems to be more efficient than Ms. Smith. On a rainy Friday when Ms. Smith was running late in getting started with her home visits, she is overhead saying to Ms. Jones, "You know your new hairstyle really looks great. You look younger and more excited about life these days." Ms. Jones replies, "Thanks, I appreciate your opinion; that makes my day." (Pause). "By the way," says Ms. Smith, "would you mind visiting Mr. Hall for me? I'll just never finish by four if I have to drive to his home. Anyway, he has always liked you better." Manipulators exploit the human desire to be needed and often feign helplessness to get what they want. Female nurses may be more inclined toward this kind of behavior because of their socialization, but men are certainly not immune to it.

Assuming Responsibility. Nurses need to resist the urge to rush in and "rescue" the situation when the other person is capable of assuming personal responsibility. For example, if a client is trying to decide how to manage the details of her recovery, she may ask the nurse, "What do you think I should do?" Responsible replies may include enabling the client to consider what alternatives are open to her and helping her solve her own problem. Nurses should not assume the decision-making role for clients, nor should they allow themselves to to be seduced into that role. Taking over may stem from an innate desire to be helpful to other people; however, every person has strengths that outnumber weaknesses, and often the way to be most helpful is to help others stand on their own feet. It generally is a disservice to do for others what they can be taught to do for themselves. Such behavior actually deprives the recipient of independence and personal integrity by conveying "I really don't think you can do . . . "

Sense of Obligation. A sense of obligation or duty can place people in vulnerable positions often subject to manipulation. Women, particularly in American culture, have been taught to feel responsible for the welfare and happiness of others. Mutual, freely accepted obligations go with any relationship, professional or personal, and nurses must not allow themselves to get out of balance in this area.

Insecurity. Insecurity occasionally makes people susceptible to manipulation. Those who know you can play on your particular fears to get agreement on any number of things. Nurses should become aware of their individual fears so they can protect themselves against those who would use fears maliciously. Common fears include fear of being replaced (the nurse may agree to all sorts of extra tasks), fear that love or approval will be withdrawn (the nurse may comply with unreasonable demands), fear of what people will think (nurses may hesitate to take risks that are in their interest), or fear of offending someone (nurses may hesitate to express their opinion even when it is needed).

Guilt. Skilled manipulators use guilt as one of their primary weapons. Feelings of guilt persuade nurses to do things they would not consider or choose otherwise. Guilt feelings, easily evoked in many nurses, make assertiveness difficult. For example, in the previous encounter between the nurses, Ms. Smith could have played on her colleague's feeling of guilt by continuing with "If you won't help me by visiting Mr. Hill, I probably will have to skip his bed bath and that sure would be a step backward in all the hard work we have done to prevent him from getting a decubitus." A nurse, troubled by dysfunctional guilt, may benefit from rethinking the ideas that underlie these feelings, which will be discussed in the later section, "Why are nurses not more assertive?"

Criticism. Criticism is probably the weapon that manipulators use with more success than all others. When one is criticized, all those old feelings of inadequacy surface from childhood. Even a mature, professional nurse who has accepted that being human also means being imperfect must relearn this lesson from time to time. However, when one's self-esteem is high, criticism can be evaluated and used for personal and professional growth and development.

Most people respond to criticism in two characteristic ways—either by denial or defense. Both responses are generally accompanied by anxiety, which blocks evaluation of the criticism. As Smith (1975) said, people need to develop skills that can minimize the typical emotional response of anxiety to criticism. They need coping behaviors to enable them to feel comfortable when they are reminded of some truth about themselves which is interpreted, explicitly or implicitly, as wrongdoing in another person's value system. Furthermore, nurses need coping skills to help them feel comfortable with their errors that may have been inefficient, wasteful, awkward, or stupid but have nothing to do with right or wrong.

According to Smith (1975), a change in external verbal behavior in the face of criticism allows for internal changes, for example, less anxiety and more assertive behavior. To facilitate such changes, Smith suggested several techniques that may be used to protect oneself from criticism.

TECHNIQUES FOR PROTECTING AGAINST CRITICISM

Fogging refers to the technique of agreeing with truth, agreeing in principle, or agreeing with the odds. It is called "fogging" because the person criticized reacts much like a fog bank—without reaction. A nurse might use such a response with a patient who complains chronically. When the patient says, "You are late getting here again. You certainly took your sweet time," the nurse might respond, "You are right. I might have gotten here earlier" (agreeing with truth). If the patient then responds, "It seems like nurses should get to the patient as soon as possible," the nurse's fogging response might be, "It certainly does seem the nurse should be there when the patient is sick" (agreeing in principle). If the patient then says, "I guess I could have died and no one would have known it," the nurse might respond, "I suppose that is possible" (agreeing with the odds).

Lange and Jakubowski (1976) question the use of fogging because it is not straight communication and could be countermanipulative if carried to extremes. They prefer a more direct assertion in the face of criticism. While their comment is worth considering, fogging does have a place in developing a repertoire of assertive skills. Although a passive way to cope with criticism, fogging is useful in situations where the criticism has been discussed repeatedly or where one just does not want to "get into it" at that time. In no case should fogging be used to prevent listening to criticism offered. For example, if an instructor or supervisor is criticizing behaviors involved in carrying out nursing actions, fogging is not usually applicable. Instructors and supervisors want to discuss, rather than avoid, the issue.

Negative assertion is a more active assertive skill described by Smith (1975). Negative assertion openly admits negative things about oneself, acknowledging that perfection is not one's goal. This technique helps change verbal behavior and modify the belief that guilt is automatically associated with making a mistake. If your supervisor says, "You did not handle that situation in a very professional manner," and you recognize the truth of the criticism, you might respond, "You're right, I was rather awkward." Professional nurses want to do what they can to rectify errors after admitting them. The skill of negative inquiry discussed in the next paragraph offers a way of discovering how the mistake can be corrected or avoided in the future.

Negative inquiry is the most assertive skill available to cope with criticism. In essence, it involves prompting further criticism of self or prompting more information about statements of wrongdoing in an unemotional, low-key manner. The criticizer can then state what is wanted through the help of the questions by the criticized person. In the example just given where the first response was negative assertion, the next response (negative inquiry) might be "What do you think I might do next time that would be more professional?" Nurses must be careful not to become sarcastic as they ask the question because verbal aggression may trigger an aggressive response. Often the tone of voice may give an aggressive ring to such a response as the example just given. The same words spoken angrily would carry a different message than if spoken with sincerity and honesty.

In professional relationships the use of negative inquiry can let the supervisor know a nurse wants to do a good job and will listen to suggestions about how to improve performance. This technique also indicates that one does not crumple under criticism but rather listens and uses the information for professional development. Negative inquiry can also be a way of soliciting regular, constructive feedback that will help improve the handling of the job.

> Supervisor: "I have been concerned, Mr. Brown, about the way you have been doing your job lately."
> Nurse: "What have your concerns been?"
> Supervisor: "I understand you have been giving the insulin injection to your diabetic patients when they come for their clinic appointments."
> Nurse: "What would be a better way for me to handle that?"
> Supervisor: "It would be more helpful to ask them to demonstrate their self-injection practices so that you can evaluate their skill and accuracy with these techniques."

Through negative inquiry the person who is criticized can learn what the specific behavior in question means to the critic and what is really wanted in the situation. Using criticism for growth is one more assertive skill to help nurses do a good job and feel good about themselves.

Assertive behavior therapy and education historically have focused on the "standing up" behaviors that help people protect their rights and prevent manipulation by others. An often neglected, though crucial, aspect of being assertive is the ability or capacity to behave in ways that build relationships and that help in approaching and getting closer to others, sometimes called "soft" assertions. Many people have great difficulty expressing affection, tenderness, appreciation, and caring. Nurses, as caring professionals, can augment their competence through verbal and nonverbal expressions of warmth and compassion.

Compliments

Giving and receiving compliments presents problems for many. To offer a compliment puts one at risk of rejection or even ridicule. For example, if you say, "You did a good job today with that client," and the response is "It was really nothing. Anyone could have done better," you might become discouraged and hesitate to voice your approval next time.

The person who receives a compliment by downgrading the giver reduces the possibility of future compliments and fails to acknowledge the giver. Both parties to the interaction probably feel vaguely uneasy and discouraged.

"Thank you" is the only necessary reply to a compliment. That response acknowledges the giver and allows the receiver to accept the compliment and be warmed by it. Of course, you may add to the "thank you" a phrase such as "I appreciate your saying that," "It feels good to know you liked that," or "I'm glad I did the job well, I've worked hard at it."

Making Conversation

Making conversation is the starting point for every relationship. Without the basic skills used in conversation people become isolated from others, personally and professionally. The first step is to speak up! Say something. The discussion in the earlier section, Speaking Clearly, applies here.

Everything that is said discloses something of the speaker and can be a conversation starter. Generally the more you disclose of yourself, the more you will receive of the other. A warning—too much too soon can frighten the listener. Few people want instant intimacy in the beginning of a relationship. The amount of self-disclosure sets the limits of intimacy and lets the other person know what is acceptable to discuss.

Every disclosure is information for the other person to use in developing the conversation. Listening for the free information, that is, information given not in response to a direct question, gives possible content for continuing the interaction. The listener then has choices about which information to respond to.

> Patient: I really wish my children could be here while I'm in the hospital, but they all live so far away and they're so busy. My son on the farm lives especially far away; it's about time for the harvest, so he couldn't possibly come. And all the grandchildren have to be taken care of."

What shall the nurse respond to when there is so much information given freely? Some possible responses might be: "Tell me more about your family." "I wonder if you're feeling a bit neglected since they aren't here?" "You want your grandchildren to come first even though you'd like your children here. How many grandchildren do you have?" "Where do your children live?" Or you might respond "So one of your children is a farmer. I grew up on a farm and I know timing is important for the harvesting." This latter response gives information about the nurse which establishes a common interest.

Developing a Support Network

The development of the social skills of conversation facilitates nurses in developing a support system—a network of relationships that builds self-esteem, provides camaraderie and companionship, and thereby nurtures the professional care giver. All people need a resource group whose presence in their lives can help them both to *be* and to *become*. A special pleasure is provided by friends—those trusted people with whom mutual give and take is experienced. As Francis Bacon (1953) said, "Friendship redoubleth joys and cutteth griefs in halves."

A functional support network may include relationships other than traditional friends. An older, more experienced nurse may become a mentor or a guide through the professional labyrinth. A mentor gives support and feedback while fledgling nurses develop professional identity and trust in their own judgment. More experienced professionals provide role models whom a novice can admire, respect, and emulate. Frequently, a professor, supervisor, or more experienced colleague fills this role. Asserting one's needs and asking for guidance may help in locating a mentor. Some supervisors are unable to serve as mentors because they are threatened by the competence of those they supervise while others are uncaring about the professional development of colleagues.

There may also be support people who challenge a nurse to grow, who believe in one's talent, and who offer encouragement as one grows and develops. Common interests also provide the base of some relationships—a colleague with whom racquetball or a passion for mystery novels, is shared. Some occasions call for a confidante who willingly offers a listening ear without judgment, who holds the mirror so oneself can be seen, and who allows the next step to be taken.

A common thread in all the different kinds of relationships nurses might have is the sense of strength that comes from the relationships. All people need others who enhance their lives through support, affirmation, sense of humor, and even challenge and caring confrontation. Nurses feel more able to cope after encounters with such people. These encounters serve as buffers between the nurse and the relationships and situations that threaten self-esteem and sense of competence.

WHY ARE NURSES NOT MORE ASSERTIVE?

The traditionally female nursing profession has defined itself in terms of the feminine cultural stereotype—passive and dependent. This belief system serves to block individual nurses and the profession as a whole. The belief of nurses (both male and female) that they are to play a secondary, subservient role retards the development of assertive behavior patterns. Early conditioning into sex roles is difficult to transcend; however, it must be done if nurses intend to take their proper place on the health care team.

Fear

Fear blocks effective functioning for many nurses. Fear of rejection and fear of inadequacy retard many nurses' ability to be actively involved in decision making in their practice. These fears may contribute to a self-defeating cycle when they inhibit assertive behavior. Nonassertive behavior is often followed by a decrease in self-esteem and an increase in anxiety. The pattern is dysfunctional to a professional nurse; it may be altered by learning more effective assertive behavior.

Anxiety

Anxiety blocks the development of assertive behavior. Because nurses deal with high-stress situations, they must learn to monitor and reduce their anxiety in both present and long-term situations.

The next chapter discusses in detail ways nurses can deal with their own anxiety and also teach clients to manage stress and anxiety. One anxiety-reducing method is progressive relaxation, a deep-muscle relaxation method developed by Jacobson (1974) and based on the tensing and relaxing of specific muscle groups. It can be used to develop awareness of early signs of tension so measures can be taken to relax (see Chapter 38 for a description of the specific process). The more nurses can be aware of their own early anxiety responses, the more they can take charge of combatting them through relaxation.

Creative imagery, another relaxation method discussed in detail in Chapter 38, focuses on releasing tensions through deep breathing and imagery, using mental scenes of pleasant places, and visualizing words such as "calm" or "relax."

Lack of clarity about the role of nurses has created confusion and anxiety in the minds of nurses, clients, and other health providers. The image of nursing must be redefined if the profession is to grow in scope of practice. A more definite assertive image—or belief about nursing as a profession—can help nurses and the public develop a more realistic view.

Belief System

The development of a positive belief system is one element in the process of becoming more assertive. Nurses must believe that "assertion, rather than manipulation, submission, or hostility enriches life and ultimately leads to more satisfying personal relationships with people" (Lange and Jakubowski, 1976, p. 55). Assertive styles of interaction that grow out of rational thinking patterns enhance professional relationships. Fortunately, nurses can identify irrational thinking patterns that underlie ineffectual behavior and can substitute more productive thought processes through conscious rethinking of their perceptions of a situation.

Ellis (1977) has made a persuasive case that faulty behavior is caused by irrational beliefs. Based on the belief that "men's minds are disturbed not by events, but by their interpretation of events," he developed a system of exploring and challenging beliefs so one can develop a rational belief system that leads to effective behavior. Believing one is "dumb," "inadequate," or "only a nurse" can block expressions of positive thoughts and feelings.

Lack of Assertiveness Skills

Lack of appropriate skill is probably the largest block to assertive behavior. Early conditioning, sex role stereotyping, peer pressure, and low self-esteem are among the factors that inhibit the development of adequate skills of interaction and assertiveness. Nurses can learn needed skills through participation in classes for that purpose, through reading, and through practice. Proficiency in any skill develops through practice. A planned program of small steps developed in a group or on your own can set the stage for the persistent practice that reaps such great rewards for nurses. The support of a network will augment a program of personal and professional growth. As they begin to take small steps, many feel more confident immediately and the confidence than encourages taking the next step. Success indeed builds on success.

HANDLING CONFLICT ASSERTIVELY

In any organization in which nurses are likely to work, conflict is inevitable. However, conflict is often viewed as a disruptive force that should be avoided whenever possible. In applying assertive skills and standing up for personal rights, conflict should not be ignored. It must be recognized, understood, and resolved. One way to do so is by using negotiation skills. Before exploring the strategy of negotiation, the nature of conflict needs to be briefly reviewed.

Conflict can be either constructive or destructive. When used solely for personal gain or to work out hidden angers or when directed toward the demise of another person, it is a destructive force. However, conflict is a clue that something is amiss and thus should generate the need for open communication and problem solving.

Conflict arises for a variety of reasons including situations in which each participant does not have the same information. One missing fact may completely alter the perception of a situation, thus clear communication, as previously mentioned, is one way to minimize conflict.

Another source of conflict lies in incompatible goals among participants. When new ideas or plans are to be implemented, it is important to have participants carefully describe their own goals for the project. This process, it must be cautioned, is complex because people tend to be guarded about some goals. When the level of trust is low or when competitiveness is particularly keen, people may be unwilling to share their own goals openly for fear of weakening their position relative to that of their opponent. Such people are said to have a "hidden agenda."

Whether conflict enhances the functioning of the involved parties, leads to a stalemate, or causes major hostilities within the group depends on how it is handled. Constructive conflict resolution can occur when participants do not feel threatened by different views and when there is a commitment to open handling of the issue. Stepsis (1974) purports that conflict resolution strategies can be categorized as avoidance, defusing (or cooling down), and confrontation. Although each strategy has both positive and negative features, confrontation seems most consistent with assertiveness skills.

Confrontation, assertiveness, and negotiation use many of the same principles for guiding behavior. Prerequisites for confrontation useful for promoting an environment of assertiveness or negotiation include the following (Thurkettle and Jones, 1978, p. 40):

1. Willingness and ability of participants to accurately identify the issue
2. Open communication, including astute, active listening
3. Focusing on the issues, not the people involved
4. Mutual responsibility for the communication outcome

Confrontation

Smoyak (1974, p. 1632) describes confrontation as a "concept, a process, and a technique" with application in nursing practice. Confrontation, like assertiveness, is not "telling the other person off" but rather is a problem-solving strategy for conflict resolution. Confrontation skills, which are briefly discussed here, are quite compatible with the negotiation process described later.

Confrontation is essentially a three-stage process: assessment, direct confrontation, and resettlement. The first step, assessment, can be carried out by asking the question in the boxed material. As can be seen from these questions, assessment includes *who* is involved,

what is the issue or problem, *what* are possible consequences, and *how* is the discussion going to be handled. Confrontation is a direct approach, like assertiveness, which deals only with the identified problem. Side issues are not drawn in nor is attention directed toward the participant's personal attributes. In confrontation all participants are apprised of the need for an open discussion about the conflict. Preplanning as to issues, participants, time, and place are part of the assessment process.

The second step, implementation or direct confrontation, is composed of basic skills of communication. Key points include sticking to the facts, handling only one subject at a time, and avoiding any interruption of other speakers. No matter how much a person may want to clarify, defend, explain, and so on, it is essential to listen carefully to what the other party has to say. People have the innate tendency to begin defending their behavior before they have heard the speaker's entire message. Once each participant has presented the issues, it is helpful to have each repeat what was heard. This form of feedback provides immediate clarification of any misperception or lack of understanding.

The last stage in confrontation, resettlement, includes agreeing that a problem exists and jointly devising a strategy for resolution. Until this point, only one participant may have perceived that a problem existed. Now it is time to take specific steps to resolve the problem.

Three students have been assigned to a work group in community health nursing. Their task is to assess a rural community near the university and establish nursing diagnoses and action plans for the community. In the first meeting the students divide the areas to be assessed and agree to meet in two weeks with their information.

During their second meeting, one of the group members, Sue, explains that she has had the flu and has not collected her community data. She assures her group that if they can give her a week's extension she will come well prepared to their next meeting. However, at the next meeting, Sue explains that her car broke down and she was unable to gather

---

Assessment Questions to Be Raised When Anticipating and Planning for Confrontation

1. What is the problem?
2. What (who) seems to be causing the problem?
3. How is it affecting me? others?
4. How and what kind of power is involved?
5. What kind of changes can be expected as a result of confrontation?
6. What are the potential consequences of a confrontation (positive and negative)?
7. What might be the cost of raising the issue?
8. What might be the cost of ignoring the issue?
9. Who is involved in the situation?

	Types of Power Useful in Negotiation

1. Power of "knowledge of needs" — what are the verbalized versus the real, yet unstated needs?
2. Power of investment — settlement often follows a substantial investment of time, energy, and money in the process of negotiation.
3. Power of rewarding or punishing — to what extent can the participants help or hinder each other?
4. Power of identification — people will identify with you if you convey knowledge, warmth, and empathy.
5. Power of morality — doing what is right.
6. Power of precedent — "we have always done it this way."
7. Power of persistence — stick to the issue.
8. Power of persuasive capacity — if you are going to persuade me, I have to know what you are saying and it must be overwhelming so that I cannot dispute it.
9. Power of attitude — keep a positive attitude with your emotions under control.

From Cohen, H.: You can negotiate anything, Secaucus, N.J., 1980, Lyle Stuart, Inc.

much information. She requests another week's extension. What should the other two members do? If they give Sue another extension are they adhering to principles of assertive behavior? Should they confront Sue now or hope she will mobilize her energies and do her part?

During the past week the other two group members had spent time assessing this situation and had decided that a problem exists. Since they have previously been in Sue's class, they know she tends to procrastinate. Thus when they raised questions such as those in the boxed material, they decided that Sue's inability to meet her acknowledged obligations was the problem. They are becoming anxious about the outcome of their project and simultaneously getting angry with Sue. They believe that the potential cost to them of Sue's behavior may be an unfinished project on the due date. They decide to confront Sue by explaining that either she will have to negotiate with them for a series of deadlines that she can meet or withdraw from the group and allow them to finish the project without her. The latter option would mean that Sue would have to discuss this situation with their instructor and request a new assignment.

Negotiation

Another strategy that uses principles of communication, conflict resolution, and assertiveness is negotiation. Ways (1979, p. 87) defines *negotiation* as "a process in which two or more parties, who have both common interests and conflicting interests, put forth and discuss explicit proposals concerning specific terms of a possible agreement." Similarly, Cohen (1980, p. 27) describes negotiation as an attempt by two parties to satisfy their mutual needs and involves time, information, and power. According to Cohen, *time* means that most people wait until the deadline is fast approaching before they commence to negotiate. *Information* means

learning as much as possible about the situation and participants before the process starts. *Power* is somewhat more complex and is the ability to use resources to achieve goals and influence people and events. Power is influenced by perception; people who believe they have power convey this notion by their actions, posture, voice tone, and so on. Cohen described nine types of power used in negotiations, and these are defined in the boxed material.

The power component of negotiation is illustrated in the dilemma of a group of students.

The student group was unable to meet the deadline for a group project because an important piece of information was not received from a publishing company in time for them to complete the project on schedule. They believe their request for an extension is legitimate, since they have been conscientious in their efforts; however, their instructor likes work turned in on schedule. The students realize they must negotiate a new deadline and, based on Cohen's power principles, plan their strategy.

First, they carefully organize their position to clearly state their request to their instructor, realizing that a positive anticipatory attitude is necessary. When they approach the instructor, they do so by setting up an appointment, selecting a spokesperson to begin the discussion, and assuming total responsibility for the delay. They present the facts regarding the needed extension, carefully sticking to the issue and posing an alternative deadline without becoming aggressive.

The instructor listens to their recommendation and agrees that situations beyond the students' control led to the delay. The students request a two-week extension which means that their project will be turned in during the first exam week. The instructor agrees with the concept of an extension but says that receiving the project during the week of final exams will create a personal burden. They brainstorm as to alternative sources of data collection for securing the missing information and agree on a 10-day extension.

In this example of negotiation no one was the loser. Actually both the students and the instructor were winners; the students received their much-needed extension and the faculty member arranged to receive the paper before the onslaught of final exam grading. This example illustrates several of Cohen's additional principles of negotiation. First, it points out that negotiation does not need to be a win-lose situation in which one party does all the giving and the other party receives the concession made. Cohen (1980, p. 119) describes a *win-lose* strategy as the "Soviet style" of negotiation, which is most effectively used when there is no continuing relationship between parties, when neither will feel remorse afterward, and when the victim is unaware of the strategy being used. These characteristics do not apply to most ongoing student-faculty interactions, since both parties may feel remorse (Cohen, 1980). Also, students are not generally in a powerful bargaining position, because they cannot reward or punish faculty. However, students can gain power in several ways, as illustrated earlier.

A more useful form of negotiation is called *win-win*, in which participants negotiate for mutual interest. As mentioned in the case of the students-instructor negotiation for turning in the paper, win-win forms of negotiation are positive for all participants. The key components of this approach are building trust, gaining commitment, and managing opposition (Cohen, 1980). In this approach participants avoid embarrassing one another in public, and each tries to remain calm and stick to the issues.

As mentioned, negotiation includes time, power, and information. In considering information, one must be aware that negotiation is a process not an event. Before beginning to negotiate participants should gather all relevant information so as not to appear confused and poorly prepared. Throughout the process it is essential to practice active listening to hear clearly what the opponent is really saying.

POTENTIAL CONSEQUENCES OF ASSERTIVE BEHAVIOR IN NURSING PRACTICE

Once community health nurses learn and become skilled in assertive techniques, it is important to remember that not everyone is going to be pleased with this behavior in nurses or clients. Not all assertive efforts are warmly and enthusiastically received. Assertive behavior can be disruptive to a relationship or environment, since it tends to affect the status quo. Virtually all change meets with some degree of resistance; people whose usual patterns are upset by new assertive actions may seek revenge. Before looking at some typical reactions to the demonstration of assertive behav-

ior, it is useful to discuss the concept of *resistance*.

According to New and Couillard (1981, pp. 17-18), people resist change for one of five reasons:

1. Threatened self-interest in which their perception of personal costs outweigh their anticipated personal benefits
2. Inaccurate perceptions where they do not understand the nature and/or implications of the change
3. Objective disagreement in which the person does not think the change will benefit the organization
4. Psychological reaction that occurs when people perceive that their personal freedom is being threatened
5. Low tolerance for change in which the person understands the change but is emotionally unable to make the transition from the old behavior or situation to the new one

All of these five forms of resistance seem to stem from fear. When one member of a family, social, or work group become more assertive, those influenced by this change wonder how they will be affected. Thus, when changing one's own behavior or teaching others to modify their behavior, it is important to assess who may be affected by these changes. What is their usual or likely reaction to any alterations? Anticipating resistance increases alertness to possible reactions and provides for early resolution of such conflicts.

Alberti and Emmons (1980) describe the most common reactions to assertiveness as being backbiting, aggression, psychosomatic reactions, and revenge. *Backbiting* occurs when someone is displeased with behavior, but rather than approaching the actor directly, the person makes comments to others such as "What's wrong with her these days?" or "Wonder who he thinks he is, anyway?" One must be careful not to respond to backbiting in like fashion but instead ignore these remarks.

Aggressive reactions to assertive behavior are usually verbal. Consider the reaction if a physician ordered a dosage of medication four times the recommended amount. You are a home health care nurse, and the client is in your caseload. Rather than give the incorrect medication, which could have serious effects on the client, you assert yourself by calling the physician and asking him to double-check the order. He immediately yells into the telephone, "No fiesty nurse is going to tell me what to do." He slams down the telephone. Instead of visiting the client you return to the office to consult with your supervisor. As might be expected, the physician has already called your supervisor *and* the director of the agency. Although you know your position was both medically and ethically correct, you begin to wonder if it was really worth all the aggravation. However, you also realize that had you given an excessive dosage of medication and had it caused the patient to have serious effects you would have been liable for your actions. Of course, this is an extreme situation, but it illustrates that nurses must not back down because of a harangue caused by actions when they are doing what is correct and necessary.

Donnelly (1979b, p.31) describes *psychosomatic responses* to assertiveness as the "weeping willow reaction." Often when one demonstrates new behaviors, others will accuse the person of giving them a headache or a backache or will indirectly complain (weep) that they are not treated fairly, that their workload gives them a headache or their back aches from lifting so many people or things without any help. Nurses do not like to think that they caused someone else to get sick. Remember, one never causes anyone else to feel a certain way. People are in charge of their responses to the behavior of others.

A final response to assertiveness is to *seek revenge*. Such reactions may be seen as public taunts about one's behavior or direct or veiled threats to retaliate. Such behavior may be demoralizing and painful, especially if people other than the two directly concerned become involved. In some cases the revenge can have serious consequences including the loss of a job or damage to one's credibility. Thus in choosing when to be assertive it is important to evaluate the potential consequences rationally.

In some instances assertiveness may influence job mobility in either a positive or negative direction. Some supervisors and administrators do not want people who can think for themselves, who behave in ways they consciously choose, and who are accountable for their actions. When supervisors are threatened by perceived competence of subordinates or when they prefer an autocratic style, assertive subordinates are usually not valued. In contrast, many administrators believe that the best run organizations are those in which coworkers are bright, assertive, skillful, and decisive decision makers. Hence, the individual nurse must critically assess the work situation and decide if the fit is a compatible one.

The emphasis on the potential negative consequences of assertiveness is not intended to belittle the positive outcomes. Many benefits of assertive behavior have been previously mentioned. However, it is important to summarize the potential positive effects on the nurse, the setting, and the client. When nurses use assertiveness, they essentially stand up for their personal rights while simultaneously respecting the rights of others. Such behavior leads to increased feelings of self-worth and personal confidence. Essentially this message is incorporated into the person's self-perception: "I am a valuable person who is entitled to say what I think and feel in a way nondetrimental to others."

Not only do clear, assertive messages enrich the nurse's self-view, but they also stimulate positive feelings among others. To be honest with another person (family, colleague, client) conveys respect for that person's worth by saying "I value you enough to be open and honest in my communications with you." Such behavior tends to keep communication patterns clear and to minimize misunderstanding and inaccurate perceptions. Being assertive with people allows them to take responsibility for their own behavior.

For example, some mothers do not clearly and specifically communicate to their children that they are expected to keep their rooms clean. Instead, coming home from a busy day at work and being greeted by two able-bodied children engrossed in television while their beds are unmade and the floor is strewn with wet towels and dirty laundry, nonassertive mothers hurry to tidy up the house while mumbling about lazy, ungrateful children. Would an assertive message be better? For example, the mother could inform the children that they may finish watching that show, but on its completion they are to turn off the television and clean their rooms. Then they may resume watching television.

In dealing with clients, there are times when the nurse may choose to refrain from being assertive *for* clients in order to teach them to be assertive. This was the case in the following example.

Mrs. Brown was being treated by Dr. Smith for hypertension. His primary approach was medication, and he had provided no specific instruction relative to diet and nutrition. When Jane, the community health nurse, made her regular visit to Mrs. Brown, who was recovering from a stroke, they discussed the implications of hypertension. Mrs. Brown told Jane that her neighbor who is also hypertensive was not taking much medication but did go to the health department every week for a nutrition and exercise class. In the past 2 months her neighbor lost 4 pounds and declared that she never felt better. Mrs. Brown wanted to attend the class too but feared that Dr. Smith wouldn't write a referral. She asked Jane to call her physician and explain the value of this program.

Jane, however, knows that Dr. Smith thinks such classes are foolish and there is nothing a nurse could teach his patients that he has not already shared with them. What should she do? Should she use assertive skills in this instance for patient advocacy? *

* Advocacy refers to "speaking in another's behalf" (Donnelly, 1979a, p.49). The community health nurse as a client advocate is described in detail in Chapter 32. This chapter defines only one time in which advocacy is not recommended. In contrast, assertive behavior refers to an attitude of self-responsibility. Thus using assertive principles to speak for others violates the basic intent unless they are unable to speak for themselves.

The most useful nursing approach at this juncture would be to teach Mrs. Brown to be assertive in this specific situation. This could be done by role-playing whereby Mrs. Brown and Jane alternate enacting the potential responses of both Dr. Smith and Mrs. Brown. Since Dr. Smith's first response may be negative, Mrs. Brown can practice using "I" messages to express clearly her desires along with a version of "broken record" where the main point is made over and over in a low-key manner. If Dr. Smith perceives that this class is really important to Mrs. Brown, he may agree.

Essentially the nurse wanted to foster Mrs. Brown's independence so she could translate the learning from this situation to other similar ones. Thus one should avoid doing for people what they can do for themselves and should reinforce independent actions. Clients may not be aware that they have rights and are entitled to be part of the decision-making process relating to their health and lives.

SUMMARY

A health promotion goal is to attain and maintain the highest possible level of human functioning. Community health nurses can enrich their own functioning and adaptation to their multienvironments as well as teach clients to do likewise by learning and practicing the skills of assertive behavior. This technique, often confused with aggressiveness, refers to clear, straightforward communication of one's needs, goals, and rights. Assertive behavior avoids using or taking advantage of others as well as being used by others. This form of communicating, behaving, and even standing, walking, and dressing conveys self-confidence and comfort with oneself as a person of value.

An assertive stance opposes the traditional female, and especially nursing, stance of subservience and deference to others. Because nurses assume responsibility for most of the health care given in all segments of the health care system, a passive posture is not in the best interests of either nurses or clients. Nurses must model and teach others to stand up for what they believe, to be clear and honest in their messages, and to learn to practice negotiation and conflict resolution so that there are no losers, only winners, in the health care system.

Specific skills are needed to be assertive. Nurses can learn communication techniques such as fogging, negative assertion, and negative inquiry to help them respond more constructively to criticism. In addition, an assertive approach includes social skills such as giving and receiving compliments, making conversation, and developing and relying on a support network.

Attainment of an assertive style may be blocked by several things. Anxiety, fear, an irrational belief system,

and lack of skill have been discussed as impediments to nurses' increased assertiveness. Many of the examples cited have directly applied to nursing practice skills so nurses could identify with them and practice the skills described. The goal has been twofold: to teach community health nurses assertive skills and to offer the potential that these skills can be taught to clients.

BIBLIOGRAPHY

Alberti, R.E., and Emmons, M.L.: Your perfect right, San Luis Obispo, Calif., 1980, Impact Publishers, Inc.

Bacon, F.: Essays: On friendship, 1625. In The Oxford dictionary of quotations, ed. 2, London, 1953, Oxford University Press.

Biddle, B.J.: Role theory: expectations, identities and behaviors, New York, 1979, Academic Press, Inc.

Branden, N.: The psychology of self-esteem, San Francisco, 1969, W.H. Freeman & Co.

Clark, C.C.: Assertiveness skills for nurses, Wakefield, Mass., 1978, Contemporary Publishers.

Clark, C.C.: Assertiveness issues for nursing administrators and managers, J. Nurs. Admin. **9**(7): 20-24, July 1979.

Clinard, M.B.: Sociology of deviant behavior, New York, 1971, Holt, Rinehart & Winston, Inc.

Cohen, H.: You can negotiate anything, Secaucus, N.J., 1980, Lyle Stuart, Inc.

Combs, A.W.: The professional education of teachers, Boston, 1965, Allyn & Bacon, Inc.

Cooley, C.H.: Human nature and the social order, New York, 1902, Charles Scribner's Sons.

Coopersmith, S.: The antecedents of self-esteem, San Francisco, 1967, W.H. Freeman & Company.

Dean, P.G.: Toward androgyny. In Muff, J., editor: Socialization, sexism and stereotyping, St. Louis, 1982, The C.V. Mosby Co., pp. 248-254.

Donnelly, G.F.: When it's best not to assert, RN **10**:49-51, Sept. 1979a.

Donnelly, G.F.: When assertiveness exacts a price, RN **10**:29-31, Oct. 1979b.

Ehrenreich, B.: The health care industry: a theory of industrial medicine, Soc. Policy **6**:4-11, Nov.-Dec., 1975.

Ellis, A.: How to live with and without anger, New York, 1977, Reader's Digest Press.

Grissum, M.: How you can become a risk-taker and role-breaker, Nursing **6**:89-98, Nov. 1976.

Grissum, M., and Spengler, C.: Womanpower and health care, Boston, 1976, Little, Brown & Co.

Horney, K.: Neurosis and human growth, New York, 1950, W.W. Norton & Co., Inc.

Jacobson, E.: Progressive relaxation, ed. 3, Chicago, 1974, University of Chicago Press.

James, W.: Principles of psychology, 2 vols., New York, 1890, Holt, Rinehart & Winston, Inc.

Kalisch, B.J., and Kalisch, P.A.: An analysis of the sources of physician-nurse conflict, J. Nurs. Admin. **7**:51-57, Jan. 1977.

Kimble, C., Yoshikawa, J., and Zehr, H.: Vocal and verbal assertiveness in same sex and mixed sex groups, J. Pers. Soc. Psychol. **40**:1047-1054, 1981.

Lange, J., and Jakubowski, P.: Responsible assertive behavior, cognitive behavioral procedures for trainers, Champaign, Ill., 1976, Research Press.

Lazarus, A.: Behavior therapy and beyond, New York, 1971, McGraw-Hill Book Co.

Mead, G.: Mind, self & society, Chicago, 1934, University of Chicago Press.

Mereness, D.: Your self-image and your practice, Am. J. Nurs. **66**:96-100. Jan. 1966.

Moniz, D.: Putting assertiveness techniques into practice, Am J. Nurs. **78**:1713, 1978.

Nesbitt, E.: Use of assertive training in teaching the expression of positively assertive behavior, Psychology Today **49**:155-161, Aug. 1981.

New J.R., and Couillard, N.A.: Guidelines for introducing change, J. Nurs. Admin. **11**:17-21, March 1981.

Pardue, S.F.: Assertivness for nursing, Superv. Nurse **11**:47-50, Feb. 1980.

Phelps, S., and Austin, N.: The assertive woman, San Luis Obispo, Calif., 1975, Impact Publishers, Inc.

Rawnsley, M.M.: The six A's of assertiveness, J. Cont. Ed. Nurs. **11**:15-18, Jan.-Feb. 1980.

Ryan, M.V.: The practice of assertiveness, Occupa. Health Nurs. **29**:7-9, April 1981.

Schill, T., Toves, C., and Ramanaiah, N.: Responsible assertion and coping with stress, Psychol. Rep. **49**:557-558, Oct. 1981.

Sewell, W.H.: Some recent developments in socialization theory and research, The Annals **349**:163-181, 1963.

Smith, M.J.: When I say no I feel guilty, New York, 1975, The Dial Press.

Smoyak, S.A.: The confrontation process, Am. J. Nurs. **74**:1632-1635, 1974.

Smoyak, S.A.: Family systems theory, Paper presented at the meeting of the Oklahoma State Nurses' Association, Oklahoma City, April 1975.

Staines, G., Tavris, C., and Jayaratne, T.E.: The Queen Bee syndrome, Psychology Today **7**:55-60, Jan. 1974.

Stepsis, J.: Conflict resolution strategies. In Jones, J.E., and Pfeiffer, J.W. The 1974 annual handbook for group facilitators, LaJolla, Calif., 1974, University Associates, p. 139.

Sullivan, H.W.: The interpersonal theory of psychiatry, New York, 1953, W.W. Norton & Co., Inc.

Thurkettle, M.A., and Jones, S.L.: Conflict as a systems process: theory and management, J. Nurs. Admin. **8**:39-43, Jan. 1978.

Ways, M.: The virtues, dangers and limits of negotiation, Fortune **99**:86-90, Jan. 15, 1979.

Wolpe, J.: The practice of behavior therapy, ed. 2, New York, 1973, Pergamon Press, Inc.

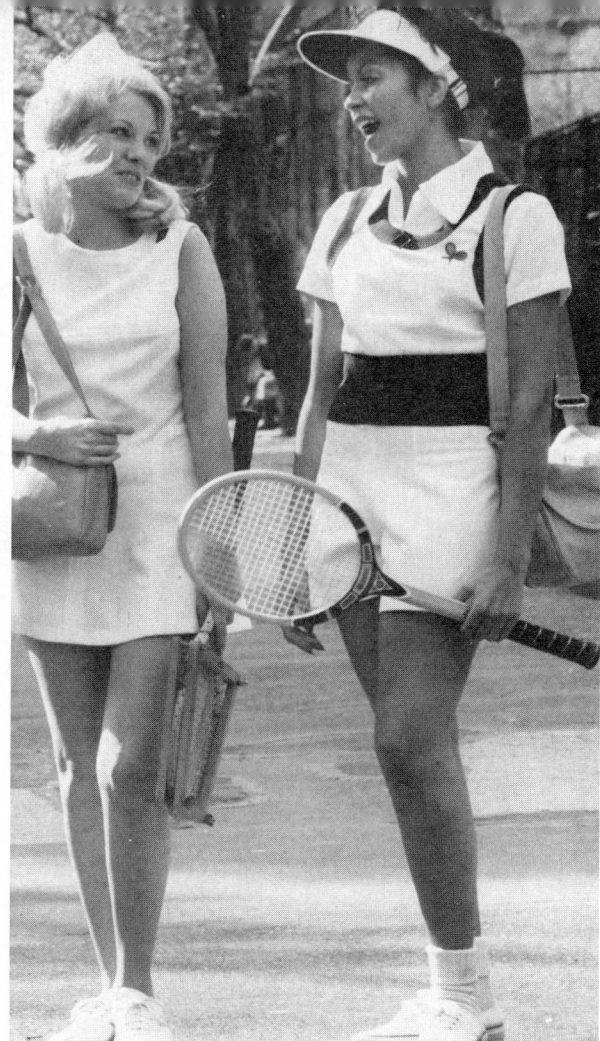

JEANETTE LANCASTER

PROMOTING HEALTH THROUGH EFFECTIVELY MANAGING STRESS

Stress and its effects on health and well-being are areas of concern for many health care providers. Stress is not new and has throughout history been a part of human existence. What does seem to be new is the amount of stress that people are confronted with currently.

Stress has been labeled the "twentieth century disease," since its effects are widespread and influential in health maintenance. To discuss fully the concept of stress and identify specific management approaches, it is necessary to briefly note key societal influences on health. The 1970s witnessed the demise of cheap energy; dreams shrunk at about the same rate as did the size of cars. For the first time in many countries it appeared that the next generation would not lead better lives than their predecessors. Half a millennium of expansion and

tremendous economic growth gave way to an era of resource contraction and scarcity.

In addition, during the 1970s the hopes and visions of modern technology were ruptured as crisis after crisis emphasized the flaws and fallibility in the hoped for progress toward a better life. In the health care arena an increasing number of questions were being raised about how adequately needs were being met. Despite skyrocketing health care costs, many preventable health problems continued to exist. Each of these factors contributed to a heightened level of stress. Sharp declines in economic growth caused by inflation, energy constraints, and rising unemployment, paralleled by a vivid realization that the expenditure of vast amounts of money had not eliminated many of the major health problems, led to an urgent need for self-analysis. The phrase, "we are what we eat, think, and do," became increasingly relevant as people recognized the necessity for interrupting risk factors that threatened health. It seemed that the way in which people responded to and managed social and economic issues would influence their health status.

Seyle (1975, p. 14), well known for his research and writing in the area of stress and the physiological response to this phenomenon, defined *stress* as "the non-specific response of the body to any demand made upon it." The demand or stressor can take a variety of forms each of which requires adaptation and readjustment. Failure to adapt to stressors can have negative and at times devastating effects. Specifically, there is an accumulating body of evidence suggesting a relation between excessive stress and the onset of major health problems.

Since stress is ever present and influences the ability to cope, adapt, and lead maximally productive lives, the nature of stress, stressors, the stress response, levels of stress, and sources of stress such as life change events and occupation have implications for community health nursing. Community health nurses must understand the effect of stress on them and be able to deal effectively with it to be a role model and teacher of clients.

Community health nurses are involved with promoting the health of individuals, families, groups, and the community as an aggregate. One way to promote health is by assessing the presence of stress in the community and monitoring its level to plan and implement appropriate interventions. Stress is generated from internal and external sources, and a major community health nursing role involves applying the nursing process to the phenomenon of community stress. Additionally, stressors can arise from developmental and maturational changes as well as from conflicting value systems, lack of basic economic resources, environmental changes, emotional traumas, and other minor and/or major demands for adaptation. Stress is present in all aspects of community health nursing.

NATURE OF STRESS

According to Selye (1965, p. 97) "*stress* is the rate at which we live at any moment." He perceived all people as being constantly under stress with all events, either pleasant or unpleasant, which accelerate life intensity as causing a temporary increase in stress and subsequent wear and tear on the body.

Hartl (1979, p. 91) defined *stress* as "that emotional and physical experience which results from a requirement to change from the condition of the moment to

any other condition." This definition emphasizes the relation between change and stress. Stress is increased when people are faced with personal, social, and environmental changes; these changes can be perceived as being either positive or negative. The key is that each change experience requires new coping abilities and often novel forms of adaptation.

Similarly, Lazarus (1980, p. 111) described stress as being dependent on the person's appraisal of a situation as being neutral, benign, or stressful. Thus Hartl and Selye equate stress with change and the individual's ability to adapt, and Lazarus added the element of appraisal.

A key factor to consider at this point is the role of perception in the experiencing of stress. What makes the same situation stressful for one person and fun or calming for another? How an event is viewed influences the response. Appraisal of a given situation is crucial to determining the potential for stress. To illustrate the role of perception, consider the varying experiences of a group of college students at a large amusement park. Many of the rides and attractions are mild, funny, and essentially nonthreatening. However, the roller coaster may arouse a variety of feelings in the students. The majority of the group may feel exhilarated over the promise of a fast, thrilling ride, whereas the "silent minority" is anxious and perhaps would prefer to avoid this ride. Because of peer pressure and the desire to be part of the group, some of the frightened members ride the roller coaster although they are afraid. Despite the varying anticipation of the ride, each of the students would have a similar bodily experience. Bounding over the loops and curves, whether finding this fun or frightening, leads to a characteristic bodily reaction.

Another aspect of perception includes the cumulative effects of stressors. Often people respond in what seems to be a disproportionate manner to a minor stressor. The observer does not know about the multiple stressors already at work in the person's life. For example, a man may go into a blind rage when his car stalls on a busy street. What would not be apparent to others is that the problem with the car is "the last straw." The man had been fired on Friday, his wife was hospitalized on Saturday, and he was on his way to the unemployment office to see if any work could be found.

The Chinese word for crisis is a combination of two symbols: one representing danger and the other opportunity. Whether a situation is a threat or a challenge is largely dependent on perception. Selye (1975) pointed out the difference between adequate stimulation and overload when he described people as being racehorses or turtles. A racehorse would be driven to distraction on a quiet beach, whereas a turtle would have considerable difficulty trying to live the life of a racehorse.

The way in which people experience stress depends to a large extent on predictability (the degree to which people can anticipate the occurrence of an event), social content (the psychosocial setting or factors present in the environment), and control (the degree to which one can alter a situation or event). The effects of stress are less disruptive if the onset is expected or preceded by some warning. The social context of a stressor influences the reaction. It is easier to tolerate loud music if it is your own rather than if it is coming from someone else's apartment. The running and yelling of small children are generally better tolerated by their parents in their own homes than in a crowded restaurant or a friend's house. In addition, the degree of perceived control influences how a situation is interpreted. For example, listening to loud music in your own automobile may be less stressful than if the music were playing in a public building where your presence was required. In your automobile you could turn the volume down, whereas in the building you might not be able to leave or adjust the volume.

How stress is experienced also depends on the ability to cope. What is stressful for one person may be energizing for another. For example, deadlines, writing papers, and public speaking affect people in highly different ways. Each person's response to stress is different because of the interplay of such factors as genetics, organ vulnerability, general state of health, fitness, sociocultural background, and previous experience with stress.

Additionally, not all stress is bad. Stress-related problems occur when the degree of stress remains high for a prolonged period of time. Stress is especially useful in times of danger when people need to mobilize physical and emotional forces for their own defense. In tolerable levels stress is a motivator; it keeps people moving toward goal accomplishment and prevents boredom and feelings of uselessness. Selye (1975) described a positive form of stress as being "eustress." The *eu* means good or positive, as in euphoria. This form of stress results from a positive occurrence or when people convert negative stress into a positive form by changing their attitudes; responses can be energizing and can increase productivity and efficiency.

CAUSES OF STRESS

According to the government publication, *Healthy People* (1979), one half of all deaths in the United States from the 10 leading causes are currently the result of unhealthy life-styles. Knowles (1980, p. 467) noted that "the health of human beings is determined by their behavior, their food, and the nature of their environment." As described in Chapter 1, the pattern of dis-

eases has changed in response to the movement from an agricultural to a technological society. Improvements in water and milk supplies, personal and food hygiene, sanitation and sewage disposal, and vaccinations all helped to reduce the incidence of infectious diseases.

In the early 1900s the infectious diseases of children and young adults accounted for the leading causes of death. By the late 1970s the major causes of mortality had shifted to cardiovascular problems, cancer, and accidents. As mentioned in Chapter 2, chronic diseases of middle and later years are the major health problems in the United States. Death and disability in middle age is premature and often preventable. For people under 44 years the leading causes of mortality are accidents, heart disease, cancer, homicide, and suicide. For people under 25 years the leading causes of death are accidents followed by homicide and suicide. Mortality figures only portray part of the story. For every death by suicide it is estimated that 10 others or 200,000 people annually have attempted suicide. Likewise, for every death caused by accidents, hundreds of others are injured, and many are prematurely disabled.

Many of the current causes of morbidity and mortality are either directly or indirectly related to stress. Since personal life-styles and environmental conditions are related to many of the major health problems, medical care today is becoming less effective in the attempt to cure or lessen illness.

In support of the contention that individual responsibility for medical care is the critical issue in improving health status, the relation between personal health practices and heart disease must be considered. Nutrition, physical activity, cigarette smoking, and psychosocial stress play substantive roles in the etiology of heart disease. Sutterly (1979) questioned whether traditional disease-oriented practices can eliminate life-style as the causative agent of diseases. Despite marvelous surgical procedures, a repaired heart is not as effective as the original one had it been kept in fine working condition. The United States is often accused of having an illness, not a health care system. However, limited attention in the past has been devoted to changing the system to a health care–oriented system. The foremost goal of health promotion is to assist people to live up to their maximum potential.

Bloom (1979) described a new paradigm for conceptualizing and delivering preventive services for mental illness, which deviates from the traditional model based on an epidemiological framework. He contended that the previous model of identification of the disease, determination of its path of transmission, and development of a prevention program have been successful with communicable diseases. However, Bloom believed that the diffuse nature of mental illness makes such a model inadequate. The new paradigm is especially applicable to a discussion of stress, since it is based on the belief that all people are to varying extents susceptible to life events. The following three steps constitute the new paradigm (Bloom, 1979, p. 183):

1. Identify a stressful life event that appears to have undesirable consequences in a significant proportion of the population. Develop procedures for reliably identifying persons who have undergone or who are undergoing that stressful experience.
2. By traditional epidemiological and laboratory methods, study the consequences of the event, and develop hypotheses related to how one might go about reducing or eliminating the negative consequences of the event.
3. Mount and evaluate experimental preventive intervention programs based on the hypotheses.

This model can be applied to many stress-related problems that are present in the community, including the death of a child or spouse, divorce, or human abuse.

STRESS RESPONSE

Stress theory is based on the concepts of adaptation and homeostatis. People strive to adapt to their stressors to maintain some semblance of balance. Stressors elicit a response from a person's entire body, including psychological and physiological components. Based on the definition of stress cited earlier, Selye (1975) identified the general adaptation syndrome (GAS). In this syndrome physiological responses in the nervous and endocrine systems alert people to the occurrence of either distress or eustress. These sensations produce a wide range of feelings varying from joy to fear and serve as an alerting mechanism so that individuals can summon their resources to fight stress. The physiological changes brought about by stress are nonspecific and affect the entire organism.

The real stress involved in the bodily reaction to a stressor is that which occurs as the body attempts to normalize once it has been disrupted from its previous state of homeostatis. When humans are in distress too long or intensively, the GAS becomes decreasingly effective and makes a person vulnerable for mental or physical health disruption. The bodily response to stress has three phases.

1. Alarm reaction—physiological indications of alertness during which defense mechanisms are mobilized
2. State of resistance—resists the alarm and fights back to normal
3. Stage of exhaustion—when stress is sustained, and adaptation energy is depleted

To minimize the effect of stress, interventions should prevent a person from ever reaching exhaustion. People need to be keenly aware of internal and external stress-producing events and recognize their personal signs of accumulating stress. Essentially stress is a response of the bodily and perceptual systems to a stressor, and the potential causative agent comes from either internal or external sources.

The bodily reaction to stress typically includes increases in the following:

1. Metabolism (oxygen consumption)
2. Blood pressure
3. Heart rate
4. Rate of breathing
5. Amount of blood pumped by the heart
6. Amount of blood pumped to the skeletal muscles

During a stress response the hypothalamus is stimulated, which in turn stimulates the autonomic nervous system (ANS) and the anterior pituitary gland. Stimulation of the ANS causes the heart to speed up, the digestive systems to slow down, and epinephrine and norepinephrine to be released. When the anterior pituitary gland is stimulated, it releases adrenocorticotropic hormone (ACTH), which subsequently stimulates the cortex of the adrenal glands and causes the release of steroids or antiinflammatory hormones. A second hormone, somatotropin (STH), is also released from the anterior pituitary gland and stimulates the growth of the body as a whole and increases the activity of proinflammatory corticoids (Selye, 1976).

When the sympathetic portion of the ANS is activated, a fight-or-flight mode of operation is seen in the accelerated heart rate, increased respiration, and redistribution of blood from peripheral areas of the body into the head and trunk. Each stressor activates the sequence just described, thereby enabling the body to fight or take flight.

The autonomic response occurs quickly and lasts only a short while; the endocrine response initiates more slowly and lasts longer. Setting off this response many times over a long period has a wear-and-tear effect on the body; eventually it lowers resistance to diseases. The hormones flowing through the system along with the accompanying tensions, also have a psychological effect. Over a period of time, the chain reaction of the stress response can cause depression, irritability, nervousness, apathy, sleep difficulties, changes in smoking, eating, and drinking habits, etc.

This whole chain reaction originally evolved to help humans escape from predators. Once safe, escapees were able to proceed with their normal routines when the physical effect wore off. Today we still trigger the same physiological response in the face of stress, but the kinds of stressors we encounter are typically different.

Burnout may occur in persons who are unable to successfully respond to stress.

BURNOUT

Some people are unable to successfully adapt to stress even with the assistance of another person. As stress increases, the person feels less able to counteract the situation. *Burnout* is the term coined to refer to this end state of stress or exhaustion. It may be observed in individuals who suffer a major loss, such as a job or a close family member, occurring within a short time span. Burnout may also be observed in persons experiencing chronic illness. Swogger (1981, p. 31) defined burnout as a "special form of stress reaction to work and organizational pressures."

The physiological concomitants of burnout include cardiac irregularities and electrolyte imbalance (hypokalemia), which may result in cardiac arrest. In other people this level of stress could lead to decreased cardiac output and the subsequent symptoms of irregular pulse, hypotension, dependent edema, decreasing kidney function with alteration in urinary output, mental confusion or forgetfulness, and weakness. Additional physical symptoms include fatigue, gastrointestinal problems, persistent colds, back pain, weight loss or gain, loss of appetite, susceptibility to infections, headaches, insominal, dyspnea, or angina.

Some or many of these physical signs are generally accompanied by several behavioral symptoms including irritability, rigid thinking and general resistance to new ideas or any threat of change, finding fault easily with other people, and often displaying a generally negative and cynical attitude. Other behavioral indicators of burnout that may be seen are absenteeism, tardiness, decreasing accuracy in work assignments, and a tendency to "take problems home."

Basically, burnout involves the loss of concern for others; nothing really matters anymore. The person approaching burnout becomes increasingly exhausted physically and emotionally, and in general, begins to show lack of respect, empathy, or warmth for others. These impersonal attitudes and feelings represent commonly observed signs of burnout and for nurses are often followed by decisions to leave the profession, go into administration, or use drugs or alcohol to cope with the stress.

Burnout, as a stress reaction in response to work or organizational pressures, is common among human service workers who spend considerable time and energy helping others. Burnout also occurs in organizational settings that lack support systems; in these settings workers do not attempt to help and encourage one another but rather seek to meet their own personal goals.

Three categories of events have been found to be instrumental in precipitating burnout among health care workers.

1. Environmental deficits such as not enough supplies or equipment, poor physical layout of the institution, and a shortage of staff.
2. Professional relationships that are characterized by ineffective communication or personality conflicts.
3. Relationships with clients and families in which the nurse identifies with the client, feels guilty that the best possible care is not being given, or sees that communication problems exist concurrently.

Strangely enough, increased knowledge can serve as a precipitator or militating factor in burnout. For example, as health care technology has improved, greater knowledge is available on preventing and treating diseases. People know what they could or should do; yet time, energy, commitment, or resources interfere with their taking the necessary actions. A failure to act leads to stress, especially if lack of action brings about untoward results. For example, a home health care nurse, Ms. Smith, was visiting an elderly client to change her indwelling catheter. Ms. Smith had one sterile catheter kit with her. She considered stopping by the office to get an extra catheter just in case she contaminated the first one. However, she was running late and decided to risk having only one cathether with her by convincing herself that she was quite skilled at changing cateters and rarely had any difficulties. As luck would have it, Ms. Smith dropped the sterile catheter just as she was about to insert it. Not only did she drop the catheter on the floor but because of her tight schedule and feeling of pressure to complete her work on time, Ms. Smith picked up the contaminated cathether and used it. The following week Ms. Smith visited this lady and saw signs indicating a urinary tract infection; she felt depressed, guilty, and overwhelmed by her inability to effectively manage her time and use good judgment. If Ms. Smith continued to have many days like the one described, she would be a likely candidate for burnout.

Burnout can also result from inadequate leadership. Controlling and authoritarian and weak or inconsistent leadership may have the same detrimental effect on the behavior, ideals, and commitment of employees. Other common causes of burnout are (1) responsibility without the necessary authority to accomplish tasks, (2) responsibility without the necessary resources to get the job done, (3) lack of meaningful recognition for efforts and accomplishments, and (4) lack of good staff communication.

Coping with burnout includes basically the same stress management techniques as those discussed later. The core of these efforts begins with self-awareness to

Self-Management for Burnout Prevention and Intervention

1. Know yourself, pay attention to your feelings to see what sets off negative feelings.
2. Delegate whenever possible, do not try to do everything for yourself and others.
3. Recognize that burnout is a function of poor situations, and work to change them.
4. Plan a variety of self-care activities to increase resistance to stress.
5. Vary the amount and type of client contact so you are not consistently caring for the same kind of people. Staff members working in tense clinical situations may plan regular, brief "time-outs" to mobilize their personal resources.
6. Keep work and home separate. Leave feelings and problems in the proper place.
7. Form a peer support group to discuss reactions and feelings about work.
8. Negotiate roles and responsibilities to do what you feel competent to do.
9. Regularly show appreciation to others; positive expressions can become contagious!

recognize accumulating stress, followed by a carefully developed intervention plan with exercise, recreation, open communication, group or individual support, outside interests and resources, and a recognition that burnout is not a function of "bad" people but rather of bad situations that need to be modified. The above box lists two general approaches for self-management of burnout, including prevention and intervention.

STRESS IDENTIFICATION

Stress cannot and should not be avoided, but rather the secret lies in successful management of stress. All machines wear out with excessive use, and the human body is no exception. Selye (1975) stated that the critical first step in managing stress is "to know thyself." Everyone is familiar with the sensation of being keyed up from nervous tension. It has been noted that this feeling has a physiochemical basis and that people respond in unique ways to stressors. It is often difficult to learn to "tune down" or decelerate the pace of life. Simple rest is no panacea for managing stress for everyone. Successful stress management judiciously balances activity and rest to meet the individual's unique requirements.

Although each person reacts in a unique way to stress, there are several commonly observed physical, behavioral, and emotional indicators of increased stress. These indicators are depicted in the following box. As noted earlier, a key part of stress diagnosis includes determining one's own way of responding to stressors. Each person demonstrates some of the indicators listed in the box.

A key part of stress diagnosis includes determining if perceptions are accurate. Occasionally, the anxiety present during a stressful time diminishes the ability to accurately perceive reality. Thus it is important to disengage from a stressful situation long enough to make certain that what is perceived is really happening. For example, passing remarks of co-workers or supervisors may be perceived negatively if people are tired and feeling worthless. Once it is determined that perceptions are accurate, the next phase of stress identification deals with targeting the stress source, and the following list of questions can be asked:

1. Is the stress work-related?
2. Is something going on in my personal life that is worrisome and unfavorable?
3. Is it a combination of demands made on me at home and at work?
4. Do I set unrealistic goals and standards for myself that make me anxious?
5. Do I resist change because it threatens me?
6. Do I feel anxious most of the time?

Fig. 38-1 is a test that can be used for personal evaluation of life-style to determine the level of health risks currently present.

Change As a General Cause of Stress

There is considerable stress in everyone's lives, and much of it results from the sheer weight of change. As discussed in Chapters 24 and 25, children experience an ongoing process of physical and emotional change as they pass through normal developmental milestones. Adults also experience increasing changes in society, values, the physical environment, organizations, and personal selves.

Holmes and Rahe (1967) developed a social readjustment rating scale in which numbers were assigned specific life changes in terms of the effect they could be expected to have on people (Table 38-1). These events were positive and negative and ranged in value from 11 (minor violations of the law) to 100 (death of a spouse). Positive events such as marriage (50 points) and outstanding personal achievement (28 points) were also included in the 42-item scale. Holmes and Rahe postulated that the more change people had, the more likely they were to get sick. They found in their research with the Life Change Test that people with over 300 life change units in a year have an 80% chance of being ill.

Text continued on p. 856.

Indicators of Stress

Physical

1. Elevated blood pressure
2. Increased muscle tension (neck, shoulders, back)
3. Elevated pulse and/or increased respiration
4. "Sweaty" palms
5. Cold hands and feet
6. Slumped posture
7. Tension headache
8. Upset stomach
9. Higher pitched voice
10. Change in appetite
11. Urinary frequency
12. Restlessness
13. Difficulty in falling asleep or waking up; frequent awakening
14. Dry mouth and throat

Behavioral

1. Decreased productivity and quality of job performance
2. Tendency to make mistakes; poor judgment
3. Forgetfulness and blocking
4. Diminished attention to detail
5. Preoccupation, daydreaming or "spacing out"
6. Inability to concentrate on tasks
7. Reduced creativity
8. Increased use of alcohol and/or drugs
9. Increased smoking
10. Increased absenteeism and illness
11. Lethargy
12. Loss of interest
13. Accident proneness

Emotional

1. Emotional outbursts and crying
2. Irritability
3. Depression
4. Withdrawal
5. Hostile and assaultive behavior
6. Tendency to blame others
7. Anxiousness
8. Feeling of worthlessness
9. Suspiciousness

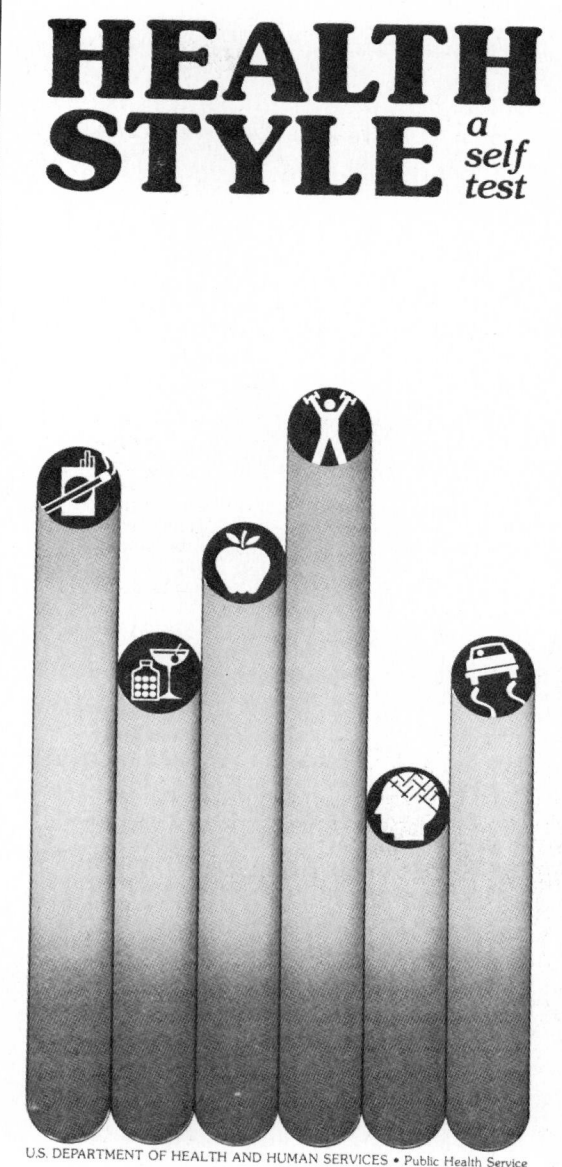

Fig. 38-1. Self-test for good health. (Adapted from Healthstyle, a self-test, DHHS Pub. No. (PHS) 81-50155, Washington, D.C., 1981, U.S. Department of Health and Human Services, Office of Disease Prevention and Health Promotion.)

Continued

How This Booklet Can Help You

All of us want good health. But, many of us do not know how to be as healthy as possible. Good health is not a matter of luck or fate. You have to work at it.

Good health depends on a combination of things . . . the environment in which you live and work . . . the personal traits you have inherited . . . the care you receive from doctors and hospitals . . . and the personal behaviors or habits that you perform daily, usually without much thought. All of these work together to affect your health. Many of us rely too much on doctors to keep us healthy, and we often fail to see the importance of actions we can take ourselves to look and feel healthy. You may be surprised to know that by taking action individually and collectively, you can begin to change parts of your world which may be harmful to your health.

Every day you are exposed to potential risks to good health. Pollution in the air you breathe and unsafe highways are two examples. These are risks that you, as an individual, can't do much about. Improving the quality of the environment usually requires the effort of concerned citizens working together for a healthier community.

There are, however, risks that you can control: risks stemming from your personal behaviors and habits. These behaviors are known as your lifestyle. Health experts now describe lifestyle as one of the most important factors affecting health. In fact, it is estimated that as many as seven of the ten leading causes of death in the United States could be reduced through common sense changes in lifestyle.

That's what the brief test contained in this booklet is all about. The few minutes you take to complete it may actually help you add years to your life! How? Well to start, it will enable you to identify aspects of your present lifestyle that are risky to your health. Then it will encourage you to take steps to eliminate or minimize the risks you identify. All in all, it will help you begin to change your present lifestyle into a new HEALTHSTYLE. If you do, it's possible that you may feel better, look better, and live longer too.

Before You Take the Test

This is not a pass-fail test. Its purpose is simply to tell you how well you are doing to stay healthy. The behaviors covered in the test are recommended for most Americans. Some of them may not apply to persons with certain chronic diseases or handicaps. Such persons may require special instructions from their physician or other health professional.

You will find that the test has six sections: smoking, alcohol and drugs, nutrition, exercise and fitness, stress control, and safety. Complete one section at a time by circling the number corresponding to the answer that best describes your behavior (2 for "Almost Always", 1 for "Sometimes", and 0 for "Almost Never"). Then add the numbers you have circled to determine your score for that section. Write the score on the line provided at the end of each section. The highest score you can get for each section is 10.

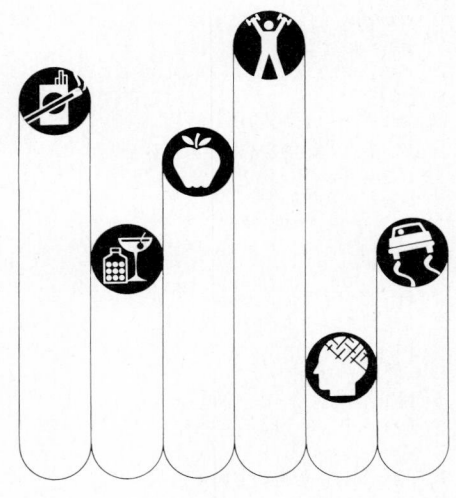

Fig. 38-1, cont'd. Self-test for good health.

A Test for Better Health

	Almost Always	Sometimes	Almost Never

If you never smoke, enter a score of 10 for this section and go to the next section on *Alcohol and Drugs*.

1. I avoid smoking cigarettes.   2 1 0

2. I smoke only low tar and nicotine cigarettes *or* I smoke a pipe or cigars.   2 1 0

Smoking Score: _____

	Almost Always	Sometimes	Almost Never

1. I avoid drinking alcoholic beverages *or* I drink no more than 1 or 2 drinks a day.   4 1 0

2. I avoid using alcohol or other drugs (especially illegal drugs) as a way of handling stressful situations or the problems in my life.   2 1 0

3. I am careful not to drink alcohol when taking certain medicines (for example, medicine for sleeping, pain, colds, and allergies).   2 1 0

4. I read and follow the label directions when using prescribed and over-the-counter drugs.   2 1 0

Alcohol and Drugs Score: _____

Eating Habits

	Almost Always	Sometimes	Almost Never

1. I eat a variety of foods each day, such as fruits and vegetables, whole grain breads and cereals, lean meats, dairy products, dry peas and beans, and nuts and seeds.   4 1 0

2. I limit the amount of fat, saturated fat, and cholesterol I eat (including fat on meats, eggs, butter, cream, shortenings, and organ meats such as liver).   2 1 0

3. I limit the amount of salt I eat by cooking with only small amounts, not adding salt at the table, and avoiding salty snacks.   2 1 0

4. I avoid eating too much sugar (especially frequent snacks of sticky candy or soft drinks).   2 1 0

Eating Habits Score: _____

Exercise/Fitness

	Almost Always	Sometimes	Almost Never

1. I maintain a desired weight, avoiding overweight and underweight.   3 1 0

2. I do vigorous exercises for 15-30 minutes at least 3 times a week (examples include running, swimming, brisk walking).   3 1 0

3. I do exercises that enhance my muscle tone for 15-30 minutes at least 3 times a week (examples include yoga and calisthenics).   2 1 0

4. I use part of my leisure time participating in individual, family, or team activities that increase my level of fitness (such as gardening, bowling, golf, and baseball).   2 1 0

Exercise/Fitness Score: _____

Fig. 38-1, cont'd. Self-test for good health.

Continued.

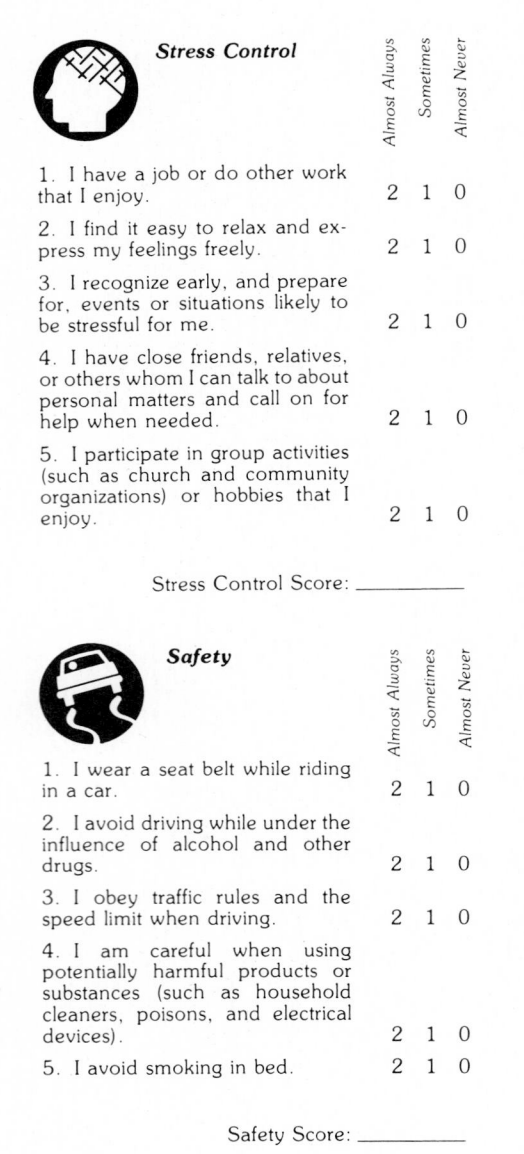

Stress Control

	Almost Always	Sometimes	Almost Never
1. I have a job or do other work that I enjoy.	2	1	0
2. I find it easy to relax and express my feelings freely.	2	1	0
3. I recognize early, and prepare for, events or situations likely to be stressful for me.	2	1	0
4. I have close friends, relatives, or others whom I can talk to about personal matters and call on for help when needed.	2	1	0
5. I participate in group activities (such as church and community organizations) or hobbies that I enjoy.	2	1	0

Stress Control Score: _____

Safety

	Almost Always	Sometimes	Almost Never
1. I wear a seat belt while riding in a car.	2	1	0
2. I avoid driving while under the influence of alcohol and other drugs.	2	1	0
3. I obey traffic rules and the speed limit when driving.	2	1	0
4. I am careful when using potentially harmful products or substances (such as household cleaners, poisons, and electrical devices).	2	1	0
5. I avoid smoking in bed.	2	1	0

Safety Score: _____

Fig. 38-1, cont'd. Self-test for good health.

Your HEALTHSTYLE Scores

After you have figured your scores for each of the six sections, circle the number in each column that matches your score for that section of the test.

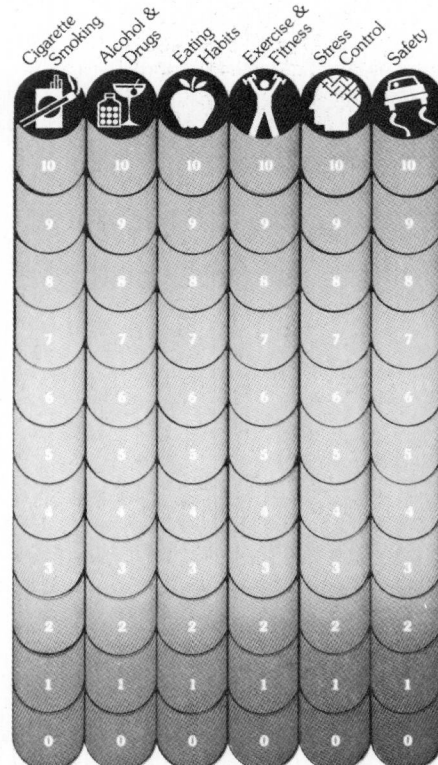

Remember, there is no total score for this test. Consider each section separately. You are trying to identify aspects of your lifestyle that you can improve in order to be healthier and to reduce the risk of illness. So let's see what your scores reveal.

What Your Scores Mean to YOU

Scores of 9 and 10

Excellent! Your answers show that you are aware of the importance of this area to your health. More importantly, you are putting your knowledge to work for you by practicing good health habits. As long as you continue to do so, this area should not pose a serious health risk. It's likely that you are setting an example for your family and friends to follow. Since you got a very high score on this part of the test, you may want to consider other areas where your scores indicate room for improvement.

Scores of 6 to 8

Your health practices in this area are good, but there is room for improvement. Look again at the items you answered with a "Sometimes" or "Almost Never". What changes can you make to improve your score? Even a small change can often help you achieve better health.

Scores of 3 to 5

Your health risks are showing! Would you like more information about the risks you are facing and about why it is important for you to change these behaviors. Perhaps you need help in deciding how to successfully make the changes you desire. In either case, help is available. See the last page of this booklet.

Scores of 0 to 2

Obviously, you were concerned enough about your health to take the test, but your answers show that you may be taking serious and unnecessary risks with your health. Perhaps you are not aware of the risks and what to do about them. You can easily get the information and help you need to improve, if you wish. A source of contact appears on the last page. The next step is up to you.

Fig. 38-1, cont'd. Self-test for good health.

YOU Can Start Right Now!

In the test you just completed were numerous suggestions to help you reduce your risk of disease and premature death. Here are some of the most significant:

 Avoid cigarettes. Cigarette smoking is the single most important preventable cause of illness and early death. It is especially risky for pregnant women and their unborn babies. Persons who stop smoking reduce their risk of getting heart disease and cancer. So if you're a cigarette smoker, think twice about lighting that next cigarette. If you choose to continue smoking, try decreasing the number of cigarettes you smoke and switching to a low tar and nicotine brand.

 Follow sensible drinking habits. Alcohol produces changes in mood and behavior. Most people who drink are able to control their intake of alcohol and to avoid undesired, and often harmful, effects. Heavy, regular use of alcohol can lead to cirrhosis of the liver, a leading cause of death. Also, statistics clearly show that mixing drinking and driving is often the cause of fatal or crippling accidents. So if you drink, do it wisely and in moderation.

 Use care in taking drugs. Today's greater use of drugs—both legal and illegal—is one of our most serious health risks. Even some drugs prescribed by your doctor can be dangerous if taken when drinking alcohol or before driving. Excessive or continued use of tranquilizers (or "pep pills") can cause physical and mental problems. Using or experimenting with illicit drugs such as marijuana, heroin, cocaine, and PCP may lead to a number of damaging effects or even death.

Continued.

Eat sensibly. Overweight individuals are at greater risk for diabetes, gall bladder disease, and high blood pressure. So it makes good sense to maintain proper weight. But good eating habits also mean holding down the amount of fat (especially saturated fat), cholesterol, sugar and salt in your diet. If you must snack, try nibbling on fresh fruits and vegetables. You'll feel better—and look better, too.

 Exercise regularly. Almost everyone can benefit from exercise—and there's some form of exercise almost everyone can do. (If you have any doubt, check first with your doctor.) Usually, as little as 15-30 minutes of vigorous exercise three times a week will help you have a healthier heart, eliminate excess weight, tone up sagging muscles, and sleep better. Think how much difference all these improvements could make in the way you feel!

 Learn to handle stress. Stress is a normal part of living: everyone faces it to some degree. The causes of stress can be good or bad, desirable or undesirable (such as a promotion on the job or the loss of a spouse). Properly handled, stress need not be a problem. But unhealthy responses to stress—such as driving too fast or erratically, drinking too much, or prolonged anger or grief—can cause a variety of physical and mental problems. Even on a very busy day, find a few minutes to slow down and relax. Talking over a problem with someone you trust can often help you find a satisfactory solution. Learn to distinguish between things that are "worth fighting about" and things that are less important.

Be safety conscious. Think "safety first" at home, at work, at school, at play, and on the highway. Buckle seat belts and obey traffic rules. Keep poisons and weapons out of the reach of children, and keep emergency numbers by your telephone. When the unexpected happens, you'll be prepared.

Fig. 38-1, cont'd. Self-test for good health.

Where Do You Go From Here?

Start by asking yourself a few frank questions:
Am I really doing all I can to be as healthy as possible? What steps can I take to feel better? Am I willing to begin now? If you scored low in one or more sections of the test, decide what changes you want to make for improvement. You might pick that aspect of your lifestyle where you feel you have the best chance for success and tackle that one first. Once you have improved your score there, go on to other areas.

If you already have tried to change your health habits (to stop smoking or exercise regularly, for example) don't be discouraged if you haven't yet succeeded. The difficulty you have encountered may be due to influences you've never really thought about—such as advertising—or to a lack of support and encouragement. Understanding these influences is an important step toward changing the way they affect you.

There's Help Available. In addition to personal actions you can take on your own, there are community programs and groups (such as the YMCA or the local chapter of the American Heart Association) that can assist you and your family to make the changes you want to make. If you want to know more about these groups or about health risks contact your local health department or mail in the card contained in this booklet. There's a lot you can do to stay healthy or to improve your health—and there are organizations that can help you. Start a new HEALTHSTYLE today!

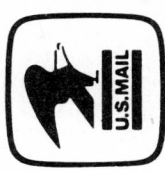
Fig. 38-1, cont'd. Self-test for good health.

Table 38-1. The social readjustment rating scale — schedule of recent experiences*

Rank	Life Event	Mean value
1	Death of spouse	100
2	Divorce	73
3	Marital separation	65
4	Jail term	63
5	Death of close family member	63
6	Personal injury or illness	53
7	Marriage	50
8	Fired at work	47
9	Marital reconciliation	45
10	Retirement	45
11	Change in health of family member	44
12	Pregnancy	40
13	Sex difficulties	39
14	Gain of new family member	39
15	Business readjustment	39
16	Change in financial state	38
17	Death of close friend	37
18	Change to different line of work	36
19	Change in number of arguments with spouse	35
20	Mortgage over $10,000	31
21	Foreclosure of mortgage or loan	30
22	Change in responsibilities at work	29
23	Son or daughter leaving home	29
24	Trouble with in-laws	29
25	Outstanding personal achievement	28
26	Wife begins or stops work	26
27	Begin or end school	26
28	Change in living conditions	25
29	Revision of personal habits	24
30	Trouble with boss	23
31	Change in work hours or conditions	20
32	Change in residence	20
33	Change in schools	20
34	Change in recreation	19
35	Change in church activities	19
36	Change in social activities	18
37	Mortgage or loan less than $10,000	17
38	Change in sleeping habits	16
39	Change in number of family get-togethers	15
40	Change in eating habits	15
41	Vacation	13
42	Christmas	12
43	Minor violations of the law	11

Reprinted with permission from Holmes, T.H., and Rake, R.H.: The Social Readjustment Rating Scale, J. Psychosom. Res. 11:213-218, 1967. By permission of Pergamon Press, Ltd.

* Directions: Add the score for all items applying to you in the past year. The number derived is a predictor of the percent of chance of hospitalization within the next year according to the following:

below 150 — 10%
between 150 and 300 — 50%
over 300 — 90%

Children's Ratings of the Stressfulness of Experiences

1. Losing a parent
2. Going blind
3. Being retained in a grade
4. Wetting in class
5. Parental fights
6. Caught in a theft
7. Suspected of lying
8. A poor report card
9. Sent to the principal
10. Having an operation (a surgical procedure)

From Yamamoto, K.: Dev. Psychol. **15:**581-582, 1979. Copyright 1979 by the American Psychological Association. Reprinted by permission of the author.

Scores between 150 and 299 units indicated a 50% chance of being ill in the near future and scores lower than 150 units decreased the chances of an illness to 30%.

Thus a job promotion with its salary and status increase, nicer office, and better fringe benefits unconsciously produces a loss. The loss may be that of the familiar. Children, like adults, experience a sense of loss produced by change. Not all family moves are unconditionally met with pleasure. Also, what may seem like relatively minor changes to adults may be perceived differently by the children who are affected. Changes in lunch programs, teachers, schools, modes of transportation, and friends potentially affect children. Yamamoto (1979) studied the perceptions of fourth, fifth, and sixth graders as to the most stressful events in their lives. The top 10 choices are seen in the above box.

STRESSORS

Stressors are defined as internal or external environmental stimuli that trigger physiological and psychological coping mechanisms. Stressors are not necessarily harmful; people need stimulation, challenges, excitement, and novel experiences to motivate and encourage new ideas and actions. Hence some stressors are positive, whereas others elicit a negative response. Similarly, what makes a stressor for one person may be energizing for another. To understand stressors, Sutterly (1979) classified them into the following two major categories: (biophysical-chemical and psychosocial-cultural.)

Biophysical-Chemical Stressors

As seen in Fig. 38-2, a variety of biophysical-chemical stressors can elicit the stress response. However, the response does not necessarily result from a cause and effect situation. For this reason nurses must carefully monitor individual responses to stress and note what provokes the stress response and in what ways stress is manifested.

The substances many people use to combat stress actually are stressors themselves. For example, coffee, cigarettes, and alcoholic beverages are often used to promote relaxation; yet these substances actually are toxic to the body and act as stressors. Similarly, overeating stresses biophysical-chemical adaptation, especially if the food taken in is composed of excessive amounts of refined carbohydrates, salt, fats, and animal protein. Foods Americans consume without awareness of the potential for generating stress include sugar, salt, caffeine, alcohol, nicotine, and food additives. When these are combined with the effects of air pollution, insecticides, and other toxins, the cumulative impact is considerable.

Physical sources of stress that are often overlooked or taken for granted include any form of trauma, accidents, weather changes, poor light, noise, physical work or living conditions, infectious agents, or inactivity. It is estimated that remaining in bed for a week generates as much stress as having a broken leg. As community health nurses, it is important to continuously estimate the cumulative stress effect on clients. For example, a bedridden person recovering from the physical stress of a stroke is more affected by an upper respiratory infection than is a relatively active, physically fit person. It is important to help clients learn what stressors are present in their lives and how to remove the optional ones as well as learn effective ways to cope with those that are inevitable. Though only a few biophysical-chemical stressors are discussed, many more exist in communities.

Living conditions affect stress. Crowded living conditions provide limited privacy, and under such conditions tempers tend to flare as people feel overstimulated by the presence of others. In an ecological analysis of Chicago, Galle et al. (1972) isolated density per room in a residential dwelling as being closely related to mortality, fertility, public assistance, juvenile delinquency, and admission to psychiatric hospitals. Based on their research, they concluded that multiple people per room led to increased stimulation, more demands on one another, and a generally increased level of frustration.

Another physical source of stress present in most communities is noise. Excessive noise is considered irritating, and in recent years data have been accumulated to indicate that it is also influential in determining how people behave. People react differently to noise. What may be pleasant to one person is often irritating to others. Consider the variable reactions of teenagers and

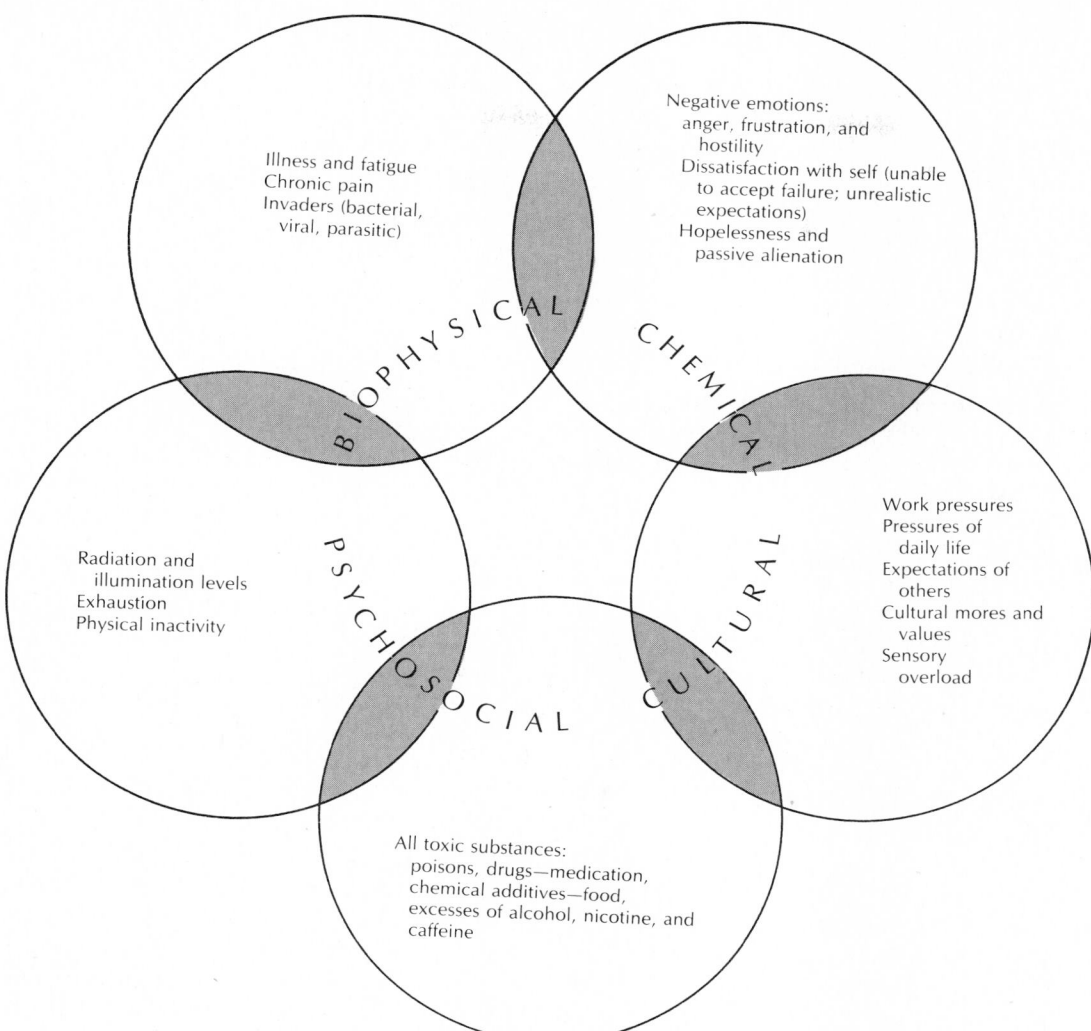

Illness and fatigue
Chronic pain
Invaders (bacterial,
viral, parasitic)

Negative emotions:
anger, frustration, and
hostility
Dissatisfaction with self (unable
to accept failure; unrealistic
expectations)
Hopelessness and
passive alienation

Radiation and
illumination levels
Exhaustion
Physical inactivity

Work pressures
Pressures of
daily life
Expectations of
others
Cultural mores and
values
Sensory
overload

All toxic substances:
poisons, drugs—medication,
chemical additives—food,
excesses of alcohol, nicotine, and
caffeine

BIOPHYSICAL CHEMICAL PSYCHOSOCIAL CULTURAL

Fig. 38-2. Multiple sources of stress: biophysical-chemical and psychosocial-cultural stressors. (Reprinted from Sutterly, D.C.: Stress and health: a survey of self-regulation modalities, Top. Clin. Nurs. **1**:1-20, April 1979. By permission of Aspen Systems Corp., © 1979.)

their parents to a loud stereo. For one group this noise is thrilling whereas to the other it is often deafening. Unpredictable noises tend to be more disruptive than steady repetitive sounds. Also, workers continuously exposed to high intensity noises show increased incidence of nervous complaints, nausea, instability, argumentativeness, sexual impotence, mood changes, and anxiety (Cohen, 1981).

To demonstrate the effect of noise on behavior, Cohen (1981) asked a colleague to walk down the street on a sunny day. Carrying a large stack of books, he walked down various streets where some people were mowing their lawns and others were walking along. Periodically he would drop several books. When the books dropped

near a lawn mower running at full speed without a muffler, only 12.5% of the other walkers offered to help, whereas 50% offered to assist him when no lawn mower was running.

Climate has historically been associated with emotions. For example, happiness is equated with sunny weather and sadness with clouds. Extremes of temperature seem to inhibit efficiency. This was particularly evident in the late 1960s when many racial riots occurred in several major cities during the hot summer months. Tempers seem to flare in exceedingly hot weather. With the advent of air conditioning and central heat people have grown accustomed to expecting predictable weather conditions and find themselves highly stressed when temperatures reach record highs and lows. Clients may need to be counseled about preparation for inclement weather conditions. Do they know where they can go to find relief when it is exceptionally hot or cold? Is it helpful to have canned foods ready if they become unable to get to the store? In addition to biophysical-chemical stressors, various psychosocial-cultural stressors influence adaptation.

Psychosocial-Cultural Stressors

As noted, a considerable amount of today's stress is brought about by the rapidly changing times, increasing technology, economic constraints, accelerated pace of living, and increased mobility. Many stressors arise at home and work. There may be conflicting values among family members causing strains and tension. Also, work situations often serve as stressors by causing people to feel overwhelmed with either the quantity or quality of work expected. People seem to cope better in work situations in which they are regarded as valuable, contributing members of the group rather than when their only value seems to revolve around the amount of output they produce. Psychosocial-cultural stressors can be thought of as arising from one of three general causes: societal, situational, and personal.

Societal Stressors

Some examples of societal causes of stress have already been identified. Others include such things as inflation, liberal attitudes about abortion. women's rights, male/female roles and relationships, dress, pornography, noise pollution, and peer pressure to behave in certain ways sanctioned by the peer group.

Situational Stressors

Examples of situational causes of stress include varying aspects of the work situation such as too much or too little structure and unclear communication or lines of authority. Changes in a person's life also prompt a stress response, especially if there is an accumulation of changes. Many of the rapid changes in society are leading to unprecedented levels of depression. Throughout history periods of social unrest and rapid change have tended to precipitate depression. Some groups are at higher risk for depression under these conditions than others. For example, the following factors seem important in the onset of stress-related depression (Jacobson, 1974, p. 12):

1. Discrete life events and ongoing stressors (including their meaning to the person)
2. Being unmarried (especially if previously married)
3. Being female
4. Belonging to the lowest socioeconomic group
5. Age (youth or elderly)
6. Family history of affective illness
7. Premorbid personality characteristics described as the dominant other

As noted previously in the Holmes and Rahe scale, it may not be the type of change per se but the amount and rapidity of change that cause stress.

French and Caplan (1980) observed that people experience more stress at work when they are not given adequate information to do their jobs and remain unclear about what is expected. This lack of clarity about role expectations is called *role ambiguity*. In contrast, role conflict occurs when information is contradictory or there are substantive differences an disagreements among workers. Likewise, role overload increases stress and generally decreases productivity. There are two general categories of role overload: qualitative and quantitative. Quantitative role overload is seen when people do not know how to do what is expected of them or do not have access to needed information, skill, and resources necessary for task completion. In contrast, quantitative role overload occurs when there is simply too much to do in too short a time.

Other work-associated causes of stress include contacts across organizational boundaries where each group may hold different goals and expectations. Familiar settings and situations generally produce greater comfort than do new situations and settings with their unique set of rules and expectations. Additionally, responsibility for people rather than things tends to be more stressful because of the potential for interruptions and human needs requiring attentions (Pope, 1982).

Major sources of situational stressors facing workers have been reported by Schwartz (1980, p. 100) as including:

1. Work overload or stagnation
2. Extreme ambiguity or rigidity
3. Extreme role conflict or too little conflict
4. Extreme amounts of responsibility
5. Cutthroat and negative competition or no competition at all
6. Constant change and daily variability
7. Ongoing contact with "stress carriers" or people who cause others to experience stress because of their unreasonable goals, expectations, or ways of speaking or responding to others.
8. The corporation (for its own survival) discouraging individuality and clearly rewarding deference of one's own goals to that of the group.

Mobility is another situational stressor that affects many individuals. When people move from one city to another, they disrupt all of their established support networks. New support systems must be developed in an unfamiliar place. Simply getting to school, work, or the grocery store is initially difficult in a new place.

Labeling and prejudice make up another situational stressor that is often present yet at times difficult to define. People tend to be appraised by others according to a wide range of specifics including race, sex, age, income, appearance, family status, and varying other personal characteristics. Many groups, including women, children, the aged, mentally ill people, minorities, and poor people, are discriminated against just for being themselves. Schecter (1979) reported that working women earn 57 cents for every dollar earned by men. She applied the term *battered women* to the new generation of working women who suffer varying abuses as they attempt to juggle multiple roles.

Economic conditions constitute an increasing source of stress for people in many parts of the world. Specifically, inflation has an insidious effect on the health of communities. Instead of an obvious change in income, people eventually realize that their buying power has slowly eroded, and their standard of living is decreasing rather the increasing. The American dream of working hard and making life better has disappeared for many. Only about 20% of Americans are socioeconomically mobile with 15% able to move up, and the remaining 5% moving downward (Johnson, 1979).

Though these stressors are observed in many work situations, some groups have unique stressors. Nursing is a stressful profession because of a variety of causes such as poor communication; politics within the organization; conflicting demands for time and attention; lack of knowledge of what is expected; underuse of skills; changes in the organization; lack of participation in making decisions; limited job progress or career advancement; relations with other nurses, supervisors, subordinates, physicians, families, and clients; role overload; and responsibility without authority (Ivancevich and Matteson, 1980, p. 19).

Willis (1979) identified the following four categories of stressors that affect pediatric nurses and are applicable to other nursing settings: (1) stressors common to institutional life, including power struggles, responsibility without adequate instruction and supervision, lack of authority, and time pressures; (2) those peculiar to the organization and administration of a given place, such as lack of recognition, incentives, difficulty in getting supplies, and lack of a competitive salary; (3) stressors peculiar to nurses involved in direct patient care; and (4) those specific to working in a given area, such as pediatrics, hospice, or psychiatry.

Personal Stressors

Personal causes of stress include low self-esteem, a need to be perfect, a need to control others, or a need to

be dominated and controlled by others. For many people irrational beliefs constitute stressful situations. People often have unrealistic personal expectations for themselves, others, and the environment. People often expect to be perfect; they indulge in considerable personal anguish when they fail to meet this expectation. Clients must be reminded that no one is perfect; everyone makes mistakes. The goal is to learn from those mistakes and not repeat the same ones.

People also tend to have unrealistic expectations of others. For example, a middle-aged widowed woman may expect that her 30-year-old married son will always do as she says and expects. She may consider it reasonable to call him two or three times a week and ask him to come over and fix something. Because of his own busy schedule and family demands, he may not always be able to comply with his mother's wishes, causing her to feel rejected. A nursing goal could be to help the mother have more realistic expectations of her son as well as develop additional support networks.

Other people have unrealistic expectations of the environment. For example, some expect that raises and promotions will automatically occur. Although this may be possible in some situations, ordinarily effort, initiative, and productivity are essential to ensure promotions.

WAYS TO MANAGE STRESS

According to Donnelly (1980a), there are basically two ways of dealing with stress: reactive and active. Reactive ways are based on the belief that stress is inevitable, and all people can do is sit back and wait for "it" to happen. This view is similar to the flight response to stress. Behaving in a reactive way, people simply take what comes along. For example, they work late when the poor planning of others causes extra work. They blame themselves for all that goes wrong at home, school, or work. When self-blame and overconscientiousness fail, the reactive person may lash out at others in an irrational or aggressive manner or may resort to personal comfort measures including drugs, alcohol, overeating, smoking, or using sleep as an escape. The reactive pattern can lead to chronic fatigue, irritability, depression, feelings of inadequacy, and finally stress-related diseases such as colitis or hypertension.

The alternative to dealing with stress in a reactive manner is to gain control and assume an active role in fighting stressors. As discussed in Chapter 37, the active role is based on an assertive posture toward self. Essentially, to respond actively to stress says, "I am responsible for what I do and how I feel. I can choose to be overly stressed or to cope adaptively and constructively."

Community health nurses can learn active stress

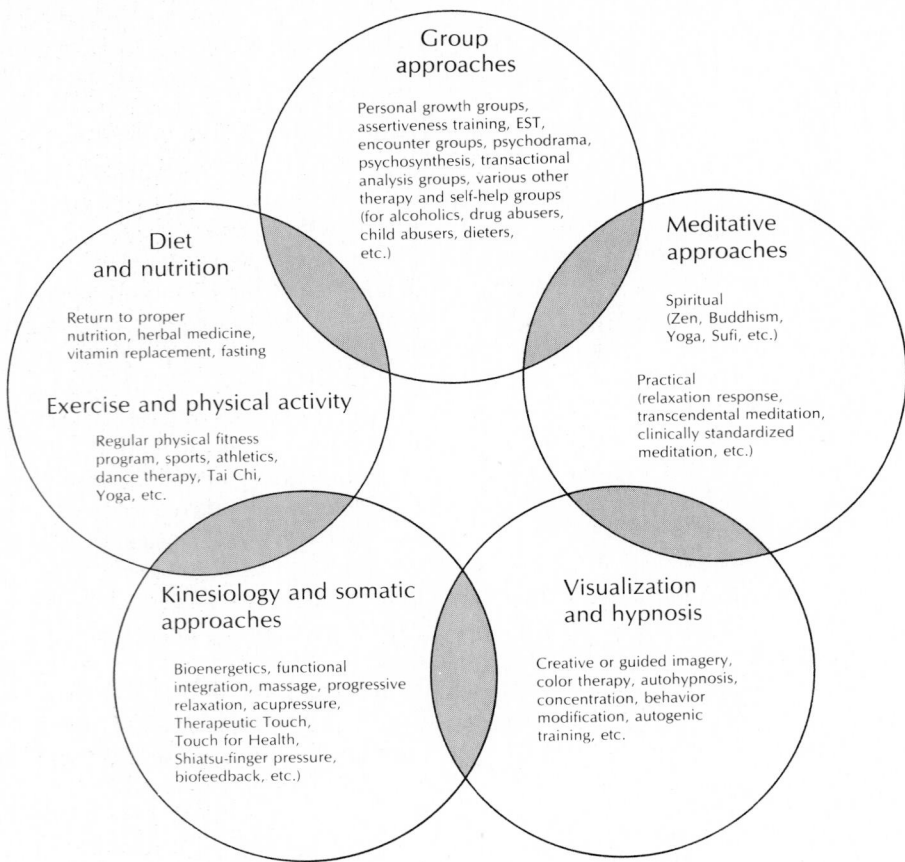

Fig. 38-3. Various approaches used in self-regulation of stress. (Reprinted from Sutterly, D.C.: Stress and health: a survey of self-regulation modalities, Top. Clin. Nurs. **1:**1-20, April 1979. Used with permission of Aspen Systems Corp., © 1979.)

management responses to promote their own health as well as that of their clients. It is difficult to teach clients about health promotion efforts that the nurse does not practice. The dangers of smoking sound shallow coming from a nurse who only speaks between puffs on a cigarette. Likewise, obese nurses do not make effective counselors on the value of a balanced diet and carefully selected exercise. Fig. 38-3 depicts a variety of approaches that can be used in the self-regulation of stress.

No one technique works for everyone; however, each person does have the potential to manage stress. The key lies in finding just the right technique for each person. Nurses cannot force clients to manage or regulate their level of stress. Such efforts require motivation and personal determination to reach a self-appointed goal. The following are the three general ways for intervening in stress:

1. Change the environment so that it is less stressful.
2. Change one's own beliefs and/or behavior so that

situations are perceived differently and are subsequently responded to in a different manner.
3. Learn to lower physiological arousal to stress by countering the long-range effects.

There are many ways to manage stress, and people have preferences in the method they find most successful. Also, certain techniques require more skill and resources than others. A variety of techniques are discussed to equip the community health nurse with many choices for developing personal stress management programs with clients. Some general principles of stress management are presented in the boxed material followed by specific and detailed techniques.

To determine the most appropriate mode of intervention for stress reduction it is important to apply the nursing process. The assessment phase begins with a series of questions that could include the following: What specific demands is the person experiencing? What are perceived as stressors? How has the person previously

---

Stress Management Tips

1. Get to know your body so that you can recognize the first signs of stress. (Have clients recall their last stressful situation and describe their physiological reaction.)
2. Learn to relax. Deep breathing is a natural relaxant.
3. Practice simple relaxing exercises.
4. Exercise. Take a brisk walk, run, play tennis, or dance to stimulate blood flow.
5. Learn to smile and laugh and to balance work and recreation. (Ask clients to recall the last time they had fun; what were they doing, and how did they feel?)
6. Learn to worry effectively by doing something about it. (Instruct people to talk out their worries with someone they trust and respect.)
7. Learn to accept things and people. Some situations are beyond your control. (Instruct people to change their attitudes about a situation or to develop a stress-reduction plan.)
8. Take one thing at a time. A sure way to become overwhelmed is to find yourself in the middle of a dozen projects.
9. Give in once in a while, and try to avoid getting angry. Once you are angry, you are conquered because the ability to think clearly and rationally is diminished in the face of anger.

---

coped with stressful situations? What support systems are available at this time, and what supports have previously been used? Other questions to be raised relate to determining what sets off a stressful situation. Is the discomfort proportional to the event, or is the person's anxiety cumulative and representative of many additive stressors? What are the person's current resources, limitations, and level of motivation?

The stress reduction plan is unique for each client depending on the level and nature of stress, the person's interest and motivation to be actively involved in reducing stress, and the comfort in practicing skills on a regular basis. As is discussed under meditation, certain personal and environmental characteristics must be present to ensure the potential for success.

Various avenues are available for implementation of a stress reduction plan including diet, exercise, changing attitudes, relaxation, creative imagery, biofeedback, hypnosis, and acupressure. Techniques such as eliciting the relaxation response, progressive relaxation, and biofeedback promote voluntary control over autonomic responses. In contrast, physical exercise can also reduce excessive stress by simply "working it off."

Nutrition

A diet that fights stress contains balanced portions of the basic four food groups with a good proportion of natural foods free from preservatives and additives (Chapter 21). The diet should also be limited in animal proteins, carbohydrates, salt, refined sugar, and alcohol. In recent years Americans have become accustomed to eating what is called the *affluent diet*. The main characteristics of this diet are high levels of fat (especially animal fats), cholesterol, and salt. To reduce stress, major changes must occur in basic eating habits.

The following changes are generally recommended in the affluent diet to make it a healthier choice of foods (Eckholm and Record, 1980, p. 135):

1. Reduce fat consumption to under 35% of total calorie intake. This often means reducing consumption of meat, dairy products, and fried foods; shifting from beef and pork to fish and chicken; and a preference for grass-fed rather than grain-fed beef.
2. Replace saturated with unsaturated fats; substitute vegetable fats (margarine) for animal fats (butter).
3. Decrease cholesterol intake (cut down on eggs).
4. Reduce sugar and salt intake.
5. Eat whole grains, potatoes and other starchy foods, fresh fruits and vegetables.
6. Balance caloric intake with energy expenditures.

Chemicals in the diet serve as stressors to the body either by stimulating bodily functioning as in caffeine or alcohol or by serving as toxins as in food additives and salt. Energy can be consumed in eating foods that are difficult to digest, such as fats and refined sugar. Given a more nutritious diet, people have greater stores of energy available to cope with stress.

Aerobic Exercise

Exercise has many benefits in fighting stress (Chapter 21). Aerobics, vigorous exercise provided by many different activities, is designed to increase the flow of blood and oxygen to all parts of the body. The primary benefits of aerobic exercise include strengthening the respiratory muscles and reducing the resistance to airflow; the heart growing stronger and more efficient, thereby increasing the blood supply to the body; muscle tone and general circulation improving, and blood

---

Relaxation Exercises

Brief relaxation should be a part of every day.

Exercise 1

1. Take 5 minutes, three times a day.
2. Sit comfortably and close your eyes.
3. Concentrate on bringing to mind a picture of the most peaceful setting you have experienced.
4. With each breath say to yourself, "Relax, relax."
5. With practice you can let your thoughts and problems float away for a few minutes.

Exercise 2

1. Sit in a comfortable position.
2. Close your eyes.
3. Inhale a deep breath through your nose — hold — exhale through your mouth. Repeat five times.
4. Breathe normally.
5. Concentrate on breathing. Each time you exhale, say the word "one" silently to yourself. Breathe in, breathe out, with "one."
6. Open your eyes.
7. Sit quietly for 1 minute.

---

pressure often being reduced; finally, the number of red blood cells and amount of hemoglobin increasing, and more oxygen being carried to the tissues.

Additionally, aerobic exercise helps to build lean muscle to replace fat, and food is absorbed more effectively, thereby using calories in a more efficient manner. Beyond the physical benefits of aerobic exercise (running, jumping rope), people report a variety of psychological benefits including clarity of thinking after the exercise and a dissipation of anger.

Certain precautions need to be taken before implementing an exercise program, including assessment of current health status, purchase of proper equipment, participation in a warm-up and cool-down period, and pacing the exercise to individual ability and condition. These precautions are discussed more fully in Chapter 21.

Group Discussion

Group discussion offers a special form of support in that it provides an unstructured, safe arena to openly share feelings, views, and perceptions. Group members can help validate the effectiveness or poor selection of a coping mechanism and assist members in learning and practicing new responses. Often people think that they have behaved so badly that no one else could possibly understand, much less accept them.

Community health nurses have for many years recognized the value of group sessions in helping clients deal with problems. Successful group experiences have included people with alcohol and/or drug dependencies, those with problems of obesity, individuals with major chronic illnesses, those suffering the loss of a child or spouse, and victims of human abuse (abusers,

too). Group approaches have historically been a significant avenue for health maintenance and promotion. Stress management groups offer a rich potential for clients and nurses. These groups can be oriented toward discussions or activities or a combination of both. Group membership is a natural and desirable social phenomenon. People are born into a group and throughout life, either consciously or unconsciously, attempt to find their place in the group. Groups can have a healing effect by providing opportunities for self-understanding and acceptance (Donnelly, 1980b, p. 32).

Nursing Implications

Consider the feelings that might be experienced if you had failed to refer a client seen in a public health clinic because you thought the complaints of chest pain were imaginary only to come to work the next day and find that the client had angina. In a group session the nurse who is feeling guilty over this experience could receive validation from other members that mistakes like this occur and that more effective ways to respond to clients rather than self-blame for faulty problem solving are necessary.

Changing Attitudes

Changing attitudes is an essential part of stress management. It is important to handle stressors as they occur and to deal directly with feelings to avoid bottling up thoughts or emotions. It is also important to find something to substitute for worrying thoughts and to chase them away. Nothing erases unpleasant thoughts more effectively than conscious efforts to focus on positive things. A process for shifting attitudes to more effectively deal with feelings can be described as the following: (Adams, 1980)

1. Notice the feeling or sensation by being consciously aware that something is occurring.
2. Give the feeling a label such as anger or happiness.
3. Make a decision as to whether or not the feeling or cluster of feelings is appropriate to the present situation being perceived in the environment.
4. Give expression to feelings in a way that is safe, will get what is wanted or needed, and will do no harm to another. That is, it is much more appropriate to talk with people about being angry than to hit them.

Relaxation

Although relaxing is a universal human ability, this activity tends to be cast aside in the busy hustle and bustle of life. For many people, relaxing is viewed as a waste of time rather than an opportunity for unwinding and passively dealing with the stresses of life. Community health nurses are in an ideal position to teach relaxation techniques by including this activity in their scope of practice. Before teaching relaxation techniques, it is useful to learn and practice them to gain comfort in this ability. Several brief relaxation exercises are included in the preceding box to provide variety in practice sessions.

Relaxation exercises are simply "journeys into self," which provide a mechanism for unwinding. The primary purpose of relaxation is to relieve muscle tension and induce a quieting response whereby the body can rebuild needed energy resources. Nurses can assist clients through teaching and role modeling to control autonomic functions by altering their state of consciousness to assume a mental state of relaxation. One form of relaxation that is discussed in some detail is progressive relaxation.

Progressive Relaxation

Progressive relaxation provides a way of reducing stress by altering the relation between muscle and psychological tension. Jacobson (1974) did extensive research on mind/muscle interaction and postulated that anxiety and relaxation are mutually exclusive. This technique was developed as a method of combating tension and anxiety by instructing clients to systematically tense and relax muscle groups. The goal of progressive relaxation is not to eliminate all stress but to allow people to monitor and control their stress levels.

Progressive relaxation, a rudimentary form of biofeedback, is based on the person's ability to differentiate tension from relaxation and to feel the difference as each of 14 major muscle groups is consecutively tensed

and then immediately relaxed. The procedure follows a systematic format moving from the feet to the head (see box on p. 864). This form of relaxation is within the scope of nursing practice and has been successful in treating clients with borderline hypertension, headaches, insomnia, and anxiety.

Specific assessment areas before instituting progressive relaxation would include, in addition to a history, a determination that the stressful situation should be treated in this manner rather than with medication. It must also be determined if any contraindications exist relative to the relaxation of certain muscle groups. For some types of low back pain, strengthening rather than relaxing certain muscle groups is preferred (Richter and Sloan, 1979). The planning and implementation phases are consistent with all other forms of relaxation. In the evaluation phase of the nursing process it is necessary to carefully observe any factors that may have compromised the effectiveness of this technique.

Bernstein and Borkovec (1973) defined the following common problems relative to progressive relaxation: (1) muscle cramps, (2) movement, (3) laughter or talking, (4) other noise, (5) intrusive thoughts, (6) sleep, (7) coughing and sneezing, (8) inability to relax certain muscle groups, (9) strange or unfamiliar feelings, (10) losing control, (11) internal arousal, (12) failure to follow instructions, and (13) problems with practicing and avoiding certain words and phrases. Many of these problems and the suggested solutions also apply to other stress reduction techniques.

In progressive relaxation cramps may occur in the neck, calves, feet, or any other muscle group held especially tense. These cramps can often be avoided by suggesting that the client reduce the tension as well as hold these muscles tense for a shorter period of time. The affected muscles can be gradually tensed and relaxed to reduce the level of strain on them. If cramps do occur, it should be suggested that the client manipulate (move or rub) the affected muscle, wait a few minutes before going on, and then continue. When progressive relaxation is practiced in a group, clients may move around excessively during the exercise, and this may be disruptive to others attempting to maintain their concentration. If comfort is a problem, the client may need some assistance in finding a desirable position. Also, it is not uncommon for participants to either laugh or talk during the early sessions because of anxiety and fear of embarrassment. Some of the muscle-tensing exercises, especially those involving facial muscles, cause participants to look "funny." They may laugh at one another or at themselves as they feel their faces assume strange positions. It is usually helpful if the nurse performs the exercises along with the client to promote a feeling of comfort and acceptance in the session.

Progressive Relaxation: Modified Approach for Community Health Nursing Practice

This activity simply involves relaxing one step at a time, as follows:

1. Sit or lie in a comfortable position.
2. Close your eyes.
3. Concentrate on breathing easily.
4. Once your body feels calm, instruct all bones and muscles of the lower body to relax in the following order:
   a. Feet   d. Knees
   b. Ankles   e. Upper legs
   c. Lower legs   f. Hips
5. Shift attention to the upper parts of your body, instructing all bones and muscles to relax in the following order:
   a. Hands   e. Upper arms
   b. Wrists   f. Neck
   c. Lower arms   g. Shoulders
   d. Elbows

By this time, your arms and legs should feel heavy and unmovable. However, if you become uncomfortable, shift your position. Then continue with step 6.

6. Spend some time concentrating on relaxing the main part of your body, instructing each organ and all muscles to be relaxed.
7. Relax your head muscles in the following order:
   a. Jaws   b. Face   c. Scalp
8. With the relaxation process complete, spend a few minutes focusing on (but not altering) your breathing, which probably has become quite shallow.
9. Gradually increase your breathing to "get the blood flowing again." To prevent dizziness, take one or two relatively deep breaths before standing up.

The ideal site for beginning progressive relaxation training is a quiet, soundproof room. Since such rooms are not always readily accessible, the best alternative is to find a quiet room that is free from distractions, especially sudden interruptions. Clocks, music, telephones, people talking, horns blowing, etc. often go unnoticed during an active day, but they are highly distracting during relaxation.

In addition to external intrusive noises, some people are disturbed by their own intrusive thoughts. One approach for dealing with this is for the nurse to increase the dialogue or assist the client in selecting a new set of relaxing thoughts. For example, the person may want to build in some pleasant imagery such as thinking of being on a raft in a calm sea with the blue sky above and the clouds gently moving.

Clients should not be encouraged to go to sleep during the relaxation exercise; the word is avoided in giving instructions in favor of a suggestion such as being "relaxed and awake." Any words or phrases that produce tension should be avoided; thus the client's reactions to the choice of words used should be noted. If people do fall asleep, they should be gently awakened and the tempo speeded up slightly to see if that helps.

Some people have difficulty tensing certain muscle groups and may need assistance in developing an alternative tensing pattern. Others have difficulty following instructions either because they were not listening carefully or they simply forgot what was said. Some people benefit from keeping their eyes open during early sessions so that they can model after the nurse, and this also may decrease their fear of the unknown (Richter and Sloan, 1979).

Other clients have strange or unfamiliar feelings during progressive relaxation such as a floating sensation. If this occurs, they may want to look away and become reoriented to their surroundings. Some people feel uncomfortable when they become relaxed because of their loss of control of the situation. If this occurs, it may be helpful to spend more time discussing the situation, introducing the steps slowly, and after the session focusing on the positive experiences that occurred. Others may feel externally relaxed at the end of a session but "uptight" inside. They need to know that internal responses are involuntarily controlled, whereas the peripheral relaxation is controlled voluntarily. Practice increases the degree of internal relaxation.

It is not uncommon for heavy smokers to have episodes of coughing, and people with colds or allergies may begin sneezing. It may be helpful to encourage less deep breathing to diminish stimulation of coughing and sneezing. Some clients have difficulty establishing a schedule for practicing, and they may need assistance with time budgeting. The following approach, meditation, is often used in combination with progressive relaxation. Additionally, progressive relaxation can be included in the creative imagery approach to reinforce the process.

Meditation

Meditation can bring about an inhibition of the sympathetic nervous system, and by doing so it reduces the effects of chronic stress by producing a state of hypometabolism (Sutterly, 1979). The physiological responses observed in meditation are opposite those seen in the fight-or-flight syndrome. One of the most widely used forms of meditation is that devised by Benson (1975). While studying the physiological results of meditation at the Harvard University laboratory, Benson demonstrated that meditation brought about reduced oxygen consumption and blood lactate levels. He was able to identify the basic elements of meditation, which he labeled the *relaxation response.*

Meditation requires (1) a quiet setting with few distractions, (2) a mental device or *mantra* such as a word or sound to be repeated mentally with each exhalation to help avoid distracting thoughts from invading the tranquility, (3) a passive attitude that allows the meditation experience to occur, and (4) a comfortable position that does not induce sleep.

Bates (1979) suggested the following instructions for the meditation process:

1. Sit quietly in a comfortable position with eyes closed.
2. Using progressive relaxation, deeply relax all muscles beginning with the feet and moving to the face.
3. Breathe through the nose being consciously aware of the breathing pattern. While exhaling, mentally say the word *one.*
4. Continue the breathing process of step three for 10 to 20 minutes, but do not set an alarm; instead open your eyes to check the time. When finished, sit for several minutes with eyes closed first and then with them open.

The value of meditation as a tool for relaxation in nursing is that it can easily and successfully be used and taught to clients in a variety of clinical settings. Modifications of this response, which are applicable to community health nursing can incorporate relaxation tapes or a personally developed schedule of steps. For example, one way to learn the relaxation process is to take 5 minutes three times a day and sit comfortably with the eyes closed and concentrate on a peaceful picture or mental image. For some people, visions of the water such as a lake or the ocean are restful, whereas other people may choose the mountains or some other unique sight. With each breath, say the word *relax.* At

first this exercise may seem unnatural, but it serves to divert the mind from the problems at hand and in essence provides a "psychological coffee break" or time out from ordinarily experienced stressors. Other mental devices include repeating the word *one* or the phrase *I am relaxed.* To practice relaxation techniques it is necessary to (1) find a comfortable place to sit; (2) place the feet flat on the floor, generally with hands in lap; (3) close the eyes; and (4) breathe steadily and with purpose for about 5 minutes while taking particular notice of the parts of the body that feel tense and willing them to relax.

Creative Imagery

Creative imagery has gained considerable attention as a way to involve people in creating a milieu for their own healing processes to occur. The concept behind creative imagery is that "the body is equipped to heal itself from every manner of disorder, and that under most circumstances the body requires no special instructions to accomplish this feat" (Achterberg and Lawlis, 1982, pp. 55-56). Mental images or internal representations of events or places use the senses to mentally and consciously alter bodily functioning (Achterberg and Lawlis, 1980). The concept of creative imagery involves any or all five of the senses, including visual, auditory, olfactory, tactile, and kinesthetic (end organs lie in the muscles, joints, and tendons, and this sense is stimulated by bodily tension). Though this concept is often used in attaining and maintaining health, its usefulness applies also to psychotherapy and spiritual care.

Creative imagery is particularly well suited to incorporation in the community health nursing role, since contact with clients often is long term allowing for the development of trust. Heidt (1979) described the use of creative imagery in conjunction with therapeutic touch and found it to aid in the formation of close relationships with clients in a shorter than usual time; it allowed them a nonthreatening means of expressing their feelings about being sick; and it encouraged clients' beliefs about their own abilities to heal. Using tape recordings to facilitate relaxation and the imagery process, clients were asked to draw a picture of their perception of their disease or discomfort and the treatment for it.

Visualization exercises help to demonstrate the relation between the mind and the body. The mind can focus on a peaceful and tranquil imaginary scene, and the body tends to respond by becoming more relaxed. Clients can be assisted to relax by suggesting that they visualize the one place they would like to be. They should become specific and thorough in the visualization to encourage active participation in the process.

For example, a client might find the seashore relaxing. First, it is suggested to the client that he imagine himself sitting beside the sea listening to the many sounds. Next, it is suggested that the client ask questions such as what kinds of sounds are most prominent at the sea, and how he feels as he sits, listens, and looks at the calm, gently moving blue sea.

The research by Simonton et al. (1978) demonstrated the use of visualization in treating cancer. They combined visualization with other methods of cancer treatment, including radiation and chemotherapy to provide patients with a mechanism for fighting rather than being consumed by the cancer. The patients are taught to visualize their concern in an attempt to combat the disease. "For many cancer patients, the body has become the enemy. It has betrayed them by getting sick and threatening their lives. They feel alienated from it and mistrust its ability to combat their disease" (Simonton et al. 1978, p. 125). These researchers devised a cancer treatment program based on the assumption that relaxation helps to reduce fear, which can itself become overwhelming. They combined the progressive relaxation technique developed by Jacobson with mental imagery. They recommended that patients practice this program three times a day for 10 to 15 minutes each time. Several principles form the foundation for the relaxation and mental imagery program developed by these researchers. By forming an image of a desired event, people can make a personal statement of what they want to occur. By repeating the statement, clients come to expect that the desired event will occur, and they begin acting in ways consistent with the achievement of the desired outcome. The following steps are recommended for dealing with pain and a variety of other ailments. (Additional steps can be found in their book for incorporation into the treatment of cancer patients.)

1. Create a mental picture of any ailment or pain that you have now, visualizing it in a form that makes sense to you.
2. Picture any treatment you are receiving and see it either eliminating the source of the ailment or pain or strengthening your body's ability to heal itself.
3. Picture your body's natural defenses and natural processes eliminating the source of the ailment or pain.
4. Imagine yourself healthy and free of the ailment or pain.
5. See yourself proceeding successfully toward meeting your goals in life.
6. Give yourself a mental pat on the back for participating in your recovery. See yourself doing this relaxation/mental imagery exercise three times a day, staying awake and alert as you do it.
7. Let the muscles in your eyelids lighten up, become ready to open your eyes, and become aware of the room.
8. Now let your eyes open and you are ready to resume you usual activities.

For example, a hypertensive person could use the creative imagery process to see the problem as being little muscles in the walls of blood vessels that clamp down under stress so that greater force is required to carry the blood to its destination. The next step would be to suggest that they visualize their medication relaxing these little muscles in the blood vessels so that the heart pumps smoothly, evenly, and with minimum resistance.

These same approaches can be used in dealing with arthritis. Clients can be instructed to picture their joints as being irritated and having many small granules on the surface. Next they are urged to see their white blood cells coming in, cleaning up the debris (including the little granules), and smoothing over the joint surfaces. Finally they visualize themselves as being active and free of joint pain.

Relaxation and mental imagery are useful, since these processes can decrease fear by allowing people to have some responsibility for and control of themselves. These processes can also bring about an attitude change moving from despair and often despondency to anticipation and the will to live. Also, physical changes can occur that enhance the immune system, and it can be a basic method for stress reduction.

Biofeedback

Biofeedback has been popular in recent years as a way to teach specific voluntary control over particular muscles or bodily responses and thereby minimize the stress response. Through this method, electronic sensors can make people aware of normally unconscious processes. Alpha brain waves, muscle tension, and skin temperature are often used to provide people with an immediate interpretation of their bodily reaction. One popular way to use biofeedback is by using an electromyograph, which is a machine designed to gauge the state of muscle tension by detecting electrical signals through the skin. Through biofeedback, people learn to reduce increasing tension as a sign of stress.

There are several simple ways that do not require any machinery to detect how people are responding to stress. It is common practice for nurses to monitor clients' reactions by noting changes in breathing, heart rate, and blood pressure. Clients can easily be taught to monitor pulse as a gauge to their emotions. The first step is to establish a baseline resting pulse. This can be done by having the person sit quietly for 5 minutes and then recording the pulse. The next step is to practice any desired type of meditation or relaxation for at least 5 minutes and record the pulse. The pulse rate should decrease; however, this does not always occur, since for some people the resting pulse is already rather low (Donnelly, 1980c).

Another simple and inexpensive type of biofeedback evaluates temperature of the extremities. Clients can be taught to use a sensitive thermometer for measuring skin temperature of the fingers while repeating the relaxation sequence described for pulse regulation. It is important to tape the thermometer firmly to the finger to obtain an accurate reading.

Another variation of temperature monitoring includes the warming of hands via biofeedback. Before warming the hands, the person's palmar skin temperature of the index finger should be measured using a standard thermometer. Readings below 85°F indicate distress. Once the temperature is recorded, the person can be taught to raise it by a variety of relaxation techniques, including sitting or lying in a comfortable position with attention focusing on slow, even breathing. The next step in warming the hands includes concentrating on and repeating the autogenic phrase, "My arms and hands are heavy and warm." As relaxation occurs, the hands begin to warm, and they may tingle as the temperature rises. The shoulders need to be relaxed throughout this process. Temperature should be recorded before and after each session to motivate and encourage participants.

Each of the following exercises demonstrates the basic principles of biofeedback: (1) monitoring a physiological index that is sensitive to stress, (2) feeding the information back to the person involved, and (3) using the information as a guide in attempting to alter the physiological state (Donnelly, 1980c). Biofeedback provides immediate confirmation of personal control of oneself. Various stress reactions have been effectively controlled with biofeedback, including excessive anxiety, phobias, tension, headaches, insomnia, essential hypertension, bruxism (teeth grinding), colitis, ulcer, or menstrual distress. Kolkmeier (1982) reported on the use of biofeedback to teach hypertensive clients to normalize their blood pressure with minimum medication. At the Biofeedback Laboratory at the Dallas Diagnostic Association, clients are taught what causes elevated blood pressure and what they can do to alter the situation. They also are counseled by a dietitian about salt restriction and weight reduction. Group support is provided to encourage compliance with the therapeutic regimen.

If the person's blood pressure is elevated considerably, medication is initially used to bring it under control before entry into the biofeedback program. Clients are aided in identifying their personal sources of stress, what physiological changes they typically experience in response to stress, and what changes can be made either in their life styles or in their responses to the stressor (See Kolkmeier [1982] for a more detailed description of this program). The main benefit is that through a reasonably simple, painless method clients can be taught to control hypertension while simultaneously reducing their reliance on drugs.

Hypnosis

It is not within the confines of this chapter to teach hypnosis either to be used by nurses or with clients but rather to briefly summarize the use of hypnosis as a stress-reducing technique. Hypnosis has been used extensively in health care often in conjunction with other treatments. Successes with hypnosis have been reported to reduce a client's fear of surgery or dental procedures and to reduce the anxiety of childbirth.

Nurses wishing to use hypnosis in their practice should become trained in this skill before practicing with clients. To stimulate interest in hypnosis as a stress-reducing effort a brief description is presented. This technique has in recent years been recognized as a medium for reducing or eliminating pain as well as managing stress. Six basic components to hypnosis include pretalk, induction, utilization, awakening, posttalk, and assessment. The basic technique can be practiced in 10 to 15 minutes in an unconditioned client who has not previously been hypnotized (Daley and Greenspun, 1979).

During the first stage, pretalk, clients are not told that they will be hypnotized, but rather the hypnotherapist simply explains the process emphasizing the need for cooperation to achieve maximum relaxation. The subjects are informed they will enter a subconscious state similar to that of being partially awake.

The induction phase usually follows a technique similar to progressive relaxation in which clients sit or lie in a comfortable position with their feet uncrossed and teeth unclenched. They loosen all restrictive clothing, and the room should be free from noise. Next, clients are directed to close their eyes, breathe deeply three times, and concentrate on relaxing each part of the body starting with the crown of the skull.

Once relaxation ensues, the stage of utilization can begin when clients are ready to receive positive reinforcement. The therapist suggests that the clients will be peaceful, tranquil, calm, and comfortable and that at a specified signal that can be given anytime in the future they will return immediately to their present level of relaxation. An example of a signal given under hypnosis might be, "at any time when I point to your forehead and say the words *deep sleep*, you will immediately return to this level of relaxation" (Daley and Greenspun, 1979, p. 63). This posthypnotic suggestion eliminates the need for lengthy subsequent inductions.

Awakening is usually a simple process that begins once the beneficial suggestions are given. The therapist might say that at the count of five the client will awake, feel calm, and be in a peaceful frame of mind. Awakening is done slowly so that clients do not experience untoward reactions such as headache, nausea, or vomiting.

The fifth stage, posttalk, begins once clients have reoriented themselves to their setting, without rushing. During this phase clients are especially susceptible and receptive, and goals should be set and agreed on, giving as much positive reinforcement as possible.

The last step, assessment, deals with the client's further needs for lessons in relaxation, and should take place 3 or 4 days after the hypnosis. Once clients learn to relax by hypnosis, a program of self-management can be developed.

Acupressure

Another form of stress reduction, acupressure, reduces tension by "reestablishing the harmony and balance of the flow of electromagnetic energy" (Sutterly, 1979, p. 12). In this process, like acupuncture, selected metabolic and circulatory processes can be stimulated by finger pressure on certain points on the body. The value of this technique lies in its use for self-regulation of chronic pain and tension. Several self-help books have been written to teach people this technique (Chan, 1974; Kurland, 1977; Thie, 1973; Warren, 1976). Of these the book by neurologist and psychiatrist Kurland is particularly useful, since it describes the use of acupressure in eliminating tension headaches.

Creating and Using Support Networks

One of the best ways of coping with stress is by seeking support from members of a reliable and caring work, family, or social group. Everyone needs someone to trust and with whom stress-producing situations can be discussed in depth without fear of rejection or retaliation. Talking with one or more members of a trusted support network provides opportunities for testing reality, obtaining feedback from someone whose opinion is valued, working through feelings, and constructively planning future actions.

In helping clients reduce stress, they should be guided in identifying the support networks currently available.

Who are the members of their support network? How many people can they call on in a crisis or a stressful situation? Seashore (1980, p. 156) described a support network as being a "resource pool drawn on selectively to support me in moving in a direction of my choice and leaves me stronger." This means that people need several options in their resource pool so they do not consistently draw on the same one and also so that the responsibility for choosing how to deal with the situation remains with the person and is not delegated to the support system.

In a support group usually a common bond exists to hold the members together. The purpose of support groups is to assist members in growing and developing through support from people who understand (often because they have lived through a similar circumstance) and who care about one another. In many support groups there are no agendas for the meeting, but rather the mission is to support, encourage, and at times challenge one another. Seashore listed four functions of a support group as the following (1980, p. 157):

1. Reestablish competence: in times of high stress people often devalue their ability and fail to recognize their own strengths.
2. Maintain high performance: in good times when excessive stress is not present, support groups help members "keep their batteries charged."
3. Gain new competencies: some members of the group may be better able to challenge, teach, or motivate others.
4. Achieve selected objectives: group membership can help in the clarification, formulation, and refinement of short-term and long-term objectives.

Support systems are useful in helping people reestablish their competence by assisting during times of high stress as well as serving as sources of strength and encouragement during ordinary situations. In using support systems, clients need to rely on them sparingly so that they are not "worn out" by giving such assistance. To maintain a support system it is useful to keep in contact in times of homeostasis as well as when under stress.

SUMMARY

Stress is a frequent and generally personal experience that can cause considerable mental and physical wear and tear. The positive aspects of stress can be maximized so that they can be used to motivate and energize people. The magnitude of the stress response to changes in life events and expectations can be minimized by a variety of stress management techniques such as relaxation, creative imagery, hypnosis, use of support networks, exercise, and diet.

People respond to stress differently based on their own needs and resources for adapting to changing life events. Stress is manifested in a variety of ways including physical, behavioral, and emotional concomitants. Interestingly, each person tends to develop a unique way of handling stress. Some bottle up their feelings and turn the stress response into physical ailments including ulcers and heart attacks, whereas other people handle stress by screaming, crying, or instituting constructive stress-reduction strategies. It is unrealistic to hope for or anticipate a "stress-free" world. There will always be stress; the key element is learning to use rather than be used and abused by it. Community health nurses can play a vital role in teaching stress-reduction techniques. Perhaps the most effective way to teach clients how to manage stress is to practice this skill and demonstrate it through formal instruction as well as through role modeling.

To assist community health nurses in recognizing the magnitude of stress in society and also to teach ways of managing this phenomenon, various contemporary stressors were identified. For example, in any community, biophysical-chemical and psychosocial-cultural stressors are present. It is the task of the nurse to assess the particular community to determine specifically what stressors are present, what populations are most affected (at risk), what resources are currently available for assisting clients to deal more effectively with stress, and finally what actions can be taken by nurses to institute new programs, assist in reducing community stress, and teach clients more effective responses. Although this chapter has focused on ways to work with individuals and families in reducing stress, it in no way discounts the vital role of community health nurses in serving as catalysts in working with the entire community to alleviate those stressors that can be altered or eliminated. Other chapters have dealt with the nurse's role in responding to the community as client and in dealing with crises.

All life situations are potential sources of stress; however, work is a major stressor for many people. Several problem areas within work settings have been mentioned to alert nurses to the potential for stress-management skills in occupational settings. A major portion of the chapter dealt with techniques for managing stress including exercise, group discussion, changing attitudes, relaxation (particularly progressive relaxation), meditation, creative imagery, hypnosis, acupressure, and creating and using support networks. The task now is to learn, practice, and teach these skills.

BIBLIOGRAPHY

Achterberg, J., and Lawlis, F.: Bridges of the body-mind: behavioral approaches to health care, Champaign, Ill., 1980, Institute for Personality and Ability Testing.

Achterberg, J., and Lawlis, F.: Imagery and health intervention, Top. Clin. Nurs. 3:55-60, Jan. 1982.

Adams, J.D.: Understanding and managing stress: a workbook in changing life styles, San Diego, Calif, 1980, University Associates.

Bates, C.: Stress and health, Health Values: Achieving High-Level Wellness, 3:136-143, May-June 1979.

Benson, H.: The relaxation response, New York, 1975, William Morrow and Co., Inc.

Bernstein, D.A., and Borkovec, T.D.: Progressive relaxation training, Champaign, Ill., 1973, Research Press.

Bloom, B.L.: Prevention of mental disorders: recent advances in theory and practice, Community Ment. Health J. 15:179-191, Fall 1979.

Chan, P.: Finger acupressure, Los Angeles, 1974, Price/Stern/Sloan Publishers, Inc.

Clemen, S.A., Eigsti, D.G., and McGuire, S.L.: Comprehensive family and community health nursing, New York, 1981, McGraw-Hill Book Co.

Cohen, S.: Sound effects on behavior, Psychology Today 15:38-46, Oct. 1981.

Cooper, K.H.: The new aerobics, New York, 1970, Bantam Books.

Daley, T.J., and Greenspun, E.L.: Stress management through hypnosis, Top. Clin. Nurs. 1:59-65, April 1979.

Donnelly, G.F.: Why you just can't take it anymore! . . . coping, RN 43:34-37, May 1980a.

Donnelly, G.F.: Remember . . . you're not in this alone! . . . how group methods can help you cope . . . and how to pick a group that's right for you, RN 43:30-33, July 1980b.

Donnelly, G.F.: How do I know I'm on the right track? . . . simple new biofeedback gadgets can help you chart your course to deep relaxation, RN 43:44-46, Sept. 1980c.

Eckholm, E., and Record, F.: The affluent diet: a worldwide health hazard. In Adams, J.D., editor: Understanding and managing stress, La Jolla, Calif, 1980, University Associates, pp. 123-138.

Flynn, P.A.R.: Holistic health and the art and science of care, Bowie, Maryland, 1980, Robert J. Brady Co.

Frain, M., and Valiga, T.M.: The multiple dimensions of stress, Topics in Clin. Nurs. 1:43-52, April 1979.

French, J.R.P., and Caplan, R.D.: Organizational stress and individual strain. In Adams, J.D., editor: Understanding and managing stress, LaJolla, Calif., 1980, University Associates, pp. 45-84.

Galle, O., Gove, W., and McPherson, J.: Population density and pathology: what are the relations for man? Science 176:23-30, April 1972.

Hartl, D.E.: Stress management and the nurse, Adv. Nurs. Sci. 1:91-100, 1979.

Healthy People: the Surgeon General's report on health promotion and disease prevention, DHEW Pub. No. (PHS) 79-55071A, Washington, D.C., 1979, Department of Health, Education, and Welfare.

Heidt, T.: Patients tell their stories, Paper presented at the second annual Conference on Imaging and Fantasy Process, Chicago, Nov. 1979. In Achterberg, J., and Lawlis, G.F.: Imagery and health intervention, Adv. Nurs. Sci. 3(4):55-60, Jan. 1982.

Holmes, T.H., and Rahe, R.H.: The Social Readjustment Rating Scale, J. Psychosom. Res. 11:213-218, 1967.

Ivancevich, J.M., and Matteson, M.T.: Nurses and stress: time to examine the potential problem, Superv. Nurse 11:17-22, 1980.

Jacobson, A.: Melancholy in the twentieth century: causes and prevention, J. Psychiatr. Nurs. 18:11-21, 1980.

Jacobson, E.: Progressive relaxation: a physiological and clinical investigation of muscular states and their significance in psychology and medical practice, ed. 3, Chicago, 1974, University of Chicago Press.

Johnson, C.L.: The American family during inflationary times, Psychiatr. Opinion **16**:13-16, Sept. 1979.

Johnson, J.W.: More about stress and some management techniques, J. School Health **51**:36-42, Jan. 1981.

Knowles, J.H.: The responsibility of the individual. In Flynn, P.A.: The health continuum: journeys in the philosophy of holistic health, Bowie, Md, 1980, Robert J. Brady Co., pp. 467-496.

Kolkmeier, L.: Biofeedback-relaxation therapy for hypertension, Adv. Nurs. Sci. **3**:69-73, Jan. 1982.

Kurland, H.D.: Quick headache relief without drugs, New York, 1977, Ballantine Books.

Lazarus, R.S., Cohen, J.B., and Falkman, S.: Psychological stress and adaptation: some unresolved issues. In Selye, H., editor: Guide to stress research, New York, 1980, Van Nostrand Reinhold Co.

Pope, R.: Identifying organizational stressors: the nurse's role, Occup. Health Nurs. **30**:34-36, March 1982.

Richter, J.M., and Sloan, R.: Stress: a relaxation response, Am. J. Nurs. **79**:1960-1964, 1979.

Schecter, D.E.: Women in the labor force: some mental health implications, Psy. Opinion **16**:17-19, Sept. 1979.

Schwartz, G.E.: Stress management in occupational settings, Public Health Rep. **95**:99-108, March 1980.

Seashore, C.: Developing and using personal support systems. In Adams, J.D.: Understanding and managing stress, LaJolla, Calif, 1980, University Associates, pp. 155-159.

Selye, H.: The stress syndrome, Am. J. Nurs. **65**:97-99, 1965.

Selye, H.: Stress without distress, Philadelphia, 1974, J.P. Lippincott Co.

Selye, H.: The stress of life, ed. revised, New York, 1978, McGraw-Hill Book Co.

Selye, H.: Stress and holistic medicine, Family and Community Health **3**(2):85-88, Aug. 1980.

Simonton, C.O., Simonton, S., and Creighton, J.: Getting well again: a step by step self help guide to overcoming cancer for patients and their families, Los Angeles, 1978, J.P. Tarcher, Inc. (Distributed by St. Martin's Press, Inc., New York.)

Sutterly, D.C.: Stress and health: a survey of self-regulation modalities, Top. Clin. Nurs. **1**:1-20, April 1979.

Swogger, G.: Toward understanding stress: a map of the territory, J. School Health **51**:29-33, Jan. 1981.

Thie, J.: Touch for health, Marina Del Ray, California, 1973, De Vorss and Co., Publishers.

Warren, F.: Freedom from pain through acupressure, New York, 1976, Frederick Fell Publishers, Inc.

Willis, R.W.: Options, in managing stress, Pediatr. Nurs. **5**:24-27, 1979.

Yamamoto, K.: Children's ratings of the stressfulness of experiences, Dev. Psychol **15**:581-582, 1979.

Appendix A

INDIVIDUAL ASSESSMENT TOOLS

DISCHARGED PATIENTS QUESTIONNAIRE *

We are asking patients and families who have recently received services from the agency to assist us in the evaluation of our programs. As a consumer of the services we offer, your answers to the enclosed questionnaire will help us determine if we are meeting our objectives as a provider of skilled nursing care in the home designed to meet the needs of residents of our county.

We would appreciate it if you could complete the questionnaire and return it to us in the envelope provided. It will not be necessary to sign the questionnaire as we are not interested in identifying a patient or the nurse who gave care.

Instructions: Please circle the *Yes* or *No* following each question below, as you feel it answers the question.

1. When the public health nurse visited your home, did you know why she was there?   Yes No

2. Did you and the nurse arrange a time for the visits that was convenient for both of you?   Yes No

3. Did the nurse do any of the following treatments?   Yes No
   - Change or irrigate catheter   Yes No
   - Irrigate colostomy or give an enema   Yes No
   - Change dressings   Yes No
   - Inject a medication   Yes No
   - Assist with exercise routine   Yes No
   - Suction or care for tracheotomy   Yes No
   - Insert a nasal-gastric tube   Yes No

   If you answered *Yes* to any of the above, did you understand what the treatment was expected to do for you?   Yes No

4. Did the nurse teach you or any member of your family to do a treatment?   Yes No

   Did you or your family learn to do the treatment yourself?   Yes No

5. Did you take medication by mouth?   Yes No

   Did you understand how to take the medication (i.e., amount to take; number of times during the day; if taken before, after, or with meals)?   Yes No

   Did the nurse help you understand what the medication was expected to do?   Yes No

6. Did the nurse examine you at any time (i.e., take blood pressure, pulse, listen to your chest with a stethoscope, examine your skin)?   Yes No

   If yes, did you understand why she was making these observations?   Yes No

7. Did the nurse help you to understand your illness?   Yes No

8. Did you understand what the nurse was planning to accomplish by visiting you?   Yes No

   Did you think it was possible to accomplish this?   Yes No

9. Did the nurse's visits make it easier for you to remain in your home and care for yourself?   Yes No

10. Did you have other problems (e.g., financial) that the public health nurse could not assist you with by herself?   Yes No

    If yes, did the nurse assist you to contact another agency that could help you?   Yes No

11. Do you feel the nursing visits were (circle one):
    Too few   Too many   Right number

12. Were you aware that the nurse was going to discharge you from her service?   Yes No

13. Did you feel you could function on your own when the nurse dismissed you from the service?   Yes No

14. If you need skilled nursing service in your home at some time in the future, will you contact the agency?   Yes No

15. If you have any comments, please write them in the space below:

* From Administrator's handbook for the structure, operation, and expansion of home health agencies, Pub. No. 21–1653 (New York: National League for Nursing, 1977), pp. 409–410. Used with permission.

HISTORY TAKING IN THE AMBULATORY SETTING*

The following is an outline of the specific information needed for a health history. The headings and questions are those traditionally used.

CHIEF COMPLAINT

Why is the child attending clinic today? Generally the answer is a simple statement in the parent's own words (e.g., "well-child care," "cold," "earache.")

PRESENT ILLNESS

What signs and symptoms of illness is the child showing? It is best to list the symptoms in order of appearance. Sometimes specific questions must be asked (e.g., Is the child coughing? When? What kind? How much? Does the child have diarrhea? When? What kind? How much? For how long?) How is the child acting otherwise? (How is his or her appetite? Bowels? Fluid intake? Sleep? Activity?) Has the child been exposed to others with illness? (Anyone in the family? Relatives? Friends? School? What type of illness was it?) What kind of treatment have the parents been giving? (Have they sought medical care before? Any medications? Any procedures?)

PAST HISTORY
Birth

Prenatal. How was the mother's health during her pregnancy with this child? Where did she receive her prenatal care and for how many months of the pregnancy? Did she have any infections? During what month? Did she have any illnesses? During which month, and how were they treated? Was she taking medications during the pregnancy? What kind and why? At what point during pregnancy? What is her blood type? What is the child's father's blood type? Does she know the child's blood type? Did she have any x-rays during her pregnancy? Was she on any special diet during the pregnancy? How nutritional was her diet? Was she hospitalized during her pregnancy? When and for what reasons? How many living children does she have? Was either she or her doctor worried about this pregnancy for any reason? Did the pregnancy last 9 months? (A report of the baby coming less than 2 weeks early or late is usually not significant unless accompanied by a history of low birth weight or neonatal problems.)

Natal. How long was the labor and were there are any problems? What type of delivery was it? What kind of anesthesia was used and were there any problems? (Such questions as Did the baby come headfirst? Did the doctor use forceps? are often helpful in eliciting this information.) Where was the baby born? What was the baby's birth weight? What was the baby's condition at birth? Did the baby cry? Was the baby blue? Did the baby need oxygen?

*From Alexander, M. M., and Brown, M. S.: Pediatric history taking and physical diagnosis for nurses, New York, 1979, McGraw-Hill Book Co., pp. 6-13. Used with permission.

Postnatal. Did the baby have any problems during the stay in the nursery? What was the length of the baby's hospital stay? Did the mother and infant come home together? Did the baby have jaundice? Was the baby ever cyanotic or blue? Were there any feeding problems during the hospitalization? Did the baby develop any rashes? How much weight did the baby lose?

Allergies

Is the child allergic to any foods? To any medications? To any insects? To any animals? At any seasons? If so, describe what happens with these allergies. Does the child ever break out in rashes? Do the parents know why?

Accidents

Has the child ever had an accident? If so, was it in the car? At home? At school? At the baby-sitter's? Can the parents describe what happened? What was the treatment? Where was the child treated? What was the child's reaction? Any residual problems?

Illnesses

Has the child had any infections? When? Where? What treatment? What follow-up? Has the child had any childhood diseases? Measles? Rubella? Roseola? Mumps? Chickenpox? Whooping cough?

Operations

Has the child ever had any operations? When? For what condition? Where? What was the outcome?

Hospitalizations

Has the child ever spent any time in a hospital? For what reason? Where? Is condition resolved? Any residual problems?

Immunizations

Has the child had any immunizations? Which kinds? Any reactions? Any boosters? (Usually a written record is the most accurate source of this information.) Has the child been tested for tuberculosis? How? When? What was the result? Has the child ever had x-rays?

FAMILY HISTORY
Family Members

What is the mother's age and state of health? What is the father's age and state of health? Are there any siblings? What ages and what sex? State of health? A diagram is of-

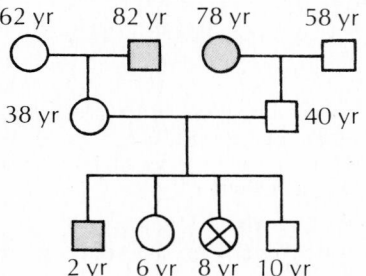

ten used to show this. A circle indicates a female and a square indicates a male; a horizontal line indicates a marriage, and a vertical line indicates a descendant. A blackened circle or square indicates that the individual is deceased. An X indicates the child with whom this particular history is concerned. The diagram above shows a maternal grandfather who died at age 82 and paternal grandmother who died at age 78, a 62-year-old maternal grandmother and a 58-year-old paternal grandfather alive, two parents alive, a 38-year-old mother and 40-year-old father, one 10-year-old brother, and one 6-year-old sister alive, and one brother who died at 2 years of age; the child about whom the history is taken is an 8-year-old girl.

Family Diseases

Within the immediate family, including both sets of grandparents and first aunts and uncles, are any of the following conditions present?

Eyes, ears, nose, and throat. Are there any nosebleeds? Sinus problems? Glaucoma? Cataracts? Myopia? Strabismus? Any other problems with their eyes, ears, nose, or throat?

Cardiorespiratory. Is there any tuberculosis? Asthma? Hay fever? Hypertension? Heart murmurs? Heart attacks? Strokes? Anemia? Rheumatic fever? Leukemia? Pneumonia? Emphysema? Any other problems with heart or lungs?

Gastrointestinal. Does anyone have ulcers? Colitis? Any other problems with stomach or intestines? Does anyone have kidney infections? Bladder infections?

Musculoskeletal. Are there any congenital dislocated hips? Muscular dystrophy? Arthritis? Club feet? Any other problems with bones or muscles?

Neurological. Does anyone have convulsions? Mental retardation? Mental problems? Comas? Epilepsy?

Special senses. Is anyone deaf? Blind?

Chronic. Does anyone have diabetes? Congenital anomalies? Cancer? Tumors? Thyroid problems?

General. Are there any other medical problems in the family that the patient thinks are important?

Social. Where does the family live? In a house? Apartment? Room? How large? Is there a yard? Are there stairs? Does anyone live with the family? Grandparents? Aunts? Uncles? Friends? What is the financial situation of the family? Does the father work? Does the mother work? What are their occupations? If no one works, how are they living? Is there any outside help? Baby-sitters? Day-care centers? Schools? What is the general relationship of the family members? Do they seem to be a happy family? Chaotic family? Sad family? Depressed family? Violent family?

REVIEW OF SYSTEMS
Skin

Does this child have any rashes?

Eyes, Ears, Nose, and Throat

Does this child have persistent nosebleeds? Frequent streptococcal sore throats? Frequent colds (more than four

a year)? Pneumonia? Frequent earaches? Do the child's eyes ever cross? Do they tear excessively?

Cardiorespiratory

Does the child have any trouble breathing? Running? Finishing a 3- to 4-ounce bottle without tiring? Does the child turn blue?

Gastrointestinal

Does the child have any problems with diarrhea? Constipation? Bleeding around the rectum? Bloody stools? Pain? Vomiting?

Genitourinary

Does the child have a straight, strong urinary stream, or does the urine just dribble out? Urinary frequency? Is there any pain? Bleeding? If an older girl, does she menstruate? What was the age of onset? How often? Any problems?

Neurological

Has the child ever had a convulsion? A fainting spell? Tremors? Twitches? Blackouts? Dizzy spells? Frequent headaches?

Musculoskeletal

Has the child ever broken any bones? Had any sprains? Complained of pain in the joints, swelling, or redness around the joints?

Special Senses

Does the child see well? Hear well? Does the child seem clumsy? Can the child see the blackboard from where he or she sits in the classroom? Is the child always falling or walking into doors?

Chronic

Any long-term diseases?

General

Any other problems?

HABITS
Eating

Is the child's appetite good? Poor? Varied? If on formula, what kind, how much, how is it mixed, and how frequently? How much does the child take in a 24-hour period? What kinds of foods does the child eat? Meat? Fruits? Vegetables? Cereals? Juices? Eggs? Sweets? Milk? Snacks? How often? What size portions? How many times a week or day does the child eat each of these? Does the child feed herself or himself? Does the child use a cup? Spoon? Knife? Fork? Is the child messy? Does the child sit with the rest of the family? Does the child take vitamins? What kind? How often? How much? What is the family attitude toward food? Is it used as a symbol of love? A bribe? A reward? What is the emotional climate of the meals? Relaxed? Tired? Rushed? Tense?

Bowels

What are the child's bowel patterns? Frequency? Consistency? Color? Any discomfort? Is the child toilet trained? Is toilet training planned? When? Any problems? If the child is toilet trained, does he or she have accidents? If so, are they during the day or night? How often? Are they frequently associated with emotional upsets?

Sleep

When does the child go to bed? Wake up? Does the child awaken during the night? How often? What happens? What does the parent do? Any nightmares? Night terrors? Does the child take naps? When? For how long? Where does the child sleep? How many hours does the child sleep in a 24-hour period? When awake, is the child alert? Or does the child seem to need more sleep than he or she is getting?

Development

How does the child compare with his or her siblings? Quicker to learn? Slower to learn? When did the child first sit? Stand? Roll over? Talk? Walk? What kinds of activities does the child do now? What is the child doing that is new since the last visit? What grade is the child in? Does the child like school? Does the child have playmates? What does the child like to do in school? What does the child like to play?

Exercise and Play

What types of play or games does the child engage in and how often? Does the older child engage in sports? Team activities? For the adolescents, do they do regular exercises? How much walking, running, or other large motor activities are involved in their daily living patterns?

Personality

What kind of personality does this child have? Is he or she quiet? Outgoing? Does the child have a temper? How does the child cope with stress? By withdrawal? By aggression? By decompensation? By symptoms of illness? How does the child handle emotions like anger, fear, jealousy, or others? Is the child able to relax well?

Family Relations

How do the members of the family get along? How do they handle disagreement within the family? How do they handle external stress? What things do they do together? How often? Do they enjoy them?

Sexuality

How much does the younger child ask about sexuality and what is the child told about it? What is the child's attitude toward it and what is the attitude of those around the child? Does the child masturbate? How is this handled by the rest of the family? What are the child's own feelings about it? What is the child's attitude and those of the family toward nudity in the home? What does the older child know about changes beginning in his or her body: early breast development, penile and testicular enlargement, pubic hair, axillary and facial hair, changes in body proportions, voice changes, menstruation, and nocturnal emissions?

Some of the questions asked when taking a complete history need to be modified for specific ages, and some areas need more detailed information if problems are encountered. Generally, if the nurse covers these six areas, he or she has a good idea about which topics may need more information. The nurse must also decide which of these areas need to be discussed at every visit, which must be investigated at regular intervals, and which need to be discussed only once. Certainly once the birth history has been taken and no problems appear, there is no reason to repeat that material at every visit. However, the habits of the child change from visit to visit, sometimes from day to day, and this may be an important area to include in every history. The review of systems can easily change, but usually it will take a longer period of time for significant change to appear. The nurse may decide to routinely take a review of systems once a year rather than monthly or weekly. The nurse must go through each category and make a decision about how frequently it will be discussed.

Health assessment for nurse-family encounters: selected ages*

Health history physical exam	Nutrition	Development	Commonly recommended laboratory procedures and immunizations
First infant encounter			
Prenatal concerns Pernatal history Birth history Neonatal history History of familial diseases Interval history Family and social history Length, weight, and head circumference Complete physical exam Discussion of normal variants and abnormal physical findings with parents	Assess caloric needs for optimum growth: 100-110 cal/kg/day Discuss need for iron, vitamins, fluoride Discuss current feeding methods	2-weeks: sucking and rooting reflexes, Moro reflex, and tonic neck reflex (TNR) Sensitive to light and noise One month: responds to bell, eyes follow to midline, regards face, lifts head when prone	Urine ferric chloride for PKU Discuss with parents Discuss immunization schedule and its importance
Health assessment at 5 to 9 weeks			
Parental concerns Interval history to include past illnesses, eating, sleeping, elimination, behavior Family and social history Length, weight, and head circumference Complete physical exam Discussion of findings with parents	Assess caloric needs for optimum growth Discuss parental attitudes and expectations re: solids Discuss need for water	5 weeks: rooting and Moro reflexes and TNR May "smile" Fist to mouth Follows light; tracks sound 9 weeks: smiles, vocalizes, hands to midline, listens, follows light past midline, holds head up 90° in prone position	Diphtheria, tetanus, pertussis vaccine (DTP) Trivalent oral polio vaccine (TOPV)
Health assessment at 2½ to 4 months			
Parental concerns Interval history Family and social history Length, weight, and head circumference Complete physical exam Discussion of findings with parents	Continued need for iron enriched formula Digestive system now mature enough to handle solids Introduction of cereal, fruits at 4 months Teething biscuits may be used; avoid wheat products	2½ mo: holds head and chest to 90° in prone position Laughs, babbles TNR and Moro reflex diminishing 4 months: holds head erect and steady in sitting position Bears weight on legs May roll over, do not leave unattended	DTP and TOPV No. 2
Health assessment at 6 months			
Parental concerns Interval history Family and social history Length, weight, and head circumference Complete physical exam including eye cover test for strabismus Discussion of findings with parents	Limit milk to 24 oz/24 hr Discuss iron-containing foods, finger foods Advise waiting to wean until after 1 year Discuss fluoride, avoidance of sugared foods Discuss cleaning of teeth Avoid all bottle propping	Laughs, babbles Passes object hand to hand and mouths objects — permit no small objects or toys Tooth eruption Turns to voice Rolls over, may get to sitting Beginning stranger anxiety Stronger attachment to mother	DTP and TOPV No. 3
Health assessment at 9 months			
Parental concerns Interval history Family and social history Length, weight, and head circumference	Advise 3 meals/day May introduce cup if child ready; advise waiting to wean until after 1 year Normal drop in appetite	Jabber, babbles Thumb-finger grasp Imitates speech sounds Plays pat-a-cake May pull to stand and/or	Hematocrit, hemoglobin, and RBC indices Sickle cell and G-6 PD screening No immunizations if up to date

*Adapted from Chow, M.P., et al.: Handbook of pediatric primary care, New York, 1979, John Wiley & Sons, Inc., pp. 73-110.

Continued.

Health assessment for nurse-family encounters: selected ages — cont'd

Health history physical exam	Nutrition	Development	Commonly recommended laboratory procedures and immunizations
Health assessment at 9 months—cont'd			
Complete physical exam including hearing assessment (infant should turn head at least 45° to locate sound) Discussion of findings with parents	Restriction of sugared foods, milk, and juices in bedtime bottles Advise to have ipecac syrup on hand	crawl — secure furniture, knickknacks; cover outlets	
Health assessment at 12 months			
Parental concerns Interval history Family and social history Length, weight, and head circumference Complete physical exam Discussion of findings with parents	Review basic food groups, table foods, and amounts appropriate for age Lessened appetite Milk limited to 16–20 oz/24 hr Avoidance of sugared foods and drinks Discuss weaning from bottle	Indicates wants Drinks from cup Pincer grasp May use spoon Ma-am, da-da Crawls, walks holding on or alone — time to childproof home	Urinalysis Hemogram if not obtained sooner Tuberculin test
Health assessment at 15 to 18 months			
Parental concerns Interval history Family and social history Height and weight Complete physical exam descussion of findings with parents	Review basic food groups Stress need for iron and avoidance of sugared foods and drinks May feed self Discuss dental care	More than 5-6 words Uses spoon Scribbles on paper Points to one or more parts of body Climbing, running	Measles, mumps, and rubella (MMR) vaccine at 15 months DTP and TOPV No. 4 at 18 months if No. 3 was given at 6 months
Health assessment at 2 years			
Parental concerns Interval history Family and social history Height, weight, and head circumference Complete physical exam Discussion of findings with parents	Review basic food groups and appropriate amounts for age Reduce milk intake to 16 oz/24 hr Discuss importance of proper snacks (low sugar, high protein) Discuss teaching use of toothbrush	May talk well and follow directions Puroseful markings on paper Balances 4 blocks Performs simple household tasks Later may throw ball overhand	Urinalysis if not done earlier
Health assessment at 3 years			
Parental concerns Interval history Family and social history Height and weight; blood pressure Complete physical exam Vision screening Hearing screening Language screening (DASE, Denver Articulation Screening Examination) Discussion of findings with parents	Review basic food groups and appropriate amounts for age Discuss proper snack foods Eating patterns are influenced by family members Discuss dental visit	Talks well, uses plurals Jumps, runs Pedals tricycle Washes and dries hands Separates from mother easily	Tuberculin skin test Urinalysis for girls Hemoglobin or hematocrit

Health assessment for nurse-family encounters: selected ages — cont'd

Health history physical exam	Nutrition	Development	Commonly recommended laboratory procedures and immunizations
Health assessment at 4 years			
Parental concerns Interval history Family and social history Height and weight; blood pressure Complete physical exam Vision screening Hearing screening Discussion of findings with parents Press (preschool, readiness)	Review basic food groups and appropriate amounts for age Continued need for iron-containing foods Avoidance of sugared snacks and drinks	Knows first and last names Copies circles and crosses Understands prepositions and opposites May dress self Separates from mother easily Heel-to-toe walk	Hematocrit and RBC indices Tuberculin skin test, if not done at 3 years
Health assessment at 5 to 10 years			
Parental and client concerns Interval history: illnesses, injuries, major changes in lifestyle Review of systems Family and social history Weight, height, blood pressure, pulse, and respiration A complete physical is done Discuss the findings with the parent and client Screening: visual acuity and audiogram, language (DASE)	Basic food groups: milk, 3 servings; meat (including poultry, fish, eggs, peanut butter, dried beans), 4 servings; fruits, vegetables, 4 servings; breads, cereals, 4 servings Food likes and dislikes Types of food used for snacking Sugar intake Other considerations: milk fortified with vitamin D; iodized salt; whole grain or enriched breads and cereals; evaluate calcium, fluoride, iron source Discuss preventive dental care	5 to 6 years: balance on one foot for 10 seconds; backward heel to toe walk; draws person with greater than 6 parts; performs self-care activities 6-9 years: latency period of physical and psychological growth; questions about sex and conception 9 to 11 years: concrete thinking continues; judges thoughts only in reference to own experience, learns by trial and error Beginning growth spurt: females at approximately 9½ years and males at approximately 10½ years Females: beginning growth of pubic hair and breast budding; tomboy activities Males: male-dominated social activity	DTP and trivalent OPV boosters are given between 4 and 6 years of age Tuberculin testing every 3 years Routine urinalysis and complete blood count if not done within the last 3 years
Health assessment at 11 to 14 years			
Past history: birth, maternal medications during pregnancy, developmental milestones, illnesses, injuries, immunizations, communicable diseases, family history Present history: client and parental concerns, history of presenting concern, nutrition; social: relationships with peers, school marks, social interests, future goals, sexual information and activity	Eating habits: number of regular meals a day, snacking pattern and types of food; use of crash diets, fasting, food fads; source of protein and iron; knowledge of balanced food choices; availability of nutritious snacking foods Discuss need for continued dental care	Hormonal influences: as a defense mechanism against changing body image there are increased somatic complaints Males: beginning growth of pubic hair, enlargement of testicles; wet dreams Females: continued breast development, growth of axillary and pubic hair Thought process: beginning of abstract thinking to manipu-	Td and TOPV boosters TB test Routine urinalysis Complete blood count (CBC) Rubella titer (females) VDRL Pap smear and gonorrhea cervical culture if sexually active (females) Sickle cell screening if indicated

Continued.

Health assessment for nurse-family encounters: selected ages — cont'd

Health history physical exam	Nutrition	Development	Commonly recommended laboratory procedures and immunizations
Health assessment at 11 to 14 years—cont'd			
Review of systems Complete physical exam is done including weight, height, blood pressure, pulse, and respiration; pelvic exam if indicated Screening: visual acuity and audiogram		late concepts outside of own experience; self-centered (egocentrism); feelings of autonomy, mood swings, antisocial behavior Family: negativism as a manifestation of rejection of parents' values and seeking own identity, testing of parental controls, beginning emancipation from family Peers: importance of peer group for psychologic support and social development	
Health assessment at 15 to 18 years			
Health history A complete physical exam, is done including weight, height, blood pressure, pulse, and respiration; pelvic exam if indicated Screening: visual acuity and audiogram	Basic food groups Eating habits Continued dental care	Hormonal influences: continued development of secondary sexual characteristics Males: increased siz of penis, testes, scrotum; growth of body hair, voice and skin changes Females: enlarged breasts, broadened pelvic bones, growth of body hair, menstruation Thought process: use of formal logic in solving problems; feelings and goals directed away from self toward idealistic causes; future goals become more clear Family: movement away from family into own relationships and activities; views family's morals and culture with criticism because of idealism Peers: regular group social activity and/or individual dating	Td and OPV boosters if not given within the last 10 years Routine urinalysis and CBC if not done within the last 3 years Rubella titer (females) VDRL Pap smear and gonorrhea cervical culture if sexually active (females) Sickle cell screening if indicated

DIET HISTORY QUESTIONNAIRE FOR INFANTS

Questionnaire I—Infants (Birth to 1 Year)

Date _____ Age _____

Name _____ Birth date _____

Please answer the following questions by checking the appropriate box or filling in the blank. Answer only those questions that apply to you or your child. All information is confidential.

1. Is the baby breast fed? Yes ___ No ___
   If yes, does he/she also receive milk or formula?
   Yes ___ No ___
   If yes, what kind? _____
2. Does the baby receive formula? Yes ___ No ___
   If yes: Ready-to-feed ___
   Concentrated liquid ___
   Powdered ___
   Evaporated milk ___
   Other _____
   How is formula prepared? _____
   Is the formula iron fortified?
   Yes ___ No ___
   Don't know ___
3. Does the baby drink milk? Yes ___ No ___
   If yes: Whole milk ___
   2% milk ___
   Skim milk ___
   Other _____
4. Does the baby drink any fluids other than milk or formula?
   Yes ___ No ___
   If yes, what? _____
5. How many times does the baby eat each day, including milk or formula feedings? _____
6. Does the baby usually take a bottle to bed?
   Yes ___ No ___
   If yes, what is usually in the bottle? _____
7. If the baby drinks milk or formula, what is the usual amount in a day?
   Less than 16 oz (2 cups) ___
   16 to 32 oz ___
   More than 32 oz (1 quart) ___
8. Does the baby take vitamin or iron drops?
   Yes ___ No ___
   If yes, how often? ___ What kind? ___
9. Is the baby on a special diet now? Yes ___ No ___
   If yes: Allergy ___
   Weight reduction ___
   Other _____
   Who recommended the diet? _____

From Bureau of Maternal and Child Health/Nutrition: Diet history questionnaire for infants, Washington, D.C., 1978.

10. Does the baby eat clay, paint chips, dirt, paper, or anything else that is not considered food?
    Yes ___ No ___
    If yes, what? _____ How often? _____
11. Do you think the child has a feeding problem?
    Yes ___ No ___
    If yes, describe _____
12. Who usually feeds the baby? _____
    Does the person have the use of:
    Working stove ___
    Refrigerator ___
    Piped water ___
13. Does the family participate in:
    Food stamp program Yes ___ No ___
    WIC program Yes ___ No ___
    Day care food program Yes ___ No ___
14. Please check which, if any, of these foods the baby eats and how often.

	Less than once a week	Not daily but at least once a week	Every day or nearly every day
Cheese, yogurt, ice cream, pudding	___	___	___
Milk or formula	___	___	___
Eggs	___	___	___
Dried beans, peas, peanut butter, nuts	___	___	___
Meat, fish, poultry, wild game	___	___	___
Bread, rice, grits, cereal, tortillas, noodles, spaghetti	___	___	___
Fruits or fruit juices	___	___	___
Vegetables (including potatoes)	___	___	___
Candy, desserts, sweets	___	___	___

15. If the baby eats fruits or drinks fruit juices every day or nearly every day, which ones does he/she eat or drink most often? (Not more than three)
    _____ _____ _____
16. If the baby eats vegetables every day or nearly every day, which ones does he/she eat most often? (Not more than three)
    _____ _____ _____
17. Does the baby eat:
    Sticky or sweet foods? Yes ___ No ___
    Salty foods? Yes ___ No ___
    If yes, what are the foods? _____

    Is salt added to the baby's food? Yes ___ No ___

18. Below list the foods and beverages the baby has had during the last 24 hours.

Time	Food eaten	Amount	How is this food prepared?

Questionnaire II—Preschool and Young School Age Child (Guardian Responds)

Date _____   Age _____

Name _____   Birth date _____

Please answer the following questions by checking the appropriate box or filling in the blank. Answer only those questions that apply to you or your child. All information is confidential.

1. Does the child drink milk? Yes ___ No ___
   If yes: Whole milk ___
             2% milk   ___
             Skim milk ___
             Other _____
   If yes: Less than 8 oz (1 cup) ___
             8-32 oz   ___
             More than 32 oz (1 qt) ___

2. Does the child drink anything from a bottle?
   Yes ___ No ___
   If yes: Milk ___
           Other _____
   Does the child take a bottle to bed? Yes ___ No ___
   If yes, what is usually in the bottle?
   _____

3. How many times a day does the child usually eat, including snacks? _____
   Does the child eat anything after he/she has gone to bed?
   Yes ___ No ___
   If yes, what? _____

4. Does the child take vitamins or iron?
   Yes ___ No ___
   If yes, how often? _____
   What kind? _____

5. Is the child on a special diet now? Yes ___ No ___
   If yes: Allergy   ___
             Weight reduction ___
             Other _____
   Who recommended the diet? _____

6. Does the child eat clay, paint chips, dirt, paper, or anything else not usually considered food?
   Yes ___ No ___
   If yes, what? _____ How often? _____

7. How would you describe the child's appetite?
   Good   ___
   Fair   ___
   Poor   ___
   Other (specify) _____

8. Who usually feeds the child? _____
   Does this person have use of:
   Working stove ___
   Refrigerator ___
   Piped water   ___

9. Does the family participate in:
   Food stamp program Yes ___ No ___
   WIC program   Yes ___ No ___
   Does the child participate in:
   School breakfast   Yes ___ No ___
   School lunch   Yes ___ No ___
   Day care food program   Yes ___ No ___
   Summer food program   Yes ___ No ___

10. Please check which, if any, of these foods the child eats and how often.

	Less than once a week	Not daily but at least once a week	Every day or nearly every day
Cheese, yogurt, ice cream, pudding	___	___	___
Milk	___	___	___
Eggs	___	___	___
Dried beans, peas, peanut butter, nuts	___	___	___
Meat, fish, poultry, wild game	___	___	___
Bread, rice, grits, cereal, tortillas, noodles, spaghetti	___	___	___
Fruits or fruit juices	___	___	___
Vegetables (including potatoes)	___	___	___
Candy, desserts, sweets	___	___	___

11. If the child eats fruits or drinks fruit juices every day or nearly every day, which ones does he/she eat or drink most often? (Not more than three)
    _____ _____ _____

12. If the child eats vegetables every day or nearly every day, which ones does he/she eat most often? (Not more than three)
    _____ _____ _____

13. Does the child usually eat between meals?
    Yes ___ No ___
    If yes, name the two or three snacks (including bedtime snacks) that the child has most often.
    _____ _____ _____

14. Does the child eat:
    Sticky or sweet foods?   Yes ___ No ___
    Salty foods?   Yes ___ No ___
    If yes, what are the foods? _____
    _____

    Is salt added to the child's food? Yes ___ No ___

15. Below list the foods and beverages the child has had in the last 24 hours.

Time	Food eaten	Amount	How is this food prepared?

Questionnaire III—School Age Child and Teenager

Date _____ Age _____

Name _____ Birth date _____

Please answer the following questions by checking the appropriate box or filling in the blank. Answer only those questions that apply to you or your child. All information is confidential.

1. Do you drink milk? Yes ___ No ___
   If yes: Whole milk ___
      2% milk ___
      Skim milk ___
      Other _____
   How often? _____
   Are there other beverages you often drink?
   Yes ___ No ___
   If yes, what? _____

2. How many times a day do you eat, including snacks?
   ___

3. Do you take vitamins or iron? Yes ___ No ___
   If yes, how often? _____ What kind? _____

4. Are you on a special diet? Yes ___ No ___
   If yes: Allergy   ___
      Weight reduction ___
      Other _____
   Who recommended the diet? _____

5. Do you eat clay, paint chips, dirt, paper, or anything else not usually considered food? Yes ___ No ___
   If yes, what? _____ How often? _____

6. Does anyone in your household participate in:
   Food stamp program Yes ___ No ___
   WIC program   Yes ___ No ___
   Do you participate in:
   School breakfast   Yes ___ No ___
   School lunch   Yes ___ No ___
   Summer food program Yes ___ No ___

7. Who usually prepares your meals? _____
   Does this person have use of:
   Working stove ___
   Refrigerator ___
   Piped water ___

8. Do you eat any:
   Sticky or sweet foods? Yes ___ No ___
   Salty foods?   Yes ___ No ___
   Do you add salt to your food? Yes ___ No ___

9. Please check which of the following foods you eat and how often:

	Less than once a week	Not daily but at least once a week	Every day or nearly every day
Cheese, yogurt, ice cream, pudding	___	___	___
Milk	___	___	___
Eggs	___	___	___
Dried beans, peas, peanut butter, nuts	___	___	___
Meat, fish, poultry, wild game	___	___	___
Bread, rice, grits, cereal, tortillas, noodles, spaghetti	___	___	___
Fruits or fruit juices	___	___	___
Vegetables (including potatoes)	___	___	___
Candy, desserts, sweets	___	___	___

10. If you eat fruits or drink fruit juices every day or nearly every day, which ones do you eat or drink most often? (Not more than three)

   _____ _____ _____

11. If you eat vegetables every day or nearly every day, which ones do you eat most often? (Not more than three)

   _____ _____ _____

12. Do you usually eat anything between meals?
   Yes ___ No ___
   If yes, name the two or three snacks (including bedtime snacks) that you have most often.

   _____ _____ _____

13. Below list the foods and beverages you have had in the last 24 hours.

Time	Food eaten	Amount	How is this food prepared?

NEEDS SATISFACTION SCALE FOR INDIVIDUALS WITH A DISABILITY

Section A: Demographic Data

Name _____

Address _____

Telephone _____

Social Security no. _____

Age _____   Birth date ____ ____ ____
                              Month Day Year

Sex ___ F ___ M

Date of interview _____

Primary disability _____

Secondary disabilities _____

Marital status

___ Married   ___ Never married
___ Separated   ___ Divorced
___ Widowed   ___ Marriage annulled

Education

___ None   ___ Attended college 1-2
___ 1-5 grade   years
___ 6-8 grade   ___ Attended college 3-4
___ 9-12 grade   years
___ High school graduate ___ 4-year college degree
___ Vocational-technical ___ Graduate degree
     without licensure/certi-   (master's)
     fication   ___ Graduate degree
___ Vocational-technical with   (doctorate)
     licensure/certification

Number of dependents

___ Self only   ___ 3
___ 1   ___ 4
___ 2   ___ 5 or more

Heritage

___ Afro-American   ___ Pacific Islander
___ Caucasian   ___ Spanish
___ American Indian   ___ Other
___ Asian

Living arrangement

___ Living alone   ___ Living with non-
___ Living with spouse   relatives
___ Living with one or both ___ Living with other rel-
     parents (including step-   atives
     parents)   ___ Other

Names and relationships of household members

_____

_____

_____

_____

Military status

___ Previous military service
___ Currently in the military
___ Never in the military

Income sources

___ Earnings   ___ Private agency
___ Interest   ___ Annuities
___ Rent   ___ Public assistance, state
___ Dividends   ___ Workman's Compensa-
___ Private insurance,   tion
     disability benefits ___ Social Security
___ Family   ___ Public assistance, federal
___ Friends

Income category

___ $0–3,000   ___ $15,000–18,000
___ $3,100–6,000   ___ $18,100–21,000
___ $6,100–9,000   ___ $21,100–24,000
___ $9,100–12,000   ___ Above $24,000
___ $12,100–15,000

Work status

___ Employed outside the home
     ___ Competitive labor market
     ___ Sheltered workshop
___ Employed, home   ___ Self-employed,
___ Unemployed   outside home
___ Self-employed,   ___ Homemaker
     home   ___ Student
                       ___ Retired

Previous occupation

___ Professional   ___ Laborer
___ Technical   ___ Semiprofessional
                       ___ Nontechnical

Currently under the services of

___ Vocational Rehabilitation Services
     ___ Regular
     ___ Homebound
___ Medicaid   ___ Crippled Children's Ser-
___ Medicare   vice

Source of transportation

___ Private automobile ___ Public
___ Private van, spe- ___ None
     cially equipped

Main care giver

___ Self   ___ Full-time attendant
___ Family member   ___ Part-time attendant

My birth order position is _____
                                    (rank)

in a family of _____
              (total no. of children)

Sexes of children in the family are: M ___   F ___
                                            (no.)   (no.)

Functional abilities	Yes	No	N/A
Dress self			
Feed self, unassisted			
Feed self with assistance			
Brush teeth			
Comb hair			
Self-help, bowel elimination			
Self-help, bladder elimination			
Bathe self			
Walk			
Other independent mobility			

Section B: Satisfaction of Needs

Directions: Please choose the response that most nearly describes your answer to the question regarding your present needs.

Basic physiological needs

1. My current state of health is ___ Poor ___ Fair
                                    1   2
   ___ Satisfactory ___ Good ___ Excellent
    3   4   5

2. Rate each of the following health needs on a scale from 1 to 5 (1—extremely problematic, 2—somewhat problematic, 3—controlled problem, 4—inactive problem, 5—no problem).

	1	2	3	4	5
a. Vision					
b. Hearing					
c. Mobility					
d. Respirations					
e. Sleep					
f. Anxiety; depression					
g. Energy level					
h. Nutrition—food intake					
i. Nutrition—fluid intake					
j. Bowel elimination					
k. Bladder elimination					
l. Exercise					
m. Recreation, play					
n. Sexual libido					

Rate the following items on a scale from 1 to 5 (1—never, 2—hardly ever, 3—sometimes, 4—often, 5—almost all the time).

	1	2	3	4	5
3. I drink 2000-3000 cc of fluid per day.					
4. I eat a well-balanced diet.					
5. I take vitamins as prescribed.					
6. I avoid smoking cigarettes, cigars, and pipes.					
7. I drink alcoholic beverages only as prescribed.					
8. I take prescribed medicines.					
9. I take patent medicines only as directed by my physician.					
10. I have ROM or other exercises daily.					
11. I get 6-8 hours sleep minimum daily.					
12. I take rest periods during the day.					
13. I experience a high energy level.					
14. My bowel elimination habits are satisfactory.					
15. My urinary elimination habits are satisfactory.					
16. I keep my immunizations up to date.					
17. I practice regular dental care daily.					
18. I watch myself for signs of cancer.					
19. I have visual examinations as suggested by physician.					
20. I am able to relax.					
21. I take special measures to conserve my health.					
22. I do not object to having to take special measures to conserve my health.					
23. I do not object to giving up things I like for the sake of my health.					
24. I am confident I can meet my future health needs.					

Need for security

	1	2	3	4	5
25. I am secure about my physical safety in my home environment.					
26. I feel secure about special precautions I take regarding physical safety.					
27. I feel secure about my financial position.					

Continued.

Need for security—cont'd

	1	2	3	4	5

28. I feel secure about meeting the expenses of my routine medicine and supplies.
29. I feel satisfied about my transportation plans.
30. I am satisfied about long term plans for my care.
31. I am satisfied with my present vocational/occupational status.

Need for love and belongingness

32. I am satisfied with the amount of love from family.
33. I am satisfied with the amount of love from friends.
34. I cope satisfactorily with stress in the home life.
35. I cope satisfactorily with stress in other aspects of life.
36. I am satisfied with my level of social effectiveness.
37. I am satisfied with my social participation.
38. I am comfortable asking for help when needed.
39. I am satisfied with the amount of religion in my life.
40. I am satisfied with family activities and traditions in which I participate.
41. I am satisfied with my role in the family.
42. I am satisfied with my level of sexual fulfillment.
43. I am satisfied with my level of knowledge about human sexuality.
44. I am satisfied with the feelings of love and belongingness I receive from others.
45. I am satisfied with the amount of love and affection I give to others.
46. I have get-togethers with friends my own age.

Need for self-esteem

47. I am satisfied with the appearance of my body.
48. I am satisfied with my intellectual functioning.
49. I am satisfied with the kind of characteristics that could be said to describe me.
50. I am satisfied with past accomplishments in my life.

Need for self-esteem—cont'd

	1	2	3	4	5

51. I am satisfied with present accomplishments in my life.
52. My predominant emotional state is happy and content.
53. I am satisfied with my level of education/occupation.

Need for self-actualization

54. I am satisfied with my state of fulfillment.
55. I am satisfied with the amount of enjoyment in my everyday life.
56. I make plans to increase my level of fulfillment.
57. I am optimistic about my potential to reach higher life.
58. I am satisfied with task accomplishment of my present life.
59. I am satisfied with my own motivational level.
60. I am satisfied with motivational level of family and friends to support my goals.
61. I am satisfied with amount of responsibilities I have in life.
62. I am satisfied with the amount of spontaneity in life.
63. I have a satisfactory level of hope in my life.
64. I have new interests in life.
65. I am satisfied with the amount of meaning and purpose in my life.
66. I am reconciled to the change in my life-style from the disability I have.
67. I am satisfied with my coping reaction to suffering.
68. I am satisfied with amount of strength (courage) I have now.

Needs	Client score	Possible score	Percentage
Basic physiological		185	
Security		35	
Love and belongingness		75	
Self-esteem		35	
Self-actualization		75	
TOTALS		405	

CLASSROOM OBSERVATION SHEET*

Teacher _____ Grade _____ Date _____

Please list the names of pupils with known or suspected health problems. These problems will be discussed at the time of the teacher-nurse conferences.

The following are conditions to record (but not limited to these):

1. Hearing problems (speaks louder than normal; turns head in direction of sound)
2. Speech problems (stuttering, lisping, difficult to understand)
3. Limited physical education
4. Dental problems (decayed teeth, missing teeth, toothache)
5. Fatigue, listlessness, inattentiveness
6. Under medical care of private physician or outpatient clinic facility
7. Vision problems (squinting, reading problems)
8. Orthopedic problems (toeing in, bowlegged, knock-kneed)
9. Allergy (hay fever), red eyes, black to bluish discoloration under eyelids
10. Extreme nervousness (constantly in motion, cries easily, irritable)
11. Known diseases such as diabetes, epilepsy, heart problems
12. Nutritional status (children who appear unusually hungry, nonbreakfast eaters)
13. Personal hygiene (more than one observation)
14. Attendance problems related to illness
15. Respiratory problems (bronchitis, asthma)

Modified from Bryan, D.: School nursing in transition, St. Louis, 1973, The C.V. Mosby Co.

*To be used with the classroom assessment by nurse and teacher, during nurse-teacher conference (planned or unplanned), or by classroom teacher.

Name	Remarks	Under care of (physician, dentist, nurse practitioner)

Appendix B

FAMILY ASSESSMENT TOOLS

FAMILY HEALTH CARE PLAN*

Goal: To reduce the risk of hypertension in the family

Objectives

To reduce by ⅓ to ½ salt (sodium) intake of both family members within 5 weeks

Target activities

a. Will use only ½ as much salt in cooking at once
b. In 1 week will no longer add salt to foods at the table
c. Will increase by 50% the use of herbs, spices, and lemon in cooking in place of salt by end of 1 week
d. Will avoid snack foods with visible salt by end of 1 week
e. Will avoid all foods prepared in brine (ham bacon, pickles, etc.) within 2 weeks
f. Will stop drinking carbonated beverages within 3 weeks
g. Will start using salt (sodium)–free vegetables (fresh, frozen, canned) after present canned vegetable supply is depleted

Formative Evaluation

Family and community health nurse together measure progress made toward accomplishing target activities at check points.

At end of week 1 measure the following
Progress toward meeting target activities *a, b, c,* and *d*
Problems encountered meeting target activities
FINDING
Husband having difficulty meeting target activity *b*
PLAN
Objective *b* modified from 1 week to 2 weeks
Plan developed for a health counseling visit
At end of week 2 measure the following
Progress made toward meeting activity *e*
Husband's progress toward meeting activity *b*
Continuing ability to meet activities *a, b* (wife), and *d*

*Sample of an approach to a health care plan for a family consisting of a middle-aged husband and wife. The family health care plan is completed by adding objectives and target activities regarding stress, weight, and exercise.

At end of week 3 measure the following
Progress made toward meeting activity *f*
Continuing ability to meet all other activities except *g* (due to canned vegetable supply on hand)
At end of week 4 measure the following
Continuing ability to meet activities

Summative Evaluation

Conducted by family and community health nurse at time when care plan fully implemented and executed. Measures extent to which the objective and target activities were met at end of 5 weeks. Also examine problems encountered in meeting target activities.

FAMILY–COMMUNITY HEALTH NURSE CONTRACT

Family health situation: Family members at high risk for hypertension
Goal: To increase the family's knowledge about hypertension and low-sodium foods

Family responsibilities (husband and wife)	Nurse's responsibilities
1. Demonstrate increased knowledge about hypertension Explain (from a lay perspective) the physiology of hypertension and attending risks Explain the relationship between preventive measures and reducing the risk of hypertension	1. Provide information to family about hypertension Provide reading materials about hypertension and related self-care Counsel with the family regarding the physiology and risks associated with hypertension; describe preventive measures (lifestyle changes, etc.)
2. Demonstrate increased knowledge about low-sodium foods Able to list common	2. Provide information to family about low-sodium foods:

high- and low-sodium foods

Modifies food purchasing habits so more low-sodium foods included and more high-sodium foods excluded

Uses low-sodium recipes

Increasingly uses low-sodium menus

Provide lists of high- and low-sodium foods

Provide low-sodium recipes and menus congruent with family's resources and life-style

Length of contract _____

Date started _____ Date concluded _____

Evaluation plan _____

_____

We mutually agree to the above goal and responsibilities. This contract may be renegotiated if it becomes necessary to do so.

Signatures:

Family members _____ Date _____

_____ Date _____

Community _____ Date _____

health nurse

FAMILY HEALTH ASSESSMENT GUIDE

General instructions: Content areas of the guide should be modified and adapted as appropriate for individual families and the circumstances of the family and/or community health nurse contact(s). The factors listed for many of the major family assessment areas are examples and should be added to or omitted as necessary.

FAMILY UNIT
Family Composition (see box below)

Extended family (parents, children, etc., outside of household)

Relationship

Place of residency

Frequency of contact

Residential history

Length of time at present address

Frequency of residential and geographical changes

Education of family member (present and/or highest level attained)

Educational level

Attending school/college

Educational goal

Vocational interests of family member

Interest

Goal

Avocational interests of family member (hobbies, other creative endeavors)

Interest

Goal

Occupation of family member

Type of work

Hours of work

Satisfaction with job

Goal(s)

Financial resources

Sources (salaries, pension, public assistance, etc.)

Total income

Distribution of income (housing, food, clothing, health/illness care, utilities, recreation, insurance, etc.)

Adequacy of income

Religious practices of family members

Religious preferences

Extent of involvement

Relative importance of religion in everyday life (influence on activities of daily living, relationships, etc.)

Rituals

Holidays and celebrations related to activities of daily living

Recreational interests of family members

Interests around home (alone and with family)

Interests outside home (alone and with family)

Activities with relatives

With friends

With community groups

What does the family do for "fun" around home? Outside of home?

Family member	Age	Sex	Ethnicity/race	Family position (e.g., mother, spouse)	Special status (e.g., adopted, single, divorced)
_____	__	__	_____	_____	_____
_____	__	__	_____	_____	_____
_____	__	__	_____	_____	_____

FAMILY ENVIRONMENT
Residence

Housing
  Type of dwelling
  Number and types of rooms
  General condition
Furnishings
  Condition
  Adequacy
Living space
  Adequate for family size
  Privacy for family members
Sleeping arrangements
  Where members sleep
  Sharing of bed(s)
  Adequacy of sleeping arrangements
Bathroom facilities
  Location
  Adequacy
  Sanitation
Food preparation arrangements
  Cleanliness
  Cooking
  Refrigeration
Eating arrangements and mealtime environment
General state of cleanliness and sanitation
Adequacy of
  Water supply and source
  Waste/garbage disposal
  Lighting
  Heating and cooling
  Ventilation
  Laundry facilities
  Telephone
Condition of yard
Pets
  Number
  Kinds
  Care
Automobile
  Number
  Conditions
Provisions for emergencies
  Smoke alarm
  Emergency numbers by telephone
Environmental stressors
  Noise
  Lack of individual territory
Environmental hazards
  Storage of medicines and household cleaners/poisons
  Sharp tools
  Fire dangers
  Unsafe toys
  Loose rugs
  Clutter
  Swimming pool
Family attitudes toward home, neighborhood, and community

GOALS FOR FUTURE
Neighborhood

Type
  Residential
  Semi-commercial
  Urban/nonmetropolitan
Dwellings
  Single-family house
  Apartment
  Combination
Age of area
  Newly constructed
  Deteriorating
  Foliage (trees, shrubbery)
Sociocultural characteristics
  Age composition
  Ethnic groups
  Employment/
    unemployment
General condition of structures, yards, streets, alleys, etc.
Traffic patterns
Efficiency of street lighting systems
Availability of fire hydrants
Resources
  Shopping
  Transportation
  Recreational
  Educational
  Religious
  Protective services
  Health/illness
  Emergency
  Human services
  Business
  Garbage/refuse disposal
Environmental stressors
  Noise
  Crime rate
  Substance abuse
  Crowding
  Poverty
Environmental hazards
  Air pollution
  Garbage/debris
  Traffic flow
  Unsafe play areas
In-migration and out-migration of residents
Neighbors' attitude toward the family
Family's involvement in the neighborhood

Community

Leadership and government
Resources (essentially the same as those listed for neighborhood)
Occupations, industries, businesses
Family's involvement in the community
  Community memberships
  Interaction with social institutions
  Use of resources

FAMILY STRUCTURE

Organization
  As a system
  Subsystems
Roles
  Roles being filled
  Satisfaction/dissatisfaction with role(s)
  Level of role functioning
  Perceptions about roles
  Acceptance of roles
  Flexibility of roles/interchangeable
Socialization processes for roles
Division of labor
  How is delegation of tasks determined?
  Who carries out which tasks?
  What is the flexibility of task responsibilities?
  What is the extent of satisfaction/dissatisfaction with task delegation and performance?
Authority and power
  Degree of autonomy for each family member
  Locus of authority
  Power relationships
  How authority is exercised
  How power is demonstrated
  Satisfaction/dissatisfaction with autonomy, authority, and power in family
Values, attitudes, and beliefs regarding family organization, roles, division of labor, autonomy, authority, and power
Stresses related to family organization, roles, division of labor, autonomy, authority, and power—how handled?

FAMILY PROCESSES
Communication

Patterns
  Ways used to communicate effectively
  Content of communications
  Interpretation of content
  Linguistic characteristics (cultural)
  Frequency of communications
  How do joy, love, anger, sadness, frustration get communicated?
  Communication patterns within family subsystems
  Effectiveness of communications—understood, clear, consistent, etc.
Satisfaction/dissatisfaction with family communication patterns
Values, attitudes and beliefs regarding family communications
Stresses related to family communications

Decision Making

How are decisions made?
  What is the process?
Who makes decisions affecting adults?
  Children?
  Entire group?

How are decisions implemented?
How are decision-making skills learned in the family?
Satisfaction/dissatisfaction with family decision-making process
Values, attitudes, and beliefs regarding family decision making
Stresses related to family decision making

Problem Solving

How are problems handled?
  What is the process?
Who is involved in the problem-solving process?
  Who provides leadership in the process?
Extent to which family can deal with problem solving and for what types of problems
Flexibility in approaches to problem solving
Ability to use information from outside family in problem-solving process
Satisfaction/dissatisfaction with family's problem-solving ability and process
Values, attitudes, and beliefs regarding family's problem solving
Stresses related to family problem solving

FAMILY FUNCTIONS
Physical

How are needs for food, shelter, clothing, etc., met?
Are physical needs being met satisfactorily? If not, what solutions have been tried by the family?
Values, attitudes, and beliefs regarding family's physical needs and functions
Stresses related to meeting family's physical needs

Emotional

Affectional relationships
  Between adults
  Between adults and children
  Between siblings
Ways of obtaining and giving emotional support: distribution of support, when given, how given, acceptance by other family member(s)
Ways in which family members do or do not assist each other in developing self-esteem
  In developing autonomy?
How do family members show respect for each other?
To what extent and how is intimacy expressed?
  Physical affection and companionship?
Satisfaction/dissatisfaction regarding how family's emotional needs are met
Values, attitudes, and beliefs regarding family's emotional needs and functions
Stresses related to family's emotional functions

Social

Goals for family and individual family members
Support for individual creativity, initiative, and leadership
Process for developing and supporting family and individual leadership

Process for strengthening family members' competency regarding adjustment in social organizations (school, etc.)

Competency regarding appropriate use of social organizations

Seeking new experiences—kind, etc.

Discipline and limit-setting practices

Individual developmental tasks (physical, affective, intellectual, language, psychosocial, sexual, moral, personality)

Level of knowledge

Seeks information as needed

Provides support

Seeks support resources as needed

Adopts socialization approaches to meet individual needs and tasks

Family developmental tasks

Level of knowledge

Seeks information as needed

Intrafamily support

Uses resources as needed

Satisfaction/dissatisfaction regarding social functions

Values, attitudes, and beliefs regarding social functions

Stresses related to social functions

COPING
Conflict

To what extent and how are conflicts expressed covertly and overtly?

Frequency of conflicts? Kinds? Attributed causes?

How are conflicts avoided? How are conflicts resolved?

Satisfaction/dissatisfaction regarding conflict resolution process

Values, attitudes, and beliefs regarding conflict resolution

Stresses related to conflicts and conflict resolution

Life Changes

Recent, present, and anticipated life changes

Impact of change(s) on family's functioning as a unit

Impact of change(s) on family roles and functions

Ability to cope with change(s): practices, behaviors, values, attitudes, beliefs

Stresses associated with change(s)

Support Systems

Resources within family—what, how used, when, effectiveness

External support systems—how used, when, effectiveness

Significant others (extended family members, friends, etc.)

Nonprofessional organizations

Professional systems

Understand how to use—seek relevant information

Availability, accessibility, use patterns

Satisfaction/dissatisfaction with support systems

Values, attitudes, and beliefs related to using support systems

Life Satisfaction

How does family feel about its quality of life?

What influences family's quality of life?

What influences the family's feelings about life?

Would the family like to change anything about its life? What? What impedes change?

What can family do? Others do?

HEALTH BEHAVIOR
Health History

Genetic or familial diseases (diabetes, heart disease, etc.)

Family history of emotional problems, suicide, etc.

Past illnesses, operations, accidents, injuries

Present illnesses and/or physical discomforts

Use of prescribed and/or over-the-counter medications

Present symptoms such as anxiety, depression, etc.

Concerns about hearing, vision, speech

Recent history regarding physical and dental examinations, immunizations, Pap smear, etc.

Health Status

Family's assessment of present health status

Concerns about present health status and/or potential health problems

Family's perceptions of vulnerability to disease/illness

What does the family perceive as a health problem?

What present and potential health problems are identified by the family? Priorities for health problems?

What is family's belief about cause of problem(s)?

What is family's belief(s) about cure/treatment for problem(s)?

Activities of Daily Living

Eating patterns and foods

Personal hygiene and daily grooming

Physical activity

Sleeping behavior

Dental practices

What are family members' daily rhythms (e.g., morning person, night person)?

How does family describe a typical weekday? A weekend?

Risk Behaviors

Inadequate nutritional behavior (overeating; undereating; irregular meals; diet high in sugar, sodium; beverages high in caffeine)

Physical inactivity

Limited sleep or irregular sleeping patterns

Smoking

Use of alcohol

Nonuse of seat belts

Excessive exposure to stress situations (family, work, social)

Health Beliefs

How does family define health? Illness?

How does family define health and illness for each family member?

What value does family assign health? Health promotion? Prevention?

What are family's perceptions about cause(s) of illness?

What are family's perceptions about control over health and illness?

What are family's perceptions about how illness/disease are cured?

What are family's health goals?

How are values, attitudes, and beliefs regarding health promotion communicated to children? What is the socialization process? How does family members' involvement in the community influence family's health values, attitudes, and beliefs?

Self-care

Knowledge

Level of knowledge regarding health promotion, preventive measures, emergency care, causes and treatment of illnesses/diseases

How is health knowledge transmitted to family members?

What are sources of health information?

How does family assess its level of health knowledge?

What would family like to know about health promotion? Prevention? Illness care?

Practices

What does family do to protect its health (physical, emotional, social, spiritual)?

What does family do to improve its health status?

What does family do to prevent illness/disease?

What does family do to generate and support health protective behaviors in family members?

What does family do to care for health problems and illnesses in the home?

How are health and illness care responsibilities distributed in the family? Is there flexibility of family roles and tasks?

What are family's perceptions regarding ability to protect family's health?

How does family care for health problems and illnesses in the home?

What are the family's values, attitudes, and beliefs regarding self-care?

Family planning

Family's values, attitudes, and beliefs regarding family planning (methods, child spacing, childlessness, appropriateness for which family members, etc.)

Decision-making process

Practices

Health Care Resources

Utilization practices regarding formal informal health and illness care systems (what systems, frequency of use, etc.)

Availability of emergency care resources

Availability, accessibility, and attractiveness of health and illness care resources

Effectiveness and efficiency with which family uses resources

How is health/illness care financed? What are other costs for family such as transportation and work time lost?

Family's knowledge about health and illness care resources

Family's perceptions of and attitudes about experiences with health/illness care resources and health care providers (nurses, physicians, etc.)

What are the family's feelings about the kinds of health services available to them in the community?

What kinds of health services would they like to receive?

What suggestions do they have about making any necessary changes in the delivery of services?

What are the family's feelings about health care providers?

What kind of relationship would the family like to have with health care providers?

What suggestions do they have about helping the health care providers to better meet the needs of the family?

Family's values and beliefs related to health/illness care resources and health care providers

Stresses related to use of health/illness care resources and interactions with health care providers

Community Health Nursing Services

Knowledge about community health nursing

Attitudes toward community health nursing services

Expectations of community health nursing services

FAMILY HEALTH ASSESSMENT SUMMARY

Family's sociodemographic profile

Family's environment—strengths and problems regarding home, neighborhood, and community

Family structure, processes, functions—strengths and limitations; existing and/or potential problems

Family's coping profile

    Conflict management—strengths and limitations

    Life changes—strengths and limitations regarding coping with changes

    Support systems—strengths and limitations

    Life satisfaction profile

Family's health behavior profile

    Health history—existing and/or potential problems

    Health status—existing and/or potential problems

    Activities of daily living—strengths and limitations/ problems

    Risk profile—for family unit and family members

    Health beliefs—profile of values, attitudes, and beliefs regarding health and illness

    Self-care—strengths and limitations

    Health care resources—adequacy of availability, accessibility, attractiveness, and use; general practices

    Community health nursing services—attitudes and expectations

FAMILY PROBLEM-SOLVING GUIDE

I. Types of family problems
   A. Problems that can be resolved by the family without the community health nurse
   B. Problems that can be resolved by the family with the community health nurse's assistance
   C. Problems that should be referred to another health care professional or other human services worker
II. Problem-solving process (family and community health nurse)
   A. Assessment of the problem
      1. Who identified problem—family, community health nurse, others?
      2. Extent of problem—is the problem a threat to the health and well-being of the family? An individual family member? Others? The community?
      3. Family's assessment of the problem—seriousness? Implications of the problem for the family? If family did not identify the problem, does the family view the situation as a problem?
      4. Community health nurse's assessment of the problem (using criteria regarding extent of problem)—if the problem is of a threatening nature but not recognized as a problem by the family, the nurse will need to assist the family to recognize and understand the implications of the problem
   B. Problem solving
      1. What is the history of the problem—when started, how started, why existing, effect on family?
      2. Is family attempting to resolve/or handle problem?
         If yes
         How? How successful is approach? If approach is succeeding, support should be given to the family to continue its efforts.
         If approach is not successful, assist family to explore possible reasons for limited or lack of resolution.
         What other possible approaches has family considered?
         Have any of these approaches been tried with the present situation or similar situations in the past? If so, how effective was the approach? If approach was successful, why? If approach was unsuccessful, why?
         Would an approach used in the past be appropriate for the present situation? Would it meet with some degree of success? Explore possibilities regarding implementation and outcomes.

If family has considered alternate approaches but has not tried them, family should be assisted to (1) think how approach could be implemented and (2) consider effectiveness of outcomes.
If family perceives that implementation and outcomes will be successful, explore why—is the reasoning realistic? If not, explore other possibilities regarding implementation and outcomes which might be more realistic and workable.
If family perceives that implementation and/or outcomes will be unsuccessful, use same exploratory process as preceding example.
The family should be assisted to explore the implications for each possible approach in order to decide on the one most effective for the problem situation and the family.
If it becomes necessary for the community health nurse to supplement the family's ideas with other suggested approaches, the same exploratory approach as in the previous example should be used by the family—and the final decision regarding a problem-solving approach resides with the family.
If no (family not attempting to resolve problem)
Must the family do something due to the nature of the problem?
What are the family's reasons for not working on the problem? For example, is there some other family situation that must be resolved first? The problem-solving process may need to refocus unless both problems can be approached simultaneously.
The family is provided with information about the resolution of the problem as well as the risks associated with neglecting the problem in order to make an informed decision about a course of action.
The family is assisted in its problem solving in the same manner as discussed previously.
   C. Evaluation (jointly by family and community health nurse)
      1. Evaluation of problem-solving process and experience.
      2. Evaluation of the implementation and outcomes of the family's selected approach to the problem.

HOME OBSERVATION FOR MEASUREMENT OF THE ENVIRONMENT

BIRTH TO THREE

Child designee _____ Date of interview _____
                 Name

Child's birthday _____ Age   Sex   Ethnicity
                                   Birth order _____
Mother's name _____ Father's name _____
Address _____

Categories

	Raw scores	Percentile scores
I. Emotional and verbal responsivity of mother	_____	_____
II. Avoidance of restriction and punishment	_____	_____
III. Organization of physical and temporal environment	_____	_____
IV. Provision of appropriate play materials	_____	_____
V. Maternal involvement with child	_____	_____
VI. Opportunities for variety in daily stimulation	_____	_____
TOTALS	_____	_____

I. Emotional and verbal responsivity of mother

                                                 Yes   No

1. Mother spontaneously vocalizes to child at least twice during visit (excluding scolding). _____ _____
2. Mother responds to child's vocalizations with a verbal response. _____ _____
3. Mother tells child the name of some object during visit or says name of person or object in a "teaching" style. _____ _____
4. Mother's speech is distinct, clear, and audible. _____ _____
5. Mother initiates verbal interchanges with observer—asks questions and makes spontaneous comments. _____ _____
6. Mother expresses ideas freely and easily and uses statements of appropriate length for conversation (e.g., gives more than brief answers). _____ _____
 * 7. Mother permits child occasionally to engage in "messy" type of play. _____ _____
8. Mother spontaneously praises child's qualities or behavior twice during visit. _____ _____
9. When speaking of or to child, mother's voice conveys positive feeling. _____ _____
10. Mother caresses or kisses child at least once during visit. _____ _____
11. Mother shows some positive emotional responses to praise of child offered by visitor. _____ _____
                                       SUBSCORE _____ _____

II. Avoidance of restriction and punishment

12. Mother does not shout at child during visit. _____ _____
13. Mother does not express overt annoyance with or hostility toward child. _____ _____
14. Mother neither slaps nor spanks child during visit. _____ _____
*15. Mother reports that no more than one instance of physical punishment occurred during the past week. _____ _____
16. Mother does not scold or derogate child during visit. _____ _____
17. Mother does not interfere with child's actions or restrict child's movements more than three times during visit. _____ _____
18. At least 10 books are present and visible. _____ _____
*19. Family has a pet. _____ _____
                                       SUBSCORE _____ _____

III. Organization of physical and temporal environment

20. When mother is away, care is provided by one of three regular substitutes. _____ _____
21. Someone takes child into grocery store at least once a week. _____ _____
22. Child gets out of house at least four times a week. _____ _____
23. Child is taken regularly to doctor's office or clinic. _____ _____
*24. Child has a special place in which to keep his toys and "treasures." _____ _____
25. Child's play environment appears safe and free of hazards. _____ _____
                                       SUBSCORE _____ _____

From Caldwell, B.: Home observation measurement of the environment, University of Arkansas Center for Child Development and Education, Little Rock, Ark.

*Items that may require direct questions.

Continued.

BIRTH TO THREE—cont'd

	Yes	No
IV. Provision of appropriate play materials		
26. Child has some muscle activity toys or equipment.	___	___
27. Child has a push or pull toy.	___	___
28. Child has stroller or walker, kiddie car, scooter or tricycle.	___	___
29. Mother provides toys or interesting activities for child during interview.	___	___
30. Provides learning equipment appropriate to age—cuddly toy or role/playing toys.	___	___
31. Provides learning equipment appropriate to age—mobile, table and chairs, high chair, play pen.	___	___
32. Provides eye-hand coordination toys—items to go in and out of receptacle, fit together toys, beads.	___	___
33. Provides eye-hand coordination toys that permit combinations—stacking or nesting toys, blocks or building toys.	___	___
34. Provides toys for literature and music.	___	___
SUBSCORE	___	___
V. Maternal involvement with child		
35. Mother tends to keep child within visual range and to look at him often.	___	___
36. Mother talks to child while doing her work.	___	___
37. Mother consciously encourages developmental advance.	___	___
38. Mother invests "maturing" toys with value via her attention.	___	___
39. Mother structures child's play periods.	___	___
40. Mother provides toys that challenge child to develop new skills.	___	___
SUBSCORE	___	___
VI. Opportunities for variety in daily stimulation		
41. Father provides some caretaking every day.	___	___
42. Mother reads stories at least three times weekly.	___	___
43. Child eats at least one meal per day with mother and father.	___	___
44. Family visits or receives visits from relatives.	___	___
45. Child has three or more books of his own.	___	___
SUBSCORE	___	___

THREE TO SIX

Date of interview _____

Child designee _____
Name

Age   Sex   Ethnicity

Child's birthday _____   Birth order _____

Mother's name _____   Father's name _____

Address _____

Categories	Raw scores	Percentile scores
I. Provision of stimulation through equipment, toys, and experiences	___	___
II. Stimulation of mature behavior	___	___
III. Provision of stimulating physical and language environment	___	___
IV. Avoidance of restriction and punishment	___	___
V. Pride, affection, and thoughtfulness	___	___
VI. Masculine stimulation	___	___
VII. Independence from parental control	___	___
TOTALS	___	___

I. Provision of stimulation through equipment, toys, and experiences

1-12 The following are present in home and either belong to child subject or he is allowed to play with them:

	Yes	No
1. Toys to learn colors, sizes, shapes—typewriter, pressouts, play school, peg boards, etc.	___	___
2. Toy or game facilitating learning letters (e.g., blocks with letters, toy typewriter, letter sticks, books about letters, etc.).	___	___
3. Three or more puzzles.	___	___

THREE TO SIX—cont'd

	Yes	No
4. Two toys necessitating some finger and whole hand movements (crayons and coloring books, paper dolls, etc.).	___	___
5. Record player and at least five children's records.		
6. Real or toy musical instrument (piano, drum, toy xylophone or guitar, etc.).	___	___
7. Toy or game permitting free expression (finger paints, play dough, crayons or paint and paper, etc.).	___	___
8. Toys or game necessitating refined movements (paint by number, dot book, paper dolls, crayons and coloring books).	___	___
9. Toys to learn animals—books about animals, circus games, animal puzzles, etc.	___	___
10. Toy or game facilitating learning numbers (e.g., blocks with numbers, books about numbers, games with numbers, etc.).	___	___
11. Building toys (block, Tinker Toys, Lincoln Logs, etc.).		
12. Ten children's books.	___	___
13. At least 10 books are present and visible in the apartment.	___	___
14. Family buys a newspaper daily and reads it.	___	___
15. Family subscribes to at least one magazine.	___	___
16. Family member has taken child on one outing (picnic, shopping excursion) at least every other week.	___	___
17. Child has been taken out to eat in some kind of restaurant three or four times in the past year.	___	___
18-20 Child has been taken by a family member to the following within the past year:		
18. Airport		
19. A trip more than 50 miles from his home (50 miles radial distance, not total distance).	___	___
20. A scientific, historical, or art museum.	___	___
21. Child is taken to grocery store at least once a week.	___	___
SUBSCORE	___	___

II. Stimulation of mature behavior

	Yes	No
22-29 Child is encouraged to learn the following:		
22. Colors		
23. Shapes	___	___
24. Patterned speech (nursery rhymes, prayers, songs, TV commercials, etc.)	___	___
25. The alphabet	___	___
26. To tell time	___	___
27. Spatial relationships (up, down, under, big, little, etc.)	___	___
28. Numbers	___	___
29. To read a few words	___	___
30. Tries to get child to pick up and put away toys after play session—without help.	___	___
31. Child is taught rules of social behavior which involve recognition of rights of others.	___	___
32. Parent teaches child some simple manners—to say, "Please," "Thank you," "I'm sorry."	___	___
33. Some delay of food gratification is demanded of the child, e.g., not to whine or demand food unless within ½ hour of meal time.	___	___
SUBSCORE	___	___

III. Provision of a stimulating physical and language environment
(Observation items, except *45*)

	Yes	No
34. Building has no potentially dangerous structural or health defect (e.g., plaster coming down from ceiling, stairway with boards missing, rodent, etc.).	___	___
35. Child's outside play environment appears safe and free of hazards (no outside play area requires an automatic "No").	___	___
36. The interior of the apartment is not dark or perceptibly monotonous.	___	___
37. House is not overly noisy—television, shouts of children, radio, etc.	___	___
38. Neighborhood has trees, grass, birds—is esthetically pleasing.	___	___
39. There is at least 100 square feet of living space per person in the house.	___	___
40. In terms of available floor space, the rooms are not overcrowded with furniture.	___	___
41. All visible rooms of the house are reasonably clean and minimally cluttered.	___	___
42. *Mother uses complex sentence structure and some long words in conversing.	___	___
43. Mother uses correct grammar and pronunciation.	___	___

*Throughout interview this refers to mother *or* other care giver who is present for interview.

Continued.

THREE TO SIX—cont'd

	Yes	No
44. Mother's speech is distinct, clear, and audible.	___	___
45. Family has TV and it is used judiciously, not left on continuously (no TV requires an automatic "No"—any scheduling scores "Yes").	___	___
SUBSCORE	___	___

IV. Avoidance of restriction and punishment
(Observation items, except *51* and *52*)

	Yes	No
46. Mother does not scold or derogate child more than once during visit.	___	___
47. Mother does not use physical restraint, shake, grab, pinch child during visit.	___	___
48. Mother neither slaps nor spanks child during visit.	___	___
49. Mother does not express over-annoyance with or hostility toward child—complain, say child is "bad" or won't mind.	___	___
50. Child is not punished or ridiculed for speech.	___	___
51. No more than one instance of physical punishment occurred during the past week (accept parental report).	___	___
52. Child does not get slapped or spanked for spilling food or drink.	___	___
SUBSCORE	___	___

V. Pride, affection, and thoughtfulness
(Observation items, except *53, 54, 55, 56, 57, 58* and *59*)

	Yes	No
53. Parent turns on special TV program regarded as "good" for children (*Captain Kangaroo, Magic Toy Shop, Walt Disney, Flipper, Lassie,* educational TV, etc.).	___	___
54. Someone reads stories to child or shows and comments on pictures in magazines fives times weekly.	___	___
55. Parent encourages child to relate experiences or takes time to listen to him relate experiences.	___	___
56. Parent holds child close 10 to 15 minutes per day, e.g., during TV, story time, visiting.	___	___
57. Parent occasionally sings to child, or sings in presence of child.	___	___
58. Child has a special place in which to keep his toys and "treasures."	___	___
59. Child's art work is displayed some place in house (anything that child makes).	___	___
60. Mother introduces interviewer to child.	___	___
61. Mother converses with child at least twice during visit (scolding and suspicious comments not counted).	___	___
62. Mother answers child's questions or requests verbally.	___	___
63. Mother usually responds verbally to child's taking.	___	___
64. Mother provides toys or interesting activities or in other ways structures situation for child during visit when her attention will be elsewhere. (To score "Yes" mother must make an active guiding gesture or suggestion to structure child's play.)	___	___
65. Mother spontaneously praises child's qualities or behavior twice during visit.	___	___
66. When speaking of or to child, mother's voice conveys positive feeling.	___	___
67. Mother caresses, kisses, or cuddles child at least once during visit.	___	___
68. Mother sets up situation that allows child to show off during visit.	___	___
SUBSCORE	___	___

VI. Masculine stimulation

	Yes	No
69. Child sees and spends some time with father or father four days a week.	___	___
70. Child eats at least one meal per day, on most days, with mother (or mother figure) and father (or father figure). (One-parent families get an automatic "No.")	___	___

71-73 The following are present in home and either belong to child subject or he is allowed to play with them:

	Yes	No
71. Ride toy (tricycle, scooter, wagon, bike with or without training wheels).	___	___
72. Medium wheel toys—trucks, doll carriage, etc.	___	___
73. Large muscle toy (jump rope, swing, ball, climbing object, etc.).	___	___
SUBSCORE	___	___

VII. Independence from parental control

	Yes	No
74. Child is encouraged to try to dress himself.	___	___
75. Child is permitted to choose some of his clothing to be worn except on very special occasions.	___	___
76. Child is permitted some choice in lunch or breakfast menu.	___	___
77. Parent lets child choose certain favorite food products or brands at grocery store.	___	___
78. Child is permitted to go to another house to play without having the caregiver accompany him.	___	___
79. Child can express negative feelings without harsh reprisal.	___	___
80. Child is permitted to hit parent without harsh reprisal.	___	___
SUBSCORE	___	___
Total score	___	

ASSESSMENT SURVEY: HOUSING FOR THE DISABLED

1. Entry
   ___ Ramp
      ___ 1 ft rise per 12 ft length
      ___ 4 ft wide
      ___ Nonslip surface
      ___ Handrail extended 18 inches beyond top and bottom step
      ___ 5 ft flat platform at top
      ___ 6 ft clearance at bottom
   ___ Elevator
   ___ Steps
   ___ Lighting
   ___ Sidewalks
   ___ Surface, level
   ___ Parking
   ___ Carport, 13-14 inches clearance space
2. Living area
   ___ Floors, nonslip
   ___ Floors, same level
   ___ Doorways, 36 inches wide, 5 ft square turning area
   ___ Doors, push handles
   ___ Mirrors, correct height
   ___ Telephone at bedside
   ___ Controls and electrical switches, 36 inches from floor
   ___ Cords, out of traffic pattern
   ___ Windows, 36 inches from floor
   ___ Carpet, secure — no scatter rugs
   ___ Linoleum, free of holes, dips
   ___ Furniture, sturdy; arranged for free movement
   ___ Lighting
   ___ Heating, location of vents and radiators
3. Kitchen
   ___ Stove, burner controls safe
   ___ Pots and pans, weight
   ___ Potholders, mitts; thickness
   ___ Dishes, accessibility
   ___ Counter space, height
   ___ Faucets, accessibility and ease of on/off
   ___ Table top equipment, clutter

4. Bathroom
   ___ Tub rails, 3-4 inches out from wall
   ___ Toilet, transfer space
   ___ Toilet, height of seat
   ___ Mirror, height
   ___ Sink, height, handles
   ___ Doorway, 36 inches wide
   ___ Floor surface, nonslip
   ___ Tub surface, nonslip
   ___ Medicine chest, height
   ___ Linen storage, height
   ___ Lighting
5. Bedroom
   ___ Space
   ___ Floor surface, nonslip
   ___ Doorway, 36 inches wide
   ___ Closet, accessibility
   ___ Lighting
   ___ Bed, ancillary equipment, e.g., side rails, trapeze
   ___ Emergency call mechanism
   General description

   Hazards identified

   Inconveniences identified

   Recommendations

6. Family members
   Names, ages, and relationships

   Source of income

   Source for medical costs coverage/payments

   Caretaker
      Schedule of care

   Contingency plans

Appendix C

COMMUNITY ASSESSMENT SOURCES

SOURCES OF SCREENING AND ASSESSMENT TOOLS

AAMD Adaptive Behavior Scale for Children and Adults, 1974 Revision

AAMD Adaptive Behavior Scale Public School Version
  Source: American Association for Mental Deficiencies
    5101 Wisconsin Avenue, N.W.
    Washington, D.C. 30016

The Denver Developmental Screening Test (DDST) by W.K. Frankenberg, J.B. Dodds, A. Fandal, E. Kazuk, and M. Cohrs (birth to 6 years)
  Source: LADOCA Project and Publishing Foundation
    East 51st Avenue and Lincoln Street
    Denver, CO 80216

The Developmental Profile by G.D. Alpern and T.J. Boll (birth to pre-adolesence)
  Source: Psychological Development Publications
    7150 Lakeside Drive
    Indianapolis, IN 46278

Education for Multi-handicapped Infants (EMI)
  Source: Department of Pediatrics
    University of Virginia
    Box 232
    Charlottesville, VA 22908

Home Observation for Measurement of the Environment (HOME), B. Caldwell (birth to 3 years, 3-6 years)
  Source: Center for Early Development and Education
    University of Arkansas
    814 Sherman Street
    Little Rock, AR 72202

Meeting Street School Screening Test—Early Identification of Children with Learning Disabilities, P.K. Hainsworth and M.L. Siqueland (5 years to 7 years, 6 months)
  Source: Crippled Children and Adults of Rhode Island, Inc.
    Meeting Street School
    333 Grotto School
    Providence, RI 02906

Peabody Individual Achievement Test (PIAT), L.M. Dunn and F.C. Markwardt, (2 years, 6 months to 18 years)
  Source: American Guidance Service, Inc.
    Circle Pines, MN 55014

The Portage Guide to Early Education, S. Blumar
The Portage Project; Cooperative Educational Service—Agency Twelve
  Source: The Portage Project
    412 East Slifer Street
    Portage, WI 53901

Slosson Intelligence Test (SIT), R.L. Slosson (birth to adult)
  Source: Western Psychological Services
    Publishers and Distributors
    12031 Wilshire Boulevard
    Los Angeles, CA 90025

Vineland Social Maturity Scale, E.A. Doll (birth to adult)
  Source: American Guidance Service, Inc.
    Circle Pines, MN 55014

The Washington Guide for Promoting Development in the Young Child, K. Barnard
  Source: University School of Nursing
    University of Washington in Seattle
    Seattle, WA 98195

Appendix D

HEALTH RISK APPRAISAL FORMS

THE LIFETIME HEALTH-MONITORING PROGRAM: RECONCILING PUBLIC-HEALTH AND PRIVATE-PRACTICE GOALS

GOALS AND PROFESSIONAL SERVICES

For each of the 10 age groups, a set of distinct health goals and professional services is desirable:

Pregnancy and Perinatal Period
Health goals

1. To provide the mother a healthy, full-term pregnancy and rapid recovery after a normal delivery.
2. To facilitate the live birth of a normal baby, free of congenital or developmental damage.
3. To help both mother and father achieve the knowledge and capacity to provide for the physical, emotional, and social needs of the baby.

Professional services

1. Prior education and appropriate counseling for parents expecting their first baby in physical, emotional and social aspects of childbearing and infant care, including family planning.
2. Antenatal and postnatal care for mother and baby, education/counseling for both parents, and risk assessment through the perinatal period as needed.
3. Delivery services, including specialized perinatal care, as needed.

Infancy (First Year)
Health goals

1. To establish immunity against specified infectious diseases.
2. To detect and prevent certain other diseases and problems before irreparable damage occurs.
3. To facilitate growth and development to the infant's optimal potential.
4. To provide a basis for lifetime emotional stability, especially through a loving relation with mother, father, and other family members.

Professional services

1. Before discharge from the hospital: tests for inherited

From Breslow, L., and Somers, A.R.: The lifetime health-monitoring program, N. Engl. J. Med. **296** (11):602-604, March 1977.

metabolic and certain other congenital disorders; parent counseling.
2. Four post-discharge professional visits with the healthy infant during the year for observation, specified immunizations and parent counseling.

Preschool Child (1 to 5 Years)
Health goals

1. To facilitate the child's optimal physical, emotional and social growth and development.
2. To begin the process of socialization through happy and effective family relations and gradual introduction to school and other facets of the outside world.

Professional services

1. Two professional visits with the healthy child and mother (ideally, the father also) at 2 to 3 years and at school entry for compliance with immunization schedule, and for observation and counseling about nutrition, activity, vision, hearing, speech, dental health, accident prevention, and general physical, emotional and social development.
2. For special high-risk groups, blood tests for anemia, lead poisoning and tuberculosis.

School Child (6 to 11 Years)
Health goals

1. To facilitate the child's optimal physical/mental/emotional/social growth and development, including a positive self-image.
2. To establish healthy behavioral patterns for nutrition, exercise, study, recreation, and family life, as a foundation for a healthy lifetime life-style.

Professional services

1. Two professional visits with the healthy child (at 6 to 7 and 9 to 10 years of age), including one complete physical/mental/behavioral/social examination, with appropriate tests for, and follow-up observation of, any physical or mental impairment, including obesity, vision and nearing defects, muscular incoordination, and learning disabilities, and completion of any necessary immunizations.
2. Mandatory school health education and individual counseling, as needed, for physical fitness, nutrition, exercise, study, accident prevention, sexual development, and use of cigarettes, drugs and alcohol.
3. Annual dental examination and prophylaxis.

Adolescence (12 to 17 Years)
Health goals

1. To continue optimal physical/mental/emotional/social growth and development.
2. To reinforce healthy behavior patterns, and discourage negative ones, in physical fitness, nutrition, exercise, study, work, recreation, sex, individual relations, driving, smoking, alcohol, and drugs, as foundation for healthy lifetime life-style, including marriage, parenthood, and career or job.

Professional services

1. Mandatory school health education and individual counseling, as needed, for the above subjects, including a course in sex, marriage and family relations as a prerequisite to graduation from high school.
2. One professional visit with the healthy adolescent (at about 13 years of age) with attention to emotional status, vision and hearing, skin, blood pressure, blood cholesterol, and contraception.
3. Annual dental examination and prophylaxis.

Young Adulthood (18 to 24 Years)
Health goals

1. To facilitate transition from dependent adolescence to mature independent adulthood with maximum physical, mental and emotional resources.
2. To achieve useful employment and maximum capacity for a healthy marriage, parenthood, and social relations.

Professional services

1. One professional visit with the healthy adult, including complete physical examination, tetanus booster if not received within 10 years, tests for syphilis, gonorrhea, malnutrition, cholesterol and hypertension, and medical and behavioral history. This visit may be provided upon entrance into college, the armed forces or first full-time job, but should be before marriage.
2. Health education and individual counseling, as needed, for nutrition, exercise, study, career, job, occupational hazards and problems, sex, contraception, marriage and family relations, alcohol, drugs, smoking and driving.
3. Dental examination and prophylaxis every 2 years.

Young Middle Age (25 to 39 Years)
Health goals

1. To prolong the period of maximum physical energy and to develop full mental, emotional and social potential.
2. To anticipate and guard against the onset of chronic diseases through good health habits and early detection and treatment where effective.

Professional services

1. Two professional visits with the healthy person—at about 30 and 35—including tests for hypertension, anemia, cholesterol, cervical and breast cancer, and in-struction in self-examination of breasts, skin, testes, neck, and mouth.
2. Professional counseling regarding nutrition, exercise, smoking, alcohol, marital, parental, and other aspects of health-related behavior and life-style.
3. Dental examination and prophylaxis every 2 years.

Older Middle Age (40 to 59 Years)
Health goals

1. To prolong the period of maximum physical energy and optimum mental and social activity, including menopausal adjustment.
2. To detect as early as possible any of the major chronic diseases, including hypertension, heart disease, diabetes and cancer, as well as vision, hearing and dental impairments.

Professional services

1. Four professional visits with the healthy person, once every 5 years—at about 40, 45, 50, and 55—with complete physical examination and medical history, tests for specific chronic conditions, appropriate immunizations and counseling regarding changing nutritional needs, physical activities, occupational, sex, marital and parental problems and use of cigarettes, alcohol and drugs.
2. For those over 50, annual tests for hypertension, obesity, and certain cancers.
3. Annual dental prophylaxis.

The Elderly (60 to 74 Years)
Health goals

1. To prolong the period of optimum physical/mental/social activity.
2. To minimize handicapping and discomfort from onset of chronic conditions.
3. To prepare in advance for retirement.

Professional services

1. Professional visits with the healthy adult at 60 years of age and every 2 years thereafter, including the same tests for chronic conditions as in older middle age, and professional counseling regarding changing life-style related to retirement, nutritional requirements, absence of children, possible loss of spouse, and probable reduction in income as well as reduced physical resources.
2. Annual immunization against influenza (unless the person is allergic to vaccine).
3. Annual dental prophylaxis.
4. Periodic podiatry treatments as needed.

Old Age (75 Years and Over)
Health goals

1. To prolong period of effective activity and ability to live independently, and to avoid institutionalization so far as possible.
2. To minimize inactivity and discomfort from chronic conditions.

3. When illness is terminal, to assure as little physical and mental distress as possible and to provide emotional support to patient and family.

Professional services

1. Professional visit at least once a year, including complete physical examination, medical and behavioral history, and professional counseling regarding changing nutritional requirements, limitations on activity and mobility, and living arrangements.
2. Annual immunization against influenza (unless the person is allergic to vaccine).

3. Periodic dental and podiatry treatments as needed.
4. For low-income and other persons not sick enough to be institutionalized but not well enough to cope entirely alone, counseling regarding sheltered housing, health visitors, home helps, day care and recreational centers, meals-on-wheels and other measures designed to help them remain in their own homes and as nearly independent as possible.
5. Professional assistance with family relations and preparations for death, if needed.

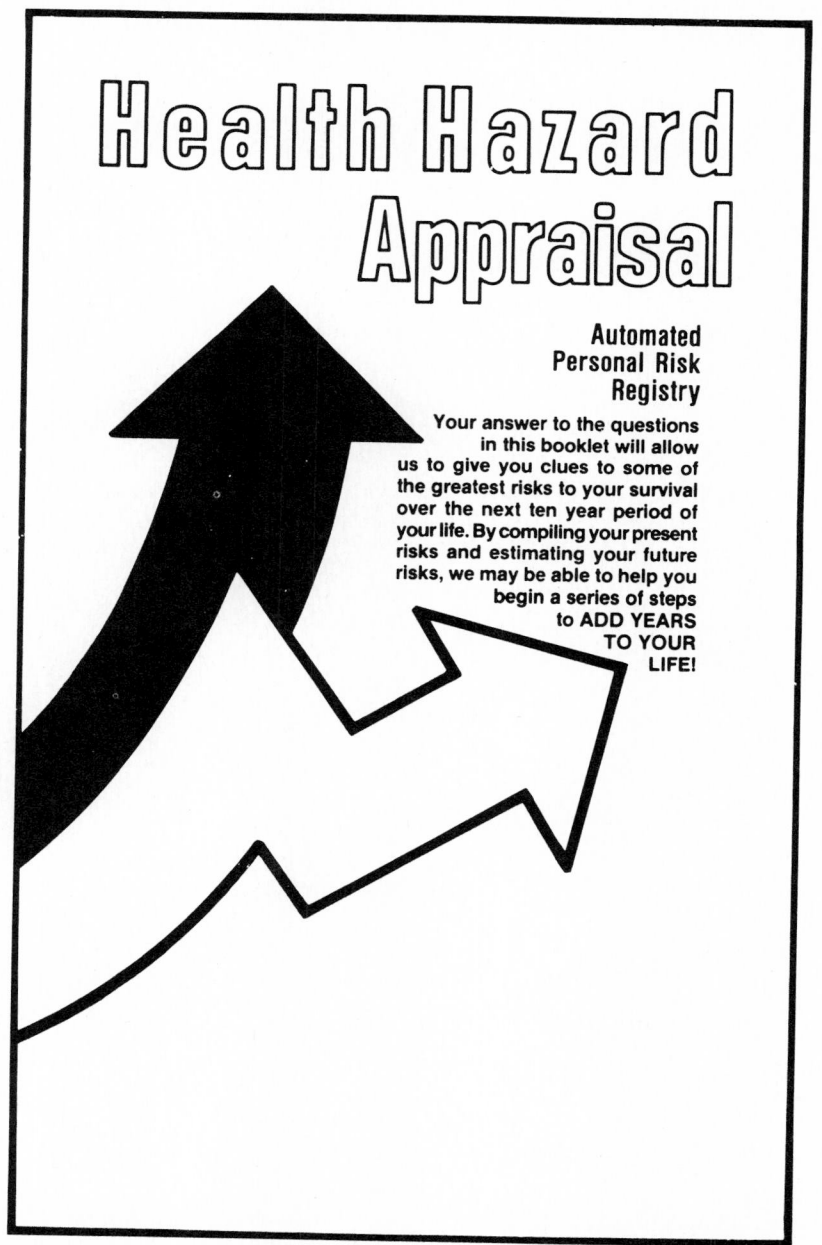

Continued.

Please answer every question. There are a few questions that inquire about race or religion. They are asked only because they are associated with different risks in certain diseases. This is your appraisal, and all answers will be completely confidential. The more honestly you answer the questions, the more accurate your appraisal will be.

PLEASE FOLLOW THESE INSTRUCTIONS:

1. Read each question thoroughly and insert the number of the most appropriate answer in the space at right.

   EXAMPLE: **An apple is red** **2**

       1. No   2. Yes   3. Do Not Know

2. In some areas of the form you will be asked to fill-in information. In these areas we ask that you **please print.**

  ★ ★ ★ ★ ★ ★ ★ ★ ★
  ★ ★ ★ ★ ★ ★ ★ ★

Social Security Number ....

Last Name

First Name, Middle Initial

Street

City

State or Province   Zip

Birth Date   MONTH   DAY   YEAR   Sex MALE/FEMALE   Race BLACK, WHITE, OTHER

Height   feet   inches   Weight   lbs.

Systolic (upper reading) Blood Pressure (if known) ....
(120 is average)

Diastolic (lower reading) Blood Pressure (if known) ....
(80 is average)

Cholesterol level (if known) ....
(210 is average)

Please list your mileage per year as both a passenger and as a driver in an automobile or any other motor vehicle. (the national average is 10,000 miles per year.) ....
THOUSAND

Do you have an annual proctosigmoidoscopy? (examination of your bowel with a lighted instrument), or screening of stool specimen is negative for blood three times a year ....

  1. No   2. Yes

Have you had any bleeding from your rectum? ....

  1. No, have not had any bleeding   2. Yes, have had some bleeding
  3. Yes, have had some bleeding, but my doctor knows about it.

Have you ever had polyps or growths in your rectum? (not piles or hemorrhoids) ....

  1. No   2. Yes   3. Do Not Know

Do you have or have you had an Ulcerative Colitis? (bloody diarrhea with pus and mucous and sores inside the rectum) ....

  1. No   2. Yes, 10 or more years   3. Yes, under 10 years

Have you had Bacterial Pneumonia? ....

  1. No   2. Yes

Have you had or do you have Emphysema? ....

  1. No   2. Yes

Have you ever had Rheumatic Fever? (Inflammation of the heart and/or joints) ....

  1. No   2. Yes, with treatment   3. Yes, without treatment

Have you ever been told that you have a Heart Murmur? ....

  1. No   2. Yes, with treatment   3. Yes, without treatment

Please list any other significant problems which you feel may affect your life expectancy.

Please continue on next page

Is your natural mother alive? · · · · · · · · · · 17
  1. No 2. Yes 3. Do Not Know

Is she now over 70, or was she at the time of death? · · · · · · · · · 18
  1. No 2. Yes 3. Do Not Know

If she is dead, did she die of Heart Disease? · · · · · · · · · 19
  1. No 2. Yes 3. Do Not Know

Is your natural father alive? · · · · · · · · · 20
  1. No 2. Yes 3. Do Not Know

Is he now over 70, or was he at the time of death? · · · · · · · · · 21
  1. No 2. Yes 3. Do Not Know

If he is dead, did he die of Heart Disease? · · · · · · · · · 22
  1. No 2. Yes 3. Do Not Know

Has any member of your immediate family (parents, brothers, sisters, or children) ever committed or attempted Suicide? · · · · · · · · · 23
  1. No 2. Yes 3. Do Not Know

Has any member of your immediate family (parents, brothers, sisters, or children) had or have Diabetes? · · · · · · · · · 24
  1. No 2. Yes 3. Do Not Know

Have you ever been told that you have Diabetes? · · · · · · · · · 25
  1. No 2. Yes with treatment 3. Yes without treatment

Approximately how much of time do you wear your seatbelt? · · · · · · · · · 26
  1. None 2. 20% 3. 40%
  4. 60% 5. 80% 6. 100%

Approximately how many alcoholic drinks do you have per week? (one drink equals 1 - 12 oz. beer, 4 oz. of wine, or 1 oz. of hard liquor) · · · · · · · 27
  1. Non Drinker 2. Have Stopped Drinking 3. 1–2 Drinks Per Week
  4. 3–6 Drinks Per Week 5. 7–24 Drinks Per Week
  6. 25–40 Drinks Per Week 7. 41 or More Drinks Per Week

Do you or have you ever taken any of the drugs or medications listed here before driving in your car? If your answer is YES, please indicate the type of drug or drugs you have taken or are presently taking · · · · · · · · · 28
  1. Do Not Take Any 2. Mood Elevators 3. Amphetamines, Diet Pills
  4. Tranquilizers, Sedatives, Sleeping Pills, Nerve Pills 5. Narcotic Pain Pills
  6. Antihistamines 7. Marijuana, LSD

Have you ever been arrested for a violent act or threat of a violent act? · · 29
  1. No 2. Yes

Do you carry a weapon? (includes carrying a weapon while at work) · · 30
  1. No 2. Yes

How much exercise do you have each day? · · · · · · · · · 31
  1. Walking less than 5 blocks or climbing up less than 5 flights of stairs. (Sedentary - No Sports)
  2. Walking 5—15 blocks or climbing up 5—15 flights of stairs. (Little - Light Sports)
  3. Walking 15—20 blocks or climbing up 15—20 flights of stairs. (Acceptable - Active Sports)
  4. Walking more than 20 blocks or climbing up more than 20 flights of stairs. (Substantial - Strenuous Sports)

Do you smoke? · · · · · · · · · 32
  1. No 2. Yes

Did you previously smoke? · · · · · · · · · 33
  1. No 2. Yes

If either of the above answers were YES, please list the amount that you now smoke per day or previously smoked per day · · · · · · · 34
  1. 40 + Cigarettes 2. 20—39 Cigarettes
  3. 10—19 Cigarettes 4. 1—9 Cigarettes
  5. Heavy Pipe 6. Light Pipe
  7. Heavy Cigar 8. Light Cigar

If you have stopped smoking, please list the number of years that you have stopped. · · · · · · · · · 35
  1. 1 yr. 2. 2 yrs. 3. 3 yrs. 4. 4 yrs.
  5. 5 yrs. 6. 6 yrs. 7. 7 yrs. 8. 8 yrs.
  9. 9 yrs. 0. More than 9 years

What would you consider your economic and social status to be? · · · · · 36
  1. Low 2. Average 3. High

Are you often depressed? · · · · · · · · · 37
  1. No 2. Yes

Do you frequently have crying spells? · · · · · · · · · 39
  1. No 2. Yes

Do you frequently think of ending your life? · · · · · · · · · 39
  1. No 2. Yes

Continued.

In the past 12 months, have you experienced any of the following:

(Insert appropriate number in each space at right)   1. No   2. Yes

Death of Spouse 49
Change in health of a family member 50
Death of a close family member 51
Death of a close friend 52
Trouble with your in-laws 53
Change in number of arguments with your spouse 54
Sexual difficulties 55
Marital separation 56
Marital reconciliation 57
Divorce 58
Marriage 59
Revision of personal habits 60
Change in sleeping habits 61
Change in eating habits 62
Minor violation of law 63
An outstanding personal achievement 64
Personal injury or illness 65
Change in responsibilities at work 66
Change in work hours or conditions 67
Trouble with boss 68
Fired from job 69
Change to a different line of work 70
Business readjustment 71
Change in your financial status 72
Change in residence 73
Change in living conditions 74
Change in number of family get-togethers 75
Begin or end school 76
Change in schools 77
Foreclosure of a mortgage or loan 78
Retirement 79
Spouse begins or stops work 80
Mortgage over $30,000 81
Mortgage or loan less than $30,000 82
Pregnancy 83
Son or daughter leaves home 84
Gain of a new family member 85
Change in social activities 86
Change in church activities 87
Change in recreation 88
Vacation 89
Christmas 90
Jail Term 91

THE FOLLOWING QUESTIONS ARE FOR FEMALES ONLY

Has your mother or any sisters or aunts ever had breast cancer? 92
1. None had   2. One had   3. Two or more had

Has your doctor ever told you that you had a lump or cyst in your breast that was NOT cancer? 93
1. No   2. Yes

Does your doctor examine your breasts at least once a year? 94
1. No   2. Yes

Do you examine your breasts at least once a month? 95
1. No   2. Yes

What is your current menstrual status? 96
1. Still menstruating   2. Natural menopause
3. Surgical menopause at under 35 years
4. Surgical menopause at over 35 years

How many times have you been pregnant? 97
1. None   2. 1–2 times   3. 3 or more times

If you have been pregnant, what was the age of your first pregnancy? 98
1. Under 20   2. 20–24   3. 25 or over

At what age did you begin to have regular sexual intercourse? 99
1. Never   2. Before 20   3. Between 20–25   4. After 25

Are you Jewish? 100
1. No   2. Yes

Has your cervix been removed? 101
1. No   2. Yes

Has your uterus been removed? 102
1. No   2. Yes

Have your ovaries been removed? 103
1. No.   2. Yes, one   3. Yes, both

Have you had any ABNORMAL vaginal bleeding in the past year? 104
1. No
2. Yes, between menstrual periods.
3. Yes, during or after sexual intercourse.
4. Yes, periods have stopped, but having bleeding every once in a while.
5. Yes, taking estrogens, bleed when off.
6. Yes, taking estrogens, bleed whether on them or off.

Please indicate the results of any Pap Smears, cancer smears, that you have by inserting the most appropriate answer 105
1. I have not had a Pap Smear in the past 5 years.
2. I have had one normal Pap Smear in the past year.
3. I have had one normal Pap Smear in the past 5 years.
4. I have had 3 normal Pap Smears in the past 5 years.
5. I have had 5 normal Pap Smears in the past 5 years.
6. I have had a Pap Smear in the past year, but it was abnormal.
7. I have had a Pap Smear in the past year, but I do not know the results.

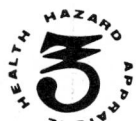

This program
is based on the
established goals of the
Society of Prospective Medicine,
to extend useful life expectancy.
The Society's logo is the symbol
of the apothecaries' ounce.
Their motto is,
"AN OUNCE OF
PREVENTION, IS WORTH A
POUND OF CURE."

**Please use the enclosed window envelope
and return this booklet to your provider as
instructed, or mail directly using sufficient
first class postage for one ounce.**

prospective
  medicine center

**prospective
medicine center**

Suite 219, 3901 North Meridian Street
Indianapolis, Indiana 46208

**RETURN THIS BOOKLET
FOR PROCESSING TO** ⬆

Continued.

HEALTH 80's QUESTIONNAIRE

1069085

```
Your Facility Name
Address
City, State
Zip
```

NOTE: *Please follow directions carefully. If you consider a question too personal, you may skip it. All information is handled confidentially.*

1-202
IDENTIFICATION

10 **Name**
   Last Name, First Name, Middle Name

11 **Today's Date**
   Mo.   Day   Yr.

12 **Date of Birth**
   Mo.   Day   Yr.

13 **Social Security Number** — —   14 **None**

15 **Female**   16 **Male**

17 **Height** ft. in.   18 **Weight** lbs.

PERMANENT HOME ADDRESS

19 **Street**

20 **City**

21 **State or Province**

22 **Zip**

23 **Country**

1-604
DEMOGRAPHIC Background

Race

10 ___ American Indian
11 ___ Black
12 ___ Caucasian
15 ___ Other

Family income level

16 ___ Low
17 ___ Middle
18 ___ High

Marital Status

19 ___ Single
20 ___ Married
21 ___ Widowed
22 ___ Separated
23 ___ Divorced

2-104
ILLNESSES and MEDICAL PROBLEMS
Check the problems you have or have had that have been diagnosed *and*
treated by a physician or other health professional.

Yes	No	Problem
10 ___	___	Alcoholism
11 ___	___	Anemia-sickle cell
12 ___	___	Bleeding trait
13 ___	___	Bronchitis, chronic
		Cancer
14 ___	___	*Breast*
15 ___	___	*Cervix*
16 ___	___	*Colon*
17 ___	___	*Lung*
18 ___	___	*Uterus*
19 ___	___	*Other cancer*
20 ___	___	Cirrhosis - liver
21 ___	___	Colitis - ulcerative
22 ___	___	Depression
23 ___	___	Diabetes
24 ___	___	Diabetes, uncontrolled
25 ___	___	Emphysema
26 ___	___	Fibrocystic breasts
		Heart problem
27 ___	___	*Heart attack*
28 ___	___	*Coronary disease*
29 ___	___	*Rheumatic heart*
30 ___	___	*Heart valve prob.*
31 ___	___	*Heart murmur*
32 ___	___	*Enlarged heart*
33 ___	___	*Heart rhythm prob.*
34 ___	___	*Other heart prob.*

Yes	No	Problem
		High blood fat, specify
50 ___	___	*Cholesterol*
51 ___	___	*Triglycerides*
52 ___	___	High blood pressure
53 ___	___	High blood pressure, uncontrolled
54 ___	___	Obesity - more than 20 lbs. overweight
55 ___	___	Pneumonia
56 ___	___	Polyps in colon
57 ___	___	Rheumatic fever
58 ___	___	Rheumatic fever, with resultant heart murmur
59 ___	___	Stroke
60 ___	___	Suicide attempt
61 ___	___	Tuberculosis

Yes	No	In the past year, have you had -
62 ___	___	Chest pain on exertion, relieved by rest?
63 ___	___	Shortness of breath lying down, relieved by sitting up?
64 ___	___	Unexplained weight loss, more than 10 lbs.?
65 ___	___	Unexplained rectal bleeding?
66 ___	___	Unexplained vaginal bleeding?

2-105
FEELINGS
Mark the frequency with which you have the feelings listed by placing a checkmark in the appropriate column.

M-Most of time   S-Some of time   R-Rarely or none

M	S	R	
10 ___	___	___	Feel sad, depressed?
11 ___	___	___	Wish to end it all?
12 ___	___	___	Feel tense and anxious?
13 ___	___	___	Worry about things generally?
14 ___	___	___	More aggressive, hard-driving than friends?
15 ___	___	___	Have an intense desire to achieve?
16 ___	___	___	Feel optimistic about the future?

FAMILY MEDICAL HISTORY (Blood Relatives)
Check items that apply for your blood relatives. Your blood relatives include your children, brothers, sisters, parents, and grandparents.

30 ___ **Do not know my family medical history.**
   (Go to next section)

Yes	No	Illness	Yes	No	Illness
31 ___	___	Anemia-sickle cell	36 ___	___	High blood press.
32 ___	___	Bleeding trait	37 ___	___	Mental illness
33 ___	___	Cancer	38 ___	___	Stroke
34 ___	___	Diabetes (sugar)	39 ___	___	Suicide
35 ___	___	Heart disease	40 ___	___	Tuberculosis

Yes	No	Check the items that apply.
50 ___	___	Father died of a heart attack before age 60?
51 ___	___	Mother died of a heart attack before age 60?
52 ___	___	Mother or sister had cancer of the breast?
53 ___	___	Did your mother take DES (diethylstilbestrol) when she was pregnant with you?

Q8020

© Medical Datamation 1980

SAMPLE QUESTIONNAIRE
2-PAGE QUESTIONNAIRE

HABITS and RISK FACTORS

Your habits influence your ability to achieve and maintain good health and long life. The questions on this page concern factors that are known to influence your health.

4-105
EATING

Yes	No	Do you usually eat the following each day?
10		Five or more servings of dairy products or red meat?
11		Five or more servings of pastries, bread, starchy foods?

EXERCISE

Specify the amount of exercise you get each day.

12 ____ None or very little

The equivalent of-

13 ____ 10 flights of stairs, or 1 mile walking
14 ____ 20 flights of stairs, or 2 miles walking
15 ____ Over 20 flights of stairs, or over 2 miles walking

SMOKING

Yes	No	Do you-
16		Smoke a pipe and inhale 5 or more times/day?
17		Smoke cigars and inhale 5 or more times/day?
18		Currently smoke cigarettes?
19		Have a history of cigarette smoking, but stopped?

If no longer smoking, specify number of years since you stopped.

20 ____ 1 yr.	23 ____ 4 yrs.	26 ____ 7 yrs.
21 ____ 2 yrs.	24 ____ 5 yrs.	27 ____ 8 yrs.
22 ____ 3 yrs.	25 ____ 6 yrs.	28 ____ 9 or more yrs.

If you have ever smoked cigarettes, specify amount and duration.

	Daily amount		Number of years
29	1/2 pack/day or less	33	Less than 1 year
30	1/2 to 1 pack/day	34	1 to 5 years
31	1 to 2 packs/day	35	5 to 10 years
32	Over 2 packs/day	36	Over 10 years

ALCOHOL

Yes	No	
37		Do you currently drink alcohol?
38		Did you formerly drink alcohol but stopped?

If you have ever drunk alcohol, specify details.

	Amount per week		Number of years
39	Less than 2 drinks/wk.	44	Less than one year
40	2 to 10 drinks/wk.	45	1 to 5 years
41	10 to 25 drinks/wk.	46	5 to 10 years
42	25 to 40 drinks/wk.	47	10 to 20 years
43	Over 40 drinks/wk.	48	Over 20 years

TRAUMA, ACCIDENTS and OTHER HAZARDS

Yes	No	Do you-
50		Know how to swim?
51		Drive after drinking or taking drugs?
52		Tend to exceed the speed limit?

How many miles do you travel in a car or other motor vehicle each year (average is 12,000 miles)?

53 ____ Up to 10,000	55 ____ 15,000 to 20,000
54 ____ 10,000 to 15,000	56 ____ Over 20,000

What percent of the time do you wear a seat belt?

57 ____ 0 to 25%	59 ____ 50% to 75%
58 ____ 25% to 50%	60 ____ 75% to 100%

What percent of the time do you wear a shoulder strap?

61 ____ 0 to 25%	63 ____ 50% to 75%
62 ____ 25% to 50%	64 ____ 75% to 100%

9-108
SELF-CARE

The early evaluation of symptoms, self-exams, and various professional health exams are important in detecting diseases. Regular medical follow-up is important in keeping problems under control and avoiding complications.

Yes	No	Have you-
10		Ever had a chest x-ray?
11		Had an abnormal chest x-ray?
12		Ever had an EKG (Electrocardiogram)?
13		Had an abnormal EKG?
14		Had a TB skin test?
15		Had a positive TB skin test?
16		Had eyes checked in past two years?
17		Had hearing tested (audiometry) in past 2 years?
18		Had dental exam in the past year?
		Do you-
19		Regularly follow your physician's advice?
20		Plan annual medical symptom review with your physician or health service?
21		Plan annual rectal exam after age 30?

WOMEN (Men go to "Tests")

Yes	No	Do you or have you-
30		Had a PAP test within past year?
31		Had at least three PAP tests in past 5 years?
32		Had an abnormal PAP test in past?
33		Plan annual PAP tests in the future?
34		Check your breasts once a month for lumps?
35		Have a breast exam by a doctor once yearly?

TESTS For these tests, if ever done, find out results from your physician. Check values shown that are closest to your own results. If measured more than once, use most recent value.

	Blood Pressure				Cholesterol	
	Systolic		Diastolic			
40	120 or less	45	82 or less	50	180 or less	
41	140	46	88	51	210	
42	160	47	94	52	240	
43	180	48	100	53	270	
44	200 or more	49	106 or more	54	300 or more	

INFORMATION

Check items for which you would like educational information.

60 ____ Alcohol	68 ____ Legal problems
61 ____ Birth Control	69 ____ Loneliness
62 ____ Diet	70 ____ Marital problems
63 ____ Drug abuse	71 ____ Medical emergencies
64 ____ Emotional problems	72 ____ Self-breast exam
65 ____ Exercise	73 ____ Sexual problems
66 ____ Financial problems	74 ____ Smoking
67 ____ Health hazards	75 ____ Venereal disease

CONCLUSION

Yes	No	
80		Do you have any other problem not covered by this questionnaire?

Please give us your opinion of this system.

81 ____ Great	83 ____ Generally good, criticism minor
82 ____ Good	84 ____ Don't like it

Thanks for completing this questionnaire. Please review for accuracy, then mail or turn in according to instructions.

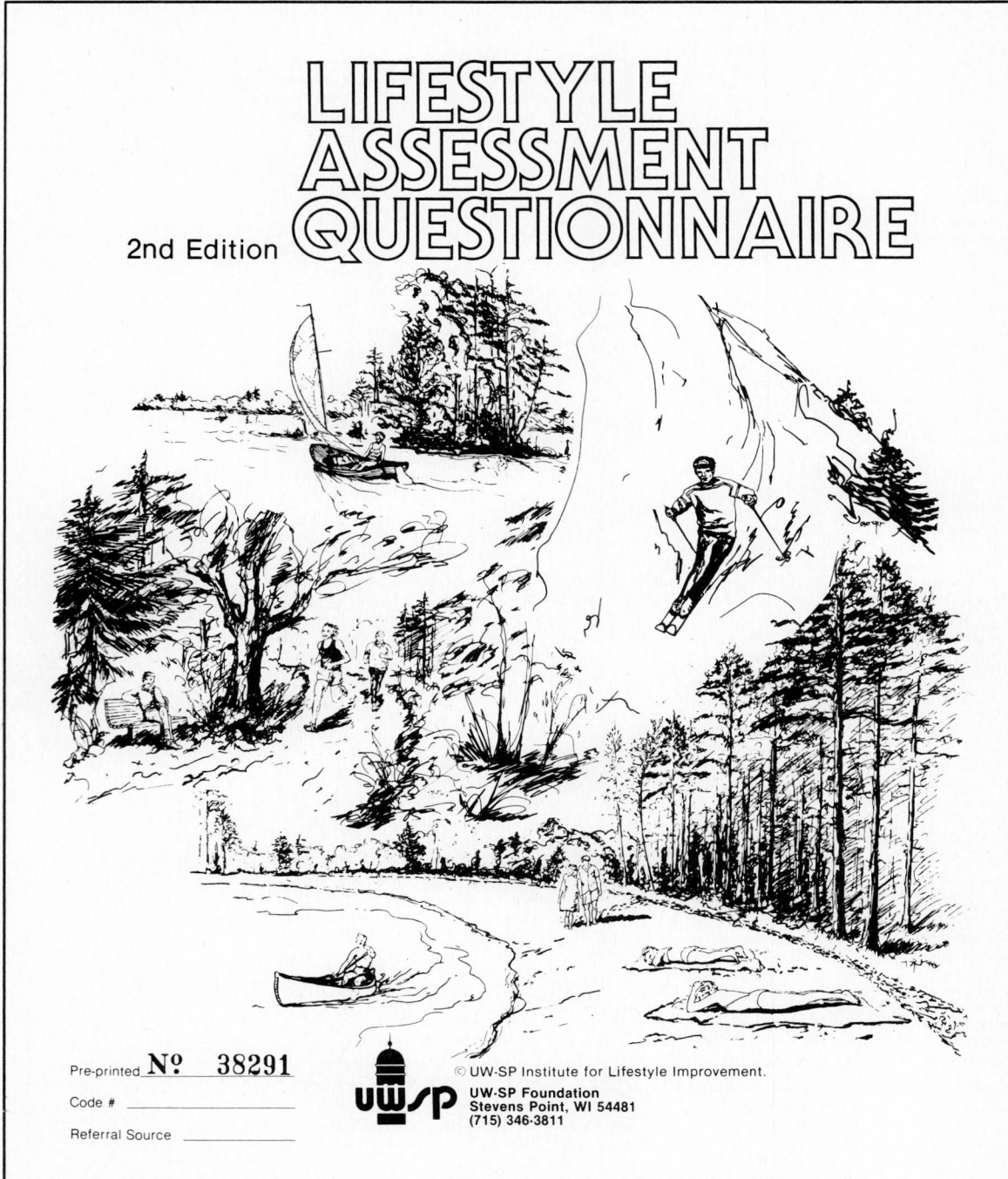

LIFESTYLE ASSESSMENT QUESTIONNAIRE

2nd Edition

Pre-printed № 38291

Code # _____

Referral Source _____

© UW-SP Institute for Lifestyle Improvement.

UW-SP Foundation
Stevens Point, WI 54481
(715) 346-3811

purpose

This Lifestyle Assessment Questionnaire is designed to help you assess your current level of wellness and the potential risks or hazards that you choose to face at this point in your life. The printouts that you will receive will reflect your strengths and the possible consequences of risks that you choose to take. The questionnaire will also assess your interest in improving the quality of your life. The printout will indicate sources of information that will help you learn more about gaining higher levels of wellness.

THE MAJOR DETERMINANT FOR JOYFUL LIVING IS YOU AND YOUR LIFESTYLE

The circle graph below indicates the factors that contribute to increasing your enjoyment and quality of life. While it is true that doctors and hospitals have a significant role to play in the quality of our lives, this graph clearly indicates that it is individuals, through the choices that they make each day, that contribute the greatest percentage toward maximizing the quality of life and health. We believe this instrument can be a useful adjunct in helping individuals identify the most likely causes of death and disability, but more importantly identify the areas of self-improvement which will lead to higher levels of joy and wellness. This instrument can be used to begin a positive, wellness approach toward living. It is our belief that this instrument can help people realize that they are the most important provider of health or "illth" care. Many of the common killers in America are the direct result of individual behaviors. We all know that our behaviors can improve our chances for leading a long useful life. Collectively, all of our behaviors can be described as our lifestyle.

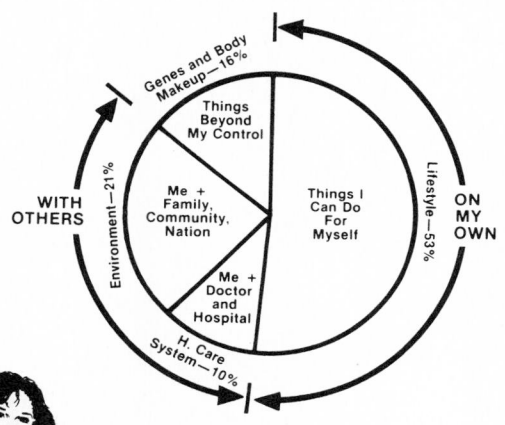

GENERAL INFORMATION CONCERNING THE LIFESTYLE ASSESSMENT QUESTIONNAIRE (LAQ)

The LAQ is organized into four sections: 1. Wellness Inventory; 2. Topics for Personal Growth; 3. Risk of Death Section, and 4. Alert Section: Medical/Behavioral/Emotional. The Wellness Inventory Section will help you identify your strengths. You will receive a printout that will indicate the percent of possible points that you gained in each topic area. The printout will also provide you with average scores for the people in your group and the total average for all people who have ever used this instrument.

The automated referral or Personal Growth section of this questionnaire will provide a printout indicating resources available for up to six topics.

The Risk of Death section will result in a printout indicating the probable number of years that you have remaining in your life, the leading causes of death for your age, race, and sex, and what behaviors could be changed to improve the chances of survival and the quality of your life.

The final section of this questionnaire entitled the Alert Section: Medical/Behavorial/Emotional will provide information which can generate a problem list for your home health record. This could also be used as part of a medical chart in a health care delivery system. We feel it will be useful for people to maintain, in their home, a current record of their immunization status and other significant problems.

It is our desire that this questionnaire be used in a positive sense to improve the understanding of self and your role in maintaining a life of high quality.

Continued.

confidentiality

The Institute for Lifestyle Improvement will maintain the confidentiality of your answers. The Institute will not permit any individually identified information from your questionnaire to be released to any person or organization other than the source from whom the LAQ was received.

Bill Hettler, M.D.
Bill Hettler, M.D.

Dennis Elsenrath
Dennis Elsenrath, Ed. D.

Fred Leafgren
Fred Leafgren, Ph.D.

THE UNIVERSITY OF WISCONSIN-STEVENS POINT INSTITUTE FOR LIFESTYLE IMPROVEMENT STEVENS POINT, WISCONSIN 54481 (715) 346-3811

The Institute for Lifestyle Improvement, which exists within the structure of the UW-SP Foundation, has three broad missions: 1. To provide health promotion services to public and private agencies; 2. To conduct research on lifestyle improvement activities; and 3. To provide continuing educational and training programs for those interested in wellness promotion strategies.

The Institute offers services in four major areas:

Lifestyle Assessment Questionnaire	Consultation and Presentation	Continuing Educational and Training Programs	Audio-Visual Materials and Self-Care Modules
—Individual and group needs assessment —Motivational tool —Health planning tool to estimate current and future disease care needs —Self-care tool to provide home health care record	—Keynote speakers for local and national meetings —Planning for community forums —Facilitators for health fairs —Speakers for corporate wellness programs —Corporate wellness program planning and evaluation —Consultation for community health promotion	—Annual wellness promotion strategies conference —Specialized conferences for target groups —On site training programs for corporations, universities or communities —In-service training for teachers and other youth workers	—Production of movies on wellness promotion topics —Production of videotapes, audio-tapes and slide/tape presentations on wellness promotion —Written materials to support wellness promotion activities —Other assessment instruments for wellness promotion —Cold self-care module

1 lifestyle assessment questionnaire

WELLNESS INVENTORY SECTION

INSTRUCTIONS:

This section will help determine the current level of wellness that you are experiencing. We hope that it will also give you ideas for areas in which you might improve. If you are uncomfortable in answering any item in this section or following sections, you may leave that item blank. Please respond to these statements using the following choices and circle your response:

A—Almost always (90% or more of the time)
B—Very frequently (approximately 75% of the time)
C—Frequently (approximately 50% of the time)
D—Occasionally (approximately 25% of the time)
E—Almost never (less than 10% of the time)
—If item does not apply to you do not mark item

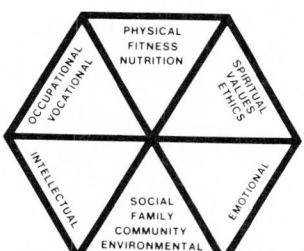

Almost always
Very frequently
Frequently
Occasionally
Almost never
If item does not apply to you, do not mark

PHYSICAL EXERCISE—Measures one's commitment to maintaining physical fitness.

1. I exercise vigorously for at least 20 minutes three or more times per week . . . .   A B C D E
2. I determine my activity level by monitoring my heart rate. . . . .   A B C D E
3. I stop exercising before I feel exhausted . . . .   A B C D E
4. I approach exercise in a relaxed manner. . . . .   A B C D E
5. I stretch before exercising. . . . .   A B C D E
6. I stretch after exercising . . . .   A B C D E
7. I walk or bike whenever possible . . . .   A B C D E
8. When feeling tired, I arrange for sufficient sleep   A B C D E
9. I participate in a strenuous sport (tennis, running, swimming, handball, basketball, etc.) . . . . .   A B C D E
10. I use foot gear of good quality, designed for the activity in which I participate . . . .   A B C D E
11. If I am not in shape, I avoid sporadic (once a week or less often) strenuous exercise. . . . .   A B C D E
12. After vigorous exercise, I "cool down" (very light exercise such as walking) for at least five minutes before sitting or lying down . . . .   A B C D E

Continued.

Almost always
Very frequently
Frequently
Occasionally
Almost never
If item does not apply to you, do not mark

PHYSICAL-NUTRITIONAL—Measures the degree to which one chooses foods that are consistent with the dietary goals of the United States as published by the Senate Select Committee on Nutrition and Human Needs.

13. When choosing non-vegetable protein, I select lean cuts of meat, poultry and fish. . . . .   A B C D E
14. I maintain an appropriate weight for my height and frame . . . .   A B C D E
15. I minimize salt intake . . . .   A B C D E
16. I eat fruits and vegetables fresh and uncooked . .   A B C D E
17. I eat breakfast . . . .   A B C D E
18. I intentionally include fiber in my diet on a daily basis . . . .   A B C D E
19. I drink enough fluid to keep my urine light yellow . . . .   A B C D E
20. I plan my diet to insure an adequate amount of vitamins and minerals. . . . .   A B C D E
21. I minimize foods in my diet that contain large amounts of refined flour (bleached white flour, typical store bread, cakes, etc.) . . . .   A B C D E
22. I minimize my intake of fats and oils including margarine and animal fats . . . .   A B C D E
23. I include items from all four basic food groups in my diet each day (fruits and vegetables; milk group; breads and cereals; meat, fowl, fish or vegetable proteins) . . . .   A B C D E
24. To avoid unnecessary calories, I choose water as one of the beverages I drink . . . .   A B C D E
25. I avoid adding sugar to my food and I minimize my intake of pre-sweetened foods such as sugar-coated cereals, syrups, chocolate milk, and most processed and fast foods.   A B C D E

PHYSICAL-SELF-CARE—Measures the behaviors that help one prevent or detect early illnesses.

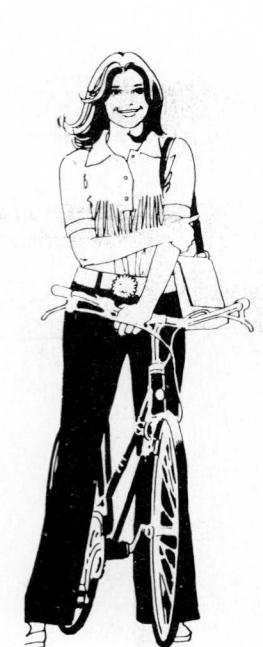

26. I maintain an up-to-date immunization record . . .   A B C D E
27. I examine my breasts or testes on a monthly basis . . . .   A B C D E
28. I have my breasts or testes examined yearly by a physician. . . . .   A B C D E
29. I have a Pap test annually (Males—do not mark).   A B C D E
30. I take action to minimize my exposure to tobacco smoke . . . .   A B C D E
31. When I'm experiencing illness or injury, I take necessary steps to correct the problem . . . .   A B C D E
32. I brush my teeth after eating. . . . .   A B C D E
33. I floss my teeth after eating . . . .   A B C D E
34. My resting pulse is 60 or less . . . .   A B C D E
35. I get an adequate amount of sleep. . . . .   A B C D E
36. I keep my blood pressure in a range that minimizes my chances of disease. (e.g., stroke, heart attack and kidney disease). . . . .   A B C D E
37. I keep my cholesterol level, high density lipids and triglycerides in a range that minimize my chances of disease . . . .   A B C D E
38. If I were to engage in sex and didn't want children at that time, I would use a contraceptive method . . . .   A B C D E
39. I take action to prevent contracting and/or transmitting venereal disease . . . .   A B C D E

1

Almost always
Very frequently
Frequently
Occasionally
Almost never
If item does not apply to you, do not mark

PHYSICAL-VEHICLE SAFETY—Measures one's ability to minimize chances of injury or death in a vehicle accident.

40. I do not operate vehicles under the influence of alcohol or other drugs .... A B C D E
41. I do not ride with vehicle operators who are under the influence of alcohol or other drugs ..... A B C D E
42. I stay within the speed limit .... A B C D E
43. I use the information I learned in a driver education or defensive driving course .... A B C D E
44. When traffic lights change from green to yellow, I prepare to stop .... A B C D E
45. I maintain a safe driving distance between cars based on speed and road conditions........... A B C D E
46. Vehicles which I drive are maintained to assure safety.. A B C D E
47. Because they are safer, I use radial tires on cars that I drive................................. A B C D E
48. I use caution when riding bicycles or motorcycles (e.g., helmets, adequate lights, etc.) ..... A B C D E

PHYSICAL-DRUG USAGE—Measures the degree to which one is able to function without the unnecessary use of chemicals.

49. I use drugs only when necessary .... A B C D E
50. I avoid the use of tobacco................... A B C D E
51. I do not consume more than two alcoholic drinks per day .... A B C D E
52. Because of the potentially harmful effects of caffeine (e.g., coffee, tea, cola, etc.), I limit my consumption .... A B C D E
53. I avoid using marijuana .... A B C D E
54. I avoid the use of hallucinogens (LSD, PCP, MDA, etc.)................................... A B C D E
55. I avoid the use of stimulants ("uppers"—e.g., cocaine, amphetamines, "pep pills", etc.) ...... A B C D E
56. I avoid the use of depressants ("downers"—e.g., barbiturates, minor tranquilizers, etc.).......... A B C D E
57. I avoid using a combination of drugs unless under medical supervision .... A B C D E
58. I follow the instructions provided with any drug I take .... A B C D E
59. I avoid using drugs obtained from unlicensed sources .... A B C D E
60. I understand the expected effect of drugs I take. A B C D E
61. I consider alternatives to drugs .... A B C D E

SOCIAL-ENVIRONMENTAL—Measures the degree to which one contributes to the common welfare of the community. This emphasizes the interdependence with others and nature.

62. I take steps to conserve energy in my place of residence .... A B C D E
63. I consider energy conservation when choosing a mode of transportation...................... A B C D E
64. I offer support to members of my family when appropriate................................. A B C D E
65. I contribute to the feeling of acceptance within my family .... A B C D E
66. I do my part to promote clean air .... A B C D E
67. When I see a safety hazard, I take action (warn others or correct the problem) .... A B C D E
68. I avoid unnecessary radiation .... A B C D E
69. I report criminal acts I observe .... A B C D E

Continued.

Almost always

Very frequently

Frequently

Occasionally

Almost never

If item does
not apply to
you, do not mark

70. I contribute time and/or money to community
projects... A B C D E
71. I actively seek to become acquainted with individuals in my community...................... A B C D E
72. I use my creativity in constructive ways........ A B C D E
73. My behavior reflects fairness and justice....... A B C D E
74. When possible, I choose an environment which
is free of noise pollution...................... A B C D E
75. When possible, I choose an environment which
is free of air pollution........................ A B C D E
76. I participate in volunteer activities benefiting
others.. A B C D E
77. I go out of my way to help others.............. A B C D E
78. I beautify those parts of my environment under
my control....................................... A B C D E

EMOTIONAL AWARENESS & ACCEPTANCE—Measures the degree to which one has an awareness
and acceptance of one's feelings. This includes
the degree to which one feels positive and enthusiastic about oneself and life.

79. I have a good sense of humor.................. A B C D E
80. I feel positive about myself.................... A B C D E
81. I feel there is a satisfying amount of excitement
in my life.. A B C D E
82. My emotional life is stable.................... A B C D E
83. I am aware of my needs........................ A B C D E
84. I trust and value my own judgment............ A B C D E
85. When I make mistakes, I learn from them...... A B C D E
86. I feel comfortable when complimented for jobs
well done.. A B C D E
87. It is okay for me to cry........................ A B C D E
88. I have feelings of sensitivity for others......... A B C D E
89. I feel enthusiastic about life................... A B C D E
90. I find it easy to laugh......................... A B C D E
91. I am able to give love......................... A B C D E
92. I am able to receive love...................... A B C D E
93. I enjoy my life................................. A B C D E
94. I have plenty of energy........................ A B C D E
95. My sleep is restful............................. A B C D E
96. I trust others.................................. A B C D E
97. I feel others trust me.......................... A B C D E
98. I accept my sexual desires.................... A B C D E
99. I understand how I create my feelings......... A B C D E
100. At times I can be both strong and sensitive..... A B C D E
101. I am aware when I feel anger.................. A B C D E
102. I can accept my anger........................ A B C D E
103. I am aware when I feel sad.................... A B C D E
104. I can accept my sadness...................... A B C D E
105. I am aware when I feel happy................. A B C D E
106. I can accept my happiness.................... A B C D E
107. I am aware when I feel frightened............. A B C D E
108. I can accept my feelings of fear.............. A B C D E

EMOTIONAL MANAGEMENT—Measures the capacity to appropriately control one's feelings and
related behaviors including the realistic assessment of one's limitations.

109. I am able to be open with those with whom I
am close.. A B C D E
110. I can express my feelings of anger............ A B C D E

1

Almost always
Very frequently
Frequently
Occasionally
Almost never
If item does
not apply to
you, do not mark

111. I can express my feelings of sadness . . . .   A   B   C   D   E
112. I can express my feelings of happiness . . . .   A   B   C   D   E
113. I can express my feelings of fear . . . .   A   B   C   D   E
114. I can compliment myself for a job well done . . . .   A   B   C   D   E
115. I accept constructive criticism without reacting defensively. . . . .   A   B   C   D   E
116. I recognize that I can have wide variations of feelings about the same person. (Such as loving someone even though you are angry with them at the moment). . . . .   A   B   C   D   E
117. I am able to develop close, intimate relationships . . . .   A   B   C   D   E
118. I make conscious decisions about my sexual activity based on personal/spiritual values. . . . . .   A   B   C   D   E
119. I stick to the limits I set for myself . . . .   A   B   C   D   E
120. I can say ''no'' without feeling guilty . . . .   A   B   C   D   E
121. I would feel comfortable seeking professional help to better understand and cope with my feelings . . . .   A   B   C   D   E
122. I set realistic objectives for myself . . . .   A   B   C   D   E
123. I can relax my body and mind (without using drugs) . . . .   A   B   C   D   E
124. I can be alone without feeling lonely . . . .   A   B   C   D   E
125. I am able to be spontaneous in expressing my feelings . . . .   A   B   C   D   E
126. I accept responsibility for my actions . . . .   A   B   C   D   E
127. I am willing to take the risks that come with making change. . . . .   A   B   C   D   E
128. I manage my feelings to avoid unnecessary suffering. . . . .   A   B   C   D   E
129. I make decisions with a minimum of stress and worry . . . .   A   B   C   D   E
130. I accept the responsibility for creating my own feelings . . . .   A   B   C   D   E

INTELLECTUAL—Measures the degree that one engages her/his mind in creative, stimulating mental activities, expanding knowledge and improving skills.

131. I read a daily newspaper. . . . .   A   B   C   D   E
132. I read twelve books or more yearly. . . . .   A   B   C   D   E
133. I read on the average one or more national magazines weekly. . . . .   A   B   C   D   E
134. When I watch TV, I choose educational programs. . . . .   A   B   C   D   E
135. I visit a museum or art show at least three times yearly. . . . .   A   B   C   D   E
136. I attend lectures, workshops and demonstrations at least three times yearly . . . .   A   B   C   D   E
137. I participate in hobbies such as photography, gardening, woodworking, sewing, painting, baking, art, music, writing, pottery, etc. . . . .   A   B   C   D   E
138. I read about local, state, national, and international political/public issues. . . . .   A   B   C   D   E
139. I make an effort to learn the meaning of new words. . . . .   A   B   C   D   E
140. I engage in some type of writing activity such as a regular journal, letter writing, preparation of papers or manuscripts . . . .   A   B   C   D   E
141. I am interested in understanding the view of others . . . .   A   B   C   D   E
142. I devote time to sharing ideas, concepts, thoughts, or procedures to advance the knowledge of others. . . . .   A   B   C   D   E

Continued.

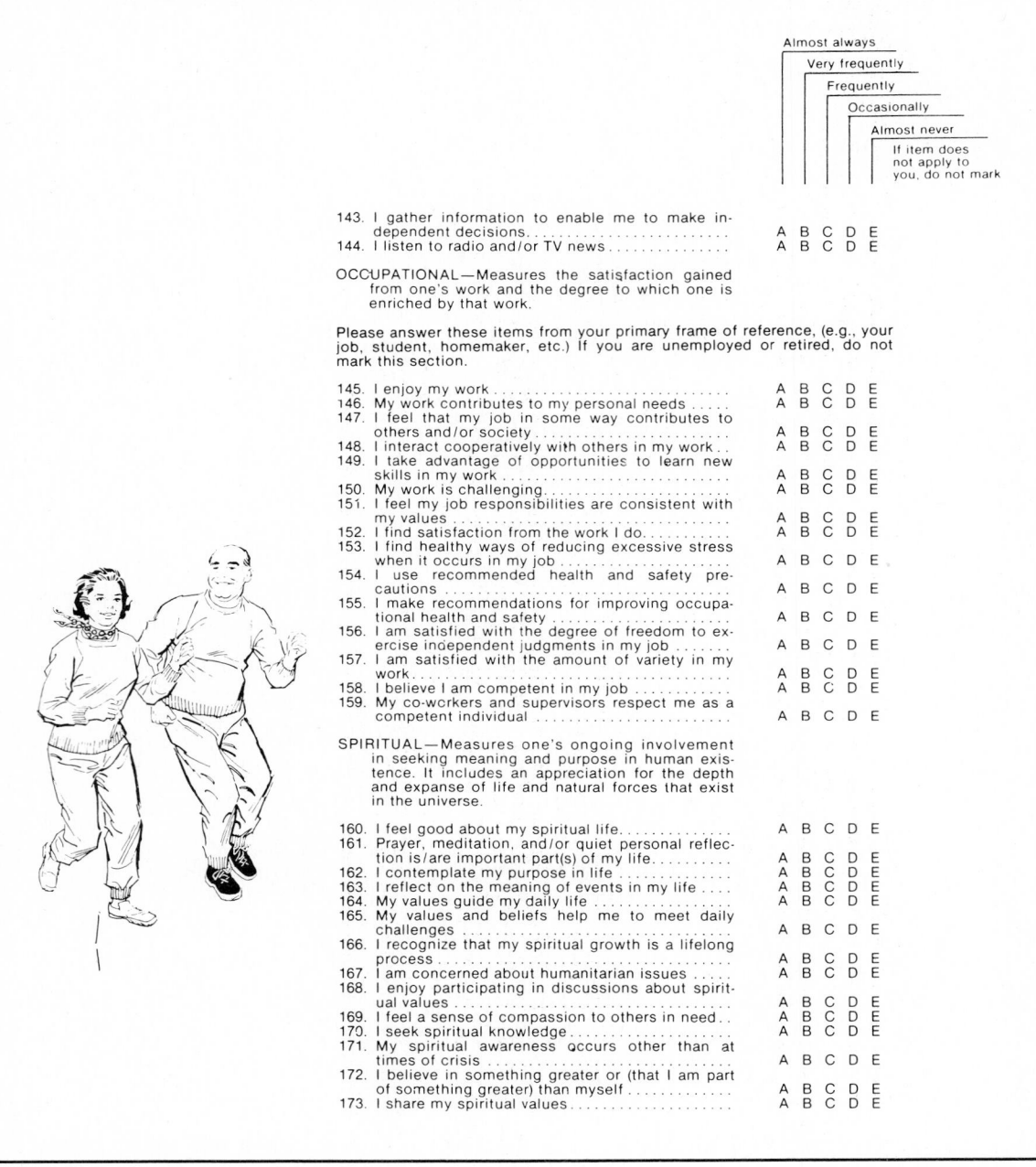

Almost always
Very frequently
Frequently
Occasionally
Almost never
If item does not apply to you, do not mark

143. I gather information to enable me to make independent decisions. . . . .   A B C D E
144. I listen to radio and/or TV news . . . .   A B C D E

OCCUPATIONAL—Measures the satisfaction gained from one's work and the degree to which one is enriched by that work.

Please answer these items from your primary frame of reference, (e.g., your job, student, homemaker, etc.) If you are unemployed or retired, do not mark this section.

145. I enjoy my work. . . . .   A B C D E
146. My work contributes to my personal needs . . . . .   A B C D E
147. I feel that my job in some way contributes to others and/or society . . . .   A B C D E
148. I interact cooperatively with others in my work . .   A B C D E
149. I take advantage of opportunities to learn new skills in my work . . . .   A B C D E
150. My work is challenging.   A B C D E
151. I feel my job responsibilities are consistent with my values . . . .   A B C D E
152. I find satisfaction from the work I do. . . . .   A B C D E
153. I find healthy ways of reducing excessive stress when it occurs in my job . . . .   A B C D E
154. I use recommended health and safety precautions . . . .   A B C D E
155. I make recommendations for improving occupational health and safety . . . .   A B C D E
156. I am satisfied with the degree of freedom to exercise independent judgments in my job . . . .   A B C D E
157. I am satisfied with the amount of variety in my work . . . .   A B C D E
158. I believe I am competent in my job . . . .   A B C D E
159. My co-workers and supervisors respect me as a competent individual . . . .   A B C D E

SPIRITUAL—Measures one's ongoing involvement in seeking meaning and purpose in human existence. It includes an appreciation for the depth and expanse of life and natural forces that exist in the universe.

160. I feel good about my spiritual life. . . . .   A B C D E
161. Prayer, meditation, and/or quiet personal reflection is/are important part(s) of my life. . . . .   A B C D E
162. I contemplate my purpose in life . . . .   A B C D E
163. I reflect on the meaning of events in my life . . . .   A B C D E
164. My values guide my daily life . . . .   A B C D E
165. My values and beliefs help me to meet daily challenges . . . .   A B C D E
166. I recognize that my spiritual growth is a lifelong process . . . .   A B C D E
167. I am concerned about humanitarian issues . . . . .   A B C D E
168. I enjoy participating in discussions about spiritual values . . . .   A B C D E
169. I feel a sense of compassion to others in need . .   A B C D E
170. I seek spiritual knowledge . . . .   A B C D E
171. My spiritual awareness occurs other than at times of crisis . . . .   A B C D E
172. I believe in something greater or (that I am part of something greater) than myself . . . .   A B C D E
173. I share my spiritual values . . . .   A B C D E

2 lifestyle assessment questionnaire

TOPICS FOR PERSONAL GROWTH SECTION

INSTRUCTIONS:

This section is intended to help you identify areas in which you would like more information or sources for group activities for continued learning or confidential personal assistance. In response to your selection from the following topics we will provide you with resources or services to meet your requests.

With regard to the following list, I would like:

	Information	Group Activities	Confidential Personal Assistance
1. Responsible alcohol use	1	2	3
2. Stop smoking programs	1	2	3
3. Sexual dysfunction	1	2	3
4. Contraception	1	2	3
5. Venereal disease	1	2	3
6. Depression	1	2	3
7. Loneliness	1	2	3
8. Exercise programs	1	2	3
9. Weight reduction	1	2	3
10. Self breast exam	1	2	3
11. Medical emergencies	1	2	3
12. Vegetarian diets	1	2	3
13. Relaxation - stress reduction	1	2	3
14. Mate selection	1	2	3
15. Parenting skills	1	2	3
16. Marital (or couples) problems	1	2	3
17. Assertive training (How to say no without feeling guilty)	1	2	3
18. Biofeedback for tension headache	1	2	3
19. Overcoming phobias (ex. high places, crowded rooms, etc.)	1	2	3
20. Educational/Career goal setting/planning	1	2	3
21. Spiritual or philosophical values	1	2	3
22. Interpersonal communication skills	1	2	3
23. Automobile safety	1	2	3
24. Suicide thoughts or attempts	1	2	3
25. Drug abuse	1	2	3
26. Test anxiety reduction	1	2	3
27. Enhancing Relationships	1	2	3
28. Time Management Skills	1	2	3
29. Nutrition	1	2	3
30. Death and Dying	1	2	3
31. Learning Skills (Speed reading, comprehension, etc.)	1	2	3

Continued.

③ lifestyle assessment questionnaire
RISK OF DEATH SECTION

INSTRUCTIONS:
This section is intended to help you identify the problems most likely to interfere with the quality of your life. This will give you a statistical assessment of the most likely causes of death facing you for the next ten (10) years. This section will also indicate what impact various personal behavioral choices have on that risk of death. Although this section will give you a printout indicating a statistical measurement of your risk based on national morbidity and mortality data, the printout will be no guarantee. Pre-existing disease or chance occurrence can completely negate the recommendations or suggestions made on this printout. We do feel, however, that it is a fairly accurate assessment of your current state of risk and offers suggestions for improving the quality of life and useful longevity.

Age in years _____

Height _____ ft. _____ inches

Weight in pounds _____

1. Sex:
   1. Male
   2. Female

2. Race:
   1. White
   2. Black
   2. Other

3. How would you describe your body build?
   1. Small
   2. Medium
   3. Large

4. What is your systolic (top number) blood pressure?
   1. 190 or more
   2. 170-189
   3. 150-169
   4. 130-149
   5. Less than 130
   Note: If you don't know your blood pressure, we will use the average for your age, race, and sex.

5. What is your diastolic (lower number) blood pressure?
   1. 103 or more
   2. 97-102
   3. 91-96
   4. 85-90
   5. Less than 85

6. What is your blood cholesterol level?
   1. 270 or more
   2. 230-269
   3. 210-229
   4. 190-209
   5. Less than 190
   Note: If you don't know your cholesterol level, we will use the average for your age, race, and sex.

7. Are you
   1. An uncontrolled diabetic
   2. A controlled diabetic
   3. Not a diabetic

8. Which of the following best describes how much physical activity you get per week including work?
   1. Climb less than 5 flights of stairs or walk less than ½ mile 4 times per week (or equivalent activity)
   2. Climb 5-15 flights of stairs or walk ½-1½ miles 4 times per week (or equivalent activity)
   3. Climb 15-20 flights of stairs or walk 1½-2 miles 4 times per week (or equivalent activity)

9. Family history of heart disease:
   1. Both parents died before age 60 of heart disease
   2. One parent died before age 60 of heart disease
   3. Neither parent died before age of 60 of heart disease

10. Do you smoke tobacco?
    1. Yes
    2. No

11. If yes, how much do you smoke per day?
    1. 2 packs of cigarettes or more
    2. 1½-2 packs of cigarettes
    3. 1-1½ packs of cigarettes
    4. ½-1 pack of cigarettes or heavy pipe or cigar
    5. Less than ½ pack of cigarettes or light pipe or cigar

12. If 10 is yes, how many years have you been smoking?
    1. Less than 2
    2. 2 - 5
    3. 5 - 10
    4. 11 - 15
    5. 16 or more

13. Are you a former smoker?
    1. Yes
    2. No

14. If yes, how much did you smoke per day?
    1. 2 packs of cigarettes or more
    2. 1½-2 packs of cigarettes
    3. 1-1½ packs of cigarettes
    4. ½-1 pack of cigarettes or heavy pipe or cigar
    5. Less than ½ pack of cigarettes or light pipe or cigar

15. How many years ago did you quit?
    1. 0-2 years
    2. 3-4
    3. 5-6
    4. 7-8
    5. 9 or more

16. Do you drink alcoholic beverages?
    1. Yes
    2. No

17. If yes to the question above, how many per week?
    1. More than 40 drinks
    2. 25-40
    3. 8-24
    4. 3-7
    5. 1-2

18. When consuming alcohol, I do not consume more than one drink per hour.
    1. Yes
    2. No

19. How many miles a year do you travel in a motor vehicle as a driver or passenger?
    1. Under 10,000
    2. 10,000-20,000
    3. 20,000-30,000
    4. 30,000-40,000
    5. Over 40,000

20. While traveling in a motor vehicle how often do you use seat belts?
    1. 20% or less of the time
    2. 20%-40%
    3. 40%-60%
    4. 60%-80%
    5. 80%-100%

21. Are you depressed much of the time?
    1. Frequently
    2. Seldom
    3. Never

22. Has anyone in your immediate family (parents, brothers, sisters) committed suicide?
    1. Yes
    2. No

23. In regard to your heart, have you had:
    1. A murmur without preventive antibiotics
    2. A murmur with preventive antibiotics
    3. No murmur

24. In regard to your heart, have you had:
    1. Rheumatic fever without preventive antibiotics
    2. Rheumatic fever with preventive antibiotics
    3. No rheumatic fever

25. To the best of your knowledge, do you have any signs or symptoms of rheumatic heart disease?
    1. Yes
    2. No

26. Have you ever been arrested for burglary, robbery, or assault?
    1. Yes
    2. No

27. Do you carry a weapon with you?
    1. Yes
    2. No

28. Have you ever had bacterial pneumonia?
    1. Yes
    2. No

29. Have you ever had emphysema?
    1. Yes
    2. No

30. Has anyone in your family (parents, brothers, sisters) had diabetes?
    1. Yes
    2. No

31. Have you ever had polyps (growth in the intestines?)
    1. Yes
    2. No

32. Have you ever had undiagnosed rectal bleeding?
    1. Yes
    2. No

33. Have you ever had ulcerative colitis?
    1. Yes, 10 or more years ago
    2. Yes, less than 10 years ago
    3. No

34. Have you had a rectal examination with a lighted instrument within the last year?
    1. Yes
    2. No

IF FEMALE, ANSWER THE FOLLOWING 9 QUESTIONS:

35. Do you perform a regular monthly self-breast examination?
    1. Yes
    2. No

36. Do you have a yearly exam by your physician?
    1. Yes
    2. No

37. How many of your blood relatives (mother, sister, aunts) have had breast cancer?
    1. 2 or more
    2. 1
    3. None

38. Have you ever had fibrocystic breast disease or other noncancerous disease?
    1. Yes
    2. No

39. Are you Jewish? (Cancer of the cervix is very rare in Jewish women)
    1. Yes
    2. No

40. Age of first intercourse. (Cancer of the cervix is more common in females who have first intercourse in teens and/or have multiple partners)
    1. Under 20 years old
    2. 20-25 years old
    3. Over 25 years old or never

41. Pertaining to a Pap smear, mark the response most accurate for you (we assume none were abnormal)
    1. Haven't had one in last five (5) years
    2. Had 1 normal within the last five (5) years
    3. Had 1 normal within last year
    4. Had 3 normal within the last five (5) years
    5. Had one normal each of the last five (5) years

42. Have you experienced undiagnosed vaginal bleeding?
    1. Yes
    2. No

43. Do you now take birth control pills?
    1. Yes
    2. No

Continued.

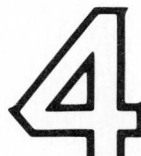

lifestyle assessment questionnaire

ALERT
SECTION

medical/behavioral/emotional

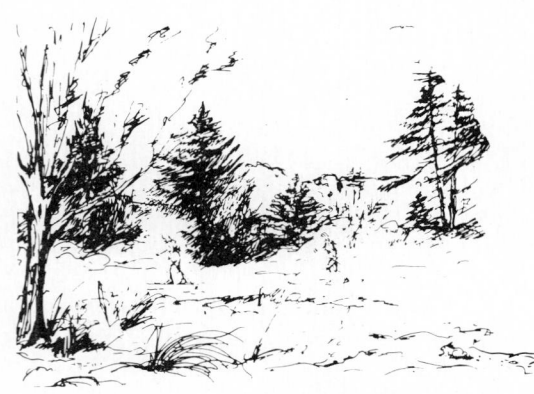

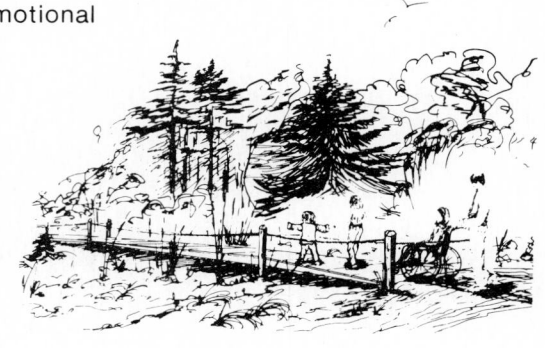

INSTRUCTIONS:

This section is intended to be used to identify high risk problems or past medical problems that we feel are important in establishing one's medical records. This can be used for a personal record by the individual or can be used by professionals as a problem list to be incorporated with the remainder of the individual's medical records. Please circle the number that is most correct in answering each question. Any question that you do not feel comfortable in answering or you think is not pertinent please leave blank.

MEDICAL

1. Do you have diabetes? . . . . **1. Yes 2. No**

2. Do you have a seizure disorder (epilepsy)? . . . . **1. Yes 2. No**

3. Do you have known heart **trouble** (acquired or congenital)? . . . . **1. Yes 2. No**

4. Did any of your blood relatives die of heart disease under the age of 50? . . . . **1. Yes 2. No**

5. Have you had major surgery? . . . . **1. Yes 2. No**

6. Do you have a physical disability that interferes with routine activities including physical fitness programs? . . . . **1. Yes 2. No**

7. Have you had a skin test for TB in the past two (2) years? . . . . **1. Yes 2. No**

8. If YES to number 7, which result did you have? . . . . **1. reaction**
no
2. reaction

9. Do you take any medication daily or several times per week? . . . . **1. Yes 2. No**

10. Do you have allergies to drugs? . . . . . . **1. Yes 2. No**

11. Are you allergic to penicillin? . . . . **1. Yes 2. No**

12. Are you allergic to sulfa? . . . . **1. Yes 2. No**

13. Are you allergic to aspirin? . . . . **1. Yes 2. No**

14. Do you have additional drug allergies not listed above? . . . . **1. Yes 2. No**

15. Do you have asthma? . . . . **1. Yes 2. No**

4

IMMUNIZATIONS

16. Did you have baby shots for DPT (diphtheria, whooping cough, and tetanus)? Ask your parents or doctor. . . . . **1.Yes 2. No**

17. Have you had a booster for tetanus in the last five (5) years? (Recommended interval is 5-10 years.). . . . . **1.Yes 2. No**

18. Have you had a form of polio vaccine? **1.Yes 2. No**

19. With regard to German measles: **1.Yes 2. No**

    1. have had a blood test showing immunity or received rubella immunization.

    2. never had a blood test or the blood test showed no immunity to rubella (German measles.)

20. Have you had a Pap test in the last year?. . . . . **1.Yes 2. No**

21. Have you ever had an abnormal Pap test?. . . . . **1.Yes 2. No**

22. Were you exposed to DES (diethylstilbesterol) while your mother was pregnant with you? (Ask your mother to check with her doctor if you are not sure.). . . . . **1.Yes 2. No**

BEHAVIORAL/EMOTIONAL

NOTE: The leading cause of death among young adults is auto accidents.

23. Do you drive a car, motorcycle, or bike after drinking alcohol?. . . . . **1.Yes 2. No**

24. Do you ride with "drinking" drivers? . . **1.Yes 2. No**

NOTE: The second leading cause of death among young adults is suicide.

25. Have you seriously considered killing yourself within the past year? . . . . **1.Yes 2. No**

26. Have you ever attempted suicide? . . . . **1.Yes 2. No**

27. Have any of your relatives committed suicide?. . . . . **1.Yes 2. No**

28. Do you frequently feel that life is not worth living?. . . . . **1.Yes 2. No**

29. Does each day look so dull that you would rather not wake up in the morning?. . . . . **1.Yes 2. No**

30. Do you feel overly tired and without motivation much of the time? . . . . **1.Yes 2. No**

31. Do you feel you have a serious emotional problem?. . . . . **1.Yes 2. No**

32. Do you have a history of/or have you recently experienced hallucinations? (Hearing or seeing things others don't.) **1.Yes 2. No**

33. Do you have difficulty feeling close to people? . . . . **1.Yes 2. No**

34. Do you worry excessively?. . . . . **1.Yes 2. No**

35. Do you feel you've had an excessive number of illnesses in the past year?. . **1.Yes 2. No**

36. Do impulsive behaviors cause you serious problems?. . . . . **1.Yes 2. No**

37. Are you unhappy too much of the time?. . . . . **1.Yes 2. No**

38. Do you cry too often? . . . . **1.Yes 2. No**

39. Do you have difficulty controlling your temper?. . . . . **1.Yes 2. No**

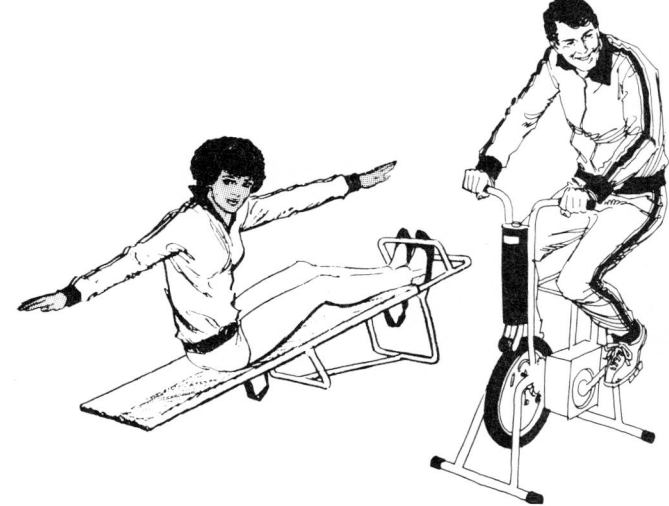

Continued.

SAMPLE PRINTOUTS

UNIVERSITY OF WISCONSIN-STEVENS POINT
LIFESTYLE ASSESSMENT RESULTS

Prepared for 9002 1 000000000

WELLNESS INVENTORY

The following scores indicate your wellness compared with average of people taking this survey with you, and averages of all the people who have taken the survey.

Catagory	Your Score	Group Average	Total Average
Physical Exercise	68	73	70
Physical Nutritional	52	67	52
Physical Self Care	46	60	48
Physical Vehicle Safety	47	75	49
Physical Drug Usage	72	95	75
Social Environmental	27	56	32
Emotional Awareness and Acceptance	20	50	24
Emotional Management	47	69	51
Intellectual	68	82	71
Occupational	73	79	73
Spiritual	65	68	66

PERSONAL GROWTH SECTION
AUTOMATED REFERRAL

EXERCISE PROGRAMS
A. Media
    1. Movies: **Coping With Life On The Run**—Sports Productions Inc.
        Run Dick, Run Jane—American Heart Association
        The Heart: An Attack—CRM
    2. Books: **Joy of Running**—Kostrubala
        Women's Running—Ullyot
        The Complete Runner—Fixx
        Stretching—Anderson
        Sheehan on Running—George Sheehan
        The Ultimate Athlete—Leonard
        Aerobics—Cooper
        Aerobics for Women—Cooper

B. Community Resources
    YMCA or YWCA programs

RISK OF DEATH SECTION

Age 40   Height 73
Race White Weight 222
Sex Male

Life Expectancy Results

    1 5 10 15 20 25 30 35 40 45

Average Years of Remaining Life in Your Sex, Age, Race Group   33 • • • • • • • • • • • • • • • • • •

Your Expected Yrs. of Remaining Life Based on your Answers   25 • • • • • • • • • • • • • •

You can achieve this expected yrs. of remaining life   38 •

RISK OF DEATH SECTION (Con't.)

Major Hazards to you
                10 year deaths
Rank Hazard per 100,000   Associated risk factors

1. Cirrhosis

	10 year deaths per 100,000	Associated risk factors
Average	304	Drinking Habits
Your	3800	
Achievable	61	

2. Arteriosclerotic Heart Disease

Average	1861	Systolic Blood Pressure
Your	2382	Diastolic Blood Pressure
Achievable	447	Cholesterol Level
		Smoking Habits
		Weight

3. Motor Vehicle Accidents

Average	339	Drinking Habits
Your	1763	Seat Belt Habits
Achievable	203	

4. Cancer of Lungs

Average	291	Smoking Habits
Your	582	
Achievable	58	

Suggestions For Increasing Your Expected Years Of Remaining Life
1. choosing non-drinking will add 8.6 exp. years of life
2. choosing non-smoking will add 2.0 exp. years of life
3. lowering cholesterol level will add 0.7 exp. years of life
4. lowering diastolic blood pressure will add 0.6 exp. years of life
5. lowering systolic blood pressure will add 0.6 exp. years of life
6. losing weight will add 0.4 exp. years of life
7. always wearing seatbelts will add 0.1 exp. years of life
8. having annual procto exam will add 0.1 exp. years of life
Total   13

Remarks:
We have had to make the following assumptions about you:

You have an average blood cholesterol level.

Hazard Summary

Based on the Lifestyle Assessment Questionnaire you have filled out, you have a health age of 48 years. If you follow all the suggestions we have given, you can reduce your health age to 35.

4

ALERT SECTION: Medical/Behavioral/Emotional

Significant Past Illnesses
1. Diabetic
2. Physical disability

Immunizations
1. Up-to-date for DPT
2. Up-to-date for polio
3. Rubella status unknown

Allergies
1. Allergic to penicillin

Emotions
1. History compatible with serious depression

WORDS FROM THE PAST

"To ward off disease or recover health, men as a rule find it easier to depend on the healers than to attempt the more difficult task of living wisely."

—Rene Dubos

"It's what you do hour by hour, day by day, that largely determines the state of your health; whether you get sick, what you get sick with, and perhaps when you die."

—Lester Breslow, M.D.

"For many years, while engaged in the practice of medicine, the author of this volume has been more and more impressed with the idea that the causes of the suffering, diseases, and premature deaths, which we witness around us on every hand, lie nearer our own doors... and that the men and women of today, are, at least, equally as responsible for existing suffering, as those who have gone before them, and often much more so. In fact, he feels satisfied that by far the greatest portion of all the suffering, disease, deformity, and premature deaths which occur, are the direct result of either the violation of, or the want of compliance with the laws of our being; calamities, which, were the requisite knowledge possessed by the community, can and should be avoided."

—taken from the Preface to **Avoidable Causes of Disease** by John Ellis, 1859.

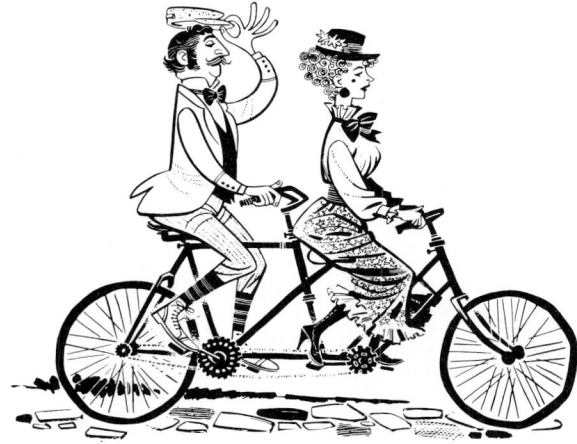

Appendix E

DRUG INFORMATION

Psychotrophic agents: antipsychotics

Generic name	Trade name	Relative potency (mg) when compared to 100 mg of chlorpromazine	Average daily dose (mg)	Dosage range per 24 hours (mg)
Phenothiazines				
Aliphatics				
Chlorpromazine	Thorazine	100	100-1500	30-1200
Triflupromazine	Vesprin	25	25-150	60-150
Piperidines				
Thioridazine	Mellaril	100	100-800	30-800
Mesoridazine	Serentil	50	100-400	100-400
Piperacetine	Quide	10	10-160	20-160
Piperazines				
Trifluoperazine	Stelazine	5	10-50	2-20
Acetophenazine	Tindal	20	40-100	40-80
Fluphenazine	Prolixin	2	6-40	1-20
Perphenazine	Trilafon	8	8-64	6-64
Prochlorperazine	Compazine	25	30-150	15-150
Butaperazine	Repoise	10	10-100	15-100
Carphenazine	Proketazine	25	50-400	75-400
Thioxanthenes				
Chlorprothixene	Taractan	100	75-600	
Thiothixene	Navane	4	10-60	
Butyrophenones				
Haloperidol	Haldol	2	2-30	
Dihydroindolones				
Molindone	Lidone Moban	20	50-200	
Dibenzoxapines				
Loxapine	Loxitane Daxolin	20	20-100	

Psychotrophic agents: antidepressants

Generic name	Trade name	Usual daily dose (mg)	Maximum daily dose (mg)	Incompatible drugs
Tricyclics				
Imipramine	Imavate Janimine Presamine SK-Pramine Tofranil	150-200	300	MAO inhibitors Alcohol Barbiturates
Desipramine	Norpramin Pertofrane	150-200	300	Central nervous system depressants
Amitriptyline	Amitril Elavil Endep	150-200	300	Thiazide diuretics Thyroid
Nortriptyline	Aventyl Pamelor	100-150	200	Vasodilators Anticholinergic agents
Doxepin	Adapin Sinequan	150-200	300	
Protriptyline	Vivactil Triptil	15-40	60	Guanethidine
Trimipramine	Surmontil	75-150	200	
Monoamine oxidase inhibitors				
Isocarboxazid	Marplan	10-20	30	Combination of any MAO inhibitors
Phenelzine	Nardil	45-60	90	Phenathiazine compounds, dopamine, methyldopa, tryptophan, antihyper- tensive and antiparkinsonian drugs, insulin
Tranylcypromine	Parnate	20	30	Thiazide diuretics Sympathomimetics including amphetamines
Tetracyclics				
Maprotiline	Ludiomil	150-200	300	

Psychotrophic agents: antianxiety

Generic name	Trade name	Hypnotic dose (mg)	Sedative dose (mg)	Half-life (hrs)
Barbiturates				
Secobarbital	Seconal	100-200	90-200	19-34
Pentobarbital	Nembutal	100-200	45-200	15-48
Amobarbital	Amytal	100-200	60-150	8-42
Butabarbital	Butisol	100-200	20-200	34-42
Phenobarbital	Barbipil and others	100-200	30-90	24-140
Benzodiazepines				
Flurazepam	Dalmane	15-30		24-100
Chlordiazepoxide	Librium and others	50-100	5-40	6-30
Diazepam	Valium	20-30	2-10	20-90
Oxazepam	Serax	30-60	10-30	3-21
Clorazepam	Tranxene and others		3.25-60	40-200
Prazepam	Verstran, Centrax	20-60	10-20	10-20
Lorazepam	Ativan	2-6	2-4	5-20

Continued.

Psychotrophic agents: antianxiety — cont'd

Generic name	Trade name	Hypnotic dose (mg)	Sedative dose (mg)	Half-life (hrs)
Nonbarbiturates/benzodiazepines				
Propanediol				
Meprobamate	Equanil, Miltown, and others	800	200-400	10
Tybamate	Solacen, Tybatran		750-2000	
Quinazolines				
Methaqualone	Quaalude, Parest, Sopor, Optimil, and others	150-300	225-300	10-14
Acetylinic alcohols				
Ethchlorvynol	Placidyl	500-1000	200-600	10-25
Piperidinedione derivatives				
Glutethimide	Doriden	250-500		5-22
Methyprylon	Noludar	200-400	150-400	
Chloral derivatives				
Chloral Hydrate	Noctec, Somnos, and others	500-2000	750-1500	
Chloral Betaine	Beta-Chlor	870-1740		
Triclofos	Triclos	750-1500		
Monoureides				
Paraldehyde	Paral	4-15 ml		
Diphenylmethanes				
Hydroxyzine	Atarax		75-400	
Hydroxyzine pamoate	Vistaril		75-400	
Benactyzine	Suavitil		3-9	
Diphenhydramine	Benadryl		25-100	

Psychotrophic agents: predicting lithium daily dosages to achieve therapeutic blood serum levels*

24-hour lithium level (mEq/L)	Total daily dosage (mg)
0.05	1200 tid
0.05-0.09	900 tid
0.10-0.14	600 tid
0.15-0.19	300 qid
0.20-0.23	300 tid
0.24-0.30	300 bid
0.30	300 qd

*Daily lithium dosages are determined by giving a primary dose of 600 mg and measuring lithium levels in the blood 24 hours later. Dosage is administered based on the above schedule. Recommended therapeutic serum lithium levels: 1—1.5 mEq/L for acute mania; 0.6—1.2 mEq/L for maintenance therapy; and 2 mEq/L as maximum.

Psychotrophic agents: commonly used antiparkinsonian agents anticholinergic

Generic name	Trade name	Usual daily dose (mg)
Anticholinergics		
Trihexyphenidyl	Artane, Pipanol, Antitrem, Tremin	2-15
Procyclidine	Kemadrin	5-20
Cycrimine	Pagitane	3.75-15.0
Biperiden	Akineton	2-6
Anticholinergic-antihistamics		
Benztropine	Cogentin	1-6
Diphenhydramine	Benadryl	25-200
Chlorphenoxamine	Phenoxene	150-400
Orphenadrine	Disipal	50-250
Ethopropazine	Parsidol	50-600
Others		
Amantadine	Symmetrel	100-400

Immunizing agents

Agent	Age to administer	Administration	Reaction and treatment
DPT: diptheria toxoid, tetanus toxoid, and pertussis vaccine	2,4,6 months; 1½ years; 4-6 years (may be given through the sixth year)	a. Primary course: three 0.5 cc doses at 8-week intervals followed by fourth 0.5 cc dose 1 year after third dose b. Booster course: one 0.5 cc dose at 4 to 6 years of age; thereafter Td 0.5 cc every 10 years *Contraindications*: (1) any acute febrile illness; (2) delete pertussis if CNS problem present or CNS disorder/symptom(s) occurs after DPT injection; (3) exposure to disease (diphtheria and pertussis): booster dose given of appropriate single antigen unless fourth dose has been given withing past year; (4) tetanus prophylaxis in wound management	a. Local reaction: induration, redness, or nodule at injection site. Treatment: warm compress to site; rotation of injection sites b. Systemic reaction: temperature elevation and irritability not lasting more than 24 to 48 hours. Treatment: acetaminophen for fever. If febrile or local reactions are severe, fractional doses should be considered
DT: pediatric — diptheria toxoid and tetanus toxoid	May be given through the sixth year	Same as DPT; indicated for use in infants and young children under 6 when pertussis vaccine is contraindicated *Contraindications*: same as for DPT	Same as DPT
Td: adult type — diptheria toxoid and tetanus toxoid	Children over 6 years; 14-16 years and every 10 years thereafter	a. Primary course: two 0.5 cc doses at 8-week interval followed by third 0.5 cc dose 6 to 12 months after second dose b. Booster course: one 0.5 cc dose at 14 to 16 years and every 10 years thereafter *Contraindications*: same as for DPT	Same as DPT
OPV: live, oral poliovirus vaccine; vaccine must be kept frozen	2,4,6 months; 1½ years, 4-6 years (do not give to persons over 18 years) Population at risk: children not vaccinated, especially a large number in 0 to 4 age group	a. Primary course: two doses at 8 week intervals in first 6 months of life with third dose at 18 months of age b. Booster course: one dose at 4 to 6 years c. Course for children or adolescents under 18 years: two doses at 8-week intervals followed by third dose in 8-14 months *Contraindications*: same as for DPT. See Chapter 23	Risk of vaccine: live virus persists in GI tract for 4 to 6 weeks after vaccination and paralytic disease can occur. Populations with immune deficiency disorders are particularly at risk, as are those over 18 years who have had no previous polio immunization and have been exposed. Use of inactivated vaccine (Salk) is recommended for these populations

Adapted from American Academy of Pediatrics: Report of the Committee on Infectious Diseases, ed. 19, Evanston, Ill., 1982.

Continued.

Immunizing agents — cont'd

Agent	Age to administer	Administration	Reaction and treatment
Measles: live attenuated virus vaccine; also available in combination as (a) measles-rubella or (b) measles-mumps-rubella	15 months of age	One subcutaneous injection of total volume of reconstituted vaccine *Contraindications*: hypersensitivity to eggs, see Chapter 23. Vaccine should be given anytime after 6 months of age if exposed to measles and repeated at 15 months *Indications* for revaccination include children vaccinated before 13 months of age, children vaccinated with simultaneous administration of gamma globulin at any age, and children for whom doubt exists about immunization status. Tuberculin testing should be done prior to, simultaneously, or 4 to 6 weeks after measles vaccine administration.	Reaction: mild noncommunicable infection with symptoms of fever, faint rash, and minor toxicity in 15% of vaccinated population. May occur 5 to 12 days after vaccination. Treatment: symptomatic
Rubella: live attenuated virus; in combination as (a) measles-rubella, (b) mumps-rubella, or (c) measles-mumps-rubella	15 months of age	Same as for measles. *Contraindications*: pregnant women. In susceptible nonpregnant females, administer if HI titer is less than 1:10 and pregnancy is not planned for 2 months	Reaction: rarely fever and rash. Treatment: symptomatic. In older age populations transient arthritis and arthralgia may occur 2 to 4 weeks after vaccination. Treatment: symptomatic
Mumps: live attenuated virus. In combination as (a) mumps-rubella or (b) measles-mumps-rubella	15 months of age	Same as measles. *Contraindications*: see Chapter 23. Indicated for use in susceptible children approaching puberty, in adolescents, and in males who have no history of mumps	Reaction: no serious side effects. Occasionally mild fever treated symptomatically

Appendix F

CONTRACTS AND FORMS: SAMPLES

COMMUNITY ORIENTED HEALTH RECORD (COHR)
COMMUNITY HEALTH ASSESSMENT MODEL

Definition of *community:* A locality-based entity—composed of systems of formal organizations reflecting societal institutions, informal groups, and aggregates, which are interdependent—whose function (expressed intent) is to meet a wide range of collective needs.

Definition of *community health:* The meeting of collective needs, through problem identifying and managing interactions within the community and between the community and the larger society. This requires commitment, self-other awareness and clarity of situational definitions, articulateness, effective communication, conflict containment and accommodation, participation, management of relations with the larger society, and machinery for facilitating participant interaction and decision making.

Community Health Assessment Guide Categories

A. Community
 1. Place
   a. Geopolitical boundaries of community
   b. Local or folk name for community
   c. Size in square miles/areas/blocks/census tracts
   d. Transportation avenues
   e. Physical environment
 2. People
   a. Number and density of population
   b. Demographic structure of population
   c. Informal groups
   d. Formal groups
   e. Linking structures
 3. Function
   a. Production—distribution—consumption of goods and services
   b. Socialization of new members
   c. Maintenance of social control
   d. Adapting to ongoing and unexpected change
   e. Provision of mutual aid
B. Community health
 1. Status
   a. Vital statistics
   b. Disease incidence and prevalence for leading causes of mortality and morbidity
   c. Health risk profiles
   d. Functional ability levels
 2. Structure
   a. Health facilities
   b. Health related planning groups
   c. Health manpower
   d. Health resource utilization patterns
 3. Process
   a. Commitment
   b. Self-other awareness and clarity of situational definitions
   c. Articulateness
   d. Effective communication
   e. Conflict containment and accommodation
   f. Participation
   g. Management of relations with the larger society
   h. Machinery for facilitating participant interaction and decision making

Community Problem List

This list and the forms for the following categories have a format similar to the sample Data Base shown on the next page. Headings of columns for the Community Problem List are Date, Number, Problem/Concern, and Supportive Data (title of appropriate section of Data Base and capsule summary of relevant data).

Community Capability List

Headings of columns for this list are Date, Number, Capability, Supportive Data (title of appropriate section of Data Base and capsule summary of relevant data).

Problem Analysis

A line labeled Problem/Statement is included at the top of the form below Name of Community. Headings of columns are Problem Correlates, Relationship of Correlates to Problem, and Data Supportive to Relationships (refer to appropriate sections of Data Base *and* relevant research findings in current literature).

Problem Prioritization

Headings of columns are Criteria, Criteria Weights (1-10), Problem, Problem Rating (1-10), Rationale for Rating, Problem Significance/(Weight X Rate).

Goals and Objectives

This form includes a line labeled Problem/Concern as well as lines for Goal Statement at the top under Name of Community. Column headings are Date, Objectives (number and statement), and By Date.

Plan

A line labeled Objective Number and Statement is included under Name of Community. Column headings are Date, Intervener Activities/Means, Value (1-10) /Probability (1-10), and Activity/Means Selected for Implementation.

Progress Notes

A line labeled Goal is included under Name of Community. Column headings are Date, Narrative, Assessment, Plan (NAP), and Budget and Time. A footnote to the second column explains the NAP procedure: Record both objective and subjective data. Interpret these data in terms of (1) whether the objectives were achieved and (2) whether the intervener activities utilized were effective. The plan is dependent on the assessment and may include both new (or revised) objectives and activities.

DATA BASE

Name of community _____

Assessment category _____   Subcategory _____

Date	Data source	Data*

*Note with an asterisk themes identified and meanings ascribed.

CONSULTATION CONTRACT

Client name _____   Consultant name _____

Address _____   Address _____

Phone _____   Phone _____

Estimated costs (external consultant only) _____
   (including phone, secretarial assistance, preparation, supplies, travel expenses and consultant sessions)

Client problem definition _____
_____
_____

Suggested intervention mode _____

Client goals

_____

_____

_____

Scope of consultation (time and no. of sessions)

_____

_____

_____

_____

Consultant resources (e.g., computer, secretary, library)

_____

_____

_____

Contract renegotiation and termination terms

_____

_____

_____

Contract limitations (e.g., who, what, when, how will data be shared)

_____

_____

_____

_____

Potential interventions (e.g., report shared with administration; meeting held with staff)

_____

_____

_____

Consultant goals

_____

_____

_____

_____

Continued.

CONSULTATION CONTRACT—cont'd

Client resources (e.g., records, secretary, copy)

_____

_____

_____

Anticipated client benefits

_____

_____

_____

Data collection methods

Interviews _____

Surveys _____

Questionnaires _____

Meetings _____

Phone _____

Contract evaluation

_____

_____

_____

CASE PRESENTATION GUIDE FOR AGENCY COMMUNICATION

1. State the problem(s).
2. Give the following identifiable information:
   A. Family composition
   B. Occupation and/or source of income
   C. Education
   D. Ethnic group
   E. Housing
   F. Family use of health care facility(ies)
3. Community assessment (as it affects the individual or family)
   A. Nutrition
   B. Mobility
   C. Recreation
   D. Religion
   E. Politics
   F. Housing
   G. Schools
   H. Economics
   I. Sanitation and pollution
4. Family history
   A. Social and medical
   B. Current estimate of each family member's present health status
   C. Current medical diagnosis
   D. Current medical treatment plan
   E. Knowledge of diagnosis, treatment, medication
   F. Obstacles to implementation
   G. Family strengths
5. Nursing interventions as they relate to the problem (brief summary)
6. Coordination of services (brief summary)
7. Continuity of services (brief summary), including referrals, resources, strengths/supports

SAMPLE NOTE TO PARENTS FROM SCHOOL NURSE

Name of School (Letterhead)

Date _____

Dear _____

In reviewing your child's record at school, we have found

that _____ needs:
                    (name of child)

_____ Medical examination
_____ Immunizations
_____ Other

If this has already been taken care of, please send a copy of the record to school. If you have further questions, please call me at the school. The telephone number is 000-0000.

Thank you,

_____
                School Nurse

REFERRAL FORM FOR SCHOOL HEALTH PROGRAM

Name of student _____

Age _____   Sex _____   Telephone _____

Address _____

Parent(s) name _____

Reason for referral _____

_____

_____

_____

Problem interventions tried by school health program

_____

_____

_____

Disposition from responding agency

_____

_____

_____

SCHOOL HEALTH RECORD

Name _____   Date of birth _____

In case of emergency call _____

Address _____   Telephone _____

Family physician _____

Family dentist _____

Family nurse practitioner _____

Existing health problem(s) _____

_____

_____

Teacher Observations

Physical: Walking gait, pimples, skin rashes, etc.

Psychological: (Please state observation as it is perceived; no labeling. For example, is the student always putting himself down?)

Sociological: (Please state observation as it is perceived; no labeling. For example, describe relationships and friendships.)

What is the educational progression of this child? (No labeling.)

Nurse's Assessment

Sex _____   Weight _____   Height _____

Immunizations:

Physical:

    Objective data _____

    Subjective data _____

    Nursing diagnosis _____

    Plan of action _____

Psychological (developmental tasks):

Sociological (developmental tasks):

    Objective data _____

    Subjective data _____

    Nursing diagnosis _____

    Plan of action _____

History of childhood diseases:

Health Risk Appraisal

Nutrition

Exercise

Accident and safety

Relaxation

Rest (sleep)

Self-care skills (self-examination of breast, self-examination of testicles for mass)

Alcohol and drugs

Smoking

Disposition _____

_____

_____

Screening

    Blood pressure

    Dental

    Vision

    Hearing

    Scoliosis

    Coordination (musculoskeletal)

Disposition _____

_____

_____

Sexuality (to include birth control information, if allowed by school district)

Peer relationships

Placement of child in family

Interests (sports, hobbies, etc.)

Disposition _____

_____

_____

Referral _____

_____

_____

Appendix G

CRITERIA AND STANDARDS FOR COMMUNITY HEALTH NURSING PRACTICE

ANA STANDARDS OF COMMUNITY HEALTH NURSING PRACTICE

Standard I

The collection of data about the health status of the consumer is systematic and continuous. The data are accessible, communicated and recorded.

Standard II

Nursing diagnoses are derived from health status data.

Standard III

Plans for nursing service include goals derived from nursing diagnoses.

Standard IV

Plans for nursing service include priorities and nursing approaches or measures to achieve the goals derived from nursing diagnoses.

Standard V

Nursing actions provide for consumer participation in health promotion, maintenance and restoration.

Standard VI

Nursing actions assist consumers to maximize health potential.

Standard VII

The consumer's progress toward goal achievement is determined by the consumer and the nurse.

Standard VIII

Nursing actions involve ongoing reassessment, reordering of priorities, new goal setting and revision of the nursing plan.

From American Nurses' Association: Standards: community health practice, Kansas City, Mo., 1973, The Association. Reprinted with the permission of ANA.

CRITERIA FOR DOCUMENTATION TO MEASURE THE QUALITY OF CARE IN THE HOME HEALTH AGENCY

1. The agency assesses the community served.
2. The agency is responsive to community health needs.
3. The agency has a legally constituted body that is responsible for the effective governing of the agency. It involves consumers in broad agency affairs.
4. Administrative responsibilities and relationships are established and clearly defined.
5. The governing body delegates to a qualified individual the authority and responsibility for overall agency administration.
6. If the agency has a person (or persons) other than the chief executive officer responsible for the administration and direction of the agency's programs, this individual (or individuals) is delegated the authority and responsibility for program administration.
7. If the agency has a person other than the chief executive officer responsible for the fiscal and business affairs of the agency, this individual is delegated the authority and responsibility for fiscal and business practices.
8. Fiscal policies and practices assure effective and efficient implementation of the program(s) of the agency.
9. The agency has agreements with organizations, agencies, and/or individuals for securing or providing services.
10. Program and fiscal management activities are coordinated to promote effective planning and implementation of programs within the agency.
11. The agency coordinates its services with other health and social agencies; consumers are kept informed of services available.
12. The agency has established programs in response to community health needs.

From National League for Nursing: Criteria and standards manual for National League for Nursing/American Public Health Association Accreditation of Home Health Agencies and Community Nursing Services. New York, 1980, Publ. No. 21-1306. Used with permission.

13. For each program and service, the agency has priorities that are responsive to agency purpose and community need.
14. The agency has policies and procedures governing programs, services, and professional practices.
15. Service records are maintained for each client.
16. All agency services are coordinated.
17. The agency has the responsibility for participation, if feasible, in the education of student health personnel.
18. The staff includes professional and nonprofessional personnel commensurate with the needs of the programs of the agency. There are written job descriptions for all classifications of personnel.
19. The agency provides consultation as needed for the administrative, supervisory, and direct-service personnel.
20. The agency has written personnel policies for all personnel.
21. The agency provides ongoing professional and/or technical supervision for all personnel.
22. The agency provides for staff development.
23. The agency has a structure and plan for evaluation.
24. The agency evaluates its organizational structure and administrative policies and practices.
25. The agency evaluates its programs.
26. The agency evaluates its staffing patterns, policies, and practices.
27. The agency establishes goals as a result of its overall evaluation. It communicates its status to the public.
28. Long-range planning is conducted by the agency to provide for future direction and viability.

Appendix H

GOVERNMENTAL INFLUENCES ON HEALTH CARE DELIVERY

SELECT MAJOR HISTORICAL EVENTS DEPICTING FINANCIAL INVOLVEMENT OF FEDERAL GOVERNMENT IN HEALTH CARE DELIVERY

1798 Marine Hospital Service Act was passed to provide medical care to Merchant Marines.

1878 Port Quarantine Act was passed to prevent epidemic diseases from entering the country through seaports.

1879 National Health Department was established by Congress with a budget of $500,000.

1887 Laboratory of Hygiene at Staten Island Marine Hospital marked the beginning of Public Health Service research activities. This bacteriologic research laboratory later evolved into the National Institute of Health.

1890 Marine Hospital Service was given authority to inspect all immigrants to bar "lunatics and others unable to care for self" from entering the country.

1902 National Health Department was renamed the Public Health and Marine Hospital Service.

1912 National Institute of Health functions were expanded to study and investigate diseases of persons and the conditions influencing the origin and spread of disease.

1912 The Public Health and Marine Hospital Service was renamed the United States Public Health Service.

1912 The Child Health Bureau was established within the USPHS.

1917 National leprosarium was established at Carville, Louisiana under the aegis of the USPHS.

1917 USPHS became responsible for the physical and mental examination of all aliens.

Sources for this listing were Hanlon, J., and Picket, G.: *Public health administration and practice,* St. Louis, 1979, The C. V. Mosby Co.; Congressional Research Service: *Summary of health legislation, 1959– 1981,* Library of Congress Pub. No. 82–127 EPW), Washington, D.C., May 7, 1981, U.S. Government Printing Office; Congressional Research Service: Major legislation of the 97th Congress, Library of Congress Pub. No. 9, Washington, D.C., Oct. 6, 1982 U.S. Government Printing Office.

1917 Congress appropriated $25,000 to USPHS to study and provide demonstration projects sharing state and federal cooperative rural health services.

1918 Because of increased venereal disease incidence during World War I, the Division of Venereal Disease was established in USPHS providing for cooperative federal and state control and prevention programs.

1921 Shepherd-Towner Maternity Infancy Act was passed to provide for the establishment of state maternal and infant programs. The Act provided for mother-child health conferences, home delivery supplies, improved prenatal care, improved infant and child care, more public health nurses, and health education.

1929 USPHS Narcotics Division was developed to provide facilities for the confinement and treatment of drug addicts (renamed Division of Mental Hygiene in 1939).

1935 Congress passed the Social Security Act. Title VI of the Act was written for the purpose of assisting states, counties, health districts, and other political subdivisions in establishing and maintaining adequate public health service, including the training of personnel for state and local health work.

1935 The Social Security Act provided for grants-in-aid to states to finance the public's health. *Grants-in-aid* resulted in increased numbers of new health departments and the strengthening and expansion of existing health departments.

1937 National Cancer Act called for the establishment of the National Cancer Institute for research into the causes, diagnosis, and treatment of cancer; for assistance to public and private agencies; and for the promotion of the most effective prevention and treatment.

1938 The second Federal Venereal Disease Control Act was passed to promote investigation and control and to provide funds for the development and maintenance of state and local programs.

1939 The Federal Security Agency was established to bring health, welfare, and education services of the federal government together.

1940   Communicable Disease Center (National Center for Disease Control) was established in Atlanta for the purpose of conducting epidemiological studies, providing health personnel training, and establishing methods of communication and education.

1940   National Office of Vital Statistics (National Center for Health Statistics) was authorized to provide data about health, illness, injuries, and death.

1941   Nurse training appropriations provided monies to nursing programs to increase enrollment and improve programs.

1943   Nurse Training Act established the U.S. Nurse Cadet Corps in USPHS to support nurse training.

1946   National Mental Health Act was passed for constructing and equipping hospitals and laboratories to stimulate research and training in mental health.

1946   Hill-Burton Act provided for hospital services and construction.

1947   National Institute of Health Division of Research Grants were established to administer and award grants for research projects and training.

1947   A permanent Nursing Corps in the Army and Navy was established.

1948   National Heart Institute was established (renamed Heart, Lung, and Blood Institute in 1976).

1948   Microbiological, Experimental Biology, and Medicine Institutes were established (renamed National Institute of Allergy and Infectious Diseases in 1955).

1948   National Institute of Dental Research was authorized.

1948   National Institute of Health became National Institutes of Health (NIH).

1949   National Institute of Mental Health was established (renamed Alcoholism, Drug Abuse, and Mental Health Administration in 1974).

1950   National Institute of Neurological Diseases and Blindness was established (renamed National Eye Institute in 1968 and the National Institute of Neurological and Communicative Disorders and Strokes in 1975).

1950   Health Manpower Training Acts evolved to provide for training of Health Personnel.

1953   National Clinical Center was founded to accelerate research and to confirm and apply research findings. A 600-bed research hospital evolved.

1954   Congress extended Hill-Burton Act to allow monies for construction of other types of health facilities, such as general, mental, tuberculosis, and chronic disease hospitals; public health centers; diagnostic and treatment centers; rehabilitation facilities; nursing homes; state health laboratories; and nurse training facilities.

1954   Taft Sanitary Engineering Center was founded in Cincinnati for research and training in environmental health.

1955   National Institutes of Health Division of Biological Standards was established to oversee the growth of the pharmaceutical industry and market.

1955   Polio Vaccination Assistance Act was passed to aid state vaccination programs.

1956   U.S. Army Medical Library was transferred to USPHS, which became the Library of Medicine at the National Institutes of Health. The library provides MEDLARS, the Medical Literature Analysis and Retrieval System.

1956   CHAMPUS program was established for dependents of military personnel.

1956   National Health Survey was established for continuous monitoring of sickness and disability in U.S.

1959   National Institute of Arthritis and Metabolic Diseases was established (renamed National Institute of Arthritis, Metabolic, and Digestive Diseases in 1981).

1960   Social Security Amendments provided grants to states for medical assistance to the aged.

1962   National Institute of Child Health and Human Development was founded.

1962   Program for state assistance in preschool vaccination programs was authorized.

1963   Aid program was established for the construction of mental retardation and community mental health facilities and the development of programs to combat health problems, e.g., maternal health, crippled children, and the mentally retarded.

1965   Heart disease, cancer, and stroke legislation was provided for the establishment of Regional Medical Programs to coordinate existing services for these three health problems.

1965   Appalachian Regional Development Act was passed to provide for construction of health services facilities in economically depressed area.

1965   Social Security Act was amended to provide for Medicare and Medicaid programs.

1966   Division of Environmental Health Services was established in Public Health Service.

1966   Partnership for health legislation consolidated pre-existing projects and *formula grants* to states through a new system of grants for comprehensive health planning. The legislation allowed health planning but did not give authority to control program development, spending, or construction of health facilities.

1968   Fogarty International Center for Advanced Study in Health Sciences was founded at NIH for international collaboration, study and research by world scholars.

1970   Occupational Health and Safety Act was passed to assure safe and healthy working conditions.

1971   Environmental Protection Agency was founded to establish an umbrella agency for all environmental programs.

1971   National Center for Toxicological Research was established at Pine Bluff, Arkansas under the aegis of the Food and Drug Administration of USPHS.

1972   National programs were established for research, screening, counseling, and treatment of sickle cell anemia and Cooley's anemia.

1972 Social Security Act amended to encourage Professional Standards Review Organizations (PSRO). PSROs were designed to review hospital services ordered by physicians to determine overuse and underuse of services for patient care.

1972 National commission was established to study and investigate causes, cures, and treatment of multiple sclerosis.

1973 Social Security Act was amended to provide for the development of health maintenance organizations (HMOs)—prepaid comprehensive health care delivery systems designed to introduce competition into the health care arena.

1973 Program of grants—contracts for establishing and operating emergency medical services systems—was authorized.

1974 National Health Planning and Resources Development Act was passed to provide a triad health planning system. The system was designed as a comprehensive planning structure to review health services and facilities and to control and limit the expenditure of federal monies by discouraging the development and continuation of unnecessary new and existing programs.

1974 National Diabetes Mellitus Research and Education Act was passed to authorize NIH to establish a National Commission on Diabetes to formulate long-range plans to combat the disease.

1974 Sudden Infant Death Syndrome Act was passed to provide a program of dissemination of research and information to the public.

1976 National Swine Flu Immunization Program was established and implemented.

1976 Toxic Substances Control Act was passed to require testing of certain chemical substances to protect human health and environment.

1977 Rural Health Clinics Services Act was passed to provide for the establishment of health clinics in rural underserved communities. The clinics were to be staffed by nurse practitioners or physician assistants. The bill marked the first national legislation passed for reimbursement of nurse practitioner and physician assistant services under Medicare and Medicaid.

1980 Civil Rights of Institutionalized Persons Act was passed to protect mentally ill, disabled, retarded, chronically ill, or handicapped persons from flagrant conditions in state-affiliated institutions.

1980 Infant Formula Act was passed to require that such formulas meet certain standards of nutrition, quality, and safety in manufacturing.

1980 Department of Health, Education, and Welfare reorganized. Department of Health and Human Services oversees the regulation of health programs.

1981 Omnibus Budget Reconciliation Act (OBRA) provided for maternal and child health block grants to states under Title V of the Social Security Act to assist the states in advancing the health of mothers and children. Legislation allows states to make decisions on how to spend monies for nine maternal-child health programs.

1981 Omnibus Budget Reconciliation Act provided preventive health services block grants to allow states to make decisions about monies spent for 10 preventive health programs like hypertensive screening, rape crisis centers, etc.

1981 Omnibus Budget Reconciliation Act provided alcohol, drug abuse, and mental health block grants for states to provide direct services through community mental health centers, and alcohol and drug abuse programs.

1981 Omnibus Budget Reconciliation Act provided primary care block grant to states for community health center funding.

1982 Defense appropriations amendments allowed for direct, independent nurse practitioner reimbursement under CHAMPUS.

1982 The Tax Equity and Fiscal Responsibility Act established reductions in Medicare and Medicaid spending, called for the development of a prospective reimbursement system, authorized Medicare payments for hospice service, and replaced PSRO with a new utilization and quality control peer review program.

SAMPLE PARTY PLATFORMS ON HEALTH
1980 DEMOCRATIC NATIONAL PARTY PLATFORM
Health

The Carter Administration and the Congress have worked closely together to improve the health care provided to all Americans. In many vital areas, there has been clear progress.

The United States spent over $200 billion for health care in 1979. Despite these high expenditures and although we possess some of the finest hospitals and health professionals in the world, millions of Americans have little or no access to health care services. Incredibly, costs are predicted to soar to $400 billion by 1984, without improvement in either access to care or coverage of costs. Health care costs already consume ten cents of every dollar spent for goods and services.

The answer to runaway medical costs is not, as Republicans propose, to pour money into a wasteful and inefficient system. The answer is not to cut back on benefits for the elderly and eligibility for the poor. The answer is to enact a comprehensive, universal national health insurance plan.

To meet the goals of a program that will control costs and provide health coverage to every American, the Democratic Party pledges to seek a national health insurance program with the following features:

Universal coverage, without regard to place of employment, sex, age, marital status, or any other factor;

Comprehensive medical benefits, including preventive, diagnostic, therapeutic, health maintenance and rehabilitation services, and complete coverage of the costs of catastrophic illness or injury;

Aggressive cost containment provision along with provisions to strengthen competitive forces in the marketplace;

Enhancement of the quality of care;

An end to the widespread use of exclusions that disadvantage women and that charge proportionately higher premiums to women;

Reform of the health care system, including encouragement of health maintenance organizations and other alternative delivery systems;

Building on the private health care delivery sector and preservation of the physician-patient relationship;

Provision for maximum individual choice of physician, other provider, and insurer;

Maintenance of the private insurance industry with appropriate public regulation;

Significant administrative and organizational roles for state and local government in setting policy and in resource planning;

Redistribution of services to ensure access to health care in underserved areas;

Improvement of non-institutional health services so that elderly, disabled, and other patients may remain in their homes and out of institutions; and

Child Health Assurance Program

We must continue to emphasize preventive health care for all citizens. As part of this commitment, we call for the enactment of legislation during the 96th Congress to expand the current Medicaid program and make an additional 5 million low-income children eligible for Medicaid benefits and an additional 200,000 low-income pregnant women eligible for pre-natal and post-natal care.

Mental Health Systems Act

We must enact legislation to help the mentally ill, based on the recommendations of the President's Commission on Mental Health. The legislation should focus on de-institutionalization of the chronically mentally ill, increased program flexibility at the local level, prevention, and the development of community-based mental health services. It is imperative that there be ongoing federal funding for the community-based mental health centers established under the 1963 Mental Health Act and that sufficient federal funding be provided for adequate staffing. We also endorse increased federal funding for ongoing training of mental health personnel in public facilities.

In the 1980's we must move beyond these existing health care initiatives and tackle other problems as well.

Long-term Care

We must develop a new policy on long-term care for our elderly and disabled populations that controls the cost explosion and at the same time provides more humane care. We must establish alternatives to the present provisions for long-term care, including adequate support systems and physical and occupational therapy in the home and the community, to make it unnecessary to institutionalize people who could lead productive lives at home.

We must support legislation to expand home health care services under Medicare and other health programs. Visits from doctors, nurses and other health personnel are a cost-effective and necessary program for the elderly who often cannot travel to medical facilities. Without home health services, many elderly citizens would be forced to give up their homes and shift their lives to institutions.

Multilingual Needs

We must support the utilization of bilingual interpreters in English-Spanish and other appropriate languages at federal and state-supported health care facilities. In addition, we support broader, more comprehensive health care for migrants.

Health Care Personnel

This nation must maintain an adequate supply of health professionals and personnel. Particular emphasis should be given to programs which educate nurses and other health professionals and related personnel, especially for the traditionally underserved rural and inner city areas.

The rising cost of education in health fields bars many who wish to enter these fields from doing so. In order to expand representation in the health professions of traditionally underrepresented groups, we support programs of financial assistance such as capitation grants. These programs must increase the presence of men and minorities in nursing, and must be targeted toward women and minorities in other health professions.

Minority and Women Health Care

We recognize the need for a significant increase in the number of minority and women health care professionals. We are committed to placing greater emphasis on enrollment and retention of minorities and women in medical schools and related health education professional programs.

We are also committed to placing a greater emphasis on medical research and services to meet the needs of minorities, women and children.

Reproductive Rights

We fully recognize the religious and ethical concerns which Americans have about abortion. We also recognize the belief of many Americans that a woman has a right to choose whether and when to have a child.

The Democratic Party supports the 1973 Supreme Court decision on abortion rights as the law of the land and opposes any constitutional amendment to restrict or overturn that decision.

Furthermore, we pledge to support the right to be free of environmental and worksite hazards to reproductive health of women and men.

We further pledge to work for programs to improve the health and safety of pregnancy and childbirth, including adequate prenatal care, family planning, counseling, and services, with special care to the needs of the poor, the isolated, the rural, and the young.

Financially Distressed Public Hospitals

Frequently, the only source of medical care for much of the inner city population is the public general hospital. The ever-increasing costs of providing high quality hospital services and the lack of insurance coverage for many of the patients served here jeopardized the financial stability of these institutions. Immediate support is required for financially distressed public hospitals that provide a major community service in urban and rural areas.

In underserved areas where public hospitals have already been closed because of financial difficulty, we must explore methods for returning the needed hospitals to active service.

We must develop financial stability for these hospitals. Our approach should stress system reforms to assure that more primary medical care is provided in free-standing community centers, while the hospital is used for referral services and hospitalization.

Medicaid Reimbursement

The Democratic Party supports programs to make the Medicaid reimbursement formulae more equitable.

Unnecessary Prescriptions

We must reduce unnecessary prescribing of drugs and guarantee the quality and safety of products that reach the market through improved approval procedures.

Substance Abuse

Alcoholism and drug abuse are unique illnesses which not only impair the health of those who abuse those products, but impose costs on society as a whole—in production losses, in crimes to supply habits, and in fatalities on the highway.

The Democratic Partnership has worked to reduce the serious national problem of substance abuse, and progress has been made.

As a result, in part, of a major adolescent drug abuse prevention campaign, levels of drug abuse among adolescents have begun to decline. However, as long as abuse still exists, we consider it a major problem requiring our attention.

Because of a coordinated, concerted attack on drug trafficking, heroin availability in the U.S. over the past four years has decreased by 44 percent; heroin-related injuries have declined by 50 percent.

Progress made since 1977 must be continued.

We must continue to focus on preventing substance abuse in the early years of adolescence by working with grassroots organizations and parent groups throughout the country.

Special efforts must be made to strengthen prevention and rehabilitation resources in the major urban areas that are so acutely affected by drug and alcohol abuse problems because of the cumulative effect of joblessness, poor housing conditions and other factors.

We must provide adequate funding for alcohol and drug abuse research and treatment centers designed to meet the special needs of women, and end the currently widespread discrimination, based on sex, race, and ethnicity, in alcohol and drug abuse programs.

We must treat addiction as a health problem and seek flexibility in administering Medicare and Medicaid for substance abuse treatment, especially alcohol and drug services.

We must reduce the availability of heroin and other illicit narcotics in this country and in the source countries.

We must conduct investigations leading to the prosecution and conviction of drug traffickers and to the forfeiture of financial and other assets acquired by their organizations.

1980 REPUBLICAN NATIONAL CONVENTION PLATFORM
Health

Our country's unequaled system of medical care, bringing greater benefits to more people than anywhere else on earth, is a splendid example of how Americans have taken care of their own needs with private institutions.

Significant as these achievements are, we must not be complacent. Health care costs continue to rise, farther and faster than they should, and threaten to spiral beyond the reach of many families. The causes are the Democratic Congress' inflationary spending and excessive and expensive regulations.

Republicans unequivocally oppose socialized medicine in whatever guise it is presented by the Democratic Party. We reject the creation of a national health service and all proposals for compulsory national insurance.

Our country has made spectacular gains in health care in recent decades. Most families are now covered by private insurance, Medicare, or in the case of the poor, the entirely free services under Medicaid.

Republicans recognize that many health care problems can be solved if government will work closely with the private sector to find remedies that will enhance our current system of excellent care. We applaud, as an example, the voluntary effort which has been undertaken by our nation's hospitals to control costs. The results have been encouraging. More remains to be done.

What ails American medicine is government meddling and the strait-jacket of federal programs. The prescription for good health care is deregulation and an emphasis upon consumer rights and patient choice.

As consumers of health care, individual Americans and their families should be able to make their own choices about health care protection. We propose to assist them in so doing through tax and financial incentives. These could enable them to choose their own health coverage, including protection from the catastrophic costs of major long-term illness, without compulsory regimentation.

Americans should be protected against financial disaster brought on by medical expenses. We recognize both the need to provide assistance in many cases and the responsibility of citizens to provide for their own needs. By using tax incentives and reforming federal medical assistance programs, government and the private sector can jointly develop compassionate and innovative means to provide financial relief when it is most needed.

We endorse alternatives to institutional care. Not only is it costly but it also separates individuals from the supportive environment of family and friends. This is especially important for the elderly and those requiring long-term care. We advocate the reform of Medicare to encourage home-based care whenever feasible. In addition, we encourage the development of innovative alternate health care delivery systems and other out-patient services at the local level.

We must maintain our commitment to the aged and to the poor by providing quality care through Medicare and Medicaid. These programs need the careful detailed re-evaluation they have never received from the Democrats, who have characteristically neglected their financial stability. We believe that the needs of those who depend upon these programs, particularly the elderly, can be better served, especially when a Republican Administration cracks down on fraud and abuse so that program monies can be directed toward those truly in need. In the case of Medicaid, we will aid the states in restoring its financial integrity and its local direction.

We welcome the long-overdue emphasis on preventive health care and physical fitness that is making Americans more aware than ever of their personal responsibility for good health. Today's enthusiasm and emphasis on staying well holds the promise of dramatically improved health and well-being in the decades ahead. Additionally, health professionals, as well as individuals, have long recognized that preventing illness or injury is much less expensive than treating it. Therefore, preventive medicine combined with good personal health habits and health education, can make a major impact on the cost of health care. Employers and employees, unions and business associations, families, schools, and neighborhood groups all have important parts in what is becoming a national crusade for better living.

Appendix I

SAMPLE GUIDES

PARTIAL LIST OF HEALTH ORGANIZATIONS USED BY COMMUNITY HEALTH NURSES

AL-ANON Family Group Headquarters, Inc.
PO Box 182, Madison Square Station, New York, NY 10010
(212) 481-6565
Founded in 1951, Al-Anon, including Alateen for teenagers, offers a self-help recovery program for relatives and friends who have been adversely affected by someone else's drinking problem. Members share experiences, strength and hope in an effort to make their own lifes manageable. Membership: 15,600 groups worldwide. Membership figure includes over 2,200 Alateen groups for teenagers.

Alcohol and Drug Problems Association of North America, Inc.
1101 15th Street, NW, Suite 204, Washington, DC 20005
(202) 452-0990
Founded in 1949, the association serves as a focal point for action and a medium of exchange for professionals in the alcohol and drug problems field at the national, state, and local governmental levels and in the private sector. Membership: 2000.

Alcoholics Anonymous
468 Park Avenue South, New York, NY 10016
(212) 686-1100
Founded in 1935. AA is a program of recovery from alcoholism. Membership: Over 1,000,000. State affiliation: 33,000 in 92 countries.

American Association for Maternal and Child Health, Inc.
PO Box 965, Los Altos, CA 94022
(415) 964-4575
Founded in 1925. Membership: 3,000.

American Association for Vital Records and Public Health Statistics
c/o Utah Dept of Health, PO Box 2500, Salt Lake City, UT 84110
(801) 533-6186
Founded in 1933, the AAVRPHS provides the only national forum for the study, discussion and solution of the problems related to programs of vital and health statistics by state and local representatives without undue influence of Federal government officials. Membership: 220.

American Burn Association
c/o William Curreri, MD, New York Hospital, Cornell Medical Center, New York, NY 10021
(212) 472-5454
Founded in 1967. Membership: 2,000.

American Cancer Society, Inc.
777 Third Avenue, New York, NY
(212) 371-2900
Founded in 1913. ACS conducts research on cause, prevention, treatment of cancer; public education programs alert Americans to protective and preventive measures; informs physicians on developments in diagnosis and treatment of cancer; provides service and rehabilitation program for patients. Membership: 2,300,000 volunteers. State affiliation: 58 divisions.

American Dental Association
211 East Chicago Avenue, Chicago, IL 60611
(312) 440-2500
Founded in 1859. The ADA is the national voluntary organization for the U.S. dental profession and is the second largest health profession in the country. It has more than 133,000 members in 54 state societies and 484 local societies. Membership: 133,000.

American Diabetes Association
600 Fifth Avenue, New York, NY 10020
(212) 541-4311
Founded in 1940. ADA funds research and conducts education programs in the field of diabetes. Publishes patient magazine and two medical journals. Membership: 130,000. State affiliation: 68 affiliates in 50 states.

American Epilepsy Society
38238 Glenn Avenue, Willoughby, OH 44094
(216) 942-9267
Founded in 1946. AES works to foster research and treatment of epilepsy in all of its phases—biological, clinical and social—and the promotion of better care and treatment of persons subject to seizures. Membership: 780.

American Fertility Society
1608 13th Avenue, Suite 101, Birmingham, AL 35205
(205) 933-7222
Founded in 1944. The primary objective of the Society is to disseminate that body of knowledge which encompasses all aspects of infertility, related endocrinology, conception control and reproductive biology. The greater emphasis is on those matters which are clinical in nature. Membership: 7,000.

American Foundation for the Blind
15 West 16th Street, New York, NY 10011
(212) 620-2000
Founded in 1921. The objective of the foundation is to stimulate, facilitate and coordinate a national effort for improving services to blind and psychological, technological/social research, gathering, preparation, publishing information to professional and general public, sponsoring workshops, seminars, conferences.

American Genetic Association
818 18th Street, NW, Washington, DC 20006
(202) 659-2096
Founded in 1903. Membership: 1,650.

American Geriatrics Society, Inc.
10 Columbus Circle, Suite 1470, New York, NY 10019
(212) 582-1333
Founded in 1942. AGS provides dissemination of information relating to the etiology, prevention, diagnosis and treatment of diseases of the aging and aged, rehabilitation of patients and problems relating to the health care of the older patient. Membership: 7000.

American Health Foundation
320 East 43rd Street, New York, NY 10018
(212) 953-1900
Founded in 1969. AHF is a unique, non-profit institution, totally committed to disease prevention and health promotion. Today, on national and community levels, AHF is achieving its goals through laboratory and clinical research, preventive health care services and public education.

American Heart Association
7320 Greenville Avenue, Dallas, TX 75231
(214) 750-5300
Founded in 1948. The AHA mission is to reduce death and disability from cardiovascular diseases. Membership: 100,000.

American Hepatic Foundation
PO Box 1005, Williamston, NC 27892
(919) 792-5279
Founded in 1973.

American Laryngological Association
110 Irving Street, NW, Washington, DC 20010
(202) 223-2676
Founded in 1878. ALA conducts annual meetings, publishes transactions in field of laryngology, rhinology, head, and neck surgery. Membership: 100.

American Liver Foundation
30 Sunrise Terrace, Cedar Grove, NJ 07009
(201) 857-2626
Founded in 1976. The ALF seeks to improve the understanding, prevention, and cure of liver diseases through professional and public education and by supporting vitally needed research training of young scientific investigators.

American Lung Association
1740 Broadway, New York, NY 10019
(212) 245-8000
Founded in 1904. ALA is primarily an educational organization to fight lung disease and work for lung health. It also works against cigarette smoking and air pollution.

American Mental Health Foundation, Inc.
2 East 86th Street, New York, NY 10028
(212) 737-9027
Founded in 1924. The AMHF is dedicated to extensive and intensive research in the theories of psychotherapy and to the implementation of needed reforms.

American Optometric Association
243 Lindbergh Boulevard, St. Louis, MO 63141
(314) 991-4100
Founded in 1898. The objectives of the AOA as stated in its constitution are: To improve the vision care and health of the public and to promote the art and science of the profession of optometry. Membership: 20,750.

American Parkinson Disease Association
147 East 50th Street, New York, NY 10022
(212) 421-5890

American Pediatric Society
David Goldring, MD, PO Box 14871, St. Louis, MO 63178
(314) 360-6880, Ext. 337
Founded in 1888. APS provides an annual scientific meeting during which short papers are presented in all the pediatric subspecialties. The subspecialty sessions are preceded by a plenary session as well as a symposium on important research achievements in pediatrics. Membership: 827.

American Physical Fitness Research Institute
824 Moraga Drive, Los Angeles, CA 90049
(213) 476-6241
Founded in 1958. APFRI provides research and development of motivational and educational information on all aspects of health, fitness, and well-being directed toward personal responsibility toward one's health.

American Psychosomatic Society, Inc.
265 Nassau Road, Roosevelt, NY 11575
(516) 379-0191
Founded in 1943. APS works to advance the research in psychosomatic medicine. Membership: 850.

American Red Cross
17th and D Streets, NW, Washington, DC 20006
(202) 737-8300
Founded in 1881. The aims of the Red Cross are to improve the quality of human life and enhance individual self-reliance and concern for others. It works toward these aims through national and chapter services governed and directed by volunteers.

American Venereal Disease Association
Box 385, University of Virginia Hospital, Charlottesville, VA 22908
(804) 924-5241
AVDA is an association of physicians, nurses and other public health professionals concerned with research, professional education, and control of sexually transmitted diseases. Publishes a quarterly journal, *Sexually Transmitted Diseases.* Membership: 700.

Arthritis Foundation
3400 Peachtree Road, NE, Atlanta, GA 30326
(404) 266-0795
Founded in 1948.

Arthritis Society

920 Yonge Street, Suite 420, Toronto, Canada M4W 3J7

(416) 967-1414

Founded in 1948. The AS is organized for the development of rheumatological manpower through associateships and fellowships; the support of research projects deemed relevant to the rheumatic diseases; and the communication about arthritis with general public and medical profession.

Association for the Care of Asthma, Inc.

Spring Valley Road, Ossining, NY 10562

(914) 762-2110

Founded in 1963. ACA conducts an annual postgraduate course in allergy and clinical immunology for the advancement of the knowledge and practice of the care and treatment of asthma, by discussion at such meetings, promoting and encouraging research and study. Membership: 100.

Association for the Care of Children in Hospitals

3615 Wisconsin Avenue, NW, Washington, DC 20016

(202) 244-1801

Founded in 1965. ACCH seeks to foster and promote the health and well-being of children and families in health care settings by education, interdisciplinary interaction and planning, and research. Membership: 2,400.

Association for Children with Learning Disabilities

4156 Library Road, Pittsburgh, PA 15234

(412) 341-1515

Founded in 1963. Membership: 60,000.

Association for Children with Retarded Mental Development, Inc.

902 Broadway, 5th Floor, New York, NY 10010

(212) 677-5800

Founded in 1951. ACRMD is a nonprofit membership corporation offering services to mentally retarded adults throughout New York City. Services include rehabilitation and sheltered workshops; day training and activities centers; day treatment centers; job placement; evening and weekend social centers; various community services. Membership: 2,000.

Association for Education of the Visually Handicapped

919 Walnut Street, 4th Floor, Philadelphia, PA 19107

(215) WA3-7555

Founded in 1853. The AEVH is a professional association interested in the progress and welfare of visually handicapped children. Membership: 2,400.

Asthma and Allergy Foundation of America

19 West 44th Street, New York, NY 10036

(212) 921-9100

Founded in 1953. The AAFA provides public education booklets and newsletters, answers inquiries on asthma and allergy; arranges for professional speakers and audio-visual materials and encourages community activities through its local chapters. Membership: 325.

Biofeedback Society of America

4200 East Ninth, C268, Denver, CO 80262

(303) 394-7054

Founded in 1969. The BSA is an interdisciplinary organization dedicated to the applied, research and educational aspects of biofeedback. Membership: 2,000.

Braille Institute

741 North Vermont Avenue, Los Angeles, CA 90029

(213) 663-1111

Founded in 1919. The institute provides training, education and special services for the blind of all ages. Membership: 3,000.

Child Abuse Listening Mediation, Inc.

PO Box 718, Santa Barbara, CA 93102

(805) 966-9762

Founded in 1971. CALM is organized for the prevention of child abuse and neglect, and provides a hot line listener, child care to reduce stress, a speakers bureau, and parent support groups.

Child Health Associate Program

4200 East Ninth Avenue, Box C219, Denver, CO 80262

(303) 394-7963

Founded in 1969. The CHAP is a training program to prepare health care professionals capable of providing a wide range of diagnostic, preventive and therapeutic services to children. Working principally in ambulatory settings as colleagues and associates of physicians, child health associates have the knowledge and skill to care for a large percentage of the patients seen in a typical pediatric practice. The training program is three years in length. Prerequisites include two years of college preparation. Membership: 80 students.

The Childrens Foundation

1420 New York Avenue, NW, 8th Floor, Washington, DC 20005

(202) 387-6119

The foundation was established in 1969 as a national, non-profit advocacy organization focusing upon the quality and availability of the federal food assistance programs for children and their families.

Committee to Combat Huntington's Disease, Inc.

250 West 57th Street, Suite 2016, New York, NY 10019

(212) 757-0443

Founded in 1967. The goals of the committee are the identification of HD families, education of the lay public and professional, the promotion and support of basic and clinical research into the causes and cure of HD, and a patient services program, coordinated with various community services. Membership: 20,000.

Council on Arteriosclerosis of the American Heart Assoc.

7320 Greenville Avenue, Dallas, TX 75231

(214) 750-5431

Founded in 1946.

Council on Education for Public Health

1015 15th Street, NW, Washington, DC 20005

(202) 789-1050

Founded in 1974. CEPH is the independent agency officially recognized by the U.S. Office of Education and the Council on Postsecondary Accreditation to accredit graduate schools of public health and certain graduate programs outside of schools of public health. Membership: 2 organizations.

Council of World Organizations Interested in the Handicapped

432 Park Avenue, South, New York, NY 10016

(212) 679-6520

Founded in 1953. The council provides a coordinating mechanism for international organizations and the UN agencies to avoid duplication of programs for disabled people. Membership: 40 organizations.

Drug Information Association, Inc.

1050 George Street, Suite 5-L, New Brunswick, NJ 08901

(201) 247-5630

Founded in 1965. The DIA is an international multidisciplinary professional association of specialists engaged in furthering modern technology of communication in medical, pharmaceutical, and allied human/animal fields. Membership: 1,000. Publishes quarterly *Drug Information Journal* as proceedings of meetings and for submitted relevant papers.

Gerontological Society

1835 K Street, NW, Suite 305, Washington, DC 20006

(202) 466-6750

Founded in 1945. The society is a national multidisciplinary organization of researchers, educators and professionals in aging devoted to stimulating and promoting research and its application to practice. Membership: 5,200. Publishes 2 bimonthly journals: *Journal of Gerontology* and *The Gerontologist*.

Goodwill Industries of America, Inc.

9200 Wisconsin Avenue, Washington, DC 20014

(301) 530-6500

Founded in 1902. Goodwill Industries provides services, materials, and information to assist member Goodwill Industries in their programs of service to handicapped people. Membership: 168.

Gray Panthers

3635 Chestnut Street, Philadelphia, PA 19104

(215) 382-3300

Founded in 1970. The Gray Panthers are people of all ages, working for social change. It tries to develop creative alternatives to the injustices in society which confront people at every phase of life. Membership: 40,000. State affiliation: 111 local networks.

Guide Dog Users, Inc.

Box 174, Central Station, Baldwin, NY 11510

(516) 223-8492

Founded in 1969. The goals of GDU are to improve the quality of the educational, cultural, employment and rehabilitation services of all blind persons, to promote the acceptance of guide dog users by federal and state agencies, employers, educational institutions, business establishments and places of entertainment. Membership: 450. National basis members at large; publication *Pawtracks* quarterly.

Health and Education Resources

4733 Bethesda Avenue, Suite 735, Bethesda, MD 20014

(301) 656-3178

Founded in 1969. HER is a non-profit organization developing programs and communications in health, education, and social services including continuing education for clinical laboratory personnel; technical assistance for implementation of a skill-and-knowledge-based task analysis method; production of audio-visual instructional materials.

Health Sciences Communications Association

2343 North 115th Street, Wauwatosa, WI 53226

(414) 258-2525

Founded in 1959. HSCA is a non-profit organization devoted to advancement of education in health sciences by means of varied contemporary educational technology. Membership: 748.

Healthright, Inc.

41 Union Square, Room 206-8, New York, NY 10003

(212) 675-2651

Founded in 1974. Healthright is a women's health education and advocacy organization which publishes a quarterly newsletter and provides a literature center with many health education pamphlets and books.

Healthy America, National Coalition for Health Promotion and Disease Prevention

1015 15th Street, NW, Suite 424, Washington, DC 20005

(202) 789-1041

Founded in 1977 the coalition is a national, non-profit organization emphasizing health advocacy, disease prevention and promotion of good health habits as means to attain lasting good health. It encourages health promotion policies and programs at all levels of government and within private sector, sponsors seminars, conferences, etc. and serves as congressional liaison for membership. Membership: 150.

International Association Cancer Victims and Friends, Inc.

7740 W. Manchester Avenue, Suite 110, Playa del Rey, CA 90291

(213) 822-5032

Founded in 1963. IACVF is a non-profit (tax exempt) corporation organized under the laws of the state of California. Its purpose is the dissemination of educational materials concerning the prevention and control of cancer through the use of non-toxic therapies. Membership: 7,500. Chapters have symposiums and seminars in their respective areas throughout the year.

International Childbirth Education Association, Inc.

8635 Fremont Avenue South, Minneapolis, MN 55420

(612) 881-9194

Founded in 1960. The ICEA promotes family centered maternity care and helps groups and individuals promote same through classes in prepared childbirth, teacher training, publications, conferences and conventions. Membership: 13,000.

International Commission for Prevention of Alcoholism

6830 Laurel Street, NW, Washington, DC 20012

(202) 723-0800

Founded in 1952. The commission is a non-government organization of the UN, focusing on prevention programming through organizing of congresses, seminars, personal contacts, educational material, and other community endeavors. Membership: 250.

International Council on Health, Physical Education and Recreation

1201 16th Street, NW, Room 417, Washington, DC 20036

(202) 833-5499

Founded in 1958. The council represents and brings together teachers, administrators, leaders, national departments of physical education and related associations in health, physical education, sports, dance and recreation into one organization at the international level. It fosters international understanding, goodwill and encourages development and expansion of educationally sound programs. Membership: 832.

The Juvenile Diabetes Foundation
23 East 26th Street, New York, NY 10010
(212) 889-7575
Founded in 1970. JDF is a non-profit voluntary agency whose prime objective is to support and fund research aimed at preventing the complications and curing the disease itself. Membership: 50,000. JDF chapters provide educational and counseling services in addition to fund raising.

W. K. Kellogg Foundation
400 North Avenue, Battle Creek, MI 49016
(616) 965-1221
Founded in 1930. The foundation is committed to the application of existing knowledge to problems of people in the areas of health, education and agriculture. It currently assists programs of four continents, including the United States and Canada, Latin America, Europe and Australia. A grant making organization, the foundation does not operate programs.

La Leche League International, Inc.
9616 Minneapolis Avenue, Franklin Park, IL 60131
(321) 455-7730
Founded in 1956. The league is a non-profit organization which provides help for breastfeeding mothers in a series of four meetings, annual seminar for physicians, biennial international conferences for parents and professionals, and a 24 hour telephone hotline. Membership: 110,000.

Leukemia Society of America, Inc.
800 Second Avenue, New York, NY 10017
(212) 573-8484
Founded in 1949. The LSA promotes and provides support into the causes, treatment and cure or control of the leukemias and related lymphomas. Membership: 1,500. Allied programs are patient service, public and professional education and community services.

The Living Bank International
PO Box 6725, Houston, TX 77005
(713) 528-2971
Founded in 1968. The LBI is an organ and body donor registry, educating the public about the importance of organ and body donations, registration, and referral of donations, at the time of death, to the appropriate medical facility closest to the point of death. Membership: 70,000.

The Lupus Foundation of America, Inc.
11673 Holly Springs Drive, St. Louis, MO 63141
(314) 872-9036
Founded in 1977. The corporation is organized exclusively for charitable, educational and scientific purposes to encourage development of research programs designed to discover the causes of, and to improve the methods of treating, diagnosing, curing and preventing Lupus Erythematosus. Membership: 19,000.

March of Dimes Birth Defects Foundation
1275 Mamaroneck Avenue, White Plains, NY 10605
(914) 428-7100
Founded in 1938. The goal of the foundation is the prevention of birth defects, our most serious child health problem, through support of research, medical services and education.

Maternity Center Association
48 East 92nd Street, New York, NY 10028
(212) 369-7300
Founded in 1918. The MCA provides complete maternity service for low-risk families; childbirth education and information service; support of nurse-midwifery education; institutes on parent education and literature on childbearing and maternity care. Membership: 1,000.

Medic Alert Foundation International
PO Box 1009, Turlock, CA 95380
(209) 632-2371
Founded in 1956. Medic Alert provides emergency medical identification in either necklace or bracelet style which includes hidden medical condition, membership number, and emergency telephone number which can be called collect. A wallet card is provided with additional emergency information. $10 membership fee includes stainless steel emblem. Membership: 925,272, U.S.; 1,475,479, international.

Mended Hearts, Inc.
721 Huntington Avenue, Boston, MA 02115
(617) 732-5609
Founded in 1951. Membership: 10,000.

Mental Health Association, National Headquarters
1800 North Kent Street, Arlington, VA 22209
(703) 528-6400
Founded in 1909. The MHA is a lay, volunteer organization which provides social action and public education in the area of mental health. Membership: 1,000,000.

Muscular Dystrophy Association
810 Seventh Avenue, 27th Floor, New York, NY 10019
(212) 586-0808
The MDA is a voluntary national health agency—a dedicated partnership between scientists and concerned citizens aimed at conquering neuromuscular diseases which affect thousands of Americans.

The Myasthenia Gravis Foundation
15 East 26th Street, New York, NY 10010
(212) 889-8157
Founded in 1952. The foundation fosters, coordinates, and supports research into the cause, prevention, alleviation, and cure of myasthenia gravis, and gives research grants to MG clinics, hospitals, medical schools throughout the United States and awards at least 10 medical student fellowships each year and a $20,000 post-doctoral fellowship.

National Association of Councils of Stutterers
Speech and Hearing Center, O'Boyle Hall, Room 100, Catholic Univ., Washington, DC 20064
(202) 635-5556
Founded in 1965. Membership: 20.

National Association for Down's Syndrome
PO Box 63, Oak Park, IL 60303
(312) 543-6060

Founded in 1960. NADS is a not-for-profit organization comprised of parents and professionals involved with the individual with Down's Syndrome. The association has a membership in excess of 1,500. Membership: 1,500.

National Association on Drug Abuse Problems, Inc.
355 Lexington Avenue, New York, NY 10017
(212) 986-1170

Founded in 1975. NADAP provides a placement service for rehabilitated drug abusers. Workshop for drug treatment counselors and corporate management.

National Association of the Physically Handicapped, Inc.
76 Elm Street, London, OH 43140
(614) 852-1664

Founded in 1958. The NAPH advances the social, economic, and physical welfare of physically handicapped. It is not a resource center for information. We give no type services; nor give financial aid. We support legislation to benefit handicapped; trying to make public aware of needs of handicapped.

National Association of Retarded Citizens
2709 Avenue E East, Arlington, TX 76011
(817) 261-4961

Founded in 1950. Membership: 300,000.

National Association for Visually Handicapped
305 East 24th Street, New York, NY 10010
(212) 889-3141

Founded in 1954. The NAVH offers guidance and counsel for all partially-seeing people and professionals and paraprofessionals working with them, informational literature. It publishes and distributes large print books, textbooks and testing material. Serves as referral agency for all services for partially seeing. Membership: 4,132. Only national health agency serving only the partially-seeing (not the totally blind).

National Ataxia Foundation
6681 Country Club Drive, Minneapolis, MN 55427
(612) 546-6220

Founded in 1957. NAF works to combat all types of hereditary ataxia and related disorders through four major objectives: education, service, prevention and research. Membership: 4,000.

National Burn Federation
3737 Fifth Avenue, Suite 206, San Diego, CA 92103
(714) 291-4766

Founded in 1975. The foundation serves as a vehicle for exchange of ideas and programs in fire safety and burn prevention; gives national focus to the burn problem, the medical resources available to treat burns, and the community prevention programs in operation which address the problem. Membership: 80.

National Committee for the Prevention of Alcoholism and Drug Dependency
6830 Laurel Street, NW, Washington, DC 20012
(202) 723-4774

Founded in 1950. The committee holds institutes and seminar-workshops throughout the U.S. periodically. It gathers and distributes information and materials concerning the effects of alcohol and other drugs on the physical, mental and moral powers of the individual citizen and promotes an educational program for prevention with visual and teaching aids throughout the country. Membership: 50. Willing to cooperate with other organizations in holding seminar-workshops in their area.

National Council on Alcoholism, Inc.
733 Third Avenue, New York, NY 10017
(212) 986-4433

Founded in 1944. The council is the only national voluntary agency founded to combat the disease of alcoholism. Membership: 87.

National Council on Drug Abuse
571 West Jackson Boulevard, Chicago, IL 60606
(312) 663-9224

Founded in 1972. NCDA is a tax-exempt not-for-profit educational and preventative organization. Our work in the fields of drug and alcohol abuse has helped thousands of professionals and laymen countrywide deter, curtail and better understand substance abuse.

National Council on Health Care Services
1200 15th Street, NW, Suite 601, Washington, DC 20005
(202) 785-4754

Founded in 1969. The council is a trade association organized to foster a better understanding of the important contribution private companies make to the nation's health care delivery system and to promote standards of quality and efficiency beneficial to both the membership and the public. Membership: 21.

National Health Council, Inc.
1740 Broadway, New York, NY 10019
(212) 582-6040

Founded in 1920. NHC is a membership organization of national voluntary, professional, and related organizations interested in improving the health of all Americans in the areas of planning, coordination, and delivery of health services. Membership: 87 organizations.

National Health Federation
PO Box 688, Monrovia, CA 91016
(213) 357-2181

Founded in 1955. Membership: 35,000.

National Hearing Aid Society
20361 Middlebelt Road, Livonia, MI 48152
(313) 478-2610

Founded in 1951. NHAS is the professional association for those engaged in fitting and selling of hearing aids. Membership: 2,000.

The National Hemophilia Foundation
25 West 39th Street, New York, NY 10018
(212) 869-9740

Founded in 1948. The foundation provides information for those interested in the field, and promotes research. Membership: 19.

National Indian Council on Aging
PO Box 2088, Albuquerque, NM 87103
(505) 766-2276

Founded in 1976. The council is a national advocacy organization to bring about improved services to

American Indian and Alaskan Native elders, including health-related services. Membership: 40 council members.

National Indian Health Board, Inc.
1602 South Parker Road, Suite 200, Denver, CO 80231
(303) 752-0931

Founded in 1972. The board provides review and comment on federal legislation that affects Indian tribes and serves as an advisory board to HEW on Indian health concerns.

National Kidney Foundation
2 Park Avenue, Room 908, New York, NY 10016
(212) 889-2210

Founded in 1958. NKF is a national voluntary health organization supporting research and public information on the diagnosis and treatment of diseases of the kidney. Membership: 3,300.

National Lupus Erythematosus Foundation, Inc.
5430 Van Nuys Boulevard, Van Nuys, CA 91401
(213) 885-8787

Founded in 1950. NLEF is a non-profit organization for the distribution of Lupus literature; compiling of information gathered from Lupus patients; funding of Lupus research, and establishing Lupus City of Hope Chapters throughout the country.

National Society for Austistic Children
1234 Massachusetts Avenue, NW, Suite 1017, Washington, DC 20005
(202) 783-0125

Founded in 1965. The NSAC is a non-profit organization of parents, professionals and other concerned citizens working for better education, research, treatment and legislation on behalf of autistic persons. Membership: 6,500.

National Spinal Cord Injury Foundation
369 Elliot Street, Newton Upper Falls, MA 02169
(617) 964-0521

Founded in 1948. The foundation addresses the needs of persons with spinal cord injuries through programs in the areas of care, cure and coping. Membership: 5,000.

National Sudden Infant Death Syndrome Foundation
310 South Michigan Avenue, Chicago, IL 60604
(312) 663-0650

Founded in 1962. Through 55 chapters in 36 states. NSIDSF provides support for SIDS research, services to families of victims of SIDS and SIDS-related disorders, and educational programs for health and emergency personnel. It also fulfills a consumer advocacy role for SIDS families.

National Tay-Sachs and Allied Disease Association
122 East 42nd Street, New York, NY 10017
(212) 661-2780

Founded in 1957. The association conducts programs in support of research, family counseling, and public and professional education into the genetic disease Tay-Sachs and many others diseases due to inborn errors of metabolism.

Pediatric Pulmonary Association of America
150 North Pond Way, Roswell, GA 30076
(404) 993-5859

Founded in 1975. PPAA works to combat chronic lung diseases in infants and children via the dissemination of knowledge of updated therapeutic techniques and through the promotion of advanced research. Also it provides a legislative base for permanent federal and state funding for meritorious programs. Membership: 300. The PPAA, through its periodical publication *The Pediatric Pulmonary Digest,* circulates the field on current news. Contributions are welcomed. Send articles to the editor.

Planned Parenthood Federation of America, Inc.
810 Seventh Avenue, New York, NY 10019
(212) 541-7800

PPF works to make effective means of birth control available for all.

The Salvation Army
120 West 14th Street, New York, NY 10011
(212) 620-4910

Founded in 1880. The Salvation Army is an international religious and charitable organization providing health and welfare services throughout the world. In the United States a wide range of services is based upon needs of community and available local resources. Membership: 396,238.

Synanon Foundation, Inc.
PO Box 786, Marshall, CA 94940
(415) 663-8111

Founded in 1958. Synanon was the first community designed for the re-education of drug addicts and other character disorders, and it continues to do that work. Since 1974 Synanon has been providing re-education for children as young as 10. Membership: 825. Facilities in Marshall, San Francisco, Los Angeles, and Badger, Calif.; Kerhonkson and New York, N.Y., Chicago, Ill., and Detroit, Mich.

United Cerebral Palsy Associations, Inc.
66 East 34th Street, New York, NY 10016
(212) 481-6300

Founded in 1948. UCP is the only nationwide voluntary organization targeting its services on the specific and multiple needs of persons with cerebral palsy and their families. UCPs more than 240 affiliates provide a variety of community services, support research and conduct programs of public education pertaining to cerebral palsy. Membership: 276.

REPORTABLE DISEASES AND CONDITIONS

Diseases Reportable in Most States

**Amebiasis
Anthrax
Aseptic meningitis
Botulism
Brucellosis
Chickenpox
*Cholera
Diphtheria
Encephalitis, primary infectious
Encephalitis, post-infectious
**Food-poisoning (outbreaks)
Hepatitis-A
Hepatitis-B
Leprosy
Leptospirosis
Malaria
Meningococcal infections
Mumps
**Pertussis
*Plague
Poliomyelitis, total and paralytic

Psittacosis (ornithosis)
Rabies in man and animals
Rubella
Rubella congenital syndrome
Salmonellosis, excluding typhoid fever
Shigellosis
*Smallpox
Tetanus
Trichinosis
Tuberculosis (new active cases)
Tularemia
Typhoid fever
Typhus, fleaborne (murine)
Typhus, tickborne (Rocky Mountain spotted fever)
Venereal diseases
Syphilis (primary and secondary)
Gonorrhea
** Other specified venereal diseases: chancroid, granuloma inguinale, and lymphogranuloma venereum
*Yellow fever

Adapted from Centers for Disease Control: Morbidity and mortality weekly report. In Annual summary, Atlanta, Ga., 1981, pp. 12-13.
*Diseases covered by International Quarantine Agreement.
**Diseases not routinely reported to Centers for Disease Control on a weekly basis.

THE MULTI-ATTRIBUTE UTILITY PLANNING METHOD APPLIED TO A HEARING SCREENING PROGRAM IN THE LOCAL SCHOOL DISTRICT

The ultimate goal of the Hearing Screening Program is to identify all elementary school children with potential hearing deficits.

STEP 1: Identify the person or aggregate whose utilities are to be maximized. The two organizations involved in the screening program are: the local public health department and the school district. The persons representing the organizations are the community health nurses and the school nurses respectively.

STEP 2: Identify the issue(s) or decisions to which the utilities are relevant. The major objectives to be met to implement the screening program are to: 1) identify the number of elementary school children with diagnosed hearing deficits and 2) identify the number of elementary school children currently requiring hearing screening.

STEP 3: Identify the entities to be evaluated.
1. School health nurse to audit health records of all children to identify target population.
2. Public health nurse to send survey to all parents of elementary school children to identify children with diagnosed hearing deficits and children who have not had prior hearing screening.
3. Teachers be asked to survey children and parents about child's hearing problems during parent teacher conferences.

STEP 4: Identify the relevant dimensions of value.

	Rank
1. Acceptable cost of surveys.	1
2. Minimal time required of community health nurse, school health nurse, teacher, or parent.	5
3. Parents' acceptance of method chosen to identify children for screening.	2
4. Acceptable level of response to chosen survey method, for example, mailed survey may only yield a 2% to 20% return.	4
5. Minimum time required to schedule parent conferences.	6
6. Children's acceptable reaction to survey.	3

STEP 5: Rank the value dimensions in order of importance. See Step 4 for ranks.

STEP 6: Rate dimensions of importance. (See Step 7.)

STEP 7: Sum the importance weights, divide each by the sum, and multiply by 100. (See below.)

Ranked dimension (5)	Raw weight (6)	Normalized weight (7)
1. Cost	50	26
2. Parents' acceptance	40	21
3. Children's reaction	40	21
4. Survey response	30	16
5. Time	20	11
6. Conference scheduling	10	5
	190	100

STEP 8: Measure the location of the entity being evaluated on each dimension. See worksheet.

STEP 9: Calculate utilities for entities. See worksheet.

STEP 10: Decide on best alternative to meet program objectives. Option 1 identified in Step 3—school health nurse audits children's health records.

Worksheet for MAUT (4, 5, 6, 7)

Entities to be evaluated (3)	Dimension to be maximized						Aggregate utility (9)	Final rank
	1	2	3	4	5	6		
Weight of dimensions	26	21	21	16	11	5		
1. School health nurse to audit children's health records								
Probability (8)	.50	.80	.00	.90	.20	.90		
Weight × probability (9)	13.0	16.8	0	14.4	2.2	4.5	50.9	1
2. Public health nurse to mail parents' survey								
Probability	.20	.50	.50	.20	.80	.50		
Weight × probability	5.2	10.5	10.5	3.2	8.8	2.5	40.7	3
3. Teachers to perform survey during parent-teacher conference								
Probability	.80	.60	.20	.50	.20	.20		
Weight × probability	2.8	12.6	4.2	8.0	2.2	1.0	48.8	2

SCHOOL AND CLASSROOM ASSESSMENT GUIDE

1. Classroom assessment for health needs
   A. People involved—classroom teacher, nurse, and student when appropriate
2. Advance preparation
   A. Health records of students in an assigned location
   B. Room and time arranged for assessment
3. Plan conference—with appropriate people
   A. When health needs are identified
   B. Include student(s), with identified health needs, in conference
4. Classroom teacher
   A. In advance, weigh and measure all children; graph results
   B. Collect all screening results and place in folder
   C. Explain to students what is about to happen
   D. Work with nurse in assessing health records
5. Nurse environmentalist
   A. Look at physical structure: Classroom—what is in it? How many students to a classroom? Cleanliness, atmosphere, arrangement of desks? Exits free from clutter, food in proper containers, refrigeration, bathrooms (soap, towel, and hot water)?
   B. Review students records with teacher

6. Nurse appropriately arranges for the following, if needed
   A. Health risk appraisal
   B. Vision screening
   C. Hearing screening
   D. Kidney screening
   E. Physical and dental examinations
   F. Follow-up of all defects
   G. Contact with parents when problems are identified
   H. Nursing assessment
   I. Blood pressure screening
   J. Scoliosis screening
7. Nurse assesses teacher's attitude toward students
   A. Use observation skills
8. School nutrition program
   A. Review menu for week
   B. Meet with school dietary staff
   C. Check to see if skimmed or low fat milk is an option
   D. Because of budget cuts, help dietary staff to make up handout to send home about nutritional brown-bag lunches
9. Nurse
   A. Assess all children in the classroom
   B. Compare growth and development of children with their peers
   C. List children with health-related problems

Health maintenance flow sheet — 2 weeks to 17 years

Procedures and ages

Assessments: 2 wk; 2, 4, 6, 9, 12, 18 mo; 2, 3, 5, 8, 11, 13, 15, 17 yr						
Date scheduled						
Date seen						
Age						
Provider						

Complete history	Date					
Complete examination	Date					

Immunizations (record dates below)

DPT										
OPV										
MMR										
Td										

Rubella serology 11 yr nonvaccinated female	Titer					
Tuberculin (tine) test 1, 3, 5, 11, 15 yr	Pos/Neg					
Hematocrit 1, 5, 13 yr	Result					
Urine culture (female) 5, 8 yr	Nl/Abn					
Blood pressure 3 yr and each subsequent visit	Result					
Development 6, 18 mo; 3, 5 yr	Nl/Abn/Q					
Hearing 6 mo; 1, 3 yr; and each subsequent visit	P/F					
Vision 4 mo; 1, 3 yr; and each subsequent visit	P/F					
Language 2, 3, 5 yr	P/F					
Dental care Each visit						
Counseling: each visit						
Nutrition						
Physical care						
Behavior/psychosocial						
Sex education						
Stimulation						
Safety						
Family planning						
Other						

From Hoole, H.A., et al.: Patient care guideline for nurse practitioners, ed. 2, Boston, 1982, Little, Brown & Co. p. 2.

REFERRAL SERVICE GUIDE

PURPOSE: To provide access to health care for students in need

PROCEDURE: Classroom teachers or any other school personnel should refer students with any of the problems listed below to the school nurse

STUDENTS

1. Any student who needs to see the nurse should come directly to the health room
2. Friends of the students may feel free to send students to the health room

CONDITIONS AND SYMPTOMS TO REFER:

1. Chronic absenteeism (other than truancy)
2. Problems with vision, hearing, or speech
3. Headache accompanied by nausea, vomiting, or blurred vision
4. Fatigue, listlessness, inattentiveness (chronic problems)
5. Allergies (i.e., red, inflamed eyes; chronic sinusitis; constant sneezing)
7. Respiratory problems such as wheezing or shortness of breath
8. Jaundice (a yellowish tint to the skin or whites of eyes)
9. Pregnant students or ones with children
10. Suspected venereal disease cases
11. Severe acne or other skin problems
12. Suspected abuse cases

EXCEPTION: The above list is not complete and teachers should not hesitate to refer other problems that they feel need attention

RELAXATION EXERCISES

EXERCISE A: relaxation techniques
1. Find a comfortable place to sit.
2. Place feet flat on the floor.
3. Close eyes.
4. Breathe steadily and with purpose for about 5 minutes.
5. Take particular notice of the parts of the body that feel tense and will them to relax.

EXERCISE B: breathing technique for relaxation
1. Close your eyes and concentrate on your breathing; exhale comfortably pulling your abdomen in. Now inhale rapidly, taking as much air into your lung as you can and filling your entire rib cage. Draw in your abdomen, forcing the accumulated air out through your mouth. Repeat 10 times.
2. This time inhale slowly so that the breath you draw in is held for 5 seconds. Hold for another 5 seconds and then exhale slowly until your lungs are completely empty. Repeat five times.

EXERCISE C: brief relaxation technique
1. Sit comfortably and close your eyes. Concentrate on bringing to mind a picture of the most peaceful setting you have experienced.
2. With each breath say to yourself, "Relax."
3. Let your mind remain free of other thoughts as your practice this for 5 minutes.

EXERCISE D: anxiety-reduction technique
1. Sit in a comfortable position with eyes closed.
2. Inhale a deep breath through your nose—hold—exhale through the mouth (5 times).
3. Breathe normally. Concentrate on your breathing. With each exhale say "one" silently. Breathe in . . . breathe out, with "one."
4. Open your eyes and sit quietly for 1 minute.

Appendix J

NURSING INTERVENTION TOOLS

Normal variations and minor abnormalities in newborn physical characteristics

Variant	Cause	Course	Nursing anticipatory guidance
Head			
Cephalhematoma	Usually caused by trauma of birth.	Soft, fluctuant, well-outlined mass of blood trapped beneath the pericranium and confined to one bone. This is a subperiosteal hematoma with no extension across suture lines.	Observe for any changes in the size or shape of the hematoma. Reassure parents.
Caput succedaneum	Caused by head pressing on the pelvic outlet in the last period of labor.	Clear fluid trapped between the scalp and bone. It is ill-defined, pits on pressure, not fluctuant. Fluid usually disappears in 1 to 2 weeks.	Explain the cause to parents and reassure them it will disappear.
Facial asymmetry	Overriding of the cranial sutures at birth caused by intrauterine molding or molding from delivery. Bones are soft and pliable.	Flattening of part of head or face. Generally disappears a few days after birth.	If the occipital area is flat because of labor and delivery, reassure parents about its disappearance in a few days. If it is caused by the "same" positioning of the child in the crib, instruct the parents to alternate the positioning of the child in the crib daily.
Asymmetry of the scalp	Usually occurs from molding during delivery or the use of forceps during delivery. Also can be caused by positioning the infant repeatedly on the same side without rotating.	Flattening of part of head.	Same as facial asymmetry.
Craniotabes	Unknown.	Softening of localized areas in the cranial bone. Sometimes found in the parietal bones at the vertex near the sagittal suture. The areas are spongelike and can be indented by the pressure of a fingertip. They resume their shape when the pressure is removed.	Usually inconsequential, but if they persist, could be indicative of a pathological cause. There is no specific treatment. It is normal for these craniotabes to persist for months. They should eventually disappear.
Fontanelle	An irregular-shaped area enclosed by a membrane which occurs where the sutures of the bone of the skull meet. These areas are called anterior fontanelle, posterior fontanelle, and temporal fontanelles.	The anterior fontanelle should be open; the posterior fontanelle may be closed.	Explain to the parents that the open fontanelle helped to protect the baby's head during the birth process. The fontanelle allows the brain to grow and will continue to do so for the next 18 months. Reassure parents that fontanelle can be touched and scalp scrubbed without ill effect.

Variant	Cause	Course	Nursing anticipatory guidance
Mouth			
Bednar's aphthae (ulcers)	Unknown. May be caused by vigorous sucking.	Usually located on hard palate posteriorly; generally bilateral.	Reassure and support parents. Explain to the parents that there is no specific treatment, and condition will disappear without any treatment.
Epstein's epithelial pearls	Small epithelial cysts.	Located along both sides of the middle of the hard palate or along the alveolar ridge.	Reassure parents that cysts will disappear. There is no specific treatment.
Bohn's pearls (nodules)	Small white papules.	Located on each side of the midline of the hard palate. They disappear spontaneously in several weeks.	Reassure and support parents. Parents sometimes think that these lesions look like thrush. Reassure that these lesions are not thrush and will go away without treatment.
High palatal arch		Of no significance if there are no other findings present.	Reassure, support, and explain the lack of significance.
Eyes			
Chemical conjunctivitis	Irritation from silver nitrate solution instilled after birth.	Eyes red with purulent exudate. Lids swollen. Onset occurs within first 24 hours and lasts about 2 to 4 days.	Cleanse eyelids with cotton balls soaked in warm saline solution. Wipe the eyes from the inner canthus out toward the outer canthus. Reassure parents that the infant's eyesight will not be affected.
Subconjunctival hemorrhage	Caused from pressure in the birth process.	Occurs at the limbus. It may be crescent shaped or may form a red halo around the iris. The hemorrhage resolves itself without any specific treatment in a few days.	Reassure parents that no residual defects occur from the hemorrhage. The blood will reabsorb itself in a few days.
Pseudostrabismus	Poor muscle coordination of the eye.	Movements of the newborn's eyes are poorly coordinated. The eyes do not necessarily move together. Very common and usually disappears spontaneously.	Reassure parents that this generally disappears spontaneously as the eye muscles strengthen and the infant's eyes continue to develop and grow.
Skin			
Vernix caseosa	Cheeselike material that sticks to the skin. Protective covering for infant in utero.	Skin of newborn covered with varying amounts of this substance.	Will dry and disappear within a few days. Discourage mother from trying to vigorously rub it off. Encourage good skin care.
Lanugo	Fine downy type of hair.	Usually found on the back, shoulders, and ear lobes.	Usually disappears in time as a result of the friction of the skin rubbing on the bassinet linens. Reassure parents.
Desquamation	Skin in the newborn is very tender and soft. Following birth, the skin reacts to the changed environment by becoming very red. When the redness subsides, desquamation of the skin tends to occur.	Shedding, flaking, or peeling of the skin. Usually occurs during the first week of life. Can vary from extensive to so slight it almost goes unnoticed.	Reassure, support, and explain the cause to parents. Encourage good skin care, which avoids overuse of lotions, oils, and powders.
Ecchymosis	Blood under the skin caused by superficial trauma to the skin.	Bruise — disappears as the blood is reabsorbed.	Provide reassurance.
Acrocyanosis	Venous stasis.	Blue hands and feet.	No specific treatment. Make sure the baby is warm and that the cause of the acrocyanosis is not from being cold.

Continued.

Normal variations and minor abnormalities in newborn physical characteristics — cont'd

Variant	Cause	Course	Nursing anticipatory guidance
Skin—cont'd			
Erythema toxicum	Unknown.	A rash consisting of small, red, flat or raised lesions. Looks splotchy and sometimes resembles chicken pox or flea bites. Usually occurs during the first 2 weeks.	No specific treatment. Reassure, support, and explain.
Nevi, pigmented Nevus spilus (hairless mole)	Increased pigmentation.	Range from smooth, flat, hairless pigmented areas to those with hair; some can look like warts.	No treatment unless for cosmetic reasons. Provide reassurance.
Nevi, telangiectatic	Widening of surface capillaries.	Small red areas due to widening of surface capillaries; disappear momentarily with blanching of skin, but usually do not disappear completely.	Provide reassurance.
Capillary Hemangiomata (sometimes called Balmar patches)	Capillary lesions of the skin.	Irregular blotchy pink spots at the nape of the neck, eyelids, globella, or lumbosacral areas. Gradually fade; usually disappear by 2 years.	Reassurance and support. No specific treatment.
Mongolian spots	Large aggregations of melanin—rich dark cells, which give the affected area a purple or blue/black color. Occur most frequently in black children but may occur in white children.	Generally found over the sacrum and coccygeal area of a large percentage of infants of black, Chicano, and Asiatic Indian origin. They do not have any significance and most disappear with time.	Explain cause and reassure parents. The spots usually disappear within the first year of life.
Mottling	Vasoconstriction—general circulatory instability.	Overall red and white coloration of the skin. Generally occurs in fair children who become chilled. Disappears when child becomes warm.	Explain causes and reassure parents; use a blanket to warm the infant.
Milia	Retained sebum in the skin.	Yellow-white, pinpoint-size lesions located on the bridge of the nose, the chin, or the cheeks. Disappear after first few weeks of life.	No specific treatment necessary. Explain to parents that lesions will disappear.
Café au lait	Variations in pigment.	Light to dark brown pigmented spots. One or two patches considered normal. If infant has several patches, may indicate fibromas or neurofibromatosis.	Assess nature of spots. If number of spots exceeds two, refer to physician or neurologist. Reassurance and support.
Accessory nipples (supernumerary nipples)	Not adequately explained (sometimes referred to as developmental cutaneous defect).	Occurs in a unilateral or bilateral distribution along the "mammary lines" from midaxilla to the inguinal area.	Reassure parents that the nipples may be excised for cosmetic reasons.
Harlequin coloring	Thought to be caused by poorly developed vasomotor reflexes.	Half of the infant's body appears red/white, the other half is pale. Transitory condition, which usually occurs when the infant cries forcefully.	Explain to parents that this is not significant. It is apparently harmless and the cause is not adequately explained.
Cyanosis (localized)	Inadequate oxygenation of tissues; localized cyanosis because of immature peripheral circulation and venous stasis.	Usually involves lips, hand and feet or cyanosis of the presenting parts. Usually present at birth and for variable number or days afterwards.	Keep child warm, cyanosis will decrease as peripheral circulation improves. Reassure and support parents. Explain cause.

Normal variations and minor abnormalities in newborn physical characteristics — cont'd

Variant	Cause	Course	Nursing anticipatory guidance
Skin—cont'd			
Cyanosis (general)	Numerous causes of general cyanosis, i.e., atelectasis, congenital heart disease, central nervous system damage, obstructed airway.	Depends on the cause.	Reassurance and support. Try to determine the relationship of cyanosis to crying, i.e., if cyanosis is relieved or improved when the child cries, then the cause may be atelectasis. Crying tends to make infants with cardiac malformations worse. Refer to physician.
Abdomen			
Umbilical cord variations	Natural process for sloughing tissues.	Blue/white at birth. Dull and yellow/brown within 24 hours, then black/brown and dry. Usually drops off at the end of the second week.	Keep cord area clean and dry. Reassure parents. Instruct parents in cord care.
Umbilical hernia	Occurs at the defect in the musculature of the abdominal wall near the umbilicus.	Skin-covered protuberance at the umbilicus. Very common in black infants and some Italian infants. Usually disappears spontaneously at the end of one year.	Reassure parents that it will probably disappear spontaneously. If it does not, it can be treated surgically when the child is older. Discourage home remedies (e.g., coin taped to hernia, binding, etc).
Other			
Vaginal discharge	Physiological manifestation of increased maternal hormonal influences.	Milky white discharge, sometimes blood tinged or whole blood. Usually disappears in 2 weeks.	Reassure mother that this is nothing to worry about. It occurs quite frequently and is considered normal. Explain that it will disappear in a few weeks.
Brachial palsy	Sometimes caused when lateral traction is exerted on the head and neck during delivery of the shoulder in a vertex presentation, or in a breech presentation when the arms are extended over the head, or when there is excessive traction on the shoulders.	Should be suspected when there is asymmetric response of the upper extremities during a Moro response. The asymmetric response occurs because there is paralysis of the muscles of the upper arm or paralysis of the entire arm. Prognosis depends on the extent of damage to the nerves.	Treatment usually consists of partial immobilization and appropriate positioning. Problem needs to be evaluated and the appropriate treatment initiated. Depending on the severity of damage, there could be complete return of function within a few months or there may be permanent damage. Teach parents the importance of carrying out the immobilization-positioning treatment on a daily basis. Reassure and support parents. Observe for any changes in the movement of the upper extremeties.

INFANT STIMULATION
Birth to 1 Month

Babies like to
  Suck
  Listen to repeated soft sounds
  Stare at movement and light
  Be *held* and *rocked*
Give your baby
  Your *talking* and *singing*
  Lamps throwing light patterns
  Your *arms*
  Rocking

1 Month

Babies like to
  Listen to your voice
  Look up and to the side
  Hold things placed in their hands
Give your baby
  A lullaby *record*
  A *mobile* overhead
  Pictures on the walls
  Your *face* near his
  A *change in scenery* and *position*

2 Months

Babies like to
  Listen to musical sounds
  Focus, especially on their hands
  Reach and *bat* nearby objects
  Smile
Give your baby
  A *music box* or a soft *musical toy*
  A soft security *cuddle toy* tied to crib
  Your *smile*
  Play time with you

3 Months

Babies like to
  Reach and *feel* with open hands
  Grasp crudely with two hands
  Wave their fists and *watch* them
Give your baby
  Musical records
  Rattles
  Dangling toys
  Textured toys

4 Months

Babies like to
  Grasp things and *let go*
  Kick
  Laugh at unexpected sights and sounds
  Make *consonant sounds*
Give your baby
  Bells
  A *crib gym*
  More *dangling toys*
  Space to kick and move

5 Months

Babies like to
  Shake, feel, and *bang* things
  Sit with support
  Play peek-a-boo
  Roll over
Give your baby
  A *high chair* with a rubber *suction toy*
  A *play pen*
  A *kicking toy*
  Toys that make noise

6 Months

Babies like to
  Shake, bang and throw things down
  Gum objects
  Recognize familiar *faces*
Give your baby
  Many *household objects*
  Tin *cups, spoons,* and pot *lids*
  Wire *whisks*
  A *clutch ball* and *squeaky toys*
  A *teether* and *gumming toys*
  Bouncing, swinging seat

7 Months

Babies like to
  Sit alone
  Use their *fingers* and *thumb*
  Notice *cause* and *effect*
  Bite on their *first tooth*
Give your baby
  Bath tub toys
  More *'things'*
  String
  More *squeaky toys*
  Finger foods

8 Months

Babies like to
  Pivot on their stomachs
  Throw, wave, and *bang* toys together
  Look for toys they have
  Make *vowel sounds*
Give your baby
  Space to pivot and creep
  2 *toys* at once to *bang* together
  Big *soft blocks*
  A *Jack-in-the-box*
  Nested plastic *cups*
  Your *conversation*

9 Months

Babies like to
Pull themselves up
Creep
Place things generally where they're wanted
Say "da-da"
Play pat-a-cake
Give your baby
A *safe corner* of the room to *explore*
Toys tied to the *high chair*
A metal *mirror*
Jack-in-the-box

10 Months

Babies like to
Poke and *prod* with their forefingers
Put things in other things
Imitate sounds

Give your baby
A big *pegboard*
Some *cloth books*
Motion toys
Textured toys

11 Months to 1 year

Babies like to
Use their *fingers*
Lower themselves from standing
Drink from a cup
Mark on paper
Give your baby
Pyramid disks
A large *crayon*
A baking *tin* with *clothespins*
Personal *drinking cup*
More *picture books*

Common concerns and problems of first year (neonate and infant)

Problem or concern	Assessment	Nursing intervention
Burping	Swallowed air bubbles trapped in stomach; occurs more frequently in bottle-fed infants who cry during feeding.	Burp frequently during feeding (i.e., before, during, and after, or after every 1 ounce of formula or after every 4-5 minutes at breast). Use upright position to burp (gently rub infant's back while baby sits on parent's knee and rests forward against parent's arm). Try to burp every 10-15 minutes while awake if not successful burping during and after feeding. Sit upright in infant seat for 30-45 minutes after feeding if awake or position with head elevated and on right side if sleeping.
Colic	Unexplained bouts of crying frequently occurring at same time of day (usually busiest) and often accompanied by abdominal distention, spasms, drawing up legs to stomach and/or passing gas. May be caused by feeding problems, maternal anxiety, allergy, and is aggravated by tension in household. Can last 3 months. Also see 3: crying.	Review basic infant needs with parents (i.e., is infant hungry, wet, have air bubble, in uncomfortable position). Review feeding method, technique and burping, review maternal diet for offending foods if breastfed. Record time when colic episodes occur. Soothe and comfort before "attack." Swaddle infant, i.e., wrap warmly and in an encompassing manner. Walk, rock, and hold infant over shoulder. Try a montonous soothing noise (music, ticking clock) or activity (ride in a car). Change infant position from stomach to side to back to sitting position. Rest infant on abdomen on warm hard surface (i.e., parent knee, warmed crib surface). Change household routine if indicated, create a quiet environment Try pacifier or sugar water; if bottle fed, try soy formula. Reassure parents that infant is not ill, that they are providing good care, and that colic will definitely go away. Provide support to parents, giving opportunity to discuss feelings. Explain theories about origin and cycle of colic.

Continued.

Problem or concern	Assessment	Nursing intervention
Crying	Periodic crying for unexplained reason; ascertain if a pattern exists for crying spells; may be related to colic; obtain a detailed history of time and length of spell; feeding frequency, method, technique and burping; stool patterns; meeting contact and sucking needs; parental handling of crying and feelings re: crying; other household factors, i.e., siblings, relative advice, parental support of each other, presence of otrher symptoms and/or allergies.	See previous section on colic. Reinforce that babies cry for a reason. Best to respond to cry versus letting baby cry it out. Crying is a release and/or exercise for infant. One or two periods a day of 5-10 minutes is normal for most infants. Assist parents to develop positive, relaxed approach. Reassure and support parents in this time of stress. Suggest parents alternate infant care and meeting infant demands.
Constipation	Consistency of stool which is hard, pebbly, rocklike. Not related to frequency, straining, grunting or number of days between stools. Ascertain color, consistency and frequency as well as presence of blood or mucus. Review infant diet and verify parent perception of constipation and expectation of normal stool patterns.	Discuss normal elimination/stool patterns for type of feeding method (i.e., breast fed stools versus bottle fed stools). Reassure that straining, grunting, infrequent number are normal. Reinforce that each infant has individual stool pattern and educate parents re: *what* constipation actually is (i.e., consistency). Discuss parents attitude regarding toilet habits and expectations about stool patterns. If constipated, increase liquids in diet; may offer water between meals. If introduced to solids too early or in too large a quantity, discontinue use until constipation clears, then begin again with smaller amounts. Karo syrup, 1 tsp/3 oz of water may be given several time a day. If appropriate for feeding stage, add prunes (up to 3 tb. or prune juice to diet.
Flatus	Air in stomach or intestines causing abdominal distress, distension and discomfort, frequently expelled through anus. May be caused by excess swallowing of air, overfeeding, underfeeding, or allergy. Ascertain details re: feeding, i.e., frequency and size of nipple, type bottle used, breast feeding technique, maternal diet, use of pacifier, propping of bottle, burping, etc.	Burp frequently during and after feedings. See first section. Calm infant when crying and burp after crying. Place on left side to ease expelling of gas. If suspect allergies, try soy formula or elimination diet (see p. 544). Reassure parents.
Hiccoughs	Sudden sharp involuntary spasms of diaphragm usually occur following a meal.	Reassure parent that infant will cry if truly distressed. Offer infant something to suck (pacifier, breast, bottle with warm water).
Pacifier	Infants demonstrate a need for non-nutritional sucking.	Assist parents to understand aspects of positive and negative use of pacifier. Positive use: indicated immediately after birth before newborn can manipulate thumb into mouth; assists in developing sucking function; contributes to establishment of breast feeding; good means of satisfying sucking need especially for bottle fed infants who need extra sucking time; does not usually become a habit unless child sucks beyond infancy; most infants substitute thumb for pacifier around 3 to 4 months. Parents should look for clues to eliminate pacifier use at this time and provide stimulation suitable for the age. Negative use: pacifiers do not replace holding; stimulation, or needs satisfaction; pacifiers should not be used constantly, especially before tending to infants needs; parents should be encouraged to discontinue use by 5 months since continued use may become a habit hard to overcome. If thumb is substituted, generally it is used less frequently than pacifier.

Common concerns and problems of first year (neonate and infant) — cont'd

Problem or concern	Assessment	Nursing intervention
Spoiling	Ascertain parent definition of spoiling. Generally it is the result of basic needs not being met in early infancy leading to a demanding, undisciplined child because need for gratification continues beyond normal time. Overgratification usually occurs then. Generally it is believed that infants cannot be spoiled under 6 months of age.	Parents require counseling and education that reinforces the following: Early infant needs must be gratified. A child cannot handle frustrations well until 8 to 9 months and is unable to delay gratification of needs until this age. A gradual and gentle approach to limits and delaying gratification is best. A relaxed, positive approach is helpful. Parents often find support groups helpful in dealing with this problem.
Biting	In first year, frequently related to teething. Particularly a problem for breast-feeding mothers. In toddlerhood related to normal aggressive impulses.	If related to teething, see later section on teething for alleviation of discomfort. Breast-feeding mothers should remove infant from breast at every occurrence and may accompany with a ''no''; should also allow time to lapse before finishing feeding. If related to impulsivity of toddlerhood, see first section of table on p. 971.
Separation anxiety	Occurs at 9-10 months as infant is learning to differentiate self from mother. Can occur again in toddlerhood as child is learning to distance and separate self from mother in attempt to establish autonomy.	Reassure mother that this is normal developmental process. Advise parents, especially mother, to do the following: Play ''peek-a-boo'' games. Allow sufficient time (30-45 minutes for child to acquaint him/herself with new person (i.e., visitor, babysitter). Avoid ''sneaking-out.'' Tell child firmly that ''mommy leaves, mommy comes back.'' Reinforce this with ''peek-a-boo'' or ''hide and seek'' games. Avoid making major changes in child's or household routines during this period (i.e., mother returning to work; changing child's room, changing regular babysitter of day care situation, etc.).
Stranger anxiety	Begins at 6 to 8 months, gradually diminishing by 18 months. Process of child development.	See preceding section on separation anxiety. Advise parents, particularly mother to: hold infant in presence of strangers. If infant is to be left, mother should spend a short time with stranger.
Infant sleep patterns	Some infants have difficulty releasing into sleep or awaken easily. Separation anxiety, teething, illness are among the common causes. Ascertain history of problem to include how long infant sleeps, what feeding schedule is, bedtime and household routines, presence of illness or teething, and how problem is handled.	Counseling should directed toward education of parents infants need gratification and normal sleep patterns, emphasizing the following: Differences in temperament and incidence of sleep problems can be related. Infants generally sleep through the night by 3 months. Infant may need help getting to sleep by rocking, holding, pacifier, walking, etc. environment and atmosphere conducive to sleep, e.g., quiet, dim, should be provided. If sleep problem is related to a physical problem, measures to remedy should be implemented.
Teething	Eruption of primary or deciduous teeth starting at about 6 months usually with lower incisors. Will continue every 2 months for first 2 years. Signs may include, but are not always present: red, swollen gums, irritable, crying and rubbing gums. Since other events in infant development are occuring simultaneously, nursing must assist parents to distinguish between these and teething as follows: Drooling, which normally occurs at 3 to 4 months and has little to do with teething, although it may persist throughout teething.	Recommend to parents hard, clean objects for baby to chew on such as rubber teething rings, or beads, hard rubber toys, cool spoon, teething biscuits or pretzels, etc. Parents should avoid use of teething toys or rings filled with liquid because plastic covers are easily broken and liquid can be ingested.

Continued.

Common concerns and problems of first year (neonate and infant) — cont'd

Problem or concern	Assessment	Nursing intervention
Teething — cont'd	Fevers do not usually accompany teething. Must be assessed separately because maternal antibody protection is diminishing and presence of fever is suspect for infectious process. Separation anxiety, sleep disturbances, or fussiness from other causes are all common developmental symptoms associated with infant age group, as is reaching for and mouthing objects.	
Diaper rashes	Rashes of varying types types occurring in diaper area. Persistent rashes which do not respond to home management or continue to occur in spite of preventive measures should be referred for medical evaluation.	Preventive measures to keep area clean, dry, and aerated: Frequent diaper changing. Cleansing with water (and mild soap after bowel movement) at each changing, dry area well. Thick diapers and/or absorbent pads are recommended; plastic or rubber pants are not suggested. A *thin* film of lubrication or powder may be used, such as A and D ointment, petroleum jelly, or Caldesene powder. Remove diapers for short periods every day. Wash diapers well as follows: 1. Soak soiled diapers in Borateen or borax solution (½ cup to 1 gallon of water). 2. Prerinse before washing. 3. Wash in full cycle with mild soap such as Ivory, Dreft, or Lux. 4. Avoid softeners and strong detergents. 5. Rinse diapers 2 to 3 times, and may be added ¼ to ½ cup vinegar to final rinse. 6. Dry in sun if possible. Home management of diaper rash: Follow preventive measures with emphasis on leaving diaper off more frequently, changing when wet, and cleaning area thoroughly during changes. Zinc oxide ointment often is helpful in checking early nonfungal rashes. Cornstarch is never recommended for rashes or their prevention. Seek medical help if rash worsens or does not improve.
Cradle cap	Form of seborrheic dermatitis in neonate characterized by scalping, flaking of scalp skin especially over anterior fontanelle. May persist beyond neonate into infancy period.	Preventive measures: Teach parents how to shampoo infant head and recommend shampooing every other day. Reassure that vigorous scrubbing will not injure fontanelle or skull. Home management for mild cases: Shampoo head daily with warm water and soap, using firm pressure on scalp. Loosen cap by applying mineral or baby oil to scalp 15 to 20 minutes before shampooing. Remove with shampoo. Comb scalp with fine comb to loosen and dislodge scaly cap. Severe cases will require medical attention and are generally managed with antiseborrheic shampoos.

Common concerns and problems of first year (neonate and infant) — cont'd

Problem or concern	Assessment	Nursing intervention
Problems related to feeding Parental concerns about overfeeding or underfeeding	Some parents find it difficult to determine appropriate amount of milk and/or solid food to give infant. Ascertain parent understanding, knowledge, and perceptions through the following: Diet history Height and weight measurement and charting on growth curve. Elimination habits and description.	Assist parents to construct a workable feeding schedule. Discuss normal feeding pattern for breast and bottle fed infants (see this chapter). Discuss infant need for nonnutrient sucking. Convey that infants will eat more than they need or require if food is offered at each cry. Offer water between feedings to postpone next feeding to reasonable time. Suggest schedule of solid food introduction (Table 26-29). Reassure parents that if infant is gaining weight he is not underfed. Explain growth and appetite spurts.
Refusal of solids	Infant may refuse new foods for a number of reasons, e.g., temperature, texture, manner presented by person feeding, or too early introduction. Ascertain through diet history which foods accepted, and likes and dislikes and parental feelings and perception regarding solid foods.	Disuss normal feeding patterns for age. Review indications for starting or not starting solid foods; No need before 4 to 6 months. Digestion begins with salivation around 4 months. Feeding of solid foods is not necessarily related to sleeping through the night. Tongue thrusting of solid food is normal and not a refusal. Discuss ways to encourage solid food acceptance: Allow infant to feed self. Avoid forcing infant to eat since this will only increase resistance. Solids may be stopped for a while, offering only ones that infant likes. Offer solid foods before milk when infant is hungriest. Offer food in calm positive manner.
Refusal of food and variations in appetite	Once solid foods have been introduced and established, infants and especially toddlers will go through periods of refusal, pickiness, and preference. Obtain diet history as reviewed in preceding section (Refusal of solids).	See preceding section (Refusal of Solids). Discuss following with parents: Refusal may be due to loss of interest in food when more active or due to form of negativism and means to control. Avoid use of food as substitute for attention or stimulation. Some degree of refusal and variation in appetite is normal for age. Try following approaches: Offer small amounts of food frequently. Emphasize favorite foods as much as possible. Use as few nonnutritive foods as possible. Allow child to feed self if child desires to and provide finger foods. Be patient as child tries to master use of utensils. Eating should be an enjoyable and sociable time. If hunger does not permit infant to wait until family dinner time, feed before and offer nibbles during family meal. Give older infant and toddler place, chair, utensils, plate at the table.
Spitting up	Regurgitation commonly following a feeding. Usually related to air swallowed with food, inability to relax esophageal sphincter, possible overfeeding, or allergy to milk. Ascertain nature of regurgitation (frequency, amount, color, consistency, etc.) as well as diet history and data regarding weight gain. Frequently outgrown by time infant is sitting well in upright position.	Reinforce the following with parents: Correct preparation of formula. Use of appropriate size nipple and nipple hole. Regular and frequent burping is needed. Place infant in an upright position for 30 minutes after feeding. Correct position of infant during feeding. Determine need to change method of feeding or formula.

Continued.

Common concerns and problems of first year (neonate and infant) — cont'd

Problem or concern	Assessment	Nursing intervention

Weaning	A transition of feeding methods. May be from bottle to cup or from breast to bottle and/or cup.
	
	Weaning from breast is difficult if parents (especially mother) have ambivalent feelings or if infant refuses alternative methods. Ascertain who wants baby weaned and why as well as schedule of feedings.
	
	Weaning from bottle should be attempted gradually, when child is ready, usually around 1 year. Ascertain who wants child weaned, what has been tried, feeding schedule and number of bottles, and ability to use cup.
		Assist parents to make decision to wean:
		  Should be discussed and decided by both parents.
		  If breast feeding, it is helpful to mother to assess every 3 months whether or not to continue nursing.
		  Positive attitude toward weaning is essential, especially for breast-feeding mothers.
		  Weaning at times of separation anxiety is not advised, especially in breast-fed infants.
		  If possible, an infant should be weaned from breast to cup. This avoids having to wean from bottle later on.
		Active weaning for breast feeding mothers:
		  start by substituting bottle or cup for breast at one feeding and allow 5-6 days before substituting second breast feeding.
		  If resistance is encountered try giving water or juice in bottle or cup before weaning starts, using nipple similar to breast or pacifier if one is used, heating milk before offering, and having someone other than mother offer bottle or cup. Keep to a schedule and be firm, positive, and patient.
		Active weaning to cup: continue preceding steps with following additions:
		  Reinforce idea of accomplishment in using a cup to child.
		  May give one bottle a day but should contain only water to avoid incidence of dental caries.
		  Avoid forcing child to wean; forcing use of cup may increase need to suck.
		Calm, relaxed, positive approach is essential.

Accident prevention

Age	Development	Major accidents	Anticipatory guidance
Neonate to 1 month	Is unable to protect self; when on abdomen can lift and turn head; dependent, requires protection; little control over body and movements	Motor vehicles	Use approved car seat Do not hold infant in lap Never leave infant in car unattended For long trips, firmly secure car bed with seat belts in back seat
		Strangulation	Spacing between crib bars should be no more than 2⅜ inches apart Avoid tying anything, including pacifiers, around neck Fasten mobiles securely
		Suffocation and injuries	Crib mattress should fit firmly to sides Do not use pillows; use bumper pads Support infant's head when lifting, holding, or bathing
		Burns including sunburn	Avoid bathing near hot water faucets Test water temperature before bath Avoid handling hot liquids and do not smoke while handling infant Keep out of direct sunlight and use sun screen Use flame-resistant clothing and furniture
2-3 months	Begins gross motor movements of wiggling, squirming, thrashing, rolling	Falls	Never leave infant unattended (at any age) for any reason Keep one hand on infant while giving care Keep crib sides up Use infant seat on floor or playpen

Age	Development	Major accidents	Anticipatory guidance
4-5 months	Mouths objects; brings hands to mouth	Aspiration and choking	Do not prop bottles (at any age) Burp well before putting infant in crib and place on stomach with head to side or propped on side Toys should be too large for infant to swallow, nonbreakable, and free of sharp edges, strings, and detachable parts Keep diaper pins closed during changing Keep small objects (e.g., buttons, coins) out of reach Use only pacifiers with a large shield
		Suffocation	Keep all plastic bags out of reach Keep stuffed animals out of crib
		Lead poisoning	Check toys and other objects for lead-free paint
6-7 months	Sits without support; has a firm grasp; rolls and creeps	Falls and falling objects	Use safety strap in stroller or high chair Use sturdy high chair or feeding table Keep doors to stairs and outside locked; use safety gates. Avoid use of hanging table-cloths Remove knickknacks and breakables
		Ingestion	Keep small objects, medicine, and plants out of reach Keep ipecac on hand and understand use Have poison control number posted Lock up medicine, cleaning agents, insecticides, etc. Keep trashcans out of reach or use locklids
		Injuries and electric shock	Cover wall outlets Place furniture so cords are inaccessible Check furniture for sharp corners — remove or pad Inspect toys for breakage Keep sharp objects out of reach
8-12 months	Pulls to stand; crawls, grabs; beginning to walk; enjoys exploring	Burns	Crawl around on floor and investigate what child could reach or get into Keep all hot food and drinks away from table edge; turn pot handles inward on stove Keep matches and lighters out of reach Keep kitchen closed up or gated Never leave child unattended near fireplace or stove Place guards around open hearths, registers, stoves, and fans Do not iron when child is crawling nearby
		Choking	Do not give child small hard foods, such as peanuts, raw vegetables, popcorn Inspect toys for broken parts Keep floors, counters, tables free of small objects
		Motor vehicles accidents	Continue use of car seat Keep doors locked
		Poisoning	See previous discussion
1-2 years	Walks up and down stairs; stoops and recovers; climbs; likes to take things apart	Falls and injuries	Supervise children in most activities, especially up and down stairs, out of doors, and at playgrounds Lock all windows; when opening, do so from top only Remove any objects or furniture in front of window that child could use as a ladder Permit climbing within child's capabilities Remove bumper pads or toys in crib which child could use to climb on

Continued.

Accident prevention — cont'd

Age	Development	Major accidents	Anticipatory guidance
1-2 years — cont'd			Check toys, expecially riding ones, for damage Keep small, pointed, or sharp objects out of reach Keep out of way of swings
		Burns	Teach child meaning of *hot* Avoid use of flowing clothing
		Drowning	Continue to supervise bath Supervise all water sport activity (e.g., swimming, boating); use floats and/or life jackets Teach child to respect water and seek swimming lessons
		Automobile-related accidents	Continue to use appropriate car seat Keep doors and windows locked Do not permit child to hang out of windows Hold onto child when crossing street or in parking lots Do not permit child to ride toys near street
		Poisoning and ingestion	Have ipecac in any household child frequents (babysitter, grandparents) Use childproof caps on medications Do not regard medicine as candy Do not give one child another's prescription
2-4 years	More adventuresome and curious; explores body orifices; more independent, with limited cognition; imitates	Falls and injuries	Teach child to be cautious around strange animals Supervise play at playground Keep out of reach small objects and foods (peanuts, beans) that can be inserted into orifices; check buttons on clothes and toys Discontinue use of crib when height of crib rail is ¾ of toddler's height Keep stairs well lighted and free of clutter Give toys a safety check Discourage running in house and limit outdoor running to safe places Teach child to respect street and cars Teach child to stay away from and out of old appliances
		Drowning	Continue to teach water safety Supervise all water activities Continue with swimming lessons
		Automobile-related accident	See previous discussion
	Play increases to include rougher games and bike riding Cognition improving and can identify good and bad	Burns	Teach child what to do if fire breaks out; hold household drills Teach child to roll and smother clothes if they catch on fire
		Drowning	Continue swimming lessons Use floats or lifejacket if child cannot swim Swim only where supervision is available (parent or lifeguard)
		Automobile-related accidents	Teach pedestrian safety, providing example for child Do not permit playing in street Use adult seat belt, if child is over 40 pounds If over 55 inches tall, use shoulder restraints

Age	Development	Major accidents	Anticipatory guidance
2-4 years — cont'd		Falls, injuries	Make periodic checks on playground or play area used frequently Check on child when out playing Instruct child in safe use of toys; keep in good condition Keep away from driveways and streets If possible, provide fenced-in play area Set a good example by using seat belt, looking before crossing street, etc.
		Burns	Teach child about danger of matches, lighters, stove Recheck radiators, space heaters, fireplaces, and protective guards
		Poisoning and ingestions	Do not become lax about keeping medication, etc., locked up Teach child to respect harmful objects and use a symbol to indicate ''danger or harmful'' to child Routinely check house, basement, and garage for harmful substances within reach
4-6 years	Continues to be curious, daring, and imitative; frequently plays out of sight		Involve child in safety discussions Continue previously described activities when using household tools and equipment

School age	Increased motor coordination and cognitive ability; increased peer and group activity and involvement in sports; assumes more responsibility for self and well-being.	Motor vehicle and bicycle accidents	Involve child in safety discussion and planning
			Assign safety responsibilities, such as checking bike
			Teach child not to ride with strangers
			Teach child how to contact police and fire department and physician
			Be certain child knows address and phone number
			Discuss bicycle and pedestrian safety
			Discuss bicycle riding rules:
			  Do not hitch ride on moving vehicles
			  Do not ride on dark street
			  Use headlight or reflector at night; wear bright clothes
			  Do not dart from behind parked cars
			  Do not carry passengers on bicycle
			  Keep bike in good repair
			Do not use street as a playground
			Use seat belts

		Injuries	Teach child to participate in sports safely using appropriate gear Permit only supervised sport activities Teach child proper use of household gadgets and equipment; supervise as necessary

		Drowning	Teach the following swimming rules:
			  Swim only where a lifeguard
			  Use buddy system
			  Know water depth before diving
			  Wear life jacket while boating or skiing or if nonswimmer
			No horseplay or call for help jokingly

		Falls	See bicycle rules
			Discuss climbing trees:
			  Avoid slippery shoes
			  Avoid weak or dead branches
			  Keep a secure handhold

Continued.

Accident prevention — cont'd

Age	Development	Major accidents	Anticipatory guidance
School age — cont'd		Burns	Continue household drills Camp with supervision Teach proper campfire and barbecue care Use safe camping gear, including flame-retardant clothes
Adolescence	Seeking identity and establishment of independence; subject to strong peer pressure; rejects unsought advice; has a need for physical activity; spends most of free time away from home	Drowning	Most important to have cooperation of adolescent when discussing and implementing safety measures See previous sections Never too late to learn to swim Enroll in lifesaving classes
		Firearms accidents	Avoid having loaded guns in household Learn safety handling if involved in sport hunting Keep guns in locked closet and ammunition in separate locked area Never assume gun is not loaded Never point gun at another
		Automobile-related accidents	Take drivers education Use seat belts for self and passengers Practice pedestrian safety Do not drive under influence of drugs or alcohol Do not hitchhike or pick up hitchhikers
		Alcohol, drugs, and tobacco	Discuss effects of substance use and abuse Assist teen to identify other ways to achieve self-esteem, independence, and peer acceptance

Infectious diseases

Disease	Presentation	Management
Viral infections		
Hepatitis	See Table 24-3	Home care and supportive treatment, including rest and well-balanced diet with sufficient calories and vitamin B complex supplements Isolation: enteric precautions Prophylaxis: Gamma globulin or hepatitis B immune globulin
Herpes simplex	Seen as gingivostomatitis in young children with reinfections being localized as "cold sores" or "fever blisters"; abrupt onset with fever, irritability, anorexia, and sore mouth; red swollen gums with small vesicles appearing on palate, tongue, and mucosa	Supportive treatment, particularly mouth care of petroleum jelly for cracking and mouth washes, rinses and analgesics for pain; secretion precautions should be observed Diet: soft, bland foods; cool liquids — avoidance of citrus juices General measures as for influenza
Herpes zoster (shingles)	Uncommon under age 10; characterized by pain and crops of vesicles confined to an area of distribution of one of spinal or cranial sensory nerves; malaise and fever may accompany vesicles	Symptomatic treatment of wet compresses, calamine lotion (for lesions), and aspirin (for pain)

Influenza	Rapid onset of chills, fever, headache, generalized aches and malaise, anorexia, and prostration; frequently young children experience vomiting and diarrhea; hacking cough and rhinitis frequently develop	Symptomatic treatment including these general measures:
		A. Fever
		  1. Antipyretic medication
		  2. Tepid sponge bath
		  3. Liberal fluid intake
		  4. Rest and limited activity

Infectious diseases — cont'd

Disease	Presentation	Management

Influenza — cont'd		B. Upper respiratory infections
		  1. Liberal fluid intake
		  2. Cool mist vaporizer
		  3. Decongestants
		  4. Warm gargle, saline mouth/throat irrigations
		  5. Cool liquids and soft foods for throat and mouth irritations
		  6. Petroleum jelly to protect nares and lips
		C. Aches and malaise
		  1. Rest and limited activity
		  2. Warm bath
		  3. Body massage
		  4. Cold compresses for headache
		  5. Analgesics
		D. Anoxeria
		  1. Small, frequent feedings of favorite foods and liquids
		  2. Relaxed approach to oral intake
		E. Rash
		  1. Proper hygiene and bathing
		  2. Cool baths, calamine lotion, mild anesthetic ointment, or systemic antihistamines
		  3. short, clean fingernails; gloves or mittens for young children
		  4. Saline mouthwashes if mucous membranes are involved

Measles (rubeola)	Malaise, fever, conjuctivitis, cough 3-4 days before appearance of red-brown or purple-red maculopapular rash, first on face, hairline, and neck, proceeding to trunk and extremities; Koplek's spots appear about 12 hours before rash on buccal mucosa; rash lasts 5-7 days	General measures as for influenza; emphasis on avoiding bright lights if photophobic and using warm water to cleanse eyes Respiratory and discharge precautions Prevention: active immunization
Mononucleosis (infectious)	Mild symptoms of headache, malaise, and fatigue; fever and sore throat, tonsils enlarged, red and covered with membrane; lymph adenopathy and splenomegaly are common	General measures as for influenza; emphasis on bed rest with gradual increase in activity; no strenuous activity while spleen is enlarged; no social contact until acute phase is over
Mumps (parotitis)	Prodrome of fever, headache, anorexia, malaise, and muscle pain. Local pain around ear and jaw within 24-48 hours, followed by swelling of parotial gland.	General measures as for influenza; emphasis on avoidance of citrus foods and fluids; alleviation of pain with aspirin and warm or cold compresses; respiratory precautions; Prevention: active immunization
Roseola (exanthem subitum)	High fever & irritability for 3-4 days followed by rose-pink, maculopapular rash, beginning on chest and spreading to trunk and face; rash lasts several hours to 2 days; fever falls to normal as rash appears	General measures as for influenza; support for parents as fever may not respond or subside for 3-5 days
Rubella (german measles)	No prodrome. Pink-red maculopapular rash first on face, progressing to neck, trunk, extremities; lasts 3-5 days	General measures as for influenza; exposure of first-trimester pregnant women to be avoided Prevention: active immunization
Varcella (chickenpox)	May have 1-2 days of fever and malaise followed by macular rash that evolves to papular to vesicles to crusts; rash appears on trunk and in crops and may progress to hairline and face; all lesions eventually dry and crust	General measures as for influenza; emphasis on skin care, alleviation of itching by cornstarch baths, systemic antipruritic medication (Benadryl) and topical lotions (calamine); general skin hygiene of bathing, changing bed linen and clothes frequently, keeping nails short and clean; isolate until vesicles dried and observe respiratory and secretion precautions

Continued.

Infectious diseases — cont'd

Disease	Presentation	Management
Bacterial infections		
Cellulitis	Affected area is warm, tender, erythematous, swollen and indurated; fever, malaise, and lymphadenopathy are present; caused by staphylococcus aureus, group A beta-hemolytic streptococci, or hemophilus influenza	Employ general measures as described under influenza; systemic antibiotic therapy; warm compresses and immobilization of affected part
Meningitis	Varies with age and causative organism	Requires medical referral and antibiotic therapy that will be determined by weight of child and depends on causative agent
	Neonates. Escherichia coli and group B streptococci common causative agents; onset is insidious: poor tone, sucking feeding difficulties, poor cry, vomiting, irritability, drowsy or irritable, jittery; tense, full, bulging fontanelle	Parent counseling regarding diagnosis and disease process is indicated as well as convalescent care and follow-up care
	Infants. Most common causative agents: hemophelus influenza, neisseria meningitides; Unexplained febrile illness preceded by respiratory or gastrointestinal infection; accompanied by irritability, fever, anorexia, vomiting, drowsiness, and high pitch cry; fontanelle may be bulging; nuchal rigidity signs may be difficult to elicit	
	Older children. Causative agent as for infants; fever, chills, vomiting, severe headache, stiff neck; nuchal rigidity and positive Kernig's and Brudzinski's signs	
	Meningococcemia. A medical emergency with rapidly developing petechial and purpuric rash, preceded by 24-hour period of fever, vomiting, irritability, and nuchal rigidity	
Scarlet fever (scarlatini)	Abrupt onset of fever, sore throat, vomiting, headache, and chills followed by bright red rash that blanches on pressure; rash has rough sandpaper texture and appears first on flexor surfaces, rapidly becoming more generalized; lasts 7 days, followed by desquamation of hands and feet.	General measures as for influenza; Penicillin is antibiotic of choice, unless allergy is present and erythromycin is indicated; prepare parents for skin desquamation; Follow-up care and throat culture is advisable as well as examination for signs of rheumatic fever and glomerulonephritis; advisable to obtain throat cultures on household contacts
Tuberculosis	Causative agents are *Mycobacterium tuberculosis* and *M. bovis*; most common portal of entry is lung where disease begins; bacilli multiply in lung parenchyma and create area of inflammatory exudate, possibly experienced as low-grade fever and productive cough; bacilli are also carried through lymphatic system to regional lymph nodes creating lymphadenopathy; hypersensitivity occurs when bacilli multiply and die as tissue reaction to bacilli changes; primary lesion becomes encapsulated and walled off; may resolve or calcify as evidenced by x-ray findings and positive tuberculin reaction	Active tuberculosis: antimicrobial therapy and general supportive measures Prevention: if positive skin test and no clinical demonstrated disease, prophylatic treatment with INH is recommended if Child is under 4 years Child has recently converted from negative to positive Skin reaction Child with positive skin test has known exposure to active TB Child with inactive primary TB has never been treated All contacts with person with active tuberculosis should be skin tested, positive reactions treated and negative skin tests retested in 6 weeks and at least every 3 months for duration of contact; infants should be removed from contact with infected person until at least 6 months after all cultures are reported as negative Prevention: tuberculin testing

Common concerns and problems of toddler and preschool years

Problem and assessment	Nursing intervention

Aggressive and negative behaviors

Biting and hitting

Temporary behaviors occurring as a result of normal aggressive impulses and most frequently happening in new or difficult situations, when tired or hungry or frustrated or when expectations are too high in terms of social behaviors (ability to play with peers); used as a means of asserting control or power

Reassure parents that behaviors are normal; discuss development and tasks child is trying to accomplish
Advise parents to
  Avoid retaliation by hitting or biting back
  Cup chin or hold hand giving reminder that biting and/or hitting is unacceptable
  Anticipate circumstances in which behaviors occur and circumvent them
  Use limits such as isolation if helpful
  Limit playmates and playtime to what is reasonable for child and his age
  Allow child and playmate to work out difficulties as much as possible, redirecting their play when necessary

Verbal negativism

Use of the word "no" as means of control in striving for independence; often used indiscriminately and inappropriately

Advise parents to
  Offer child a choice when possible, making alternatives simple
  Avoid bargaining and arguments
  If no choice is available, do not offer one — approach with a matter-of-fact attitude
  Develop strategy for times when child will choose and then change his mind

Temper tantrums

Developmental behavior directed at gaining control; Frequently triggered by unmet needs (tired, hungry), frustration and/or overgratification and need for limits; ascertain when tantrums occur and how they are handled

Management by parents should be directed at finding cause and prevention; counseling is directed toward approaches to discipline and limit setting (see section on discipline) and the following:
  Discussion of child's need for limits at this age
  Diary can be kept to identify pattern when tantrums occur
  Intervention is made before tantrum begins

Should tantrum occur, possible approaches include the following:
  Calm, matter-of-fact approach by parents
  Isolation of child by removal to neutral room until control is achieved
  Hold and comfort child until control is achieved, possibly offering substitute for desired object or activity that triggered tantrum
  Use of corporal punishment (spanking) to achieve control

Discipline

Discipline is guidance offered by parents to assist child in demonstrating correct, acceptable safe behaviors; discipline is based on the parent's concepts, feelings, and attitudes regarding desirable behaviors and rules of conduct for them; mechanisms of discipline will set limits and control undesirable behaviors

Advise parents regarding different approaches to discipline:
  Permissiveness
  Overpermissiveness
  Authoritarianism
Advise parents that setting limits should permit self-respect and protection of parent and child integrity; parents should be aware that discipline is essential to healthy growth
Parent techniques include the following:
  Set examples of desirable behaviors (honesty, unselfishness, good manners)
  Be fair, clear, and consistent
  Agree on methods of discipline
  Give simple clear directions; bend a little by giving warnings
  Allow child to express feelings
  Respect your child; be sure to praise, show approval, and encourage
  Be realistic in behaviors expected
  Avoid arguing, threatening, promising, sermonizing, overpermissiveness, and an overauthoritarian manner
  Discipline (punishing the act)

Continued.

Problem and assessment	Nursing intervention

Punishment

A method of controlling behaviors when limits are exceeded and based on child being made to feel guilty for misdeed; guilt will eventually inhibit impulse to commit act; punishment may be verbal, restrictive, or physical and should always be appropriate to the act; most punishment is the result of parent loss of temper

Advise parents to
  Allow a cooling-off period
  Direct anger at situation or act, not child
  Avoid retaliation by hitting, belittling, sarcasm, ridicule, humiliation, or shame
  Avoid sending to bed or going without food
  Avoid depriving child of love to examine their feelings and experiences regarding punishment. Remind them that it can be an effective method of discipline with appropriate motivation and intent
Review points discussed in discipline section

Breathholding

A high indicator of a disturbed parent-child relationship, this symptom may be caused by overprotection, a tense rigid daily schedule, or prematurely enforced toilet training regime; it has a high familial incidence and is characterized by a preceding temper tantrum, with child holding breath and turning blue

Ascertain circumstances that trigger episodes and how handled by parents

Counseling directed toward guidance and education regarding parent-child relationship; parents will need reassurance and support as they attempt to
  Ignore breathholding in an attempt to prevent child satisfaction in gaining control
  Redirect relationship with child emphasizing meeting of his needs in a positive way, reinforcing desireable behaviors

See section on discipline

Rocking, head banging, bed shaking

Forms of self-stimulation as a result of undergratification; frequently occurs at bedtime; ascertain how child's needs are met

Counseling directed toward advising parents regarding
  Gratification of needs
  Avoidance of letting child "cry it out"
  Provision of comfort and extra stimulation time
  Provision of relaxed, calm atmosphere through holding, singing, music

Masturbation

A normal reaction, which is an exploration of body that results in stimulation of pleasurable sexual feelings; generally occurs at bedtime and starts accidentally becoming more purposeful and frequent around 4 years

Ascertain frequency, how parents handle, and their attitude and feelings.

Advise parents that masturbation is normal and that censoring of open masturbation is appropriate; otherwise parents should convey to child that they are aware of and understand the behavior
Avoidance of placing excessive importance on masturbation which may only encourage it; it is best to ignore it and/or set limits as appropriate to situation
A punitive attitude should be avoided

Persistent thumb sucking

A form of self-comfort occuring in times of stress and persisting beyond 3 to 4 years; generally sporadic sucking is harmless and regular sucking until 2 or 3 is considered normal

Assist parents to identify source of stress and ways to alleviate it.
  Reassure and support parents when thumb sucking is within normal range
  Suggest parents remove fingers or thumb from mouth after asleep
  Suggest parents avoid constant nagging and reminding; pulling thumb from mouth; use of restraints, foul-tasting medications, or bandages

Feeding-related problems

Loss or variations of appetite; refusal of food
Common problems related to: "too busy to eat," development of food preferences; a normal decrease in amount of food required and/or an attempt to control and assert independence

See pp. 577-579 for anticipatory guidance

Sleep-related problems

Nightmares
Problems may follow a tiring busy day, be associated with illness, or be the result of working things out in dreams
Nightmares are frightening dreams that awaken child who feels fear and helplessness; they generally occur as a result of increased aggressive urges

Review normal sleep patterns with parents (Table 23-6)
Reassure parents that dreams and terrors are normal and tend to disappear spontaneously
Parents should comfort child when awakened by dream — may attempt to explain they are not "real"
Parents should avoid making a fuss over these sleep problems

Night terrors
These are dreams, generally frightening in nature, from whch a child does not awaken; after acting out dream and/or a period of disorientation, child returns to sleep

Common concerns and problems of toddler and preschool years—cont'd

Problem and assessment	Nursing intervention

Toilet training

Achievement of control over bodily elimination; development of habits that make child self-sufficient in toileting; parents need to understand child's development and readiness before instituting a toilet training regime (see following); parent must ascertain attitude and expectations regarding toilet training as well as measures previously used

Indicators of readiness to toilet train	Approximate age (yr)
1. Manipulates sphincter muscles	1½-2
2. Manual dexterity needed to manipulate clothing	2-2½
3. Can hold urine for up to 4 to 5 hours	2-2½
4. Can understand simple directions	1½-2
5. Can communicate needs using words or gestures	1½-2
6. Developed a sense of self	1-2
7. Demonstrates trust in mother and desire to please	1½-2
8. Demonstrates sense of independence and a desire to do for self	2-2½
9. Is proud of own accomplishments	2-2½
10. Demonstrates behavioral control	2-2½

Direct counseling toward parental understanding of realistic expectations, readiness of child, types of toilet training and frequent problems encountered

Types of toilet training:

A. Early training from ages 10 months to 15 months; Points to emphasize:
   1. Child is not physiologically able to use toilet at this age
   2. Parents may be ready to train child, but they will be the ones who will have to pick up signals, put child on toilet, undress and redress, etc.; therefore, they should be highly motivated
   3. Bowel training may be accomplished but accidents will happen and will be due to trainer (parent), not trainee (child)
   4. Training should not be stressful for parent or child

B. Training at 18-30 months; points to emphasize:
   1. Review readiness signs and check off which ones child has accomplished. If the majority have been achieved, probably appropriate to start training
   2. Select a good time such as when
      There are no major changes in household and child has shown some interest after observing others
      Nursery school friends are trained
      Child is aware of wet and dirty versus dry and clean
   3. Select a method and stick to it
   4. Training should not be stressful; if child resists it is best to forget for awhile then try again
   5. Accomplishment of training is variable; It may be a few days or several weeks or months
   6. Parents need to develop a relaxed, positive attitude
   7. Alternative methods include
      Place child on own potty chair at given intervals during the day
      Place child on potty before elimination is expected
      Place child on potty when parent goes
      Always positively reinforce a successful attempt

C. "Natural" toilet training (children training themselves), points to emphasize:
   1. Toileting is brought to child's attention when readiness is indicated
   2. Child handles situation by himself
   3. Child needs to know parents are willing to help
   4. Although enjoying a sense of independence and accomplishment, child also needs limits set at this age

Problems are frequently encountered; reassure parents about naturalness, normalcy and transient nature of these problems:
   1. Problem with sitting or standing for boys; suggest starting training with sitting progressing to standing
   2. Problem using large toilet; suggest potty chair with portable seat which can be taken on excursions
   3. Regression; suggest reinforcing as little as possible; depending on severity may require going back to diapers for awhile
   4. Need help with wiping; suggest allowing child to try if wants to clean self
   5. Being able to communicate toilet needs to others; suggest parents make sure other caretakers are aware of child's progress in training, how he communicates need, what words and what degree of independence have been achieved
   6. Child does not wish to flush bowel movements; suggest this point not be emphasized; flush toilet later
   7. Playing with feces; suggest play with clay or fingerpaints; parent should matter-of-factly state displeasure when this occurs

Health problem	Etiology	Incidence	Assessment	Management	Prevention
Urinary tract infections	Bacteria enter urinary tract through urethra	5% to 10% of girls and 1% of boys experience a UTI before 18 years	History of signs and symptoms urgency frequency burning, dribbling, foul-smelling urine, fever, irritability, GI symptoms; *may be asymptommatic*	2-week medication course based on causative organism, age, weight of child, sensitivity of organism to drug and previous occurrences	Routine urine screening, particularly for girls early in life (1-2 years)
	Predisposing factors include Short female urethra Obstruction Foreign body Poor hygiene and/or fecal contamination Incomplete bladder emptying resulting in urine stasis Chemical irritants Pinworms Indwelling catheters or catheterization Sexual intercourse Pregnancy	More frequent in girls than boys	Laboratory signs: bacteria on urine culture of greater than 100,000 colonies of a single bacteria per ml of urine confirms infection in symptommatic child.	Medication frequently used: Sulfisoxiazole (Gantrisin) Ampicillin Nitrofurantoin (Furandantin) Cephalexin (Keflex)	Hygiene education: Wipe front to back Frequent voiding (3-4 hours) with complete bladder emptying Avoid bubble baths and harsh detergents Use cotton versus nylon panties Avoid tight clothing Adequate fluid intake
	Causative organisms: Escherichia coli accounts for 80% to 85% of cases) Gram-positive organisms (Staphylococcus aureus) Klebsiella, enterobacteria, Pseudomonas, and Proteus			Increased fluid and rest	Prompt attention for recurrent symptoms
				Symptomatic measures for generalized signs Follow-up is essential: Urine culture 48-72 hours after medication is instituted Urine culture on completion of medication Further follow-up at 1 month (U/A culture); 3 months; 6 months; 12 months (physical exam); 18 months; 24 months (physical exam); annually	

Health problems of school age child — cont'd

Health problem	Etiology	Incidence	Assessment	Management	Prevention
Bacterial infections					
Impetigo	Superficial skin lesion invaded by staphyloccoci or streptococci, spread by direct contact with incubation of 2-10 days	Potential risk for glomerulonephrites	Appearance of discolored spots that form vesicles or bullae; these vesicles break and form yellow, honey-colored seropurulent lesions Most frequently on hands, face, or perineum and accompanied by regional lymphadenopathy Culture fluid from lesion or at base of lesion	Topical treatment with Bacitracin or neomycin ointment after soaking with warm compresses. Systemic antibiotic if numerous lesions are present Follow-up if not improved with 3 days	Teach child not to pick or scratch insect bites, healing lesions, etc. Keep nails short and clean Frequent handwashing Isolate child's washing and bed linen, drinking glass, and clothes Inspect other family members Adequate rest and nutrition
Cellulitis	Bacterial invasion of skin (both dermis and subcutaneous tissue) caused by Staphylococcus aureus, group A beta-hemolytic streptococci, or Hemophilus influenza Less communicable than impetigo but suspect throughout infection; more apt to lead to septicemia	Frequently a secondary infection to impetigo or other skin lesions	Warm tender, erythematous, swollen, and indurated area on skin Lymphangitis seen on extremeties Fever, malaise, lymphadenapathy often present	Warm compresses Immobilization of affected part Rest and symptomatic measures Systemic antibiotic therapy	Prevention as for impetigo All family members should be cultured and those with positive cultures treated
Streptococcal pharyngitis	Group A-Beta hemolytic streptococcus	Increased incidence in winter and spring 30-50% of cases appear in school-age children At risk for complications of cervical adenitis, otitis media, peritonsillar abscess, sinusitis, acute glomerulonephritis, acute rheumatic fever	Must differentiate from viral pharyngitis Obtain throat culture	10-day course of penicillen when strep confirmed by culture Repeat culture at end of medication course Symptomatic treatment for fever reduction; normal saline gargles, hard sour candy for sore throat; hot or cold compresses for tender cervical nodes	Culture all symptommatic exposed family contacts Avoid contact with infected child and his eating/drinking utensils Education regarding illness and necessity of full treatment course of medication

Continued.

Health problems of school age child — cont'd

Health problem	Etiology	Incidence	Assessment	Management	Prevention
Bacterial infections—cont'd					
Tuberculosis	Communicated through sputum and cough spray of infected person Causative organism are Mycobacterium tuberculosis and M. bovis Incubation range is 2 to 10 weeks	Most at risk in first 3 years and the second year preceding puberty For children of all ages, an average of 4,000 new cases are reported annually Predisposing factors include state of health and nutrition; age; environmental and socioeconomic circumstances (crowding, poor sanitation); virulence and number of bacilli	Development of overt symptoms occurs in small percentage Demonstrated systemic hypersensitivity as evidenced by positive skin test Chest x-ray to determine presence and extent of active lesions Sputum smears	Rest, adequate diet, and gradual return to normal activity; prevention of other infection Drug therapy Counseling and support	Screening tests particularly for at risk population Identify, screen, and treat contacts Hygiene and sputum precautions/measures
Parasitic infections					
Scabies	Caused by parasite, female mite that burrows into stratum corneum of skin and lays eggs in the tunnel Transmitted by direct contact with infected person; can be contracted from infected bedding and clothing	Pandemic in U.S. since 1974	Vesicular or papulovesicular rash occurring typically on genitals, buttocks, between fingers and in folds of wrist, elbows, armpits, and at beltline Appear as fine wavy line; gray to pink in color Pruritus is worse at night Skin scrapings from over lesion reveal mite presence under microscope	Scabecide (Kwell) applied to affected areas; one application is generally sufficient — may be repeated Clothing and bedding should be washed	Avoid contact with infected person's bedding and clothing Family members should do self-skin inspection
Tinea capitis (scalp), corporis (body), pedis (foot)	Fungal infection frequently transmitted by dogs and cats; caused by Microsporum canis or by Trichophyton transmitted by humans	Increased incidence in puberty Permanent baldness may occur with severe capitis	Capitis: bald patches with erythema, gray scaling, and crusting Corporis: macule that enlarges peripherally, healing in center to present as scaly, circular lesions found on face, upper extremities, and trunk; may have mild pruritus	Capitis: grisofulvin — follow-up cultures should be done Corporis: tolnaftate (tinactin) 1% solution or cream Pedis: tolnaftate (Tinactin) solution or cream and Desenex or tinactin powder prophylactically	Capitis: avoid exchange of head gear; avoid/treat infected animal; wash scalp after haircuts; avoid use of infected person's personal care articles Corporis: preceding plus avoiding exchange of clothing and community showers or bathing places

Health problem	Etiology	Incidence	Assessment	Management	Prevention
Parasitic infections—cont'd					
Tinea capitis — cont'd			Pedis: vasicular eruptions with skin maceration between toes Laboratory procedures: (1) microscopic exam with KOH; (2) ultraviolet light fluoresces Microsporum infections; (3) microscopic culture		Pedis: preceding plus thoroughly dry between toes; use cotton socks and change frequently wear well ventilated shoes; air feet; wear rubber sandals in community showers
Dental					
Caries	Progressive lesions of calcified dental tissue characterized by tooth structure loss Bacteria, carbohydrates, and plaque are definite factors producing tooth decay	50%-97% of children have 1 or more cavities by 6 years of age Greatest incidence occurs between 4 to 8 years and 12 to 18 years	Characterized as discolored areas or actual lesion in fissures of chewing surfaces of teeth May be visible on inspection Dental equipment and x-rays most reliable in detecting caries	Dental referral Prevention	Preventive measures: Early institution of dental care and visits Brushing and flossing after every meal Water fluoridation; oral supplemental fluorideif indicated; fluoride rinses Topical fluoride application and use of toothpaste fluoride containing fluoride. Limited carbohydrate content of diet (see Table 25-12)
Malocclusion	Irregularities of tooth alignment and improper fitting of teeth Causative factors: abnormal jaw alignment; abnormal muscle function; incompatibility of tooth and jaw size creating abnormal spacing, crowding or teeth irregularities; delayed permanent teeth eruption; prolonged retention of primary teeth; neglected teeth; prolonged occurrence of lip biting, mouth breathing, tongue twisting, teeth grinding, thumb sucking	Most frequently recognized in early school age years Not common in deciduous teeth	Variation of normal occlusion of top molars meeting firmly on opposing bottom posterior teeth with upper incisors barely overlapping and touching bottom anterior incisors	Dental referral Prevention	Preventive measures: Meeting early sucking needs Avoidance of prolonged use of bottle over 2 years Weaning to cup at 1 year to promote jaw and mouth development after sucking Gentle reminder about finger/thumb sucking, lip biting, etc. Remove finger, thumb from mouth when child is sleeping

Continued.

Health problems of school age child — cont'd

Health problem	Etiology	Incidence	Assessment	Management	Prevention
Obesity					
	Causes are related to organic problem and imbalance between caloric intake and energy expenditure Influencing factors: Genetic Activity patterns Metabolic rate Number and size of fat cells Nutritional habits Attitude about feeding Quantity of food ingested	Approximately 10% to 30% of American children are considered obese	Clinically children with weight 20% above the mean for their age and height are obese with those 10% to 20% over mean defined as overweight Organic problems must be ruled out Nutritional status and diet history (see Tables 23-19 and 24-6 and pp. 616-618	Referral if organic problem indicated Weight control or reduction plan that modifies eating habits, reduces caloric intake, increases energy expenditure, and promotes sense of well-being and self-esteem Early prevention	Preventive measures: Encourage breast feeding Avoid overfeeding in infancy/early childhood including milk Teach nutritional needs to parents Encourage healthful eating habits Avoid extra caloric foods (sweetened water, candy as reward) Delay early introduction of solids Encourage home-prepared baby foods and meals for older children Avoid commercially prepared baby dinners and meals for older children Encourage physical activity

Common behaviors of school age child and adolescent

Behavior	Development	Guidance
School age		
Cheating	Testing right and wrong; generally follow parents' rules and authority but may succumb to peer pressure to "break rules"; becoming more aware of their parents "cheating" in different ways	Assist parents to 　Reinforce positive "good" behaviors 　Maintain limits and discipline standards 　Recognize that most children confess or are caught and that disciplinary action must be immediate 　Identify what prompted cheating
Lying	Differentiating between fantasies and realities; use of untruth to avoid the unpleasant; becoming more aware of parents not always telling the truth	Confront and assess problem with assistance from teacher and involvement of child Reassure child that a real world of absolute truthfulness does not exist Point out to child untruths that are fantasies, emphasizing the real component Use discipline for act and discuss meaning of untruths Reinforce honest behaviors positively
Stealing	Curiosity about other possessions; continue to learn and internalize concept of "mine" versus "yours"; not easy to resist temptation; limited idea of property	Act as role model; respect child's property and spouse's property; ask before use Reinforce concept of property and ownership verbally as well as behaviorally Discipline for petty acts, e.g., have child return or pay back item; use verbal disapproval Assess, help, and seek referral if problem is persistent
Fighting	More boys than girls fight; siblings usually fight; an attempt to establish position for self; may be result of frustration	Act as role model; parents who verbally and physically fight indicate behavior is acceptable Establish behaviors that are acceptable as vents for frustration/and anger Emphasize the need to share, exchange, and interact in positive manner

Behavior	Development	Guidance
School age—cont'd		
Fighting — cont'd		Separate siblings when fighting; then allow them to work out differences once composure is regained
		Avoid condoning physical assault as a means of retaliation with peers; assist child to find other solutions
		Discover reason for fighting if it is continual
Scatology	Uses dirty words as means of attention and testing parents; frequently has no understanding of meaning	Set an example; do not use dirty words in front of child
		Indicate unacceptability of dirty words; remind when child uses
		Avoid a struggle, argument, or excessive discipline unless profound problem exists
		Seek help if persistent
Fears	Often learned from parents; indicative of struggle to cope with unknown or unpleasant experience; may be result of learning right from wrong.	Deal with each fear separately
		Avoid overemphasis of own fear
		Identify what specifically about situation evokes fear
		Reassure child; reinforce that some fears are healthy and protective in nature
		Seek help if fears interfere with daily life
Adolescent		
Moodiness/non-communicative	Result of emotional conflicts of establishing an identity, developing sexually, and worries over body image and social relationships	Assist adolescent and parents to:
		Feel reassured about normalcy of wanting to be alone, mood swings, and fears
		Recognize and discuss family conflicts and possible solutions
		Recognize and discuss importance of communication and need to validate feelings
Preoccupation with body image and sexuality	Physical changes are dramatic; need to be the same as peers; sexual fantasies and erotic urges and behaviors are heightened with physiological changes	Recognize normalcy of feelings and preoccupation
		Understand normal physical growth, physiological changes, and individual patterns
		Accept self; develop constructive coping behaviors (e.g., sublimate into activity; need to verbalize feelings)
		Identify other resources of information: courses at school books, etc.
		Encourage physical activity as tension release.
Rebellion	Need to establish own value and belief system	Alleviate conflicts through open communication and validation of feelings
		Roleplay and offer reflective feedback to each other
		Focus on individual needs and place value and pressure from others in perspective
Conformity	Need for allegiance and belonging; assists in challenge of authority and developing of self; serves as validation mechanism	Reinforce positive aspects of peer group and what is taught by them
		Recognize normalcy of need
		Find solutions when conformity interferes with adolescents and family's goals
Inferiority feelings	Result of feelings of loneliness and being different when unable to conform to peer group	Relate importance of social involvement to individual goals
		Explore interest and participation in after-school activities
		Recognize feelings about self (what he/or she likes/and dislikes and what are desired changes)
		Identify solutions to problem behaviors identified
Poor study habits	May result from disinterest, preoccupation, excessive parent expectations	Identify cause of poor habits; may need remedial help or assistance in developing constructive habits
		Avoid nagging or conflict over issue
		Identify constructive solutions
		Identify feelings and attitudes
		Discuss individual goals, methods of meeting goals as related to ability and consequences.
Ambivalence	An attempt to identify dependent versus independent needs; reflects conflict between parental rules and own wishes	Identify conflict and possible solutions
		Maintain a system of accountability for behavior and compliance with rules of system
		Deal with feelings constructively (e.g., verbally, physical exercise)
		Recognize importance and normalcy of behavior

ACNE ASSESSMENT QUESTIONNAIRE

History

1. How long have you had acne? _____
2. Did your parents or siblings have acne? _____ How long? _____
3. Are there seasonal variations in your skin? _____ What kind? _____
4. Do you find sunlight is beneficial? _____ Do you use a sunlamp? _____
5. Do you rub your face often? _____
6. Do you use sweatbands? _____ Football helmet? _____ Shoulderpads? _____ Tight collars or turtlenecks? _____ Tight hats? _____
7. Describe changes, if there are any, in your skin that accompany your menstrual period.
8. Are there certain foods that aggravate your skin? _____ If so, list them: _____ What happens? _____
9. Do you feel guilty when you eat certain foods? _____
10. Do your parents and/or friends say eating affects the skin? _____

Hygiene

1. How often do you wash your face? _____
2. What kind of soap: _____ What kind of shampoo and how often? _____
3. How do you wash your face? _____
4. After washing, does your face feel clean? ___ How long do you feel clean? _____
5. Do your parents nag you about washing? _____
6. How often do you pick your pimples? _____ With what? _____
7. What kind of cosmetics do you use? _____ Any moisturizing cream or lotion? _____
8. Do you use pomade on your hair? _____

From Stone, A.C.: Facing up to acne, Pediat Nurs. **8**:229-237, July-Aug. 1982, p. 231.

Medical

1. Have you ever used medication for your skin? _____If so, what have you used? _____ Results? _____ What are you currently using? _____ What is the dose and how often do you use it? _____ Who selected the present treatment? _____
2. List any other medications you take (including birth control pills and over-the-counter preparations). _____
3. Name any other medical problems. _____

Social

1. What is your occupation? _____
2. How many are in your family? . Whom do you live with? .
3. How do you spend leisure time? _____ Favorite hobby? _____
4. If in school, are you satisfied with your performance there? .
5. Whom are you emotionally closest to? _____ What do they say about your skin? _____
6. Describe any changes, if there are any, in your skin when you're upset. _____
7. Most teen-agers have acne. (True—False)
8. Masturbation has no effect on acne. (True—False)
9. Dirty thoughts cause acne. (True—False)
10. My skin makes my life harder. (True—False)
11. I believe I will be successful no matter how I look. (True—False)
12. Clear skin is necessary to be really happy. (True—False)
13. What do your parents and friends say cause acne? _____
14. What bothers you most about your body? _____If you could change your body, what would you do first? _____
15. Do friends tease you about your skin? _____
16. Name something you are good at doing. _____

Appendix K

SCREENING TOOLS

NEONATAL PERCEPTION INVENTORY*

The Neonatal Perception Inventory is easily and quickly administered by telling the mother: "We are interested in learning more about the experiences of mothers and their babies during the first few weeks after delivery. The more we can learn about mothers and their babies, the better we will be able to help other mothers with their babies. We would appreciate it if you would help us to help other mothers by answering a few questions."

The procedures are identical for administering the Average Baby form of the NPI on the first or second postpartum day and the NPI at 1 month of age. The mother is handed the Average Baby form while the individual administering the inventory says: "Although this is your first baby, you probably have some ideas of what most little babies are like. Will you please check the blank you *think* best describes what *most* little babies are like."

The tester waits until the mother has completed the Average Baby form and takes it from the mother and then hands the mother the Your Baby form.†

The procedure for administering the Your Baby forms of the NPI is the same at Time I and Time II. However, the instructions given to the mother vary slightly to take into account the time factor. At Time I the tester tells the mother: "While it is not possible to know for certain what your baby will be like, you probably have some ideas of what your baby will be like. Please check the blank you *think* best describes what *your* baby will be like."

At Time II, she says:

"You have had a chance to live with your baby for a month now. Please check the blank you think best describes your baby."

---

*Information regarding the NPI can be obtained from Broussard, E.R., and Hartner, S.: Further considerations regarding maternal perception of the first born. In Hellmuth, J. editor: Exceptional infant: studies in abnormalities, vol. 2, New York, 1971, Brunner/Mazel.

†The tester remains with the mother during the entire administration procedure.

Method of Scoring

The Average Baby Perception form elicits the mother's concept of the average baby's behavior. The Your Baby Perception form elicits her rating of her own baby. Each of these instruments consists of six single item scales. Values of 1-5 are assigned to each of these scales for each of the inventories. The blank signified none is valued as 1 and a great deal has a value of 5. The lower values on the scale represent the more desirable behavior.

The six scales are totaled with no attempt at weighting the scales for each of the inventories separately. Thus a total score is obtained for the Average Baby and a total score is obtained for the Your Baby.

The total score of Your Baby Perception form is then subtracted from the Average Baby Perception form. The discrepancy constitutes the Neonatal Perception Inventory score.

The inventories have shown both construct and criterion validity.

NEONATAL PERCEPTION INVENTORY I
Average Baby

Although this is your first baby, you probably have some ideas of what most little babies are like. Please check the blank you think best describes the average baby.

How much crying do you think the average baby does?

a great deal	a good bit	moderate amount	very little	none

How much trouble do you think the average baby has in feeding?

a great deal	a good bit	moderate amount	very little	none

How much spitting up or vomiting do you think the average baby does?

a great deal	a good bit	moderate amount	very little	none

How much difficulty do you think the average baby has in sleeping?

a great deal	a good bit	moderate amount	very little	none

How much difficulty does the average baby have with bowel movements?

———— ———— ———— ———— ————
a great deal   a good bit   moderate amount   very little   none

How much trouble do you think the average baby has in settling down to a predictable pattern of eating and sleeping?

———— ———— ———— ———— ————
a great deal   a good bit   moderate amount   very little   none

Your Baby

While it is not possible to know for certain what your baby will be like, you probably have some ideas of what your baby will be like. Please check the blank that you think best describes what your baby will be like.
How much crying do you think your baby will do?

———— ———— ———— ———— ————
a great deal   a good bit   moderate amount   very little   none

How much trouble do you think your baby will have feeding?

———— ———— ———— ———— ————
a great deal   a good bit   moderate amount   very little   none

How much spitting up or vomiting do you think your baby will do?

———— ———— ———— ———— ————
a great deal   a good bit   moderate amount   very little   none

How much difficulty do you think your baby will have sleeping?

———— ———— ———— ———— ————
a great deal   a good bit   moderate amount   very little   none

How much difficulty do you expect your baby to have with bowel movements?

———— ———— ———— ———— ————
a great deal   a good bit   moderate amount   very little   none

How much trouble do you think the average baby has in settling down to a predictable pattern of eating and sleeping?

———— ———— ———— ———— ————
a great deal   a good bit   moderate amount   very little   none

NEONATAL PERCEPTION INVENTORY II

NOTE: Same inventory for average baby is given again.

Your Baby

You have had a chance to live with your baby for a month now. Please check the blank you think best describes your baby.
How much crying has your baby done?

———— ———— ———— ———— ————
a great deal   a good bit   moderate amount   very little   none

How much trouble has your baby had feeding?

———— ———— ———— ———— ————
a great deal   a good bit   moderate amount   very little   none

How much spitting up or vomiting has your baby done?

———— ———— ———— ———— ————
a great deal   a good bit   moderate amount   very little   none

How much difficulty has your baby had in sleeping?

———— ———— ———— ———— ————
a great deal   a good bit   moderate amount   very little   none

How much difficulty has your baby had with bowel movements?

———— ———— ———— ———— ————
a great deal   a good bit   moderate amount   very little   none

How much trouble has your baby had in settling down to a predictable pattern of eating and sleeping?

———— ———— ———— ———— ————
a great deal   a good bit   moderate amount   very little   none

Degree of Bother Inventory

Listed below are some of the things that have sometimes bothered other mothers in caring for their babies. We would like to know if you were bothered about any of these. Please place a check in the blank that best describes how much you were bothered by your baby's behavior in regard to these.

Crying
———— ———— ———— ————
a great deal   somewhat   very little   none

Spitting up or vomiting
———— ———— ———— ————
a great deal   somewhat   very little   none

Sleeping
———— ———— ———— ————
a great deal   somewhat   very little   none

Feeding
———— ———— ———— ————
a great deal   somewhat   very little   none

Elimination
———— ———— ———— ————
a great deal   somewhat   very little   none

Lack of a predictable schedule
———— ———— ———— ————
a great deal   somewhat   very little   none

Other (specify):
———— ———— ———— ————
a great deal   somewhat   very little   none

————————
———— ———— ———— ————
a great deal   somewhat   very little   none

————————
———— ———— ———— ————
a great deal   somewhat   very little   none

————————
———— ———— ———— ————
a great deal   somewhat   very little   none

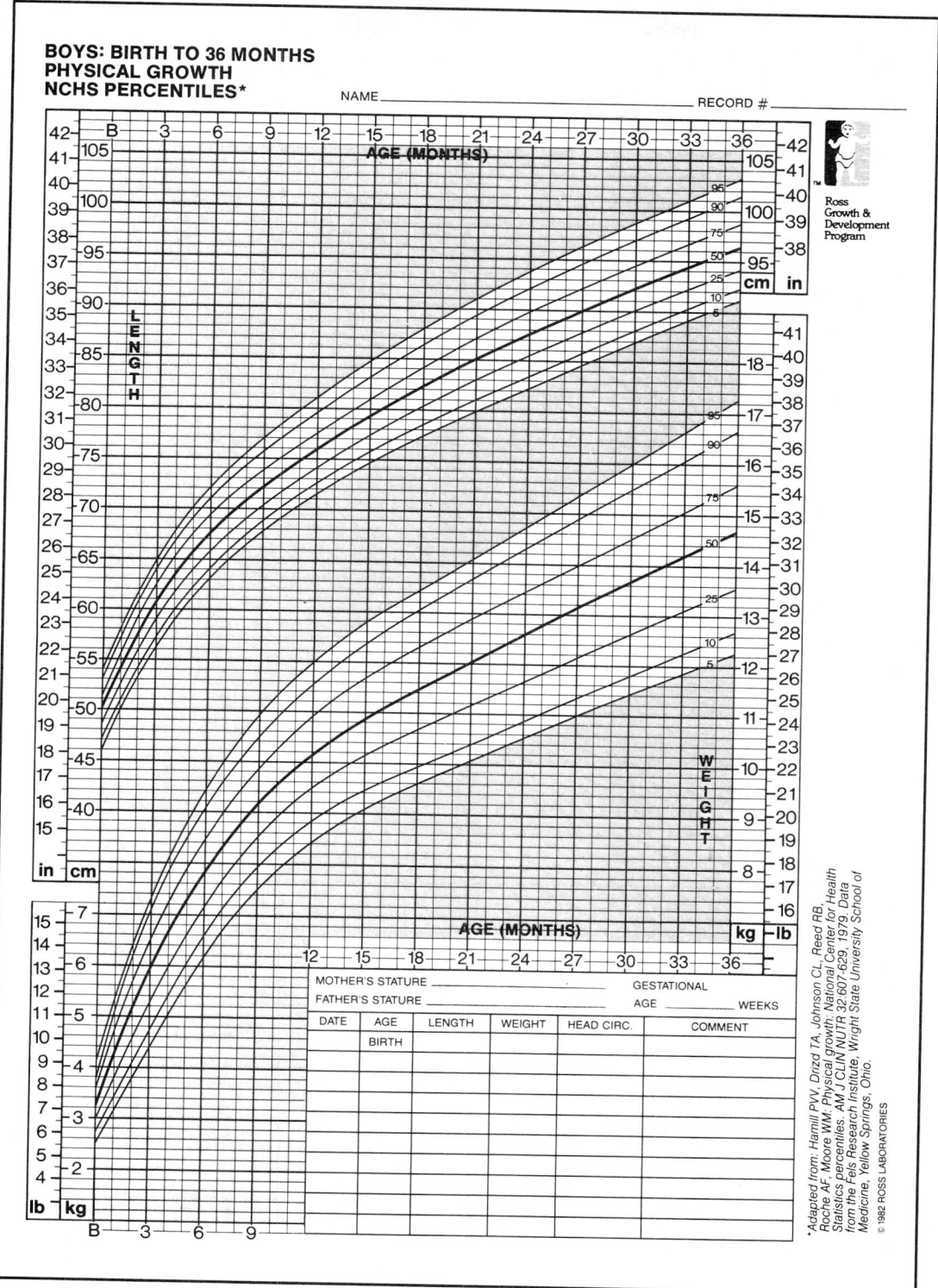

BOYS: BIRTH TO 36 MONTHS
PHYSICAL GROWTH
NCHS PERCENTILES*

NAME_____ RECORD #_____

Ross
Growth &
Development
Program

MOTHER'S STATURE _____ GESTATIONAL
FATHER'S STATURE _____ AGE _____ WEEKS

DATE	AGE	LENGTH	WEIGHT	HEAD CIRC.	COMMENT
	BIRTH				

*Adapted from: Hamill PVV, Drizd TA, Johnson CL, Reed RB, Roche AF, Moore WM: Physical growth: National Center for Health Statistics percentiles. AM J CLIN NUTR 32:607-629, 1979. Data from the Fels Research Institute, Wright State University School of Medicine, Yellow Springs, Ohio.

© 1982 ROSS LABORATORIES

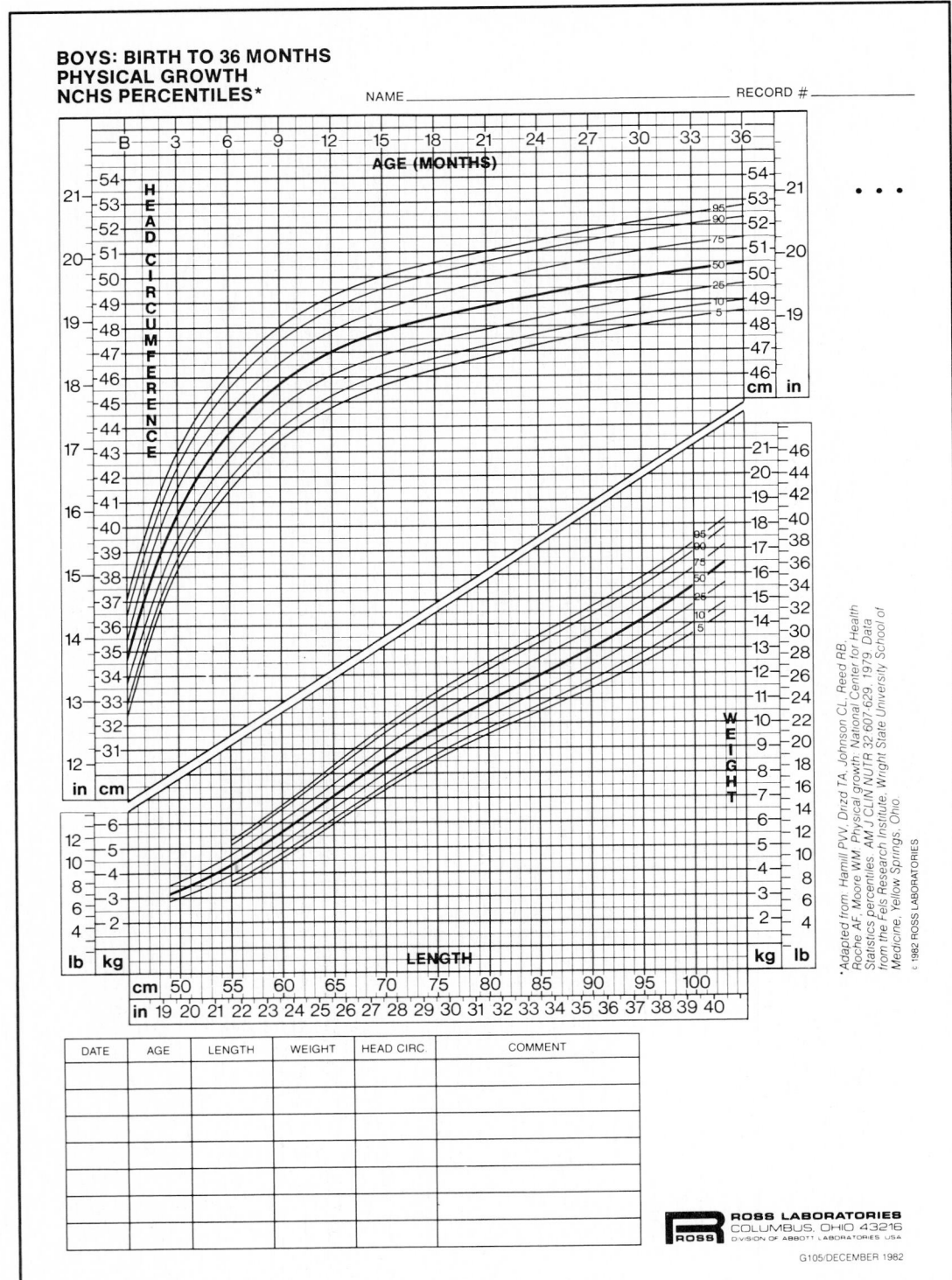

**BOYS: BIRTH TO 36 MONTHS
PHYSICAL GROWTH
NCHS PERCENTILES***

NAME _____   RECORD # _____

AGE (MONTHS)

HEAD CIRCUMFERENCE

WEIGHT

LENGTH

DATE	AGE	LENGTH	WEIGHT	HEAD CIRC.	COMMENT

*Adapted from Hamill PVV, Drizd TA, Johnson CL, Reed RB, Roche AF, Moore WM. Physical growth: National Center for Health Statistics percentiles. AM J CLIN NUTR 32:607-629, 1979. Data from the Fels Research Institute, Wright State University School of Medicine, Yellow Springs, Ohio.

© 1982 ROSS LABORATORIES

ROSS LABORATORIES
COLUMBUS, OHIO 43216
DIVISION OF ABBOTT LABORATORIES USA

G105/DECEMBER 1982

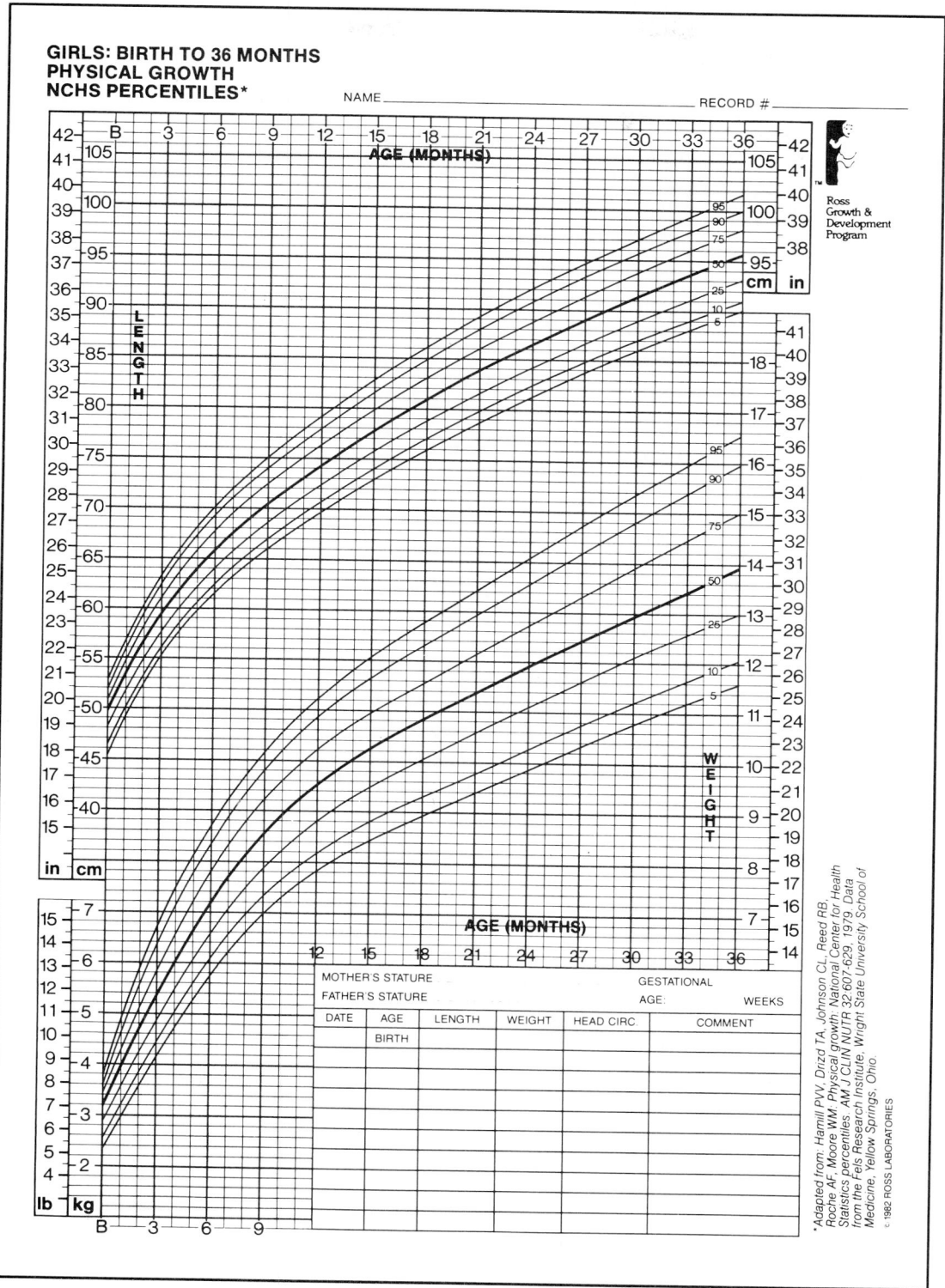

GIRLS: BIRTH TO 36 MONTHS
PHYSICAL GROWTH
NCHS PERCENTILES*

NAME _____   RECORD # _____

Ross
Growth &
Development
Program

*Adapted from: Hamill PVV, Drizd TA, Johnson CL, Reed RB, Roche AF, Moore WM. Physical growth: National Center for Health Statistics percentiles. AM J CLIN NUTR 32:607-629, 1979. Data from the Fels Research Institute, Wright State University School of Medicine, Yellow Springs, Ohio.

© 1982 ROSS LABORATORIES

DATE	AGE	LENGTH	WEIGHT	HEAD CIRC.	COMMENT
	BIRTH				

MOTHER'S STATURE
FATHER'S STATURE
GESTATIONAL AGE: _____ WEEKS

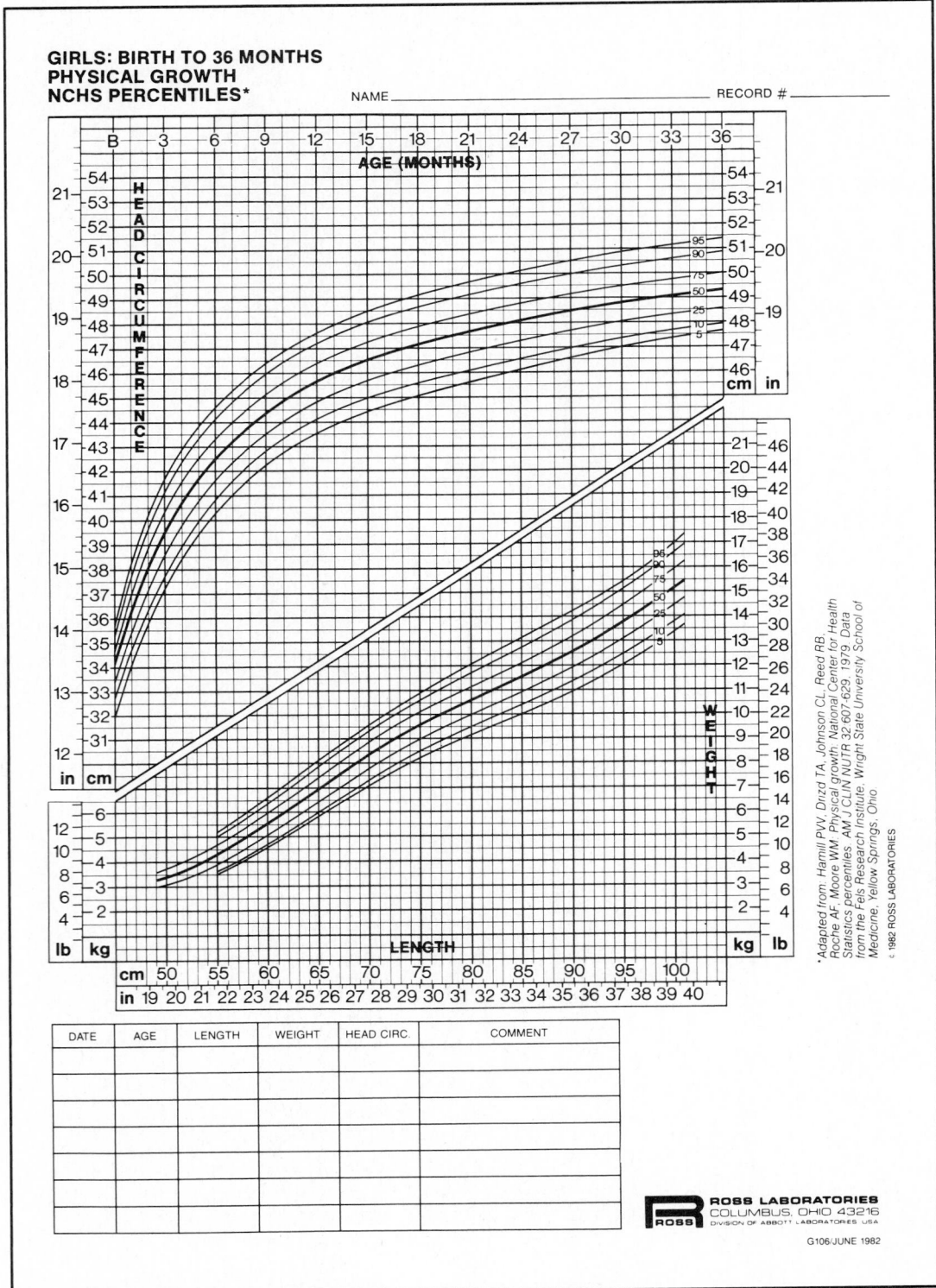

GIRLS: BIRTH TO 36 MONTHS
PHYSICAL GROWTH
NCHS PERCENTILES*

NAME _____ RECORD # _____

*Adapted from: Hamill PVV, Drizd TA, Johnson CL, Reed RB, Roche AF, Moore WM. Physical growth: National Center for Health Statistics percentiles. AM J CLIN NUTR 32:607-629, 1979. Data from the Fels Research Institute, Wright State University School of Medicine, Yellow Springs, Ohio.

© 1982 ROSS LABORATORIES

DATE	AGE	LENGTH	WEIGHT	HEAD CIRC.	COMMENT

ROSS LABORATORIES
COLUMBUS, OHIO 43216
DIVISION OF ABBOTT LABORATORIES USA

G106/JUNE 1982

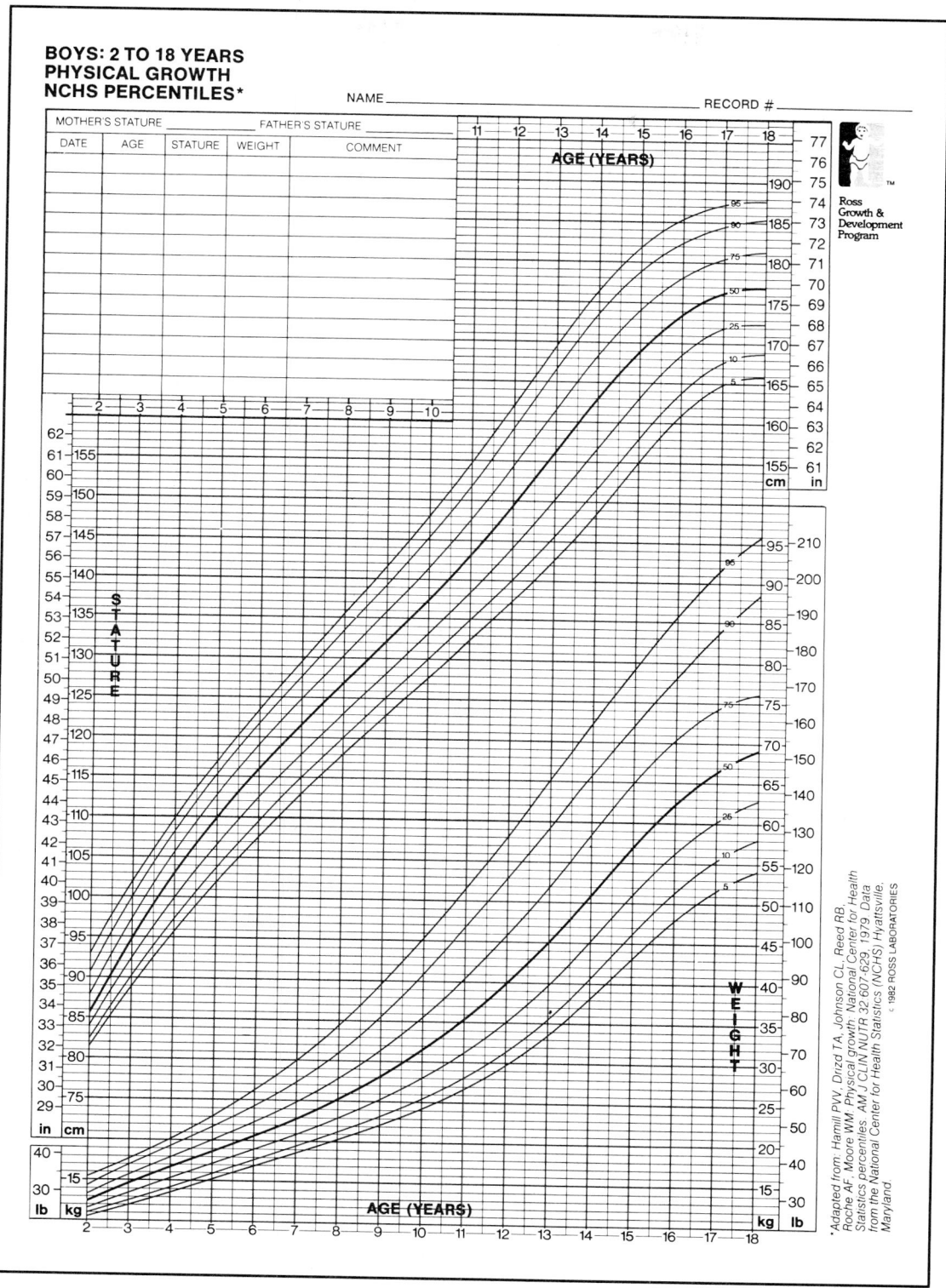

BOYS: 2 TO 18 YEARS
PHYSICAL GROWTH
NCHS PERCENTILES*

NAME _____ RECORD # _____

Ross
Growth &
Development
Program

*Adapted from Hamill PVV, Drizd TA, Johnson CL, Reed RB,
Roche AF, Moore WM. Physical growth: National Center for Health
Statistics percentiles. AM J CLIN NUTR 32:607-629, 1979. Data
from the National Center for Health Statistics (NCHS) Hyattsville,
Maryland.
© 1982 ROSS LABORATORIES

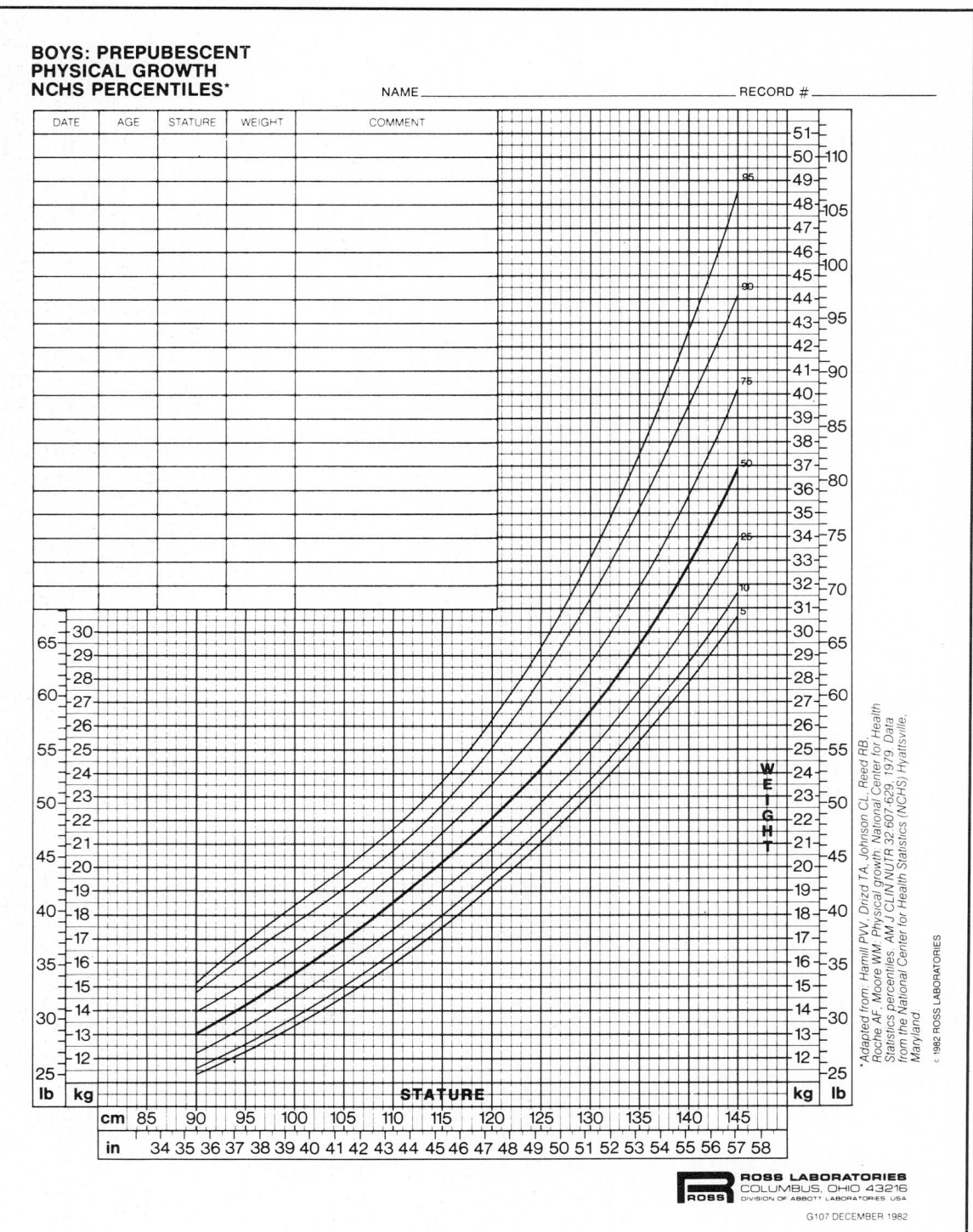

BOYS: PREPUBESCENT PHYSICAL GROWTH NCHS PERCENTILES

NAME _____   RECORD # _____

DATE	AGE	STATURE	WEIGHT	COMMENT

STATURE

cm 85 90 95 100 105 110 115 120 125 130 135 140 145

in 34 35 36 37 38 39 40 41 42 43 44 45 46 47 48 49 50 51 52 53 54 55 56 57 58

WEIGHT

*Adapted from Hamill PVV, Drizd TA, Johnson CL, Reed RB, Roche AF, Moore WM. Physical growth: National Center for Health Statistics percentiles. AM J CLIN NUTR 32:607-629, 1979. Data from the National Center for Health Statistics (NCHS) Hyattsville, Maryland.

© 1982 ROSS LABORATORIES

ROSS LABORATORIES
COLUMBUS, OHIO 43216
DIVISION OF ABBOTT LABORATORIES USA

G107 DECEMBER 1982

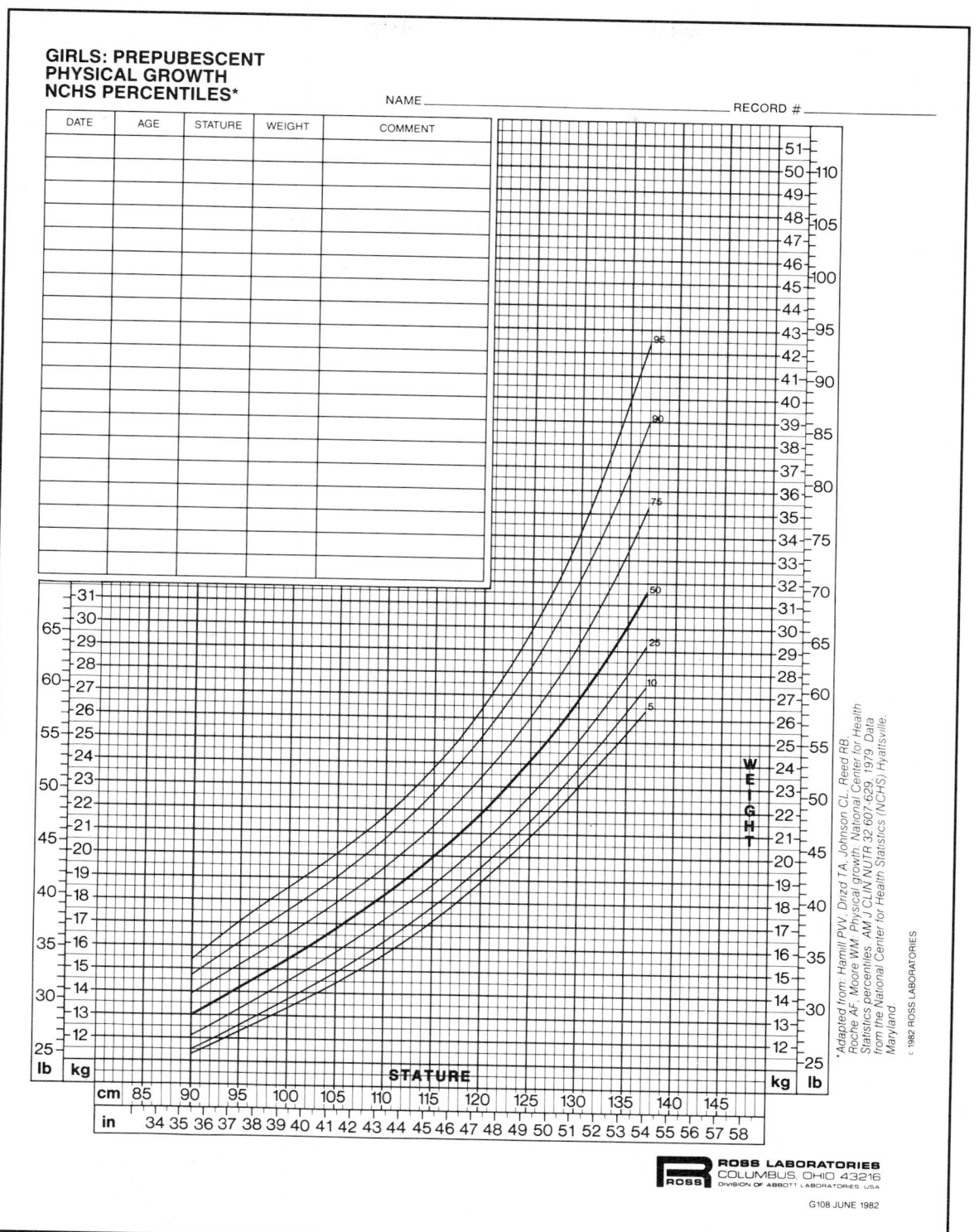

**GIRLS: PREPUBESCENT
PHYSICAL GROWTH
NCHS PERCENTILES***

NAME _____ RECORD # _____

DATE	AGE	STATURE	WEIGHT	COMMENT

STATURE

cm 85 90 95 100 105 110 115 120 125 130 135 140 145

in 34 35 36 37 38 39 40 41 42 43 44 45 46 47 48 49 50 51 52 53 54 55 56 57 58

WEIGHT

*Adapted from: Hamill PVV, Drizd TA, Johnson CL, Reed RB,
Roche AF, Moore WM. Physical growth: National Center for Health
Statistics percentiles. AM J CLIN NUTR 32:607-629, 1979. Data
from the National Center for Health Statistics (NCHS), Hyattsville,
Maryland.

© 1982 ROSS LABORATORIES

ROSS LABORATORIES
COLUMBUS, OHIO 43216
DIVISION OF ABBOTT LABORATORIES, USA

G108 JUNE 1982

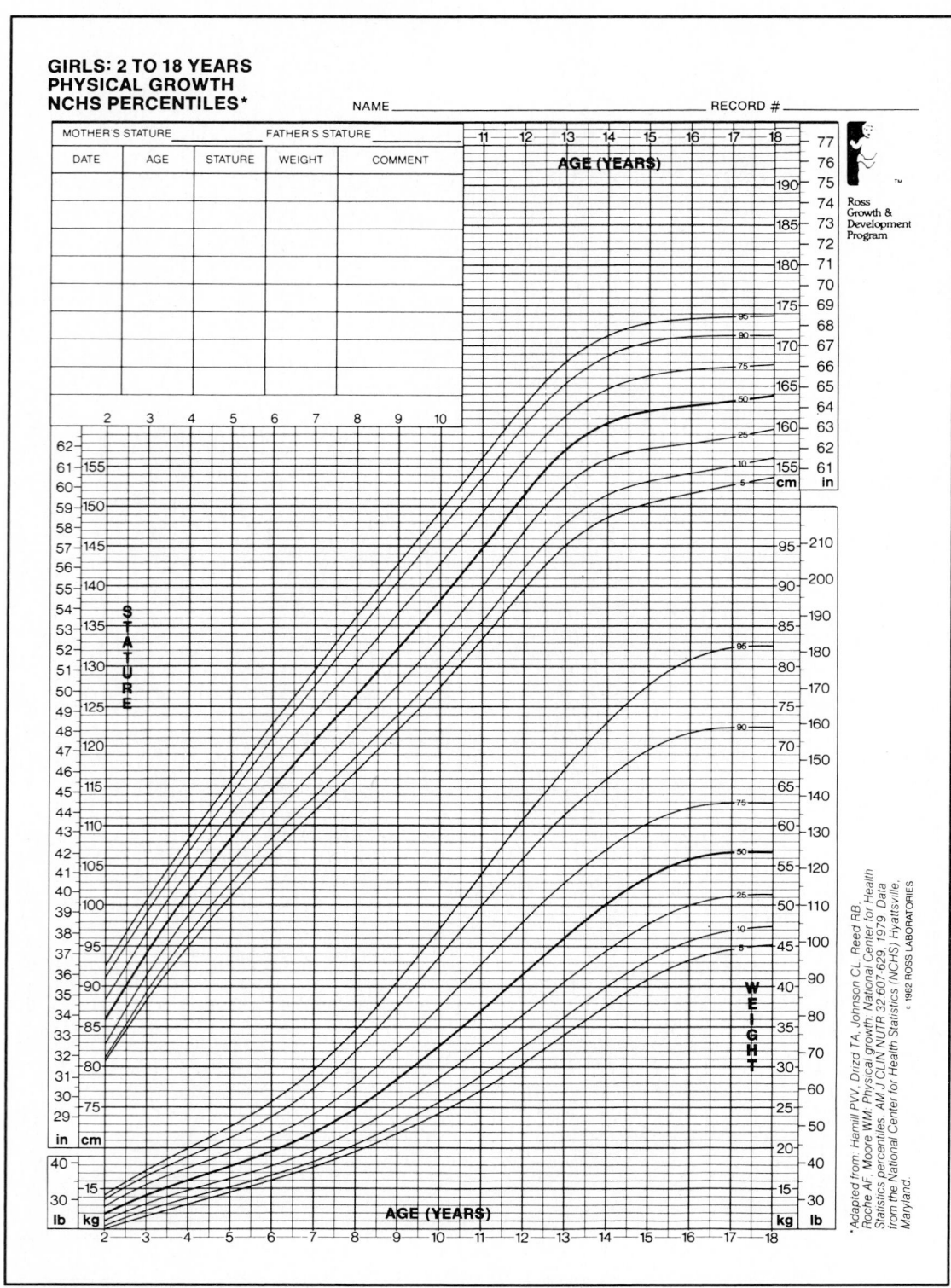

GIRLS: 2 TO 18 YEARS
PHYSICAL GROWTH
NCHS PERCENTILES*

NAME _____ RECORD # _____

* Adapted from: Hamill PVV, Drizd TA, Johnson CL, Reed RB, Roche AF, Moore WM: Physical growth: National Center for Health Statistics percentiles. AM J CLIN NUTR 32:607-629, 1979. Data from the National Center for Health Statistics (NCHS), Hyattsville, Maryland.

c 1982 ROSS LABORATORIES

Ross
Growth &
Development
Program

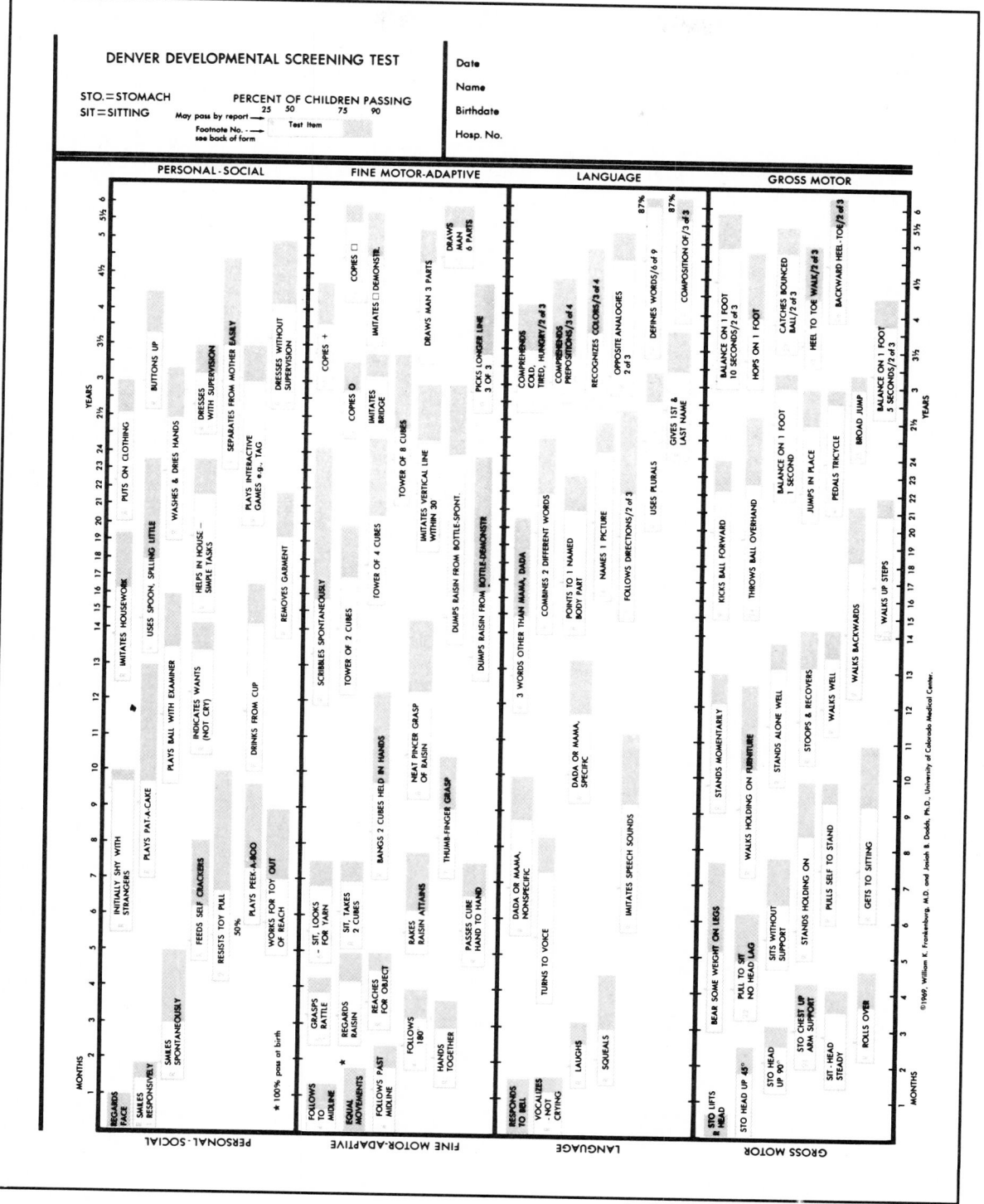

Continued.

DIRECTIONS

DATE

NAME

BIRTHDATE

HOSP. NO.

1. Try to get child to smile by smiling, talking or waving to him. Do not touch him.
2. When child is playing with toy, pull it away from him. Pass if he resists.
3. Child does not have to be able to tie shoes or button in the back.
4. Move yarn slowly in an arc from one side to the other, about 6" above child's face.
   Pass if eyes follow 90° to midline. (Past midline; 180°)
5. Pass if child grasps rattle when it is touched to the backs or tips of fingers.
6. Pass if child continues to look where yarn disappeared or tries to see where it went. Yarn
   should be dropped quickly from sight from tester's hand without arm movement.
7. Pass if child picks up raisin with any part of thumb and a finger.
8. Pass if child picks up raisin with the ends of thumb and index finger using an over hand
   approach.

9. Pass any en-
   closed form.
   Fail continuous
   round motions.

10. Which line is longer?
    (Not bigger.) Turn
    paper upside down and
    repeat. (3/3 or 5/6)

11. Pass any
    crossing
    lines.

12. Have child copy
    first. If failed,
    demonstrate

When giving items 9, 11 and 12, do not name the forms. Do not demonstrate 9 and 11.

13. When scoring, each pair (2 arms, 2 legs, etc.) counts as one part.
14. Point to picture and have child name it. (No credit is given for sounds only.)

15. Tell child to: Give block to Mommie; put block on table; put block on floor. Pass 2 of 3.
    (Do not help child by pointing, moving head or eyes.)
16. Ask child: What do you do when you are cold? ..hungry? ..tired? Pass 2 of 3.
17. Tell child to: Put block on table; under table; in front of chair, behind chair.
    Pass 3 of 4. (Do not help child by pointing, moving head or eyes.)
18. Ask child: If fire is hot, ice is ?; Mother is a woman, Dad is a ?; a horse is big, a
    mouse is ?. Pass 2 of 3.
19. Ask child: What is a ball? ..lake? ..desk? ..house? ..banana? ..curtain? ..ceiling?
    ..hedge? ..pavement? Pass if defined in terms of use, shape, what it is made of or general
    category (such as banana is fruit, not just yellow). Pass 6 of 9.
20. Ask child: What is a spoon made of? ..a shoe made of? ..a door made of? (No other objects
    may be substituted.) Pass 3 of 3.
21. When placed on stomach, child lifts chest off table with support of forearms and/or hands.
22. When child is on back, grasp his hands and pull him to sitting. Pass if head does not hang back.
23. Child may use wall or rail only, not person. May not crawl.
24. Child must throw ball overhand 3 feet to within arm's reach of tester.
25. Child must perform standing broad jump over width of test sheet. (8-1/2 inches)
26. Tell child to walk forward,   heel within 1 inch of toe.
    Tester may demonstrate. Child must walk 4 consecutive steps, 2 out of 3 trials.
27. Bounce ball to child who should stand 3 feet away from tester. Child must catch ball with
    hands, not arms, 2 out of 3 trials.
28. Tell child to walk backward,   toe within 1 inch of heel.
    Tester may demonstrate. Child must walk 4 consecutive steps, 2 out of 3 trials.

DATE AND BEHAVIORAL OBSERVATIONS (how child feels at time of test, relation to tester, attention
span, verbal behavior, self-confidence, etc,):

Vision and hearing screening procedures

Method	Age	Procedure	Normal response
Vision			
Following	Infancy	Shine light or hold bright object directly in front of infant's line of vision; move slowly from side to side.	Follows light or bright object up to 180 degrees
Turn to light response	Infancy	Hold back of head to bright light source.	Eyes turn toward source of light
Optokinetic drum	Infancy	Twirl drum with stripes slowly in front of infant's eyes.	Nystagmus occurs
Herschberg reflex (corneal light reflex)	Infancy through adolescence	Shine penlight into child's eyes; note where light reflex falls. For older children: have child focus and stare at point 14 inches and then 20 inches away before shining light into eyes.	Light reflex falls in same position in eye
Cover test	Toddler through adolescence	Have child focus on specified spot first 14 inches, then 20 inches away. While child is focusing, one eye is completely covered for 5 to 10 seconds. Cover is then removed and eye observed for movement. Procedure repeated for other eye.	No wandering or sharp jerky movement of eyes noted, indicating ability to focus
Snellen E	Preschool	Child is instructed to point finger in direction that the E or table legs are pointing from a distance of 20 feet. Test each eye separately, then together. Test as far down on chart as child can go.	Visual acuity of 20/30
Snellen alphabet	School age through adolescence	Child stands 20 feet from chart and reads letters. Each eye is tested separately and then together. Testing usually started at 20/30 or 20/40 line and child allowed to test as far down chart as possible. Passing score consists of reading majority of letters (or Es) on each line.	Visual acuity of 20/20
Hearing			
Startle reflex	Newborn	Loud noise or bang made near infant's ears.	Jumps at noise, blinks, cries or widen eyes
Tracks sound	3-6 months	Make noise, call name or sing.	Eyes shift toward sound; responds to mother's voice coos to verbalization
Recognizes sound	6-8 months	As preceding, from out of line of vision.	Turns head toward sound; responds to name, babbles to verbalization
Localization of sound	8-12 months	Call name, or use tuning fork or say words.	Localizes source of sound; turns head (and body at times) toward sound, repeats words
Pure tone screening—play	Toddler to preschool	Demonstrate to child by putting headphones on and making believe you hear sound. As you say "I hear it," put a block in box or ring on holder. Put headphones on child and give block or ring to use. Sound a 50 dB tone at 1000 Hz and guide child's hand with block to box. When child can do this alone, begin screening. Set at 25 dB at 1000 Hz. If child responds, go to 2000, 4000, and 6000 Hz. Praise child and place new block in hand. Switch to other ear and test.	Should respond at 25 dB at any frequency
Pure tone audiometry	School age through adolescence	Explain procedure to child. Place headphones on ears. Test 1 ear at a time in sequence as preceding (i.e., 25 dB at 1000, 2000, 4000 and 6000 Hz). Have child raise hand to indicate sound is heard.	Should respond at 25 dB at any frequency

Continued.

Vision and hearing screening procedures — cont'd

Method	Age	Procedure	Normal response
Hearing—cont'd			
Tuning fork test	Some preschoolers; school age through adolescence		
A. Weber test		Strike tuning fork to make it vibrate and place the stem in midline of scalp. Ask child if sound is same in both ears or louder in either ear.	Sound heard equally well in both ears
B. Rinne test		Strike tuning fork until it vibrates, place stem on child's mastoid until he no longer hears it. Then place vibrating fingers of fork 1 to 2 inches in front of concha. Ask child if he can still hear sound.	Sound from fingers of fork vibrating in air should be heard when child can no longer hear sound with stem against mastoid, i.e., air conduction is greater than bone conduction

Screening for common orthopedic problems in infancy and childhood

Deformity	Screening	Deformity	Screening
Congenital hip dislocation (CHD)			
Complete or partial displacement of femoral head out of the acetabulum	Barlow's maneuver (for dislocation of femoral head): flex hip to 90 degrees grasp symphysis in front and sacrum in back with one hand; with other hand, apply lateral pressure to medial thigh with thumb and longitudinal pressure to knee with palm; abduct flexed hip. A positive sign is sensation of abnormal movement. Reverse hands for examining other hip. See Fig. K-10.		jects further anteriorly, femur is longer; if one knee is higher, the tibia is longer. 2. With child on back, back, both legs are extended out with pressure on knees. Heels are matched and observed for equal or unequal length. 3. Trendelenburg sign: with child standing on one leg, observe pelvis. When child stands on abnormal leg, the pelvis drops on normal side. See Fig. K-13.
	Ortolani's maneuver (for reduction of femur): abduct hip to 80 degrees, lifting proximal femur anteriorly with fingers placed on lateral thigh. A positive sign is sensation of a jerk or snap with reduction into socket. See Fig. K-11.	**Metatasus adductus (Varus)**	
	Limited full abduction of hips: with child flat on back, abduct hips one at a time, then together. See Fig. K-12 for degrees of hip abduction.	Adduction or turning in of forefoot with high longitudinal arch and wide space between fist and second toes. Commonly associated with tibial torsion	Test foot for flexibility and elicit tonic foot reflexes. Rigidity is indicated by eversion or inversion when foot does not move beyond neutral position or does not respond to toe grasping or by dorsiflexing. Signs of metatarsus adductus are illustrated in Fig. K-14.
	Apparent shortening of femur: 1. Allis sign: with child lying on back, pelvis flat, knees flexed and feet planted firmly, observe knees. If the knee pro-		

Continued.

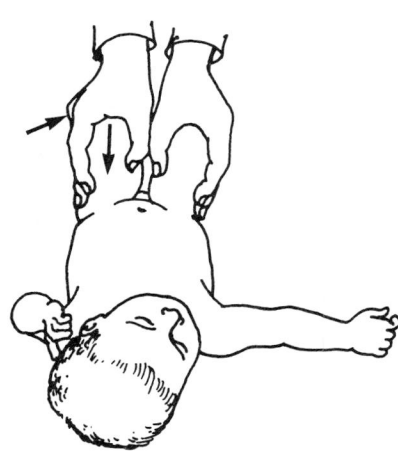

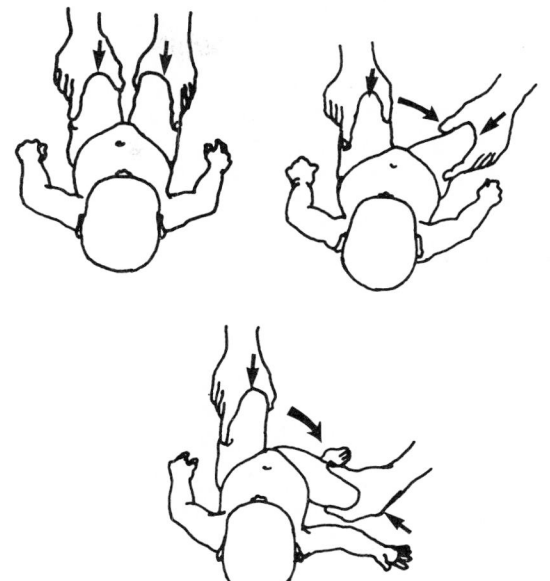

Fig. K-10. Barlow test. The baby's thighs are grasped as shown. The thigh is adducted toward the midline with gentle lateral pressure placed on the midthigh with the thumb. In a dislocatable hip, the femoral head can be displaced from the acetabulum. (From Barnard, M.U., 1981, et al.: Handbook of comprehensive pediatric nursing, New York, 1981, McGraw-Hill Book Co., p. 67. Used with permission.)

Fig. K-11. Ortolani test. With the baby on a firm surface, each hip is examined separately. The hip and knee are flexed 90° with the examiner's index or middle fingers over the two greater trochanters and the thumb midthigh (see 1). One leg is then gently abducted (see 2 and 3). In a positive finding, the examiner senses a hip click by palpation or audibly as the femoral head slips from its dislocated posterior position into the acetabulum. (From Barnard, M.U., et al.: Handbook of comprehensive pediatric nursing, New York, 1981, McGraw-Hill, p. 66, as adapted from Stanisauljeuic, S.: Diagnosis of congential hip pathology in the newborn, Baltimore, 1964, The Williams & Wilkins Co.)

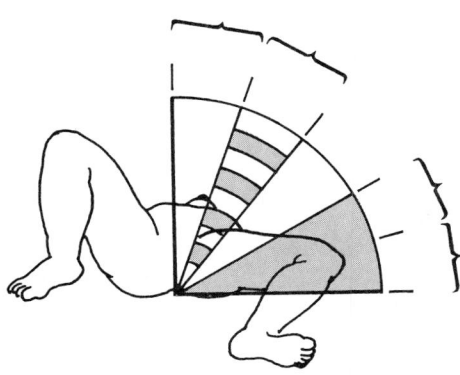

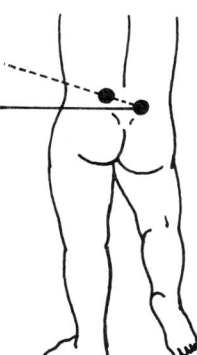

Fig. K-12. Degrees of abduction of the hip: (a) normal limits, (b) abnormal (suspicious) limits, (c) positive sign for CHD. (From Chow, M., et al.: Handbook of pediatric primary care, New York, 1979, John Wiley & Sons, p. 700, as adapted from Tachdjian, M.O., Pediatric orthopedics, vol. 1, Philadelphia, 1972, W.B. Saunders Co. p. 136.)

Fig. K-13. Positive Trendelenburg sign. (From Chow, M., et al.: Handbook of pediatric primary care, New York, 1979, John Wiley & Sons, p. 701, as adapted from Lowell, J. D., et al., Congenital hip dysplasia, Clin Pediatr 3:279-287, May 1964, p. 282).

Screening for common orthopedic problems in infancy and childhood—cont'd

Deformity	Screening	Deformity	Screening
Pes planus (flat feet)			
When child is weight bearing, longitudinal arch of foot appears flat on floor	1. Observe feet in weighted and unweighted position		3. Observe space between ankles from front and back. Normal spacing between medial malleoli at heel is 2 inches.
(1) Pseudo flat feet: very common until ages 2 to 3; created by plantar fat pad. Feet are flexible, exhibit hypermobility of joint, and have a low arch	2. Stand child on toes. Arch disappears with weight bearing in flexible flat foot and reappears when on toes. See Fig. K-15 3. Elicit dorsal and plantar flexion to rule out tight heel cord. 4. Elicit eversion and inversion flexion to rule out tarsal coalition.	**Genu Varum (bowlegs)** Deviant axis of thighs and calves which is (1) Physiological: normal until ages 2 to 3; occurs with internal tibial torsion and genu valgum (2) Pathological	Same for genu valgum
(2) Rigid flat feet: Uncommon; created by tightness of heel cord or tarsal coalition (a cartilaginous fibrous or bony connection between bones)	Same as for preceding No. 1 (pseudo flat feet)	**Internal tibial torsion** Twisting or torsion of tibia usually accompanied by metatarsus adductus	1. Examine legs for range of motion, flexibility of ankle and elicit tonic foot reflexes. 2. Holding knee firmly with foot in neutral position, observe medial and lateral mallioli. The normal angle between them is approximately 15 to 20 degrees. See Fig. K-17.
Genu Valgum (knock-knees) A deviant axis of thighs and calves of more than 10 to 15 degrees; (normal from ages 2-6)	1. Observe axis of thighs and calves with child standing. Normally axis are parallel with 10 to 15 degrees deviance. See Figure K-16 2. Observe space between the knees from front and back. Normal spacing is 1½ inches.		3. Have child sit on examining table and draw a circle over patellar and external mallioli. With patella facing forward only anterior edge of malleolar circle should be seen. See Fig. K-18.

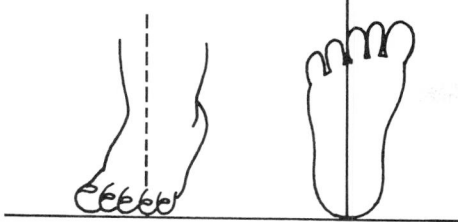

Fig. K-14. Signs of metatarsus adductus: (a) convex lateral border of foot, (b) concave medial border of foot with possible wrinkling, (c) space may exist between the large toe and second toe, (d) midline bisects third and fourth toes. (From Chow, M., et al.: Handbook of pediatric primary care, New York, 1979, John Wiley & Sons, p. 704.)

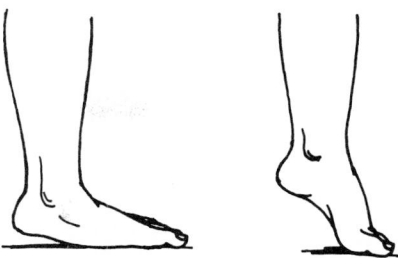

Fig. K-15. Pseudo flat feet. The flat arch disappears with child on toes. (From Chow, M., et al.: Handbook of pediatric primary care, New York, 1979, John Wiley & Sons, p. 706, as adapted from Ducroquet, R. J., et al.: La marche et les boîteries, Paris, 1965, Masson.)

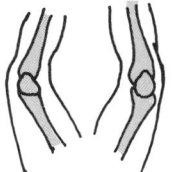 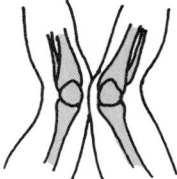 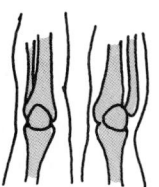

Fig. K-16. Axis of thigh and calf: (a) normal axis, (b) deviant axis exhibiting knock-knees (genu valgum), (c) deviant axis exhibiting bowlegs (genu varum). (From Chow, M., et al.: Handbook of pediatric primary care, New York, 1979, John Wiley & Sons, p. 707, as adapted from Ducroquet, R.J., et al.: La marche et les boîteries, Paris, 1965, Masson.)

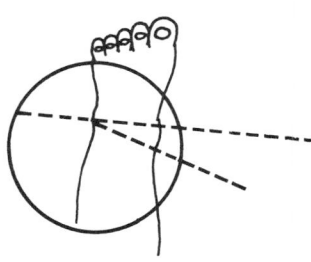

Fig. K-17. Normal angle between medial and lateral malleolus. (From Chow, M., et al.: Handbook of pediatric primary care, New York, 1979, John Wiley & Sons, p. 709.)

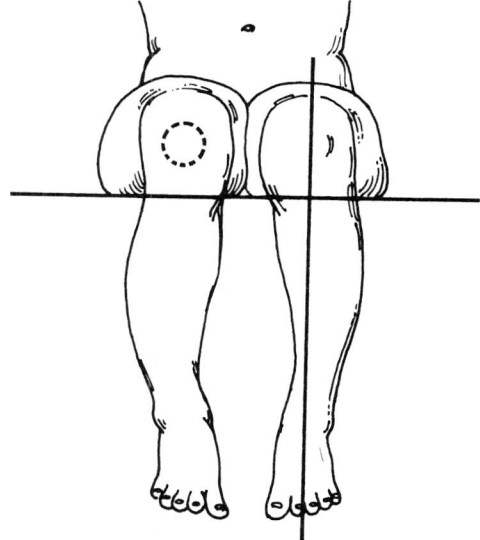

Fig. K-18. Examiner testing for tibial torsion. (From Alexander, M.M., and Brown, M.S.: Pediatric history taking and physical diagnosis for nurses, New York, 1979, McGraw-Hill Book Co., p. 205. Used with permission.)

DENVER ARTICULATION SCREENING EXAM
for children 2 1/2 to 6 years of age

Instructions: Have child repeat each word after you. Circle the underlined sounds that he pronounces correctly. Total correct sounds is the Raw Score. Use charts on reverse side to score results.

NAME

HOSP. NO.

ADDRESS _____

Date: _____ Child's Age: _____ Examiner: _____ Raw Score: _____
Percentile: _____ Intelligibility: _____ Result: _____

1. table	6. zipper	11. sock	16. wagon	21. leaf
2. shirt	7. grapes	12. vacuum	17. gum	22. carrot
3. door	8. flag	13. yarn	18. house	
4. trunk	9. thumb	14. mother	19. pencil	
5. jumping	10. toothbrush	15. twinkle	20. fish	

Intelligibility: (circle one)   1. Easy to understand   3. Not understandable
     2. Understandable 1/2   4. Can't evaluate
     the time.

Comments:

Date: _____ Child's Age: _____ Examiner: _____ Raw Score _____
Percentile: _____ Intelligibility: _____ Result: _____

1. table	6. zipper	11. sock	16. wagon	21. leaf
2. shirt	7. grapes	12. vacuum	17. gum	22. carrot
3. door	8. flag	13. yarn	18. house	
4. trunk	9. thumb	14. mother	19. pencil	
5. jumping	10. toothbrush	15. twinkle	20. fish	

Intelligibility: (circle one)   1. Easy to understand   3. Not understandable
     2. Understandable 1/2   4. Can't evaluate
     the time.

Comments:

Date: _____ Child's Age: _____ Examiner: _____ Raw Score _____
Percentile: _____ Intelligibility: _____ Result: _____

1. table	6. zipper	11. sock	16. wagon	21. leaf
2. shirt	7. grapes	12. vacuum	17. gum	22. carrot
3. door	8. flag	13. yarn	18. house	
4. trunk	9. thumb	14. mother	19. pencil	
5. jumping	10. toothbrush	15. twinkle	20. fish	

Intelligibility: (circle one)   1. Easy to understand   3. Not understandable
     2. Understandable 1/2   4. Can't evaluate
     the time.

Comments:

Copyright 1971. Amelia F. Drumwright   University of Colorado Medical Center

To score DASE words: Note Raw Score for child's performance. Match raw score line (extreme left of chart) with column representing child's age (to the closest previous age group). Where raw score line and age column meet number in that square denotes percentile rank of child's performance when compared to other children that age. Percentiles above heavy line are ABNORMAL percentiles, below heavy line are NORMAL.

PERCENTILE RANK

Raw Score	2.5 yr.	3.0	3.5	4.0	4.5	5.0	5.5	6 years
2	1							
3	2							
4	5							
5	9							
6	16							
7	23							
8	31	2						
9	37	4	1					
10	42	6	2					
11	48	7	4					
12	54	9	6	1	1			
13	58	12	9	2	3	1	1	
14	62	17	11	5	4	2	2	
15	68	23	15	9	5	3	2	
16	75	31	19	12	5	4	3	
17	79	38	25	15	6	6	4	
18	83	46	31	19	8	7	4	
19	86	51	38	24	10	9	5	1
20	89	58	45	30	12	11	7	3
21	92	65	52	36	15	15	9	4
22	94	72	58	43	18	19	12	5
23	96	77	63	50	22	24	15	7
24	97	82	70	58	29	29	20	15
25	99	87	78	66	36	34	26	17
26	99	91	84	75	46	43	34	24
27		94	89	82	57	54	44	34
28		96	94	88	70	68	59	47
29		98	98	94	84	84	77	68
30		100	100	100	100	100	100	100

To Score intelligibility:

	NORMAL	ABNORMAL
2 1/2 years	Understandable 1/2 the time, or, "easy"	Not Understandable
3 years and older	Easy to understand	Understandable 1/2 time Not understandable

Test Result: 1. NORMAL on Dase and Intelligibility = NORMAL

2. ABNORMAL on Dase and/or Intelligibility = ABNORMAL

* If abnormal on initial screening rescreen within 2 weeks. If abnormal again child should be referred for complete speech evaluation.

GLOSSARY

academic degree Static credential that indicates successful completion and graduation from an educational program.

accommodation Ways in which children modify their conception of the world as they have new experiences that influence their responses.

accountability Being answerable to someone for something one has done.

    moral Being answerable to someone for how moral requirements of nursing practice have been carried out.

    legal Being answerable to someone for how legal requirements of nursing practice have been carried out.

accreditation Mechanism for assessing the quality of educational programs.

acculturation Adaptation and incorporation of ideas, values, behaviors, customs, and certain aspects of the majority culture concurrent with maintaining aspects of the traditional or primary culture. Learning one's culture through a process of acquiring knowledge and internalizing values.

achievable age Risk age, expressed in years, individuals can attain if they comply with suggested medical therapies and life-style changes. Synonymous with survival advantage and compliance age.

acid rain Caused by ozone depletion.

active immunization Administration of all or part of a microorganism to stimulate active response by the host's immunological system, resulting in complete protection against a specific disease.

activity theory of aging The premise of older adults maintaining previous middle years' activity levels.

acupressure Form of stress reduction whereby selected metabolic and circulatory processes are stimulated by finger pressure on certain points of the body.

acupuncture Insertion of needles into selected parts of the body to control pain.

administrative law Branch of law dealing with administration of the executive branch of government (e. g., licensing boards).

adult day care center Congregate facility for activities such as socialization, eating, and supervised care of older adults during specified day hours with the person returning home for the evening hours.

adult nurse practitioner Registered nurse with additional education through a master's degree program in nursing or through a nondegree certificate continuing education program preparing the nurse to deliver primary health care to adults.

adversary Litigant opponent, the opposing party in a writ or action.

advocacy Pleading the cause of another.

advocate One who pleads the cause of another.

aerobics Form of exercise designed to increase the flow of blood and oxygen to all parts of the body.

affective disorder One of the most common psychiatric syndromes, essentially of three types: depressive, manic, and bipolar (manic and depressive alterations).

affective domain Deals with changes in interests, attitudes, values, and the development of appreciations and adequate adjustments.

agency Includes every relation in which one person acts for or represents another by the latter's authority.

agent Causative factor invading a susceptible host through a favorable environment to produce disease.

aggregate Individuals or parts of a whole who have in common one or more personal or environmental characteristics.

aggressive behavior Pressing of one's own behavior in such a way as to infringe on the rights of others.

aging Process of changes; biological, psychological, and sociological, occurring from conception to death.

akathisia Inability to sit down because the thought of doing so causes severe anxiety. A feeling of restlessness and an urgent need of movement with complaints of feelings of muscular quivering.

Alanon Organization of relatives of alcoholic individuals operated in many communities within the structure of Alcoholics Anonymous.

Alateen Self-help program for children of alcoholics; provides a forum for discussing family stressors, learning coping skills, and gaining support and encouragement from knowledgeable peers.

Alcoholics Anonymous Lay, self-help group that practices a 12-step approach to recovery.

alcoholism Disease characterized by the repetitive and compulsive ingestion of any sedative drug (ethanol representing but one of this group) in such a way as to result in interference with some aspect of the person's life.

allegation Charge, assertion.

ambulatory clinic Health care facility, generally associated with a hospital, providing follow-up care after hospitalization. Clients are seen for nonemergency problems.

analysis Fourth level of cognitive learning that requires the learner to break down communication into constituent parts to distinguish between the parts and understand the relationship among them.

analytic epidemiology Second stage of epidemiological investigation that focuses on testing etiological hypotheses using observational studies.

andragogy Helping people learn.

antabuse Drug used as a deterrent to alcohol consumption; when alcohol and antabuse are mixed, the person experiences a variety of unpleasant physiological reactions.

antagonism Factors acting in opposition.

anthrax Illness with varying symptoms caused by a spore-forming organism. May be endemic to many agricultural areas.

antianxiety agent Agent affective against anxiety.

anticholinergic Agents impeding the impulses or action of the fibers of the parasympathetic nerves; provides cholinergic blocking action.

anticipatory guidance Counseling related to expected developmental or therapeutic manifestations and/or responses.

antidepressants Agents effective in relieving depression.

antipsychotics Drugs effective in controlling psychotic behaviors.

antitoxin Solution of antibodies derived from the serum of animals immunized with specific antigens (e. g., diphtheria, tetanus) used to achieve passive immunity.

anxiety Troubled feeling that may be a sense of dread or fear over a real or imagined threat to one's mental or physical well-being.

appeal Complaint to a superior court to reverse or correct an injustice or alleged error committed by an inferior court.

appellate court Judgments of trial courts are reviewed or appealed.

application Third level of cognitive learning; means the learner takes the information provided and uses it in new, particular, and concrete situations.

appraised age Total health risk, expressed in years, experienced by an individual. Determined by adjusting the average risk of death from selected causes for the individual's age, sex, and racial group to his own risk.

appropriations Actual amount of monies approved for a program authorized by law.

arachnicide Chemical pesticide used to kill spiders.

artificial acquired immunity Immune state that results from immunization or vaccination to a specific disease.

ascariasis (roundworm infection) Largely asymptomatic disease caused by injection and multiplication of a nematode, *Ascaris lumbricoides.*

assault Threat to do bodily harm.

assertiveness Standing up for personal rights, thoughts, feelings, and beliefs in a direct and honest manner that does not violate the rights of others.

assertiveness training Teaching people how to honestly and directly express themselves by identifying what is blocking such behavior and by setting goals for increasing personal assertive behavior.

assessment Systematic, organized evaluation of an individual's biological, psychological, and sociological functions.

assessment of community resources Procedure similar to the process used on behalf of individual clients. The scope of the investigation is more detailed and includes examination of data from health planning groups, including the number of public health facilities, availability of health personnel, availability of funds, and a multitude of other statistics like those on mortality and morbidity.

assessment of need Verifying and mapping out the extent and location of a problem and its attendant target population.

assimilation Process of a minority group becoming absorbed into the dominant or majority culture by adopting its behaviors. Also, the process of responding to the environment in accordance with a person's cogniture structures so that elements in the environment are incorporated into the child's cognitive structures.

atropine psychosis Produced by excessive anticholinergic agent usage.

attitude Persistent disposition to act either positively or negatively toward a person, group, object, situation, or value.

attributable risk Statistical measure that estimates the reduction in the occurrence of a particular disease, which could be affected by elimination of a specific causal agent.

attribute Any physical, psychological, or social characteristic describing an individual.

authorization Process of placing a ceiling on monies to be requested for a program.

battered women Physically and/or emotionally abused by a spouse.

battery Committing bodily harm.

BCG vaccines Several different vaccines that vary in their ability to induce active immunity and therefore prevent tuberculosis.

bioenergetics Series of exercises designed to bring about natural healing based on bringing into harmony the natural environment and body rhythms.

biofeedback Process in which delicate physiological monitoring instruments serve as teaching tools by helping people become aware and learn to consciously control many physiological variables previously thought to be automatic.

biological hazards Disease-producing agents primarily consisting of bacteria, viruses, and other microorganisms and parasites.

biological plausibility A reasonable physiological mechanism to explain how a causal factor could operate to bring about a particular disease.

biosphere World of living things.

"BLACK LUNG" Disease common among coal miners, characterized by a large solid black lung mass caused by deposits of black mining dust in the lungs.

blacking out Central nervous system effect of excessive alcohol intake whereby the person experiences a period of total amnesia yet may not appear at the time to be under the influence of alcohol.

breach of contract Unjustified failure to perform the terms of a contract as agreed on or when performance is due.

brucellosis Infectious disease of nonhuman mammals, which is contagious to humans.

burnout Special form of stress reaction to work and organizational pressures.

byssinosis Type of lung disease common among cotton mill workers, similar to nonoccupational bronchitis.

capitation Payment of tax of a fixed amount per person.

carboxyhemoglobin Formed when carbon monoxide bumps oxygen molecules out of red blood cells.

carcinogenic agent Single cancer-inducing substance that triggers the change in behavior of cells, resulting in uncontrolled growth.

case finding Careful, systematic observations of children to identify those with present or potential problems.

case law Decisions by the courts; judicial opinions.

catalytic intervention mode Situation whereby the consultant assists clients to broaden their view of an existing situation by gaining additional information or by unifying existing data.

catchment area Designated service area for a community mental health center consisting of between 75,000 and 200,000 people.

cause Stimulus that produces an effect or outcome.

cause of action Averment of allegations or facts sufficient for defendant to respond.

Congressional Budget Office (CBO) Advises and assists Congress in evaluating costs and economic impact of budget proposals on taxpayers.

celebration Methods in group work for acknowledging accomplishment of group goals.

Centers for Disease Control Branch of the U.S. Public Health Service in which primary responsibility is to propose, coordinate, and evaluate changes in the surveillance of disease in the United States.

certificate of need Determination in any given community of the need for new health care facilities based on the currently available resources and the anticipated demands for use.

certification One mechanism, usually by written examination, to provide an indication of professional competence in a specialized area of practice.

chamber Legislative division commonly known as the House and/or Senate.

change To make different or alter.

characteristics of crisis Psychological and physiological changes of individuals in crisis.

charter Mechanism by which a state government agency under state laws grants corporate status to institutions with or without rights to award degrees.

chemical additive contamination Either deliberately or incidentally added to food.

child abuse Neglect or active forms of maltreatment against children.

child neglect Physical or emotional. Physical neglect refers to failure to provide adequate food, clothing, shelter, hygiene, or necessary medical care, whereas emotional neglect refers to the omission of basic nurturing, acceptance, and caring essential for healthy development.

childbirth center Health facility where prenatal care and delivery services are provided to low risk pregnant women by a team of nurse-midwives, obstetricians, pediatricians, and ancillary health personnel.

chiropractic System of manipulative treatment, which teaches that all diseases are caused by infringement on spinal nerves and can be corrected by spinal adjustments.

chiropractor One who practices chiropractic methods.

chlorine Toxic gas used in the chemical and paper industry.

civil law Concerned with the legal rights and duties of private persons.

client community Target of service; that is, the population group for whom healthful change is sought.

clinical disease Stage in the natural history, which begins when sufficient anatomical or functional changes have occurred to produce recognizable signs and symptoms of a disease.

clinical horizon Imaginary line dividing the point at which there are and are not detectable signs and symptoms of disease.

cocaine One of several alkaloids found in the leaves of the coca plant; can be fatal when injected in impure or large doses; is a central nervous system stimulant.

code of ethics Statements encompassing rules that apply to people in professional roles.

cognitive learning Acquisition of facts dealing with recall and recognition of information.

cognitive restructuring Strategy for self-modification that depends on rational self-statements and evaluations before or during a given event.

cognitive uncertainty Inability to predict the outcome of a situation because of a lack of available information.

cohort Group of people born during the same era, who are influenced by some of the same biological, psychological, and social factors.

collaboration Mutual sharing and working together to achieve common goals in such a way that all persons or groups are recognized, and growth is enhanced.

collaborative practice Professionals working together in a collegial relationship to provide primary health care to a given population.

common fate, principle of Tendency to see objects moving in the same direction as a perceptual unit.

common law Derived from judicial decisions.

communicable disease Primarily infectious in nature and requiring interaction between the host, agent, direct or indirect transmission from the agent reservoir in the environment, and a host that can provide adequate living conditions for the infectious agent.

communication Interactive process of sharing or transmitting thoughts and feelings.

communication structure Arrangement of group member positions according to their place in the communication network.

community Locality-based entity composed of systems of formal organizations reflecting societal institutions, informal groups, and aggregates. These organizations are interdependent, function to meet a wide variety of collective needs, and are the target of community-oriented practice.

community attitudes Information gathered from professionals and lay people who work with health-related services in the community.

community health Meeting collective needs through problem identifying and managing interactions within the community and larger society. The goal of community-oriented practice.

community health capabilities Resources available to meet community health needs.

community health nurses' goal Contribute to a comprehensive effort that provides continuity of services to clients as groups, individuals, families, or communities.

community health nursing Synthesis of nursing and public health practice applied to promoting and preserving the health of populations. The practice is general and comprehensive with the dominant responsibility to the population as a whole.

community health problems Needs for action. Discrepancies between the nurse's and community's concepts of community health and what is found in the data base.

community health services Directed to meet the needs of groups, and tend to reflect a public health orientation of health promotion and maintenance.

community insurance rates Method used to establish similar premium rates for all subscribers, regardless of illness risk.

community mental health Orientation toward health care, which seeks to provide a program of continuing and comprehensive mental health care to a specific population.

comparative negligence, doctrine of Negligence of the plaintiff and defendant is compared, and apportionment of damages is made based on the acts the parties are found to have committed.

compensatory damages Amounts of money for proven loss.

compost Aerobic process whereby bacteria, especially fungi, feed on organic material; uses a 30:1 carbon to nitrogen ratio.

comprehension Second level of cognitive learning; to grasp the meaning of the known information.

Comprehensive Health Planning and Public Health Services Amendments of 1966 (CHP) Emphasized regional planning, and represented landmark legislation establishing the first time each person's "right to health care" was acknowledged.

compromise Two or more people or groups with goals that cannot be met without modification of the positions of each person or group (implies "give and take" in the negotiating process).

concept Category or class of objects or phenomena that represents either an abstract version of the real world (such as an ideal) or a concrete idea such as a chair or bench.

conceptual framework Group of concepts plus a set of propositions that spell out the relationships between them.

conceptual model Set of concepts and those assumptions that integrate them into a meaningful configuration.

concrete operation Children can think about those things they can see; a level of cognitive development.

concurrent resolution Document expressing the principles, opinions, and purposes of Congress on matters affecting the operation of both houses. They originate separately in either chamber. Concurrent resolutions are not usually legislative in character.

conditioning Strategy for self-modification that depends on shaping a client's behavior by rewarding changes toward the goal in the intended direction.

confidential communication Information passing between individuals in a fiduciary relationship who have a duty not to reveal the contents.

confrontation Three-phase process including assessment, direct confrontation, and resettlement, which is a problem-solving strategy for conflict resolution.

congressional record Document published daily by the Superintendent of Documents reporting on public proceedings whenever at least one house of Congress is in session.

connectionism in stimulus-response theories The connection is the neural joining between a stimulus and the response.

consistency of the association Degree to which findings of various studies investigating the relation between a particular factor and a disease outcome are consistent.

constitutional law Branch dealing with organization and function of government.

constraints Investigation of services, resources, and facilities; may highlight problems that could potentially impede the planning of programs to meet consumer needs.

constructs Conceptual components that are not directly observable; deliberately created ideas or references that cannot actually be seen but allow for explanation and analysis.

consultant One who gives professional advice, services, or information.

consultation Interactional or communication process between two or more persons, one of whom is a consultant, and the other is considered a consultee. The consultant seeks to help the consultee solve a problem or improve or broaden skills.

consultee Person seeking the help of an outside, usually impartial person in problem resolution.

consumer Receiver of services or products.

consumer sovereign power Consumer control in determining the behavior of products.

consumerism Belief that the recipients of a service should be informed and responsible in seeking that service, and belief that their needs should be a high priority in the goals of the provider.

continuity, principle of Tendency to respond to trends and themes running through a series of objects and to perceive all corresponding to that trend or theme as being part of the same perceptual unit.

continuity of care Series of client care activities rendered to the client in three situations (before, during, and after hospitalization); a basic objective of discharge planning.

contract Promissary agreement between two or more persons that creates, modifies, or destroys a legal relation. Also, it is a legally enforceable promise between two or more persons to do or not to do something. Or it can be any working agreement continuously renegotiable between the nurse and family.

contributory negligence Act or omission amounting to want of ordinary care on the part of the complaining party, which concurring with defendant's negligence, is the proximate cause of injury.

coordination Conscious activity of assembling and directing the work efforts of a group of health providers so that they can function harmoniously in the attainment of the objective of client care.

correctness of temporality Evidence that exposure to a causal factor occurs before the onset of the disease.

corroboration Strengthens or adds to credibility by adding or confirming facts or evidence.

cosmic radiation Emanates from the sun and other parts of the earth and consists of many types of particulate and electromagnetic radiation.

cost accounting Studies finding the actual budgetary cost of a program, procedure, or technique.

cost benefit Studies assessing the desirability of a program, procedure, or technique by placing a specific quantifiable value, a dollar amount, on all costs and benefits of the variable to be evaluated.

cost effectiveness Studies measuring the quality of a program, procedure, or technique as relative to cost.

cost efficiency Studies analyzing the actual costs of performing a number of services at different volumes when the same standards are applied.

cost plus reimbursement Method of payment to an agency for actual costs of services delivered plus added allowable expenses such as depreciation of facilities, equipment, and administrative costs.

counselor One who helps others arrive at workable solutions to their problems.

credentialing Mechanism that seeks to produce performance of acceptable quality by individuals and programs of education and service. The four fundamental features of credentialing are quality, identity, protection, and control.

crisis Upset in a steady state, disequilibrium.

crisis intervention Short-term therapeutic modality to assist those in crisis to resolve problems and restore equilibrium at least at the level of functioning before crisis.

crude rates Statistical rates in which the events in the numerator and denominator refer to the entire population.

cultural Relating to the underlying common attitudes, values, customs, and beliefs of a particular group.

culture Standards for decisions on what is, what can be, how to feel about it, and how to do it.

culture bound Illnesses specific to a particular culture (e. g., *mal ojo* [evil eye] in the Mexican American culture).

culture shock Feelings of helplessness, discomfort, and disorientation experienced by a person attempting to understand or effectively adapt to a different cultural group because of dissimilarities in practices, values, and beliefs.

curriculum vitae (resume) Summary of past education, professional experiences, activities, and honors to be used during employment-seeking endeavors.

data collection Process of acquiring existing information or developing new information.

data gathering Acquisition by the information collector of existing, readily available data, usually statistical in nature.

data generation Development of data, frequently qualitative rather than numerical.

data interpretation Process of analyzing and synthesizing data that culminate in the identification of community health problems and capabilities.

decibels (dB) Measure of the magnitude of noise.

deductive approach Quantifies data; hypothesis testing is used.

deinstitutionalization Effort to move long-term psychiatric patients out of the hospital and back into their own community.

delirium tremens Severe reaction to alcohol withdrawal characterized by disorientation, paranoia, and outbursts of irrational behavior; symptoms also may include tachycardia, fever, rapid breathing, sweating, vomiting, and diarrhea.

democratic leadership Cooperative structure that promotes and supports member's functioning in all aspects of decision making and planning.

deontology Doctrine that moral duty or obligation is binding. Also, what makes acts right are nonconsequential characteristics such as fidelity, veracity, justice, and honesty.

depression Mental state characterized by dejection, lack of hope, and absence of cheerfulness.

dereflection Logotherapeutic technique, used in the fight for something; not simply taking a person's mind off the goal but a positive redirection to another goal. Such action often results in accomplishment of the original goal. A technique to direct focus away from the problems at hand and to focus instead on assets and abilities.

DESC scripting A way of negotiating for positive changes in a humane, open, and assertive manner by *describing* the unwanted behavior, *expressing* feelings about it, and *specifying* what change can be made, such as spelling out the *consequences* of abiding by the contract.

descriptive epidemiology First stage of epidemiological investigation that focuses on describing disease distribution by characteristics relating to time, place, and person.

detoxification Gradual withdrawal from an abused substance; best achieved in a controlled hospital setting.

developmental crisis Upset in a steady state, disequilibrium occurring at a predictable transition in life.

developmental theory Aging theory based on the premise of continuation into later years of earlier developed traits and characteristics.

dichotomy planning Events preparing for clients' ongoing and future needs for health care resources as they move along the health/illness continuum toward their maximum potential.

dioxin Ingredient in the defoliant Agent Orange, which can kill and cause birth defects, cancer, and problems of the liver, kidney, nervous system, and skin.

direct causal association Relationship in which a factor causes a disease with no other factors intervening in the process.

direct provider reimbursement Method of payment to a provider for services delivered (e.g., fee-for-service).

disability Degree of physical or mental impairment, which is observable and measurable.

discharge planning Event often planned by a multidisciplinary team within a given setting, which enhances the client's ability to return to an optimum life-style.

disease prevention Activities that seek to protect clients from potential or actual health threats and their harmful consequences.

disengagement theory Aging theory postulated on the premise of older people withdrawing from society.

distress Unpleasant and avoided emotional and/or physiological response to a stressor.

dust Solids suspended in air, resulting from fragmentation of matter.

duty Conduct based on moral or legal obligation or as required by or relating to one's occupation or position. Moral duty is based on moral principles and may or may not be supported by law and may even be prohibited. Legal duty is that which is required by law.

absolute Cannot be overridden by any other duty; intrinsically right or wrong.

advocacy Moral obligation to speak, write, or take action in support of the client or client populations.

veracity Obligation to tell the truth and not lie or deceive people.

dystonias Impaired or disordered tonicity, especially muscle tone.

early adopters Individuals and/or groups who adopt new ideas from mass media rather than face-to-face information sources; those with specialized rather than global goals.

ecological fallacy Erroneous assumption that associations of the presence of a hypothetical causal agent and a disease observed in populations can be assumed to reflect a causal role for that factor in an individual.

ecology Study of the interaction among living organisms and their environment.

economics Social science concerned with the problems of using or administering scarce resources in the most efficient way to attain maximum fulfillment of society's unlimited wants.

ecosystem Sum total of all living and nonliving parts that support a chain of life events within a selected area.

educator Vehicle for transmitting knowledge.

efficacy Ability of an intervention to produce desired results.

emancipated Free from parental care and control.

emergency nurse practitioner Registered nurse with additional education through a master's degree program in nursing or through a nondegree/certificate continuing education program preparing the nurse to deliver primary care within an emergency room setting.

emotional abuse Extreme debasement of a person's feelings so that he feels inept, uncared for, and worthless.

enculturation Process of acquiring knowledge and internalizing values, or individuals learning their culture.

endemic Usual frequency of occurrence of a disease.

enterobiasis Pinworm infestation.

entitlement theory People have rights to resources as determined by the natural lottery and may increase their possessions in any way possible (by purchase, gift, or legitimate exchange), as long as they do not cheat others or acquire them in an unjust manner.

environment All external conditions and influences affecting the life of living things.

environmental health Aspect of community health concerned with those forms of life, substances, forces, and conditions in the surroundings of people that may exert an influence on their health and well-being.

epidemic Occurrence of any given disease phenomenon in excess of normal expectation.

epidemiology Study of the distribution of states of health and the determinants of deviations from health in populations.

equalitarian theory Doctrine that takes the needs of all people into account equally.

equilibration Way in which children seek a balance with the environment. As they become capable of thinking, they are able to respond to increasingly complex situations.

erythema Reddened raised area on the skin produced by a tissue response to small doses of antigenic substances.

ethical principles Abstract guides that serve as foundations for moral rules.

    autonomy To respect people and their rights to make choices and act according to individual determinations.

    beneficence To do good and prevent or avoid doing harm.

    justice Equals should be treated the same, and those unequal in similar respects should be treated differently according to their similarities.

ethical theories Collection of principles and rules providing theoretical foundations for deciding what to do when moral principles or rules conflict.

ethics Science or study of moral values; a code of principles and ideals that guide action.

ethnic collectivity Group with common origins, a sense of identity, and shared standards for behavior.

ethnicity Group membership and affiliation of people sharing common heritage and practices.

ethnocentrism Belief that one's own group or culture is superior to others.

eustress Positive form of stress occurring when people convert negative stress into a positive form by changing their attitudes.

evaluation Collection of methods, skills, and sensitivities necessary to determine whether or not a human service is needed and likely to be used, is conducted as planned, and actually does help people in need. Also, provision of information through formal means such as criteria, measurement, and statistics for making rational judgments necessary in decision-making situations.

excess mortality Premature death, that occurring before the average-life expectancy for persons of the same sex.

existential vacuum Feeling of emptiness and meaninglessness; apathy toward life; an inner void.

experience insurance rates Method used to establish a premium rate for a subscriber based on an estimate of the risk of claims by that subscriber.

experimental epidemiology Third stage of epidemiological investigation, which uses experimental design for studies to confirm the causal nature of relationships identified through observational studies.

extrapyramidal side effects Group of side effects produced by the blockage of dopamine receptor sites in the extrapyramidal system tract.

faith healing Belief in the healer's power to cause a cure to or recovery from illness and that God gives the healer this power.

family Basic human unit with generic properties; the coexistence of more than one human, involving continuous, presumably permanent sharing of living facilities, perceiving of reciprocal obligations, sensing of commonness, and sharing of certain obligations toward others.

family assessment Systematic collection, classification, and analysis of family data for the purpose of identifying the family's health-related strengths and problems.

family health Includes the promotion and maintenance of physical, mental, spiritual, and social health for the family unit and for individual family members.

family nurse practitioner/clinician Registered nurse with additional education through a master's degree program in nursing or a nondegree/certificate continuing education program preparing the nurse to deliver primary health care to individuals, groups, and communities of all ages.

family planning nurse practitioner (obstetric/gynecological nurse practitioner) Registered nurse with additional education through a master's degree program in nursing or a nondegree/certificate continuing education program preparing the nurse to deliver obstetrical and gynecological primary care to women.

family self-care Decision-making process that involves the family in self-observation, symptom perception and labeling, judgment of severity, and choice and assessment of treatment options.

family strengths Those factors or forces that contribute to family unity and solidarity and foster the development of the potentials inherent within the family.

federal register Document published each official federal working day to inform the public of executive regulations, presidential orders, organization changes, hearings, meeting schedules, and other administrative matters.

fee-for-service benefit schedule List of physician services with monetary or unit values attached that specify the amount third parties must pay for a specific service.

fee screen system Usual, customary, and reasonable charge, based on regional evaluation in all specialties, that allows physicians to set their own reimbursement level for units of service.

feedback Translation of a message into action.

fetal alcohol syndrome May occur when a pregnant woman has consumed alcohol regularly (about six drinks per day). Infants tend to be of low birth weight, mentally retarded, and may have behavioral, facial, limb, genital, cardiac, or neurological impairments.

field theory Belief that the environment consists of interdependent events.

figure-ground relationship Perceptual field is divided into an object of focus (figure) and a diffuse background (ground).

fiscal year Annual operating year of the government, October 1 to September 30 of the next year.

fitness Attainment of wellness on a continuing basis. See WELLNESS.

fogging Assertiveness technique of agreeing with truth in principle or with the odds.

formal communication Organization of channels for transmitting and receiving information within a network—social, professsional, political, and economic.

formal group Persons having a defined membership and specified purpose. The group may or may not have an official or public place in the community's organization.

formal operations Level of cognitive development in which thoughts are independent of physical experience and allow children to deal with hypothetical questions.

free radical Theory of aging based on the premise of an imbalance between the production and elimination of free radicals as contributory to aging.

Freon Hydrocarbon gas often used as a propellant and refrigerant.

fulfilment Perception of harmony in life when the individual has found meaning and is leading a purposeful life.

function Responsibilities and tasks associated with a particular role.

fungicide Chemical agent that kills or retards the growth of fungi.

general adaptation syndrome Manifestations of stress in the whole body, as they develop in time. This happens in three stages: (1) alarm reaction, (2) resistance, and (3) exhaustion.

geriatric day care Ambulatory health care facility for elderly people; it uses a broad range of professional and community services to maximize functional independence for this age group in the home and community.

geriatric nurse practitioner Registered nurse with additional education through a master's degree program in nursing or a nondegree/certificate continuing education program preparing the nurse to deliver primary health care to older adults.

Gestalt German word meaning pattern or configuration.

goal Global or specific statement of the desired outcome.

goal of coordination To maximize the collaborative effort of health providers while minimizing friction among them in the attainment of the client care objectives.

green box Large metal box with a capacity of 4 to 12 cubic yards located at a road intersection or near a service station or grocery store for the collection of solid waste.

gross national product (GNP) Equals the total value of all final goods and services produced in the country in one year.

group Three or more individuals functioning interdependently to meet a common goal.

group cohesion Measurement of attraction between members and toward the group.

group norms Unwritten and often unspoken standards for group members that guide their behavior and influence their attitudes and perceptions.

hallucinosis Can result from alcohol withdrawal; the person remains oriented and rational but may be confused about time.

handicap Extent to which an impairment and disability affect one's living pattern.

hazard Likelihood that a substance will cause injury in a given environment or situation.

health Balanced state of well-being resulting from harmonious interaction of body, mind and spirit.

health care Product of health services delivered through personal or public health services.

health care system Totality of resources that a population or society distributes in the organization and delivery of health services.

health contracts Usually a written agreement between client and health care provider, which identifies and assigns priorities for health goals and includes measurable criteria to be met within a designated time frame.

health culture Society's beliefs and practices concerning health and illness.

health economics Branch of economics concerned with the problems of producing and distributing the health care resources of the nation in a way that provides maximum benefit to the most people.

health education Any combination of learning experiences designed to facilitate adaptations of behavior conducive to health.

health maintenance Activities that individuals perform to maintain their current health status.

health maintenance organization (HMO) Public or private organized system of health care that provides comprehensive services to a voluntarily enrolled population for a per capita fee.

health promotion Advancement of activities such as disease prevention services, environmental protection, and health education that are devoted to the attainment of optimum physical, social, and emotional well-being for individuals, families, communities, and society at large.

health risk appraisal Process that allows for data gathering, analyzation, and comparison of an individual's prognostic characteristics of health with a standard age group, thereby providing a prediction of a person's likelihood of developing prematurely the health problems that have high morbidity and mortality in this country.

health risk/health risk factor Disease precursor in which the presence is associated with higher than average morbidity and/or mortality. Disease precursors include demographic variables, certain individual behaviors, positive individual and/or family history, and some physiological changes.

health risk reduction Application of selected interventions to control or reduce risk factors and minimize the incidence of associated disease and premature mortality. Risk reduction is reflected in greater congruence between appraised and achievable ages.

health services Personal and public services performed by individuals or institutions for the purpose of maintaining or restoring health.

health systems agency Federally funded agency that plans and approves the development of health care facilities in a community.

health workforce shortage area Determined by the federal government to have too few health professionals to provide adequate health care for the population.

helminth Wormlike animal.

herbicide Chemical agent used to destroy unwanted plants.

heroin Drug leading to serious addiction; treated most effectively with methadone.

Hill-Burton Act First U. S. legislation to focus on planning as a major area of concern. Its primary purpose was to provide for a more equal distribution of hospitals across the nation by matching federal funds for one third to two thirds of the total cost of the facility.

HMO Act Legislation enacted in 1973 to provide a demonstration program for the development of health maintenance organizations.

holistic health Integrated state of wellness that includes the mind, body, spirit, and environment.

holistic health care centers View health as a positive state and seek to teach people ways to be responsible for their physical, psychological, and spiritual needs.

homeopathy Belief that herbs, drugs, and chemicals, when used in small quantities, can cure or prevent a disease ordinarily caused by a larger dose of the same substance.

homicide Any violent death that is neither a suicide nor an accident.

hospice Palliative system of health care for terminally ill people; takes place in the home with family involvement under the direction and supervision of health professionals, especially the visiting nurse. Hospice care takes place in the hospital when severe complications of terminal illness occur, there is family exhaustion, or there is loss of commitment.

host Human or animal that provides adequate living conditions for any given infectious agent.

human abuse The misuse of people, or treating them in an injurious way.

human ecology Study of the interrelationships between individuals and their environments as well as among the individuals in the environment.

hydrocarbons Family of compounds containing carbon and hydrogen.

hyperintention Excess concentration on an objective, which ironically inhibits its accomplishment.

hyperreflection Compulsion to observe oneself; excess attention to oneself.

hypnosis Technique for reducing stress; a trancelike condition that may be psychically induced by another person and characterized by loss of consciousness and a greater or lesser degree of responsiveness to the suggestions of the hypnotist.

hypothesis Relationship between two or more variables.

iatrogenesis Physician-induced illness. Clinical iatrogenesis, the most familiar, includes illnesses created as by-products of medical intervention (e.g., infections caused by antibiotics that alter the body's normal bacterial flora).

iatrogenic guilt Engendered at the time of illness because of assignment of blame for the illness by the care provider to the patient. For example, the patient with heart disease may be told by his physician, "You could have avoided this by not smoking, exercising regularly, and eating a diet low in animal fats."

identification of target market The identification of a specific geographical area and the boundaries that define the market area, constituting a selected group of residents.

imagery Creation of pictures through the use of mental processes; can be spontaneously or deliberately created and used for many purposes.

immune globulin (IG) Sterile solution containing antibodies from human blood. IG is primarily indicated for routine maintenance of certain immunodeficient individuals and for passive immunization.

immunity Natural or acquired ability to ward off disease.

immunization Process of effecting an immune or resistant state in a given host.

immunological theory Aging theory based on the premise that normal cells are unrecognized as such, thereby setting off an immune reaction.

impairment Disturbance in structure or function resulting from anatomical, physiological, and/or psychological abnormalities.

implementation Transforming a plan for improved community health into the actual achievement of goals and objectives.

implementation mechanism Vehicle or mode by which innovations are transferred from the planners to the units of service.

incest Sexual abuse among family members.

incidence rates Measures of the rate of newly occurring cases of a disease in a population over a defined period of time.

incidental additives Food additives from the use of pesticides, herbicides, or chemical changes brought about by processing methods.

incineration Burning of wastes.

inclusiveness, principle of Tendency to respond to objects in the environment that contain the largest number of stimuli.

incubation period Time beginning with host exposure to an infectious agent and continuing until the organism multiplies to sufficient numbers to produce a host reaction and clinical symptoms.

independent practice Private practice of a professional who works independently from other professionals.

indirect provider reimbursement Method of payment to an agency for services delivered by health providers, such as nurses.

inductive approach Qualitative data are analyzed, and practice problems are examined within their own context rather than from some predetermined theoretical or conceptual basis.

infection Complex interaction between a host and a specific agent that entails the replication of organisms in the tissue of the host.

infectivity Organism's ability to spread rapidly from one host to another.

informal communication Interaction channels that arise out of the interpersonal relationships of network parts.

informal group Persons having no articulated membership and purpose.

informed consent Client has received sufficient information concerning the health care proposed, its incumbent risks, and the acceptable alternatives.

injunction Court order to stop a party in the contract from performing the specific promise or act under other circumstances.

insecticide Chemical pesticide used to control insects.

intent of law Legislative language of a law, which provides general guidelines for the writing of specific regulations.

intentional additives Substances deliberately added in food processing to enhance or conserve nutritional value or to improve or maintain flavor, color, texture, or consistency.

interacting group Those clusters of individuals who are linked by personal relationships; links may be either primary such as the family or secondary such as the voluntary association.

interiority Assessment and reformulation of self as valuable and self-determined rather than determined by others.

interiorization Merging of reflex and cognitive processes as a response to the environment.

intervention activities Means or strategies by which objectives are achieved and change is effected.

introspection Process of an individual's inward examination of traits, habits, and qualities.

invasion of privacy Right to be left alone to live in seclusion without being subjected to unwarranted or undesired publicity.

invasiveness Agent's ability to spread within the host.

inversion Reversal of the normal atmospheric gradient.

involuntary smoking Inhaling of tobacco combustion products in a smoke-filled atmosphere by a nonsmoker.

joint practice Professionals who work together in a complementary and consultative manner.

joint resolution Form of legislation similar to a bill; it contains a resolving clause as prescribed by law in 1871. The term joint does *not* signify simultaneous introduction by both houses. It becomes law in the same manner as a bill.

judge Officer who guides court proceedings to ensure impartiality and sees that the rules of evidence are observed. The trial judge determines the applicable law and instructs the jury; the appellate judge hears appeals and renders decisions about the correctness of actions of the trial judge, the law of the case, and the sufficiency of the evidence.

jurisdiction Court has the authority to hear the case.

kawasaki disease (mucocutaneous lymph node syndrome) Acute febrile illness that occurs predominately in children under 5 years of age. No causative agent has been identified.

kinesiology Study of movement that applies principles of anatomy, physiology, and physics.

knowledge Lowest level of cognitive knowing, recalling or bringing to mind the appropriate material.

korsakoff's psychosis results from excessive alcohol consumption and is characterized by disorientation and a memory defect whereby people fill in the gaps by making up forgotten information.

landfill Low-lying area on which trash and garbage is burned between layers of earth.

law Sum total of rules and regulations made by humans by which society is governed in a formal and legally binding manner.

law witness One who testifies to what he has seen, heard, or otherwise observed.

lay advisors Individuals who are influential in approving or disapproving new ideas and who seek advice and information from others about these things.

lead Guide or direct a course of action.

learning Change in behavior, which persists over time and is practiced and repeatedly reinforced.

legal Permitted or authorized by law.

legionnaires' disease (legionellosis) Pneumonia-like communicable disease caused by *Legionella pneumophila.* Mode of transmission is presumed to be airborne.

legislative counsel Consultants in the House and Senate available to assist in the framing of ideas in suitable legislative language and form for introduction.

liaison Position or responsibility within an organization for maintaining communication links with external individuals or organizations.

licensure Legal sanction to practice a profession after attaining the minimum degree of competence to ensure protection of public health and safety.

life space Term coined by Kurt Lewin to describe the simultaneous influences on a person at a given time. Those things that could affect behavior are considered psychological facts, and their totality make up the life space.

life-style change Alteration in such personal behaviors and habits as diet, use of cigarettes, alcohol consumption, and exercise.

life-style–induced health problems Diseases with natural histories that include conscious exposure to certain health-compromising or risk factors. For example, heart disease is life-style–induced; that is its onset is generally preceded by smoking, unwise eating, failing to exercise, and sustaining unbuffered stress.

litigation Trial in court to determine legal issues and the rights and duties between the parties.

logotherapy Treatment modality based on a blend of humanistic and existential psychology, which assists the client in finding meaning and purpose in life and in unique life experiences.

long-term care facility (nursing home) Typically for the older adult, where individuals can receive minimum to maximum skilled nursing care, depending on the type of facility and the need of the client.

macro level interventions Health-generating changes carried out at the societal level.

mainstream smoke Inhaled and exhaled by the smoker.

maintenance functions Behaviors that provide physical and psychological support and therefore hold the group together.

maintenance norms Create group pressures to ensure affirming actions for members and are helpful in maintaining comfort.

majority party Political party holding the most number of seats in the House and the Senate.

malpractice Professional misconduct, improper discharge of professional duties or a failure to meet the standard of care by a professional, which results in harm to another.

management Planning, organizing, directing, and controlling of time, money, and material and human resources.

mandatory credentialing Requires statutory law (e.g., State Nurse Practice Acts).

marijuana Derived from cannabis and can lead to a variety of short-term effects including reddening of the eyes, drying of the mouth, and dose-related distortions of sensory information.

markup Line-by-line review of a bill by a committee for the purpose of changing the wording or amending the intent.

massage Systematic method of applying pressure and touch to relieve tension, enhance flexibility, and create greater coordination between mind and body.

mass media Communication source that is impersonal, institutional, and formal.

maturational crisis Occurs at times of natural transitions in the developmental process.

maximin theory Distribution of goods and resources to maximize the minimum position in society, while at the same time allowing free exercise of liberty on the part of all people.

mediating structures Institutions standing between the individual in private life and the larger institution of public life, such as one's neighborhood, family, church, and voluntary associations.

Medicaid Federally and state funded insurance plan that provides financial assistance for health care for people who are handicapped or can otherwise demonstrate a need for financial aid.

medical care Subset of health care; organization, financing, and delivery of personal or individually oriented illness services.

medical technology Set of techniques, drugs, equipment, and procedures used by health care professionals in delivering medical care to individuals and the system within which such care is delivered.

Medicare Federally funded insurance plan whereby Social Security funds are used to provide health care services primarily to people over 65 years of age.

meditation State of consciousness in which stimuli are eliminated from awareness so that the mind can focus on only one thing, thus providing for rest and relief of stress.

mental health Complex process whereby people maintain at least a moderate degree of adaptation to the environment and are able to function in everyday activities and cope with daily stressors.

mental illness Occurs when people cease to be able to maintain a state of equilibrium with the environment and thereby become unable to function effectively in daily activities.

message Expression or content of the client situation.

microbiological food contamination Results from toxins deposited in food.

micro level interventions Health-generating changes performed at the individual level. Examples are cognitive restructuring, self-confrontation, modeling, conditioning, and stimulus control.

middle adult Individual who is in a transitional stage between young adulthood and old age; people in the 36-64 year-old age group whose psychosocial task is generativity versus stagnation.

middlescence Intermediate stage of life between young adulthood and old age, marked by physical, psychological, and social changes; the developmental task is generativity.

minority party Political party holding the least number of seats in the House and the Senate.

model Analogies that help to depict complex situations in a simplified way.

modeling Strategy for self-modification that depends on the client's observing the behavior of others who have realized the goal the client has identified as his own.

molds Toxic chemical that exists as a fungi; it deteriorates food fiber, induces plant disease, and can cause pulmonary and invasive disease.

monoamine oxidase inhibitor Group of drugs effective in treating depression.

morale/cohesion problem Occurs when the client has lost confidence in his ability to solve problems and feels powerless to institute corrective action.

moral obligation Duty to act in a particular way in response to moral norms.

moral virtue Ideal standard of human behavior or thinking; excellence in response to moral norms, such as goodness.

morbidity Relative disease rate; usually expressed as incidence or prevalence of a disease.

mortality Relative death rate, the proportion of deaths at a particular time and place.

mycotoxin Toxic metabolite that can be produced by food molds.

National Health Planning and Resources Development Act of 1974 (P.L. 93-641) Set forth to coordinate and direct national health policy via state and regional regulatory agencies; its major goal was to establish a nationwide network of health systems agencies.

National Health Service Corps Program established in 1970 by the Public Health Service to recruit health providers to health work force shortage areas.

National Joint Practice Commission Organization established by the American Nurses' Association and the American Medical Association to promote collaborative efforts between medicine and nursing; disbanded in 1981.

National Labor Relations Act Passed in 1935 and known as the Wagner Act; protected employees' rights to organize and to join unions and also provided for action against unfair labor practices of employers.

national labor relation act amendments of 1974 (P.L. 93-360) Amended the Taft Hartley Act of 1947 by extending the rights to organize collectively for matters concerning wages, hours, and working conditions to all employees of nonpublic health care facilities.

National Labor Relations Board Administrative agency for implementing federal policy affecting labor relations.

natural history Process of development and progression of a disease without intervention by humans.

natural law Doctrine holding that there is a natural moral order or natural moral law inherent in the structure of the universe, which can be known by human reason.

natural radiation Comes from the soil and certain rocks, body potassium, and loss of protection caused by ultraviolet sun rays.

negative assertion Open admission about oneself, acknowledging that perfection is not a goal.

negative inquiry Prompting further criticism of self or prompting more information about statements of wrongdoing in an unemotional, low-key manner.

negative right Claim to other peoples' forbearances.

negligence Failure to act as an ordinary prudent person; conduct contrary to that of a reasonable person under a specific circumstance.

negotiation Bargaining between people to reach a mutually desirable goal; takes place in an atmosphere of openness and trust.

nematocides Chemical pesticide used to kill worms.

"Nightingalism" Ideology emphasizing self-sacrifice on the part of the nurse when the primary concern of the nurse is the welfare of the client with minimum attention to personal economic and general welfare needs.

nitrogen oxide Comes primarily from automobile exhaust or by-products of industry.

noise Any unwanted sound within the environment.

Noise Control Act Passed by Congress in 1972 to identify major sources of noise, establish noise emission standards, and provide a mechanism for people to take civil action in their own behalf when a person or agency violates the Act.

nonassertive behavior Denial of one's own rights by failing to express thoughts, beliefs, and feelings honestly.

noncausal association Relationship in which a factor varies systematically with a causal factor and therefore with the occurrence of the disease, but the factor is not a cause of the disease.

noogenic neurosis Mental health problem caused by spiritual (not religious) problems or moral conflicts; a type of mental conflict in which values are not clarified.

norms Standards that guide, control, and regulate individuals and communities.

nosocomial infection In the episodic setting an infection that is not present or incubating at the time of admission. In the distributive setting any infection that is not present or incubating at the time the client is initially admitted for care by a given agency or service.

nuclear family A small group consisting of parents and their non-adult children living in a single household.

nurse as advocate One who acts in the client's best interest.

nurse-midwife Registered nurse with certificate or master's level advanced education in the areas of health assessment, diagnosis, and treatment at they relate to the primary obstetrical and gynecological care of women, including the labor and delivery of normal pregnancies.

nurse practitioner Nursing role that includes a primary care component that focuses on health maintenance, disease prevention, and client counseling.

nursing centers Health care facilities in which the primary aim is to offer nursing services, including health assessment, promotion, screening, and health teaching.

nursing process Organized, systematic, deliberate act of moving through a series of interdependent, developmental stages (assessing, planning, implementing, evaluating) toward goal achievement.

objective Precise, behavioral statement; achievement of which will accomplish partial or total realization of the goal. There is a specified date by which achievement is expected.

occupational health Worker's ability to function at an optimum level of well-being (see HEALTH) at the worksite and is reflected by higher employee productivity, increase in work attendance, reduction in workers' compensation claims, and an increase in longevity in employment status.

occupational medicine Special field of preventive medicine concerned with the medical problems and practices relating to occupation and especially to employees of industry.

occupational socialization Orientation into a given job-related set of behaviors; that is, the set of expected behaviors that accompanies a specific job.

Older American's Act Legislation enacted in 1965 to mandate and provide funds for services, programs, and activities deemed essential to accomplish certain goals for older Americans meeting specified criteria.

OMB (White House Office of Management and Budget) Advises the President on the budget and financial affairs of the nation.

operant behavior Not elicited by a known stimulus but simply emitted by the organism.

ozone Unstable colorless gas with an oxidizing power surpassed only by fluorine.

pancreatitis Results from excessive alcohol consumption; symptoms range from gastritis-like sensations to severe pain with nausea, vomiting, and rigidity of the abdomen.

pandemic Epidemics that include widespread geographical areas of the world.

paradoxical intention Logotherapeutic technique whereby the client is encouraged to do what he fears and in fact to exaggerate it to the point of humor; useful in the treatment of phobias.

parens patria Duty of state to protect its citizens.

parkinsonism Symptoms of Parkinson's disease; fine, slowly spreading tremor, muscular weakness, rigidity, and a peculiar gait.

participant observation Conscious and systematic sharing in the life activities and occasionally in the interests and affects of a group of persons; observational method of assessment.

partnership Informed, flexible, and negotiated distribution of power among all participants in the process of change for community health.

passive immunization Administration of a preformed antibody to a susceptible host.

paternal leadership Wins respect and dependence from followers by parent-like devotion to members' needs at the leader's own expense.

pathogenicity Refers to the agent's relative ability to produce disease.

patriarchal leadership Often controls membership through rewards and threats, keeping members in the dark about goals and rationale behind prescribed actions.

pedagogy Art and science of teaching children; based on belief that the purpose of education is the transmittal of knowledge.

pediatric nurse practitioner Registered nurse with certificate or master's level advanced education in the areas of health assessment, diagnosis, and treatment. Program preparing the nurse to deliver primary health care to infants and children.

pediculosis Infestation of various hairy body sites by different subspecies of *Pediculus humanus* or lice.

perception Process of acquiring knowledge about oneself and the surrounding environment, which results in a personal definition of the world in which the individual resides as well as the meaning assigned to specific situations. The way people view everything around them.

perceptual constancy According to Gestalt theory, an object is seen in the same way under varying circumstances.

periodontal disease Bacterial plaque causing disease of gum tissue and resulting in gingivitis (inflammation of the gums) and periodontitis (destruction of supporting bones and ligaments resulting in loose or drifting teeth). The leading cause of loss of teeth after age 35.

periodontoclasia Loosening of permanent teeth.

peripheral polyneuropathy Affliction of several nerves, which usually results from nutritional deficiencies associated with excessive alcohol consumption and characterized by weakness, numbness, partial paralysis of extremities, pain in the legs, and impaired sensory reactions and motor reflexes.

personal health services Directed toward the maintenance of the health status of individuals.

person-year Statistical measure representing one person at risk of developing a disease for one year.

phases of crisis Occurrence of a significant stressor event, onset of disequilibrium, rise in tension levels, decrease in levels of functioning, and resolution with equilibrium reestablished.

phi phenomenon Experience of apparent motion that is cause by lights flashing on and off at a certain frequency.

photosynthesis Formation of carbohydrates by chlorophyll-containing plants exposed to the sun.

physical abuse One or more episodes of extreme disciplining or displaced aggression or frustration, often resulting in serious physical damage to the internal organs, bones, central nervous system, or sense organs.

physician assistant New health practitioner created in the 1960s to free physician's time by completing tasks such as taking medical histories and conducting physical examinations.

physician extender Non-physician health care provider who performs medical activities typically performed by physicians.

plaintiff Party who brings a civil suit seeking damages or other legal relief.

plan Operationalization of goals; action-oriented approach to solving the identified problem or obtaining the designated goal.

planning Conscious design of a desired future state, which includes a description of the selection of alternative means to achieve and the activities necessary to attain the future state.

pneumoconiosis Lung disease associated with dusts.

pocket veto President allows a bill to lay on his desk for 10 days after Congress has adjourned. Thus without his signature the bill dies.

polarity therapy Based on an understanding of the positive and negative energy patterns of the body, which allow massage to be used to reestablish bodily harmony.

policies Guidelines within which employees of an institution must operate.

policy Principles that govern action towards given ends.

politics Art of influencing policy and decision making.

pollutants Exist as gases or fine particles and exert their effects by either depressing or stimulating normal functioning.

pollution Addition of something that changes the natural qualities.

position (status) Location in a social structure. Occupants of positions are collective categories of people who differ from the general public in some specified shared attribute or behavior.

position power Formal authority associated with an individual's position in the organization.

positive right Claim to other peoples' positive actions.

power Ability of individuals or groups to require others to act as the power holder desires.

power/authority issue Question of who has the right to be in charge and who has the right to make decision.

practice setting Context and/or environment within which nursing care is given.

precedent Previous adjudged decision that serves as the authority in a similar case.

precursor or disease precursor Prognostic characteristic or feature of personal health history, health behavior or habit, physical examination, and laboratory and x-ray film findings associated with a higher or lower risk of death than the average.

prescriptive intervention mode Requires less collaboration between consultant and client because the consultant explicitly tells the client how to solve the problem.

presymptomatic disease Early stages of disease when physiological changes have begun but no signs or symptoms are present.

prevalence rate Measures the number of existing cases of a disease present in a defined population at a given time.

prevention, level of
    primary General health promotion.
    secondary Identification and prevention of disease and health problem for those who are likely to develop them.
    tertiary Health restoration and maintenance.

prima facie duty Moral or legal duty that may be overridden when in conflict with other duties that are morally stronger.

primary care Accessible, comprehensive, coordinated, and continuous care provided by accountable care givers.

primary health care team Health care providers with specialized and complementary skills who function together as a team to provide primary health care services.

primary nursing Modality for delivering nursing care in which the client contributes to and receives care, and the provider is not only available but has authority, autonomy, and accountability.

primary prevention Activities directed toward intervening in the natural history of disease before any pathological changes occur in a host; these activities seek to keep the agent away from the host or to increase host resistance.

probability Likelihood that an intervention activity can be implemented.

problem analysis Process of identifying problem correlates and interrelationships and substantiating them with relevant data.

problem prioritization Evaluation of problems and establishment of priorities according to predetermined criteria.

professional socialization Process by which a person acquires the knowledge, skills, and sense of occupational identity characteristic of members of a given profession.

professional standards review organization Reviews the use of institutional services by physicians to determine if health care meets predetermined standards.

program Standing arrangement that provides for a social service. Set of activities occurring within the health care system, which have specific inputs, with organization and processes for establishing relationships among the inputs and outputs which can be evaluated against standards. Organized response to reduce or eliminate one or more problems.

program evaluation Collection of methods, skills, and sensitivities necessary to determine whether a human service is needed, likely to be used, conducted as planned, and actually does help people.

progressive relaxation Technique for combating tension and anxiety by systematically tensing and relaxing muscle groups.

proportional mortality Statistical measure that relates the number of deaths from a particular condition to all deaths for the same period of time.

propositions Statements that specify and describe the relation between two or more concepts.

prospective medicine Early identification of pathological or potentially pathological processes and the prescription of intervention to stop the processes at this point.

prospective reimbursement Method of payment to an agency for services to be delivered based on predictions of what an agency's costs will be for the coming year.

protocol Outline or plan for a procedure, written and signed by a physician.

protocols (algorithms) Written, standing orders that have been mutually agreed on by the nurse practitioner and physician. The nurse practitioner uses them as a guide to manage certain illnesses or conditions.

proximate cause Legal concept of cause and effect; the injury would not have occurred from the particular cause; causal connection.

proximity, principle of Objects that are close together are seen as a perceptual unit.

psittacosis Acute febrile illness that is transmitted to humans by various species of birds.

psychomotor domain Includes observable performance of skills that requires some degree of neuromuscular coordination.

psychosis Mental disorder often characterized by delusions and hallucinations.

psychotic Pertaining to or affected by psychosis.

psychotropic drugs Affect psychic function, behavior, or experience.

quality assurance Monitoring of the activities of client care to determine the degree of excellence attained in the implementation of the activities.

radiation Sending out of rays.

radioisotope Radioactive isotope.

rape Natural or unnatural sexual intercourse forced on an unwilling person by threat of bodily injury or loss of life.

rapid eye movement (REM) Movement of the closed eyes observed or recorded during sleep, occurring while the subject is dreaming.

rate Statistical measure with the frequency of an event as the numerator and the number of persons among whom the event occurred as the denominator.

ratio Statistical measure in which the numerator is not included in the denominator.

reasonable care Degree of skill and knowledge customarily used by a competent health practitioner or student of similar education and experience in treating and caring for the sick and injured in the community in which the individual is practicing.

reasonably prudent person doctrine Requires a person of ordinary sense to use ordinary care and skill.

recognition Process whereby one agency accepts the credentialing status of and the credentials conferred by another.

Red Squill Used as a poison for rodents. Since rats cannot regurgitate, Red Squill is lethal, whereas it acts as an enteric for humans.

referral Involves action that guides clients toward and assists them in using resources available to resolve their problems.

reflexology Systematic massage of the soles of the feet; uses principles similar to acupressure.

regional medical programs (RMP) Health, Disease, Cancer and Stroke Amendments of 1965 broadened the focus of planning to include all medical resources available in a region, which were considered essential in meeting a specific medical objective.

rehabilitation Restore to a former state of functioning or limit impairment and disability to the least possible level.

relative risk ratio Statistical measure of how much the risk of acquiring a particular disease increases with exposure to a specific causal agent or risk factor.

REM (roentgen equivalent man) Measure of the amount of radiation absorbed in human tissues.

representative group Type of community group whose members are elected, appointed, or selected from various community sectors.

respite time Relief time from responsibilities of the care of an older adult provided for the caretaker.

respondeat superior Employer is responsible for the legal consequences of the acts of the servant or employee while employee acts within scope of employment.

respondent behavior Elicited by a known stimulus.

retirement Period following the termination of major, gainful employment during which the individual is eligible for certain benefits based on the previous employment.

retrospective cost reimbursement Method of payment to an agency based on units of service delivered.

reversibility Once something is thought, it can be mentally undone.

right That to which a person has a just claim.

　legal Claim recognized as valid by a legal system.

　moral Claim recognized as valid by moral principles that in turn may or may not be recognized by legal rules.

right to health Right to not have one's health affected by others (a negative right).

right to health care Right to goods, resources, and services to maintain and improve one's state of health (a positive right).

risk Probability of an unfavorable event such as developing a disease.

risk appraisal and reduction Ways of assisting individuals and groups in developing a portion of their self-health care agendas; often professionally determined and/or controlled.

risk factor Disease precursor the presence of which is associated with higher than average mortality. Disease precursors include demographic variables, certain everyday health practices, family history of disease, and some physiological changes.

risk management Intervention designed to induce and/or sustain changes in health-compromising behaviors, such as counseling, mass media campaigns, or increased production of low fat dairy goods.

rodenticide Chemical pesticide used to kill rodents.

role Identifiable social position associated with a set of behavioral expectations.

role conflict Presence of contradictory and often competing role expectations.

role overload Occurs when there is insufficient time in which to carry out all of the expected role functions.

role strain Results from situations requiring complex role demands and the fulfillment of multiple roles.

role structure Arrangement of group member positions according to the expected functions of members.

rule of confidentiality Nondisclosure of personal information about others, such as clients, to those not authorized to know this information; also, a rule grounded in the principle of autonomy.

rule of utility Derived from the principle of beneficence. Includes the moral duty to weigh and balance benefits and reduce the occurrence of harms.

rules Guides, principles, or regulations that govern conduct.

> **legal** Established by legal principles.
> **moral** Established by moral principles.

rules and regulations Clear and concise statements mandating or prohibiting certain activity in an institution.

Rural Health Clinic Act Legislation enacted in 1978 to provide for the development of rural health clinics staffed by new health professionals in existing medically underserved areas of the United States.

sanitary landfill Method of solid waste disposal where waste is taken to canyons, swamps, and ravines; compacted by heavy machines; and covered with earth before rodent infestation occurs.

satellite clinic Health care facility generally operated under the auspices of a large institution but situated in a location away from the large facility.

schizophrenia Large group of disorders, usually of psychotic proportion, manifested by characteristic disturbances of thought, mood, and behavior.

school nurse practitioner Registered nurse with certificate or master's level advanced education in the areas of health assessment, diagnosis, and treatment who is prepared to deliver primary health care to school age children.

screening Method of dividing people into categories on the basis of the measurement of some characteristic.

secondary analysis Method of assessment in which existing data are used.

secondary prevention Activities directed toward early detection and treatment of disease.

selective inattention Screening out the part of the message the listener does not want to hear.

self-confrontation Strategy for self-modification that depends on clients' recognition of and dissatisfaction with inconsistencies in their own values, beliefs, behaviors or between their own personal system and that of an admired other.

self-diagnosis Lay assessment of individual health illness status.

self-health care Activities, continuous and episodic, volitional and unintentional, which people can do for themselves, individually or collectively, in a variety of health and illness matters.

self-transcendence Ability to get outside oneself, to focus attention on doing something for the sake of others or for the world, as opposed to self-actualization in which doing something for or to oneself is the end goal.

serendipity Accidental discovery.

serum sickness Reaction to various serum substances, which consists of rash, urticaria, arthritis, adenopathy, and fever occurring hours or days after the initial injection.

sexual abuse Ranges from fondling to rape and robs children of feeling in control of themselves; emphasizes their vulnerability.

shaping Altering the behavior by supplying step-to-step reinforcement of actions consistent with desired behavior.

sidestream smoke Generated by the cigarette while it smolders.

similarity, principle of Objects that are similar to one another are organized into one perceptual unit.

simple resolution Document used by only one chamber to deal with issues affecting the operation of the house in which they are introduced.

situational crisis Upset in a steady state, disequilibrium, which follows an unanticipated and significant stressor event.

skill Ability to apply knowledge to the performance of some task.

social Relating to the interpersonal relationships among people.

socialization Process in which people acquire the skills, knowledge, attitudes, and values necessary for performing their social roles.

socratic dialogue Logotherapeutic technique using self-discovery discourse; engaging in thought-provoking conversation with a client to create new insight and to change attitudes.

specific immune globulin Special preparations obtained from human blood preselected for its high antibody count against a specific disease (e.g., varicella zoster immune globulin).

specific rates Statistical rates in which both the events in the numerator and the denominator are restricted to a specified subgroup of the population.

specificity of the association Uniqueness of a relationship between a causal factor and occurrence of the disease.

staff review committees Designed to monitor client-specific aspects of care appropriate for certain levels of care.

standard of care Those acts performed or omitted that an ordinary prudent person in the defendant's position would or would not have done; a measure by which the defendant's conduct is compared to ascertain negligence.

standardized rates (adjusted rates) Artificial rates that are calculated to allow comparison of rates of disease in populations with differing distribution of characteristics such as age or race.

standards Criteria of measuring and conformity to established practice.

statute of limitations Legal limit on the time one has to file suit in civil matters, usually measured from the time of the wrong or from the time a reasonable person would have discovered the wrong.

statutes Legislative enactments; act of legislative declaring, commanding, or prohibiting something.

stereotypes Exaggerated beliefs and images that are generally false and serve to obscure important differences among members of a group and exaggerate the differences between groups.

stimulus control Strategy for self-modification that depends on manipulating the antecedents of behavior to increase goals and/or behaviors desired by the client and to decrease undesired ones.

stimulus-generalization Conditioning whereby the reaction to one stimulus is reinforced to allow transfer of reaction to other occurrences.

strategy Premeditated approach or method of dealing with a situation.

strengthening In stimulus response it is an increase in the probability that a response will be made when the stimulus recurs.

strength of the association Degree of a relationship between a causal factor and disease occurrence, usually measured by the relative risk ratio.

stress General nonspecific response by the body to demands made on it.

stressors Internally or externally generated agents that make demands on individuals.

structure In groups describes the particular arrangement of group parts that help to describe the group as a whole.

subpoena Court order requiring a person to come to court to give testimony; failure to appear results in punishment by the court.

substance abuse Use of chemicals having actual or potential undesirable effects.

substantive epidemiology Body of knowledge derived from epidemiological studies; for each disease it includes the natural history of the disease, patterns of occurrence, and factors associated with high risk for developing the disease.

suicide Killing oneself.

sulfur oxide Gives off bluish-white fumes and reduces visibility; generated by burning wood, coal, and petroleum products.

supervision Denotes line responsibility with active involvement in decision making and implementation activities in an ongoing relationship, which is the antithesis of consultation.

supplemental security income Monies awarded to an individual with insufficient resources for the purpose of increasing the income level to a minimum standard.

surveillance Process of monitoring a given population for the occurrence of disease.

survey Method of assessment in which data from a sample of persons are reported to the data collector.

susceptibility Potential to be affected by an agent.

synergism Factors that reinforce one another.

synthesis Fifth level of cognitive learning in which learners are required to build on the previous four by putting the parts or elements together into a unified whole.

system Complex of elements in interaction.

tabula rasa Blank state view of the mind.

Taft-Hartley Act Passed in 1947 and was a revision of the Wagner Act of 1935; included in the 1947 law was a provision that professional employees should not be organized in the same bargaining unit with nonprofessionals unless a majority of the professional employees voted for such an inclusion.

tardive dyskinesia Slow, rhythmical, automatic stereotyped movements, either generalized or in single muscle groups.

target of service Population group for whom healthful change is sought.

task Function but with work or labor overtones assigned to or demanded of the person.

task functions Behaviors that focus or direct movement toward the main work of the group.

task norms Strength of this standard determines the intensity with which the group keeps to its work.

territory Area of expertise or space over which an individual or group exerts control.

tertiary prevention Activities directed toward limitation of disability or restoration of function.

testimony Oral statement of a witness given under oath at a trial.

theories of justice Doctrines that indicate how to distribute goods and resources to the people.

theory Set of interrelated construct (concept) definitions and propositions that present a systematic view of phenomena by specifying relations among variables with the purpose of explaining and predicting the phenomena.

theory-principles intervention mode Requires the client to be taught theories and their application to problem solving.

therapeutic community Institution that treats and rehabilitates people with relatively severe behavioral problems like drug addiction and alcoholism.

therapeutic touch Method of healing that uses a meditative state to enter another person's energy field and passively visualize or free the flow of energy from practitioner to recipient to promote healing.

third party payer Government program or private health insurance plan that represents a client in the monetary transaction between a health care provider and consumer.

threshold limit values Maximum concentration of a chemical to which workers can be exposed for 8 hours per day without developing disease.

tobacco withdrawal syndrome Occurs with cessation or reduction in nicotine and includes the following: changes in mood and performance as seen in temper outbursts; lack of tolerance for people, events, and things; impaired performance because of a lack of concentration; episodes of daydreaming; anxiety.

tolerance Need to continually increase the dosage of a drug or alcohol to achieve the desired effects.

tool Mechanism used to accomplish some task or goal.

tort Legal or civil wrong committed by one person against the person or property of another.

toxicity Ability of a substance to cause injury to biological tissues.

toxoid Modified bacterial toxin that has been made nontoxic but retains the ability to stimulate the formation of anti-toxin used to produce active immunity.

triage Deciding which individuals need the most immediate attention and by whom.

triangulation Use of multiple assessment methods.

tuberculin skin test Substance injected in minute doses intradermally to detect or confirm mycobacterial infection.

unit of service Entity—individual, family, aggregate, organization, or community—to whom nursing care is given. The level at which service is delivered. The entity from which healthful changes are sought.

utilitarianism Doctrine that the purpose of all action should be to bring about the greatest happiness for the greatest number of people; also, that the value of anything is determined by its utility.

utilitarian theory Claims that the best way to distribute resources among people is to decide how expenditures or the use of resources will bring about the greatest net total of good and serve the largest number of people.

utilization review Directed toward assuring that care is actually needed and the cost is appropriate for the level of care provided.

vaccine Suspension of attenuated live or killed microorganisms. Vaccination or administration of a vaccine is given to induce immunity and therefore prevent infectious disease.

value Likelihood that an intervention activity will achieve the objective and contribute to problem resolution.

values Beliefs about how one should or should not behave. Values are organized into value systems, and individual value systems reflect culture, reference groups, and personal needs.

variable Concept that takes on more than one value.

variables Key characteristics of the problem under study.

vector Agent that actively carries a germ to a susceptible host.

verdict Formal declaration of the jury of its findings of fact, which is signed by the jury foreman and presented to the court.

vertical coordination Community health nurses serve as links between their level in the organization and those above and below them. They also serve as links between the agency and the client.

veto President returns a bill to the chamber of origin without a signature and accompanied by written objections.

violence Excessive display of physical or emotional force or roughness.

virulence Ability to produce severe disease.

voluntary agency Relies on staff and volunteers to provide a wide range of services; must seek operating funds from a variety of sources including gifts, dues, and fees.

voluntary credentialing Performed by an agency or institution (e.g., certification examinations offered to nurses by the American Nurses' Association.

web of causation Interrelationships among multiple factors that contribute to the occurrence of a disease.

wellness Dynamic state of health in which individuals progress toward a higher level of functioning, thus maximizing their potential in the environment.

Wernecks's encepholopathy Neurological disorder caused by excessive alcohol consumption characterized by ophthalmoplegia, nystagmus atoxia, apathy, drowsiness, confusion, and inability to concentrate.

windshield survey Observation from an automobile of many dimensions of a community's life and environment. An observational method of assessment.

young adult Individual in the 20 to 35-year-old age group whose psychosocial task is intimacy versus isolation.

Index